Endodontics

Endodontics

Principles and Practice

SIXTH EDITION

South Asia Edition

Mahmoud Torabinejad, DMD, MSD, PhD

Affiliate Professor of Endodontics, Department of Endodontics, University of Washington Seattle, WA, USA
Adjunct Professor, Department of Endodontics
School of Dentistry, Loma Linda University, Loma Linda, CA, USA
Adjunct Professor, Department of Endodontics
University of Pacific Arthur A. Dugoni School of Dentistry;
Adjunct Professor, Department of Preventive and Restorative Dentistry, Section of Endodontics
University of California in San Francisco School of Dentistry
San Francisco, CA, USA

Ashraf F. Fouad, DDS, MS

Freedland Distinguished Professor
Vice-chair, Division of Comprehensive Oral Health
Adams School of Dentistry, University of North Carolina
Chapel Hill, NC, USA

Shahrokh Shabahang, DDS, MS, PhD

Associate Professor
Department of Endodontics
School of Dentistry
Loma Linda University
Loma Linda, CA, USA

ELSEVIER

ELSEVIER

RELX India Pvt. Ltd.
Registered Office: 818, Indraprakash Building, 8th Floor, 21, Barakhamba Road, New Delhi-110001
Corporate Office: 14th Floor, Building No. 10B, DLF Cyber City, Phase II, Gurgaon-122 002, Haryana, India

Endodontics: Principles and Practice, 6e, Mahmoud Torabinejad, Ashraf F. Fouad, Shahrokh Shabahang.

First edition 1989, Second edition 1996, Third edition 2002, Fourth edition 2009, Fifth edition 2015.

ISBN: 978-0-323-62436-7.

This adapted reprint of Endodontics: Principles and Practice, 6e, by Mahmoud Torabinejad, Ashraf F. Fouad, Shahrokh Shabahang was undertaken by RELX India Private Limited and is published by arrangement with Elsevier Inc.

Endodontics: Principles and Practice, 6e – South Asia Edition, Mahmoud Torabinejad, Ashraf F. Fouad, Shahrokh Shabahang.

Adapted Reprint ISBN: 978-81-312-6287-0.

Notice

Practitioners and researchers must always rely on their own experience and knowledge in evaluating and using any information, methods, compounds or experiments described herein. Because of rapid advances in the medical sciences, in particular, independent verification of diagnoses and drug dosages should be made. To the fullest extent of the law, no responsibility is assumed by Elsevier, authors, editors or contributors in relation to the adaptation or for any injury and/or damage to persons or property as a matter of products liability, negligence or otherwise, or from any use or operation of any methods, products, instructions, or ideas contained in the material herein.

Although all advertising material is expected to conform to ethical (medical) standards, inclusion in this publication does not constitute a guarantee or endorsement of the quality or value of such product or of the claims made of it by its manufacturer.

Online resources are not available with this reprint. To access any or all of these assets, the original edition must be purchased by the individual user.

This publication is licensed for sale in Bangladesh, Bhutan, India, Maldives, Nepal, Pakistan and Sri Lanka only. Circulation of this version outside these territories is unauthorized and illegal.

Content Strategist: Ruchi Mullick
Content Project Manager: Supriya Barua Kumar

Printed in India by Sanat Printers, Kundli, Haryana

Contents

Foreword

Almost three decades ago, I was working as an assistant professor at Manipal College of Dental Sciences, Mangalore, under Dr Premanand Kamath one of the finest teachers and mentors I had the privilege of working with. One day, a graduate student came to us and talked about a new cement being developed by Dr Mahmoud Torabinejad, that she thought would revolutionize endodontics. That material was MTA. It had not yet been commercially launched, but she was keen to do a study on it. We advised her to get in touch with Dr Torabinejad, which she did and then we waited. To our utter amazement his reply came in the form of a container full of MTA, maybe 25–30 grams and his best wishes for the study!!

As I write this foreword to the sixth edition of Dr Torabinejad's seminal textbook *Endodontics—Principles and Practice*, I still remember his remarkable generosity in sharing a material which was not yet commercially available.

I have always been a great admirer of this book even earlier for its emphasis on diagnosis especially the endodontic–periodontic continuum. This edition continues in the same vein, solid on science and a clinical focus which is very helpful for the practicing dentist.

In the sixth edition of this book, he is joined by Ashraf F. Fouad and Shahrokh Shabahang, both noted experts in their field who bring years of research and experience to this project.

They are ably aided by a galaxy of researchers and clinicians from all over the world who have contributed to specific chapters dealing with their area of expertise.

The overall result is a comprehensive textbook which in every way reflects what they set out to do, create a text which is concise, current, and easy to follow. It is comprehensive and up to date, while at the same time not too verbose and complex. The design, layout, and graphics make it easy on the eye and eminently readable.

This book has been written for the dental students and the general dentist. It is specifically designed with a focus on helping anyone who wants to incorporate endodontics in their practice. And for those working toward competitive entrance exams, there is a wonderful set of MCQs with answers at the end of each chapter. All in all, a book I would highly recommend for students and clinicians alike.

Dr Arvind Shenoy
Professor,
Bapuji Dental College and Hospital, Davangere.
Editor- Philips Science of Dental Materials
South Asian Edition

Preface

The primary responsibility of dentists has always been to relieve dental pain and prevent tooth loss. Despite their efforts, many teeth develop caries, suffer traumatic injury, or are impacted by other disorders that may require endodontic care. Endodontics is a discipline of dentistry that deals with the morphology, physiology, and pathology of the human dental pulp and periapical tissues, as well as the prevention and treatment of diseases and injuries related to these tissues. Its scope includes diagnosis and treatment of pain of pulpal and/or periapical origin, vital pulp therapy, regenerative endodontic procedures, nonsurgical root canal treatment, surgical or non-surgical retreatment of cases with persistent disease and internal bleaching of discolored teeth. Ultimately, the primary goal of this discipline is to preserve the natural dentition. Root canal treatment is a well-tested procedure that has provided pain relief and has restored function and esthetics to patients for decades. Millions of patients expect preservation of their natural dentition. When root canal treatment is indicated, patients should be aware that the procedure is safe and has a high success rate, if properly performed.

As with other dental specialties, the practice of endodontics has two inseparable components: art and science. The *art* consists of executing technical procedures during root canal treatment. The *science* includes the basic and clinical sciences related to biological and pathological conditions that guide the art of endodontics through the principles and methods of evidence-based treatment. Evidence-based treatment integrates the best clinical evidence with the practitioner's clinical expertise and the patient's treatment needs and preferences. A principal objective of *Endodontics: Principles and Practice* is to incorporate recent evidence-based information regarding technological and scientific advances in the field of endodontics when available and when appropriate.

There are not enough endodontists to manage the endodontic needs of the public, so general dentists must assist endodontists to preserve natural dentition. Their responsibility is to diagnose pulpal and periapical diseases and to perform uncomplicated root canal treatments. In fact, most of the endodontic procedures are performed by generalists. Our textbook, written specifically for dental students and general dentists, focusses on clinical content and contains the information necessary for those who would like to incorporate endodontics in their practice. This includes diagnosis and treatment planning as well as management of pulpal and periapical diseases. In addition, the general dentist must be able to determine the case complexity and whether she or he can perform the necessary treatment or if referral is the better option.

The new edition of this book focuses on clinical content and has removed some of the basic science since the readers have already studied the basic sciences related to endodontic practice. We have also overhauled the table of contents with many new contributors to combine and / or eliminate chapters to be more updated and have newer clinically relevant information.

This edition contains information regarding the pathogenesis of pulp and periapical diseases, systemic consideration for patients who need endodontic intervention, endodontic radiology including the use of CBCT, diagnosis and treatment planning, differential diagnosis of pain and radiolucencies of non-pulpal origin, endodontic case complexity and when to refer to an endodontist, endodontic instruments, local anesthesia, emergency treatment, management of vital pulp including regeneration of pulp-dentin complex, traumatic injuries, root canal anatomy, access preparations, cleaning and shaping, obturation, and temporization as well as restoration of endodontically treated teeth and bleaching. In addition, it covers etiology, prevention, and treatment of accidental procedural errors, as well as treatment of cases with persistent disease using nonsurgical and surgical approaches and their treatment outcomes that provide guidelines regarding the assessment of these procedures.

Endodontics: Principles and Practice is not intended to include all background information on the art and science of endodontics. At the same time, it is not designed to be a "cookbook" or a preclinical laboratory technique manual. The purpose of this textbook is to provide the reader with the basic information to perform root canal treatment and to give the reader background knowledge in related areas. It should be used as a building block for understanding the etiology and treatment of teeth with pulpal and periapical diseases; then the reader can expand her or his endodontic experiences with more challenging cases. Providing the best quality of care is the guiding light for treatment planning and performing appropriate treatment.

We would like to thank the contributing authors for sharing their materials and experiences with our readers and with us; their contributions improve the quality of life for millions of patients. In addition, we acknowledge our colleagues and students who provided cases and gave us constructive suggestions to improve the quality of our book.

Mahmoud Torabinejad
Ashraf F. Fouad
Shahrokh Shabahang
2020

List of Contributors

The editors would like to acknowledge and offer grateful thanks for the input of all previous editions' contributors, without whom this new edition would not have been possible.

Hamid Abedi, DDS MS MBA
Clinical endodontist, Irvine, CA, USA

Kenneth Abramovitch, DDS, MS
Professor and Chair, Department of Oral Pathology, Radiology and Medicine, University of Missouri – Kansas City, School of Dentistry, Kansas City, MO, USA

Anita Aminoshariae, DDS, MS
Associate Professor, Endodontics, CWRU School of Dental Medicine, Cleveland, OH, USA

Ana Arias, DDS, MS, PhD
Professor of Conservative Dentistry, School of Dentistry, Complutense University, Madrid, Spain

Adham A. Azim, BDS
Division Head and Director of the Post-Graduate Program, Periodontics and Endodontics, University at Buffalo, Buffalo, New York, NY, USA

Brooke Blicher, DMD, Certificate in Endodontics
Clinical Endodontist, Upper Valley Endodontics, White River Junction, Vermont;
Clinical Instructor, Department of Restorative Dentistry and Biomaterials Science, Harvard School of Dental Medicine, Boston, MA, USA;
Assistant Clinical Professor, Department of Endodontics, Tufts University School of Dental Medicine, Boston, MA, USA;
Dental Staff, Department of Oral Surgery, Dartmouth Hitchcock Medical Center, Lebanon, VT, USA

Tatiana Botero, DDS, MS
Clinical Associate Professor, Cariology Restorative Sciences and Endodontics, Ann Arbor, MI, USA

Sami Chogle, BDS, DMD, MSD
Chair and Program Director, Graduate Endodontics, Boston University, Boston, MA, USA;
Adjunct Associate Professor, Graduate Endodontics, Case Western Reserve University, Cleveland, OH, USA

William Herbert Christie, DMD, MS, FRCD(C)
Retired Professor, Senior Scholar, Department of Restorative Dentistry, University of Manitoba, Winnipeg, Manitoba, Canada

Blaine Cleghorn, DMD, MS
Professor and Assistant Dean, Faculty of Dental Clinical Sciences, Dalhousie University, Halifax, Nova Scotia, Canada

Anibal Diogenes, DDS, MS, PhD
Professor and Vice Chair, Department of Endodontics, University of Texas Health Science Center at San Antonio, San Antonio, TX, USA

Melissa Drum, DDS, MS
Professor, Advanced Endodontics Director, Division of Endodontics, College of Dentistry, The Ohio State University, Columbus, OH, USA

Brad Eli, DMD, MS
Staff, Department of Dentistry, Scripps Memorial Hospital, La Jolla, CA, USA

Mohamed I. Fayad, DDS, MS, PhD
Clinical Associate Professor, Director of Research, Department of Endodontics, University of Illinois, College of Dentistry, Chicago, IL, USA

Natasha M. Flake, DDS, PhD, MSD
Associate Professor, Department of Endodontics, University of Washington, Seattle, WA, USA

Ashraf F. Fouad, DDS, MS
Freedland Distinguished Professor, Vice-chair, Division of Comprehensive Oral Health, Adams School of Dentistry, University of North Carolina, Chapel Hill, NC, USA

Brian Goodacre, DDS, MSD
Assistant Professor, Department of Prosthodontics, School of Dentistry, Loma Linda University, Loma Linda, CA, USA

Charles J. Goodacre, DDS, MSD
Distinguished Professor, Department of Restorative Dentistry, School of Dentistry, Loma Linda University, Loma Linda, CA, USA

Robert Handysides, DDS
Dean, Department of Endodontics, School of Dentistry, Loma Linda University, Loma Linda, CA, USA

Brad Johnson, DDS, MHPE
Professor and Head, Director of Postdoctoral Endodontics, Department of Endodontics, University of Illinois at Chicago, Chicago, IL, USA

James David Johnson, DDS, MS
Clinical Professor and Chair, Department of Endodontics, University of Washington School of Dentistry, Seattle, WA, USA

Mo Kang, DDS, PhD
Professor and Chairman, Department of Endodontics, UCLA School of Dentistry, Los Angeles, CA, USA

Philip Michaelson, MS, DMD
Private Practice, Endodontics, Professional Endodontics, Inc., Chagrin Falls, OH, USA

W. Craig Noblett, DDS, MS
Volunteer Faculty, University of California, San Francisco, CA; Private practice, Fresno, CA

Ali Nosrat, DDS, MS, MDS
Clinical Assistant Professor, Department of Endodontics, School of Dentistry, University of Maryland, Baltimore, MD, USA;
Private Practice, Centreville, VA, USA

John M. Nusstein, DDS, MS
Professor and Chair, Division of Endodontics, College of Dentistry, The Ohio State University, Columbus, OH, USA

Avina Paranjpe, BDS, MS, MSD, PhD
Associate Professor, Department of Endodontics, University of Washington, Seattle, WA, USA

Masoud Parirokh, DMD, MSc
Distinguished Professor, Department of Endodontics, School of Dentistry, Kerman University of Medical Sciences, Kerman, Islamic Republic of Iran;
Distinguished Professor, Endodontology Research Center, Kerman University of Medical Sciences, Kerman, Islamic Republic of Iran

Ove A. Peters, DMD, MS, PhD
Professor and Discipline Lead, Endodontics, School of Dentistry, The University of Queensland, Brisbane, Qld, Australia

Al Reader, DDS, MS
Professor, Division of Endodontics, College of Dentistry, The Ohio State University, Columbus, OH, USA

Ilan Rotstein, DDS
Professor and Chair, Endodontics, Orthodontics and General Practice Residency, Herman Ostrow School of Dentistry of USC, University of Southern California, Los Angeles, CA, USA;
Associate Dean, Continuing Education, Herman Ostrow School of Dentistry of USC, University of Southern California, Los Angeles, CA, USA

Richard A. Rubinstein, DDS, MS, FACD
Adjunct Clinical Associate Professor, Cariology, Restorative Sciences and Endodontics, University of Michigan, Ann Arbor, MI, USA

Nikita B. Ruparel, MS, DDS, PhD
Associate Professor, Department of Endodontics, UTHSCSA, San Antonio, TX, USA

Mohammed Sabeti, DDS, MA
Clinical Professor, PRDS, University of California at San Francisco, San Francisco, CA, USA

Nasser Said-Al-Naief, DDS, MS
Professor and Chair, OMFP Laboratory Director, Pathology and Radiology, OHSU, Portland, OR, USA;
Hospital Staff, OMFS, School of Medicine, OHSU, Portland, OR, USA;
Professor, Anatomic Pathology, School of Medicine, OHSU, Portland, OR, USA

Christine Sedgley, MDS, MDSc, FRACDS, MRACDS(ENDO), PhD
Professor and Chair, Department of Endodontology, Oregon Health and Sciences University, Portland, OR, USA

Frank Setzer, DMD, PHD, MS
Assistant Professor, Endodontic Clinic Director, and Predoctoral Endodontic Program Director, Department of Endodontics, University of Pennsylvania, Philadelphia, PA, USA

Shahrokh Shabahang, DDS, MS, PhD
Associate Professor, Department of Endodontics, School of Dentistry, Loma Linda University, Loma Linda, CA, USA

Renato Silva, DDS, MS, PhD
Associate Professor, Department of Endodontics, University of Texas Health Science Center at Houston, Houston, TX, USA

Tory Silvestrin, DDS, MSD, MSHPE
Chairman and Graduate Program Director, Department of Endodontics, School of Dentistry, Loma Linda University, Loma Linda, CA, USA

Fabricio B. Teixeira, DDS, MS, PhD
Professor and Chair, Department of Endodontics, University of Iowa, Iowa City, IA, USA

Yoshitsugu Terauchi, DDS, PhD
President, Endodontics, CT and MicroEndodontic Center, Yamato-shi, Kanagawa, Yamato City, Japan

Mahmoud Torabinejad, DMD, MSD, PhD
Affiliate Professor of Endodontics, Department of Endodontics, University of Washington Seattle, WA, USA;
Adjunct Professor, Department of Endodontics, School of Dentistry, Loma Linda University, Loma Linda, CA, USA;
Adjunct Professor, Department of Endodontics, University of Pacific Arthur A. Dugoni School of Dentistry;
Adjunct Professor, Department of Preventive and Restorative Dentistry, Section of Endodontics, University of California in San Francisco, School of Dentistry, San Francisco, CA, USA

Marco Aurelio Versiani, Lt. Col., DDS, MSc, PhD
Associate Researcher, Department of Restorative Dentistry, Dental School of Ribeirão Preto, University of São Paulo, Ribeirão Preto, São Paulo, Brazil

Richard Walton, DMD, MS
Professor Emeritus, Department of Endodontics, University of Iowa, Iowa City, IA, USA

Shane N White, BDentSc, MS, MA, PhD
Professor, UCLA School of Dentistry, Los Angeles, CA, USA

Anne E. Williamson, DDS, MS
Associate Professor, Endodontics, University of Iowa, Iowa City, IA, USA

1

Pathogenesis of Pulp and Periapical Diseases

CHRISTINE SEDGLEY, RENATO SILVA, AND ASHRAF F. FOUAD

CHAPTER OUTLINE

LEARNING OBJECTIVES

After reading this chapter, the student should be able to:

1. Describe the histology and physiology of the normal dental pulp.
2. Identify etiologic factors causing pulp inflammation.
3. Describe the routes of entry of microorganisms to the pulp and periapical tissues.
4. Classify pulpal diseases and their clinical features.
5. Describe the clinical consequences of the spread of pulpal inflammation into periapical tissues.
6. Describe the histopathological diagnoses of periapical lesions of pulpal origin.
7. Identify clinical signs and symptoms of acute apical periodontitis, chronic apical periodontitis, acute and chronic apical abscesses, and condensing osteitis.
8. Discuss the role of residual microorganisms and host response in the outcome of endodontic treatment.
9. Describe the steps involved in repair of periapical pathosis after successful root canal treatment.

Histology and Physiology of Normal Dental Pulp

The dental pulp is a unique connective tissue with vascular, lymphatic, and nervous elements that originates from neural crest cells. It resides inside the tooth in a chamber with rigid walls.

The pulp contains odontoblasts, highly specialized cells with a secretory function, which not only form dentin, but also interact with dental epithelium early in tooth development to initiate the formation of enamel. The pulp also contains fibroblasts, undifferentiated mesenchymal cells, collagen type I and II, proteoglycans, glycoproteins, and water[1] (Fig. 1.1).

The histologic structure of the pulp is important, because it reflects a unique architecture suited for the formation of dentin and defense against invading pathogens. Odontoblasts form a palisading layer that lines the walls of the pulp space, and their tubules extend about two thirds of the length of the dentinal tubules. The tubules are larger at a young age and eventually become more sclerotic as the peritubular dentin becomes thicker. The odontoblasts are primarily involved in production of mineralized dentin. They are connected by gap junctions that allow them to form a semipermeable membrane. In addition, odontoblasts play an important role in defense as they express Toll-like receptors (see later), cytokines, and defensins, among other immunologic mediators.

Two main types of sensory fibers innervate the pulp: Aδ-fibers in the periphery and C-fibers in the central pulp. The Aδ-fibers are responsible for the sharp response to thermal changes. They extend between the odontoblasts, lose their myelin sheath, and extend to a distance of 100 to 200 μm into the dentinal tubules. The C-fibers are unmyelinated and are responsible for the dull

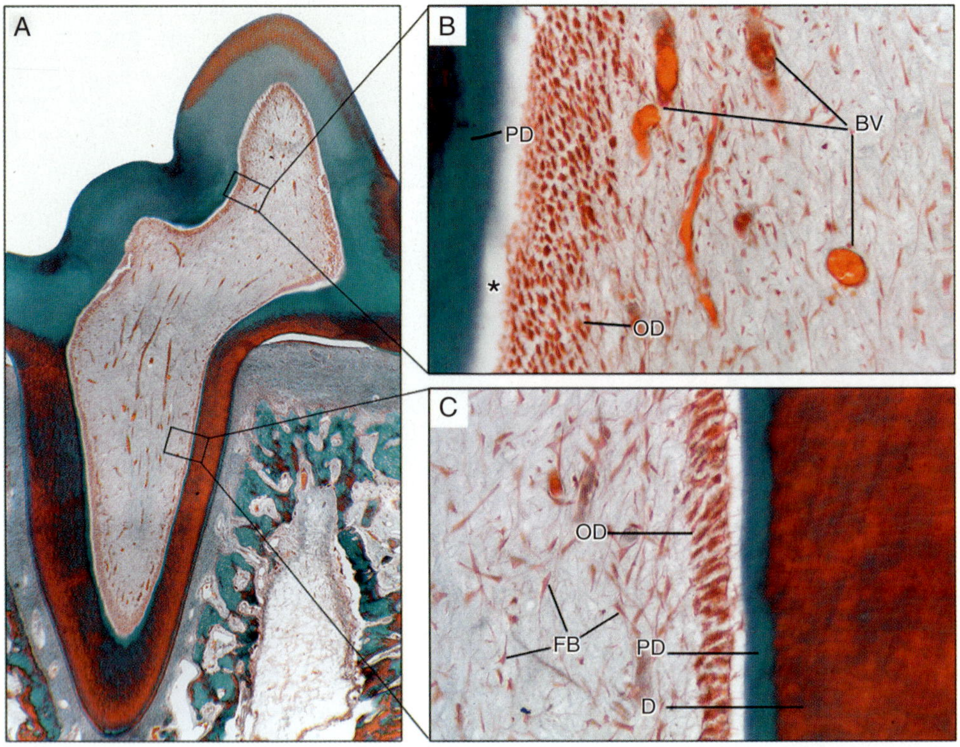

• **Fig. 1.1** Histologic section of **(A)** rat molar tooth showing coronal **(B)** and **(C)** radicular dental pulp in higher magnification. Masson-Goldner trichrome staining. *BV*, Blood vessels; *D*, dentin; *FB*, fibroblasts; *OD*, odontoblasts in odontoblastic layer; *PD*, predentin. An artifact *(*)* separating the predentin from the odontoblastic layer. (Courtesy Dr. Claudia Biguetti.)

ache that affects patients with symptomatic irreversible pulpitis. The pulp may also have Aβ-fibers and sympathetic fibers in the walls of arterioles.

The pulp vasculature plays a critical role in its response to irritation. When the tooth first erupts into the oral cavity, the root apex is immature, and there is ample blood supply to the pulp. Eventually, the apex matures, and the ability of the pulp to withstand external irritation, such as from trauma or caries, diminishes. However, the pulp of the mature tooth has mechanisms to cope with increased blood flow during inflammation, such as arteriovenous anastomoses and loops that can circulate and increase volume of blood when the need arises. The pulp also contains an elaborate network of arterioles and capillaries around the odontoblasts, which are high-metabolic-rate cells, commonly known as the *terminal capillary network*.

Etiology of Pulpal and Periapical Diseases

Injury or irritation of pulpal or periapical tissues can result in inflammation. The reactions of the dental pulp to irritants are largely dictated by the type and duration of a stimulus. These irritants can be broadly classified as nonliving (mechanical, thermal, or chemical) or living (microbial).

Mechanical Irritants

The potential for pulp irritation increases as more dentin is removed during deep cavity preparations because dentinal permeability is greater closer to the pulp[2] (Fig. 1.2). The removal of tooth structure without proper cooling may also cause pulp inflammation. Deep scaling and curettage may injure apical vessels and nerves, resulting in pulpal damage.[3]

Pulpal damage can occur because of impact injuries. Teeth undergoing mild to moderate trauma and those with immature apices have a better chance of pulpal survival in comparison with those suffering severe injury or those with closed apices. Intrusion injuries are more likely to lead to pulp necrosis than are lateral or extrusion injuries[4] (Fig.1.3).

Periapical tissues can be mechanically irritated and inflamed by impact trauma, hyperocclusion, overinstrumentation of root canals, perforation of the root, and overextension of root canal filling materials (Fig. 1.4). Inaccurate determination of root canal length is usually the cause of overinstrumentation and subsequent inflammation. In addition, lack of an adequate apical resistance form created during cleaning and shaping can cause overextension of filling materials into the periapical tissues, causing physical and chemical damage (Fig. 1.5).

Application of forces beyond the physiologic tolerance of the periodontal ligament (PDL) during orthodontic tooth movement results in disturbance of the blood and nerve supply of the pulp tissue.[5,6] In addition, orthodontic movement may initiate resorption of the apex, usually without a change in vitality.

Chemical Irritants

Antibacterial agents, such as silver nitrate, phenol with and without camphor, and eugenol, have been used to "sterilize" dentin after cavity preparations. The effectiveness of many of these products is questionable,[7] and their cytotoxicity can cause inflammatory changes in the underlying dental pulp.[8] Other irritating agents include cavity cleansers, such as alcohol, chloroform, hydrogen peroxide, and various acids; chemicals present in desensitizers, cavity liners and bases; and temporary and permanent restorative materials.

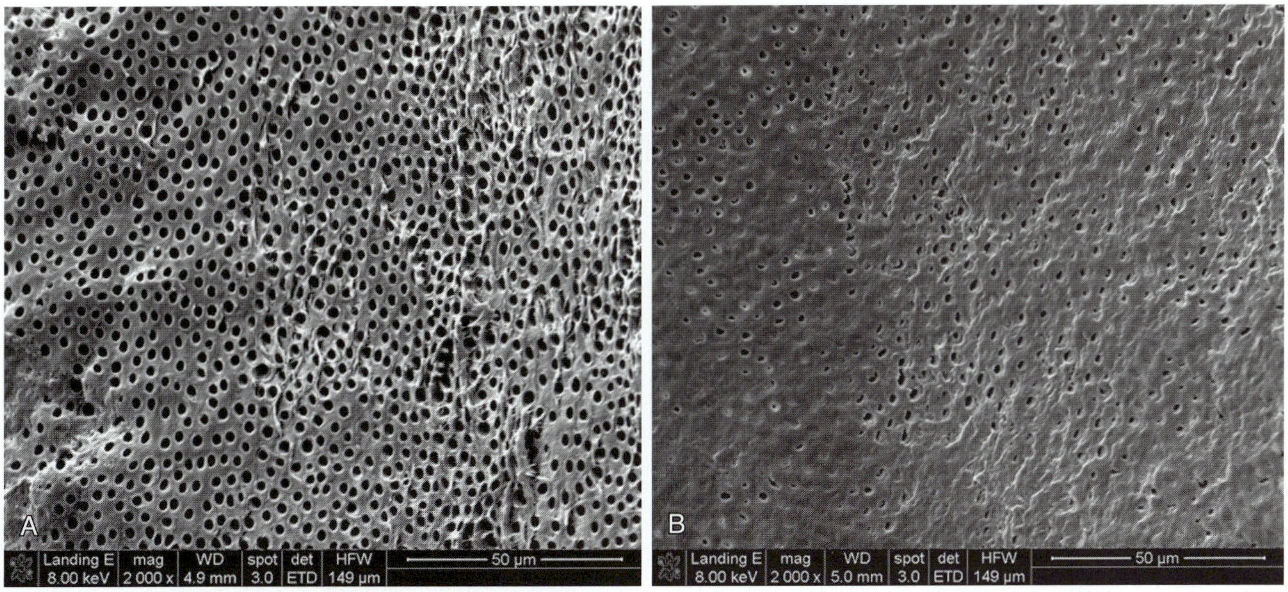

• **Fig. 1.2** Scanning Electron Microscopy of Human Dentin. Dentinal permeability is greater closer to the pulp **(A)** than near the dentinoenamel junction **(B)** or the cementodentinal junction due to the higher number of tubules per unit and bigger tubule diameter. Therefore the potential for pulp irritation increases as more dentin is removed.

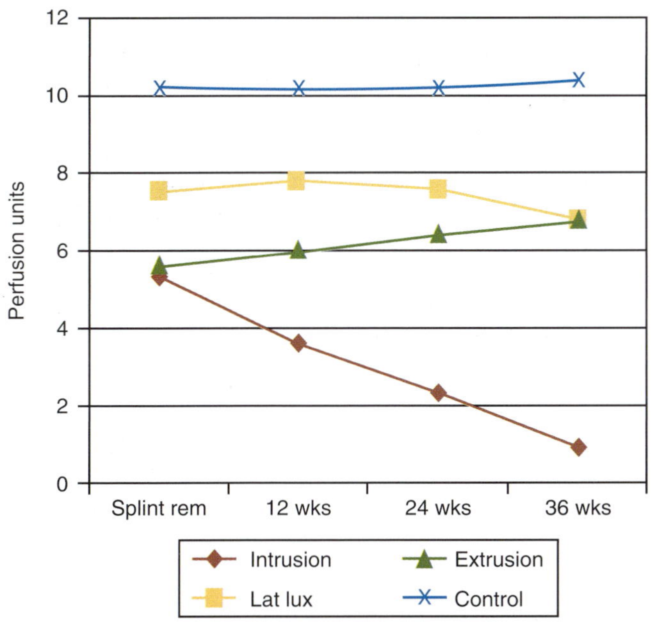

• **Fig. 1.3** Graphic representation of pulpal circulation subsequent to various types of luxation injuries to teeth. Pulp circulation is measured in perfusion units over a 36-week observation period.

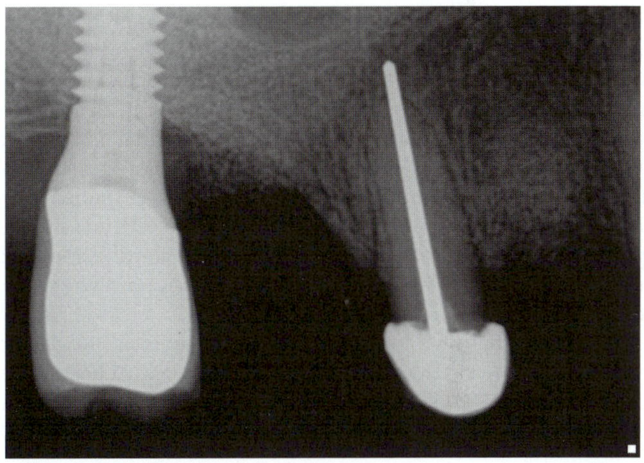

• **Fig. 1.4** Periapical radiograph showing overextension of root canal filling material.

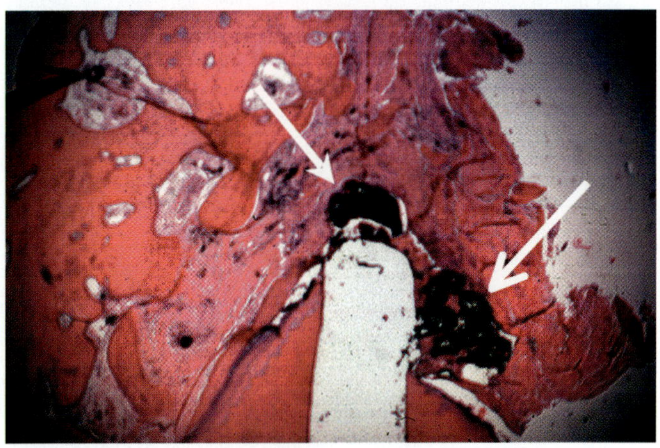

• **Fig. 1.5** Improper instrumentation and extrusion of filling materials into the periapical tissues causes periradicular inflammation *(arrows)*.

Antibacterial irrigants used during cleaning and shaping of root canals, intracanal medications, and some compounds present in obturating materials are examples of potential chemical irritants to periapical tissues.[9,10] When testing the effects of antimicrobial medications on dental pulp cells, researchers showed that calcium hydroxide and lower concentrations of antibiotic pastes are conducive to cell survival and proliferation, but more concentrated forms of antibiotic pastes have detrimental effects.[11]

Microbial Irritants

Although mechanical and chemical irritations are predominantly transient in nature, the most significant cause of inflammation is microbial. Studies have shown that even superficial carious lesions in enamel are capable of attracting inflammatory cells in the pulp.[12,13] The initial reaction of the pulp to these irritants is mediated through the innate immune response. This early response to caries results in focal accumulation of chronic inflammatory cells, such as macrophages, lymphocytes, and plasma cells.[14] As caries progresses toward the pulp, the intensity and character of the infiltrate change. Pulpal tissue may remain inflamed for long periods and may undergo eventual or rapid necrosis. This change depends on several factors: (1) the virulence of the microorganisms; (2) the ability to circulate inflammatory fluids to avoid a marked increase in intrapulpal pressure; (3) host resistance, including genetic variations; (4) the amount of circulation and (5) an important factor, lymphatic drainage. Subsequently, microorganisms or their byproducts and other irritants from the necrotic pulp diffuse from the canal to the periapical region, resulting in the development of an inflammatory lesion (Fig. 1.6).

Pulpal and periapical pathoses do not develop without the presence of bacterial contamination.[15,16] Kakehashi and collaborators created pulp exposures in conventional and germ-free rats.[15] In the germ-free rats, minimal inflammation only occurred throughout the 72-day observation period. Further, pulpal tissue in these animals was not devitalized but rather showed calcific bridge formation by day 14, with normal tissue apical to the dentin bridge (Fig. 1.7, *A*). In contrast, infection, pulpal necrosis, and abscess formation occurred by the eighth day in conventional rats (Fig. 1.7, *B*). The bacteriological investigation by Sundqvist examining the flora of human necrotic pulps supports the findings of Kakehashi and collaborators[15] and Möller and coworkers.[16] Sundqvist examined previously traumatized intact teeth with necrotic pulps, with and without apical pathosis. The root canals of teeth without apical lesions were aseptic, whereas those with periapical pathosis had positive bacterial cultures.[17]

Several mechanisms have been proposed for identification of microorganisms as irritants by the immune system. Detection of these pathogens can occur via interaction between pathogen-associated molecular patterns (PAMPs) and specific receptors broadly identified as pattern recognition receptors (PRRs).[18] PRRs recognize PAMPs and initiate host defenses. G-protein coupled receptors and Toll-like receptors (TLRs) are part of the innate immune response and activate phagocytic functions to allow microbial ingestion. G-protein coupled receptors bind to chemokines, lipid mediators (e.g., platelet-activating factor, prostaglandin E2, and leukotriene B_4) or bacterial proteins, causing extravasation of leukocytes and production of bactericidal substances. TLRs are transmembrane proteins that are expressed by cells of the innate immune system playing a central role in the initiation of cellular innate immune responses.[19] These receptors recognize invading microbes and activate signaling pathways that launch immune and inflammatory responses to destroy the invaders. At least 13 TLRs have been discovered to date with different recognition abilities. Table 1.1 presents some of the currently identified TLRs and their specific interactions.

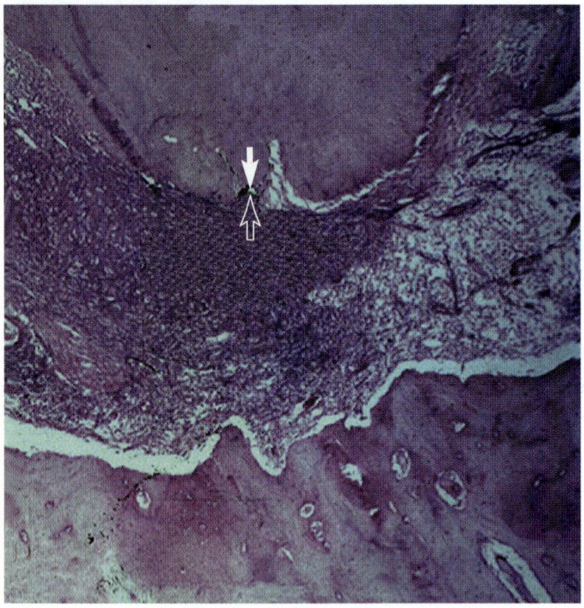

• **Fig. 1.6** Egress of irritants *(closed arrow)* from the root canal into the periapical tissue causes inflammation *(open arrow)* and replacement of normal periapical structures with a granulomatous tissue.

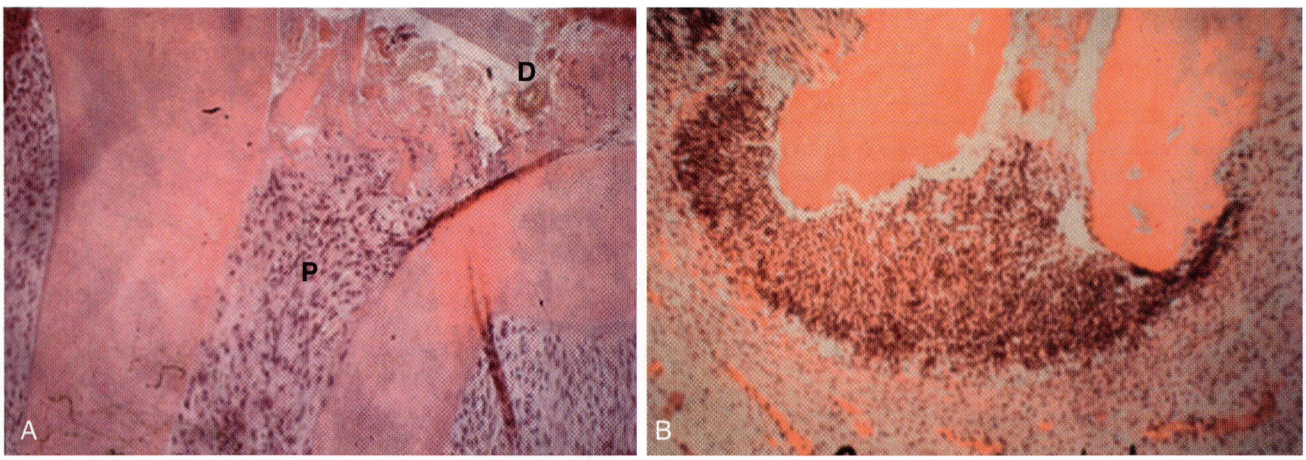

• **Fig. 1.7** **A**, No inflammation is seen in an exposed pulp *(P)* of a germ-free rat. Food particles and other debris *(D)* are packed into the chamber. **B**, Periapical lesion is apparent in a conventional rat after pulp exposure. (Courtesy Dr. H. Stanley.)

TABLE 1.1 Examples of Toll-Like Receptors (TLRS) and Associated Activators

PAMP	PRR	Pathogen
LPS, Lipid A	TLR4	Gram-negative bacteria
Flagellin	TLR5	Bacteria, flagellum
dsRNA	TLR3	Virus
RNA	TLR7,8	Virus
CpG DNA	TLR9	Bacteria, DNA
PAMP	PRR	Pathogen

PAMP, Pathogen-associated molecular patterns; *PRR,* pattern recognition receptors.

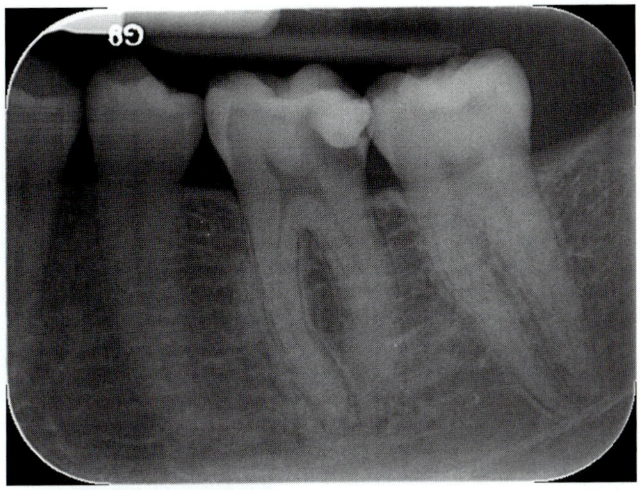

• **Fig. 1.8** Radiograph showing pulp exposure as a result of caries.

Microbiology of Root Canal Infections

Routes of Root Canal Infection

Under normal conditions, the dental pulp and dentin are isolated from oral microorganisms by overlying enamel and cementum. When the integrity of these protective layers is breached (e.g., as a result of caries, trauma-induced fractures and cracks, restorative procedures, congenital anomalies of teeth, scaling and root planing, attrition, or abrasion) or naturally absent (e.g., because of gaps in the cementoenamel junction at the cervical root surface), the dentin-pulp complex becomes exposed to the oral environment. The pulp then becomes at risk of infection by oral microorganisms present in caries, saliva, and dental plaque. The risk increases with the depth of lesions due to the diameter of dentinal tubules increasing as they approach the pulp (see Fig. 1.2).

Caries are the most common cause of pulpal exposure (Fig. 1.8). However, microorganisms may also reach the pulp via direct pulpal exposure as a result of iatrogenic restorative procedures, as a result of trauma, and through a periodontal pocket extending to the apical foramen or lateral canal. After pulp necrosis, microorganisms can invade the entire root canal system uninhibited by host defense mechanisms. As a consequence of the interaction between microorganisms and the host defenses, inflammatory changes take place in the periapical tissues and give rise to the development of apical periodontitis.

Endodontic infections can be classified according to their anatomic location as intraradicular or extraradicular. Microorganisms that initially invade and colonize the necrotic pulp tissue cause primary intraradicular infections. Microorganisms that were not present in the primary infection but were introduced into the root canal system during or after initial treatment cause secondary infections. Secondary infections are suspected when a preoperative infection heals after treatment and then recurs at a later time. Persistent infections are caused by microorganisms from a primary infection that resisted intracanal antimicrobial procedures and remained in the prepared root canal system. Persistent and secondary infections are responsible for several clinical problems, including persistent exudation, continuation of symptoms, interappointment flare-ups, and failure of the endodontic treatment.

The goal of root canal treatment is to *remove* microorganisms from the root canal system. However, in the absence of a strict aseptic technique, microorganisms from caries and dental plaque can be introduced into the canal system *during treatment* because of lack of rubber dam usage or leakage of the rubber dam. Contaminated endodontic files and instruments, including delivery systems for antimicrobial agents, are additional potential sources for the introduction of microorganisms into the root canal system during treatment.

Microorganisms can enter the root canal system *between appointments* via loss or leakage of temporary restorative materials, fracture of the tooth structure, and teeth left open for drainage. Entry of microorganisms *after root canal filling* occurs by loss or leakage of temporary or permanent restorative materials, during preparation of posts or other intracanal restorations without the rubber dam, fracture of the tooth structure, and by recurrent caries that expose the root canal filling material. Leakage after completion of root canal treatment is more likely to occur if the placement of the permanent restoration is delayed.

Extraradicular infection is characterized by microbial invasion and proliferation into the inflamed periapical tissues and is almost invariably a sequel to intraradicular infection. Once the intraradicular infection is properly controlled by root canal treatment or tooth extraction and drainage of pus, the extraradicular infection can be addressed by the host defenses and usually subsides (Fig. 1.9).

Endodontic Infections Are Biofilm Infections

The role of microorganisms as the primary etiologic agents of root canal infections was established in seminal studies published several decades ago.[15,16,20] In these and subsequent microbiological analyses of samples recovered from root canal infections, species were isolated and identified by using planktonic (liquid) culture techniques. During the past two decades, it became apparent that microorganisms exist in the root canal system not as planktonic cultures, or as single species, but rather as multispecies biofilm communities composed of microcolonies irreversibly attached to a substratum, to an interface like dentin, and to each other.[21,22] All anatomic areas of the infected root canal system can harbor microbial cells organized as highly variable biofilm structures[22,23] (Fig. 1.10).

Biofilm formation encompasses attachment of microbial cells to a surface, followed by cell proliferation, adherence to other microorganisms, production of matrix, and microcolony maturation. Dispersal of cells allows the formation of new biofilm microcolonies.[24] Microbial cells occupy only a small proportion of the biofilm. Quorum sensing is the expression of specific microbial proteins after the bacterial cells reach a threshold number. It

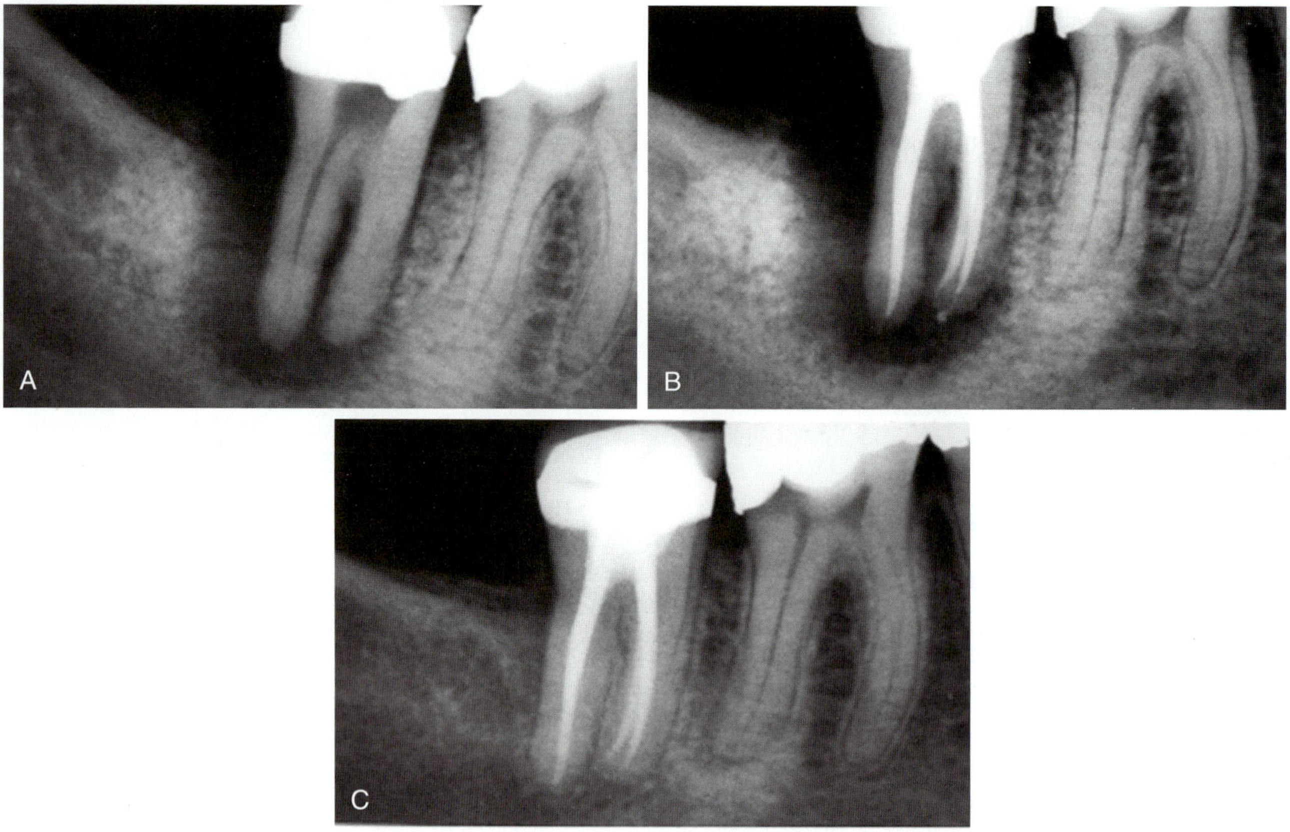

• **Fig. 1.9** **A**, Preoperative radiograph of a second molar with pulpal necrosis and evidence of chronic apical periodontitis. **B**, Postoperative radiograph of the tooth. **C**, Postoperative radiograph 2 years after root canal therapy shows complete resolution of the periradicular pathosis.

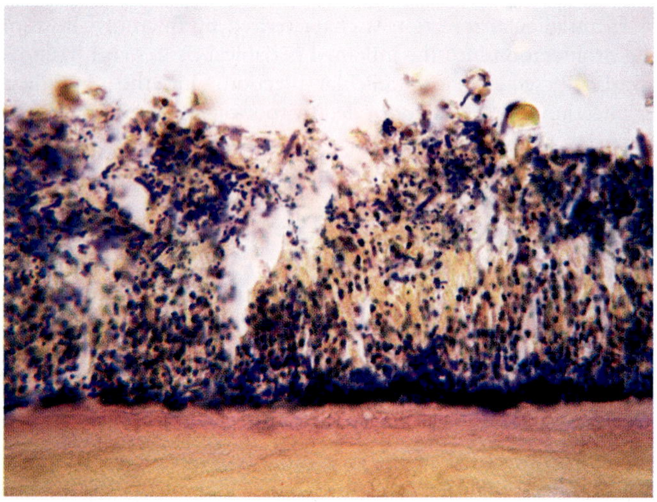

• **Fig. 1.10** Intracanal Biofilms With Predominance of Cocci. Note the high concentration of cells at the bottom of the biofilm and in direct contact with the root canal wall. (From Ricucci D, Siqueira JF Jr: Biofilms and apical periodontitis: study of prevalence and association with clinical and histopathologic findings, *J Endod* 36(8):1277–1288, 2010.)

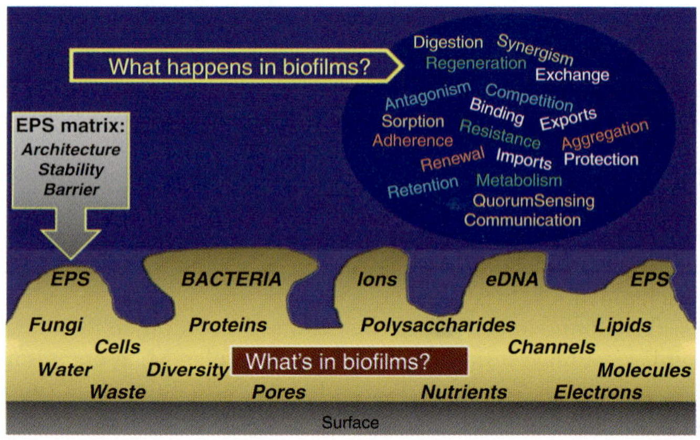

• **Fig. 1.11** Properties of biofilms emerging from life in the extracellular polymeric substance (EPS) matrix. (From Flemming HC: EPS-then and now, *Microorganisms* 4[4]:pii: E41, 2016 Nov 18.)

allows the coordinated regulation of expression of these proteins by microorganisms in biofilms to regulate population density and possibly virulence.[25] The majority of the biofilm structure is a highly heterogeneous matrix composed of extracellular polymeric substances (EPSs) produced by cells within the biofilm. The EPS matrix provides multiple functions (Fig. 1.11). From a clinical perspective, the EPS can act as a physical barrier to antimicrobial agents such as antibiotics and disinfectants.[26] Microbial organization into multispecies biofilm communities results in increased pathogenic effects on the host.[27]

The Microbiome of Endodontic Infections

The identity of specific microorganisms in root canal infections has been a major focus of interest for more than a century.[28] Studies using culture-dependent approaches have recovered several species

TABLE 1.2 Bacterial Genera Represented in Endodontic Infections

GRAM-NEGATIVE BACTERIA		GRAM-POSITIVE BACTERIA	
Anaerobes	**Facultatives**	**Anaerobes**	**Facultatives**
Rods		**Rods**	
Dialister	*Capnocytophaga*	*Actinomyces*	*Actinomyces*
Porphyromonas	*Eikenella*	*Pseudoramibacter*	*Corynebacterium*
Tannerella	*Haemophilus*	*Filifactor*	*Lactobacillus*
Prevotella		*Eubacterium*	
Fusobacterium		*Mogibacterium*	
Campylobacter		*Propionibacterium*	
Pyramidobacter		*Eggerthella*	
Catonella		*Olsenella*	
Selenomonas		*Bifidobacterium*	
Centipeda		*Slackia*	
		Atopobium	
		Solobacterium	
		Lactobacillus	
Cocci		**Cocci**	
Veillonella	*Neisseria*	*Parvimonas*	*Streptococcus*
Megasphaera		*Peptostreptococcus*	*Enterococcus*
		Finegoldia	*Granulicatella*
		Peptoniphilus	
		Anaerococcus	
		Streptococcus	
		Gemella	
Spirilla			
Treponema			

that have been identified as putative endodontic pathogens. The microbiome of carious dentin causing pulpitis and subsequent endodontic infection includes significant numbers of lactobacilli,[29] gram-negative bacteria,[30] and species from the Firmicutes, Actinobacteria, and Proteobacteria phyla.[31] Primary root canal infections harbor a multispecies population of facultative and strict anaerobic gram-positive and gram-negative bacteria, spirochetes, yeasts, Archaea, and other unidentified species.[32-36] In addition, Epstein-Barr virus may be associated with irreversible pulpitis and apical periodontitis,[37] and papilloma virus and human herpes virus have been found in exudates from acute apical abscesses.[38]

Microorganisms have been traditionally characterized in terms of their morphology (rods, cocci, spirilla), cell wall characteristics (gram-positive and gram-negative), and oxygen tolerance (anaerobic and facultatively anaerobic). Genera cultured from symptomatic and asymptomatic root canal infections include *Prevotella, Porphyromonas, Fusobacterium, Peptostreptococcus, Streptococcus, Lactobacillus, Enterococcus, Actinomyces, Propionibacterium,* and *Candida.*[20,39] (Table 1.2)

More recently, the microbiome of endodontic infections has been redefined using culture-independent molecular biology techniques. These studies have both confirmed the findings from culture studies and greatly expanded knowledge. Many species that had already been considered putative pathogens because of their frequency of detection, as reported by culture-dependent methods, have been found in a similar or even higher prevalence by using molecular approaches, strengthening associations with causation of apical periodontitis. Molecular technology has enabled the recognition of many new putative pathogens that had not previously been found in samples from endodontic infections.[40,41] A review of 12 studies that used next-generation DNA sequencing (pyrosequencing) methods to evaluate the microbiome of endodontic infections has corroborated previous multiple reports of microbial diversity. The most abundant phyla were Firmicutes, Actinobacteria, Bacteroidetes, Proteobacteria, and Fusobacteria. The most frequently detected genera were *Prevotella, Fusobacterium, Porphyromonas, Parvimonas,* and *Streptococcus.*[42] (Fig. 1.12)

Many microorganisms isolated from endodontic infections have also been identified as commensals in the oral cavity. The transition from oral "commensal" to root canal "pathogen" likely reflects an innate ability to switch on genes that enable survival and propagation in a different environment and encode a range of virulence factors (Fig. 1.13). The first reported virulence factor associated with endodontic infections was lipopolysaccharide ("endotoxin"), a virulence factor produced by gram-negative bacteria.[43]

It has been suggested that symptoms increase when certain microbial species are part of the infective endodontic microbiome. Nevertheless, the same species can be found in asymptomatic cases with prevalence comparable to that of symptomatic cases; this apparent discrepancy could be explained in part by the variations in expression of virulence factors by different strains of the same species. Protein analyses (the metaproteome) of endodontic infections, along with the host response, are future steps toward better understanding of interactions between the microbiome of endodontic infections and the host throughout the infection and healing process.[44,45]

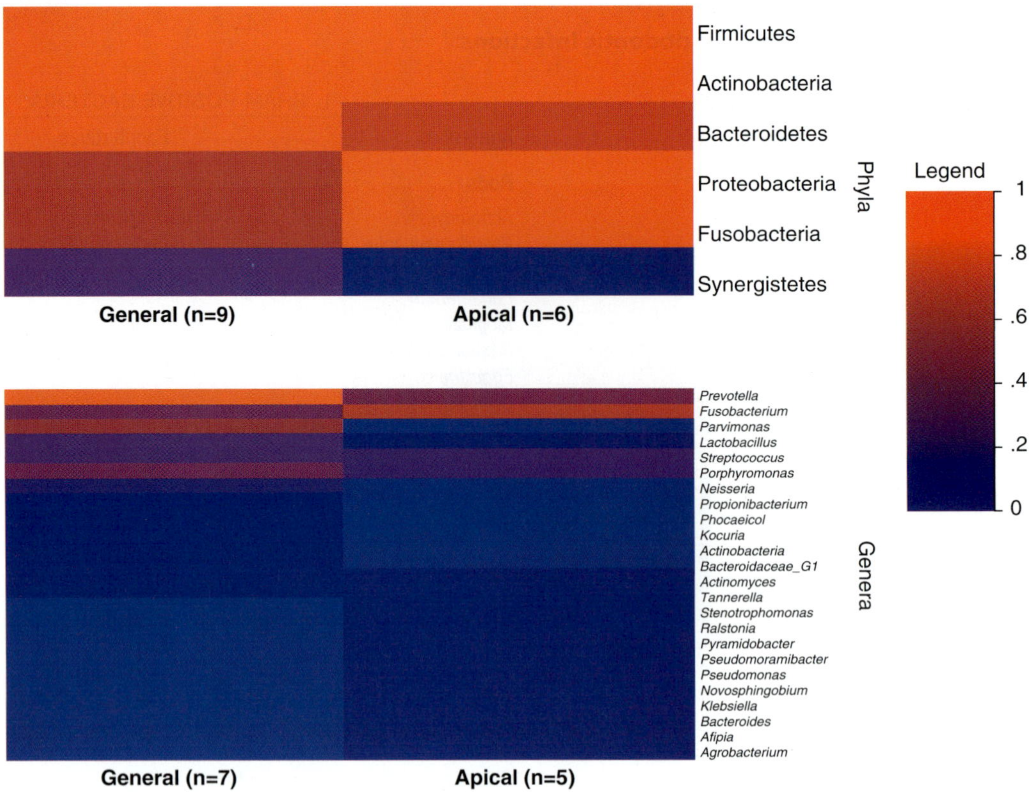

• **Fig. 1.12** A heat map of root canal community profiles based on bacterial prevalence in 15 groups of root canal microbiomes gathered from 12 studies using next-generation DNA sequencing. Microbiome profiles are divided into general (entire root canal) and apical samples. Heat map scale ranges from 0 to 1 by taxa where "1" indicates that all samples had that specific taxa as their top 5 phyla or genera. A "0" score indicates that taxa did not appear as a top 5 phyla or genera. (From Shin JM, Luo T, Lee KH, et al: Deciphering endodontic microbial communities by next-generation sequencing, *J Endod* 44[7]:1080–87, 2018.)

Pulpal Diseases

Host Response in the Dental Pulp

The response of the dental pulp to microbial and other physical and chemical irritants is similar to the response in other connective tissues. An inflammatory process starts in the pulp and corresponds to the location where the irritation reaches it. For example, in an incipient carious lesion at the depth of an occlusal fissure, the pulp at the end of the affected dentinal tubules is seen to have a small inflammatory process histologically. This inflammation progresses throughout the coronal pulp as the carious lesion penetrates deeper in dentin, until the microbial irritants eventually invade the pulp in large numbers and cause severe inflammation (Fig. 1.14).

However, unlike other connective tissues, the dental pulp lacks collateral circulation and is confined within rigid dentinal walls. Therefore at a specific point in the disease process, the inflammation changes from reversible (one that would respond favorably to conservative methods of treatment and eventually heal) to irreversible pulpitis. The transition of reversible to irreversible pulpitis is important to identify clinically because it determines the optimal procedure that should be employed to treat it.

Studies have shown that the inflammatory response in the pulp is associated with several cellular and molecular changes. The degree of irritation appears to trigger a corresponding level of inflammation. This titration of the inflammatory response to the level of irritation is orchestrated by a balance of proinflammatory and antiinflammatory factors in the pulp. The condition of the pulp deteriorates or improves based on the reaction of pulpal factors to the external environment. Cellular responses include the increase in inflammatory cells, most notably neutrophils, lymphocytes, macrophages, plasma cells, mast cells, and dendritic cells (Figs. 1.15 to 1.17). The inflammatory cell response correlates in its intensity with the depth of the carious lesion.[46] Noninflammatory cells, such as odontoblasts and fibroblasts, do contribute to the inflammatory response. Odontoblasts have been shown to express TLRs, cytokines, chemokines, and defensins.[47] However, the degree to which noninflammatory cells contribute to the inflammation is much less than inflammatory cells like neutrophils and macrophages. A recent study showed reasonably good agreement between clinical signs and symptoms, and the histologic condition of the pulp in cases with caries.[48] In this study, microbial ingress into the pulp, which is indicative of severe pathosis, seemed to be confined to cases diagnosed clinically as irreversible pulpitis.

In recent years there has also been considerable interest in molecular mediators of pulpal inflammation. Some inflammatory mediators have been shown to correlate directly with increased pulpal pain and the clinical diagnosis of symptomatic irreversible pulpitis. These mediators include prostaglandins, neuropeptides, bradykinin, cytokines, chemokines, and matrix metalloproteinases.[49,50] The dental pulp is heavily innervated by

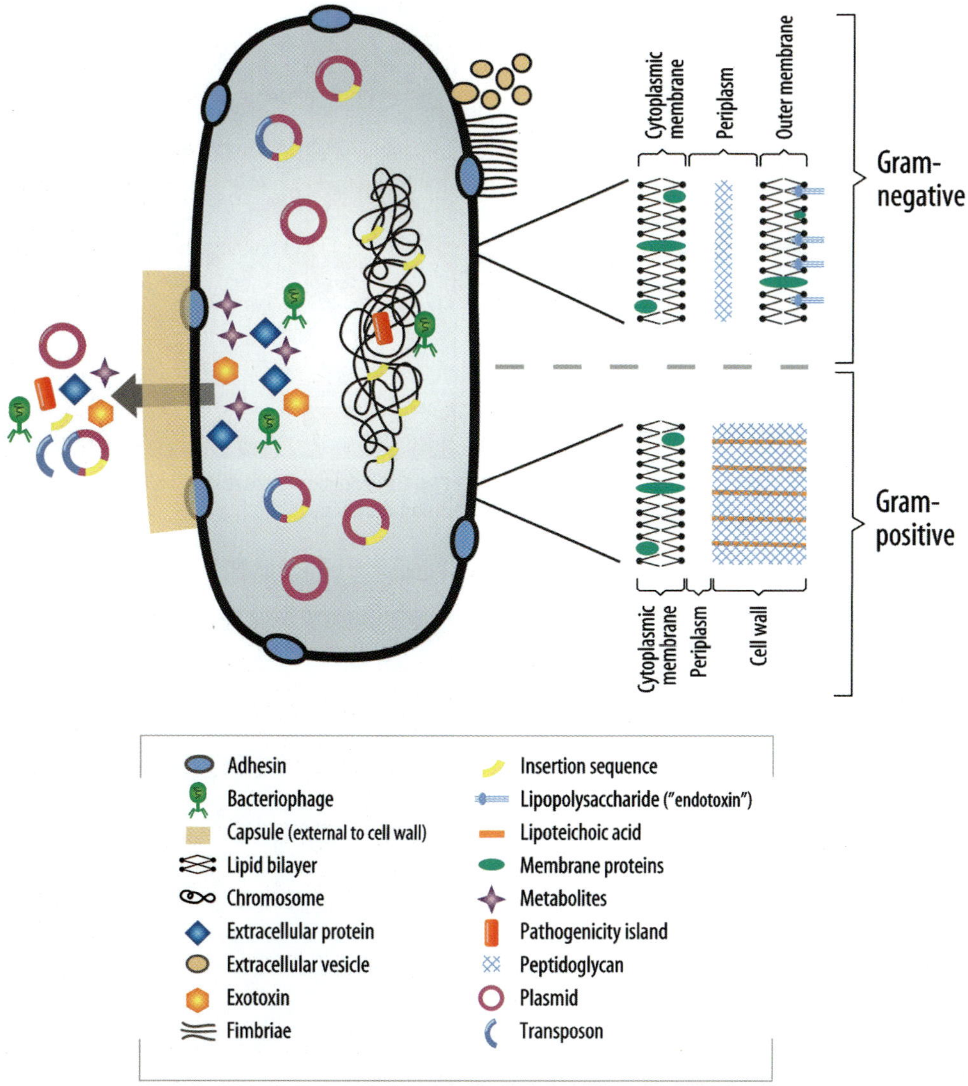

• **Fig. 1.13** Potential Virulence Factors Associated With a Bacterial Cell. (From Sedgley CM. Virulence of endodontic bacterial pathogens. In Fouad AF, editor: *Endodontic microbiology*, Ames, IA, 2009, Wiley-Blackwell Publishing, pp. 130–151.)

sensory fibers. During the inflammatory process, there is sprouting of pulp nociceptors, with an increase in secretion of neuropeptides like substance P and CGRP. These mediators lower the pain threshold and increase the permeability of blood vessels to inflammatory cells.

The compromised ability of the pulp to survive severe forms of inflammation, in comparison with other connective tissues, is illustrated by the differences in response to trauma between teeth with immature apex and those with mature apex. After luxation injuries, such as extrusion, intrusion, or even total avulsion and replantation, the tooth with immature apex is much more likely to retain (or revascularize) a vital pulp than a tooth with mature apex. This difference is primarily related to the increased collateral circulation in the immature teeth that can take advantage of the wide apical foramen.

Occasionally, radiographic analysis of the dental pulp reveals an increase in mineralization and deposition of hard dentinal tissues. Increased mineralization occurs gradually due to deposition of secondary dentin throughout life. However, as a result of traumatic injuries, a substantial increase in mineralization may occur in the tooth or teeth that were traumatized. Increased areas of mineralization, commonly known as *pulp stones*, are also associated with caries or deep restorations. Excessive pulp stones have also been associated with cardiovascular diseases,[51] and with intake of statin medications.[52] Increased mineralization of the pulp, even when obliterating the entire canal space (Fig. 1.18), in the absence of symptoms or apical pathosis, is not considered pathologic. However, if pulpal disease arises in these conditions, root canal treatment may become very challenging.

Less frequently, the pulp may undergo internal resorptive defects (Fig. 1.19). The cells that typically initiate the resorption, the osteoclasts or odontoclasts, are not normal inhabitants of the healthy pulp. These cells, which arise from monocytes, are normal mediators of bone turnover and are present in the PDL and alveolar bone. When resorptive lesions are detected clinically (internally or externally), they have usually attained a large size and are considered pathologic, even in the absence of symptoms.

• BOX 1.1 Review Study Questions

1. Which of the following is a condition that can be described as irreversible pathosis of the pulp:
   a. Dentin hypersensitivity
   b. Pulp canal obliteration (total calcification)
   c. Internal resorption
   d. Sharp, brief pain with thermal changes
2. The following inflammatory mediator(s) is/are not elevated in the pulp, in cases with symptomatic irreversible pulpitis:
   a. Prostaglandins
   b. Leukotrienes
   c. Bradykinin
   d. Neuropeptides
   e. Matrix metalloproteinases
3. The following cytokine acts to control the expansion of periapical lesions:
   a. IL-1
   b. IL-8
   c. IL-10
   d. TNF-alpha
   e. IL-17
4. Root canal infections are best described as:
   a. Single-species biofilms, predominantly microorganisms
   b. Single-species biofilms, predominantly extracellular matrix
   c. Multispecies biofilms, within an extracellular matrix, predominantly microorganisms
   d. Multispecies biofilms, within an extracellular matrix, predominantly matrix
5. Compared with bacteria in suspension (planktonic), microorganisms in biofilms:
   a. Are less resistant to antimicrobial agents
   b. Can resist alkaline stress better
   c. Have a decreased potential for cell-to-cell interaction
   d. A and C

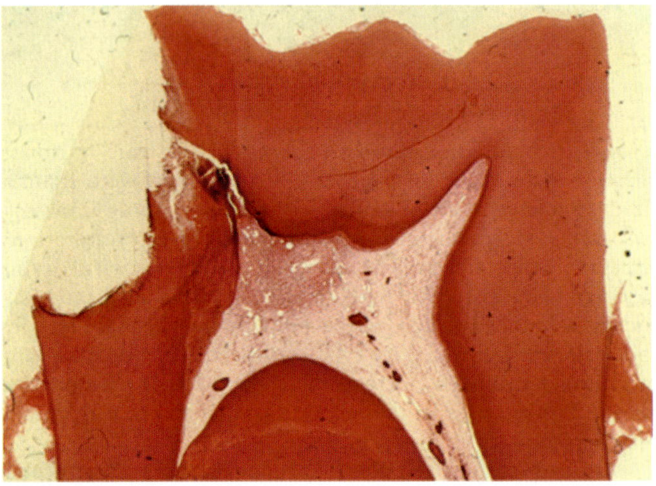

• **Fig. 1.14** A localized inflammatory reaction containing mainly polymorphonuclear leukocytes (PMNs) at the site of a carious pulpal exposure. The remainder of the coronal pulp is almost free of inflammatory cells. (Courtesy Dr. J.H. Simon.)

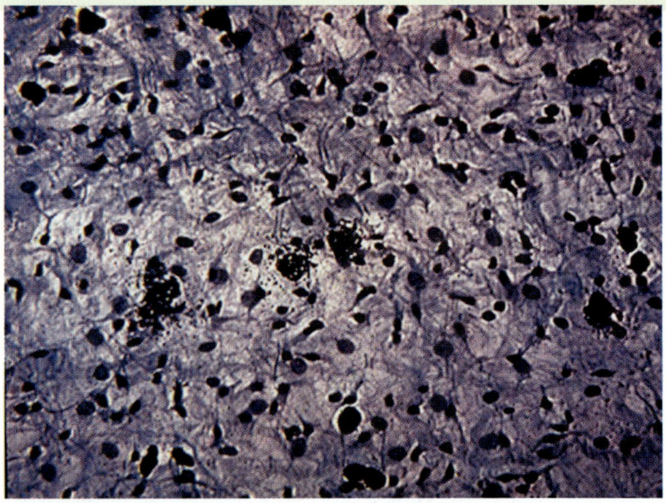

• **Fig. 1.15** Mast cells are readily visible as dark-stained cells in this inflamed human dental pulp.

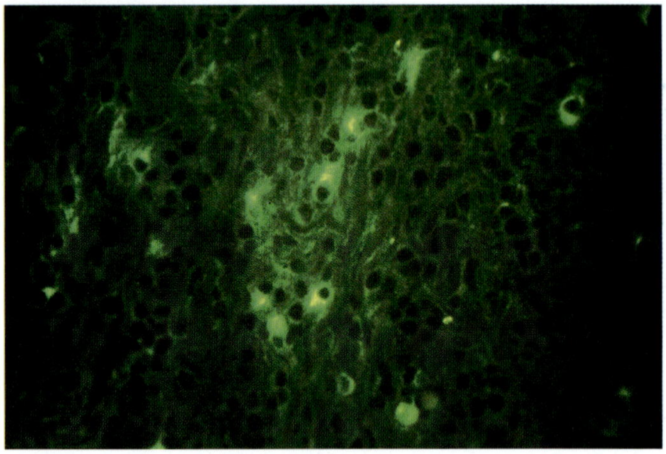

• **Fig. 1.16** Some plasma cells stain positively for IgM in inflamed human dental pulp, indicating immunologic activity.

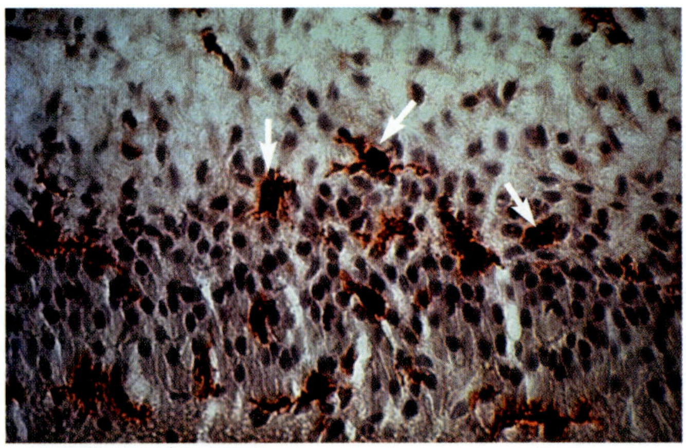

• **Fig. 1.17** Many dendritic cells *(arrows)* are present in an inflamed dental pulp. (Courtesy Dr. M. Jontell.)

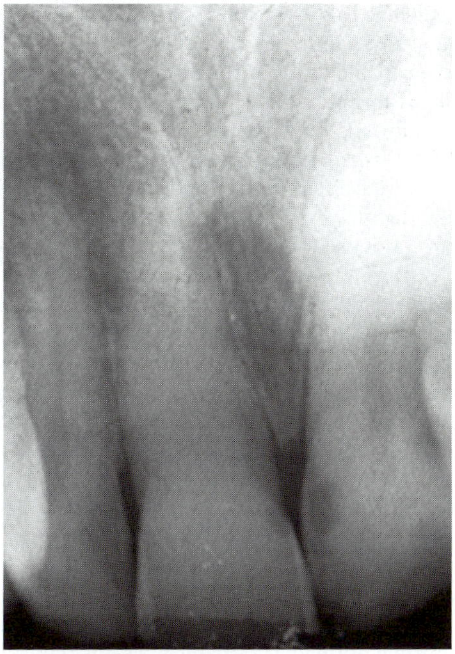

• **Fig. 1.18** Calcific metamorphosis does not represent pathosis per se and may occur with aging or low-grade irritation. It also may occur subsequent to a traumatic injury to the tooth.

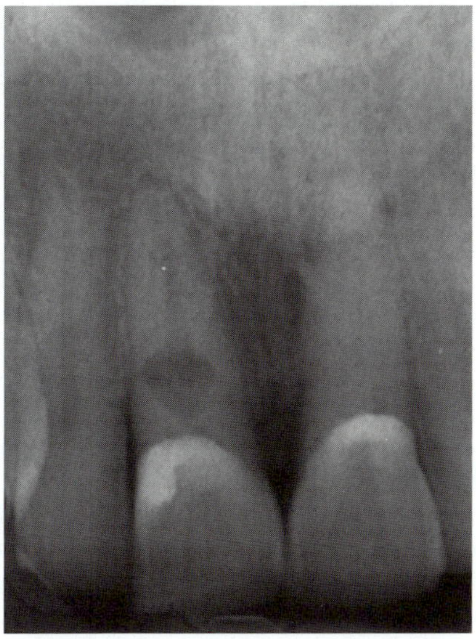

• **Fig. 1.19** Hard tissue resorption that causes disappearance of normal radiographic evidence of the root canal *usually* indicates an internal resorption defect.

Clinical Classification of Pulpal Conditions

The dental pulp is encapsulated by hard tissues and therefore is not amenable to direct visual or tactile examination, or sampling for biopsy. The clinician must rely on signs and symptoms of disease, the results of clinical testing, and radiographic imaging to reach a pulpal diagnosis (see Chapter 4). A diagnosis must be obtained before any endodontic procedure is contemplated. Here the general classification and features of different pulpal conditions will be described to introduce the reader to the disease progression in the dental pulp. Histological examination of the pulp in various stages of disease, except for total necrosis, reveals that different areas of the pulp may have different stages of normalcy, inflammation, or necrosis. Indeed, the progression from reversible pulpitis to irreversible pulpitis and then to necrosis is gradual and occurs in small compartments of the pulp at any one time, thereby complicating the clinical diagnosis.

Normal Pulp

As noted previously, normal pulp is histologically characterized by the presence of an intact odontoblastic layer, a cell-free zone, a cell-rich zone, and the absence of inflammation or necrosis. The odontoblasts may be interspersed with dendritic cells or nerve endings. Occasionally, inflammatory cells such as lymphocytes, neutrophils, or macrophages may be seen, but they are sporadic and located in the central pulp. However, the pulp tissue is primarily composed of fibroblasts, vascular elements, stem cells, and myelinated and unmyelinated nerve fibers.

Reversible Pulpitis

Pulpal inflammation begins with the onset of a carious lesion, or other irritation, such as a crack, cervical abrasion, crown attrition or fracture, or in response to a dental procedure on an intact tooth. These external stimuli lead to biological or physical irritation of the pulp and result in an increased area of inflammatory response in close proximity to the area of irritation. An example of this response may be dentin hypersensitivity in relation to cervical abrasion or attachment loss treated with scaling and root planing. Clinically, the patient with reversible pulpitis usually has no symptoms, or may have mild hyperalgesia of the pulp. The latter is expressed as increased sharp pain (with thermal changes) that is short in duration. Correction of the clinical problem that caused reversible pulpitis, such as with a restoration of a carious lesion or desensitization of hypersensitive dentin, results in healing and resolution of symptoms.

Irreversible Pulpitis

The transition from reversible to irreversible pulpitis is gradual and may or may not be associated with changes in symptoms. Irreversible pulpitis is characterized histologically by the presence of areas of severe inflammation and partial necrosis in the pulp, commonly in proximity to an area of carious exposure. There is typically microbial invasion of a portion of the pulp, with intense inflammatory response that is attempting to wall off the microbial infection. The rest of the pulp tissue typically has mild inflammation or no inflammation and therefore, is responsive to clinical vitality testing. Irreversible pulpitis may be associated with severe spontaneous and lingering pain, or with milder symptoms or no pain. Because the association of pain with irreversible pulpitis is not consistent, the diagnosis of irreversible pulpitis may be challenging (see Chapter 4).

Two additional conditions are usually diagnosed as irreversible pulpitis: cases with internal resorption, with a vital (responsive) pulp (Fig. 1.19) and cases with hyperplastic pulpitis (pulp polyp) (Fig. 1.20). The latter represents a proliferative response that is occasionally seen in the pulp of children, that has been exposed to the oral cavity, and in which the pulp tissue may be covered by desquamated epithelium from oral mucosa.

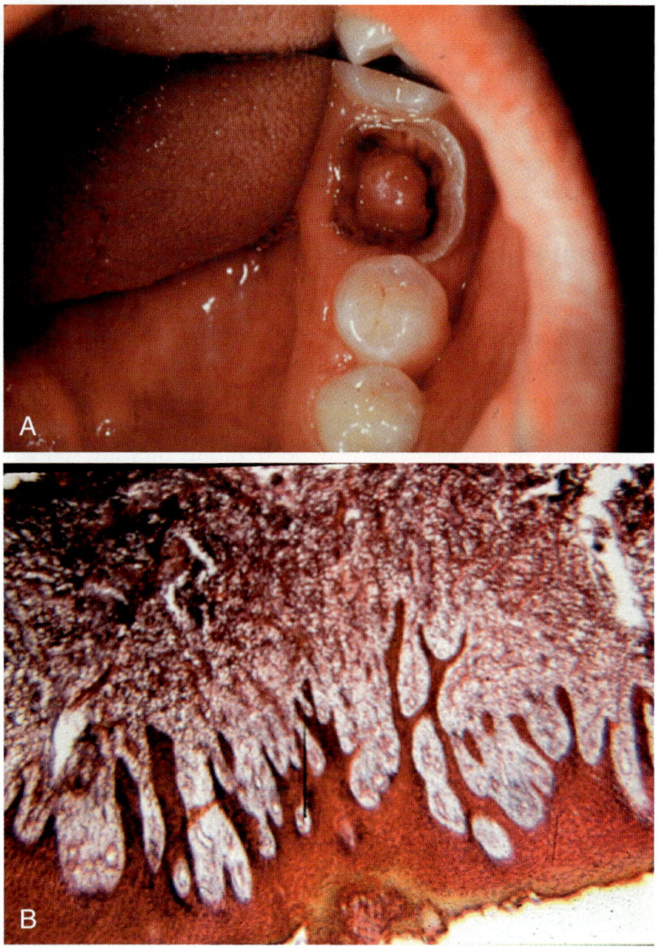

• **Fig. 1.20** **A**, Pulp polyp, also known as *hyperplastic pulpitis.* The involved tooth is usually carious with extensive loss of tooth structure; the pulp remains vital and proliferates from the exposure site. **B**, Histologic examination of hyperplastic pulpitis shows surface epithelium and underlying inflamed connective tissue.

Pulp Necrosis

In about 40% of cases, irreversible pulpitis develops into pulp necrosis without symptoms.[53] In this condition, the dental pulp degenerates completely and is replaced by serous or purulent fluid or by dry necrotic tissue. The root canal environment contains microbial biofilms that vary in their composition, location, and thickness, depending on nutritive factors, pH, oxygen tension, and continued access to the oral cavity. In addition, the biofilm invades dentinal tubules, which are wide enough to accommodate microbial cells, especially in young patients with larger dentinal tubules.[54]

Pulp necrosis is asymptomatic, because the nerve endings supplying the pulp are no longer present. However, clinically, there are instances when the patient can feel endodontic instruments that are exploring the necrotic pulp space. This sensation may be due to remaining pulpal nerve fibers or fluid pressures that stimulate apical nociceptors. In addition, pulp necrosis may be associated with several apical conditions that are symptomatic (see later section).

Periapical Diseases

As the inflammation progresses throughout the radicular pulp, it gradually starts to affect the periapical tissues. The progression of the pulp disease into the periapical tissues presents a major biological challenge to those tissues. The PDL is a very thin, highly fibrous tissue that is confined within the bony crypt. As such, these tissues are not capable of mounting an immune response that can stop the advancing microbial ingress. Therefore the hallmark of apical periodontitis is bone resorption to accommodate the formation of a soft tissue lesion, in which the immunologic reactions that can stop the advancing infection can be concentrated.

Animal studies have shown that apical bone resorption and inflammatory response starts soon after the initiation of pulpal inflammation. In one study, researchers found that the pathogenesis of pulpitis and apical periodontitis in the initial phases, and in the absence of severe virulent bacteria, is primarily coordinated by innate rather than adaptive immune responses.[55] In another study, adaptive responses were found to be critical in preventing disseminated infections if a significant microbial load of virulent species is introduced.[56] As noted before, a variety of microbial factors are important in development of periapical lesions, such as lipopolysaccharides (LPSs), lipoteichoic acid, bacterial enzymes, adhesion factors, toxins, etc. (Fig. 1.13). Although LPS is a well-characterized irritant that can induce pulpal and periapical lesions even in the absence of live bacteria,[57,58] periapical lesions have been induced in animal models that do not respond to LPS in a similar manner to normal animals.[59] Periapical lesions typically take 5 to 8 weeks in large animal models to be visible radiographically.[60]

The inflammatory response in the periapical lesion is similar to that in the pulp, except that bone resorption is now a critical component of the host response. Numerous studies have documented the tightly regulated process of periapical bone loss that correlates with the degree of the advancing microbial irritation and the balance of proinflammatory and antiinflammatory factors. Important cytokines in bone resorption include IL-1, IL-6, IL-11, IL-17, and TNF-alpha. Cytokines that limit bone resorption include IL-4 and IL-10. Another key protein that plays a major role in bone resorption is nuclear factor-κB ligand (RANKL). RANKL binds to its receptor (RANK), resulting in osteoclast differentiation. This interaction is inhibited by osteoprotegerin (OPG), a decoy protein that binds to the receptor. Levels of RANKL and the ratio of RANKL to OPG both peak at 2 to 3 weeks, concurrent with the progression of periapical bone destruction. RANKL production tapers off between weeks 4 and 8, whereas production of OPG increases during this time, creating a negative feedback loop that limits the amount of bone destruction caused by bacterial infection.[61] The RANKL-RANK interaction is involved in both physiologic and pathologic bone resorption. In periapical tissues, a significant increase in RANKL levels has been found in granulomatous lesions compared with healthy controls.[62,63] Finally, T-reg lymphocytes have been shown to control the size of periapical lesions in a significant manner.[64]

Histologically, periapical lesions have traditionally been classified into granulomas, cysts, or apical abscesses. A granuloma has a collection of inflammatory cells, such as lymphocytes, plasma cells, macrophages, and mast cells, that are arranged in a granular manner, thus the name *granuloma*. Occasionally, there are multinucleated giant cells and foam cells that may represent osteoclasts or engorged macrophages, respectively. A periapical cyst arises in a part of a granuloma and thus has a granuloma as part of its wall. A cyst represents a proliferation of the epithelial rests of Malassez, which are vestigial embryonic cells that remain after the disintegration of the epithelial root sheath of Hertwig after root development. Cysts may be formed by one of several mechanisms. Either the epithelial strands proliferate to surround an area of the granuloma, restrict the blood supply, and cause degeneration of the central tissue, or the epithelial mass widens to the extent that

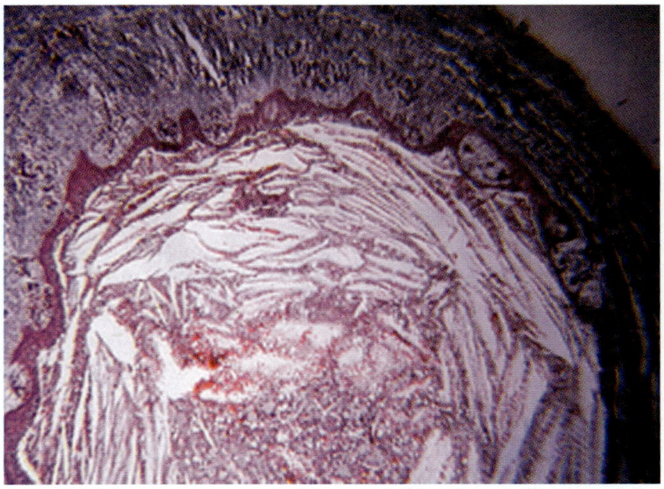

• **Fig. 1.21** A region of human apical cyst consists of a central cavity filled with eosinophilic material *(EM)* and a wall lined with epithelium.

central cells degenerate due to their distance from the sources of nutrition. Cysts contain clear cyst fluid that may be filled with eosinophilic material and cholesterol crystals (Fig. 1.21).

The literature shows that the incidence of granulomas and cysts varies considerably. Most of these studies are from pathology services, in which only a select number of cases are submitted for examination, typically when the practitioner suspects nonendodontic pathosis. The sources may be extracted teeth that may or may not have had endodontic treatment, lesions recovered during apical surgery, or lesions in edentulous areas, suspected to have been associated with previously extracted teeth. The tissue may or may not be the complete lesion, and the pathologist may or may not perform serial sectioning to diagnose the entire lesion. In addition, many pathologists would diagnose a cyst upon identifying any epithelial tissue in the lesion, and some pathologists need to see evidence of cyst lining and lumen before making the same diagnosis. Finally, some of the larger studies have documented a high percentage of nonendodontic lesions (27% in one study[65]) that are submitted for examination, thus raising the possibility that some of these cases may not adhere to other characteristics of apical pathosis. With this diversity, the incidence of cysts has been reported to be from 7% to 54% of apical lesions.

Two types of apical radicular cysts have been described in the literature: true cysts and pocket (or bay) cysts. True cysts are those that do not communicate directly with the apical foramen of the offending tooth but are separated from it by an area of the lesion. Pocket or bay cysts are those in which the root apex and apical foramen open directly into the lumen of the cyst. This distinction between the types of cysts was proposed as a rationale for an argument that true cysts would not respond to nonsurgical treatment and would require surgical enucleation.[66] However, there has never been direct evidence to support this hypothesis.[67,68]

A large body of literature has examined the differences between cysts and granulomas in inflammatory cells or molecular mediators and whether they can be distinguished clinically without obtaining a biopsy. However, it is now thought that cysts arise from granulomas of long standing and in conditions that are conducive to the proliferation of the epithelial rests. It is also generally accepted that the differentiation of cysts and granulomas is not critical, because both can heal equally well after surgical or nonsurgical treatment,[68] provided that bacterial irritants have been controlled.[67] The clinical importance of apical radicular cysts (or large granulomas) may be in the differential diagnosis from other nonodontogenic lesions (see later section). Cysts may also push roots, causing malalignment of teeth.[69]

An apical abscess is characterized histologically by the presence of an intense inflammatory response surrounding areas of tissue necrosis. If bacterial stains are used, then bacteria may be physically present in these areas of necrosis. If bacterial invasion is extensive and prolonged, particularly in patients who are immunocompromised, osteomyelitis may develop. Histologically, areas of necrotic bone with empty lacunae are seen surrounded by intense inflammatory response. Microbial presence in asymptomatic apical lesions is relatively infrequent.[70,71] However, studies have shown that about 50% of cases with persistent disease after endodontic treatment may have bacterial presence in the lesion.[72] Occasionally the predominant bacterial colony is from the *Actinomyces* spp.[73] This organism is filamentous in nature, and the histologic picture is characteristically described as actinic rays (Fig. 1.22)

Clinical Classification of Periapical (Apical) Conditions

Normal Periapex

In this clinical condition, there is no evidence of apical pathosis clinically or radiographically, and the tooth is asymptomatic to percussion and apical palpation. In these cases, it is thought that the inflammation of the pulp has not yet reached the apical tissues but may do so if the pulpal condition is not addressed.

Symptomatic Apical Periodontitis

In this condition, the tooth is tender to percussion and/or apical palpation. This condition is also referred to as *mechanical allodynia* of the involved tooth. The inflammation has progressed in this case to the apical tissues, and therefore the pulpal pathosis is considered irreversible in nature. It is noteworthy, however, that after restorative procedures on a vital normally responsive pulp, if the occlusion on the tooth is inadvertently left high, the tooth is rendered tender to percussion. In these cases, the occlusion needs to be adjusted, and the pulpal condition is considered reversible.

Cases with symptomatic apical periodontitis may have widened PDL space on the periapical radiograph (Fig. 1.23), or a small radiolucency on the cone beam computed tomography (CBCT). However, there are also many cases with asymptomatic apical periodontitis, in which an apical lesion is evident radiographically, that eventually develop clinical symptoms and become symptomatic. It is not clear why asymptomatic lesions occasionally exacerbate and become symptomatic; however, it is thought that this change may be due to changes in the microbial composition of the infected root canal causing an increase in virulent strains, an increase in microbial load, or a disruption of the host response that favors a more pathogenic infection.

Asymptomatic Apical Periodontitis

In these conditions, an apical radiolucent lesion is evident radiographically and associated with a necrotic pulp (Fig. 1.24). The lesion is typically associated with one or more roots of the tooth and occasionally extends to the furcation area as well. In fact, the lesion is associated with any area of the root in which there is the

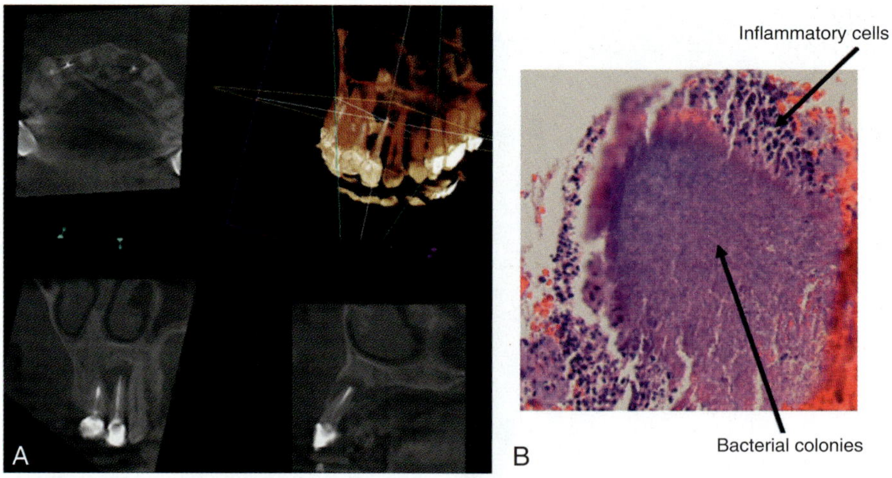

• **Fig. 1.22** Apical Actinomycosis. Cone beam computed tomography (CBCT) in **(A)** is of a patient with persistent apical periodontitis related to previously treated tooth #10. After root end resection and filling, the biopsy result was apical actinomycosis. Photomicrograph of the lesion is shown in **(B)**.

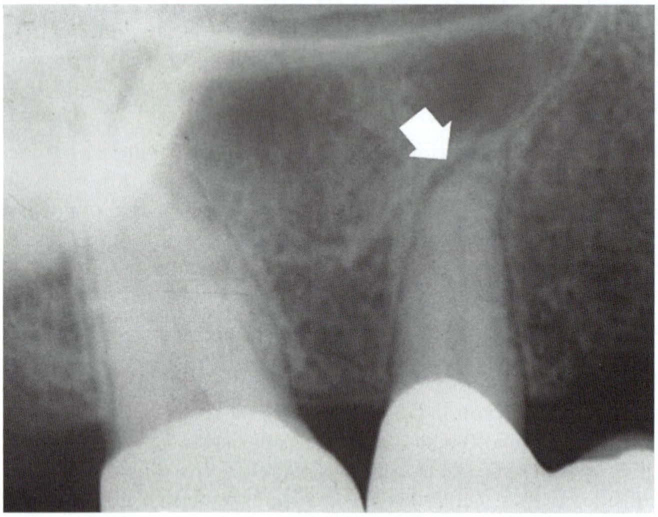

• **Fig. 1.23** After cementation of a three-unit bridge, the premolar developed clinical signs and symptoms of acute apical periodontitis. Radiograph shows a widened periodontal ligament space *(arrow)*.

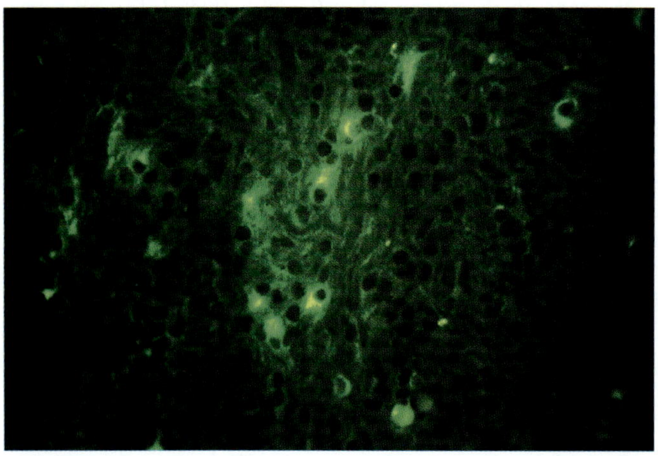

• **Fig. 1.24** Some plasma cells stain positively for immunoglobulin M (IgM) in inflamed human dental pulp, indicating immunologic activity.

foramen of the main, lateral, or accessory canals. Occasionally, the presence of the lesion indicates the location of a foramen of a large lateral canal that cannot be seen radiographically and may not be treatable directly due to its location and size. Asymptomatic apical periodontitis may remain asymptomatic for years and may reach very large sizes. In these cases, the lesion is detected if the dentist develops a suspicion to image for apical pathosis or as an incidental finding on an intraoral or extraoral radiograph taken for other purposes. These lesions may be granulomas or cysts, but this distinction cannot be determined clinically.

Acute Apical Abscess

This condition is the most serious clinical diagnosis in endodontics. It indicates that virulent bacterial infection has invaded the periapical tissues in sufficient numbers to cause pain and swelling related to the offending tooth (Fig. 1.25). An acute apical abscess ranges in severity from a small localized swelling in the attached gingiva that is not associated with constitutional symptoms, to a large swelling that invades fascial spaces and causes severe morbidity or even mortality of the patient. Microorganisms from the root canal environment are capable of raising systemic immunoglobulins, acute phase proteins, and systemic cytokines such as IL-1.[74-77]

Chronic Apical Abscess

This condition is less severe than an acute apical abscess, although it is biologically very similar to it. The pulp necrosis in this case is the source of virulent bacteria that invade the apical tissues and cause purulent drainage through a sinus tract, typically in the attached gingiva surrounding the involved tooth. The drainage may also occur through an isolated periodontal pocket that communicates with the apical lesion. The path of the sinus tract is determined by the path of least resistance. In rare instances, the sinus tract travels beyond the insertion of facial muscles and opens on the skin of the patient's face or chin area. A sinus tract, regardless of location and duration, spontaneously heals once the source of the microorganisms, namely the infected root canal environment, is effectively treated through root canal treatment or tooth extraction.

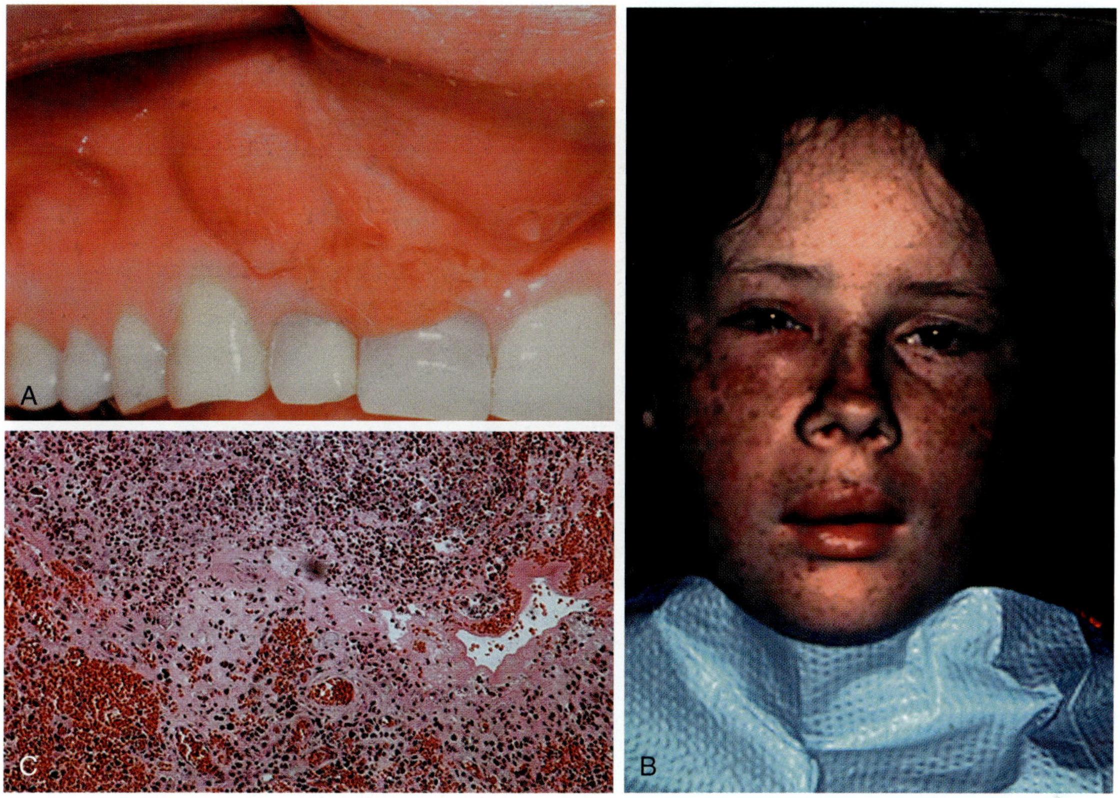

• **Fig. 1.25** **A**, Localized vestibular swelling resulting from the necrotic pulp in the right lateral incisor. **B**, An acute apical abscess (AAA) has created diffuse facial swelling. **C**, Histologic examination of the AAA shows edematous tissue heavily infiltrated by degenerating polymorphonuclear leukocytes (PMNs).

Condensing Osteitis

This condition represents a radiographic feature of the periapex of some teeth with pulpal pathosis. In these cases, the bone surrounding the apical region is more sclerotic than that surrounding neighboring teeth. The pulpal condition may have any of the pathologic conditions described earlier in this chapter. It is thought that low-grade irritation of the bone may result in sclerosis rather than in resorption. In the absence of irreversible pathosis of the pulp, there is no need to address condensing osteitis. Condensing osteitis is often confused with enostosis (sclerotic bone), a nonpathologic entity that may be associated with teeth with normal pulp.

Nonendodontic Pathosis

Benign lesions with radiographic appearances like periapical lesions include (but are not limited to) the initial stages of periapical cemental dysplasia (Fig. 1.26), early stages of fibrous dysplasia, ossifying fibroma, odontogenic keratocyst, lateral periodontal cyst, dentigerous cyst, median maxillary or mandibular cyst, traumatic bone cyst, central giant cell granuloma, central hemangioma, hyperparathyroidism, myxoma, and ameloblastoma. Usually (but not always), radiographically the lamina dura around the root apices is intact, and responses to pulp tests are normal. The final diagnosis of these lesions is often based on surgical biopsy and histopathologic examination.

Malignant lesions that may simulate periapical lesions of pulpal origin and are often metastatic include lymphoma (Fig. 1.27), squamous cell carcinoma, osteogenic sarcoma, chondrosarcoma, and multiple myeloma. Unlike endodontic lesions, these lesions are usually associated with rapid and extensive hard tissue (bone and tooth) destruction. Ordinarily, the teeth in the affected region remain responsive to vitality tests, although occasionally the pulps or sensory nerves are disrupted and nonresponsive. The patient may also experience numbness rather than pain in these situations.

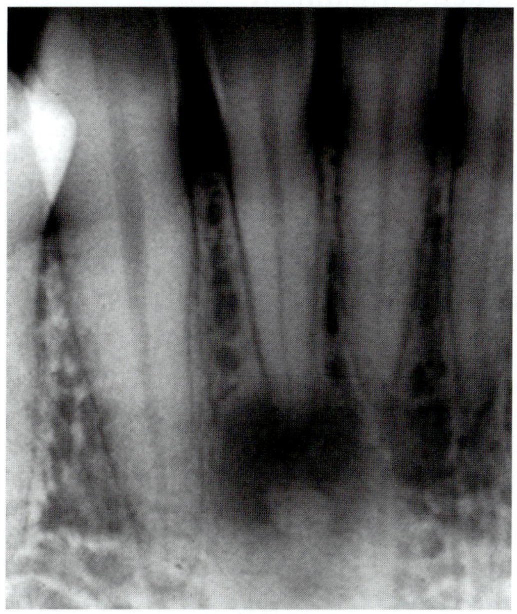

• **Fig. 1.26** A periapical radiolucency in the early stages of cementoma can simulate a periapical lesion of pulpal origin. However, the pulps' responses are within normal limits.

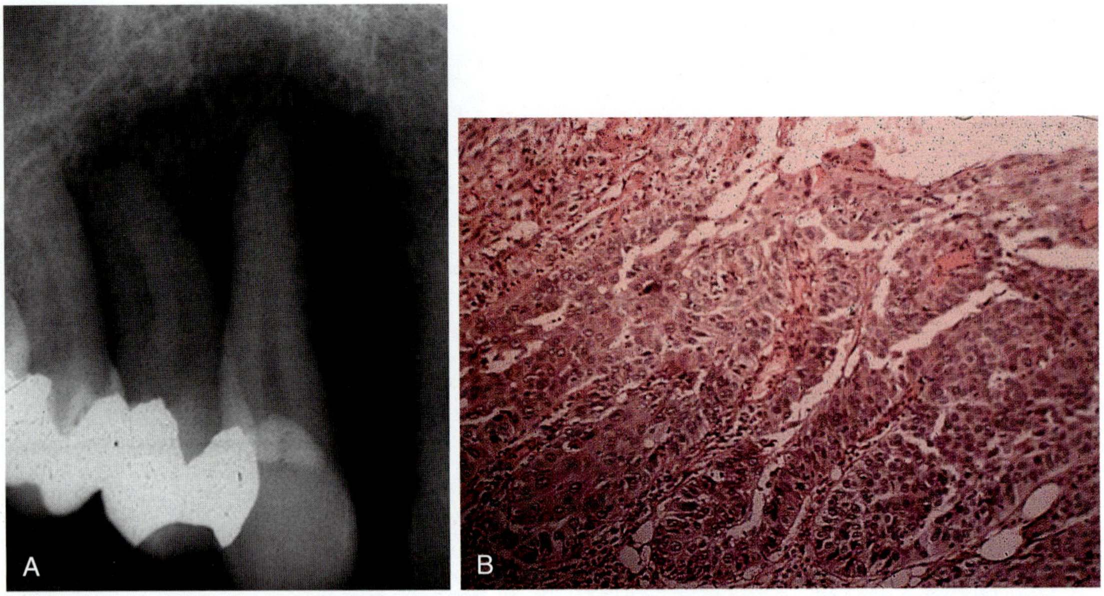

• **Fig. 1.27** **A**, Periapical radiolucent lesion of nonpulpal origin. **B**, Positive results of vitality tests and histologic examination of the tissue confirmed a diagnosis of carcinoma.

The percentages of different histopathologic diagnoses have been presented in one of the largest studies to document endodontic and nonendodontic apical pathosis submitted for biopsy[65] (Fig. 1.28).

Role of Residual Microorganisms in the Outcome of Endodontic Treatment

Root canal treatment aims to eliminate necrotic pulp tissue, biofilm, and debris from the root canal system. However, several obstacles to optimal root canal disinfection can exist, resulting in persistent infections, or infections arising from members of the original microbiome that have survived root canal treatment.[78] These obstacles include the anatomic complexities of the root canal system, the buffering effects of dentin, and the physical barrier to antimicrobials provided by the EPS matrix of the biofilm. As a consequence, some species survive endodontic treatment procedures, and persistent infection can ensue.[79,80] Microbial products from persistent infections diffusing into the apical tissues through root canal ramifications and exposed dentinal tubules can induce an inflammatory response with consequent release of cytokines that activate resorption mechanisms (Fig. 1.29).

The primary cause of endodontic treatment failure has been attributed to intraradicular infections, usually in the form of biofilms.[81] Microorganisms present in the apical portion of the root canal, apical deltas, and lateral canals have the potential to sustain long-standing infections.[22] Those microorganisms that survive need to be able to resist periods of starvation and withstand possible disruption of the EPS matrix. If communication with the apical tissues is present, then the biofilm is likely to have access to a source of nutrients that facilitates growth and a subsequent host response that sustains or exacerbates periapical inflammation and avoids healing.

Extraradicular infections have been associated with cases of long-standing lesions and persistent root canal infections.[82] It is generally accepted that *Actinomyces* spp. and *Propionibacterium propionicum* are involved in periapical lesions refractory to endodontic treatment because of their ability to evade the host response, survive in the apical tissues, and prevent apical healing (Fig. 1.22). However, there is no clear evidence that apical actinomycosis is actually independent of the intraradicular infection.[73] In these cases surgical management that includes root end resection and removal of the infected tissue typically provides a successful outcome.

Healing of Pulp and Periapical Tissues

Regeneration is a process by which altered tissues are completely replaced by tissues native to their original architecture and function. Repair is a process by which altered tissues are not completely restored to their original structures. Inflammation and healing are not two separate entities; in fact, they constitute part of one process in response to tissue injury. On the molecular and cellular levels, they are inseparable. Inflammation dominates the early events after tissue injury, shifting toward healing after the early responses have subsided. The level of healing is proportional to the degree and extent of tissue injury and the nature of tissue destruction.

Process of Pulp Healing

In the absence of irritants, a healthy pulp has tremendous capacity to heal. Odontoblasts are the first cells to encounter the invading microorganisms and their components, as well as to detect dentin matrix constituents released during demineralization.[83] Together with pulp fibroblasts,[84] they are capable of orchestrating an inflammatory response, contributing to the recruitment of immune system cells and releasing cytokines and chemokines.[85,86]

Human dental pulp stem cells (hDPSCs) are ectodermal-derived stem cells, originating from migrating neural crest cells, and possess mesenchymal stem cell (MSC) properties. It has been reported in the literature that stem/progenitor cells from inflamed human dental pulp retain tissue generation potential.[87] Pulp capping materials may also contribute to pulpal stem cells' differentiation and repair.[88,89] Andelin and associates used immunostaining with dentin sialoprotein (DSP) to determine the type of tissue

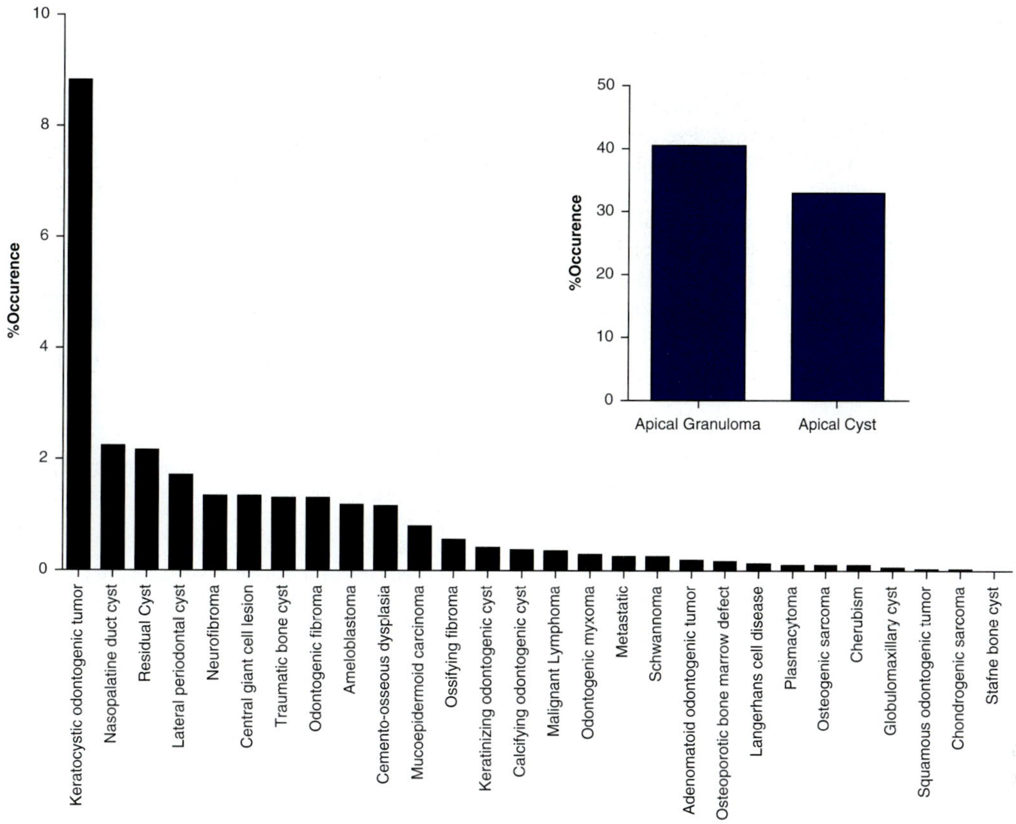

• **Fig. 1.28** Lesions associated with crowns of unerupted teeth (dentigerous cysts, hyperplastic follicle) which would not be confused with ones from endodontic origin, have been excluded from this list (*n* = 9.723). Apical cysts and granulomas were the most common, comprising 73% of the considered jaw lesions. Ameloblastomas were reported 144 times (1.2%). Squamous odontogenic tumors and chondrogenic sarcomas were reported twice (0.02%) and a Stafne bone cyst was reported once (0.01%). (From Koivisto T, Bowles WR, Rohrer M: Frequency and distribution of radiolucent jaw lesions: a retrospective analysis of 9,723 cases, *J Endod* 38[6]:729–32, 2012.)

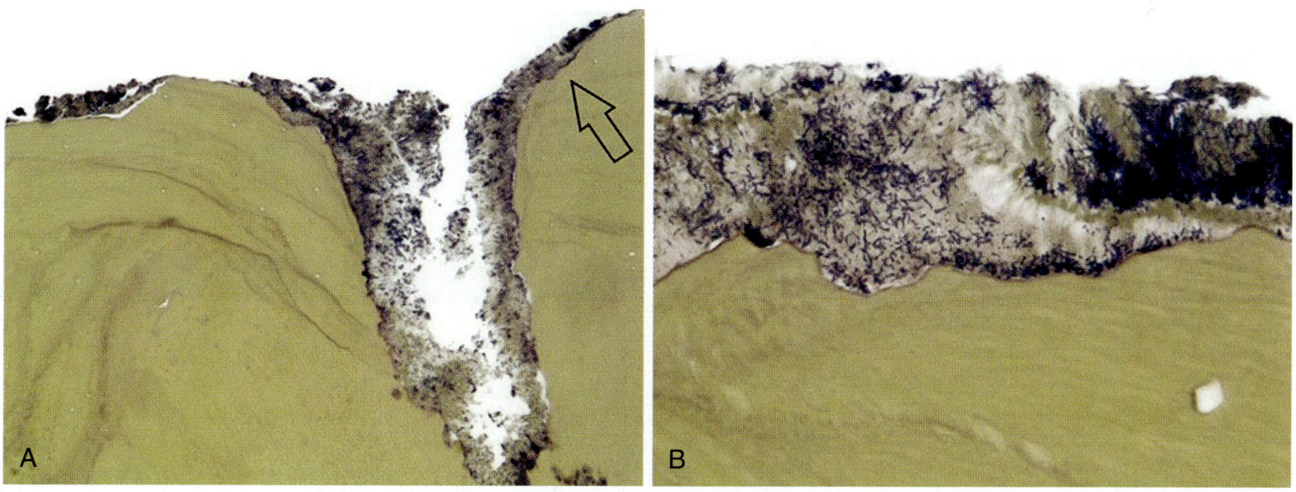

• **Fig. 1.29** Apical Foramen and External Surface of Tooth With Persistent Root Canal Infection. **A**, Longitudinal section cut through the foramen, which appears clogged with a biofilm, extending on the outer apical surface (Taylor-modified Brown-Brenn, original magnification 50). **B**, High-power view of the external apical surface indicated by the arrow in (**A**) showing different concentrations of bacteria within the biofilm, which appears firmly attached to the resorbed cementum (original magnification × 400). (From Ricucci D, Loghin S, Gonçalves LS, et al: Histobacteriologic conditions of the apical root canal system and periapical tissues in teeth associated with sinus tracts, *J Endod* 44[3]:405–413, 2018.)

that forms after pulp capping procedures.[88] DSP is present in both bone and dentin but is expressed at an approximately 400-fold higher level in dentin than in bone.[90] Depending on the capping material used, dentin healing may occur through regeneration of dentin (identified through heavy DSP staining; Fig. 1.30, *A*) or through repair with an amorphous mineralized scar tissue (light DSP staining; Fig. 1.30, *B*).

Mild injury to the pulp and endothelial cells stimulates stem-cell recruitment, and proliferation of dental stem cells can be stimulated by platelet-derived growth factor BB (PDGF-BB), vascular endothelial growth factor (VEGF), insulin-like growth factor 1 (IGF-1), and transforming growth factor β1 (TGF-β1).[91] On the other hand, prolonged injury (e.g., as seen in microbial infections) results in stem-cell apoptosis and impairment of these cells' function and ability to repair the pulp.[92]

Process of Periapical Healing

The sequence of events leading to resolution of periapical lesions has not been studied extensively. Based on the processes involved in the repair of extraction sites,[93] after removal of irritants, inflammatory responses decrease, and tissue-forming cells (fibroblasts and endothelial cells) increase; finally, tissue organization and maturation ensue. Bone that has resorbed is replaced by new bone; resorbed cementum and dentin are repaired by cellular cementum. The PDL, which is the first tissue affected, is the last to be restored to normal architecture (Fig. 1.31). Histologic examination of healing of periapical lesions shows evidence of healing in the form of cementum deposition, increased vascularity, and increased fibroblastic and osteoblastic activities.[94] Studies have shown that some cytokines, MMPs and TIMP1, HSP27, and Serpine1 play an important role during healing of periapical lesions.[95-98] MSCs' mobilization also results in the attenuation of apical periodontitis progression associated with immunosuppressive and prohealing mechanisms.[99]

Some lesions do not completely regain all the original structures. Variations are seen in different fiber or bone patterns. These variations may be obvious radiographically with a widened lamina dura or altered bony configuration. Certain factors, such as the size of the defect or the extent of injury to the underlying stroma, may affect complete regeneration of the original tissue architecture.

Factors Influencing Healing

Other factors that may affect the healing of periapical lesions include inherent host factors (e.g., leukopenia, impairment of blood supply, inadequate nutrition), corticosteroids, and other systemic diseases. For instance, patients with diabetes mellitus have a significantly lower healing rate after root canal therapy of teeth with apical lesions than do nondiabetic patients.[100] Uncontrolled hyperglycemia may also affect pulp healing. In a pulp capping model using streptozotocin-induced diabetes in rats, Garber and coworkers found significant impairment of dentin bridge formation compared with that of normal rats.[101] Impairment of dentin bridge formation was directly correlated with the amount of pulp inflammation.

It has been suggested that genetic predisposition can contribute to an individual's susceptibility to pulpal inflammation and apical periodontitis and that a complex signaling network operates in the determination of the nature and extent of their progression, as well as the associated bone-destructive process. In recent years, polymorphisms in a few genes (*IL1B, MMP2, MMP3, HSPA1L,* and *HSPA6*) mostly belonging to immune response–related pathways, have been shown to be associated with pulpal inflammation and apical periodontitis.[102-105] Differential methylation profiles of immune response–related genes, such as *FOXP3*[106] and microRNAs,[107] may also have an influence on individual susceptibility to pulpal and apical inflammation and patient treatment outcomes through their potential contributions to altered expression of disease-relevant genes.

• BOX 1.2 Study Questions

6. Biofilms have been observed on the apical root surface of teeth with persistent apical periodontitis:
   a. True
   b. False
7. Direct pulp exposure to microorganisms is not a prerequisite for pulpal response and inflammation
   a. True
   b. False
8. The process by which altered or damaged pulp tissues are completely replaced by tissues native to their original architecture and function is described as
   a. Repair
   b. Revascularization
   c. Regeneration
   d. Calcification
9. Which of these sentences is considered wrong in regard to the process of pulp healing?
   a. In the absence of irritants, a healthy pulp has tremendous capacity to heal.
   b. DSP is present in both bone and dentin but is expressed at an approximately 400-fold higher level in bone than in dentin.
   c. Mild injury to the pulp and endothelial cells stimulates stem cell recruitment and proliferation of dental stem cells.
   d. Prolonged injury results in stem cell apoptosis and impairment of these cells' function and ability to repair the pulp.
10. Genetic predisposition to pulpal and periapical inflammation has been reported in the literature as an important factor that can influence healing. Which of the genes listed is considered a good candidate gene for the investigation of individual's susceptibility to develop pulpal and periapical inflammation?
   a. TGFB
   b. IL1B
   c. OPG
   d. IL10

ANSWERS

Answer

1 c. Internal resorption
2 b. Leukotrienes
3 c. IL-10
4 d. Multispecies biofilms, within an extracellular matrix, predominantly matrix
5 b. Can resist alkaline stress better
6 a. True
7 a. True
8 c. Regeneration
9 b. DSP is present in both bone and dentin but is expressed at an approximately 400-fold higher level in bone than in dentin
10 b. IL1B

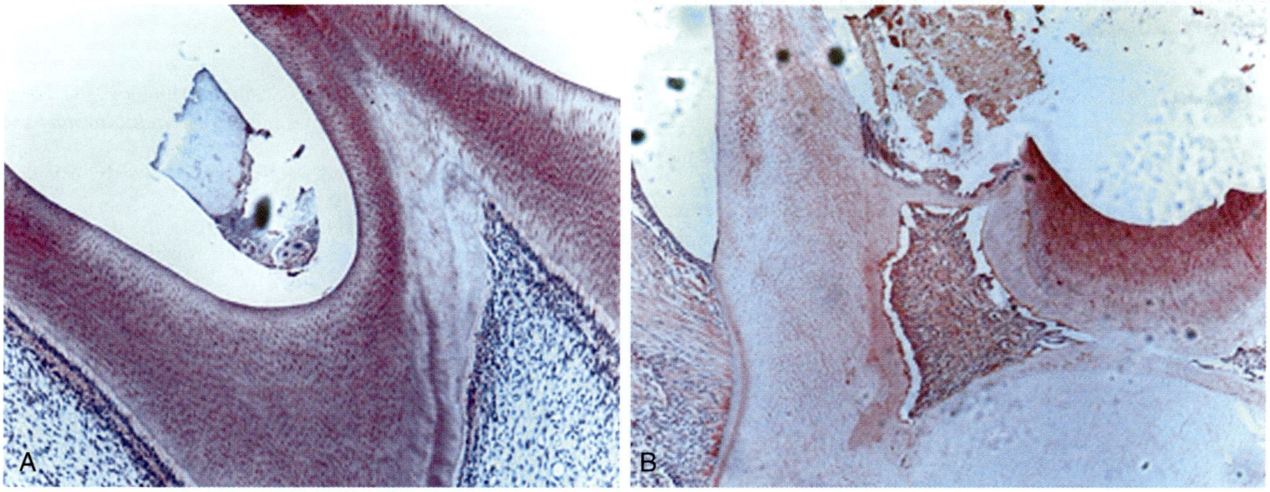

• **Fig. 1.30** **A**, Sclerotic dentin, which appears as an irregularly organized, mineralized tissue and stains lighter than normal tubular dentin with antibody against dentin sialoprotein (DSP). **B**, Dentin bridge; also, secondary dentin, deposited along canal wall after a pulp capping procedure, which shows a tubular structure and stains similarly to the primary dentin with antibody against DSP.

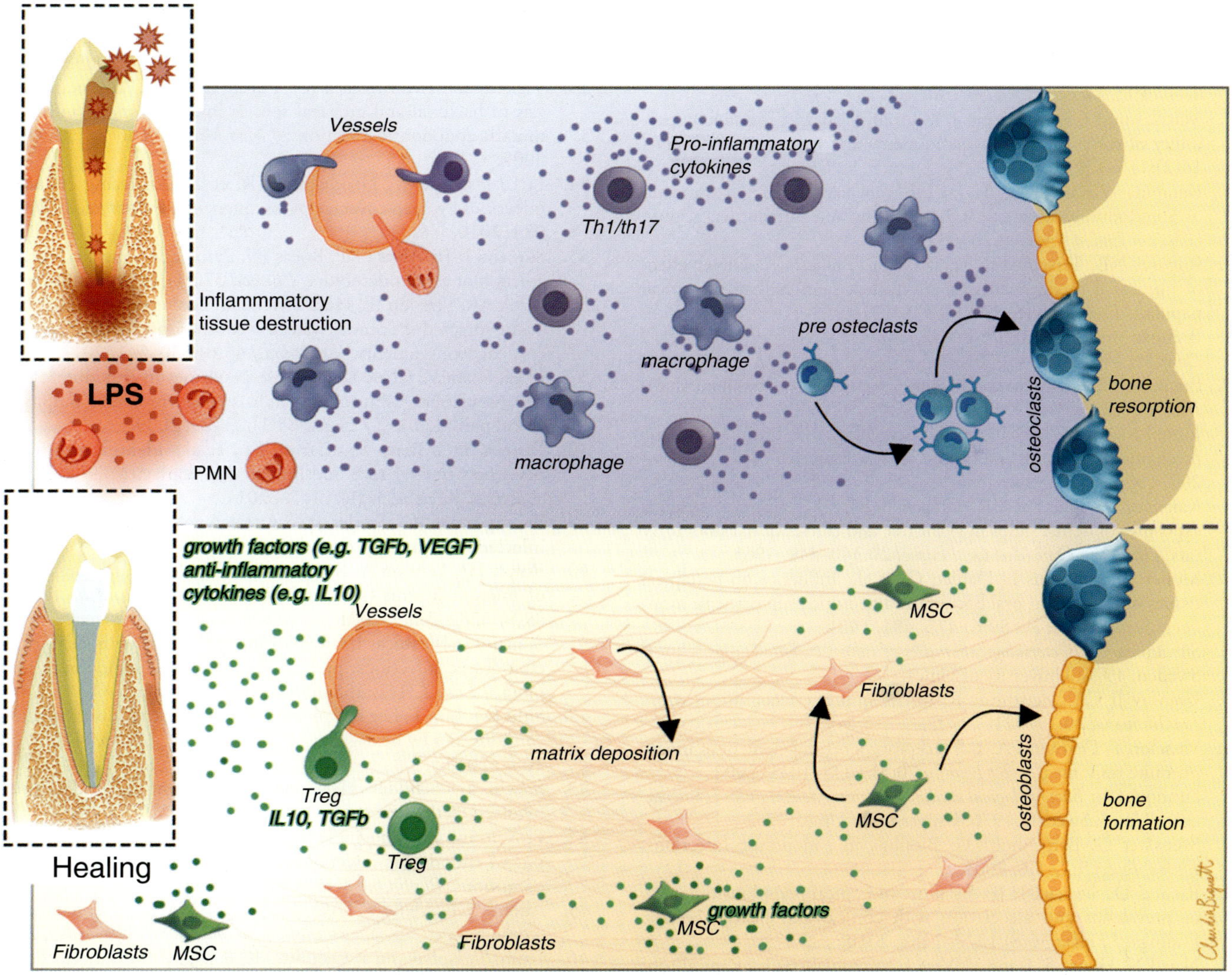

• **Fig. 1.31** Schematic Illustration of Wound Healing of Periapical Tissues After Endodontic Therapy. Apical periodontitis is an inflammatory lesion caused by microorganisms and their byproducts derived from an infected root canal system. It also represents an important host defense mechanism with the participation of inflammatory cells such as polymorphonuclear leukocytes (PMNs), macrophages, and lymphocytes (Th1/Th17). These cells express several proinflammatory cytokines that will activate osteoclasts contributing to bone resorption. After successful endodontic therapy, T regulatory cells (Tregs), mesenchymal stem cells (MSC), connective tissue fibroblasts, and osteoblasts will initiate the healing/repair process, releasing growth factors and antiinflammatory cytokines, resulting in matrix deposition and new bone formation. *IL10*, Interleukin 10; *LPS*, lipopolysaccharides; *TGFb*, transforming growth factor beta; *VEGF*, vascular endothelial growth factor. (Courtesy Dr. Claudia Biguetti.)

References

1. Yu C, Abbott PV: An overview of the dental pulp: its functions and responses to injury, *Aust Dent J* 52(Suppl 1):S4–16, 2007.
2. Garberoglio R, Brännström M: Scanning electron microscopic investigation of human dentinal tubules, *Arch Oral Biol* 21(6):355–362, 1976.
3. Bergenholtz G, Lindhe J: Effect of experimentally induced marginal periodontitis and periodontal scaling on the dental pulp, *J Clin Periodontol* 5(1):59–73, 1978.
4. Strobl H, Haas M, Norer B, et al.: Evaluation of pulpal blood flow after tooth splinting of luxated permanent maxillary incisors, *Dent Traumatol* 20(1):36–41, 2004.
5. Kayhan F, Küçükkeleş N, Demirel D: A histologic and histomorphometric evaluation of pulpal reactions following rapid palatal expansion, *Am J Orthod Dentofacial Orthop* 117(4):465–473, 2000.
6. Taşpinar F, Akgül N, Simşek G, et al.: The histopathological investigation of pulpal tissue following heavy orthopaedic forces produced by rapid maxillary expansion, *J Int Med Res* 31(3):197–201, 2003.
7. Messer HH, Chen RS: The duration of effectiveness of root canal medicaments, *J Endod* 10(6):240–245, 1984.
8. Langeland K: Management of the inflamed pulp associated with deep carious lesion, *J Endod* 7(4):169–181, 1981.
9. Masillamoni CR, Kettering JD, Torabinejad M: The biocompatibility of some root canal medicaments and irrigants, *Int Endod J* 14(2):115–120, 1981.
10. Karapinar-Kazandağ M, Bayrak OF, Yalvaç ME, et al.: Cytotoxicity of 5 endodontic sealers on L929 cell line and human dental pulp cells, *Int Endod J* 44(7):626–634, 2011.
11. Ruparel NB, Teixeira FB, Ferraz CC, Diogenes A: Direct effect of intracanal medicaments on survival of stem cells of the apical papilla, *J Endod* 38(10):1372–1375, 2012.
12. Brännström M, Lind PO: Pulpal response to early dental caries, *J Dent Res* 44(5):1045–1050, 1965.
13. Baume LJ: Dental pulp conditions in relation to carious lesions, *Int Dent J* 20(2):309–337, 1970.
14. Jontell M, Okiji T, Dahlgren U, Bergenholtz G: Immune defense mechanisms of the dental pulp, *Crit Rev Oral Biol Med* 9(2):179–200, 1998.
15. Kakehashi S, Stanley HR, Fitzgerald RJ: The effects of surgical exposures of dental pulps in germ-free and conventional laboratory rats, *Oral Surg Oral Med Oral Pathol* 20:340–349, 1965.
16. Möller AJ, Fabricius L, Dahlén G, et al.: Influence on periapical tissues of indigenous oral bacteria and necrotic pulp tissue in monkeys, *Scand J Dent Res* 89(6):475–484, 1981.
17. Sundqvist G: *Bacteriological studies of necrotic dental pulps*, Umeå, Sweden, 1976, University of Umeå.
18. Janeway Jr CA, Medzhitov R: Innate immune recognition, *Annu Rev Immunol* 20:197–216, 2002.
19. Vasselon T, Detmers PA: Toll receptors: a central element in innate immune responses, *Infect Immun* 70(3):1033–1041, 2002.
20. Sundqvist G: *Bacteriological studies of necrotic dental pulps [Dissertation]*, Umeå, Sweden, 1976, University of Umeå.
21. Svensäter G, Bergenholtz G: Biofilms in endodontic infections, *Endod Topics* 9:27–36, 2004.
22. Ricucci D, Siqueira Jr JF: Biofilms and apical periodontitis: study of prevalence and association with clinical and histopathologic findings, *J Endod* 36(8):1277–1288, 2010.
23. Nair PN, Henry S, Cano V, Vera J: Microbial status of apical root canal system of human mandibular first molars with primary apical periodontitis after "one-visit" endodontic treatment, *Oral Surg Oral Med Oral Pathol Oral Radiol Endod* 99(2):231–252, 2005.
24. McDougald D, Rice SA, Barraud N, et al.: Should we stay or should we go: mechanisms and ecological consequences for biofilm dispersal, *Nat Rev Microbiol* 10(1):39–50, 2012.
25. Parsek MR, Greenberg EP: Sociomicrobiology: the connections between quorum sensing and biofilms, *Trends Microbiol* 13(1):27–33, 2005.
26. Flemming HC, Wingender J: The biofilm matrix, *Nat Rev Microbiol* 8(9):623–633, 2010.
27. Siqueira Jr JF: Rôças IN: Community as the unit of pathogenicity: an emerging concept as to the microbial pathogenesis of apical periodontitis, *Oral Surg Oral Med Oral Pathol Oral Radiol Endod* 107(6):870–878, 2009.
28. Miller WD: An introduction to the study of the bacterio-pathology of the dental pulp, *Dental Cosmos* 36(7):505–528, 1894.
29. Chhour KL, Nadkarni MA, Byun R, et al.: Molecular analysis of microbial diversity in advanced caries, *J Clin Microbiol* 43(2):843–849, 2005.
30. Martin FE, Nadkarni MA, Jacques NA, Hunter N: Quantitative microbiological study of human carious dentine by culture and real-time PCR: association of anaerobes with histopathological changes in chronic pulpitis, *J Clin Microbiol* 40(5):1698–1704, 2002.
31. Rôças IN, Alves FRF, Rachid CTCC, et al.: Microbiome of deep dentinal caries lesions in teeth with symptomatic irreversible pulpitis, *PLoS One* 11(5):e0154653, 2016, https://doi.org/10.1371/journal.pone.0154653.
32. Waltimo TM, Sen BH, Meurman JH, et al.: Yeasts in apical periodontitis, *Crit Rev Oral Biol Med* 14(2):128–137, 2003.
33. Vickerman MM, Brossard KA, Funk DB, et al.: Phylogenetic analysis of bacterial and archaeal species in symptomatic and asymptomatic endodontic infections, *J Med Microbiol* 56(Pt 1):110–118, 2007.
34. Li L, Hsiao WW, Nandakumar R, et al.: Analyzing endodontic infections by deep coverage pyrosequencing, *J Dent Res* 89(9):980–984, 2010.
35. Siqueira Jr JF, Alves FRF, Rôças IN: Pyrosequencing analysis of the apical root canal microbiota, *J Endod* 37(11):1499–1503, 2011.
36. Ozok AR, Persoon IF, Huse SM, et al.: Ecology of the microbiome of the infected root canal system: a comparison between apical and coronal root segments, *Int Endod J* 45(6):530–541, 2012.
37. Li H, Chen V, Chen Y, et al.: Herpesviruses in endodontic pathoses: association of Epstein-Barr virus with irreversible pulpitis and apical periodontitis, *J Endod* 35(1):23–29, 2009.
38. Ferreira DC, Paiva SS, Carmo FL, et al.: Identification of herpesviruses types 1 to 8 and human papillomavirus in acute apical abscesses, *J Endod* 37(1):10–16, 2011.
39. Baumgartner JC, Falkler Jr WA: Bacteria in the apical 5 mm of infected root canals, *J Endod* 17(8):380–383, 1991.
40. Rolph HJ, Lennon A, Riggio MP, et al.: Molecular identification of microorganisms from endodontic infections, *J Clin Microbiol* 39(9):3282–3289, 2001.
41. Siqueira Jr JF, Rôças IN: Exploiting molecular methods to explore endodontic infections: part 2—redefining the endodontic microbiota, *J Endod* 31(7):488–498, 2005.
42. Shin JM, Luo T, Lee KH, et al.: Deciphering endodontic microbial communities by next-generation sequencing, *J Endod* 44(7):1080–1087, 2018.
43. Schein B, Schilder H: Endotoxin content in endodontically involved teeth, *J Endod* 1(1):19–21, 1975.
44. Provenzano JC, Siqueira Jr JF: Rôças IN, et al: Metaproteome analysis of endodontic infections in association with different clinical conditions, *PLoS One* 8(10):e76108, 2013.
45. Alfenas CF, Mendes TAO, Ramos HJO, et al.: Human exoproteome in acute apical abscesses, *J Endod* 43(9):1479–1485, 2017.
46. Izumi T, Kobayashi I, Okamura K, Sakai H: Immunohistochemical study on the immunocompetent cells of the pulp in human non-carious and carious teeth, *Arch Oral Biol* 40(7):609–614, 1995.
47. Horst OV, Horst JA, Samudrala R, Dale BA: Caries induced cytokine network in the odontoblast layer of human teeth, *BMC Immunol* 12:9, 2011.

48. Ricucci D, Loghin S, Siqueira Jr JF: Correlation between clinical and histologic pulp diagnoses, *J Endod* 40(12):1932–1939, 2014.
49. Zanini M, Meyer E, Simon S: Pulp inflammation diagnosis from clinical to inflammatory mediators: a systematic review, *J Endod* 43(7):1033–1051, 2017.
50. Mente J, Petrovic J, Gehrig H, et al.: A prospective clinical pilot study on the level of matrix metalloproteinase-9 in dental pulpal blood as a marker for the state of inflammation in the pulp tissue, *J Endod* 42(2):190–197, 2016.
51. Edds AC, Walden JE, Scheetz JP, et al.: Pilot study of correlation of pulp stones with cardiovascular disease, *J Endod* 31(7):504–506, 2005.
52. Pettiette MT, Zhong S, Moretti AJ, Khan AA: Potential correlation between statins and pulp chamber calcification, *J Endod* 39(9):1119–1123, 2013.
53. Michaelson PL, Holland GR: Is pulpitis painful? *Int Endod J* 35(10):829–832, 2002.
54. Kakoli P, Nandakumar R, Romberg E, et al.: The effect of age on bacterial penetration of radicular dentin, *J Endod* 35(1):78–81, 2009.
55. Fouad AF: IL-1 alpha and TNF-alpha expression in early periapical lesions of normal and immunodeficient mice, *J Dent Res* 76(9):1548–1554, 1997.
56. Teles R, Wang CY, Stashenko P: Increased susceptibility of RAG-2 SCID mice to dissemination of endodontic infections, *Infect Immun* 65(9):3781–3787, 1997.
57. Dahlén G, Bergenholtz G: Endotoxic activity in teeth with necrotic pulps, *J Dent Res* 59(6):1033–1040, 1980.
58. Warfvinge J, Dahlén G, Bergenholtz G: Dental pulp response to bacterial cell wall material, *J Dent Res* 64(8):1046–1050, 1985.
59. Fouad AF, Acosta AW: Periapical lesion progression and cytokine expression in an LPS hyporesponsive model, *Int Endod J* 34(7):506–513, 2001.
60. Fouad AF, Walton RE, Rittman BR: Induced periapical lesions in ferret canines: histologic and radiographic evaluation, *Endod Dent Traumatol* 8(2):56–62, 1992.
61. Kawashima N, Suzuki N, Yang G, et al.: Kinetics of RANKL, RANK and OPG expressions in experimentally induced rat periapical lesions, *Oral Surg Oral Med Oral Pathol Oral Radiol Endod* 103(5):707–711, 2007.
62. Sabeti M, Simon J, Kermani V, et al.: Detection of receptor activator of NF-kappa beta ligand in apical periodontitis, *J Endod* 31(1):17–18, 2005.
63. Vernal R, Dezerega A, Dutzan N, et al.: RANKL in human periapical granuloma: possible involvement in periapical bone destruction, *Oral Dis* 12(3):283–289, 2006.
64. Francisconi CF, Vieira AE, Biguetti CC, et al.: Characterization of the protective role of regulatory t cells in experimental periapical lesion development and their chemoattraction manipulation as a therapeutic tool, *J Endod* 42(1):120–126, 2016.
65. Koivisto T, Bowles WR, Rohrer M: Frequency and distribution of radiolucent jaw lesions: a retrospective analysis of 9,723 cases, *J Endod* 38(6):729–732, 2012.
66. Nair PN: New perspectives on radicular cysts: do they heal? *Int Endod J* 31(3):155–160, 1998.
67. Lin LM, Huang GT, Rosenberg PA: Proliferation of epithelial cell rests, formation of apical cysts, and regression of apical cysts after periapical wound healing, *J Endod* 33(8):908–916, 2007.
68. Lin LM, Ricucci D, Lin J, Rosenberg PA: Nonsurgical root canal therapy of large cyst-like inflammatory periapical lesions and inflammatory apical cysts, *J Endod* 35(5):607–615, 2009.
69. Natkin E, Oswald RJ, Carnes LI: The relationship of lesion size to diagnosis, incidence, and treatment of periapical cysts and granulomas, *Oral Surg Oral Med Oral Pathol* 57(1):82–94, 1984.
70. Ramachandran Nair PN: Light and electron microscopic studies of root canal flora and periapical lesions, *J Endod* 13:29–39, 1987.
71. Ricucci D, Pascon EA, Ford TR, Langeland K: Epithelium and bacteria in periapical lesions, *Oral Surg Oral Med Oral Pathol Oral Radiol Endod* 101(2):239–249, 2006.
72. Sunde PT, Olsen I, Göbel UB, et al.: Fluorescence in situ hybridization (FISH) for direct visualization of bacteria in periapical lesions of asymptomatic root-filled teeth, *Microbiology* 149(Pt 5):1095–1102, 2003.
73. Ricucci D, Siqueira Jr JF: Apical actinomycosis as a continuum of intraradicular and extraradicular infection: case report and critical review on its involvement with treatment failure, *J Endod* 34(9):1124–1129, 2008.
74. Ren YF, Malmstrom HS: Rapid quantitative determination of C-reactive protein at chair side in dental emergency patients, *Oral Surg Oral Med Oral Pathol Oral Radiol Endod* 104(1):49–55, 2007.
75. Gomes MS, Blattner TC, Sant'Ana Filho M, et al.: Can apical periodontitis modify systemic levels of inflammatory markers? A systematic review and meta-analysis, *J Endod* 39(10):1205–1217, 2013.
76. Torabinejad M, Theofilopoulos AN, Ketering JD, Bakland LK: Quantitation of circulating immune complexes, immunoglobulins G and M, and C3 complement component in patients with large periapical lesions, *Oral Surg Oral Med Oral Pathol* 55(2):186–190, 1983.
77. Svetcov SD, DeAngelo JE, McNamara T, Nevins AJ: Serum immunoglobulin levels and bacterial flora in subjects with acute oro-facial swellings, *J Endod* 9(6):233–235, 1983.
78. Siqueira Jr JF, Rôças IN: Clinical implications and microbiology of bacterial persistence after treatment procedures, *J Endod* 34(11):1291–1301.e3, 2008.
79. Sundqvist G, Figdor D, Persson S, Sjögren U: Microbiologic analysis of teeth with failed endodontic treatment and the outcome of conservative re-treatment, *Oral Surg Oral Med Oral Pathol Oral Radiol Endod* 85(1):86–93, 1998.
80. Hancock 3rd HH, Sigurdsson A, Trope M, Moiseiwitsch J: Bacteria isolated after unsuccessful endodontic treatment in a North American population, *Oral Surg Oral Med Oral Pathol Oral Radiol Endod* 91(5):579–586, 2001.
81. Ricucci D, Siqueira Jr JF, Bate AL, Pitt Ford TR: Histologic investigation of root canal-treated teeth with apical periodontitis: a retrospective study from twenty-four patients, *J Endod* 35(4):493–502, 2009.
82. Wang J, Jiang Y, Chen W, et al.: Bacterial flora and extraradicular biofilm associated with the apical segment of teeth with post-treatment apical periodontitis, *J Endod* 38(7):954–959, 2012.
83. Cooper PR, Takahashi Y, Graham LW, et al.: Inflammation-regeneration interplay in the dentine-pulp complex, *J Dent* 38(9):687–697, 2010.
84. Jeanneau C, Lundy FT, El Karim IA: About I: Potential therapeutic strategy of targeting pulp fibroblasts in dentin-pulp regeneration, *J Endod* 43(9S):S17–S24, 2017.
85. Veerayutthwilai O, Byers MR, Pham TT, et al.: Differential regulation of immune responses by odontoblasts, *Oral Microbiol Immunol* 22(1):5–13, 2007.
86. Staquet MJ, Durand SH, Colomb E, et al.: Different roles of odontoblasts and fibroblasts in immunity, *J Dent Res* 87(3):256–261, 2008.
87. Alongi DJ, Yamaza T, Song Y, et al.: Stem/progenitor cells from inflamed human dental pulp retain tissue regeneration potential, *Regen Med* 5(4):617–631, 2010.
88. Andelin WE, Shabahang S, Wright K, Torabinejad M: Identification of hard tissue after experimental pulp capping using dentin sialoprotein (DSP) as a marker, *J Endod* 29(10):646–650, 2003.
89. Bakhtiar H, Nekoofar MH, Aminishakib P, et al.: Human pulp responses to partial pulpotomy treatment with theracal as compared with biodentine and proroot MTA: a clinical trial, *J Endod* 43(11):1786–1791, 2017.
90. Qin C, Brunn JC, Cadena E, et al.: Dentin sialoprotein in bone and dentin sialophosphoprotein gene expressed by osteoblasts, *Connect Tissue Res* 44(Suppl 1):179–183, 2003.

91. Leprince JG, Zeitlin BD, Tolar M, Peters OA: Interactions between immune system and mesenchymal stem cells in dental pulp and periapical tissues, *Int Endod J* 45(8):689–701, 2012.
92. Kobayashi C, Yaegaki K, Calenic B, et al.: Hydrogen sulfide causes apoptosis in human pulp stem cells, *J Endod* 37(4):479–484, 2011.
93. Amler MH: The time sequence of tissue regeneration in human extraction wounds, *Oral Surg Oral Med Oral Pathol* 27(3):309–318, 1969.
94. Fouad AF, Walton RE, Rittman BR: Healing of induced periapical lesions in ferret canines, *J Endod* 19(3):123–129, 1993.
95. Danin J, Linder LE, Lundqvist G, Andersson L: Tumor necrosis factor-alpha and transforming growth factor-beta1 in chronic periapical lesions, *Oral Surg Oral Med Oral Pathol Oral Radiol Endod* 90(4):514–517, 2000.
96. Leonardi R, Lanteri E, Stivala F, Travali S: Immunolocalization of CD44 adhesion molecules in human periradicular lesions, *Oral Surg Oral Med Oral Pathol Oral Radiol Endod* 89(4):480–485, 2000.
97. Cavalla F, Biguetti C, Jain S, et al.: Proteomic profiling and differential messenger RNA expression correlate HSP27 and serpin family B member 1 to apical periodontitis outcomes, *J Endod* 43(9):1486–1493, 2017.
98. Letra A, Ghaneh G, Zhao M, et al.: MMP-7 and TIMP-1, new targets in predicting poor wound healing in apical periodontitis, *J Endod* 39(9):1141–1146, 2013.
99. Araujo-Pires AC, Biguetti CC, Repeke CE, et al.: Mesenchymal stem cells as active prohealing and immunosuppressive agents in periapical environment: evidence from human and experimental periapical lesions, *J Endod* 40(10):1560–1565, 2014.
100. Fouad AF, Burleson J: The effect of diabetes mellitus on endodontic treatment outcome: data from an electronic patient record, *J Am Dent Assoc* 134(1):43–51, 2003. quiz 117-8.
101. Garber SE, Shabahang S, Escher AP, Torabinejad M: The effect of hyperglycemia on pulpal healing in rats, *J Endod* 35(1):60–62, 2009.
102. Morsani JM, Aminoshariae A, Han YW, et al.: Genetic predisposition to persistent apical periodontitis, *J Endod* 37(4):455–459, 2011.
103. Menezes-Silva R, Khaliq S, Deeley K, et al.: Genetic susceptibility to periapical disease: conditional contribution of MMP2 and MMP3 genes to the development of periapical lesions and healing response, *J Endod* 38(5):604–607, 2012.
104. Dill A, Letra A, Chaves de Souza L, et al.: Analysis of multiple cytokine polymorphisms in individuals with untreated deep carious lesions reveals IL1B (rs1143643) as a susceptibility factor for periapical lesion development, *J Endod* 41(2):197–200, 2015.
105. Maheshwari K, Silva RM, Guajardo-Morales L, et al.: Heat Shock 70 protein genes and genetic susceptibility to apical periodontitis, *J Endod* 42(10):1467–1471, 2016.
106. Campos K, Franscisconi CF, Okehie V, et al.: FOXP3 DNA methylation levels as a potential biomarker in the development of periapical lesions, *J Endod* 41(2):212–218, 2015.
107. Zhong S, Zhang S, Bair E, et al.: Differential expression of microRNAs in normal and inflamed human pulps, *J Endod* 38(6):746–752, 2012.

2

Systemic Health Considerations in the Endodontic Patient and Geriatric Endodontics

ANITA AMINOSHARIAE AND ASHRAF F. FOUAD

CHAPTER OUTLINE

LEARNING OBJECTIVES

After reading this chapter, the student should be able to:

1. Recognize the various ways in which endodontic pathosis and systemic disease interact and some of the mechanisms of such interactions.
2. Identify general consideration for the safe management of the endodontic patient with systemic disease.
3. Identify the effects of diabetes mellitus, smoking, genetic predisposition, irradiation, sickle cell disease, and viral infections on the pathogenesis of endodontic pathosis and endodontic treatment outcomes.
4. Determine the potential for acute and chronic endodontic infections to cause or contribute to systemic disease.
5. Discuss the prognosis of the endodontic treatment in relation to the systemic condition.
6. Identify age changes in the anatomy and physiology of the older dental pulp and periapical tissues, as well as differences in pathogenesis of disease and response to treatment.
7. Identify factors that complicate case selection and discuss the differences in treatment between older and younger patients.
8. Identify those elderly patients who should be considered for referral.

Health and Medical History

Successful dental management of a patient with extensive medical history depends on a thorough evaluation of the patient and on determining the diagnosis and treatment plan that takes risks and benefits into consideration. It is essential to determine and identify modifications to the dental treatment for a medically complex patient. Thorough discussion of the dental management and risk assessment of medically complex patients is beyond the scope of this chapter. However, some of the common illnesses will be explained. In patients with serious disorders, referral to an endodontic specialist may be appropriate. Specialist care is generally more expedient and offers better prevention and management of treatment complications (see Chapter 6).

The Systemic Health Assessment of the Endodontic Patient

In the review of the medical history and during clinical examination and treatment of the endodontic patient, the clinician needs to be keenly aware of specific areas in which systemic health affects the management of the patient. Importantly, endodontic patients should be managed in a manner that assures their safety, comfort, and well-being during and after the procedure.

Patients should be asked whether they have received prior endodontic treatment and how they view and feel about this form of dental treatment. Previous experiences or information that patients have from other sources may render them especially anxious about this procedure. Many patients have severe apprehension about having endodontic treatment, and their care may need premedication, sedation, or other auxiliary methods that facilitate the experience for them. Occasionally, especially in the case of children, moderate to deep sedation or general anesthesia may be the only practical approach to treating them.

Endodontic patients especially should be asked about the history of chronic pain of any type. These patients are at an increased risk of postoperative and of persistent pain, and this aspect should be reviewed with them during the informed consent process (see Chapter 5).

Endodontic treatment involves the effective use of local anesthesia (see Chapter 8), adjunctive analgesics, and antibiotics. Therefore complete history of cardiovascular, endocrine, respiratory, hepatic, and renal systems should be obtained. Preoperative vital signs, such as blood pressure, pulse, and respiration, should be recorded. Occasionally, preoperative glycemia (blood glucose measurement or glycated hemoglobin [HbA_{1c}]) are needed to assess the control of glycemia for diabetics or the need for referral to a physician in patients at high risk of diabetes. International normalized ratio (INR) is required for the patient on Coumadin (warfarin), especially before surgical treatment. The INR is a standardized way of expressing the prothrombin time test (PT). Heparin is an anticoagulant that will prolong partial thromboplastin time, activated PTT (PTT, aPTT). Detailed lists of medications, allergies, previous hospitalizations, medical and surgical treatments, and previous untoward reactions should be collected. Like any dental procedure that results in risk of bacteremia, the risk of infective endocarditis or of late artificial joint infection should be identified, and appropriate antibiotic coverage should be instituted whenever indicated according to current guidelines. The American Dental Association has recently provided guidelines for the use of systemic antibiotics for endodontic patients (see https://ebd.ada.org/en/evidence/guidelines/antibiotics-for-dental-pain-and-swelling?utm_source=EBDsite&utm_content=guidelines for guidelines).

Allergies to specific materials or reagents used in endodontics are rare. Reports of hypersensitivity to gutta percha, amide-based local anesthetic agents, sodium hypochlorite, and nickel (present in nickel titanium files) should be considered in the treatment of the endodontic patient. Consultations with a medical specialist in hypersensitivity reactions should be made before treatment decisions are made. Referral to an endodontist would be indicated for management of patients with true allergy to any endodontic materials.

Physical Examination: Vital Signs

Vital signs are an important component of patient treatment and give the health care provider information regarding the current medical status of that patient (see Chapter 4). Blood pressure, heart rate, respiratory rate, and temperature should be recorded. In some cases, fasting blood glucose and/or the values of HbA_{1c} are recorded or documented, too. This information helps the clinician better understand the patient's physiological state.

Systemic Considerations

Dentists are members of the health team whose role ultimately is to ensure that the patient's health, including oral health, is maintained at an optimal level. Over the past two to three decades, the close relationship between oral health and systemic health has gained much attention, and many advances in this area have been achieved. In the early part of the 20th century, endodontic infections were thought to be a focus of infection that may lead to a variety of ailments and chronic diseases in the body. Although the systemic spread of acute oral infections is clear, recent objective research has identified compelling associations between systemic disease and chronic oral infections, including endodontic infections. The available evidence on the relationship between endodontic pathosis and systemic disease is presented here.

Endodontics and Systemic Disease

With regard to the relationship between endodontic pathosis and systemic disease, the practitioner needs to be aware of three factors: systemic diseases that mimic endodontic pain or periapical radiolucency (see Chapters 4 and 5), systemic diseases that may accelerate or potentiate pulpal pathosis or influence treatment outcomes, and conditions in which the endodontic infection may initiate or contribute to an infection in a distant site or another systemic disease.

Systemic Diseases That May Influence Endodontic Pathosis or Its Treatment

Certain systemic conditions were reported to be associated with pathogenesis of endodontic lesions in a recently published systematic review.[1] Specifically the authors found that there was a moderate risk for and association of cardiovascular disease and diabetes with endodontic pathosis. In another systematic review, the authors investigated the interaction of systemic disease with endodontic healing and reported that certain systematic diseases are associated with endodontic healing.[2] Patients with medical conditions that compromise their immune response may have a less favorable endodontic treatment outcome. Though the mechanism or pathway for this interaction remains speculative at this time, it is critical to note that the patient's medical condition is preemptive to his or her dental care and prognosis.

Endodontic Disease May Initiate or Contribute to Systemic Diseases

The oral cavity is the first component of the digestive system and has a large component of the human microbiome (as noted in Chapter 1). The diversity of microorganisms in the mouth is related to its exposure to dietary and environmental factors and to the unique characteristics of the oral environment. Deleterious effects of these microorganisms are prevented by an intact mucosal lining, which is capable of a formidable immune response, and by oral hygiene measures that limit the progression of oral microbial biofilms. The dental pulp is protected from bacteria by intact enamel and dentin, whereas the periodontium is protected by periodontal attachment and sulcular epithelium. With marginal periodontitis or pulpal pathosis, these barriers are absent, and the oral microflora may have free access to the periodontium or periapical tissues; in this way, microorganisms that are normally commensals become pathogenic.

Acute Endodontic Infections

There is no doubt that bacteria from acute endodontic infections can cause bacteremia and can migrate to local lymph nodes and fascial spaces. Case reports have documented the association of acute endodontic infections with brain abscess,[3-5] mediastinitis,[6,7] and fatal necrotizing fasciitis.[8] In fact, researchers reported that about 8000 patients in the United States are hospitalized annually for periapical abscesses, some of whom have comorbid conditions such as diabetes or hypertension.[9] Therefore it is essential for the practitioner to obtain adequate diagnostic data for patients with acute endodontic infections and to evaluate their progress carefully, in case they need referral for management in a hospital setting. Patients with abscesses should have their temperature measured, and they must be evaluated for lymphadenopathy, malaise, and fascial space infection. These patients should receive prompt and complete elimination of local irritants, including drainage of the swelling. Those with a fascial space infection (cellulitis) also should be treated with adjunctive antibiotics and, most important, should be monitored carefully until their condition improves (see Chapter 9).

Chronic Endodontic Infections

The evidence for the presence of bacteria in periapical lesions and their escape systemically in chronic endodontic infections is less conclusive. Animal[10,11] and human[12,13] studies show that this is infrequent in primary lesions (Fig. 2.1). Studies have found that the number of bacteria in persistent periapical lesions after unsuccessful treatment may be much higher.[14,15] Teeth with chronic apical abscesses and sinus tracts have been reported to have very complex bacteriologic conditions with biofilm attached to the outer root surfaces in 17 out of 24 teeth.[16]

One way to investigate this potential for bacteria in chronic infections to travel from the endodontic environment to participate in the pathogenesis of systemic disease is to determine the

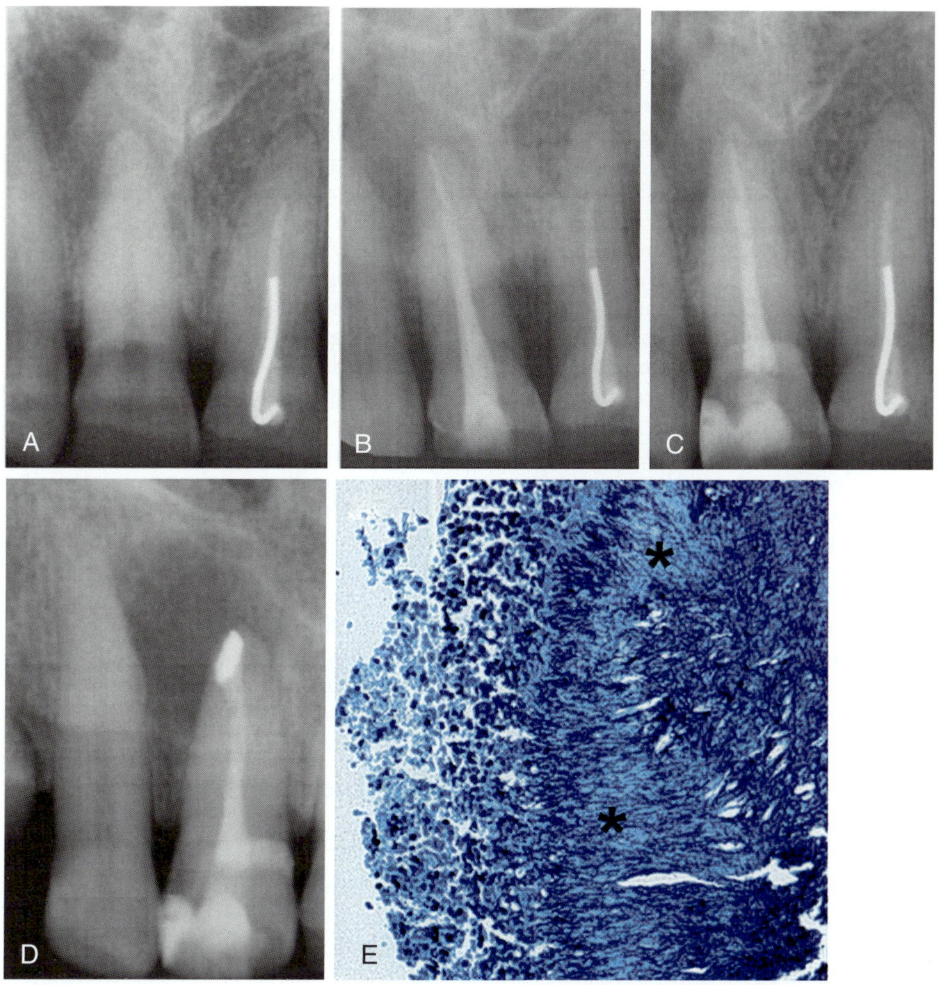

• **Fig. 2.1** Periapical Actinomycosis. **A,** Preoperative radiograph shows tooth #8 presenting with signs of pulp necrosis and chronic apical abscess. **B,** Root canal treatment was completed. **C,** Recall in 6 months revealed a persistent sinus tract. **D,** Root-end surgery was completed, and tissues were submitted for biopsy. **E,** Biopsy result revealed actinic filaments *(*)* surrounded by a severe inflammatory reaction. (Courtesy Dr. Blythe Kaufman.)

epidemiologic associations between the two forms of disease. One report associated periapical lesion-years (the number of years with a periapical lesion) and incident coronary heart disease in men younger than age 40.[17] Another study of patients with myocardial infarction (MI) reported a significantly higher number of patients with missing teeth and teeth with periapical lesions in the MI group compared with controls.[18] An additional large cohort study of male health professionals showed that the presence of coronary heart disease was significantly associated with the presence of one or more root canal–treated teeth (as a marker of pulpal and periapical disease).[19] In a systematic review of longitudinal cohort studies, the authors reported a moderate risk of causation.[20] However, they raised questions about the interrelationship of these different diseases, warranting further animal and human studies. Interventional studies would be required to prove causation, and those are clearly difficult to perform, given the ethical issues involved.

Diabetes Mellitus

Diabetes mellitus is one of the most significant chronic diseases that affects humans worldwide. In the United States about 30.3 million people, or 9.4% of the U.S. population, had diabetes in 2015. This total included 30.2 million adults age 18 or older, or 12.2% of all U.S. adults. About 7.2 million of these adults had diabetes but were not aware that they had the disease or did not report that they had it.[21] Diabetes is not curable, and it has serious complications, including cardiovascular disease, neuropathy, renal disease, blindness, limb amputations, and periodontal disease.

Health care practitioners generally know that diabetics have a higher prevalence of teeth with periapical lesions.[1,22-25] The longitudinal treatment outcome is generally not different for diabetics and nondiabetics.[26,27] However, if the outcomes of cases with and without preoperative periapical lesions are separated, a notable difference is observed. In cases with preoperative lesions, diabetics are significantly less likely to have successful treatment than do nondiabetics, especially when controlling for several other confounding factors.[28,29]

People with diabetes may have compromised healing, particularly those with higher glycemic rates and with preoperative endodontic infection, for several reasons. These individuals may select for specific microorganisms that may be more virulent.[30] They may have a variant of inflammatory cells, such as monocytes, characterized by excessive secretion of inflammatory mediators, including bone resorptive cytokines, that are critical for the development of periapical lesions.[31] The increased glycemia may also spontaneously result in excessive production of advanced glycation end products (AGEs). AGEs interact with their receptors (RAGEs), resulting in the production of bone resorptive mediators, which may lead to persistence of the periapical lesions.[32]

Hypertension

Hypertension is a sign of cardiovascular disease that may indicate a variety of underlying conditions and comorbidities, including diabetes. Hypertension appears to be associated with reduced survival (meaning continued presence of the tooth in the mouth) of endodontically treated teeth. In a study of the Indian Health Service in two U.S. states, 4500 patients were examined.[33] It was found that patients who had diabetes and/or hypertension had a significantly reduced chance of retention of endodontically treated teeth within a period of 10 years. In another cohort that included more than 49,000 teeth followed for about 2 years, researchers found that the presence of diabetes and/or hypertension resulted in significant reduction in tooth retention.[34] It is noteworthy, however, that the study of tooth survival in the absence of exact endodontic diagnosis and assessment of periapical health is confounded by the fact that diabetes and cardiovascular diseases are also associated with periodontal disease, which may have played an important role in the loss of these teeth.

Risk for Osteoradionecrosis or Osteonecrosis of the Jaw

Patients who have undergone radiation therapy for the treatment of malignancies in the craniofacial area are at risk of osteoradionecrosis at the site of a surgical procedure such as tooth extraction. Therefore many of these patients have teeth that would ordinarily not be amenable to treatment but that are retained with endodontic treatment to avoid the risk of osteoradionecrosis. A report documented the treatment outcome in 22 patients treated endodontically after having received 50 Gy irradiation in the area within the preceding 6 months.[35] After a mean of 19 months, successful treatment was found in 91% of the patients, which was consistent with treatment averages for normal patients in other studies. However, treatment of patients who have undergone radiation therapy is frequently complicated by fibrotic tissues that do not permit adequate mouth opening (Fig. 2.2). About 66 to 70 Gy of radiotherapy has been reported to result in progressive decrease in pulp vitality testing and electric pulp testing at 12 months.[36] Also, dry mouth results in recurrent caries, compromising the prognosis.

Over the past decade, it has been recognized that patients undergoing bisphosphonate therapy may be at risk for bisphosphonate-related osteonecrosis of the jaw (BRONJ). This risk is greater in patients receiving intravenous (IV) bisphosphonates, particularly if more than one agent is used simultaneously, and the risk increases with the duration of bisphosphonate use and with surgical procedures, such as extractions.[37] Although rare, BRONJ may occur after endodontic treatment[38] or endodontic surgery.[39] When nonsurgical endodontic treatment is performed on a patient receiving IV bisphosphonates, care should be taken not to injure the soft tissue. For example, the clamps should be carefully placed to avoid injury to the soft tissues and alveolar bone[40].

Oral bisphosphonates pose a much lower risk of BRONJ. Endodontic outcomes are not different between patients taking oral bisphosphonates and other patients.[41]

Viral Infections

HIV/AIDS

When the human immunodeficiency virus (HIV) was first identified, practitioners were concerned that patients with HIV infection would be so compromised that severe complications would ensue with endodontic disease and/or endodontic treatment, particularly in patients whose cluster of differentiation 4 (CD4+) cell count had dropped below 200/mL. However, a cohort study of patients with acquired immune deficiency syndrome (AIDS) who had received various oral health procedures documented that the patients did not

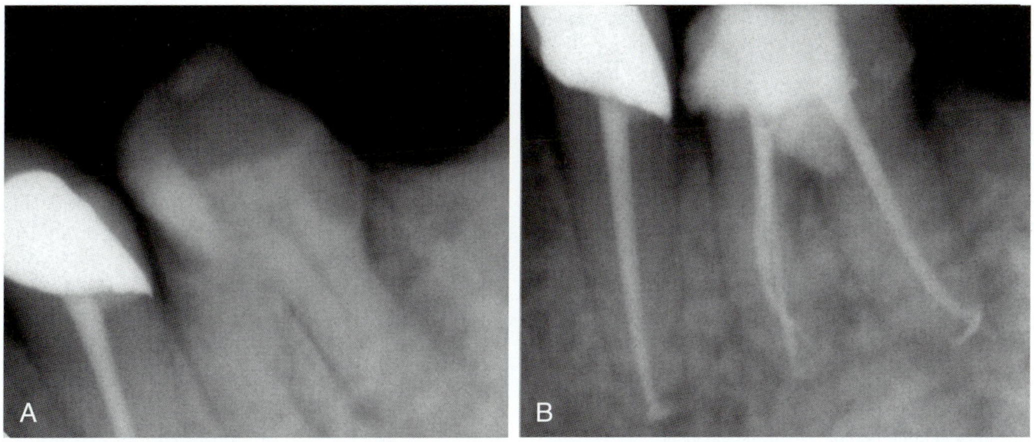

• **Fig. 2.2** A compromised case of an older adult patient who had had a hemimandibulectomy on the right side to treat oral cancer, together with radiation therapy; that treatment resulted in severe restriction in mouth opening. The patient could open her mouth only about 15 mm at the incisors, making the introduction of radiographic sensors, mirrors, and dental instruments very difficult. **A,** A poor-quality preoperative radiograph shows a previous restoration that compromised pulp health and led to a periradicular lesion. **B,** Treatment was attempted to prevent osteoradionecrosis and save the tooth for function. Complications arose in the furcation area, because the clinician was unable to use the mirror and the handpiece together for access preparation.

appear to suffer any undue pain or infection with endodontic treatment.[42] In addition, 1 year after treatment, no difference was seen in the outcomes of treatment between patients who were HIV positive and those who were not infected with the virus.[43]

Herpes Viruses

There are many different types of herpes viruses that affect humans. These types include varicella zoster virus (VZV), which causes herpes zoster infection; human herpes viruses (HHV1-8); human cytomegalovirus (HCMV); and Epstein-Barr virus (EBV).

Herpes zoster infections frequently represent a diagnostic dilemma, because after the herpetic blisters heal, the patient may suffer from postherpetic neuralgia, which mimics endodontic pain. Careful documentation of the medical history and diagnostic tests should help the practitioner identify this condition and make the right decisions and/or referrals. However, herpes zoster infection may also induce spontaneous pulpal pathosis.[44-48]

Periapical lesions in patients infected with HCMV and/or EBV, but not herpes simplex viruses, may be larger and more painful. In addition, irreversible pulpitis or acute endodontic infections may be associated with a higher incidence of EBV or the HHV pathogens.[49,50] However, it is not yet conclusively known whether the viral association potentiates the development of more aggressive forms of endodontic pathosis or whether the findings of the small studies and case reports available were merely coincidental. One systematic review has not identified significant associations between HCMV or EBV and symptomatic endodontic pathosis.[51]

Sickle Cell Anemia

Sickle cell anemia is characterized by a congenital abnormality of red blood cells that results in deficient oxygenation of the blood. A milder form of the disease, known as *sickle cell trait,* results from homozygous transmission of the affected gene. Oral findings of sickle cell anemia include the radiographic "stepladder" trabecular pattern of bone, enamel hypomineralization, calcified canals, increased overbite, and overjet.[52] An older case series showed the spontaneous development of pulpal pathosis in some noncarious teeth in patients with sickle cell anemia.[53] More recently, it was shown that patients with sickle cell anemia have a significantly higher incidence of orofacial pain than controls and have pulp necrosis in 6% of their teeth that have no other apparent etiologies in comparison with none in the controls.[54]

Smoking

The oral health problems of smoking, including the increase in periodontal disease, mucositis, and oral premalignant and malignant lesions, have been well documented. Recently, there has been an interest in the association of smoking with pulpal and periapical diseases. Smoking is also associated with a high prevalence of periapical lesions[55-57] and with incident root canal treatment as a marker of pulpal and periapical diseases.[58] The incidence of root canal treatment (as a marker of endodontic disease and its treatment) was also increased with the duration of smoking and reduced in smokers who stopped smoking more than 9 years before the evaluation time. Smoking was also shown to increase the incidence of pain and/or swelling after endodontic surgery.[59] Smoking has been reported to change the immunoregulatory function of the cytokines and chemokines in dental pulps.[60] In addition, smokers tend to have more postsurgical infections than do nonsmokers.[59]

Genetic Predisposition

Several gene polymorphism associations have been made with endodontic treatment outcomes. Thus interleukin (IL)-1β allele 2 was found to be associated with reduced healing after endodontic treatment.[61] Gene polymorphism in IL-1β, IL-6, and IL-8 have been reported to be associated with apical periodontitis.[62,63]

It is noteworthy, however, that these associations do not prove causation and that studies with large sample sizes are needed to confirm these initial findings.

• BOX 2.1 Review Study Questions

1. Why is it important to be familiar with the patient's medical history?
   a. Most patients require antibiotic treatment. Thus the clinician needs to premedicate most patients.
   b. Most patients are in pain and need to be premedicated with antibiotics, analgesics, and narcotics.
   c. As with any invasive procedure, there is a high prevalence for bacteremia.
   d. The clinician needs to be keenly aware of the patient's systemic health as it affects the dental management.
2. Reports of hypersensitivity to gutta percha, amide-based local anesthetic agents, sodium hypochlorite, and nickel (present in nickel titanium files) have been reported, but it is rare.
   a. True
   b. False
3. Diabetes has which of the following complications:
   a. Neuropathy
   b. Liver dysfunction
   c. Blood disorder
   d. Hepatitis
4. There are several reasons why diabetics may have compromised healing. All the following are reasons except one. Which one is the EXCEPTION?
   a. Impaired immunologic cells
   b. More virulent microorganisms
   c. Variant inflammatory cells
   d. Reduced glycemia
5. What dose of radiotherapy has been reported to result in progressive decrease in pulp vitality testing and electric pulp testing at 12 months?
   a. 10 to 20 Gy
   b. 30 to 40 Gy
   c. 50 to 55 Gy
   d. 66 to 70 Gy

Presentation of Endodontic Disease in the Older Adults

Endodontic considerations in older adult patients are similar in many ways to those in younger patients, but there are some notable differences.

The number of persons age 65 or older in the United States exceeds 39 million, and they are expected to comprise 20% of the population by 2020. Their dental needs will also continue to increase.[64-66] More older adult patients will not accept tooth extraction unless there are no alternatives.[67] They have a high utilization rate of dental services.[68] The expectations for dental health parallel their demands for quality medical care. An even more important consideration is that these dentitions will continue to experience caries[69] and decades of dental disease, in addition to restorative[65] and periodontal procedures specifically[70] (Fig. 2.3). These factors all have compound adverse effects on the pulp and periapical and surrounding tissues (Fig. 2.4). In other words, the more injuries inflicted, the greater the likelihood of irreversible disease, and thus the greater the need for treatment. The number of older adult endodontic patients is increasing and will continue to do so.[71]

The combination of an increase in pathosis and dental needs, coupled with greater expectations, has resulted in more endodontic procedures among aging patients (Fig. 2.5). Furthermore, expanded dental insurance benefits for retirees and more disposable income have made complex treatment more affordable.[72] Other means will likely be available to finance the costs of oral health care in the future.[73]

Endodontic considerations in older patients include physical, biologic, medical, and some psychologic differences from young patients, in addition to treatment complications.

Physical Limitations

If a patient cannot be suitably reclined or if the mouth opening is limited, referral should be considered.

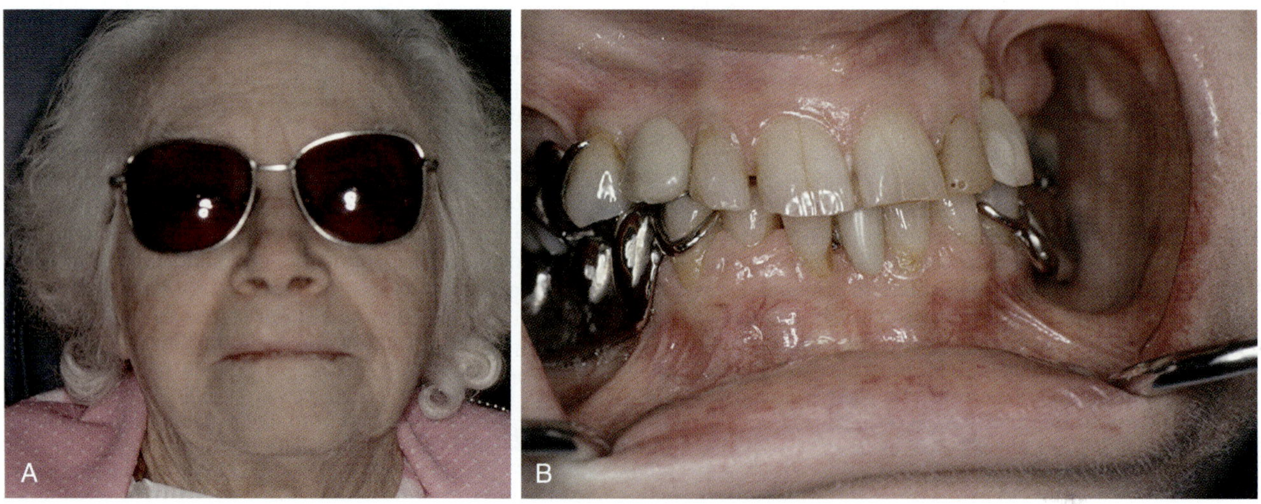

• **Fig. 2.3 A,** This 87-year-old woman has Alzheimer's disease. **B,** Her dentition shows diverse problems caused by many years of disease, restorations, and oral and systemic changes. Diagnosis is challenging, and the dentition will be difficult to restore to acceptable function and esthetics, particularly in a patient with mental impairment.

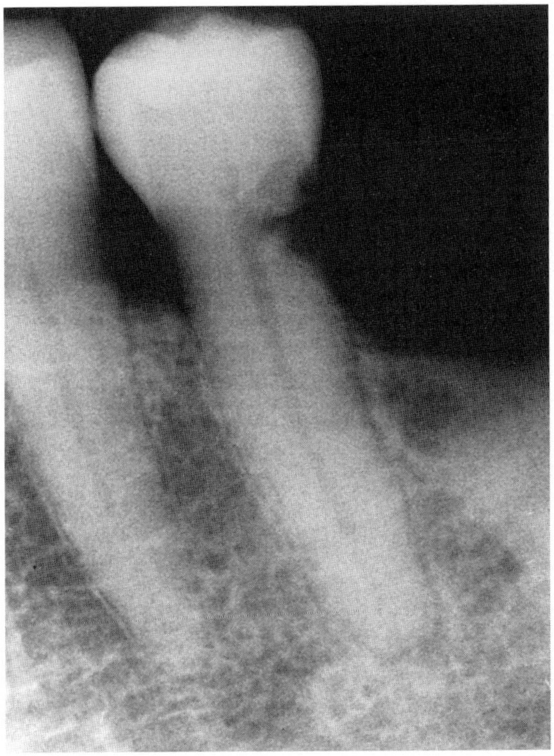

• **Fig. 2.4** Cervical External Resorption Exposing the Pulp. A free-end removable partial denture has settled posteriorly, exerting pressure on the gingiva and inducing inflammation and root resorption. (From Walton RE: Endodontic considerations in the geriatric patient, *Dent Clin North Am* 41(4):795–816, 1997.)

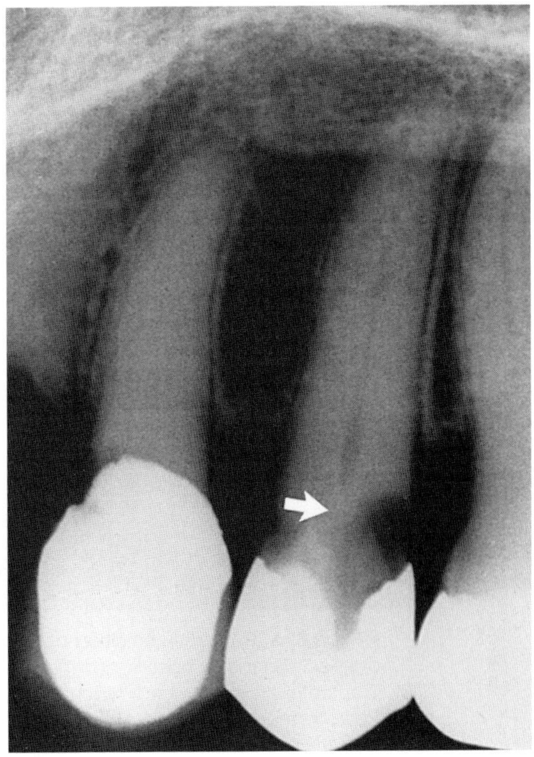

• **Fig. 2.5** Restorations, caries, and time have resulted in dentin formation. The first premolar shows calcific metamorphosis (a very small pulp space is present). The second premolar has dentin formation *(arrow)* in response to recurrent caries. Both are difficult to treat and restore. (From Walton RE: Endodontic considerations in the geriatric patient, *Dent Clin North Am* 41(4):795–816, 1997.)

Restorative Considerations

Severe caries or fractures from trauma may render the tooth difficult to isolate or restore.

Biologic Considerations

Biologic considerations are both systemic and local. In the older patient, systemic or local changes unique to endodontics are not different from those for other dental procedures. Similarly, the response of the pulp and periapical tissues is not markedly different.

Anatomy

Pulp Chamber

As a tooth ages, pulp chamber space decreases. Chamber size and pulp stones, in addition to the extent of calcifications in the canal system, must be considered.

Canal Calcification (Calcific Metamorphosis)

Secondary and perhaps tertiary dentin formation leads to narrowing of the canals, sometimes to an extent that they are not visible radiographically (Figs. 2.6 and 2.7).

Calcifications include denticles (pulp stones) and diffuse (linear) calcifications.[74] Pulp stones tend to be found in the coronal pulp, and diffuse calcifications are found in the radicular pulp. It has been speculated that the nidi of calcification arise from degenerated nerves or blood vessels, but this has not been proved. Another common speculation is that pulp stones may cause odontogenic pain; however, this is not true. Pulp stones were shown to increase in patients with cardiovascular disease and those on statins.[75]

Pulp Response

Changes With Age

Two considerations are important in age-related changes in pulp response: (1) structural (histologic) changes that take place as a function of time and (2) tissue changes that occur in response to irritation from injury. These changes tend to have similar appearances in the pulp. In other words, injury may prematurely "age" a pulp. Therefore an "old" pulp may be found in a tooth of a younger person (e.g., a tooth that has experienced caries, restorations, etc.). Whatever the etiology, these older (or injured) pulps react somewhat differently than do younger (or uninjured) pulps. The aging pulp may be less resistant to injury, although this may be due to the cumulative effect of irritation, which increases with age, rather than the effect of age. Stem cells were shown to be present in periapical tissues of older adults.[76] This is not necessarily the case with the young immature tooth (open apex) in which pulps have indeed been shown to be more resistant to injury. There is a theory that pulps in older teeth may in fact be *more* resistant because of decreased permeability of dentin.[77] However, this resistance to injury in old teeth has not been proved.[78] Therefore the

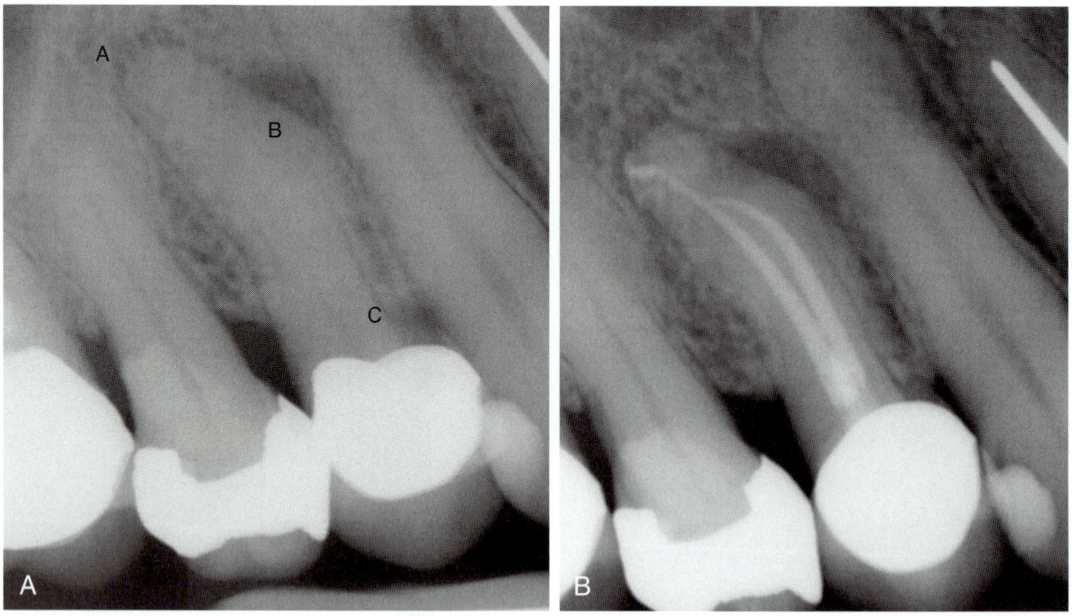

• **Fig. 2.6 A,** Periapical radiolucency *(A)* and mesial radiolucency in the apical third *(B)*. The canals are calcified, the root is narrow, and there is a hint of a significant mesial concavity in the coronal third *(C)*. The tooth is also crowned, which increases access complexity. This is considered a high-risk case. **B,** Postoperatively, the mesial radiolucency resulted from the buccal root exiting several millimeters shorter than the palatal root, with a significant distal curvature. The practitioner must be prepared to manage the unexpected should problems arise during treatment.

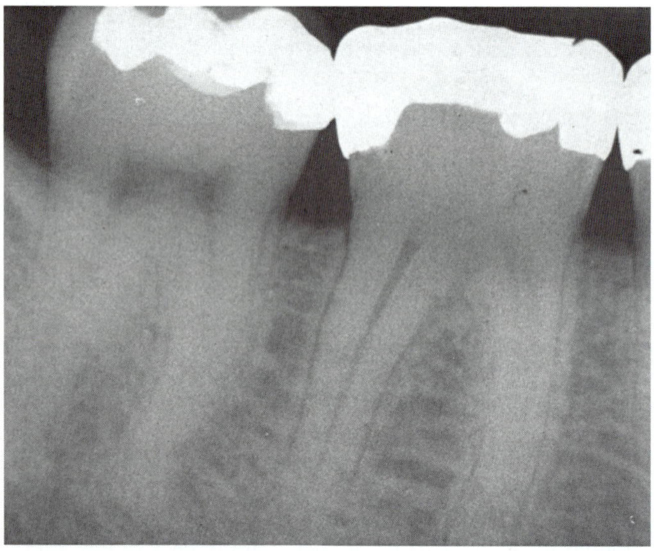

• **Fig. 2.7** Pulp chamber and root canals show calcific metamorphosis; this situation is rated as extreme risk.

dental pulp in older patients require more care in preparation and restoration; this response to irritation is probably the result of a history of previous irritation rather than age per se.

Chronologic Versus Physiologic

Does a pulp in an older individual react differently to injury compared with pulp in a younger individual? This question has not been answered definitively. A previously injured pulp (from caries, restoration, and so on) in a younger person probably has *less* resistance to injury than an undamaged pulp in an older individual. At a histologic level, there are some consistent changes in the older pulps and in irritated pulps.

Structural

The pulp is a dynamic connective tissue. With age, there are changes in cellular, extracellular, and supportive elements. There is a decrease in cells, including both odontoblasts and fibroblasts. There are also fewer supportive elements (i.e., blood vessels and nerves).[79,80] Fewer and smaller vessels result in a decrease in blood flow in the pulp; the significance of this decrease is unknown. Capillaries show somewhat degenerative changes in the endothelium with age.[81] There is presumably an increase in the percentage of space occupied by collagen but less ground substance.[82]

Dimensional

In general, pulp spaces progressively decrease in size and often become very small,[83] a phenomenon known as *calcific metamorphosis* or pulp canal obliteration.[84] Dentin formation may be accelerated by irritation from caries, trauma, abrasion, restorations, and periodontal disease and is not uniform. For example, in molar pulp chambers there is more dentin formation on the roof and floor than on the walls.[79] The result is a flattened (disk-like) chamber (Fig. 2.8).

Nature of Response to Injury

The older patient does tend to have more severe pulpal reactions to irritation than the reactions that occur in the younger patient. The reason for these differences is not fully understood, but the more severe reactions probably result from a lifetime of cumulative injuries.

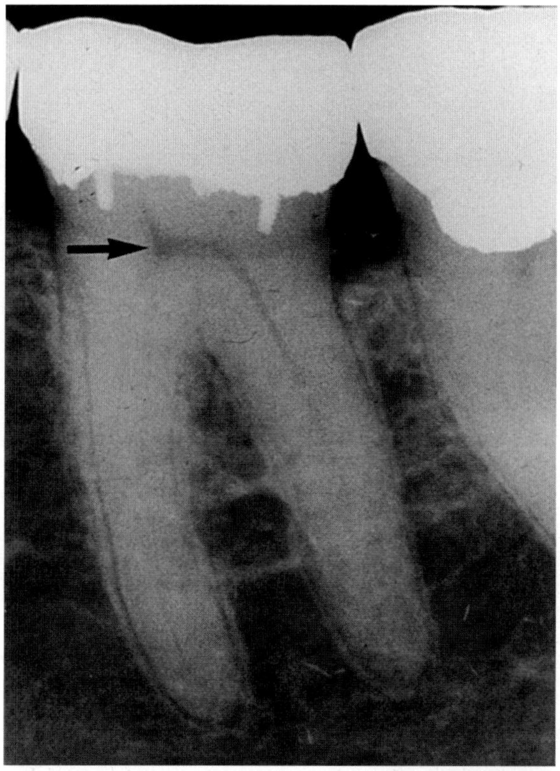

• **Fig. 2.8** Disk-like Chamber *(arrow).* The chamber is flattened because of dentin formation on the roof and floor. These chambers and canals are a challenge to locate. (From Walton RE: Endodontic considerations in the geriatric patient, *Dent Clin North Am* 41(4):795–816, 1997.)

Irritation

There are reasons for pulp pathosis after restorative procedures. First, the tooth may have experienced several injuries in the past. Second, the tooth is likely to have undergone more extensive procedures that involve considerable tooth structure, such as crown preparation. Multiple potential injuries are associated with a full crown, such as foundation placement, bur preparation, impressions, temporary crown placement (temporary crowns may leak), cementation, and unsealed crown margins. The cause of final demise, or "coup de grâce," of a pulp that is already stumbling along may be that final restoration.

Systemic Conditions

There is no conclusive evidence that systemic or medical conditions directly affect (decrease) pulp resistance to injury. One proposed condition is atherosclerosis, which has been presumed to directly affect pulp vessels[85]; however, the phenomenon of pulpal atherosclerosis could not be demonstrated.[86] There may be differences among patients due to gene polymorphism that lead to faster or slower pulp necrosis. For example, one study showed that two heat shock protein gene variations were significantly associated with whether deep carious lesions were related to the presence of vital pulp versus a periapical lesion.[87]

Periapical Response

Little information is available on changes in bone and soft tissues with age and how these changes might affect the response to irritants or to subsequent healing after removal of those irritants. There is some indication that relatively little change occurs in periapical cellularity, vascularity, or nerve supply with aging.[88] Therefore it is unlikely that there are significantly different periapical responses in older patients compared with younger individuals.

Additional Considerations

In treatment planning for older patients, the tendency is to plan according to anticipated longevity.[89] It is natural to assume that procedures need not be as permanent because the patient may not live very long. The concept that treatment should not outlast the patient is not accepted by many elder patients, who desire health care equivalent to that rendered to younger patients. Esthetic and functional concerns may not differ.

Root Canal Treatment

Treatment Considerations

Time Required

On average, longer appointments are necessary to accomplish the same procedures in older adult patients, for the reasons discussed earlier.

Anesthesia

Primary Injections

The need for anesthesia is somewhat less in older patients with pulp necrosis and an increased risk to local anesthetic toxicity.[90] It is necessary for vital pulps but is often unnecessary for pulp necrosis, obturation appointments, and retreatments. Older patients tend to be less sensitive and are more likely to prefer procedures without anesthetic. Also, they tend to be less anxious and therefore have a higher threshold of pain. Although there are no differences in effectiveness of anesthetic solutions, various systemic problems or medications may preclude the use of vasoconstrictors.

Supplemental Injections

Intraosseous, periodontal ligament (PDL), and intrapulpal forms of anesthesia are effective adjuncts if the primary anesthesia is not adequate. Certain cardiac conditions may preclude the use of epinephrine, particularly with the intraosseous and PDL techniques. The duration of anesthesia is considerably decreased without a vasoconstrictor, and reinjection during the procedure may be required.

Procedures

Isolation

Isolation is often difficult because of subgingival caries or defective restorations. However, placement of a rubber dam is imperative and often requires ingenuity (see Chapter 13).

Access Preparation

Achieving good access that enables the clinician to locate and then negotiate canal orifices is challenging in older teeth because of the internal anatomy (Fig. 2.9). Radiographs are helpful. A slightly larger, rather than a too small, access opening is preferable, particularly through large restorations such as crowns. Magnification is also helpful, either from a microscope or from other visual aids.

A supererupted tooth, as a result of caries or restoration, has a short clinical crown, requiring a less deep access preparation. The distance from the reference cusp to the chamber roof should be measured on the bur radiographically. A very small or invisible chamber may be an indication to begin the access without the

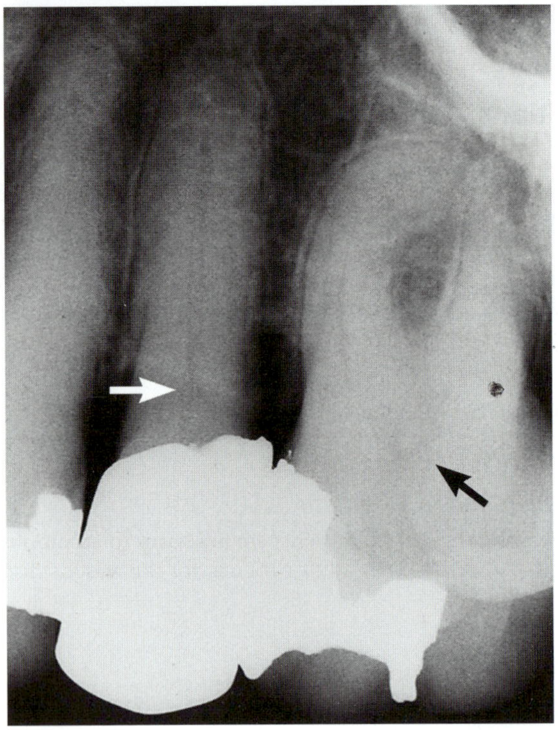

• **Fig. 2.9** Age, caries, and restorations have resulted in small chambers *(arrows).* Either would be a challenge to access, and referral should be considered.

rubber dam; this helps the clinician parallel to the long axis of the tooth (Fig. 2.10). Once the canal has been located, the rubber dam is immediately placed, before working length radiographs are made.

Locating canal orifices is often fatiguing and frustrating for both the clinician and the patient. Although a reasonable time should be allocated for this, there is a limit. It may be best to stop and have the patient return for another appointment. Often the canals are readily located at a subsequent visit. This circumstance also is a time to consider a referral because imaging with cone beam computed tomography (CBCT) and/or another procedure, such as surgery, may be indicated.

Working Length

There are some differences in working length for the older patient.[91] Because the apical foramen varies more widely (Fig. 2.11) than in the younger tooth and because of the decreased diameter of the canal apically, it is more difficult to determine the preferred length.[92] In teeth of any age, materials and instruments are best confined to the canal space. One millimeter short of the radiographic apex is the preferred working and obturation length[93]; this length should be decreased if an apical stop is not detected.Electronic apex locators are also useful, particularly when there is difficulty obtaining adequate working-length radiographs.[94]

Cleaning and Shaping

A common challenge is a much smaller canal that requires more time and effort to enlarge. A very small canal may be more easily negotiated and initially prepared with a lubricant, such as glycerin, RC-Prep, or Glyde. This process may be used through two or three smaller sizes of files to facilitate enlargement and to reduce the risk of binding and separation. The same principles of débridement and adequate shaping are followed. Glide path 0.02 taper instruments such as PathFiles or ProGlider (Sirona/Dentsply) may be helpful in these situations (see Chapter 14).

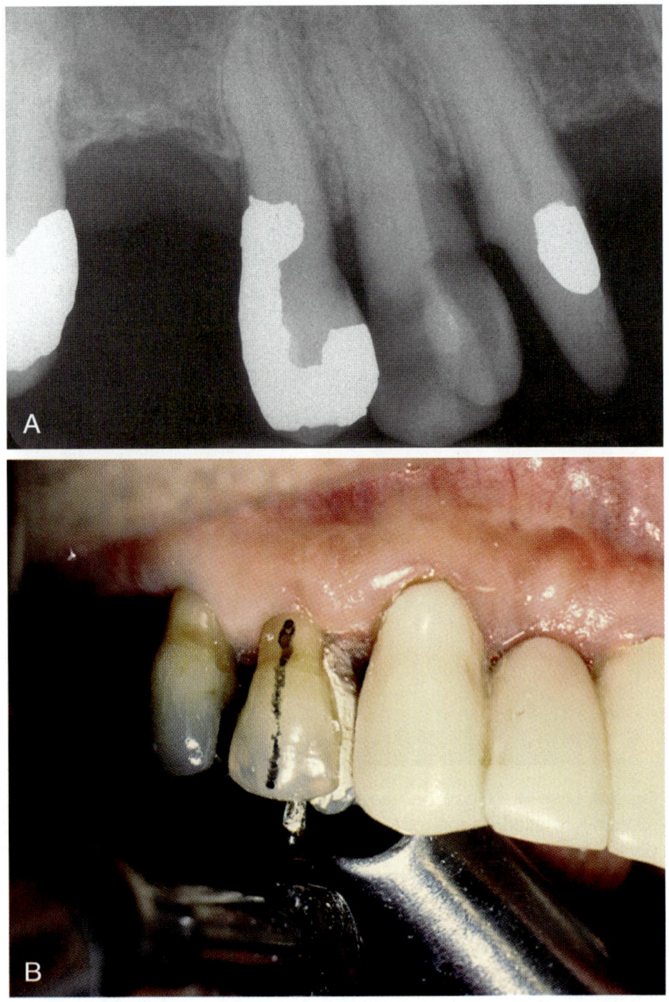

• **Fig. 2.10 A,** The first premolar is tilted and has a "receded" pulp chamber. **B,** Aids in orientation during access. The preparation is initiated without the rubber dam in place. A pencil mark is placed on the crown to guide the bur in the long axis of the root. (From Walton RE: Endodontic considerations in the geriatric patient, *Dent Clin North Am* 41(4):795–816, 1997.)

Intracanal Medicaments

Intracanal medicaments are not useful, with the exception of calcium hydroxide. This chemical is antimicrobial, inhibits bacterial growth between appointments, and possibly reduces periapical inflammation.[95] Its use is indicated if the pulp is necrotic and the canal preparation is essentially complete.

Obturation

There is no demonstrated preferred approach, although cold-lateral and warm-vertical gutta-percha obturations are the most commonly used and their use the best documented.

Effect of Restoration

In general, the larger and deeper the restoration, the more complicated the root canal treatment would be. The old tooth is more likely to have a full crown. There are two concerns when there is a crown: (1) potential damage to retention or components of the crown and (2) blockage of access and poor internal visibility.

The porcelain-fused-to-metal (PFM) crown is more common than a full metal crown and creates additional problems. Porcelain may fracture or craze during access preparation. This problem is minimized by using burs specifically designed to prepare through

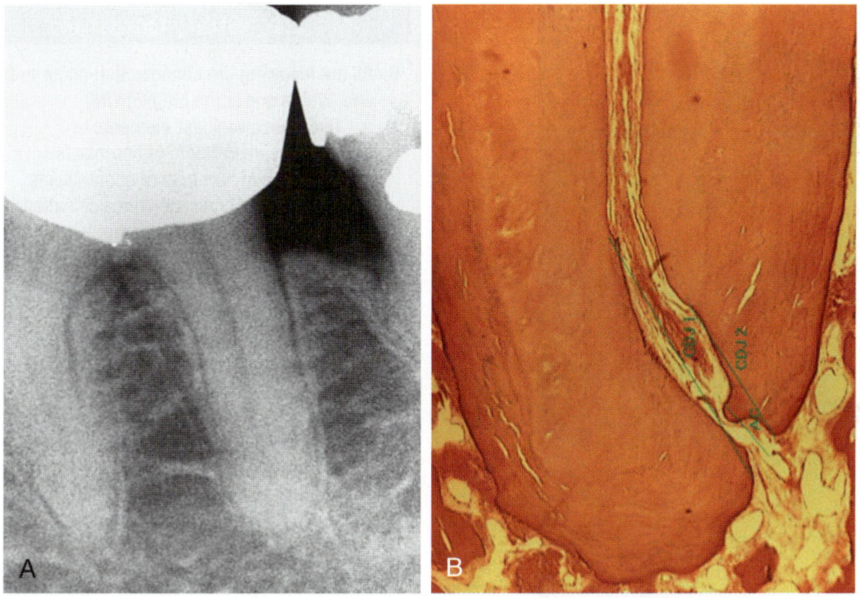

• **Fig. 2.11** Variability in Apical Foramen Location. **A,** The foramen is not visible radiographically. **B,** Histologically, the distal root shows the foramen to be well short of the apex. (From Walton RE: Endodontic considerations in the geriatric patient, *Dent Clin North Am* 41(4):795–816, 1997.)

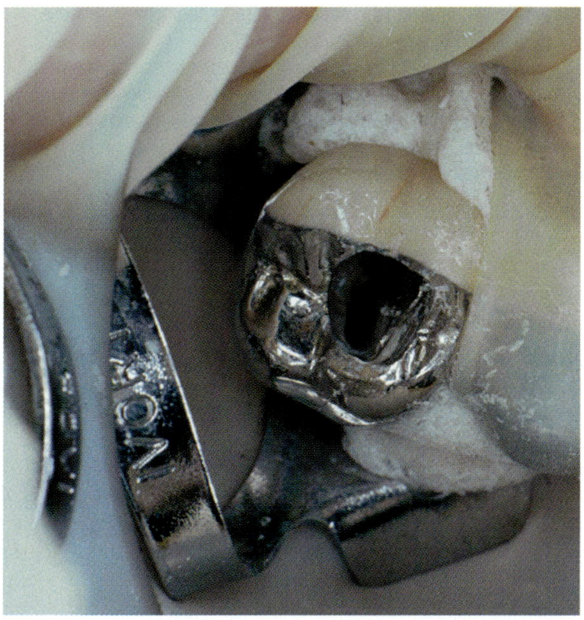

• **Fig. 2.12** Access Through a Porcelain-Fused-to-Metal Crown. The outline is large for visibility. Also, the preparation does not extend to the porcelain to avoid fracture of the porcelain. (From Walton RE: Endodontic considerations in the geriatric patient, *Dent Clin North Am* 41(4):795–816; 1997.)

porcelain,[96] combined with slow cutting and copious use of water spray. Occlusal access is wide (Fig. 2.12). Metal should not be removed after the chamber has been opened to prevent metal shavings from entering and blocking canals. Access through a PFM or gold crown (either anterior or posterior) that is to be retained is best permanently repaired with amalgam. Anterior nonmetallic crowns may be repaired with composite.

Retreatment

Factors that lead to failure tend to increase with age; thus retreatment is more common in older patients. Retreatment at any age is often complicated and should be approached with caution; these patients should be considered for referral. Retreatment procedures and outcomes are similar in older and younger teeth (see Chapter 19).

Endodontic Surgery

Considerations and indications for surgery are similar in older adult and younger patients. These indications include incision for drainage, periapical procedures, corrective surgery, root removal, and intentional replantation. Overall, the incidence of most of these factors increases with age. Small nonnegotiable canals, resorptions, and canal blockages occur more often with age. Perforation during access or preparation, ledging, and instrument separation are related to restorative and anatomic problems.

Medical Considerations

Medical considerations may require consultation and are a concern but generally do not contraindicate a surgical approach.[97] This contraindication is particularly true when extraction is the alternative; surgery is often less traumatic.

Excessive hemorrhage during or after surgery is a concern; many older adult patients are receiving anticoagulant therapy. Interestingly, recent studies examined bleeding patterns in oral surgery patients taking low-dose aspirin[98] and prescribed anticoagulants.[99] The findings were that anticoagulant therapy should not be altered and that hemorrhage was controllable by local hemostatic agents.[100] Consultation with the physician and maintenance of the INR at the 2- to 3-unit range are appropriate in these cases. It is important to note that patients undergoing antithrombotic therapy, patients with previous history of MI, patients with history of renal disease, or patients with severe asthma should not receive nonsteroidal antiinflammatory drugs.[101]

Biologic and Anatomic Factors

Bony and soft tissues are similar and respond the same in older and younger patients. There may be somewhat less thickness of overlying soft tissue; however, alveolar mucosa and gingiva seem to be

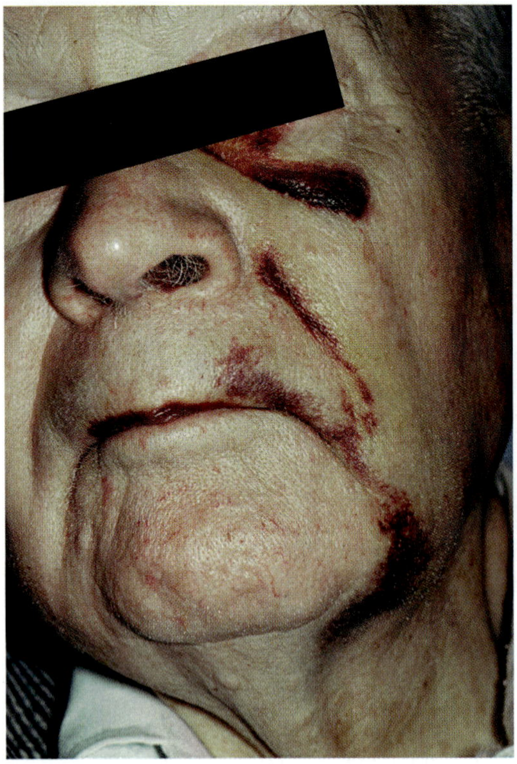

• **Fig. 2.13** Postsurgical Ecchymosis. Root-end surgery of a maxillary lateral incisor resulted in widespread migration of hemorrhage into the tissues, with resultant discoloration. This is not an uncommon occurrence in older adult patients. No treatment is indicated, and the problem resolves in 1 to 2 weeks.

structurally similar. Anatomic structures, such as the sinuses, floor of the nose, and location of neurovascular bundles, are essentially unchanged. Often, periodontal and endodontic surgery must be combined. In addition, crown-to-root ratios may be compromised because of periodontal disease or root resorption.

Healing After Surgery

Hard and soft tissues heal as predictably in older patients as they heal in younger ones, although somewhat more slowly.[102-104] Postsurgical instructions should be given both verbally and in writing to minimize complications. If the patient has cognitive problems, instructions are repeated to the person accompanying the patient. Even very old patients have good healing, provided they follow posttreatment protocols and have no underlying immunologic problems. Ice and pressure (in particular) applied over the surgical area reduce bleeding and edema and minimize swelling. Overall, older patients experience no more significant adverse effects from surgery than do younger patients. Outcomes depend more on oral hygiene than on age, as has been shown in periodontal surgery patients.[105]

One problem that seems to be more prevalent in older patients is ecchymosis after surgery. This is hemorrhage that often spreads widely through underlying tissue and commonly presents as discoloration (Fig. 2.13). Patients are informed that this may occur and that it should not be a concern. Normal color may take 1 to 2 weeks or longer to return. In addition, the discoloration may go through different color phases (purple, red, yellow, green) before disappearing.

• BOX 2.2 Study Questions

6. All the following are changes that occur in the pulp with age except one. Which one is the EXCEPTION?
   a. Decreased vascular elements
   b. Increase in numbers of fibroblasts
   c. Decrease in numbers of odontoblasts
   d. Increase in occurrence of calcifications
7. Which of the following statement is true regarding calcifications in the pulp space?
   a. Pulp stones are found frequently in the radicular pulp.
   b. Pulp stones are associated with odontogenic pain.
   c. Calcification increases with both age and irritation.
   d. Diffuse calcifications are mostly commonly found in the pulp chamber.
8. With age, which of the following describes the dimensional changes in the pulp space?
   a. Pulp space progressively decreases in size in occlusal-apical dimension.
   b. Pulp space decreases primarily in a mesiodistal dimension.
   c. The volume remains the same.
   d. Pulp space increases in size in response to irritation; hence called *inflammation.*
9. Epinephrine should be used with caution particularly in patients with
   a. Hepatic disease
   b. Renal disease
   c. Cardiovascular disease
   d. Diabetes
10. Working length determination in older adult patients may be more difficult because of which of the following?
    a. Increased bone density, making radiographs harder to interpret
    b. Increased cementum deposition, modifying the apical anatomy
    c. Differences in tissue electrical resistance, making apex locators less accurate
    d. Patient's inability to withstand and sit still for radiograph

ANSWERS

Answer Box 2

1 d. The clinician needs to be keenly aware of the patient's systemic health as it affects the dental management.
2 a. True
3 a. Neuropathy
4 d. Reduced glycemia
5 d. 66 to 70 Gy
6 b. Increase in numbers of fibroblasts
7 c. Calcification increases with both age and irritation
8 a. Pulp space progressively decreases in size in occlusal-apical dimension
9 c. Cardiovascular disease
10 b. Increased cementum deposition, modifying the apical anatomy

Identifying Patients for Referral

The AAE Endodontic Case Difficulty Assessment Form and Guidelines is a great tool for decision-making regarding case selection. In general, those patients with complex medical history, serious illness, or disability (American Society of Anesthesiologists Classes 3–5) should be referred. On that list, there are also those patients who are difficult to anesthetize, uncooperative, have limitation in opening, have extreme gag reflex that has compromised past dental care, and/or have severe pain or swelling.

Other considerations include difficult diagnosis, extreme curvature of the roots, extensive pretreatment modification required for rubber dam isolation, significant deviation from normal tooth due to crown morphology to root morphology, indistinct canal morphology, extensive resorption, concurrent severe periodontal disease, cracked teeth, and endodontic surgery.

References

1. Khalighinejad N, Aminoshariae MR, Aminoshariae A, et al.: Association between systemic diseases and apical periodontitis, *J Endod* 42:1427–1434, 2016.
2. Aminoshariae A, Kulild JC, Mickel A, Fouad AF: Association between systemic diseases and endodontic outcome: a systematic review, *J Endod* 43:514–519, 2017.
3. Greenstein A, Witherspoon R, Leinkram D, Malandreni M: An unusual case of a brain abscess arising from an odontogenic infection, *Aust Dent J* 60:532–535, 2015.
4. Aldous JA, Powell GL, Stensaas SS: Brain abscess of odontogenic origin: report of case, *J Am Dent Assoc* 115:861–863, 1987.
5. Antunes AA, de Santana Santos T, de Carvalho RW, et al.: Brain abscess of odontogenic origin, *J Craniofac Surg* 22:2363–2365, 2011.
6. Bonapart IE, Stevens HP, Kerver AJ, Rietveld AP: Rare complications of an odontogenic abscess: mediastinitis, thoracic empyema and cardiac tamponade, *J Oral Maxillofac Surg* 53:610–613, 1995.
7. Furst IM, Ersil P, Caminiti M: A rare complication of tooth abscess—Ludwig's angina and mediastinitis, *J Can Dent Assoc* 67:324–327, 2001.
8. Stoykewych AA, Beecroft WA, Cogan AG: Fatal necrotizing fasciitis of dental origin, *J Can Dent Assoc* 58:59–62, 1992.
9. Allareddy V, Lin CY, Shah A, et al.: Outcomes in patients hospitalized for periapical abscess in the United States: an analysis involving the use of a nationwide inpatient sample, *J Am Dent Assoc* 141:1107–1116, 2010.
10. Fouad AF, Walton RE, Rittman BR: Induced periapical lesions in ferret canines: histologic and radiographic evaluation, *Endod Dent Traumatol* 8:56–62, 1992.
11. Walton RE, Ardjmand K: Histological evaluation of the presence of bacteria in induced periapical lesions in monkeys, *J Endod* 18:216–227, 1992.
12. Ramachandran Nair PN: Light and electron microscopic studies of root canal flora and periapical lesions, *J Endod* 13:29–39, 1987.
13. Ricucci D, Pascon EA, Ford TR, Langeland K: Epithelium and bacteria in periapical lesions, *Oral Surg Oral Med Oral Pathol Oral Radiol Endod* 101:239–249, 2006.
14. Ricucci D, Siqueira Jr JF, Lopes WS, Vieira AR: Rocas IN: Extraradicular infection as the cause of persistent symptoms: a case series, *J Endod* 41:265–273, 2015.
15. Sunde PT, Olsen I, Gobel UB, et al.: Fluorescence in situ hybridization (FISH) for direct visualization of bacteria in periapical lesions of asymptomatic root-filled teeth, *Microbiology* 149:1095–1102, 2003.
16. Ricucci D, Loghin S, Goncalves LS, Rocas IN, Siqueira Jr JF: Histobacteriologic conditions of the apical root canal system and periapical tissues in teeth associated with sinus tracts, *J Endod* 44:405–413, 2018.
17. Caplan DJ, Chasen JB, Krall EA, et al.: Lesions of endodontic origin and risk of coronary heart disease, *J Dent Res* 85:996–1000, 2006.
18. Willershausen B, Kasaj A, Willershausen I, et al.: Association between chronic dental infection and acute myocardial infarction, *J Endod* 35:626–630, 2009.
19. Joshipura KJ, Pitiphat W, Hung HC, et al.: Pulpal inflammation and incidence of coronary heart disease, *J Endod* 32:99–103, 2006.
20. Aminoshariae A, Kulild JC, Fouad AF: The impact of endodontic infections on the pathogenesis of cardiovascular disease(s): a systematic review with meta-analysis using grade, *J Endod* 44:1361–1366, e3, 2018.
21. Centers for Disease Control and Prevention: *National diabetes statistics report*, 2017. Atlanta, GA, 2017, Centers for Disease Control and Prevention, U.S. Dept of Health and Human Services.
22. Britto LR, Katz J, Guelmann M, Heft M: Periradicular radiographic assessment in diabetic and control individuals, *Oral Surg Oral Med Oral Pathol Oral Radiol Endod* 96:449–452, 2003.
23. Falk H, Hugoson A, Thorstensson H: Number of teeth, prevalence of caries and periapical lesions in insulin-dependent diabetics, *Scand J Dent Res* 97:198–206, 1989.
24. López-López J, Jané-Salas E, Estrugo-Devesa A, et al.: Periapical and endodontic status of type 2 diabetic patients in Catalonia, Spain: a cross-sectional study, *J Endod* 37:598–601, 2011.
25. Segura-Egea JJ, Martín-González J, Cabanillas-Balsera D, et al.: Association between diabetes and the prevalence of radiolucent periapical lesions in root-filled teeth: systematic review and meta-analysis, *Clin Oral Investig* 20:1133–1141, 2016.
26. Doyle SL, Hodges JS, Pesun IJ, et al.: Factors affecting outcomes for single-tooth implants and endodontic restorations, *J Endod* 33:399–402, 2007.
27. Ng YL, Mann V, Gulabivala K: A prospective study of the factors affecting outcomes of nonsurgical root canal treatment: part 1: periapical health, *Int Endod J* 44:583–609, 2011.
28. Arya S, Duhan J, Tewari S, et al.: Healing of apical periodontitis after nonsurgical treatment in patients with type 2 diabetes, *J Endod* 43:1623–1627, 2017.
29. Fouad AF, Burleson J: The effect of diabetes mellitus on endodontic treatment outcome: data from an electronic patient record, *J Am Dent Assoc* 134:43–51, 2003; quiz 117-8.
30. Fouad AF, Kum KY, Clawson ML, et al.: Molecular characterization of the presence of Eubacterium spp and Streptococcus spp in endodontic infections, *Oral Microbiol Immunol* 18:249–255, 2003.
31. Salvi GE, Beck JD, Offenbacher S: PGE2, IL-1 beta, and TNF-alpha responses in diabetics as modifiers of periodontal disease expression, *Ann Periodontol* 3:40–50, 1998.
32. Lalla E, Lamster IB, Schmidt AM: Enhanced interaction of advanced glycation end products with their cellular receptor RAGE: implications for the pathogenesis of accelerated periodontal disease in diabetes, *Ann Periodontol* 3:13–19, 1998.
33. Mindiola MJ, Mickel AK, Sami C, et al.: Endodontic treatment in an American Indian population: a 10-year retrospective study, *J Endod* 32:828–832, 2006.
34. Wang CH, Chueh LH, Chen SC, et al.: Impact of diabetes mellitus, hypertension, and coronary artery disease on tooth extraction after nonsurgical endodontic treatment, *J Endod* 37:1–5, 2011.
35. Lilly JP, Cox D, Arcuri M, Krell KV: An evaluation of root canal treatment in patients who have received irradiation to the mandible and maxilla, *Oral Surg Oral Med Oral Pathol Oral Radiol Endod* 86:224–226, 1998.
36. Gupta N, Grewal MS, Gairola M, et al.: Dental pulp status of posterior teeth in patients with oral and oropharyngeal cancer treated with radiotherapy: 1-year follow-up, *J Endod* 44:549–554, 2018.
37. Badros A, Weikel D, Salama A, et al.: Osteonecrosis of the jaw in multiple myeloma patients: clinical features and risk factors, *J Clin Oncol* 24:945–952, 2006.
38. Sarathy AP, Bourgeois Jr SL, Goodell GG: Bisphosphonate-associated osteonecrosis of the jaws and endodontic treatment: two case reports, *J Endod* 31:759–763, 2005.
39. Katz H: Endodontic implications of bisphosphonate-associated osteonecrosis of the jaws: a report of three cases, *J Endod* 31:831–834, 2005.
40. Kyrgidis A, Arora A, Antoniades K: Rubber dam clamp trauma, root canal therapy, and osteonecrosis of the jaw, *J Oral Maxillofac Surg* 69(7):1854–1855, 2011.
41. Hsiao A, Glickman G, He J: A retrospective clinical and radiographic study on healing of periradicular lesions in patients taking oral bisphosphonates, *J Endod* 35:1525–1588, 2009.

42. Glick M, Abel SN, Muzyka BC, DeLorenzo M: Dental complications after treating patients with AIDS, *J Am Dent Assoc* 125:296–301, 1994.
43. Quesnell BT, Alves M, Hawkinson Jr RW, et al.: The effect of human immunodeficiency virus on endodontic treatment outcome, *J Endod* 31:633–636, 2005.
44. Goon WW, Jacobsen PL: Prodromal odontalgia and multiple devitalized teeth caused by a herpes zoster infection of the trigeminal nerve: report of case, *J Am Dent Assoc* 116:500–504, 1988.
45. Gregory Jr WB, Brooks LE, Penick EC: Herpes zoster associated with pulpless teeth, *J Endod* 1:32–35, 1975.
46. Sigurdsson A, Jacoway JR: Herpes zoster infection presenting as an acute pulpitis, *Oral Surg Oral Med Oral Pathol Oral Radiol Endod* 80:92–95, 1995.
47. Ferreira DC, Paiva SS, Carmo FL, et al.: Identification of herpesviruses types 1 to 8 and human papillomavirus in acute apical abscesses, *J Endod* 37:10–16, 2011.
48. Li H, Chen V, Chen Y, et al.: Herpesviruses in endodontic pathoses: association of Epstein-Barr virus with irreversible pulpitis and apical periodontitis, *J Endod* 35:23–29, 2009.
49. Sabeti M, Slots J: Herpesviral-bacterial coinfection in periapical pathosis, *J Endod* 30:69–72, 2004.
50. Slots J, Nowzari H, Sabeti M: Cytomegalovirus infection in symptomatic periapical pathosis, *Int Endod J* 37:519–524, 2004.
51. Jakovljevic A, Andric M: Human cytomegalovirus and Epstein-Barr virus in etiopathogenesis of apical periodontitis: a systematic review, *J Endod* 40:6–15, 2014.
52. Taylor LB, Nowak AJ, Giller RH, Casamassimo PS: Sickle cell anemia: a review of the dental concerns and a retrospective study of dental and bony changes, *Spec Care Dentist* 15:38–42, 1995.
53. Andrews CH, England Jr MC, Kemp WB: Sickle cell anemia: an etiological factor in pulpal necrosis, *J Endod* 9:249–252, 1983.
54. Demirbas Kaya A, Aktener BO, Unsal C: Pulpal necrosis with sickle cell anaemia, *Int Endod J* 37:602–606, 2004.
55. Bahrami G, Vaeth M, Kirkevang LL, et al.: *The impact of smoking on marginal bone loss in a 10-year prospective longitudinal study*, Community Dent Oral Epidemiol, 2016.
56. Lopez-Lopez J, Jane-Salas E, Martin-Gonzalez J, et al.: Tobacco smoking and radiographic periapical status: a retrospective case-control study, *J Endod* 38:584–588, 2012.
57. Segura-Egea JJ, Castellanos-Cosano L, Velasco-Ortega E, et al.: Relationship between smoking and endodontic variables in hypertensive patients, *J Endod* 37:764–767, 2011.
58. Krall EA, Abreu Sosa C, Garcia C, et al.: Cigarette smoking increases the risk of root canal treatment, *J Dent Res* 85:313–317, 2006.
59. García B, Penarrocha M, Martí E, et al.: Pain and swelling after periapical surgery related to oral hygiene and smoking, *Oral Surg Oral Med Oral Pathol Oral Radiol Endod* 104:271–276, 2007.
60. Ghattas Ayoub C, Aminoshariae A, Bakkar M, et al.: Comparison of IL-1beta, TNF-alpha, hBD-2, and hBD-3 expression in the dental pulp of smokers versus nonsmokers, *J Endod* 43:2009–2013, 2017.
61. Morsani JM, Aminoshariae A, Han YW, Montagnese TA, Mickel A: Genetic predisposition to persistent apical periodontitis, *J Endod* 37:455–459, 2011.
62. Salles AG, Antunes LAA, Kuchler EC, Antunes LS: Association between apical periodontitis and interleukin gene polymorphisms: a systematic review and meta-analysis, *J Endod* 44:355–362, 2018.
63. Aminoshariae A, Kulild JC: Association of functional gene polymorphism with apical periodontitis, *J Endod* 41:999–1007, 2015.
64. Meskin L, Berg R: Impact of older adults on private dental practices, 1988-1998, *J Am Dent Assoc* 131:1188–1195, 2000.
65. Lloyd PM: Fixed prosthodontics and esthetic considerations for the older adult, *J Prosthet Dent* 72:525–531, 1994.
66. Hiltunen K, Vehkalahti MM, Mantyla P: Is prosthodontic treatment age-dependent in patients 60 years and older in Public Dental Services? *J Oral Rehabil* 42:454–459, 2015.
67. Marcus SE, Drury TF, Brown LJ, Zion GR: Tooth retention and tooth loss in the permanent dentition of adults: United States, 1988-1991, *J Dent Res* 75(Spec No):684–695, 1996.
68. Warren JJ, Cowen HJ, Watkins CM, Hand JS: Dental caries prevalence and dental care utilization among the very old, *J Am Dent Assoc* 131:1571–1579, 2000.
69. Tan HP, Lo EC, Dyson JE, et al.: A randomized trial on root caries prevention in elders, *J Dent Res* 89:1086–1090, 2010.
70. Ramsay SE, Papachristou E, Watt RG, et al.: Socioeconomic disadvantage across the life-course and oral health in older age: findings from a longitudinal study of older British men, *J Public Health (Oxf)*, 2018.
71. Goodis HE, Rossall JC, Kahn AJ: Endodontic status in older U.S. adults. Report of a survey, *J Am Dent Assoc* 132:1525–1530, 2001. quiz 95–96.
72. Berkey DB, Berg RG, Ettinger RL, Mersel A, Mann J: The old-old dental patient: the challenge of clinical decision-making, *J Am Dent Assoc* 127:321–332, 1996.
73. Jones JA: Financing and reimbursement of elders' oral health care: lessons from the present, opportunities for the future, *J Dent Educ* 69:1022–1031, 2005.
74. Sayegh FS, Reed AJ: Calcification in the dental pulp, *Oral Surg Oral Med Oral Pathol* 25:873–882, 1968.
75. Pettiette MT, Zhong S, Moretti AJ, Khan AA: Potential correlation between statins and pulp chamber calcification, *J Endod* 39(9):1119–1123, 2013.
76. Chrepa V, Henry MA, Daniel BJ, Diogenes A: Delivery of apical mesenchymal stem cells into root canals of mature teeth, *J Dent Res* 94:1653–1659, 2015.
77. Ketterl W: Age-induced changes in the teeth and their attachment apparatus, *Int Dent J* 33:262–271, 1983.
78. Murray PE, Stanley HR, Matthews JB, et al.: Age-related odontometric changes of human teeth, *Oral Surg Oral Med Oral Pathol Oral Radiol Endod* 93:474–482, 2002.
79. Bernick S, Nedelman C: Effect of aging on the human pulp, *J Endod* 1:88–94, 1975.
80. Ikawa M, Komatsu H, Ikawa K, et al.: Age-related changes in the human pulpal blood flow measured by laser Doppler flowmetry, *Dent Traumatol* 19:36–40, 2003.
81. Espina AI, Castellanos AV, Fereira JL: Age-related changes in blood capillary endothelium of human dental pulp: an ultrastructural study, *Int Endod J* 36:395–403, 2003.
82. Stanley HR, Ranney RR: Age changes in the human dental pulp. I. The quantity of collagen, *Oral Surg Oral Med Oral Pathol* 15:1396–1404, 1962.
83. Morse DR, Esposito JV, Schoor RS, et al.: A review of aging of dental components and a retrospective radiographic study of aging of the dental pulp and dentin in normal teeth, *Quintessence Int* 22:711–720, 1991.
84. McCabe PS, Dummer PM: Pulp canal obliteration: an endodontic diagnosis and treatment challenge, *Int Endod J* 45:177–197, 2012.
85. Bernick S: Age changes in the blood supply to human teeth, *J Dent Res* 46:544–550, 1967.
86. Krell KV, McMurtrey LG, Walton RE: Vasculature of the dental pulp of atherosclerotic monkeys: light and electron microscopic findings, *J Endod* 20:469–473, 1994.
87. Maheshwari K, Silva RM, Guajardo-Morales L, et al.: Heat Shock 70 protein genes and genetic susceptibility to apical periodontitis, *J Endod* 42:1467–1471, 2016.
88. Van der Velden U: Effect of age on the periodontium, *J Clin Periodontol* 11:281–294, 1984.
89. Braun RJ, Marcus M: Comparing treatment decisions for elderly and young dental patients, *Gerodontics* 1:138–142, 1985.
90. Waldinger R, Weinberg G, Gitman M: Local Anesthetic Toxicity in the Geriatric Population, *Drugs Aging*. doi: 10.1007/s40266-019-00718-0. [Epub ahead of print].
91. Stein TJ, Corcoran JF: Anatomy of the root apex and its histologic changes with age, *Oral Surg Oral Med Oral Pathol* 69:238–242, 1990.

92. Zander HA, Hurzeler B: Continuous cementum apposition, *J Dent Res* 37:1035–1044, 1958.
93. Wu MK, Wesselink PR, Walton RE: Apical terminus location of root canal treatment procedures, *Oral Surg Oral Med Oral Pathol Oral Radiol Endod* 89:99–103, 2000.
94. Real DG, Davidowicz H, Moura-Netto C, et al.: Accuracy of working length determination using 3 electronic apex locators and direct digital radiography, *Oral Surg Oral Med Oral Pathol Oral Radiol Endod* 111:e44–e49, 2011.
95. Law A, Messer H: An evidence-based analysis of the antibacterial effectiveness of intracanal medicaments, *J Endod* 30:689–694, 2004.
96. Haselton DR, Lloyd PM, Johnson WT: A comparison of the effects of two burs on endodontic access in all-ceramic high lucite crowns, *Oral Surg Oral Med Oral Pathol Oral Radiol Endod* 89:486–492, 2000.
97. Campbell JH, Huizinga PJ, Das SK, et al.: Incidence and significance of cardiac arrhythmia in geriatric oral surgery patients, *Oral Surg Oral Med Oral Pathol Oral Radiol Endod* 82:42–46, 1996.
98. Ardekian L, Gaspar R, Peled M, et al.: Does low-dose aspirin therapy complicate oral surgical procedures? *J Am Dent Assoc* 131:331–335, 2000.
99. Blinder D, Manor Y, Martinowitz U, Taicher S: Dental extractions in patients maintained on oral anticoagulant therapy: comparison of INR value with occurrence of postoperative bleeding, *Int J Oral Maxillofac Surg* 30:518–521, 2001.
100. Jeske AH, Suchko GD: Lack of a scientific basis for routine discontinuation of oral anticoagulation therapy before dental treatment, *J Am Dent Assoc* 134:1492–1497, 2003.
101. Aminoshariae A, Kulild JC, Donaldson M: Short-term use of nonsteroidal anti-inflammatory drugs and adverse effects: an updated systematic review, *J Am Dent Assoc* 147:98–110, 2016.
102. Holm-Pedersen P, Loe H: Wound healing in the gingiva of young and old individuals, *Scand J Dent Res* 79:40–53, 1971.
103. Rapp EL, Brown Jr CE, Newton CW: An analysis of success and failure of apicoectomies, *J Endod* 17:508–512, 1991.
104. Stahl SS, Witkin GJ, Cantor M, Brown R: Gingival healing. II. Clinical and histologic repair sequences following gingivectomy, *J Periodontol* 39:109–118, 1968.
105. Lindhe J, Socransky S, Nyman S, et al.: Effect of age on healing following periodontal therapy, *J Clin Periodontol* 12:774–787, 1985.

3

Endodontic Radiology

KENNETH ABRAMOVITCH AND MOHAMED I. FAYAD

CHAPTER OUTLINE

LEARNING OBJECTIVES

After reading this chapter, the student should be able to:

1. Differentiate between stochastic and deterministic dental x-radiation biorisks and recognize which poses the greatest endodontic patient risk.
2. Understand the basic design of a wall mounted x-ray unit and why it is preferred to hand-held x-ray units.
3. Contrast and compare the differences between the indirect PSP plate sensors, the CCD solid state direct sensors and the CMOS solid state direct sensors used for intraoral endodontic radiography.
4. Understand how shifting horizontal angles of the intraoral x-ray beam can be used to localize the relative buccal vs. lingual/palatal locations of superimposed root canals or jaw pathoses that superimpose teeth.
5. Recognize FOV dimension measurements and how these relate to the coverage needed for most endodontic scan indications.
6. Understand how voxel size affects storage space, uploading, downloading and transmission of CBCT volumes.
7. Differentiate between DICOM file data and proprietary file data and how these interplay with various CBCT viewer software programs.
8. Recognize how beam hardening and scatter artifacts degrade CBCT image quality.
9. Review indications where CBCT imaging provides diagnostic and treatment advantages over the standard endodontic image requirements.

Prologue

Dr. William Herbert Rollins was already an established Harvard-trained physician and dentist when x-rays were discovered in 1895. Dr. Rollins, like his contemporaries, was fascinated by the usefulness of x-ray images. However, he was also one of the first to recognize the poorly understood—but genuine—risks associated with x-ray imaging.

Suffering radiation erythema to his hand in January 1898, and having seen the lethal effects of x-rays in his guinea pig experiments, Rollins attempted to caution his contemporaries of its dangers; however, the enthusiasm for the new x-ray technology was blinding radiographers to its morbid hazards. By the late 1920s, it was clear that there were biorisks associated with x-rays as the ranks of prominent radiographers in the New England area had been thinned. Further demonstrating this risk was the fact that at radiology meetings in the 1920s, roast beef was rarely served because the radiographers wore gloves to hide their scars and, by doing so, could not cut the roast beef with the cutlery provided.[1]

It was not until the post-World War II atomic era, that the scientific community again began to heed the warnings of Rollins from a half century earlier.[1]

Introduction

By virtue of its ability to image beyond the scope of the intraoral examination, radiography is an indispensable part of the diagnostic process in dentistry. Within this scope of oral health care, endodontics makes full use of this most useful of diagnostic techniques.

Imaging in the 21st century no longer relies solely on the use of x-rays for diagnostic imaging. Other imaging modalities from which dental care now benefits include optical scan imaging, magnetic resonance imaging, and on the frontier, ultrasound imaging.[2,3] However, with the advent of digital technology, x-ray imaging remains progressive with constant innovation. These innovations keep x-ray imaging an integral and up-to-date part of the diagnostic process for endodontic care.

The use of sensors in dental imaging has changed dramatically, from the earliest days of photographic emulsion on glass plates, to the development of plastics to support radiographic emulsion (i.e., film). In the 1980s, intraoral digital sensors were introduced by Dr. Frances Mouyen.[4] Endodontics eventually embraced this technology because digital sensors dramatically facilitated the efficiency at which endodontic procedures could be completed.[5]

In the 1960s endodontics became the eighth recognized dental specialty of the American Dental Association. At the same time, extraoral panoramic imaging became the exhilaration of dentistry with its ability to image large areas of the jaws in a single exposure. However, extraoral imaging was not as beneficial to the intricacies of endodontic patient care until the introduction of cone beam computed tomography (CBCT). In the 21st century, CBCT is a digital extraoral imaging modality that has greatly facilitated endodontic care. This chapter outlines the utility of radiographic imaging for endodontic patient care with the continued use of intraoral radiography as well as the progressive advances initiated with extraoral CBCT.

Radiation Biology

Contemporary clinicians must still deal with the reality that there are long-term risks that may be realized from exposure to x-radiation. Endodontic care will typically lead to multiple patient x-ray exposures. The radiation dosage to oral and other tissues has been calculated to be very low and extrapolated to cause minimal (but some) risk.[6,7] Table 3.1 illustrates the effective doses of various dental imaging procedures. This table provides the reader with a measure of the biorisk from intraoral exposures in relation to other dental imaging procedures. A more detailed radiation dosimetry review is available elsewhere.[8,9]

In the early days of x-ray imaging, deterministic biorisks, such as skin burns, scarring, and cataracts, were prominent, and the stochastic risks of malignancy (skin cancers and leukemias, etc.) were also very high. The reality of deterministic risks is negligible today, but the morbidity risk from x-ray–induced malignancies (i.e., stochastic risks) remains.[10,11] Practitioners must also be cognizant of the fact that the probability of getting an x-ray–induced malignant disease increases with increased numbers of exposures. With each exposure from each new endodontic procedure, small but cumulative increases in the probability of suffering an x-ray–induced malignancy exist. However, the endodontist must also remember that the overall patient x-ray biorisk is not merely from endodontic x-ray procedures. Risk will increase and be added to from additional endodontic procedures, such as other dental or medical imaging needs (e.g., dental implants, cardiovascular imaging, brain scanning, gastrointestinal [GI] series, orthopedic imaging, etc.). Therefore the risks remain real, and the need for vigilance to keep radiation exposures as low as reasonably achievable (i.e., ALARA) remains forever present.[12] The value of imaging for any endodontic diagnosis or treatment indication should be determined on an individual basis to assure that the benefit-to-risk assessment supports the use of imaging.[13]

In pediatric patients, the biorisks from the x-radiation are greater than the adult risks for a given radiation dose. This increased risk is due to the pediatric patient's inherently greater radiosensitivity and because children have more remaining years of life during which a radiation-induced malignant neoplasm could develop.[14] Hence, as with any imaging modality, the decision to use any diagnostic x-radiation is an objective-laden thought process where the benefits of the information obtained must outweigh the risks of the x-radiation.

TABLE 3.1 Differential Diagnosis for the Most Common Injuries to the Periodontium

Type of Radiographic Exam	Medain Effective Dose (µSv)	Days of Equivalent Background Radiation
Rectangular Collimation BW PSPP	5	0.6
FMX PSP	40	4
FMX CCD	20	2.5
Round Collimation FMX D-speed	400	48
FMX PSP -	200	24
FMX CCD -	100	12
Panoramic	20	–2.5
Cephalometric	5	0.6
CBCT - large FOV (craniofacial)	120	15
CBCT - medium FOV (full arch; dentoalveolar)	100	12
CBCT -small FOV (~3-5 teeth; <6.0cm. dia.)	50	6

Equipment for 2D Image Capture

Intraoral X-ray Units

Standard Wall-Mounted Units

Dental x-ray units have changed very little over the years since David Coolidge designed the first enclosed x-ray tube and tube head, the Victor CDX, in 1919.[15]

Exposure times have decreased to less than 20% of the exposures from as little as three decades ago. Because of this, the need for large x-ray tube heads housing the larger generators needed to produce kV potentials greater that 70 kV has decreased. The need for high milliamperage (i.e., mA settings greater that 10 mA) is also no longer indicated with the shorter exposure times needed for digital receptors. Most contemporary x-ray tube heads are smaller with kV potentials between 60 and 70 kV and mA in the 6- to 8-mA range. With some exposure times now less than 0.10 seconds, most units have digital microprocessor timers that can reproducibly generate direct current (DC) exposures in the 0.05- to 0.10-second range. These smaller x-ray units produce adequate x-radiation to expose contemporary digital receptors, including American National Standards Institute (ANSI) F speed film, and reduce patient radiation dose with the shorter exposure times

Another option available in dental x-ray units is the recessed x-ray tube. Instead of the x-ray tube placed adjacent to the window within the tube head and the position indicating device (PID), contemporary x-ray tube heads have the x-ray tube recessed further away from the window (Fig. 3.1). The recessed tube produces a longer focal distance (x-ray source-to-object distance), which projects a sharper image outline. With an increased focal distance, the inverse square law dictates that the exposure must be increased. However, even though the exposure needs to be greater to obtain a diagnostic image density, the patient dose is actually decreased, which is an added benefit of the recessed x-ray tube. This benefit is because the increased distance will prevent many of the low-energy x-ray photons in the beam from reaching the patient. Thus the recessed x-ray tube acts as a distance filter, which will decrease the patient dose.

Handheld Units

In the past decade, handheld x-ray units for dental imaging have become very popular in clinical practice.[16,17]

Handheld units were originally designed for the benefit of mobility to provide dental imaging in remote locations where standard equipment is not available or for nonambulatory patients in need of dental services who cannot access standard dental facilities. Because these units are made for portability, they have become more popular in regular office designs and are used as a single unit for multiple standard operatories. Image quality is generally acceptable; however, due to the portability, the maximum kV and mA are less than those possible with standard units. The biggest issue with handheld units is the radiation dose to the operator if used without proper training. However, units have been shown to have adequate shielding to protect the operator if used properly with a backscatter shield.[18-20]

Proper usage includes assuring that backscatter shields are attached to the units so that the operators can keep their bodies within the protective range of the shield (Fig. 3.2).

Because of their convenience and popularity, several handheld units are now commercially available. There is concern that some newer units do not have the same degree of protective operator shielding.[21] This aspect is a critical feature when considering a handheld unit of choice.

Despite their convenience for remote venues, the units lack the power of the wall-mounted units. However, smaller power packs are necessary to keep the unit at an appropriate lighter weight for the handheld use of the typical office staff member. Hence, remote charging and reinserting battery packs become an additional maintenance task. Care must also be taken when lifting and handling the nonergonomic units to avoid shock damage.

Furthermore, there is concern that the features of portability do present challenges for optimal image quality and safety. Consequently, unless clinical facilities demonstrate distinct advantages of handheld units over wall-mounted units where the latter installations are possible, the routine practice of using handheld units over wall-mounted units is not always a recommended guideline.[22]

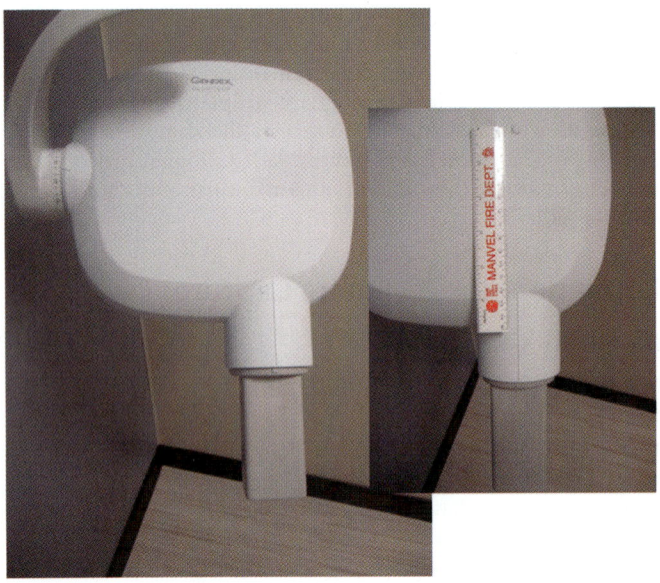

• **Fig. 3.1** X-ray tube head with position dot indicating the position of the focal spot that is inside the x-ray tube head *(red arrow)*. The inset image demonstrates the increased length of the focal distance. This increased length offers sharper image outlines and reduced patient dose.

Intraoral Image Receptors

As described in this chapter's introduction, the types of sensors used in dental imaging have changed dramatically. Digital sensors are the preferred type of sensor for endodontic management. Although it has been shown that the digital image quality has no major advantages over film images,[23-28] digital sensors are by far more practical than film. Digital sensors are advantageous in that there is reduced patient radiation exposure, with increased speed of image acquisition, storage, retrieval, and transmission. An additional advantage of digital sensors over film is that digital sensors forego the arduous chemical film processing, which takes longer and also requires the use of a darkroom. Digital sensors have dramatically facilitated the efficiency at which endodontic procedures can be completed.

Types of Digital Image Receptors

Digital image formats include indirect photostimulable phosphor (PSP) plates and the direct solid-state sensors that may either be

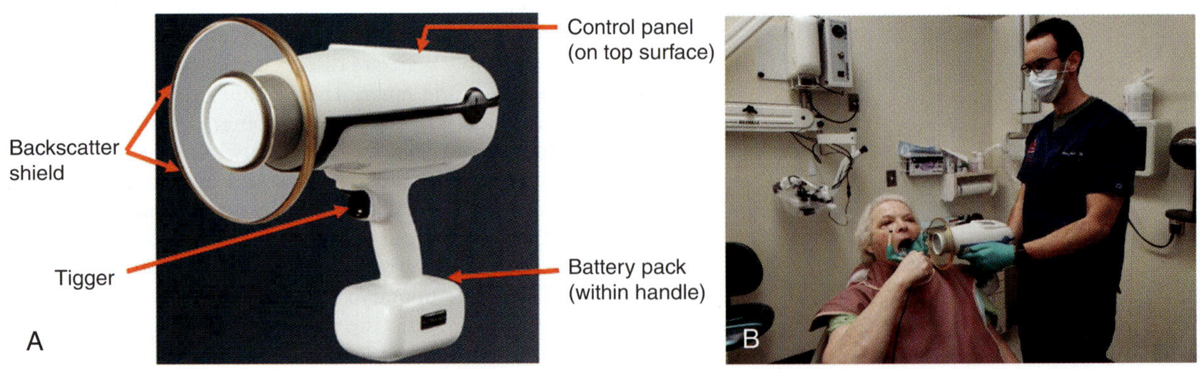

• **Fig. 3.2** **A**, KaVo™ NOMAD Pro 2™ handheld x-ray unit. **B**, Proper operator position for handheld x-ray unit which maximizes operator protection from backscatter radiation. All operator body parts are within the shields protective range. (A, Courtesy KaVo, Charlotte, NC. USA; www.kavo.com)

the charge-coupled device (CCD) sensor or the complementary metal-oxide semiconductor (CMOS) active pixel sensor. The latter is also abbreviated as CMOS-APS.

Photostimulable Phosphor Plates

The PSPs are considered indirect because, after exposure, the sensor must be removed from the patient's mouth and transferred to a laser scanner so that the stored latent electronic charges of the pixels on the sensor's surface can be scanned with a laser light to generate an electrical signal. The digital process includes assigning a numerical value to the electrical signal strength of each of the pixels. These numerical values are then assigned a gray-scale value to be used by the imaging software for display on a monitor.

Solid-State (Direct) Sensors

The solid-state direct sensors transmit the electronic signal straight from the sensor directly to a computer so the image can be displayed in as little as 3 to 5 seconds or less, depending on the computer processing speed and the server's size and efficiency.

At this time, the CMOS is the predominantly used direct sensor. They are generally less expensive to manufacture and are faster in transmitting the electronic signal for processing and require a simple USB connection to a computer. Despite the improved CCD sensitivity to x-radiation, their slightly greater manufacturing costs and their more cumbersome digital processing sequences have now decreased their commercial availability.

Despite the advantages and increased preference for direct digital sensors, there remain some disadvantages, which delay an industry-wide total conversion to these sensors. Direct digital sensors are thicker (5 to 8 mm)[29] and less comfortable than the thinner and more flexible traditional film or PSPs. Because of this discomfort, not all patients tolerate imaging procedures with direct sensors. Although the direct digital sensors have the approximate height and width of conventional film sensors, the actual active sensor area is smaller, ranging among different manufacturers from 20% to 25% reduction of the image surface area compared with conventional film or PSPs.[29,30]

This problem creates issues with cut-off apices from the compromised vertical dimension and missing apices when the horizontal dimension is compromised, and horizontal angulation is needed to image the multiple root apices of multirooted teeth.

Dental Film

For those clinicians still using dental film, "F"-speed film is the film recommended for endodontic use. However, the slower "D"-speed film is still available, the increased radiation exposure and slightly higher contrast are not of any added benefit for endodontic imaging. Although the active surface areas are larger on film (as previously discussed), this technology is being replaced by direct sensor technology. For clinicians still using dental film, a more detailed discussion of their use and chemical film processing is discussed in other reference sources.[31-33]

Techniques for Intraoral Image Capture

Periapical Imaging

The main image capture techniques for periapical imaging are the paralleling technique and the bisecting angle technique. These techniques are amply described in main radiology textbooks.[33-35] For the paralleling technique, the receptor is ideally positioned parallel to both the long axis and the mesiodistal plane of the tooth being evaluated. The beam is then directed perpendicular to the plane of the receptor. It is necessary to stabilize the receptor in this planned position. When it is not possible to place the receptor parallel to the tooth, the bisecting angle technique may then be applied. With this technique, the receptor is stabilized against the lingual side of crown and the adjacent palatal/lingual mucosa. Because the receptor no longer parallels the long axis of the tooth, it is necessary to project the vertical angle of the x-ray beam perpendicular to the plane that bisects the angle formed by the intersecting planes of the long axis of the tooth and the vertical axis of the receptor. Frequently, clinicians choose to align all these planes freehand, with the use of simple receptor bite blocks or with other simple holding instruments (modified hemostats, Snap-a Ray devices, etc.), but without the aid of beam alignment devices (Fig. 3.3, *A* and *B*). However, for more predictable imaging, receptor stabilizing–beam alignment devices are available for this purpose. These instruments are preferred for best image quality with minimal projection artifact, such as cone cutting, foreshortening, elongation, and so on (Fig. 3.3, *C*).

When working length images or master cone images are needed, the rubber dam clamp does make it more cumbersome to position the receptor. Again, the use of the receptor stabilizing–beam alignment devices best facilitate obtaining the most favorable images. Specially adapted instruments are made with appropriate bite block modifications to accommodate the rubber clamp and endodontic files positioned in the canals (Fig. 3.3, *D*).

Due to the variability of human nature, it is not always possible to get patient cooperation to tolerate the placement of the instruments necessary for beam alignment. This difficulty is especially true for the "working" radiographs taken during an endodontic treatment with the rubber dam in place. Sometimes, it may require cooperation by the patient if they hold the sensor in position. In these scenarios, trying the *modified paralleling* technique is recommended.[36] Essentially, the sensor is not parallel to the tooth, but the central beam is oriented at right angles to the receptor surface. In endodontic working radiographs, a further modification is made by varying the horizontal beam angle.

Tube Shift

Modification of the horizontal angle of the x-ray beam becomes a necessary modification to separate structures that superimpose one another on the 2D image. Principles of relative movement of structures and sensor orientation are applied to the differentiation of object position, as demonstrated in Figs. 3.4 and 3.5.[37-39]

These principles of tube shift have been adapted to object localization of structures in the nonvisible buccolingual dimension of 2D radiography. One of the most useful techniques in endodontics is the SLOB Rule.[38] SLOB is an acronym—**S**ame **L**ingual **O**pposite **B**uccal, as first described by Richards.[38]

When two objects and the sensor are in a fixed position buccal and lingual from each other, and the radiation source is moved in a horizontal or vertical direction, the images of the two objects move apart in opposite directions (Fig. 3.6).

One way to visualize this effect is to close one eye and hold two fingers directly in front of the open eye so that one finger is superimposed on the other. By moving the head one way and then the other, the position of the fingers relative to each other shifts. The same effect is produced with two superimposed roots (the fingers) and the way in which they move relative to the radiation

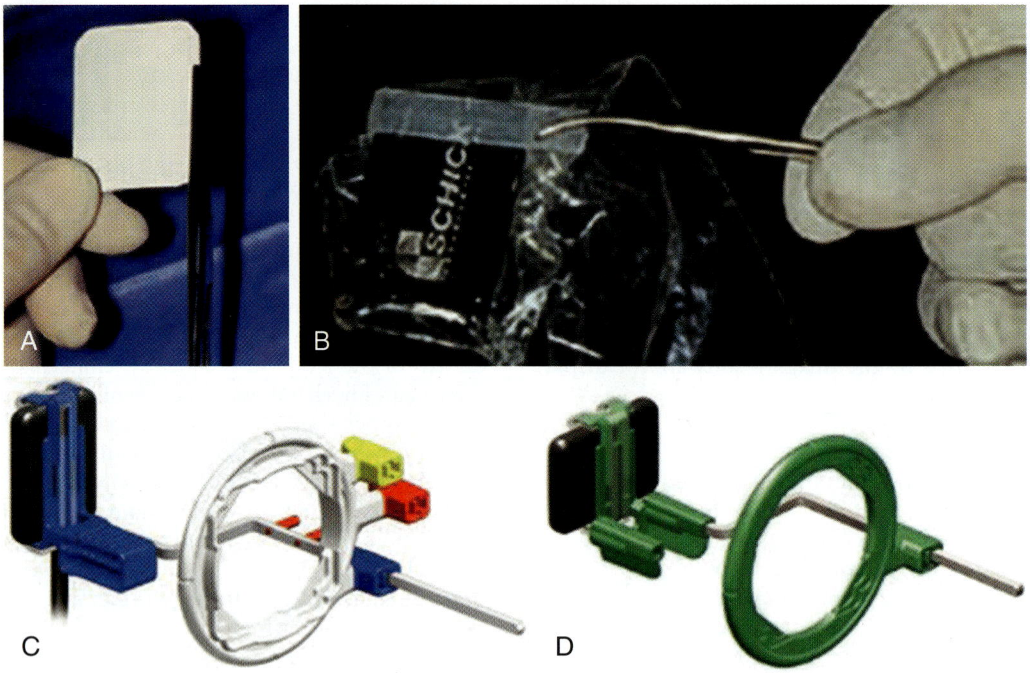

• **Fig. 3.3** Receptor Stabilizing Devices for Intraoral Imaging. **A**, A hemostat is used for grasping film or a PSP plate and does help orient the x-ray beam. **B**, A hemostat holds a plastic holder for a solid-state digital sensor. **C**, The Rinn XCP-DS ORA receptor stabilizing-beam alignment device is used for standard periapical projections. **D,** The XCP-DS FIT Universal Sensor Holder and beam alignment device for working endodontic radiographs. This sensor holder stretches to fit all types of receptors including solid state sensors. (**C**, Courtesy Dentsply Sirona, York, PA; **D**, Courtesy Dentsply Sirona, York, PA)

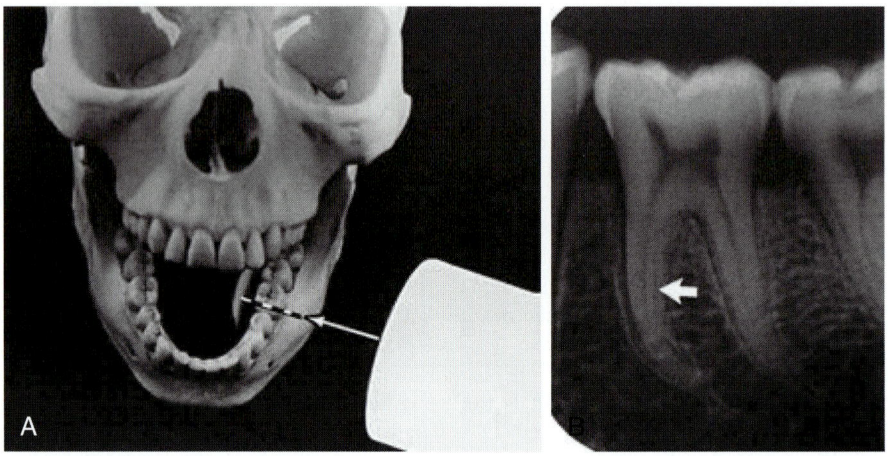

• **Fig. 3.4** **A**, The receptor is positioned parallel to the plane of the arch. The central ray *(arrow)* of the x-ray beam is directed toward the receptor at right angles. This is the basic beam–receptor relationship used for horizontal or vertical angulations. **B**, There is a clear outline of the first molar but limited information about superimposed structures (canals that lie in the buccolingual plane). The *arrow* points to a periodontal ligament space adjacent to a superimposed root bulge, not to a second canal. (From Walton RE: Endodontic radiographic techniques, *Dent Radiogr Photogr* 46(3):51–59, 1973.)

source (the eye) and the central beam (the line of sight). When the cone-shift technique is used, it is critical to know in which direction the shift was made and to determine what is buccal and what is lingual. Otherwise, serious errors may occur. Fig. 3.7 demonstrates how the horizontal angle is shifted to accomplish these localization techniques.

This horizontal tube-shifting technique can be used to separate superimposed root canals and superimposed roots or to separate roots of teeth from adjacent superimposing anatomy, such as the mental foramen in the mandible or the zygomatic process of the maxilla in the maxillary arch. Examples of this tube shift are demonstrated in Fig. 3.11, *A–F*, of the next section.

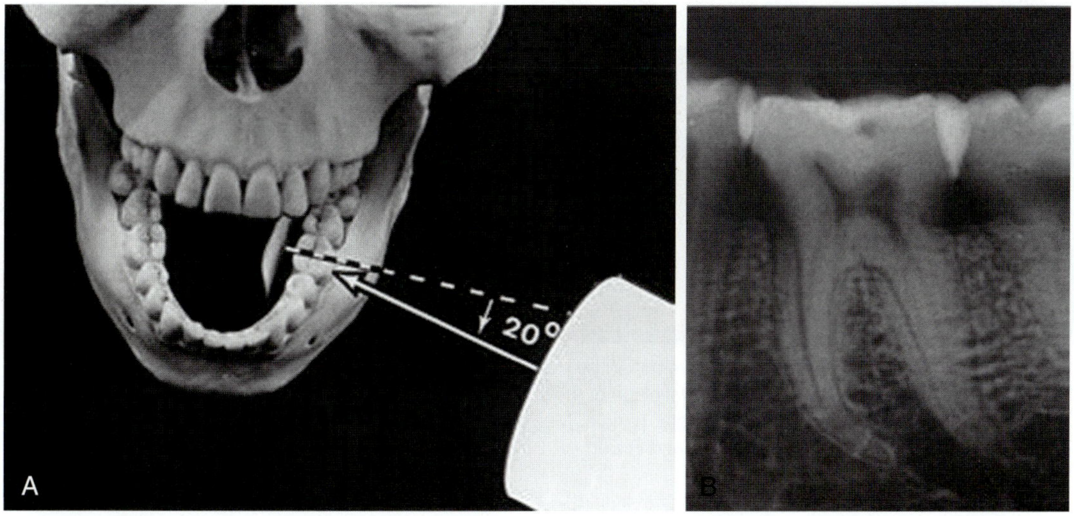

• **Fig. 3.5** **A,** The horizontal angulation of the cone is 20-degrees mesial from the parallel, right-angle position (mesial projection). **B,** The resultant radiograph demonstrates the morphologic features of the root or canal in the third dimension. For example, two canals are now visible in the distal root of the first molar. (From Walton RE: Endodontic radiographic techniques, *Dent Radiogr Photogr* 46(3):51–59, 1973.)

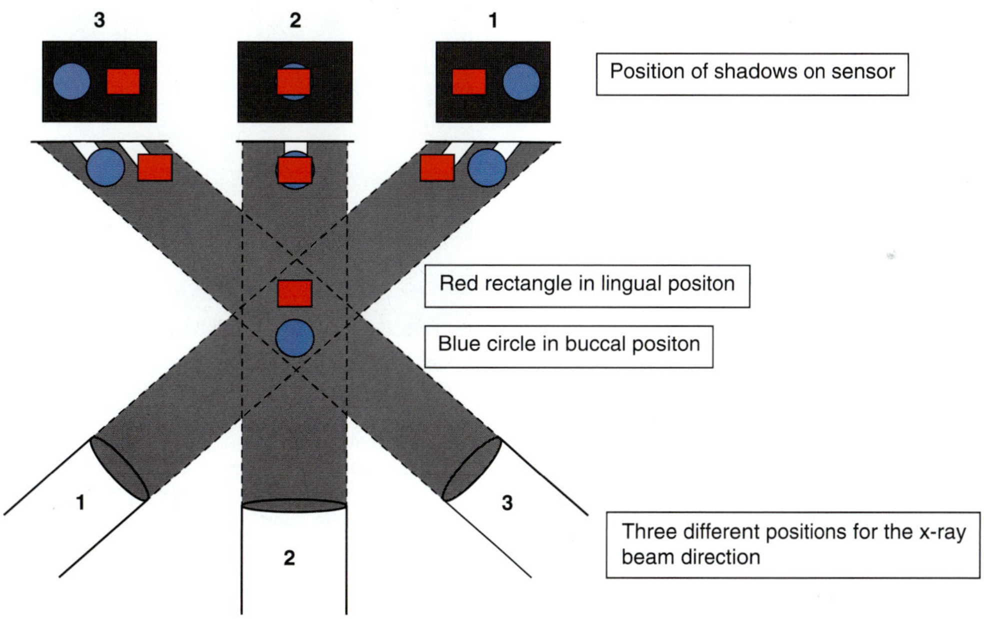

• **Fig. 3.6** This schematic demonstrates the projected images of the blue circle (buccal) that is closest to the x-ray source and the red rectangle that is further from the x-ray source and closest to the receptor (lingual). In Position 2 of the x-ray beam, the objects superimpose on the Sensor 2 projected image. When the object superimposes on this single 2D image, it is not possible to tell which of the objects is positioned in the buccal or lingual position. When the beam is projected from Position 1 (i.e., left of Position 2), the objects are separated on the projected Sensor 1 image. The resulting image on Sensor 1 shows the red rectangle lingual object moved in the same left direction as the beam and the blue circle buccal object moved in the opposite direction of the beam to the right; hence, the acronym SLOB—**S**ame **L**ingual **O**pposite **B**uccal. When the beam is projected from Position 3 (i.e., right of Position 2), the objects are separated on the projected Sensor 3 image. The resulting image on Sensor 3 shows the red rectangle lingual object moved in the same right direction as the beam and the blue circle buccal object moved in the opposite direction of the beam to the left, hence the SLOB rule applies again. (Modified from: Abramovitch K. Imagery Chapter 5. In *Impacted teeth*, Alling III CC, Helfrick JF and Alling RD. WB Saunders, Philadelphia, 1993, pp. 110–116.[39])

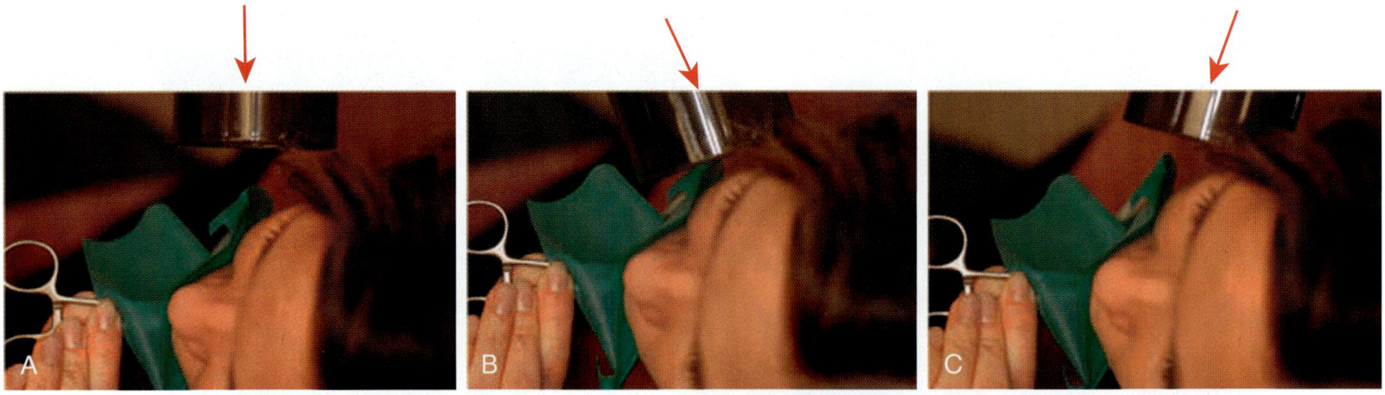

• **Fig. 3.7** Horizontal angulation is determined by looking down from the top of the patient's head. **A,** The position is set by aligning the horizontal plane of the position indicating device (PID) indicated by the arrow, parallel to the long axis of the hemostat handle. Mesial **(B)** and distal **(C)** horizontal angulations are then varied accordingly. (From Walton RE and Fouad AF, 2014.)

Study Questions

1. The major biorisk from x-rays used for endodontic imaging is:
   a. Deterministic
   b. Traumatic
   c. Cyclic
   d. Stochastic
2. A disadvantage of digital solid-state sensors for periapical imaging is the:
   a. Smaller area for image capture
   b. Projection of double images
   c. Greater propensity for dimensional distortion
   d. Inferior diagnostic sensitivity to dental film
3. In comparison with handheld x-ray units, wall-mounted x-ray units:
   a. Are more durable
   b. Have greater portability
   c. Produce less image distortion
   d. Process digital images more quickly
4. Handheld x-ray units:
   a. Improve image resolution
   b. Increase biorisk to the radiographer
   c. Require shorter exposure times
   d. Are used only with digital sensors
5. Tube shifting is a
   a. CBCT technique that improves image resolution
   b. A method of directing the rotational path in a CBCT scanner
   c. Beam alignment method that minimizes root canal length distortion
   d. Technique used to localize the buccal and lingual position of objects

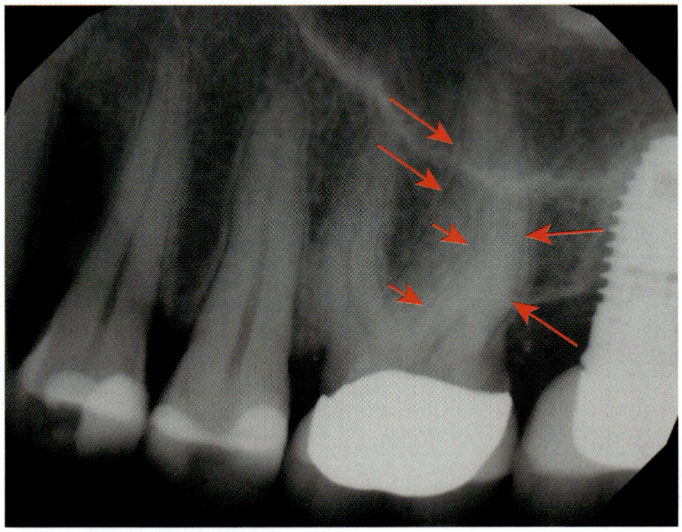

• **Fig. 3.8** This standard periapical projection shows the root surface outlines with the periodontal ligament space and the adjacent lamina dura around the roots of the premolars and first molar. Even with the superimposition of the palatal and distobuccal roots, the root surface outlines *(short, thick arrows)* and the periodontal ligament space *(longer, thick arrows) and* adjacent lamina dura *(long, thin arrows)* still project, and the clinician must visualize these structures to evaluate periapical health.

Endodontic Imaging Needs

There are numerous indications in endodontic patient management where imaging plays a vital role in decision making and treatment rendering. These indications range from diagnosing a treatment indication, to rendering the treatment, and then to follow-up of the treatment. These situations are outlined later in this section.

Disease Diagnosis

Before diagnosing any disease process, the clinician must be able to distinguish the normal anatomic range of structures in the dentoalveolar complex and its supporting structures. This range would include the root and pulp anatomy of any affected dentition and their relationship to adjacent structures, whether maxillary molar roots adjacent the zygomatic process and maxillary sinus in the maxilla or the apices of mandibular premolars adjacent the mental foramen. Pulp chambers are identified within the dental crown, and the root canals will extend from the pulp chamber to its specific root apex. The periodontal ligament (PDL) space is differentiated from the pulp chamber as it follows the outline of roots and has a consistent narrow width (<1.0 mm) around the roots. It also will have a peripheral thin radiopaque lamina dura adjacent to it (Fig. 3.8).

Identifying Pathosis

The recognition of disease requires an understanding of the pulpal, periodontal, or periapical changes that may arise in

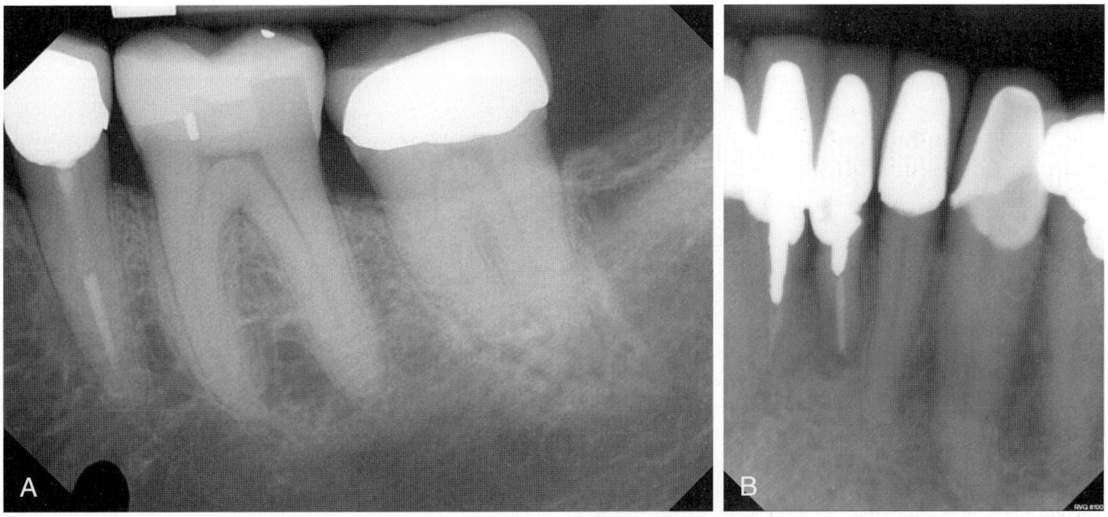

• **Fig. 3.9** **A,** Physiologic apical periodontal ligament (PDL) outlines are present on the mesial and distal roots of tooth #19. Note the position of the retentive pin adjacent the mesial pulp horn which was the cause of the patient's odontalgia. **B,** Note the altered apical PDL and external resorption on #24 that is occurring in the absence of symptoms. These changes and the periodontal bone loss compromise this tooth's prognosis.

the presence of disease and how these changes can affect the identification of the normal anatomic outlines. Similarly, an understanding of systemic or local hard tissue pathologic processes that affect the jaws is also necessary to recognize these processes as they present. The more astute clinicians recognize these changes in their earliest stages of tissue alteration. It is also important to remember that pathologic processes in their earliest stages are often symptomatic before the development of prominent radiographic signs or clinical signs or symptoms (Fig. 3.9).

The presence and nature of lesions that may arise on routine or follow-up radiographs must be evaluated on any images taken during the course of treatment or follow-up. These lesions may be periapical, periodontal, or nonendodontic. It is important to repeat that such lesions frequently present with no overt signs or symptoms and may be detectable only radiographically (Fig. 3.10). A more detailed discussion of pathologic changes is given in Chapters 1 and 4.

Moving Superimposed Structures

Radiopaque anatomic structures often overlay and obscure roots and apices. Using special cone angulations, these radiopaque structures can be "moved" to give a clear image of the apex. The zygomatic process of the maxilla is one such structure[40] (Fig. 3.11, *A* and *B*). The mental foramen on the buccal surface of the mandibular basal bone can be positioned on radiographs to superimpose in the vicinity of the mandibular second premolar apex. In these instances, it can simulate apical periodontitis. Again, a horizontal shift of the beam angulation can separate the two structures for a better evaluation of the premolar apices (Fig. 3.11, *C* and *D*).

Locating Roots and Canals

Canal location is obviously essential to success. Standard and horizontal beam-shifting techniques allow the practitioner to determine the position of canals either not located on a standard periapical image or possibly even missed during access (Fig. 3.11, *E* and *F*).

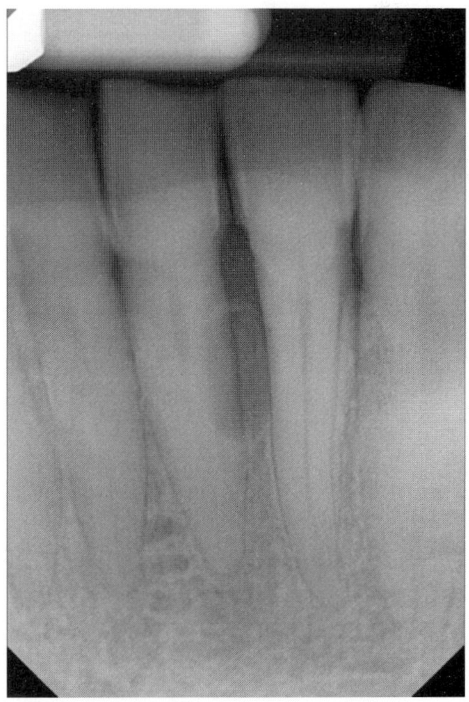

• **Fig. 3.10** This 60-year-old female patient presented with asymptomatic gingival swelling. There were no signs of pulpal disease on any of her radiographs. A lateral periodontal cyst is present in the #23/#24 interradicular bone.

Evaluating Treatment Progress

During endodontic treatment, "working" radiographs are needed usually with a dental rubber dam and clamp in place. These images are needed at various stages during the treatment phase. These include the (1) initial assessment of working length; (2) determining the working length; (3) fitting the master cone; and (4) evaluating the obturation made while the dental dam is in place

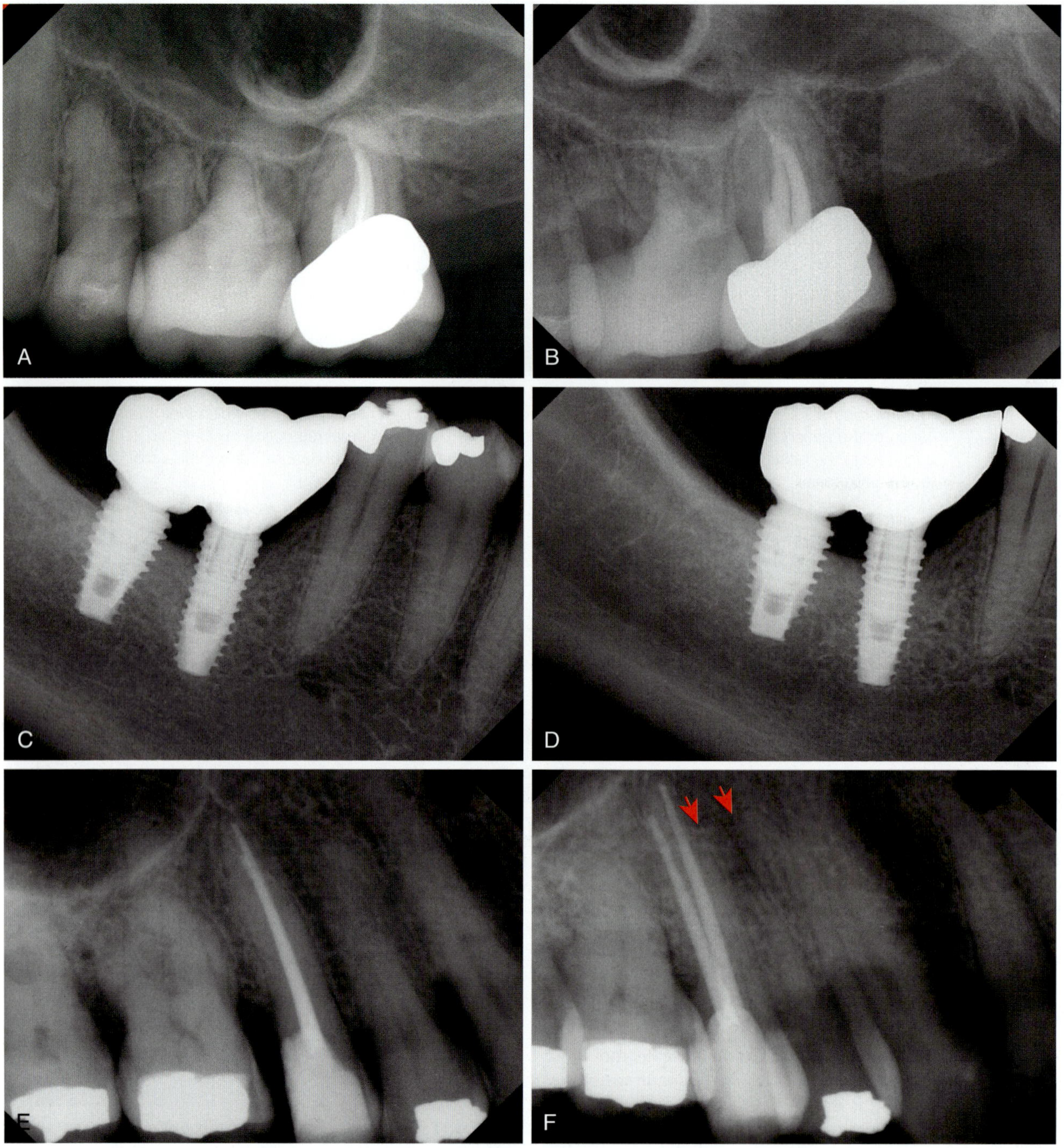

• **Fig. 3.11** A, The #14 palatal root apex is difficult to evaluate. **B**, By changing the horizontal angle by 20 degrees to the distal, the buccally positioned zygomatic process moves mesial (opposite the direction of the tube shift), and the palatal root can be evaluated better when isolated from the zygomatic process. **C**, Radiolucent area over the apex could be mistaken for pathosis. **D**, Pulp testing (vital response) and a more distal horizontal and increased vertical angulation show the radiolucency to be the buccal positioned mental foramen. With this distal angulation, the #29–#30 interproximal contact opens and the mental foramen moved more mesial and inferior to the #29 apex. **E** and **F**, The first premolar root outlines are not clear. By shifting the horizontal angle by 20 degrees to the distal, the outlines of the palatal and buccal roots are identified. The buccal root has moved mesially (opposite the direction of the tube shift), and the palatal root has moved distally (the same direction as the tube shift). Arrows point to the palatal and buccal apices. (Courtesy Dr. Jason Fowler, Loma Linda, CA.)

(intermediary fill radiograph), which creates problems in film placement and cone positioning. These radiographs are exposed during the treatment phase and the special tube-shifting technique applications discussed earlier in this chapter may then be necessary to accomplish diagnostic images.

Initial Assessment of Working Lengths

The distance from a reference point to the radiographic apex is determined precisely. This determination establishes the distance from the apex at which the canal is to be prepared and obturated[41] (Fig. 3.12).

Determining Working Length

In general, establishment of working length should require only a single exposure. If a root contains or may contain two superimposed canals, either a mesial or distal angle projection is absolutely necessary; the straight facial view is not particularly helpful.[42] Additional working length radiographs may be required later for confirmation of working lengths to detect the presence or lengths of newly discovered canals or for reexposure if an apex has been cut off in the first radiograph. The length from the apex, density, taper, and outline of the root canal's shape are constantly evaluated with these images.

Master Cone

The same principles used with working length films apply. With proper technique, only one radiograph is necessary to evaluate the length of the master gutta-percha cone. The master cones should extend to, or very close to, the corrected working length (Fig. 3.13, *A*) Procedures for the fitting of master cones are discussed in Chapter 15.

Evaluating the Obturation (Intermediary Fill and Final Radiographs)

After canal obturation, postoperative radiographs provide considerable information on the general quality of obturation in terms of the overall density and presence of voids and quality of fill to the level of the apical foramen, which are determined from these radiographs (Fig. 3.13, *B*).

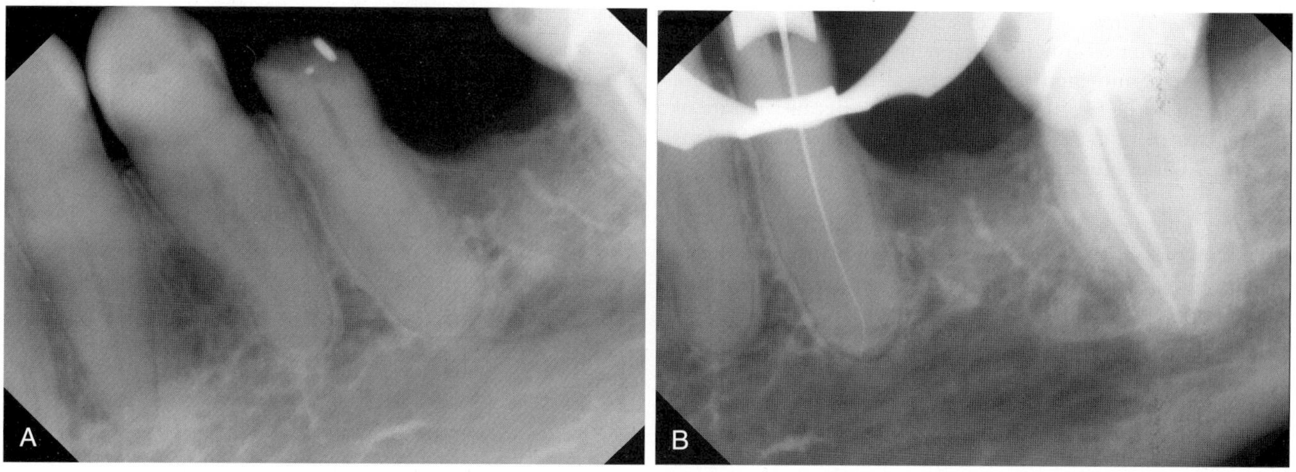

• **Fig. 3.12 A,** An initial assessment of working length. Note the tip of the endodontic file and its distance relationship with the radiographic apex. **B** and **C**, The preliminary radiograph and then the working length assessment with the tip of the endodontic file at the radiographic apex. This particular tooth and the adjacent premolar have hypercementosis on the root. There is no contraindication to nonsurgical root canal therapy (NSRCT) in roots with this condition.

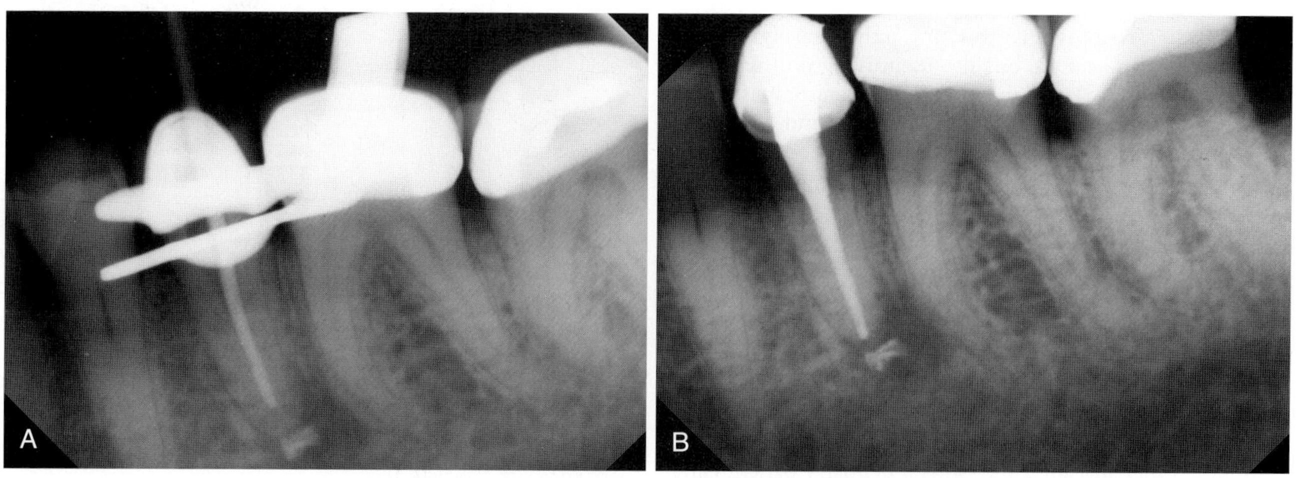

• **Fig. 3.13** Fitting of the master cone **(A)** and final obturation **(B)** evaluations

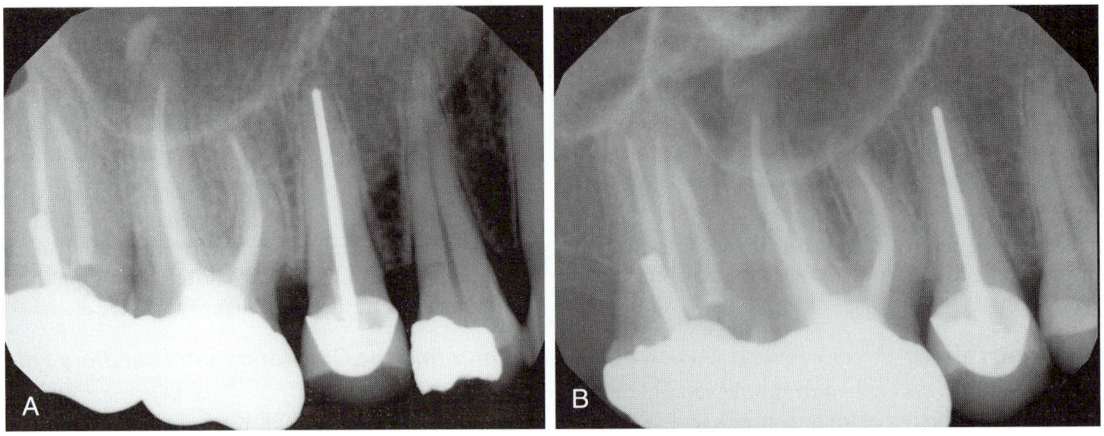

• **Fig. 3.14** **A**, On the 2-year posttreatment follow-up, healing is noted at the three apices of the first molar. **B,** The 6-year follow-up demonstrates a periapical lesion on the mesial buccal (MB) root. The patient did report mild, transient symptoms. The premolar and second molar continue to show no signs of recurrent disease in this 6-year time interval.

Follow-up of Treatment Outcomes

Ultimate success of treatment is verified at specified intervals of months or years after treatment. Generally, the first follow-up is done at 6 months, and then annually for 2 to 4 years until the final disposition of the treatment is determined. Because failure of endodontic treatment can occur before the development of signs or symptoms, follow-up radiographs are essential to evaluate the periapical status[43] (Fig. 3.14).

The same exposure and projection principles used for diagnostic and treatment-evaluation radiographs remain applicable to any of the follow-up or recall radiographs. Exposure factors typically follow the x-ray unit and sensor manufacturer's recommendations. However, these factors can always be tweaked, pending the preference of the clinician, so that the image quality is acceptable and that the exposure parameters do not exceed the recommended dose limits set by the state or any other regulatory agencies.

Pretreatment lesions should be healing or should have healed. In a successfully treated case, reestablishment of the PDL, lamina dura, and trabecular bone is expected to reestablish apical health (Fig. 3.14, *A*). However, if the treatment is deemed to be questionable (missed canals, inadequate fill, root fracture, etc.) or if there is disease recurrence (Fig. 3.14, *B*), additional angled radiographs may become necessary.

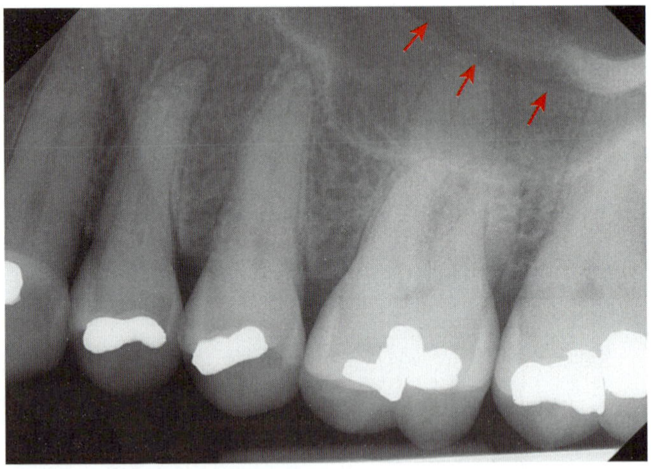

• **Fig. 3.15** The curvilinear radiolucent structure adjacent the molar roots and within the superimposing the sinus lumen *(red arrows)*, is the anomalous presence of the posterior superior alveolar canal that courses its way anteriorly in the lateral wall of the maxillary sinus. The presence of this structure on periapical radiographs is dependent on numerous factors in the patient's anatomy and the projection angle of the x-ray beam. If seen unilaterally, it should not be misinterpreted as pathologic.

Determining Root and Pulpal Anatomy

Determining the anatomy involves not only identifying and counting the roots and canals, but also identifying unusual adjacent anatomy (Fig. 3.15) or anomalous tooth anatomy, such as dens invaginatus and a C-shaped configuration,[44] and determining curvatures, canal relationships, and canal location.[45,46]

Cone Beam Computed Tomography

Equipment and Principles for 3D Image Capture

CBCT was introduced two decades ago as a new dental technology for the 21st century[47,48] that has certainly had a dramatic and highly positive effect on endodontic care. The dental marketplace is very competitive, with new units and complementary software programs continuously being developed for CBCT applications in endodontic, other specialty, and general dentistry patient care. Except for the size of the receptor opposite the x-ray tube, CBCT units look similar to panoramic x-ray machines (Fig. 3.16).

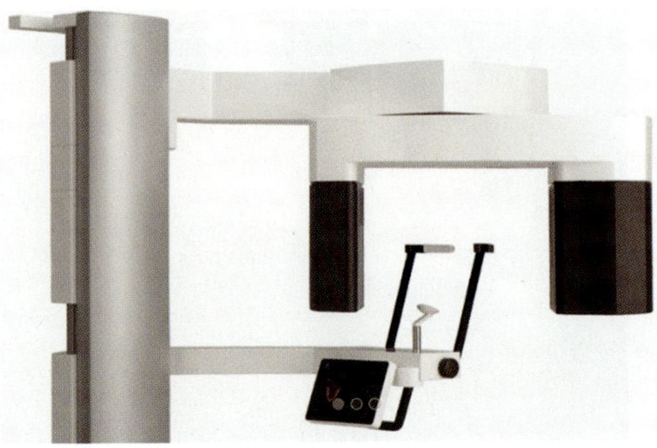

• **Fig. 3.16** An example of a cone beam computed tomography (CBCT) unit with small field of views (FOVs) more typically used for endodontic evaluations. Note the flat panel detector *(red arrow)* on the left side of the gantry opposite the x-ray tube head. Veraview X800. (Courtesy J. Morita USA, Inc., Irvine, CA.)

Field of View

The size of the scanned object volume is called the field of view (FOV). The FOV for CBCT units with a flat panel detector is a cylindrical shape. The CBCT scanning controls are programmed to scan FOVs within the limits of the size of the flat panel as determined by the manufacturer. The dimensions of a flat panel detector's FOV are expressed by the height of the cylinder (H) and the diameter of the base (D) (Fig. 3.17, *A*).

The FOV is a very flexible option in contemporary scanners. The range of commercially available FOVs for flat panel detectors can be

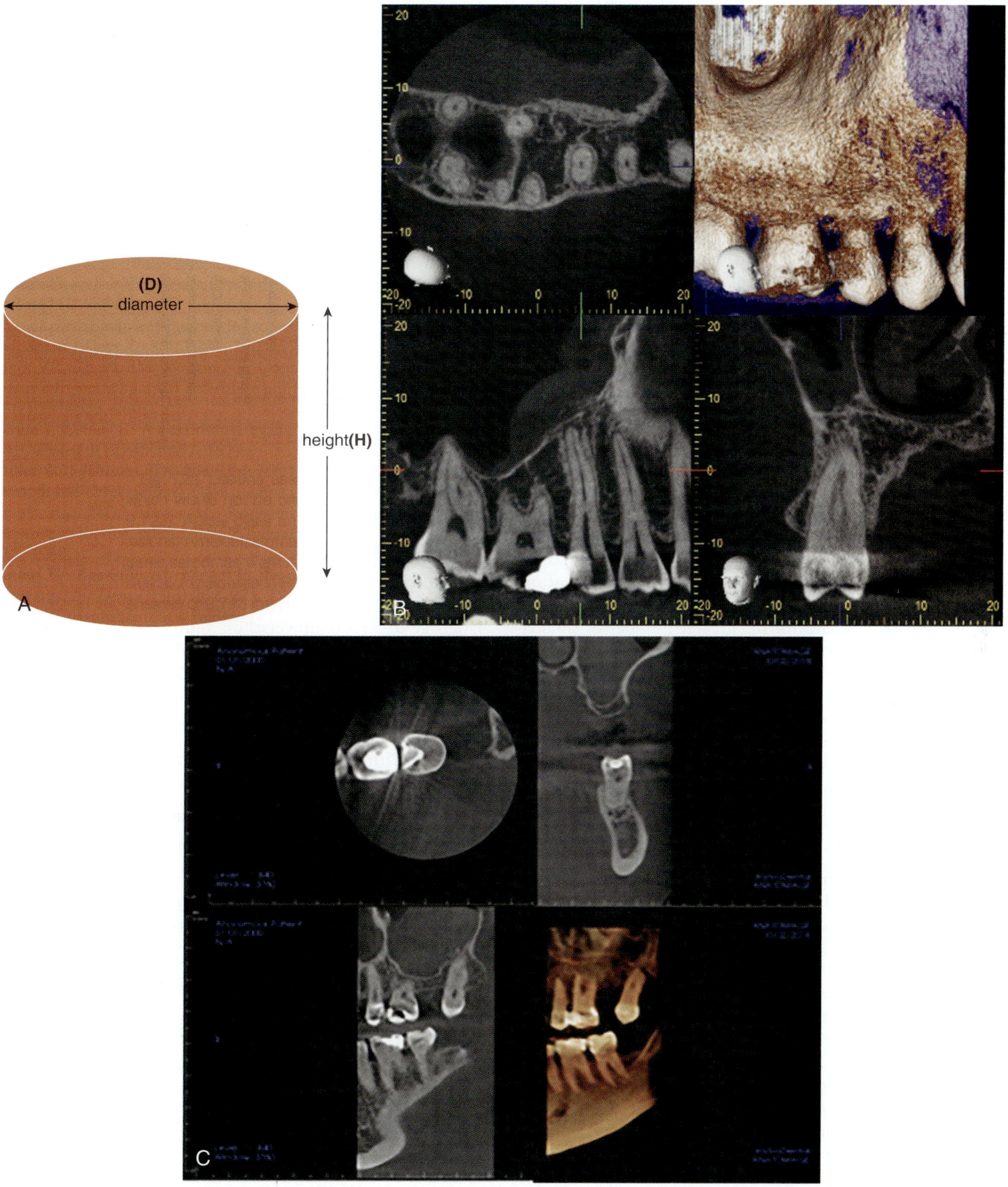

• **Fig. 3.17** **A**, Cylindrical shape of the field of view (FOV) for cone beam computed tomography (CBCT) units with flat panel detectors. **B**, 40 mm × 40 mm FOV multiplanar image reconstruction. **C,** 40 mm × 80 mm FOV multiplanar image reconstruction.

from 30 mm (D) × 30 mm (H) to 240 mm (D) × 165 mm (H). For endodontic purposes, the smaller FOV options are typically used. These smaller FOVs are dependent on the size of the detector units but typically range from 40 mm × 40 mm (three to five teeth in one jaw arch) to 40 mm × 80 mm (which will include similar numbers of maxillary and mandibular teeth (Fig. 3.17, *B* and *C*). Although these larger FOVs are available, they are more expensive and not really indicated for the smaller field sizes needed for endodontic purposes. Smaller FOV units which image three to five teeth in a jaw (maxilla or mandible) are therefore the preferred FOV for endodontic evaluations. The area covered in these smaller volumes is adequate for a thorough 3D periapical evaluation of the selected teeth, alveolar bone, and the limited amount of maxillary or mandibular basal bone. Flat panel detectors are the most used detector for CBCT units.

Voxel Size and Bit Depth

Voxel size and bit depth are two components of CBCT imaging not germane to standard intraoral imaging. Voxels are the cubic-shaped elements that store the 3D object density information in the volumetric data. The smaller the voxel size at which the object is scanned, the higher the resolution of the object. Due to the indications for endodontic CBCT imaging (early-stage apical periodontitis, vertical root fractures [VRF], complex root anatomy, etc.), smaller voxel sizes are preferred. Voxel sizes for endodontic reasons are typically in the range of 0.075 mm^3 (75 µm) to 0.125 mm^3 (125 µm). Most other CBCT applications do not require this degree of resolution. For these other indications (implants, large pathologic lesions, etc.), voxel sizes are in the range of 0.20 mm^3 (200 um) to 0.40 mm^3 (400 µm). Although voxel sizes less than 0.075 mm^3 (75 µm) are possible, there is an increase in image graininess that offsets the benefit of the increased resolution.

Because smaller voxel sizes provide more density information of the object, the radiation exposure needs to be higher to generate adequate x-ray photons for the greater number of smaller voxels in the volumetric data. Intuitively, more x-ray photons in the radiation beam are needed to provide the signal to the greater number of smaller voxels that compose the volumetric data of the object. The scan time will be longer, and the frame rate of basis image capture will be higher. This increase in the frame rate causes an increase in the radiation dose for small FOV scans. Consequently, although the radiation dose for endodontic CBCT scans is lower due to the smaller FOV, this dose-lowering is offset by the greater radiation dose needed when the smaller voxel sizes are employed. This paradox with respect to voxel size explains the large dose range for small FOV scans (Table 3.1). It also explains the dose overlap of small FOV scans with the intermediate and large FOV scans. Large FOV scans have a larger dose due to the larger body part being scanned. The option of large FOV scans with small voxels sizes are not typically a setting on CBCT units. The higher frame rate, processing time, RAM, and storage memory are beyond the capacity of larger commercially available CBCT units.

Another property of the image detector is the bit depth. The bit depth is an exponential binary property expressing the total number of gray shades the detector is able to discriminate. A 16-bit detector (i.e., 2^{16}) can display 65,536 shades of gray. The range of bit depth of commercial CBCT units is between 12 and 16 bits (4096 and 65,536 shades of gray), indicating the wide range of contrast discrimination capability. Although the detector is capable of this degree of gray scale discrimination, limiting features to the contrast resolution include the lower bit depth of the imaging software and the monitor display, and the eye perception of the viewing clinician. Even though bit depth is important for contrast resolution, the American College of Radiology has concluded that there is no added benefit to diagnostic interpretations by the use of higher than 8-bit depth in the viewing computer's operating system.[49]

Volumetric Data and Projection Data

During a CBCT scan, image capture software, usually proprietary to each machine manufacturer, will capture multiple "basis" images at the various angles in the scan rotation. The number of basis images per scan ranges from 300 to 600 images. The complete set of basis images is called the *projection data*, which is then used by the software to construct a 3D volumetric data set. This processed data is then accessed by image reconstruction software programs to "construct" the primary multiplane images or multiplanar reconstructions (MPR) for display, as previously seen in Fig. 3.17, *B* and *C*. The MPRs are often derived from the proprietary software that comes with the particular CBCT scanner. However, because of the versatility of independent "third-party" imaging software to also construct multiple kinds of secondary reconstructions (panoramic, temporomandibular joint, implant planning, etc.), clinicians may prefer to view the scan data in these other software programs. Third-party imaging software is software not associated with the capture and proprietary software of the CBCT scanner. Currently, a variety of third-party software programs are commercially available for image reconstruction of CBCT volumetric data sets. Some examples are listed in Table 3.2.

Image File Format

If third-party software is being used, the file format of the volume set must be converted from the proprietary file format or file language to a more universal or common digital file format. This common digital file format must conform to the Digital Imaging and Communications in Medicine (DICOM) standard (National

TABLE 3.2 Third-party software available for imaging DICOM CBCT data sets

Software	Manufacturer
NobelClinician	Nobel Biocare USA, LLC Yorba Linda, CA
CareStream 3D	CareStream Dental Rochester, NY
Dolphin 3D	Dolphin Imaging Chatsworth, CA
InVivoDental	Anatomage Inc. San Jose, CA
OnDemand3D	Cybermed Inc. Irvine, CA
OsiriX	Pixmeo SARL Berne, Switzerland
Xelis™ Dental	Infinitt NA, Phillipsburg, NJ

Electrical Manufacturers Association [NEMA] Standard PS3 2018, i.e., the current DICOM standardized file format.)[50] This format is the International Organization for Standardization (ISO) referenced standardized digital file format for medical images and related information (i.e., ISO 12052.) To facilitate access to health care, multiple imaging modalities used in medicine and dentistry (x-ray, visible light, ultrasound, etc.), all must be compliant with ISO 12052.

Scatter and Beam Hardening Artifacts

During image reconstruction of a data set, dense metal structures in the FOV often cause scatter and beam hardening artifacts on the image reconstructions. Gutta-percha and silver point endodontic filling materials, cement overfills, metal posts, silver amalgam, dental implants, and metal alloys used in coronal restorations all create artifacts that present either as light or dark scatter lines (streaking), or as a dark periphery adjacent to metallic borders (beam hardening). The streaks often superimpose regular anatomy and significantly degrade image quality. The main types of beam hardening are the dark streaks or the dark bands that present adjacent radiopaque restorations in the image reconstructions. The latter often simulates disease, such as recurrent caries or fractures in endodontically treated teeth (Fig. 3.18, *A* and *B*). In other instances, beam hardening can also give the illusion of extra root canals, which, if not properly interpreted, can lead to inappropriate endodontic treatment (Fig. 3.18, *C–E*).

These artifacts are prominent problems for dental applications with CBCT as root canal treatment (RCT) fillings and coronal metallic restorations are often within the FOV of most dental and endodontic patient CBCT scans. The metallic restorations then cause the resultant beam hardening and streak artifacts, which then compromise the image quality. To repeat, the examples in Fig. 3.18 illustrate how harmful these artifacts are at degrading image quality and making image assessments very difficult.

Software correction algorithms that minimize these metallic artifacts have been reported.[51,52] However, they have not been demonstrated to be any more beneficial than noncorrected software programs when evaluating peri-implant and periodontal disease[53] or root fractures.[54] Differences in root fill materials also have no effect on minimizing the effects of these artifacts.[55] Consequently, there are no immediate methods to correct or minimize these prominent artifacts. The best way to avoid streaking and beam hardening is to try to keep the FOV as small as possible in an attempt to minimize the number of metals within the scan's FOV.

Indications and Special Applications

The American Association of Endodontists (AAE) and the American Academy of Oral and Maxillofacial Radiology (AAOMR) wrote a joint position paper in 2011.[56] They made several evidence-based guidelines for CBCT use in endodontic patient care. This joint position paper was subsequently updated in 2015,[57] and the key recommendations from this latest publication are outlined in the remainder of this chapter.

1. 2D Imaging remains the initial imaging procedure of choice

Endodontic diagnosis depends on evaluation of the patient's chief complaint, the medical and dental history, and the clinical and radiographic examination. According to these AAE/AAOMR recommendations, 2D intraoral imaging remains the imaging procedure of choice for these initial evaluations and most endodontic imaging needs (Recommendation 1).

Only if the 2D evaluation leaves the diagnosis or the treatment in question does CBCT with its advanced capabilities become indicated. These situations will arise as 2D radiographs have inherent limitations due to the manner in which anatomic structures in three dimensions are compressed onto a 2D image. Interpreting 2D images continues to be a somewhat subjective process. Goldman et al.[58] showed that the agreement between six examiners was only 47% when evaluating healing of periapical lesions using 2D periapical radiographs. In a follow-up study, Goldman et al.[59] also reported that when examiners evaluated the same images at two different times, they had only 19% to 80% agreement with their previous interpretations. Agreement among six observers for detecting periradicular radiolucencies with 2D digital images was less than 25%; whereas the agreement for five of six observers was approximately 50%.[60] Several studies have shown where CBCT overcomes many of the 2D imaging limitations.[61-67]

2. Limited FOV CBCT is indicated for cases with contradictory or nonspecific clinical signs and symptoms associated with endodontically untreated or previously treated teeth

This indication is the main premise of AAE/AAOMR Recommendation 2. CBCT imaging has the ability to detect periapical pathology before it is apparent on 2D radiographs[68] (Fig. 3.19). This capability was validated in clinical studies in which the sensitivity of detecting apical periodontitis on intraoral radiographs versus CBCT images was 20% and 48%, respectively.[69] Ex vivo studies in which simulated periapical lesions were created showed a similarly greater CBCT sensitivity than did intraoral radiography.[70,71]

The inability to determine the etiology of persistent dentoalveolar pain can be attributed to the limitations in both clinical vitality testing and intraoral radiography. Atypical odontalgia (AO) is a persistent dentoalveolar pain without the evidence of periapical bone destruction.[72] The diagnostic yield of CBCT compared with intraoral radiographs was 17% greater in definitively diagnosing apical periodontitis from suspected AO.[73]

3. Limited FOV CBCT should be considered the imaging modality of choice for initial treatment of teeth with the potential for extra canals and suspected complex morphology

The efficacy of CBCT as a modality to accurately explore tooth anatomy and identify the prevalence of extra or atypical canals is the premise of Recommendation 3. The greater sensitivity at identifying a second mesiobuccal canal (MB2) in maxillary molars with CBCT in comparison with the gold standard (clinical and histologic sectioning) has been well documented.[74,75] Fig. 3.20 demonstrates a recurrent case of apical periodontitis in a maxillary first molar initially diagnosed and treated with periapical imaging. The recall radiograph with the persistent disease is seen in Fig. 3.20, *A*. Fig. 3.20, *B–D* demonstrates the MB2 canal in the multiplanar reconstructions. The MB2 was not seen when tooth #14 was diagnosed and treated with periapical radiographic imaging. The final postoperative periapical radiograph Fig. 3.20, *E* shows the obturated MB1 and MB2 canals.

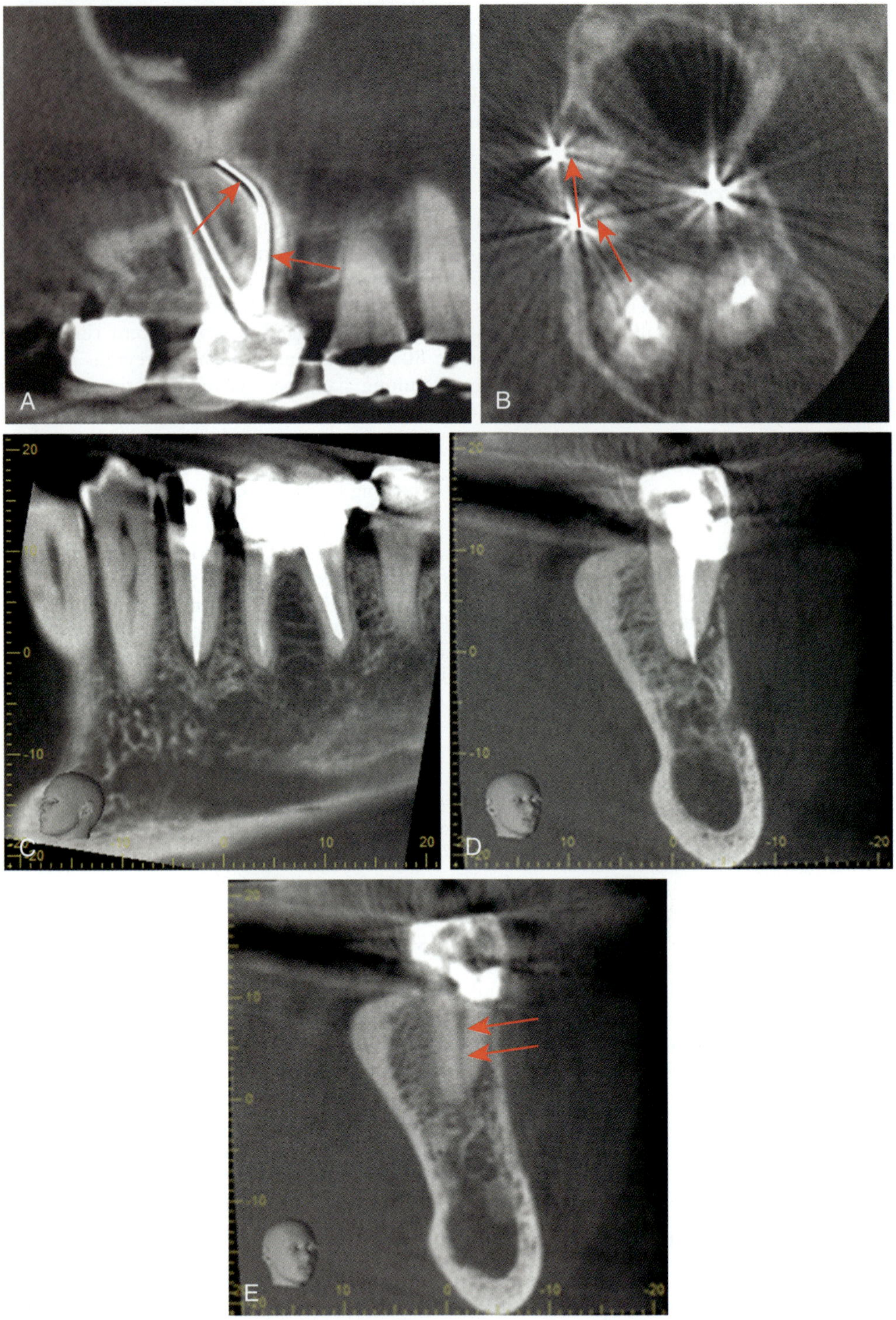

• **Fig. 3.18** Beam Hardening Artifact and Streaking Adjacent the #5 Root Canal Treatment (RCT). **A**, Parasagittal reconstruction with beam hardening artifact adjacent the #3 MB RCT. **B**, Radiolucent and radiopaque streak artifact radiates from the #3 MB and #3 DB root fills. Note how the former often simulate fracture lines *(arrows)*. **C**, Parasagittal reconstruction evaluating the persistent pain on #20. **D**, Cross-section of #20 oriented through the root canal filling. Note the fill overextension and the ~2.0 mm widening of the apico-buccal periodontal ligament (PDL) that is not apparent on 2D imaging. **E**, Cross-section of #20 oriented between the root canal filling and the distal proximal surface. Note the beam hardening artifact of the RCT filling that simulates a second unfilled canal.

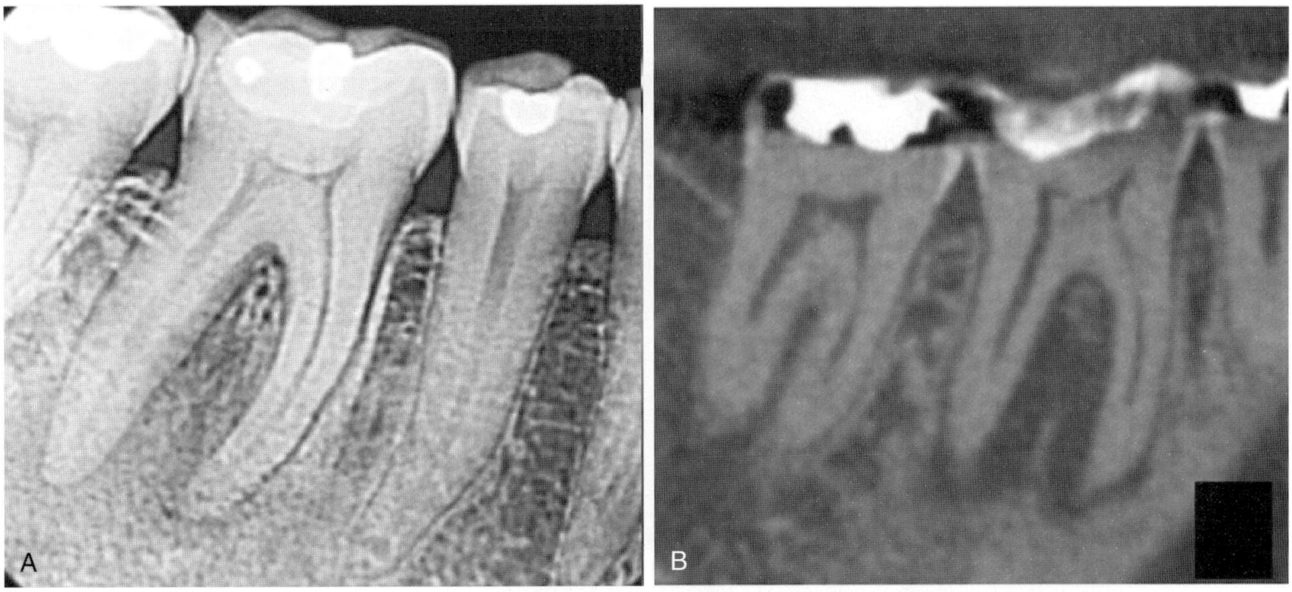

• **Fig. 3.19** This patient presented with pain to percussion and no response to cold testing on #30. Periodontal probing depths were within normal limits. Root canal therapy was indicated based on the cone beam computed tomography (CBCT) radiographic findings and the clinical tests. **A,** Periapical radiograph of tooth #30. **B,** 2D parasagittal CBCT reconstruction. The periapical radiolucency is better delineated demonstrating involvement of the furcation and both the mesial and distal root periapices.

CBCT showed higher mean values of specificity and sensitivity in comparison with intraoral radiographic assessments in the detection of the MB2 canal.[76]

4. Limited FOV CBCT should be used for the detection of VRF

A thorough dental history, pain symptoms, clinical signs of swelling, a sinus tract, and/or an isolated deep periodontal pocket are suggestive of a VRF. Radiographically, a combination of a periapical and a lateral root radiolucency "halo" (or J-shaped) appearance is also suggestive of VRF. Any combination of these clinical and radiographic findings may be present to establish a presumptive diagnosis of VRF.[77] The following five CBCT findings were found to be consistent in confirmed cases of VRF[78]:

1. Loss of bone in the midroot area with intact bone coronal and apical to the defect
2. Absence of the entire buccal plate of bone in MBR
3. Radiolucency around a root where a post terminates
4. Space existing between the buccal/or lingual plate of bone and fractured root surface
5. Visualization of the VRF on the CBCT multiplanar views.

Fig. 3.21 shows an example of the sensitivity of CBCT in detecting a VRF. The application of a dye during surgical exploration is still the gold standard for VRF diagnosis.[79]

Several studies have demonstrated the validity of using CBCT to detect VRFs when 2D imaging is inconclusive (Recommendation 6). In a study comparing the sensitivity and specificity of CBCT with those of 2D radiography in detecting VRF, the sensitivity and specificity were 79.4% and 92.5%, respectively, for CBCT and 37.1% and 95%, respectively, for 2D imaging.[80] This same study reported that the specificity of CBCT was reduced in the presence of root canal filling material.[80] Higher sensitivity and specificity were observed in a clinical study in which the definitive diagnosis of VRF was confirmed at the time of surgery to validate CBCT findings, with sensitivity being 88% and specificity 75%.[81] In vivo and laboratory studies[82-83] evaluating CBCT in the detection of VRF agreed that sensitivity, specificity, and accuracy of CBCT were generally higher and reproducible. The detection of fractures was significantly higher for all CBCT systems compared with that of intraoral radiographs.

However, any radiographic assessment of fracture must be interpreted with caution because the detection of VRF is dependent on the size of the fracture and the spatial resolution (voxel size) of the CBCT.[84] Consequently, this affects the sensitivity in not being able to detect a fracture that may actually be present (false negative finding). The beam hardening and streaking artifacts discussed previously also make it difficult to discern these VRF, either by obscuring or by simulating fracture lines. The former may also contribute to a false negative finding. The latter would affect the specificity and lead to a false positive finding if in fact a fracture was not present. These VRF diagnostic dilemmas come to light more often in teeth with posts because these teeth have more potential for root fracture and the metallic posts and metallic coronal restorations contribute to the streaking artifact, which would then affect both the sensitivity and the specificity of VRF diagnosis.

5. Utilization of Limited FOV CBCT in non-surgical retreatment, surgical treatment planning, assessment of endodontic treatment complications or retreatment of treatment complications:

Accurate diagnostic data leads to better treatment decisions and potentially more predictable outcomes.[85] The use of CBCT has been recommended for treatment planning of endodontic surgery (Recommendation 7).[86-88]

CBCT was a more accurate imaging modality for the diagnosis and subsequent treatment planning of endodontic pathology compared with the diagnosis and treatment decisions using only periapical radiographs. An accurate diagnosis was reached in 36.6% to 40% of the cases when using periapical radiographs in comparison with 76.6% to 83.3% of the cases when using CBCT.[89] This high level of misdiagnosis is potentially clinically relevant, especially in cases of invasive cervical root resorption and VRF, when a lack of

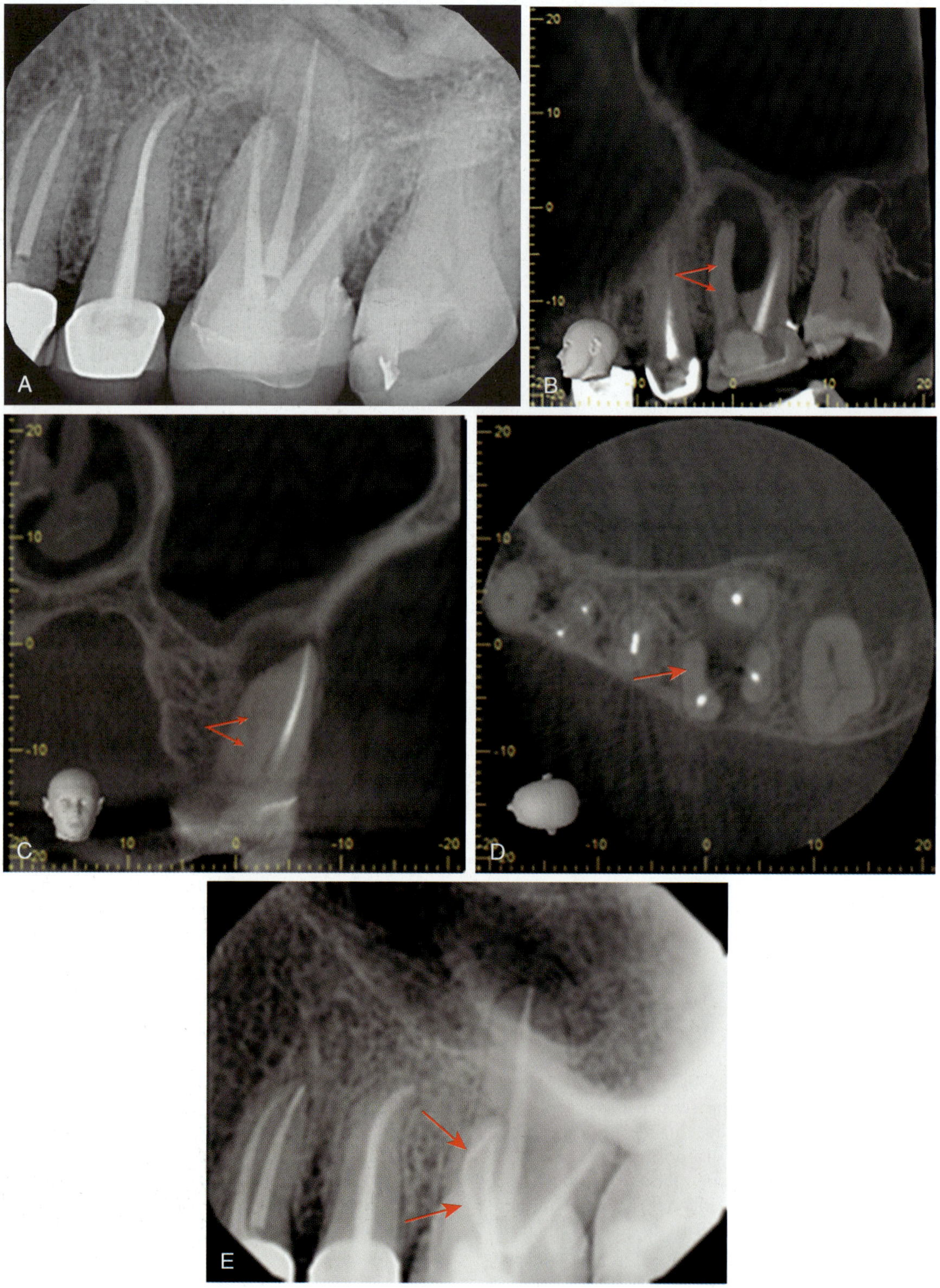

• **Fig. 3.20** **A**, A follow up 2D periapical image on #14 demonstrates recurrent apical periodontitis. **B–D**, The sagittal, coronal, and axial cone beam computed tomography (CBCT) reconstructions further document the recurrent #14 apical periodontitis and the unfilled palatal canal in the mesiobuccal root (MB2). **E**, The 2D periapical image of the retreatment demonstrates the filled MB2 canal (see *arrows*). (**A**, Courtesy Dr. Janelle Silvers, Redlands, CA; **E**, Courtesy Dr. Janelle Silvers, Redlands, CA.)

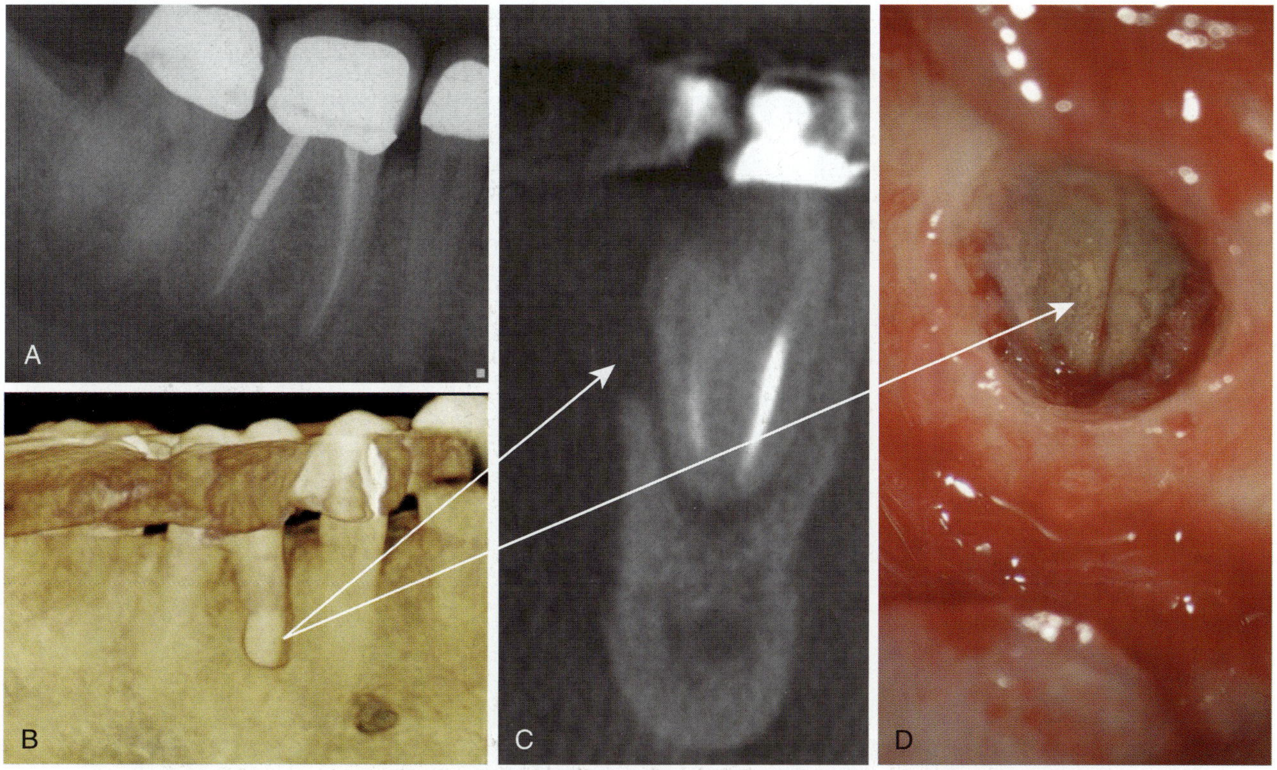

• **Fig. 3.21** **A**, Periapical radiograph of tooth #30; **B**, 3D reconstruction demonstrating midroot buccal plate fenestration of the mesial root. **C**, 2D coronal reconstruction demonstrating the midroot buccal fenestration *(arrow)*. **D**, Surgical curettage and degranulation of the defect demonstrating the mesial root's vertical fracture *(arrow)*.

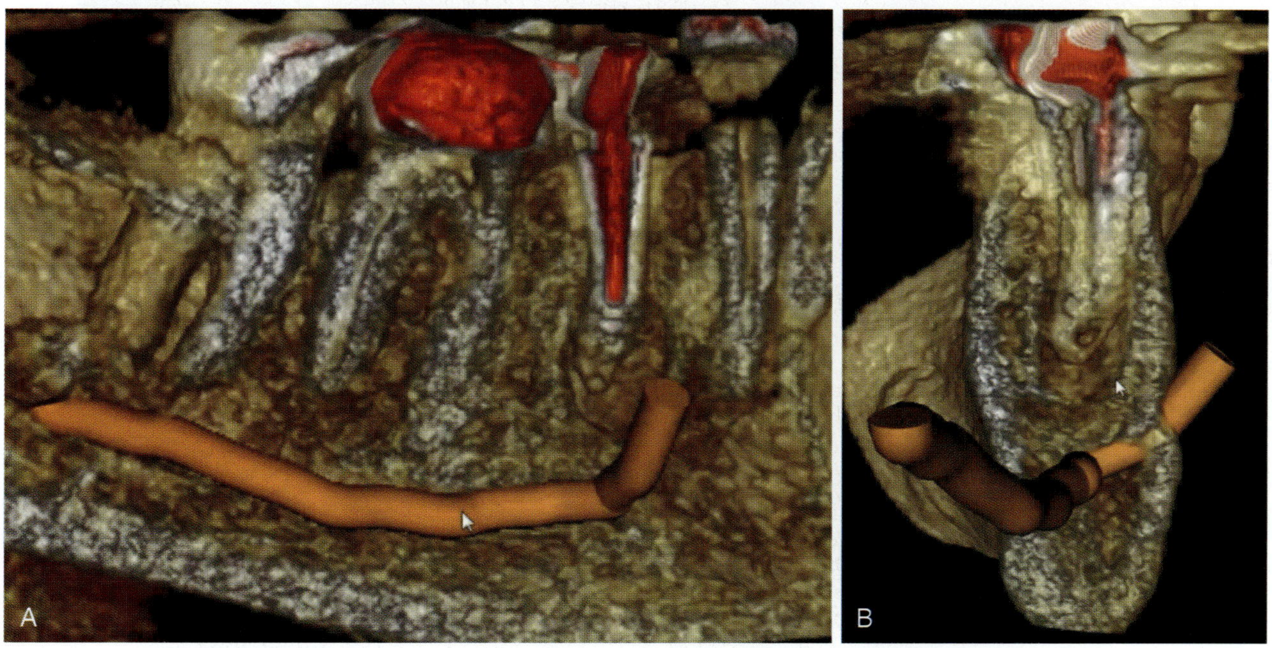

• **Fig. 3.22** **A**, 3D rendering demonstrating the relation of the inferior alveolar nerve (IAN) to the periapical defect at the #29 periapical lesion. **B**, A cropped 3D coronal rendering demonstrating the mental foramen and the IAN in relation to the base of the periapical defect *(arrow)*. Note the apical root resorption.

early detection could lead to unsuccessful treatment and tooth loss. The previous study also demonstrated that the treatment plan may be directly influenced by information gained from CBCT studies as the examiners altered their treatment plan after viewing the CBCT scan in 56.6% to 66.7% of the cases overall (Recommendation 8). This high number indicates that CBCT had a significant influence on the examiners' treatment plan.

6. Use of limited FOV CBCT to localize root apex/apices and to evaluate the proximity to adjacent anatomic structures

CBCT visualization of periapical disease proximity to vital structures and anatomic landmarks is superior to that of periapical images. Therefore it is recommended for surgical treatment planning where such proximity is suspected (Recommendation 9). Figs. 3.22 and 3.23 exemplify the use of CBCT

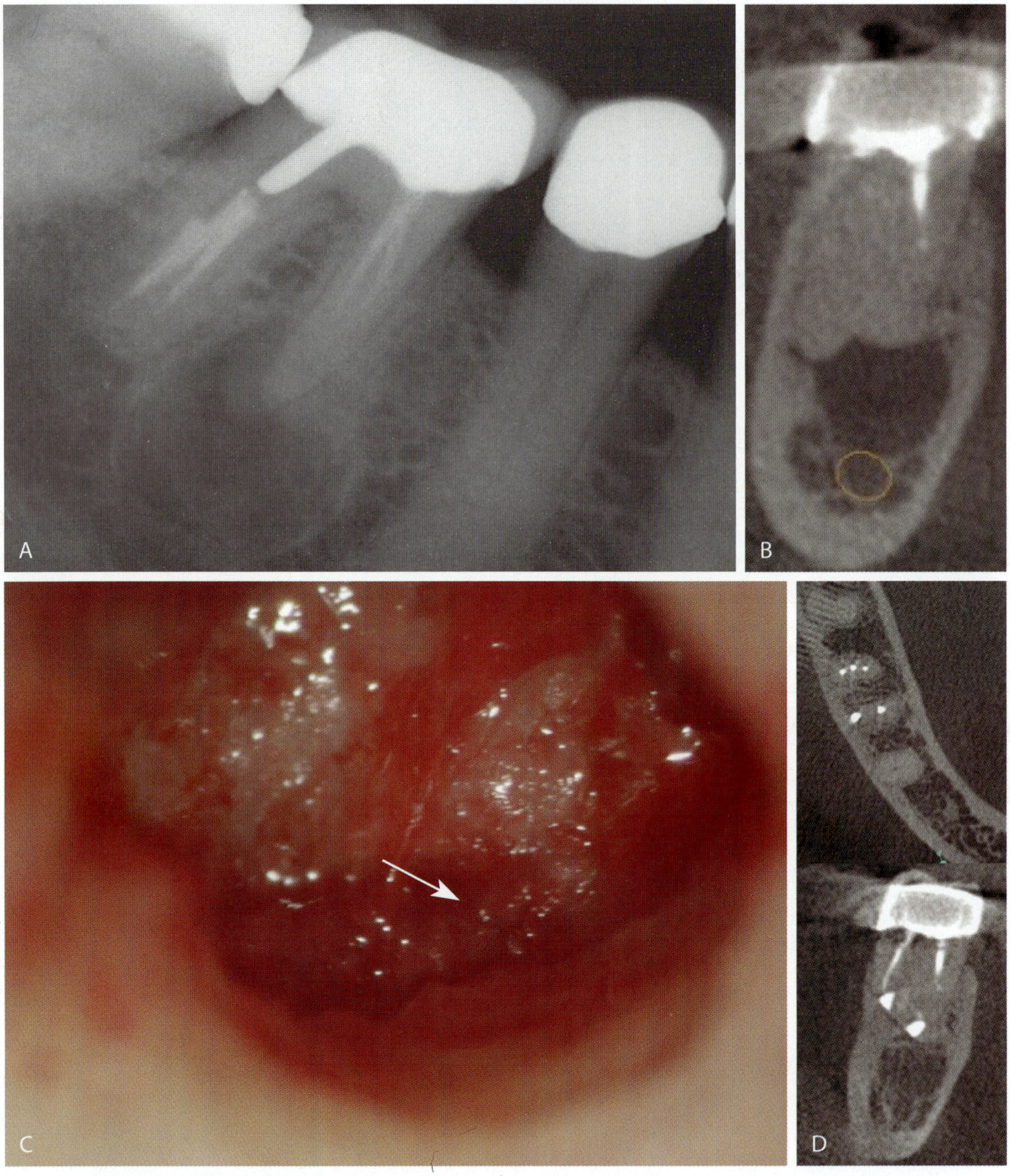

• **Fig. 3.23** **A**, Periapical radiograph of tooth #30. This tooth was referred for periapical surgery after non-surgical retreatment was unsuccessful. An untreated third distal canal was identified and treated, and the mesial canals were blocked. **B**, Cone beam computed tomography (CBCT) coronal reconstruction of #30 mesial root demonstrating the communication of the periapical defect with the inferior alveolar canal. **C**, Surgical view of the mesial root apex after curettage and degranulation of the defect. The inferior alveolar nerve was uncovered immediately inferior to the base of the defect *(white arrow)*. **D**, Axial and coronal views of tooth #30 at the 24-month recall demonstrating complete remodeling of the defect and restoration of the surgically defect in the buccal cortical plate.

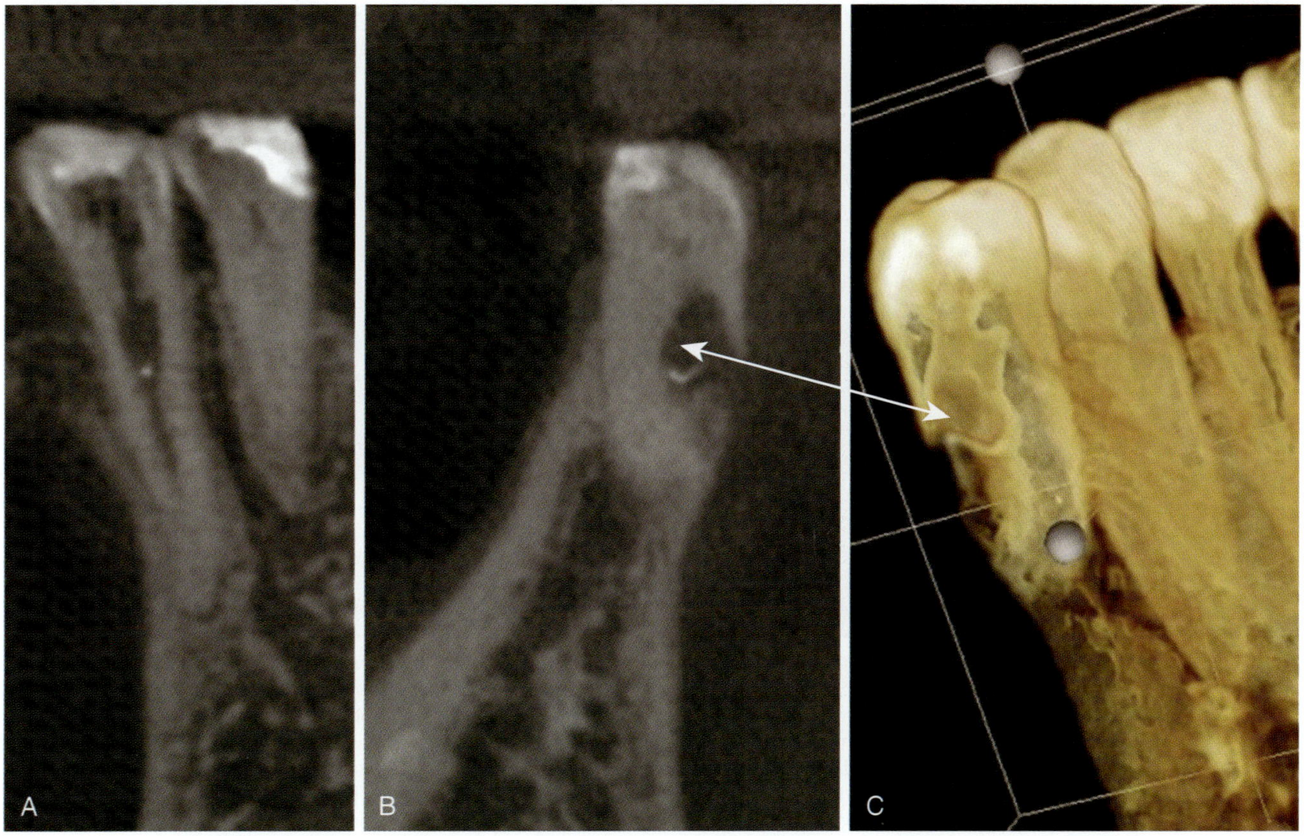

• **Fig. 3.24** This patient was referred for evaluation and treatment of an internal resorptive defect on #21. **A**, Parasagittal view of tooth #21 demonstrating the external/internal resorptive defect. **B**, Cross-sectional view of tooth #21 also demonstrating the external/internal resorptive defect. **C**, 3D reconstruction of the resorptive defect. In addition to the resorptive defects, images **(B)** and **(C)** demonstrate a buccal root perforation *(white arrow)*. This cone beam computed tomography (CBCT) finding rendered tooth #21 nonrestorable, and this changed the endodontic treatment plan.

imaging in surgical treatment planning of cases with proximity to vital structures.

7. Use of CBCT in endodontic diagnosis and detection of resorptive defects

Diagnosis and detection of root resorption is often challenging owing to the quiescent onset nature and varying clinical presentation. Because CBCT is a better imaging option than periapical imaging for resorptive defects,[90,91] it is the AAE/AAOMR Recommendation 12. There is now a 3D classification for external cervical resorption (ECR) that takes into account lesion height, degree of circumferential spread, and proximity to the root canal.[92] This novel and clinically relevant classification that relies on CBCT better facilitates the objective description of ECR progression or resolution. It is also expected to facilitate effective communication of ECR between colleagues. Fig. 3.24 shows an example where CBCT imaging facilitated the diagnosis and treatment planning of inflammatory resorptive defects.

8. Use of CBCT in endodontic diagnosis and detection of traumatic dental injuries (TDI)

Radiographic assessment is important to identify the location, type, and severity of TDI. In the 2012 International Association of Dental Traumatology guidelines,[93] a series of periapical radiographs from different angulations and an occlusal film are recommended for evaluation of TDI. However, 2D imaging has limitations in the evaluation of TDI due to projection geometry, magnification, superimposition of anatomic structures, distortion, and projection errors. The use of CBCT for TDI is now a recommendation of the AAE/AAOMR (Recommendation 11), particularly traumatic or horizontal root fractures (HRFs) and lateral luxations, for monitoring of healing and or any related complications.

In the diagnosis of HRF using 2D imaging, the fracture line will be detected only if the x-ray beam passes directly through it. The 2D nature limits the accuracy in the diagnosis of the location, severity, and extent of HRF. The risk of misdiagnosis of the location and extent of the fracture by using only 2D intraoral radiography could lead to improper treatment and an unfavorable outcome. Because of the limitations of intraoral radiography, CBCT was suggested as the preferred imaging modality for diagnosis of HRF.[94]

CBCT overcomes several of the limitations of 2D imaging by providing a considerable amount of 3D information about the nature and extent of the HRF. The significant difference in the nature of HRF when assessed with 2D radiographs compared with CBCT has been reported.[95] Fig. 3.25 demonstrates a case where CBCT imaging is advantageous in the diagnosis, prognosis, treatment planning, and treatment follow-up of an HRF case.

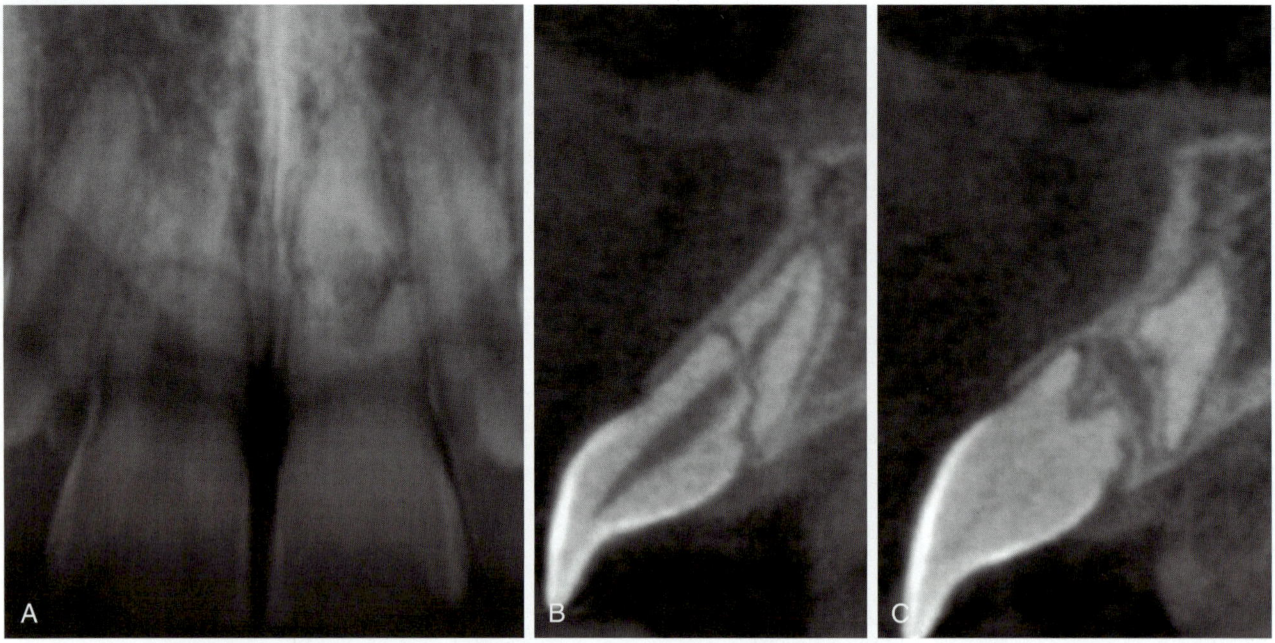

• **Fig. 3.25** A 15-year-old patient with a history of trauma to the anterior maxilla was referred for consultation of teeth #8 and #9. Tooth #8 had a grade I mobility and tooth #9 had a grade II+ mobility. **A**, Periapical radiograph of teeth #8 and #9 demonstrated midroot horizontal root fractures in both teeth. Periodontal probing depths were within normal limits. The marginal and attached gingiva demonstrated normal color and architecture. **B** and **C** are the sagittal views of teeth #8 and 9, respectively. Note the oblique nature of the root fractures and bone fill between the coronal and apical segments in **(C)**. Because the patient was asymptomatic and cone beam computed tomography (CBCT) revealed no periradicular pathosis, a palatal splint was suggested to address the mobility, but no endodontic intervention was recommended at the time.

Study Questions

6. In CBCT scanning, generally the smaller the voxel size, the __________ the image resolution.
   a. darker
   b. higher
   c. lower
   d. worse
7. "Beam hardening" effects seen on CBCT reconstructions
   a. Occur when the mA settings are high
   b. Compromise diagnostic image quality
   c. Improve the outlines of endodontic treated canals
   d. Occur less with restorative materials in the FOV
8. The AAE/AAOMR joint position paper on the CBCT applications for endodontic patient care is highly valued because:
   a. Many endodontists follow the recommendations.
   b. The recommendations are evidence based.
   c. The use of CBCT images can shorten the duration of RCT treatment.
   d. CBCT images are the most definitive for posttreatment follow up evaluations.
9. The imaging procedure of choice for most endodontic evaluations is:
   a. Limited CBCT FOV with a large voxel size
   b. Periapical intraoral imaging
   c. Any size CBCT FOV with high resolution
   d. The procedure favored by the treating endodontist
10. Consistent CBCT findings for a VRF include all of the following EXCEPT:
   a. Loss of bone at the mid root level with intact bone apical and coronal to the defect
   b. Apical radiolucency around a root with a restorative post
   c. Absence of cortical bone in the 3D multiplanes
   d. Actual visualization of the VRF in the CBCT multiplanes
11. CBCT is a preferred imaging modality for evaluating
   a. HRF
   b. Carious dental lesions approaching the pulp
   c. Posttreatment recalls of more than 5 years
   d. All maxillary first molars in need of endodontic treatment

ANSWERS

Answer Box 3

1 d. Stochastic
2 a. Smaller area for image capture
3 a. Are more durable
4 b. Increase biorisk to the radiographer
5 d. Technique used to localize the buccal and lingual position of objects
6 b. Higher
7 b. Compromise diagnostic image quality
8 b. The recommendations are evidence based
9 b. Periapical intraoral imaging
10 b. Apical radiolucency around a root with a restorative post
11 a. HRF

References

1. Gittinger JW: Inside out: early investigations of x-ray by two Harvard-educated physicians revealed the technology's benefits—and dangers, *Harvard Med Alum Bull* http://alumnibulletin.med.harvard.edu/bulletin/spring2008/insideout.php, 2008.
2. Cotti E, Esposito SA, Musu D, et al.: Ultrasound examination with color power Doppler to assess the early response of apical periodontitis to the endodontic treatment, *Clin Oral Investig* 22(1):131–140, 2018.
3. Musu D, Rossi-Fedele G, Campisi G, Cotti E: Ultrasonography in the diagnosis of bone lesions of the jaws: a systematic review, *Oral Surg Oral Med Oral Pathol Oral Radiol* 122(1):e19–29, 2016.
4. Mouyen F, Benz C, Sonnabend E, Lodter JP: Presentation and physical evaluation of RadioVisioGraphy, *Oral Surg Oral Med Oral Pathol* 68(2):238–242, 1989.
5. Ong EY, Pitt Ford TR: Comparison of radiovisiography with radiographic film in root length determination, *Int Endod J* 28(1):25–29, 1995.
6. Danforth R, Torabinejad M: Estimated radiation risks associated with endodontic radiography, *Endod Dent Traumatol* 6:21, 1990.
7. Torabinejad M, Danforth R, Andrews K, Chan C: Absorbed radiation by various tissues during simulated endodontic radiography, *J Endod* 15(6):249, 1990.
8. Mallya SM, Lam EWN: *White and Pharoah's oral radiology: principles and interpretation*, ed 8, St. Louis, 2019, Elsevier.
9. Ludlow JB, Davies-Ludlow LE, White SC: Patient risk related to common dental radiographic examinations: the impact of 2007 International Commission on Radiological Protection recommendations regarding dose calculation, *J Am Dent Assoc* 139:1237–1243, 2008.
10. Tang FR, Loke WK, Khoo BC: Low-dose or low-dose-rate ionizing radiation–induced bioeffects in animal models, *J Radiat Res* 58(2):165–182, 2017.
11. De Gonzales AB, Salotti JA, McHugh K, et al.: Relationship between paediatric CT scans and subsequent risk of leukaemia and brain tumours: assessment of the impact of underlying conditions, *Br J Cancer* 114(4):388–394, 2016.
12. National Council on Radiation Protection and Measurements: *Dental x-ray protection*, Report 145. Bethesda, MD, 2003, National Council on Radiation Protection and Measurements.
13. Farman AG: ALARA still applies, *Oral Surg Oral Med Oral Pathol Oral Radiol Endod* 100:395–397, 2005.
14. Brenner DJ, Hall EJ: Computed tomography—an increasing source of radiation exposure, *N Engl J Med* 357:2277–2284, 2007.
15. Fortier P, Glover Jr JA: Origins of dental radiology. In Goaz PW White SC, editor: *Oral radiology: principles and interpretation*, ed 1, St. Louis, 1982, C.V. Mosby Company, pp 3–14.
16. Van Dis ML, Miles DA, Parks ET, Razmus TF: Information yield from a hand-held dental x-ray unit, *Oral Surg Oral Med Oral Pathol* 76:381–385, 1993.
17. Essig SL: New York moves to facilitate the use of hand-held X-ray devices, *N Y State Dent J* 75(57), 2009.
18. Makdissi J, Pawar RR, Johnson B, Chong BS: The effects of device position on the operator's radiation dose when using a handheld portable X-ray device, *Dentomaxillofac Radiol* 45(3):20150245, 2016.
19. Rottke D, Gohlke L, Schrodel R, et al.: Operator safety during the acquisition of intraoral images with a handheld and portable X-ray device, *Dentomaxillofac Radiol* 47(3):20160410, 2018.
20. Gray JE, Bailey ED: Ludlow JB: Dental staff doses with handheld dental intraoral x-ray units, *Health Phys* 102(2):137–142, 2012.
21. Thatcher A: *Comparison of Four Handheld X-Ray Devices Preliminary results, Equipment Audits.* Office of Radiation Protection Washington State Division of Environmental Health, 2018.
22. Berkhout WER, Suomalainen A, Brüllmann D, et al.: Justification and good practice in using handheld portable dental X-ray equipment: a position paper prepared by the European Academy of DentoMaxilloFacial Radiology (EADMFR), *Dentomaxillofac Radiol* 44(6):20140343, 2015.
23. Akdeniz B, Sogur B: An ex vivo comparison of conventional and digital radiography for perceived image quality of root fillings, *Int Endod J* 38:397, 2005.
24. Bhaskaran V, Qualtrough A, Rushton VE, et al.: A laboratory comparison of three imaging systems for image quality and radiation exposure characteristics, *Int Endod J* 38:645, 2005.
25. Kositbowornchai S, Hanwachirapong D, Somsopon R, et al.: Ex vivo comparison of digital images with conventional radiographs for detection of simulated voids in root canal filling material, *Int Endod J* 30:287, 2006.
26. Burger C, Mork T, Hutter J, et al.: Direct digital radiography versus conventional radiography for estimation of canal length in curved canals, *J Endod* 25:260, 1999.
27. Holtzmann D, Johnson W, Southard T, et al.: Storage-phosphor computed radiography versus film radiography in the detection of pathologic periradicular bone loss in cadavers, *Oral Surg Oral Med Oral Pathol* 86:90, 1998.
28. Sullivan J, Di Fiore P, Koerber A: Radiovisiography in the detection of periapical lesions, *J Endod* 26:32, 2000.
29. Al-Rawi W, Teich S: Evaluation of physical properties of different digital intraoral sensors, *Compend Contin Educ Dent* 34(8), 2013.
30. Christensen GC: Digital radiography sensors. which is best? *Clinicians Report* 4(9):1–3, 2011.
31. Iannucci JM, Howerton LJ: *Dental radiography: principles and techniques*, ed 5, St Louis, 2017, Elsevier, pp 72–103.
32. Thomson EM, Johnson ON: *Essentials of dental radiography for dental assistants and hygienists*, ed 10, New York, 2018, Pearson Education Inc., pp 78–105.
33. Mallya SM, Lam EWN: *White and Pharoah's oral radiology: principles and interpretation*, ed 8, St. Louis, 2019, Elsevier, pp 89–118.
34. Iannucci JM, Howerton LJ: *Dental radiography: principles and techniques*, ed 5, St Louis, 2017, Elsevier, pp 152–196.
35. Thomson EM, Johnson ON: *Essentials of dental radiography for dental assistants and hygienists*, ed 10, New York, 2018, Pearson Education Inc., pp 158–194.
36. Forsberg J: Radiographic reproduction of endodontic "working length" comparing the paralleling and the bisecting-angle techniques, *Oral Surg Oral Med Oral Pathol* 64:353, 1987.
37. Walton RE: Endodontic radiographic techniques, *Dent Radiogr Photogr* 46(3):51–59, 1973.
38. Richards AG: The buccal object rule, *Dent Radiogr Photogr* 53:37, 1980.
39. Abramovitch K: Imagery Chapter 5. In Alling III CC, Helfrick JF Alling RD, editors: *Impacted teeth,* Philadelphia, PA, 1993, WB Saunders, pp 110–116.
40. Tamse A, Kaffe I, Fishel D: Zygomatic arch interference with correct radiographic diagnosis in maxillary molar endodontics, *Oral Surg Oral Med Oral Pathol* 50:563, 1980.
41. Stein TJ, Corcoran JF: Radiographic "working length" revisited, *Oral Surg Oral Med Oral Pathol* 74:796, 1992.
42. Klein R, Blake S, Nattress B, et al.: Evaluation of x-ray beam angulation for successful twin canal identification in mandibular incisors, *Int Endod J* 30:58, 1997.
43. Zakariasen K, Scott D, Jensen J: Endodontic recall radiographs: how reliable is our interpretation of endodontic success or failure and what factors affect our reliability? *Oral Surg Oral Med Oral Pathol* 57:343, 1984.
44. Lambrianidis T, Lyroudia K, Pandelidou O, et al.: Evaluation of periapical radiographs in the recognition of C-shaped mandibular second molars, *Int Endod J* 34:458, 2001.
45. Serman N, Hasselgren G: The radiographic incidence of multiple roots and canals in human mandibular premolars, *Int Endod J* 25:234, 1992.
46. Sion A, Kaufman B, Kaffe I: The identification of double canals and double rooted anterior teeth by Walton's projection, *Quintessence Int* 15:747, 1984.
47. Mozzo P, Procacci C, Tacconi A, et al.: A new volumetric CT machine for dental imaging based on the cone-beam technique: preliminary results, *Eur Radiol* 8(9):1558–1564, 1998.
48. Arai Y, Tammisalo E, Arai Y, et al.: Development of a compact computed tomographic apparatus for dental use, *Dentomaxillofac Radiol* 28(4):245–248, 1999.
49. Andriole KP, Ruckdeschel TG, Flynn MJ, et al.: ACR-AAPM-SIIM practice guidelines for digital radiography, *J Digit Imaging* 26(1):26–37, 2013.
50. National Electrical Manufacturers Association, Digital Imaging and Communications in Medicine (DICOM), PS 3 2018. Rosslyn (VA): *National*

Electrical Manufacturers Association (NEMA). Available from http://dicom.nema.org/medical/dicom/current/output/html/part01.html, 2018.
51. Bechara B, McMahan CA, Geha H, et al.: Evaluation of a cone beam CT artefact reduction algorithm, *Dentomaxillofac Radiol* 41(5):422–428, 2012.
52. Bechara B, Moore WS, McMahan CA, et al.: Metal artefact reduction with cone beam CT: an in vitro study, *Dentomaxillofac Radiol* 41(3):248–253, 2012.
53. Kamburoglu K, Kolsuz E, Murat S, et al.: Assessment of buccal marginal alveolar peri-implant and periodontal defects using a cone beam CT system with and without the application of metal artefact reduction mode, *Dentomaxillofac Radiol* 42(8):20130176, 2013.
54. Bechara B, McMahan CA, Moore WS, et al.: Cone beam CT scans with and without artefact reduction in root fracture detection of endodontically treated teeth, *Dentomaxillofac Radiol* 42(5):20120245, 2013.
55. Zhang W, Makins SR, Abramovitch K: Cone Beam Computed Tomography (CBCT) artifact characterization of root canal filling materials, *J Investigative Dent Sci* 1(1):1–4, 2014.
56. Use of Cone Beam Computed Tomography in Endodontics: Joint Position Statement of the American Association of Endodontists and the American Academy of Oral and Maxillofacial Radiology, *J Endod* 37(2):274–277, 2011.
57. Use of Cone Beam Computed Tomography in Endodontics 2015 Update: Joint Position Statement of the American Association of Endodontists and the American Academy of Oral and Maxillofacial Radiology, *J Endod* 41(9):1393–1396, 2015.
58. Goldman M, Pearson AH, Darzenta N: Endodontic success: who's reading the radiograph? *Oral Surg Oral Med Oral Pathol* 33(3):432–437, 1972.
59. Goldman M, Pearson AH, Darzenta N: Reliability of radiographic interpretation, *Oral Surg Oral Med Oral Pathol* 38(3):287–293, 1974.
60. Tewary S, Luzzo J, Hartwell G: Endodontic radiography: who is reading the digital radiograph? *J Endod* 37:919–921, 2011.
61. Patel S, Durack C, Abella F, Shemesh H, Roig M, Lemberg K: Cone beam computed tomography in endodontics: a review, *Int Endod J* 48:3–15, 2015.
62. Cotton TP, Geisler TM, Holden DT, et al.: Endodontic applications of cone-beam volumetric tomography, *J Endod* 33:1121–1132, 2007.
63. Patel S, Dawood A, Whaites E, Pitt Ford T: New dimensions in endodontic imaging: part 1. Conventional and alternative radiographic systems, *Int Endod J* 42:447–462, 2009.
64. Patel S: New dimensions in endodontic imaging: part 2. Cone beam computed tomography, *Int Endod J* 42:463–475, 2009.
65. Scarfe WC, Farman AG, Sukovic P: Clinical applications of cone-beam computed tomography in dental practice, *J Can Dent Assoc* 72:75–80, 2006.
66. Nair MK, Nair UP: Digital and advanced imaging in endodontics: a review, *J Endod* 33:1–6, 2007.
67. Setzer FC, Hinckley N, Kohli MR, Karabucak B: A survey of cone-beam computed tomographic use among endodontic practitioners in the United States, *J Endod* 43:699–704, 2017.
68. De Paula-Silva FW, Wu MK, Leonardo MR, da Silva LA, Wesselink PR: Accuracy of periapical radiography and cone-beam computed tomography scans in diagnosing apical periodontitis using histopathological findings as a gold standard, *J Endod* 35(7):1009–1012, 2009.
69. Patel S, Wilson R, Dawood A, Mannocci F: The detection of periapical pathosis using periapical radiography and cone beam computed tomography—part 1: preoperative status, *Int Endod J* 8:702–710, 2012.
70. Sogur E, Grondahl H, Bakst G, Mert A: Does a combination of two radiographs increase accuracy in detecting acid-induced periapical lesions and does it approach the accuracy of cone-beam computed tomography scanning, *J Endod* 38(2):131–136, 2012.
71. Patel S, Dawood A, Mannocci F, Wilson R, Pitt Ford T: Detection of periapical bone defects in human jaws using cone beam computed tomography and intraoral radiography, *Int Endod J* 42(6):507–515, 2009a.
72. Nixdorf D, Moana-Filho E: Persistent dento-alveolar pain disorder (PDAP): Working towards a better understanding, *Rev Pain* 5(4):18–27, 2011.
73. Pigg M, List T, Petersson K, et al.: Diagnostic yield of conventional radiographic and cone-beam computed tomographic images in patients with atypical odontalgia, *Int Endod J* 44(12):1365–2591, 2011.
74. Blattner TC, George N, Lee CC, et al.: Efficacy of CBCT as a modality to accurately identify the presence of second mesiobuccal canals in maxillary first and second molars: a pilot study, *J Endod* 36(5):867–870, 2010.
75. Michetti J, Maret D, Mallet J-P, Diemer F: Validation of cone beam computed tomography as a tool to explore root canal anatomy, *J Endod* 36(7):1187–1190, 2010.
76. Vizzotto MB, Silveira PF, Arús NA, et al.: CBCT for the assessment of second mesiobuccal (MB2) canals in maxillary molar teeth: effect of voxel size and presence of root filling, *Int Endod J* 46(9):870–876, 2013.
77. Tsesis I, Rosen E, Tamse A, et al.: Diagnosis of vertical root fractures in endodontically treated teeth based on clinical and radiographic indices: a systematic review, *J Endod* 36:1455–158, 2010.
78. Fayad MI, Ashkenaz PJ, Johnson BR: Different representations of vertical root fractures detected by cone-beam volumetric tomography: a case series report, *J Endod* 10:1435–1442, 2012.
79. Walton RE: Vertical root fractures: factors related to identification, *J Am Dent Assoc* 148(2):100–105, 2017.
80. Hassan B, Metska ME, Ozok AR, et al.: Detection of vertical root fractures in endodontically treated teeth by a cone beam computed tomography scan, *J Endod* 35:719–722, 2009.
81. Edlund M, Nair MK, Nair UP: Detection of vertical root fractures by using cone-beam computed tomography: a clinical study, *J Endod* 37(6):768–772, 2011.
82. Metska ME, Aartman IH, Wesselink PR, Özok AR: Detection of vertical root fracture in vivo in endodontically treated teeth by cone-beam computed tomography scans, *J Endod* 38(10):1344–1377, 2012.
83. Brady E, Mannocci F, Wilson R, et al.: A comparison of CBCT and periapical radiography for the detection of vertical root fractures in non-endodontically treated teeth, *Int Endod J* 47(8):735–746, 2014.
84. Melo SLS, Bortoluzzi EA, Abreu M, et al.: Diagnostic ability of a cone-beam computed tomography scan to assess longitudinal root fractures in prosthetically treated teeth, *J Endod* 36:1879–1882, 2010.
85. Liang YH, Li G, Wesselink PR, Wu MK: Endodontic outcome predictors identified with periapical radiographs and cone-beam computed tomography scans, *J Endod* 37:326–331, 2011.
86. Venskutonis T, Plotino G, Tocci L, et al.: Periapical and endodontic status scale based on periapical bone lesions and endodontic treatment quality evaluation using cone-beam computed tomography, *J Endod* 41(2):190–196, 2015.
87. Bornstein MM, Lauber R, Pedram Sendi P, Arx T: Comparison of periapical radiography and limited cone-beam computed tomography in mandibular molars for analysis of anatomical landmarks before apical surgery, *J Endod* 37(2):151–157, 2010.
88. Low KM, Dula K, Bürgin W, Arx T: Comparison of periapical radiography and limited cone-beam tomography in posterior maxillary teeth referred for apical surgery, *J Endod* 34(5):557–562, 2008.
89. Ee J, Fayad MI, Johnson BR: Comparison of endodontic diagnosis and treatment planning decisions using cone-beam volumetric tomography versus periapical radiography, *J Endod* 40:910–916, 2008.
90. Estrela C, Bueno MR, De Alencar AH, et al.: Method to evaluate inflammatory root resorption by using cone beam computed tomography, *J Endod* 35(11):1491–1497, 2009.
91. Durack C, Patel S, Davies J, et al.: Diagnostic accuracy of small volume cone beam computed tomography and intraoral periapical radiography for the detection of simulated external inflammatory root resorption, *Int Endod J* 44(2):136–147, 2011.
92. Patel S, Foschi F, Mannocci F, Patel K: External cervical resorption: a three dimensional classification, *Int Endod J* 51(2):206–214, 2018.
93. Diangelis AJ, Andreasen JO, Ebeleseder KA, et al.: International association of dental traumatology guidelines for the management of traumatic dental injuries: 1—fractures and luxations of permanent teeth, *Dent Traumatol* 28:2–12, 2012.
94. May JJ, Cohenca N, Peters OA: Contemporary management of horizontal root fractures to the permanent dentition: diagnosis—radiologic assessment to include cone-beam computed tomography, *J Endod* 39(3 Suppl):S20–S25, 2013.
95. Iikubo M, Kobayashi K, Mishima A, et al.: Accuracy of intraoral radiography, multidetector helical CT, and limited cone-beam CT for the detection of horizontal tooth root fracture, *Oral Surg Oral Med Oral Pathol Oral Radiol Endod* 108:e70–74, 2009.

4

Endodontic Diagnosis and Treatment Planning

BROOKE BLICHER, RICHARD E. WALTON, AND MAHMOUD TORABINEJAD

CHAPTER OUTLINE

LEARNING OBJECTIVES

After reading this chapter, the student should be able to:

1. Recognize that diagnosis and treatment planning for pulpal and periapical conditions should be part of a broader examination and treatment plan.
2. Understand the importance of the medical and dental histories to endodontic diagnosis.
3. Conduct comprehensive extraoral and intraoral examinations of both hard and soft tissues, including the application of pulp sensitivity tests.
4. Develop the knowledge base to order and interpret appropriate diagnostic radiographs.
5. Consolidate all data from the history, clinical examination, and radiographic examination to form a diagnosis of pulpal and periapical conditions using appropriate terminology.
6. Diagnose adjunctive conditions to the typical endodontic diagnosis, including resorption, fractures, and endodontic–periodontic interrelationships.
7. Recognize when orofacial pain and infections are not of endodontic origin.
8. Identify conditions for which root canal treatment is indicated and contraindicated; understand alternative treatments.
9. Integrate the endodontic diagnosis and treatment plan into an overall treatment plan.
10. Understand which procedures are ordinarily not within the graduating dentist's realm of training or experience and which patients should be considered for referral.

Introduction

Accurate diagnosis is paramount to appropriate care. Endodontic diagnosis and treatment planning generally occur in two basic scenarios. In the first scenario, the emergency patient presents with pain and possibly swelling, or with a displaced, fractured, or avulsed tooth. In the second, pulpal or periapical disease is detected incidentally; endodontic care is expected. Emergency situations demand an accurate and timely diagnosis. Missteps in diagnosis will result in continued morbidity. Errors in diagnosis may result in the addition of unnecessary treatment with increased cost and suffering for the patient (Fig. 4.1), In the short term, misdiagnosis can result in unsatisfied patients and clinical frustration for the provider. In the long term, uncontrolled infections may have serious consequences to systemic health and affect the prognosis of future treatments.

Even nonemergent situations require care in confirming the appropriate diagnosis, because nuances to the diagnosis can render traditional nonsurgical root canal therapy ineffective. For example, a tooth that has developed pulpal and periapical pathosis secondary to a coronal fracture with root involvement might not survive in the long term after endodontic therapy. Additionally, other normal and pathological entities can mimic endodontic pathosis; these entities are discussed in Chapter 5.

Diagnosis is the science of recognizing and identifying disease by means of signs, symptoms, and tests. The basic elements of diagnosis are data gathering and analysis to develop a differential diagnosis, a definitive diagnosis, and a treatment plan. This chapter will focus on the appropriate means to obtain an accurate endodontic diagnosis, including the specifics of the examination process, the appropriate terminology to describe endodontic pathosis, and a discussion of

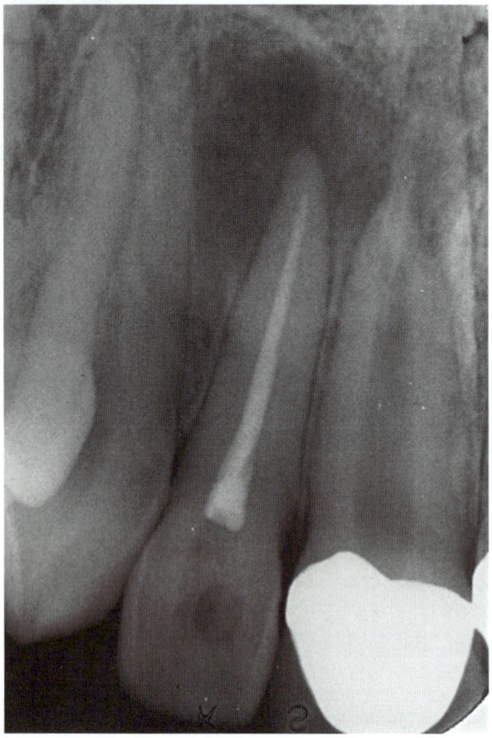

• **Fig. 4.1** A reliance on "clinical experience" rather than on adequate tests resulted in the wrong treatment. The dentist relied on a radiograph only (no tests) and concluded that the lateral incisor was the painful problem tooth. After treatment, with no change in the level of pain, the patient was referred for root-end surgery. Examination of preoperative and postoperative radiographs, as well as clinical tests, showed that treatment had been performed on a tooth with normal pulp. The central incisor was found to have pulp necrosis and an acute apical abscess. Immediate pain relief followed root canal treatment on the correct tooth.

definitive care to be delivered based on the findings and their interpretation.

Examination

Subjective Examination

Chief Complaint

The chief complaint is the first verbal information from the patient. The chief complaint is often volunteered without a question and is recorded in the patient's own words. Close attention is paid to this statement.

Dental History

Dental history is divided into the present dental illness, also referred to as the history of the chief complaint, and the past dental history. Once the patient has described why he or she is seeking care, details are established by methodical questioning. There are a limited number of complaints of endodontic consequence. If there are two or more concurrent complaints, such as pain and swelling, then the history of each complaint should be obtained.

Beyond gathering a list of reported symptoms, questions are asked regarding their timeline and quality. As pain is the most common reason for seeking endodontic care, this symptom is questioned directly. Some patients supply a detailed history of pain; others require guidance to determine the location, onset, duration, quality, intensity, and exacerbating or relieving factors.

TABLE 4.1 Example Questions to Guide a Patient Through the History of the Chief Complaint

Location	Where is the pain located? Is it always in the same spot?
Onset	When did your symptoms start? Did or does anything initiate the pain?
Duration	When you have pain, how long does it last? When did your symptoms last occur? Is the pain continuous or intermittent?
Quality	How would you describe your pain? (For example, dull/achy or sharp/electrical)
Intensity	On a 0–10 scale, where would you rate your pain at its worst?
Exacerbating factors	Does anything make your pain worse? (For example, cold, heat, or biting.)
Relieving factors	Does anything make your pain better? (For example, cold, pressure, or analgesics.)

Directive questions should be open-ended when possible to avoid any influence on the patient's answers. In the early stages of a pulpitis, pain may be difficult to localize, thus nonlocalizable pain raises suspicion. Certain referral patterns of odontogenic pain are common, such as pain from a pulpitis in a mandibular molar commonly referring to the ear. Similarly, certain referral patterns for nonodontogenic pain are common and will be discussed in Chapter 5. Examples of questions to obtain a detailed history of the chief complaint are in Table 4.1.

Patients will often falsely report presence or a history of swelling. True swelling must be associated with pulp necrosis, though patients may perceive swelling even with symptomatic irreversible pulpitis.

Although localized acute apical abscesses do not associate with systemic symptoms,[1] endodontic infections rarely can spread with serious sequelae. Patients with swelling require further questioning about the onset and duration, changes over time, and effects on jaw opening, swallowing, or breathing. Although rare, any rapidly progressive swelling, accompanied by trismus, dysphagia, or dyspnea is considered a progressive cellulitis (space infection) necessitating prompt referral to an oral surgeon or hospital for intravenous antibiotics and probable extraoral incision and drainage. The nature of the swelling, whether indurated or soft, and associated drainage may be reported by the patient. With cellulitis, the patient should also be examined for signs of systemic involvement such as fever, malaise, or lymphadenopathy, all of which might prompt the use of systemic antibiotics.[2,3] More information on dental emergencies and indications and contraindications for systemic antibiotics are in Chapter 9.

Traumatic dental injuries require their own workup, including an assessment for comorbid injuries, such as concussion, jaw fractures, soft-tissue lacerations, or involvement of other teeth, as well as lapses in tetanus immunity. More information specific to the workup related to traumatic dental injuries is in Chapter 11.

Patients presenting with endodontic pathosis will usually have a history of dental procedures. Prior pain is even considered a risk factor for current endodontic pathosis.[4] Patients are asked about overall oral health, including recent dental procedures, a history of trauma, and previous issues with temporomandibular dysfunction. Patients may report cracks or fractures that prompted prior restorative care. Other findings during the objective portion of the examination prompt further questioning. For example, if soft-tissue scarring is seen, a patient may be asked about a history of oral surgical care.

Medical History

An updated picture of the patient's health is obtained at each visit, including a complete medical history, list of active medical issues, medications, and allergies.

Certain health issues are of concern in endodontic diagnosis. For example, acute respiratory infections, particularly of the maxillary sinus, often produce toothache-like symptoms. Pain-modulating conditions, such as fibromyalgia, may have atypical pain presentations. Treatment options may be affected. Bisphosphonates, biologics, and chemotherapy agents are associated with osteonecrosis of the jaw and can limit a patient's options for surgical or extraction alternatives in favor of root canal therapy.[5] Radiation therapy to the head and neck limits these more invasive treatment options due to risks of osteoradionecrosis.

A complete list of medications and allergies is needed to ensure that drug interactions and adverse events will not occur during treatment. The need for antibiotic prophylaxis related to cardiac conditions, prosthetic joints, and certain immune deficiencies are considered. A comprehensive review of medical conditions that can affect endodontic care, as well as discussion of antibiotic prophylaxis, are in Chapter 2. Whenever doubt exists as to limitations for care or the need to premedicate, consultation should be had with the patient's treating physicians.

Objective Examination

Vital Signs

Vital signs, including blood pressure, respiratory rate, and pulse, should be obtained as part of the examination process. In addition, in patients reporting swelling or signs and symptoms of infection, including suspected fever, malaise, or lymphadenopathy, an oral temperature reading should be taken.

Extraoral Examination

General appearance, skin tone, facial asymmetry, swelling, discoloration, redness, extraoral scars or sinus tracts, and lymphadenopathy are indicators of the physical status of the patient. Aberrant findings are suggestive of related orofacial infections or inflammation (Fig. 4.2).

Intraoral Examination

Soft Tissue

Examination of the intraoral soft tissues includes a thorough visual, digital, and probing examination of the lips, oral mucosa, cheeks, tongue, palate, muscles, and periodontium for abnormalities. Particular focus should be paid to the alveolar mucosa and attached gingiva adjacent to a suspicious tooth for the presence of discoloration, inflammation, ulceration, and sinus tract formation. A stoma or parulis is the visible point of drainage of a sinus tract, and usually indicates the presence of a necrotic pulp and chronic apical abscess (Fig. 4.3). Sinus tracts may also occur secondary to nonendodontic pathology such as a periodontal abscess, vertical root fracture (VRF), or even osteomyelitis; thus, the source of drainage should always be determined. Sinus tracts may be traced radiographically with gutta-percha, or cone beam computed tomography (CBCT) imaging may show their point of origin.

A limited periodontal examination should occur as part of any endodontic workup. Periodontal probing depths should be measured, because localized attachment loss can indicate not only the presence of periodontal disease that might affect the overall prognosis and affect treatment planning but can also suggest the presence of additional pathology. Fractures, whether originating coronally, or involving root structure, may present with localized deeper probing depths when a root is involved.[5-7] Endodontic–periodontic lesions will typically present with a wider area of attachment loss (Fig. 4.4).

Mobility should be measured, as extreme mobility usually indicates limited periodontal support or an underlying root fracture. In addition, a periapical lesion may occasionally alter the periodontal support; mobility should decrease dramatically after successful root canal treatment.

Hard Tissue

A visual examination assesses for discolorations, fractures, abrasion, erosion, caries, defective restorations, or other abnormalities. Use of a pointed explorer can help detect caries, failing restorative margins, and sometimes subgingival root resorption. A discolored crown is often pathognomonic of pulpal pathosis or may be the sequela of earlier root canal treatment. The most common etiologies of pulpal involvement are caries, fractures, or historically deep restorations; a visual examination will help elicit the cause of pathosis. Teeth that lack extensive restorations, or have small, class 1 nonbonded restorations in place, may suffer from pulpitis secondary to marginal ridge fractures extending deep into pulp or even root structure.[8,9]

Clinical Tests

Objective tests are applied to both suspect and control teeth. These tests have limitations; some cannot be used on each tooth, and results are often inconclusive. The data they provide must be interpreted carefully and in conjunction with all other information available. Importantly, these are *not* tests of *teeth;* they are tests of a patient's *response* to a variety of applied stimuli, which may be highly variable. Tests on control teeth educate the patient on which response to expect and provide a "calibrated" baseline for responses on suspect teeth.

Periodontal Inflammation Tests

Percussion, palpation, and bite testing can detect inflammation of the periodontium. Percussion testing is commonly performed by tapping on the incisal or occlusal surface of the tooth, with the end of a mirror handle parallel or perpendicular to the crown. This test is preceded by gentle digital pressure to detect teeth that are very tender and should *not* be tapped with the mirror handle, which could be very painful.

Palpation testing is performed by application of firm fingertip pressure on the buccal or facial mucosa overlying the apex. Palpation testing additionally allows for careful detection of intraoral swelling or bony expansion. When pain on chewing is reported, bite testing should replicate symptoms. Bite testers include cotton rolls, cotton swabs, or commercially available plastic testers that can isolate individual cusps (Fig. 4.5).

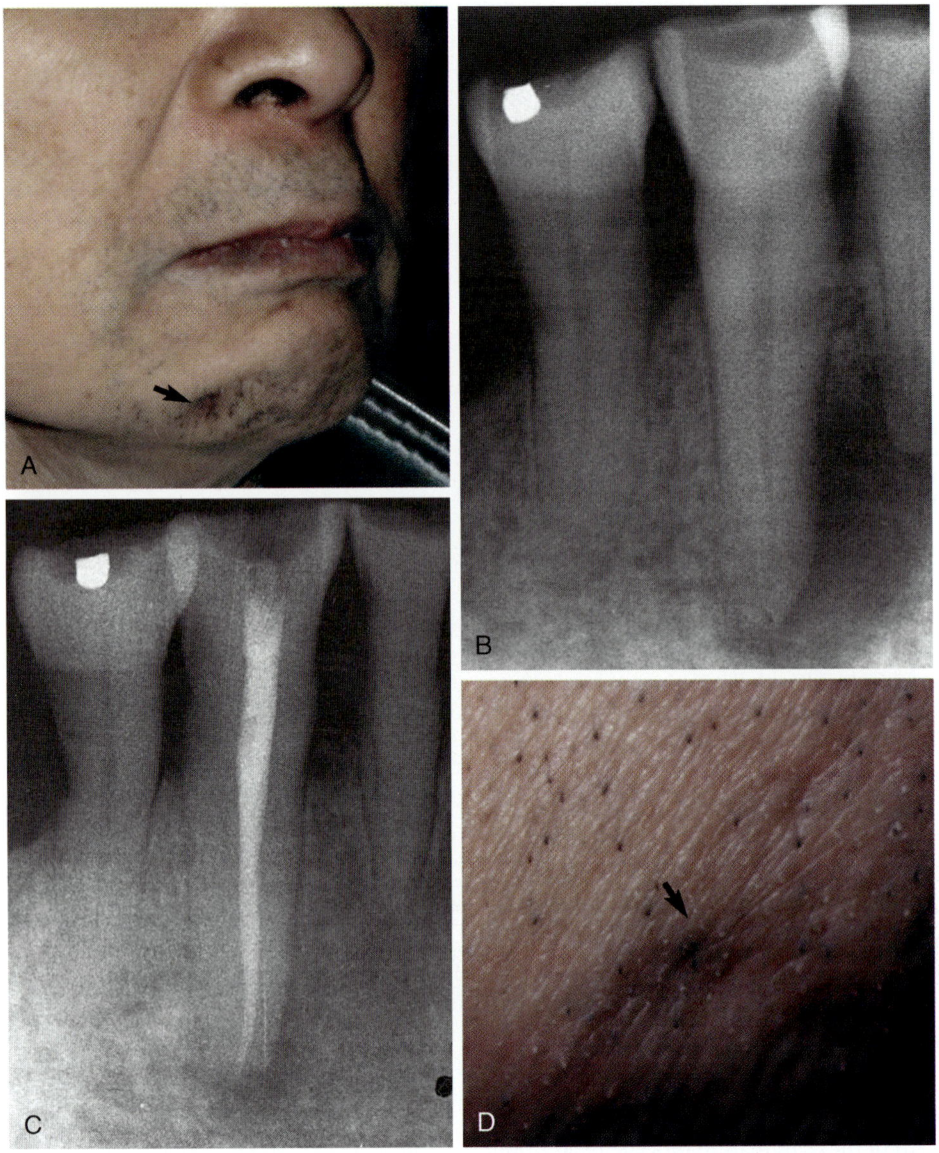

• **Fig. 4.2** Extraoral Sinus Tract. **A,** This surface lesion *(arrow)* was misdiagnosed and treated unsuccessfully by a dermatologist for several months. Fortunately, the patient's dentist then recognized it to be a draining sinus tract and its source was a mandibular anterior tooth. **B,** The pulp was necrotic because of severe attrition with pulp exposure. **C,** After proper root canal treatment only, **D,** the sinus tract and surface lesion resolved completely *(arrow)*.

If a marked painful response is elicited, some degree of periapical inflammation is assumed. Pain on biting can also indicate the presence of a coronal fracture, possibly hidden beneath a large occlusal restoration. Often, teeth adjacent to the diseased tooth may be tender because of the local spread of cytokines and neuropeptides that lower the pain threshold. Periapical inflammation may also be nonendodontic, due to traumatic dental injuries, occlusal trauma, or periodontal disease.

Pulp Sensitivity Tests

Determination of the vitality status of the pulp, whether normal, pulpitis, or pulpal necrosis, is critical. Absolute measures of pulp vitality are not yet clinically accurate. Measures to detect vascular components using beams of light in dual wavelength spectrophotometry,[10] pulse oximetry,[11] or laser Doppler flowmetry[12] are, however, on the horizon. Currently, these approaches are more experimental than clinically practical, and the devices are expensive. As the technology improves and cost decreases, their use in the future is likely.

Until then, conduit measures of pulp sensitivity via nervous system response and replication of symptoms include thermal, direct dentin, and electric stimuli. Though no currently available test reflects the true histologic status of the pulp with absolute accuracy,[13] reasonable agreement occurs.[14,15]

All tests are subject to errors and false responses,[16] and certain teeth cannot be tested by all means. For example, immature teeth lack fully developed Aδ fibers, which are the responding fibers in currently available pulp sensitivity tests; thus, testing is unreliable until full root maturation occurs.[17] The choice of which test to use should factor in reliability as well as the presenting chief complaint. All aspects of the clinical and radiographic examination are assessed to define a pulpal diagnosis. The definitive diagnosis might change when the pulp is accessed and visualized.

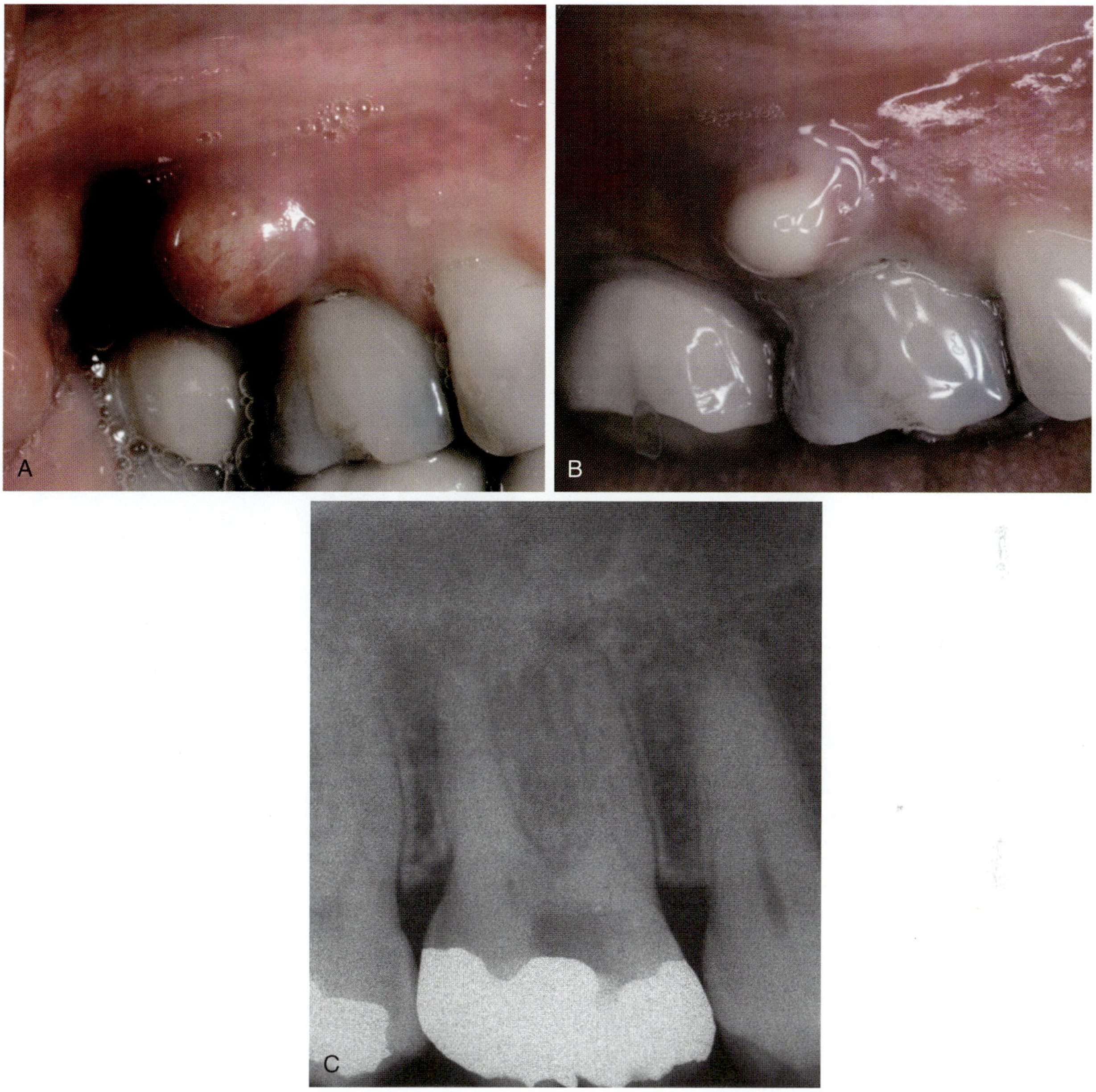

• **Fig. 4.3** Sinus Tract and Parulis. **A,** Asymptomatic, intraoral swelling on mucosa near first molar. **B,** Purulence can be expressed. **C,** The first molar is nonresponsive to pulp sensitivity testing and there is a radiolucency apical to the mesiobuccal root.

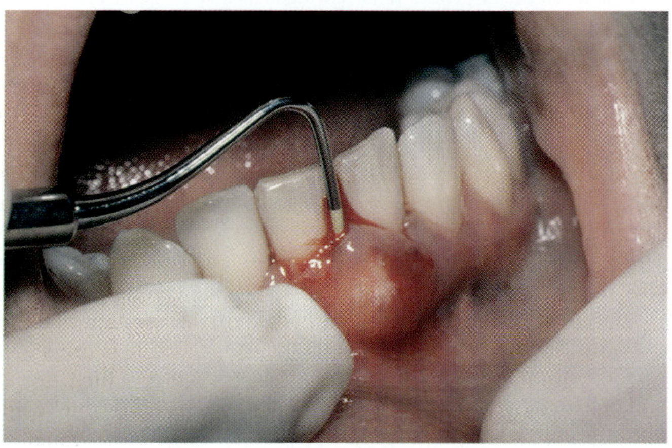

• **Fig. 4.4** Periodontal probing reveals a deep defect. Pulp necrosis suggests that this lesion is endodontic and not periodontic.

Cold Testing

Although no currently available test has absolute accuracy, cold testing is considered the most reliable measure.[16] Often, cold sensitivity is the chief complaint of a painful pulpitis, and replication of symptoms will point to the offending tooth. Although alternative means exist for cold testing, including the use of ice sticks, carbon dioxide, or dry ice, refrigerant sprays are considered the most convenient and reliable means of cold testing.[18,19] Additionally, refrigerant sprays provide the most accurate results in testing through porcelain-fused-to-metal restorations[20] (Fig. 4.6).

Cold testing relies on outward hydrodynamic fluid flow to stimulate Aδ fibers in the pulp.[21] Because inflammation associated with pulpitis can cause both allodynia and hyperalgesia of these fibers, the cold response may be heightened. A normal cold response is typically sharp and quick but should be comparable to responses for adjacent and contralateral control teeth.

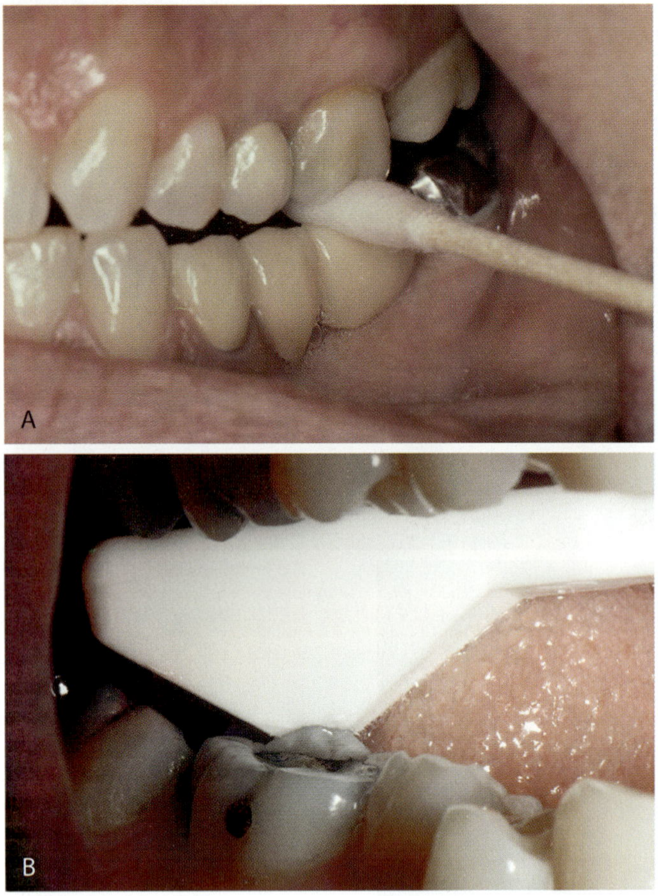

• **Fig. 4.5** **A**, Biting test. Firm pressure on a cotton swab that produces definite pain is a good indicator of apical periodontitis. **B**, Special diagnostic "biting" instruments, such as a Tooth Slooth, are placed on one cusp at a time while the patient grinds with opposing teeth. Sharp pain on pressure or release may indicate a cusp fracture or cracked tooth.

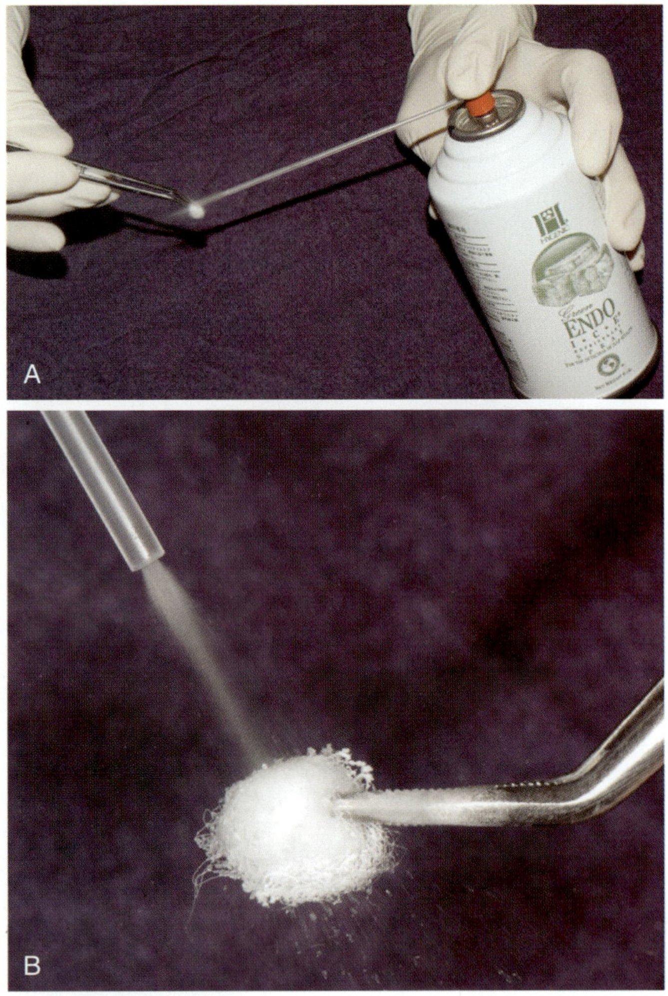

• **Fig. 4.6** **A**, Refrigerant is available in a pressured can. **B**, Refrigerant sprayed on a large cotton pellet is convenient and effective for determining pulp responsiveness.

A heightened and lingering response to cold is very suggestive of symptomatic irreversible pulpitis. No response usually suggests pulpal necrosis.

A *false-negative* response is common when cold is applied to teeth with calcific metamorphosis presumably due to reduction in hydrodynamic fluid flow.[22] A *false-positive* response may result if cold contacts gingiva or is transferred to adjacent teeth with vital pulps. Surprisingly, gingival recession and attachment loss decrease the sensitivity to cold testing.[23]

Heat Testing

Heat testing is reserved for use when the chief complaint includes heat sensitivity; results are less reliable than cold and electric pulp testing (EPT).[16] Various techniques and materials can be used. Heated gutta-percha applied directly to the buccal or facial crown surface, either by use of a Bunsen burner or a commercially available welled tip for a System B device, can be utilized.[24] Use of a dry rubber prophy cup rotated on the surface of a tooth to create frictional heat is a safe alternative (Fig. 4.7). Heated metal instruments or hot water can be damaging to the dental pulp and their use should be avoided.[24]

Like cold testing, heat testing relies on hydrodynamic fluid flow causing Aδ fiber stimulation, this time in a pulpward direction away from the stimulus.[21] As with cold, a sharp and nonlingering pain response to heat indicates a vital pulp; however, false negatives are common. Heat responses may occur in previously treated teeth as a result of untreated anatomy.[25] Diagnostic heat testing usually results in replication of the pain and corresponds to a diagnosis of symptomatic irreversible pulpitis.

Electric Pulp Testing

EPT is a useful adjunct. It is less accurate than cold testing and does not differentiate between normal pulp and that with a pulpitis. All electrical pulp testers are used in a similar manner. It is important to clean, dry, and isolate the teeth. The surface is scrubbed with a cotton roll, isolated with the same roll, and dried thoroughly with the air syringe. A small amount of toothpaste is placed on the electrode. The electrical circuit is completed by using a lip clip or having the patient touch the metal handle. The electrode is placed on the facial or lingual surface of enamel or dentin (Fig. 4.8), and the level of current is gradually increased until a response is reported by the patient.

Electric pulp testers cannot contact composites or metallic restorations, including crowns.

EPT produces a high-frequency electric current that creates ionic changes in dentinal fluid, which stimulates the Aδ fibers in the pulp.[26] Because it does not rely on the hydrodynamic fluid flow of the thermal tests, EPT may be more accurate with calcific

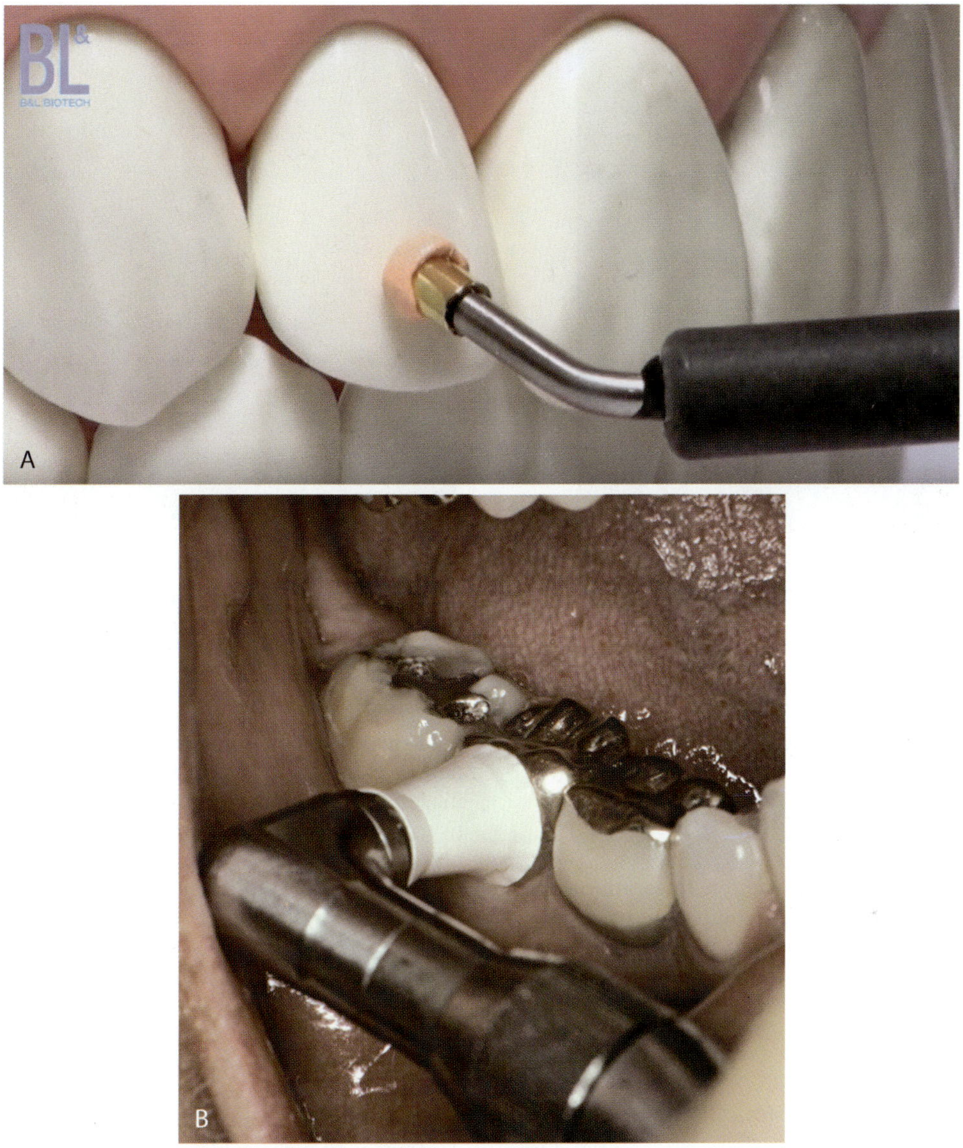

• **Fig. 4.7** A, Heated gutta-percha via a welled tip used with an obturation device (photo of welled System B tip courtesy B&L Biotech), and **B**, a prophy cup run at high speed produce controlled heat for pulp sensitivity testing.

metamorphosis.[22] High readings tend to indicate necrosis. Low readings indicate vitality. Testing normal control teeth establishes the approximate boundary between the two conditions. The exact number of the reading is of no significance and does not detect subtle degrees of vitality, nor can EPT indicate inflammation.[27]

Adjunctive Tests

Usually, this sequence of subjective and objective testing together with the radiographic examination will allow for accurate diagnosis. Occasionally, inconsistent findings will be found, or the question will remain as to whether endodontic pathosis is indeed present. Dentin stimulation (the stimulating of dentin without anesthesia) is often applied when traditional pulp sensitivity tests are inconclusive. A test cavity (or scratching exposed dentin or cementum) producing sensitivity is an indicator of pulp vitality. Several adjunctive means of examination are available, including caries removal, selective anesthesia, transillumination, and staining.

Caries Removal

Determination of the depth of caries is often necessary to make a definitive pulpal diagnosis, particularly in asymptomatic cases with deep decay as seen on a radiograph. A soft carious pulp exposure after complete excavation of caries, in an otherwise asymptomatic tooth with normal responses to clinical testing, is asymptomatic irreversible pulpitis.

Selective Anesthesia

The use of local anesthetic to selectively anesthetize and narrow the focus of pain can be especially helpful when a patient cannot identify the offending tooth. When aiming to determine whether a pain source is maxillary or mandibular in origin, the maxilla is generally anesthetized first using local infiltration. The technique should begin with anesthesia in the mesial most suspected location, working distally as needed to broaden the scope of anesthetized tissues. If maxillary teeth have been ruled out, then mandibular techniques, again moving mesially to distally, can be

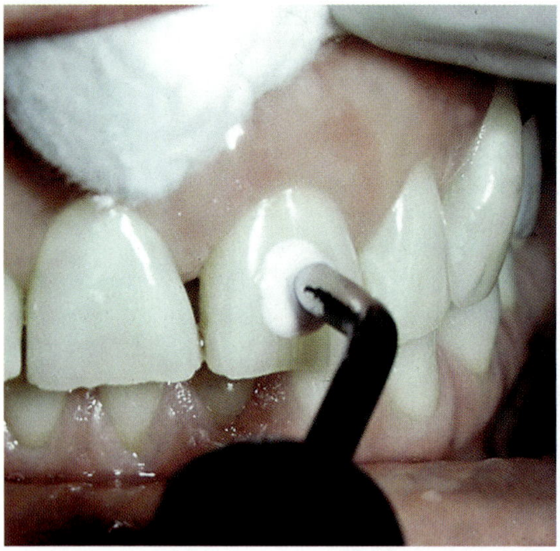

• **Fig. 4.8** The tooth surface is carefully scrubbed, dried, and isolated. A small spot of conductive medium is placed on the electrode, which is applied to tooth structure.

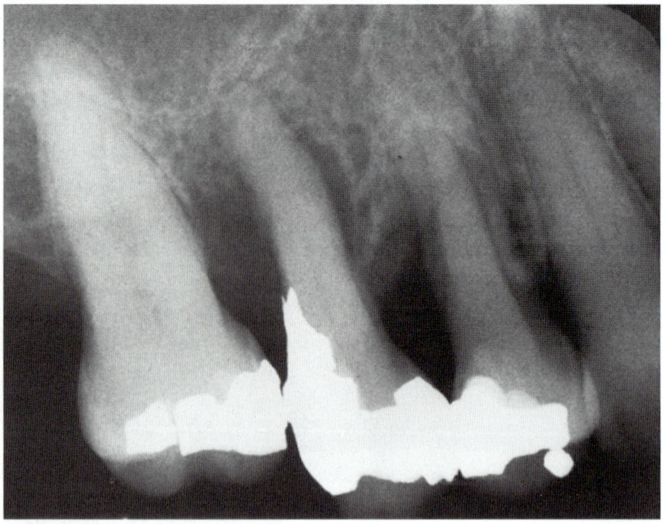

• **Fig. 4.9** Horizontal, as well as vertical, bone loss is evident in this quadrant. All teeth are responsive to vitality tests; therefore the resorptive defects represent a severe periodontal condition and not pulp or apical pathosis. Root canal treatment is not indicated.

used, with administration of block anesthesia as the last line in the anesthesia of posterior mandibular teeth. Periodontal ligament (PDL) injections will often anesthetize several teeth and are not considered useful for this purpose.[28]

Radiographic Examination

Radiographs detect carious lesions, defective restorations, previous root canal treatments, abnormal pulpal and periapical appearances, impacted teeth, the relationship among teeth and the adjacent neurovascular bundle and maxillary sinuses, and bone loss from periodontal disease. They may also reveal structural changes and bony disease unrelated to the pulp (Fig. 4.9).

Selection of Appropriate Imaging Modality

A high-quality, properly aligned periapical image is essential. Bitewing radiographs are helpful in the determination of bone heights when considering restorability and when evaluating for caries depth, restoration integrity, occlusion, and periodontal health.

Although not yet the standard of care, CBCT imaging has increasingly become routine. CBCT imaging eliminates the anatomic noise that limits two-dimensional imaging,[29] particularly in areas of structural overlap, such as the maxillary posterior.[30] CBCT images can detect periapical pathosis in an earlier stage of disease than can two-dimensional imaging techniques[31] (see Chapter 3). As extraoral images, they can be readily used when otherwise limited by oral structures or a prominent gag reflex. CBCT imaging does, however, have disadvantages, including increased radiation exposure, as well as cost and availability. Images require a longer duration of time that a patient must be still, which can itself be a limiting factor.

CBCT imaging should be considered as an aid in difficult diagnoses, such as when there are contradictory clinical signs and symptoms, as a treatment aid related to complex anatomy, in previously endodontically treated teeth to assess for untreated anatomy, in evaluating for prior treatment complications, in assessing potential surgical cases, and in the workup of cases of trauma or resorption.[32]

Periapical Lesions

Periapical inflammation results in bone resorption and the resultant periapical radiolucency. Although small radiolucent lesions may be present with irreversible pulpitis, especially with the sensitive images of CBCT, a sizable radiolucency with a vital pulp is not endodontic. It is impossible to determine whether a lesion is cystic by radiographs alone; rather, surgical access, biopsy, and histologic analysis are necessary for identifying the true nature of pathosis.[33-38]

Periapical lesions of endodontic origin generally have the following four radiographic characteristics:

1. The lamina dura is absent apically.
2. The radiolucency remains at the apex in radiographs made at different cone angles, as well as on CBCT imaging.
3. The radiolucency resembles a hanging drop.
4. There is an identifiable etiology that caused the pulpal necrosis.

Radiopaque changes can also occur.[35-38] Condensing osteitis is a reaction to pulpal or periapical inflammation and results in adjacent increased density of trabecular bone,[39] presenting as a diffuse circumferential medullary pattern with indistinct borders (Fig. 4.10). It is differentiated from the well-circumscribed, more homogeneous enostosis or sclerotic bone commonly found in the mandibular posterior region, and other nonendodontic radiopacities associated with the roots of teeth with normal pulp tissue.

Radiographs are often the only means to detect root resorption. External root resorption, including apical, lateral, and invasive cervical forms, can be detected by changes in root size and shape. CBCT imaging is essential to determine the nature and location these lesions.

Pulpal Lesions

Careful visualization of the pulpal space allows for detection of pathologic and nonpathologic conditions. Extensive diffuse calcification in the chamber, or pulp canal obliteration, may indicate long-term, low-grade irritation related to deep restorative treatment or trauma and is not usually pathologic.[40] Pulp stones are discrete calcified bodies found in pulp chambers and are sometimes visible

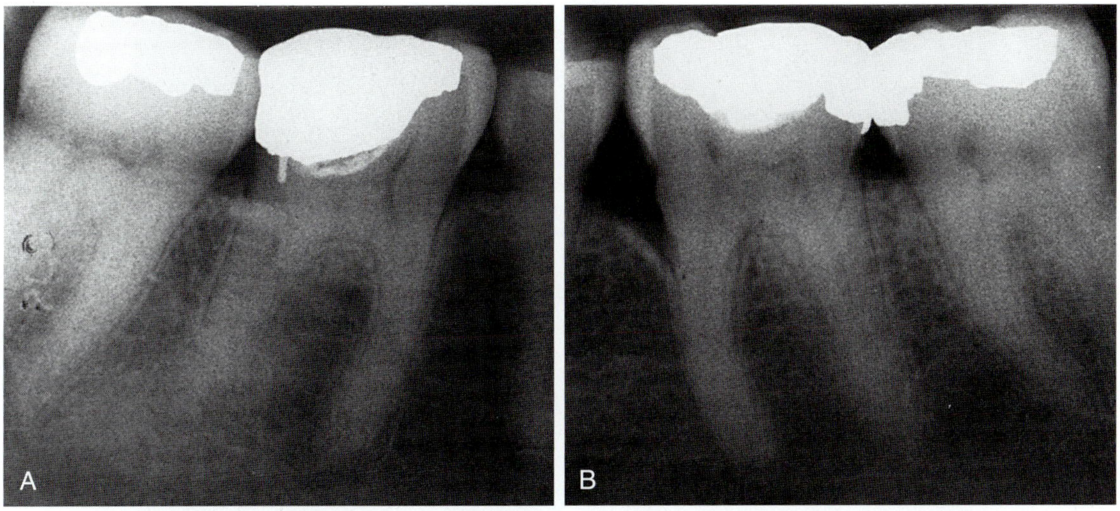

• **Fig. 4.10** Condensing Osteitis. **A,** Surrounding the distal root apex is diffuse trabeculation. **B,** This contrasts with the contralateral molar, which demonstrates a normal, sparse trabecular pattern.

on radiographs. They are not considered pathologic, but they have been associated with cardiovascular disease,[41] gout, hypercalcemia, end-stage renal disease,[42] dentinogenesis imperfecta,[43] and certain medications, including statins[44] and corticosteroids.[45]

Internal root resorption is an abnormally altered pulp space enlargement due to localized pulpal inflammation with resultant dentinoclastic activity,[46,47] (Fig. 4.11). As in external resorption, CBCT imaging can determine the location and extent of these lesions.

Study Questions

1. A patient history should include which of the following?
   a. Chief complaint
   b. Past dental history
   c. Medical history
   d. Social history
   e. A, B, and C
2. A visible sinus tract usually indicates…
   a. Endodontic–periodontic pathosis
   b. Resorption
   c. Chronic apical abscess
   d. Sinus infection
   e. Cracked tooth
3. No response to cold testing indicates pulpal necrosis…
   a. Always
   b. Sometimes
   c. Never
4. CBCT imaging is the standard of care for identifying suspected longitudinal fractures.
   a. True
   b. False
5. Pulp stones indicate endodontic pathosis.
   a. True
   b. False

Diagnosis

Developing a Diagnosis

Endodontic pathosis is never without a cause (Fig. 4.12) and is usually dental in origin. Rarely, expansive tumors of the jaw can occur with resultant pulpal pathosis. Spontaneous pulpal necrosis has been reported due to sickle cell anemia[48,49] or zoster.[49]

Endodontic pathosis is often discovered incidentally on routine examinations. Pulpal or periapical pathosis is frequently without marked signs and symptoms at time of examination or in the past[50]; thus, the development of associated periapical pathosis may also go unnoticed by the patient. A detailed discussion of nonendodontic sources of pain and pathology can be found in Chapter 5 (Fig. 4.13).

In the development of any diagnosis, it is helpful when subjective and objective findings are consistent. Whenever inconsistencies are encountered, additional testing modalities can be used, including the use of the adjunctive tests like selective anesthesia described in the earlier section titled Adjunctive Tests. Analgesics, such as ibuprofen, have been shown to affect the results of cold, percussion, and palpation testing[51]; thus, retesting on another date might allow for more reliable results. Referral to a specialist who has additional testing and imaging modalities, not to mention experience in elucidating the difficult diagnosis, should be considered.

Endodontic Terminology

A limited number of possible diagnoses exist for pulp and periapical conditions.[52] The pathosis of these conditions is described in Chapter 1.

Pulpal Diagnosis

Normal or Reversible Pulpitis

Generally, normal responses to pulp sensitivity testing compared with control teeth indicate a healthy, vital pulp. Slight hypersensitivity to cold can occur in cases of reversible pulpitis, and these cases will resolve with removal of the causative irritant.

Asymptomatic Irreversible Pulpitis

A carious exposure will cause inflammatory changes to the adjacent pulp, often without symptoms or aberrant clinical testing. Novel techniques propose vital pulp therapy using calcium silicate–based materials such as mineral trioxide aggregate (MTA) as a viable means of definitive treatment as discussed in Chapter 10; however, root canal therapy or extraction may be warranted depending on the extent of inflammation observed at the time of treatment, or due to developing pathosis down the line.

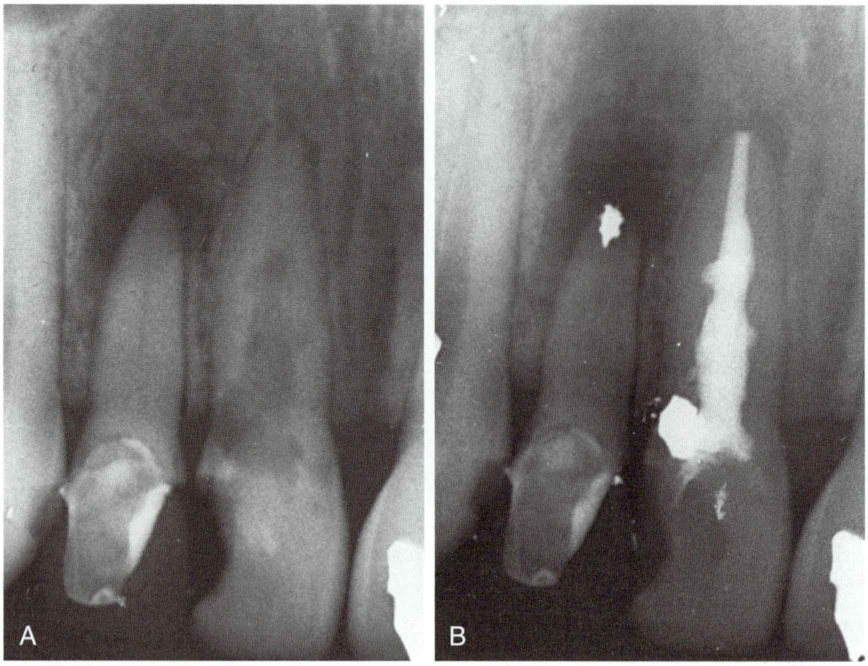

• **Fig. 4.11** Differing Pulp Responses to Injury. **A,** Central incisor shows extensive, perforating internal resorption; the lateral incisor has calcific metamorphosis. **B,** Special techniques manage these problems with both surgical and nonsurgical treatment.

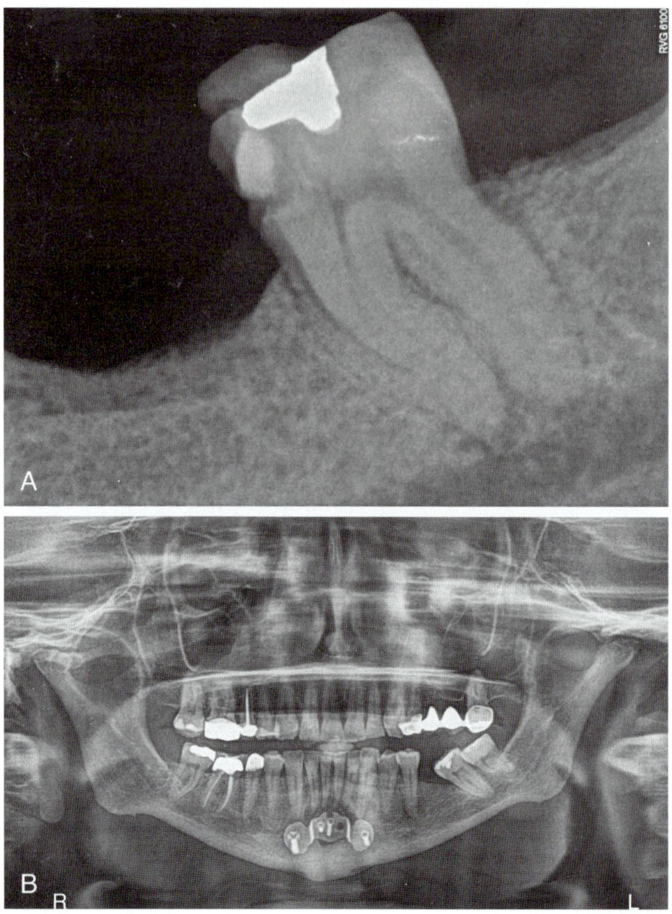

• **Fig. 4.12** Common and Uncommon Etiologies of Endodontic Pathology. A combination of recurrent caries and fracture led to endodontic pathosis in #18 **(A)**. A failing chin implant with associated abscess damaged the blood supply and led to pulpal necrosis in the mandibular anterior teeth **(B)**.

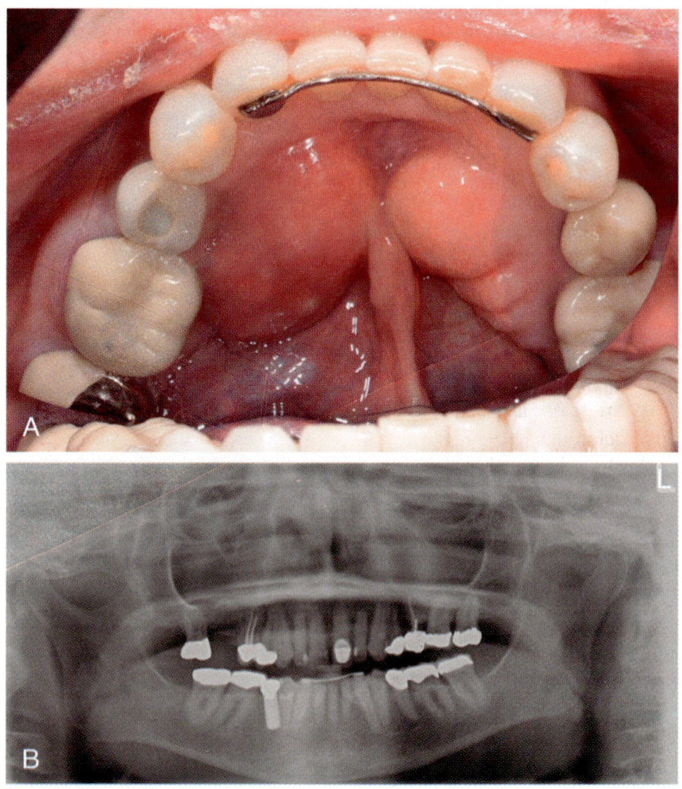

• **Fig. 4.13** A and **B,** A case of an infected torus mimicking endodontic pathology. (Courtesy Dr. Michael Melkers.)

Symptomatic Irreversible Pulpitis

Painful pulpitis should correspond to replicable symptoms on clinical testing. Typically, cold testing results in a heightened and lingering response. Heat testing will mimic presenting symptoms. Root canal therapy or extraction is indicated.

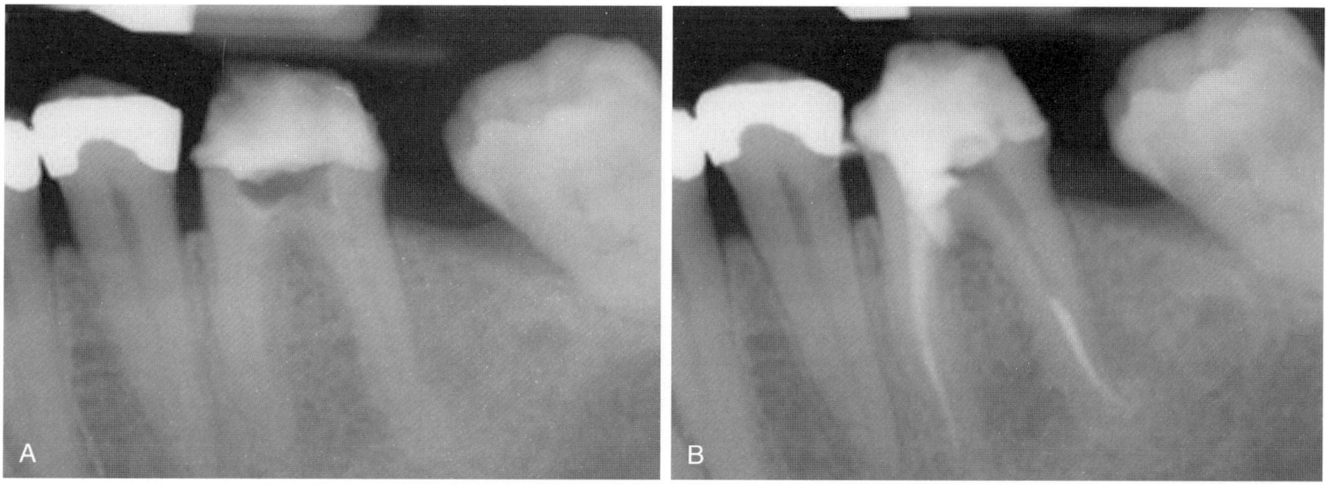

• **Fig. 4.14** A and **B,** Before referral, a furcal perforation occurred in this case of previously initiated treatment, necessitating perforation repair with mineral trioxide aggregate before definitive root canal therapy.

Necrosis

Though pain associated with periapical pathosis may be present, the necrotic pulp is typically nonpainful and nonresponsive to pulp sensitivity testing. Root canal therapy or extraction is indicated.

Previously Initiated Treatment

Evidence of endodontic access, either by pulpotomy or pulpectomy, requires definitive care. Intracanal medicaments may be in place. Assessment should be made as to the extent of prior treatment and any anatomic alterations or procedural errors that might require additional treatment or affect the prognosis. Definitive treatment includes root canal therapy or extraction (Fig. 4.14).

Previously Treated

This circumstance represents previous treatment with placement of some sort of obturation material. Included are nonsurgical or surgical root canal retreatment. As to management, the choice between nonsurgical and surgical root canal retreatment depends on many factors involving the restoration and accessibility to remove prior obturation material in an orthograde fashion, feasibility of surgical access, patient preference, and provider preference related to the reasons for failure. The prognosis depends on whether the etiology of failure can be identified, and whether deficiencies in prior treatment can be corrected. Extraction is an alternative. For example, previously treated teeth with failure due to VRF will have a hopeless prognosis and should be considered for extraction or root removal. These cases of failed treatment are complex and should be considered for referral.

Periapical Diagnosis

Normal

Normal periapical tissues are associated with teeth with either normal pulps, or those with pulpal disease. No periodontal ligament-mediated symptoms, such as percussion, palpation, or bite sensitivity are expected, and radiographic changes are absent

Symptomatic Apical Periodontitis

Inflamed or necrotic pulp tissue will usually result in periapical inflammation that may present with pain on pressure. When confined to bone, the diagnosis is symptomatic apical periodontitis. Clinical tests will result in replicable sensitivity to percussion, palpation, or bite testing, though neither swelling nor signs of drainage will be present. Radiographic findings may be present or absent. Root canal therapy or extraction is indicated.

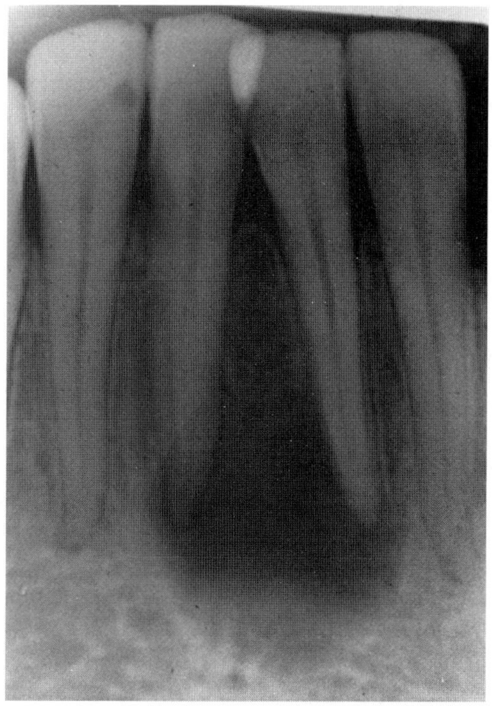

• **Fig. 4.15** Because of its size, this lesion is likely to be an apical radicular cyst. The lesion is related to pulp necrosis in the left central incisor. Although superimposed over the apex of the adjacent incisor, the pulp is not affected and therefore does not require treatment. Proper root canal treatment of the left incisor would lead to resolution without surgery.

Asymptomatic Apical Periodontitis

Pain does not always accompany periapical inflammation. When radiographic signs of periapical disease are present, but clinical findings are unremarkable in regard to percussion, palpation, and bite testing, the diagnosis is asymptomatic apical periodontitis. Though emergency treatment is not required, definitive management includes root canal therapy or extraction. The size of the lesion seen on radiograph is of little concern. Lesions of different sizes will usually heal after appropriate treatment (Fig. 4.15). However, the mere presence of a radiographic apical lesion results in a reduced prognosis.[52a]

Acute Apical Abscess

When swelling is present, regardless of size, the diagnosis is acute apical abscess. The basic treatment is similar, with the addition that drainage of the abscess is attempted either through the tooth or by incision of the soft tissue. Occasionally, such drainage cannot be achieved, so resolution of symptoms is slow.

Chronic Apical Abscess

When drainage of an abscess is via a sinus tract, the diagnosis is chronic apical abscess. Confirmation of the source of the sinus tract may be facilitated via gutta percha tracing or CBCT imaging. The treatment for chronic apical abscess is the same as for the previous diagnoses except that drainage has already been established naturally. The sinus tract requires no treatment and resolves after appropriate débridement and obturation.

Condensing Osteitis

As described radiographically, condensing osteitis is an inflammatory reaction in the periapical bone secondary to pulpal or periapical pathosis. This entity requires no special treatment. Because it occurs with different pulp conditions, treatment will vary. Condensing osteitis resolves in approximately 50% of teeth after *successful* root canal treatment.[53] Because there is no apparent problem if the condensing osteitis does *not* resolve, no further treatment is required unless there are other findings suggestive of failure.

Adjuncts to the Endodontic Diagnosis

Certain disease entities can coexist with pulpal and periapical diagnoses that can modify their presentations and therefore treatment. These adjunctive diagnoses include longitudinal fractures, trauma, resorption, and endodontic–periodontic pathosis.

Longitudinal Fractures

These fractures represent diagnostic and treatment challenges. Fractures present with a variety of signs, symptoms, and radiographic changes that require a careful differential diagnosis and accurate classification for appropriate management. Clinicians must determine the extent and nature of the fracture to decide whether a restoration should be placed, or if root canal therapy or even extraction is indicated.[54] Crack detection is one aspect of a thorough evaluation, but the presence of a crack alone does not provide information on the status of the pulp or periapical tissues; other tests and findings will determine a diagnosis. Because of their complex nature in terms of identification, diagnosis, and management, referral should be considered.

Some teeth with fractures can be managed and saved; others cannot. The key factors are knowing:

1. How to identify and classify cracks
2. The characteristic signs and symptoms of each
3. How to detect the crack early in development, if possible

Diagnosis of Longitudinal Fractures

If a fracture is suspected, several steps are taken. These steps include obtaining a chief complaint and subjective history, followed by objective testing, probing, clinical and radiographic examination, restoration removal, transillumination, wedging forces, and possibly staining, or a surgical assessment if VRF is suspected.

Transillumination can be a useful aid because visualization of the full extension of a crack or fracture is difficult with the naked eye. A fracture line will not transmit light.[55,56] Shining a fiber-optic light will illuminate the proximal portion of the tooth, whereas the distal portion of the tooth will remain dark (Fig. 4.16).

Beyond transillumination, *staining* with methylene blue, iodine, or caries-detection dyes may also disclose fracture lines.[56] A cotton pellet soaked with dye is placed against the fractured tooth structure. The dye is then washed away, revealing the extent of the crack (Fig. 4.17). Improved visualization is enhanced by combining dyes and magnification via loupes or a surgical operating microscope.

Longitudinal Fracture Types[57]

The term *longitudinal* is used because it describes the vertical extensions of fractures that tend to grow and change over distance and time. Longitudinal fractures can further be divided into (1) craze lines; (2) fractured cusp; (3) cracked tooth; (4) split tooth; and (5) VRF. The first four types initiate from the occlusal, are primarily mesial-distal in orientation, and extend in a cervical/apical direction with time. VRFs are very different, as they initiate and are confined to the root and are facial-lingual.

Craze lines affect only the enamel, whereas other types involve other hard and soft tissues. The deeper fractures are a pathway for bacterial penetration, sometimes very deep, resulting in pulpal, periapical, and often periodontal pathosis. Because fractures are difficult or impossible to visualize on initial examination, their diagnosis may be confused with other etiologies. If the fracture has extended to the pulp, there may be signs and symptoms of pulp and periapical pathosis; thus, a careful and systematic differential diagnostic procedure is necessary.

Classification of Fracture Types

Craze Lines

Most adult teeth have craze lines. In posterior teeth, craze lines are common and usually evident crossing marginal ridges or extending along buccal and lingual surfaces. Long vertical craze lines commonly appear on anterior teeth. Craze lines affect only the enamel, are not symptomatic, and require no treatment.[58] Craze lines may be confused with cracks, which are more extensive, but can be differentiated by transillumination. If the fracture is confined to enamel, the light passes through. If in dentin, the light is blocked because of the dentinal crack.

Fractured Cusp

This fracture is a complete or incomplete fracture initiated from the crown and extending subgingivally, usually directed mesiodistal or buccolingual. A single cusp or both cusps may be involved. Cusp fractures are more likely to occur in teeth with extensive caries or restorations undermining cusps.[59] Treatment depends on the findings. If the fracture is complete (reaches surfaces in all directions), the fractured segment must be removed. Root canal treatment or vital pulp therapy is necessary if the pulp has been exposed, creating an irreversible pulpitis. If the fracture is incomplete, the tooth must be restored with preferably a full cast crown to hopefully stop the progression of the fracture.

Cracked Tooth

In this case, an incomplete fracture (meaning it does not reach a surface in all areas) initiates from the crown and extends

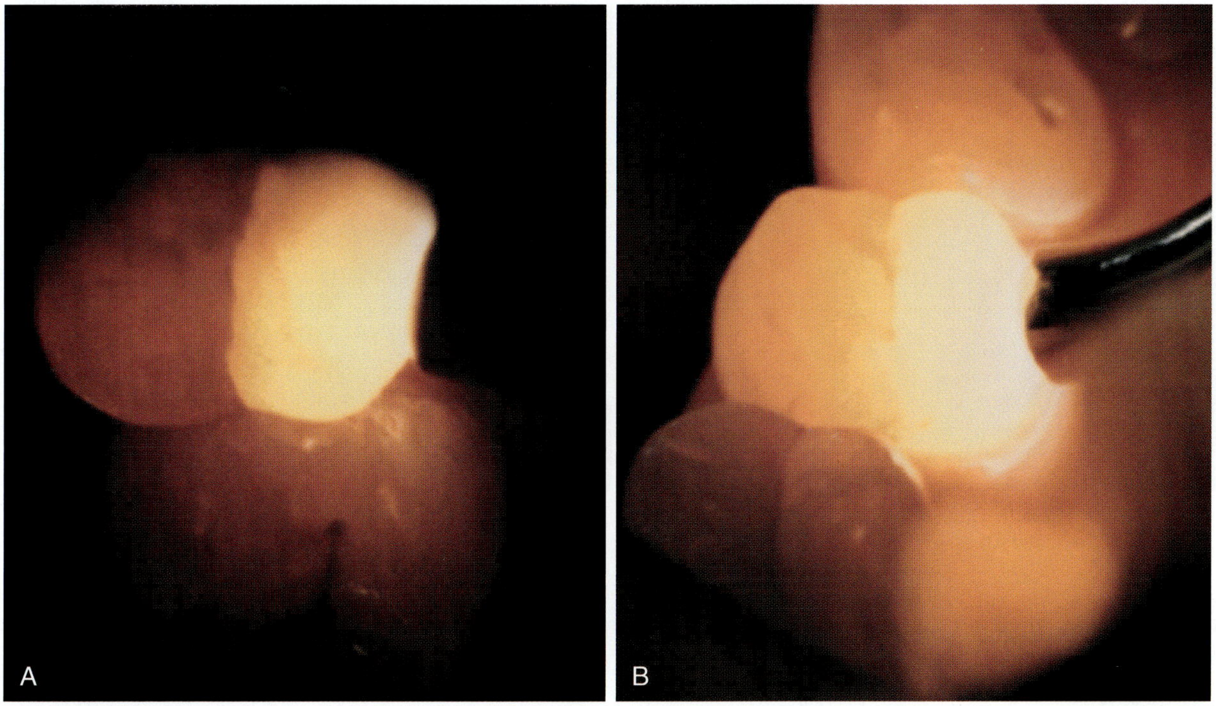

• **Fig. 4.16** Cracked Tooth. **A,** Fracture through dentin reflects transilluminated light showing abrupt change in brightness. **B,** For comparison, an adjacent noncracked premolar with a craze line transmits light readily.

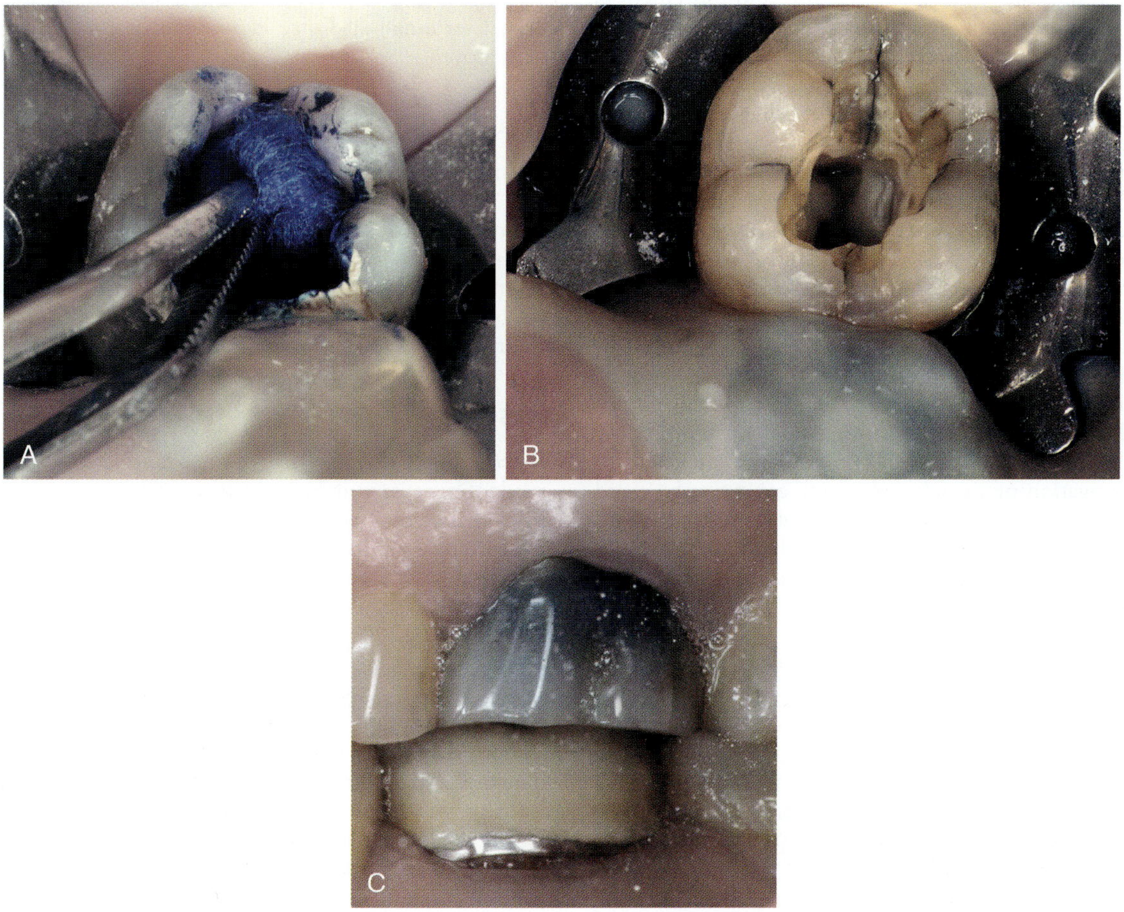

• **Fig. 4.17** **A,** Disclosing solution on a cotton pellet (in this case, methylene blue) is placed in the cavity for a few minutes or sealed in for a week. **B,** This technique may clearly disclose the fracture and its extent. **C**, Staining solutions may discolor the tooth.

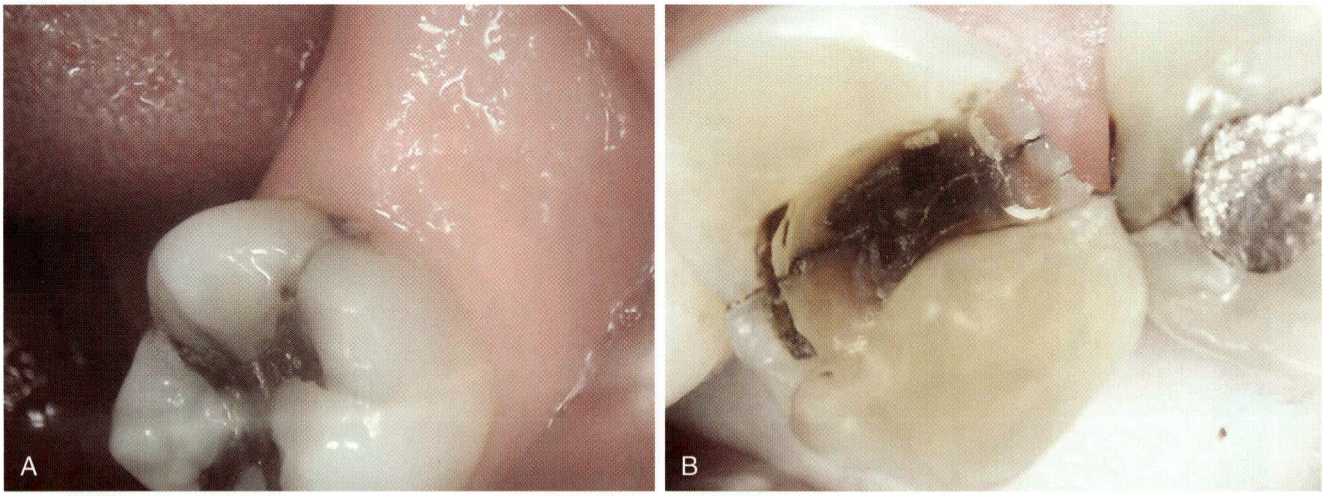

• **Fig. 4.18** Cracks may be seen visually on coronal structure **(A)**, or sometimes once a restoration is removed **(B)**.

subgingivally and mesio-distally (Fig. 4.18). The fracture may extend through either or both marginal ridges and down the proximal root surface. This fracture is more centered and is more likely to expose the pulp than a cusp fracture would. If there is a restoration, it should be removed for visualization. If a crack is detected, wedging determines the degree of separation of segments: little or no separation indicates incomplete fracture, and movement is more likely to be split tooth. Treatment will vary depending on the location and extent of the crack. Root canal treatment may be indicated based on signs and symptoms, as well as results of clinical testing, and is often successful.[60] It usually involves access preparation for better visualization. If the fracture extends to the floor or into a canal, and there is a deep probing defect, the prognosis is poor and the tooth should be extracted. At best, the prognosis is always questionable, as the fracture may continue to propagate. However, with cracks presenting with a vital pulp, the chance of success is considerably improved.[61]

Split Tooth

The split tooth is the result of a fracture that reaches all surfaces; the tooth is in two separate segments. A split tooth is an extension and end result of a cracked tooth. The split may occur suddenly after a traumatic biting incident but is more likely the result of long-term propagation of a crack. Split teeth can never be saved intact; if the fracture extends beyond the cervical third, the tooth must be extracted. The tooth may be saved if the fracture is more cervical; the smaller segment is removed, and the remainder of the tooth salvaged.

Vertical Root Fracture[62]

This type is a complete or incomplete facial-lingual fracture initiated on the root at any level. It extends to the PDL and causes considerable soft- and hard-tissue damage to the surrounding periodontium due to bacteria within the fracture and canal space.[63] Patients generally have minimal signs and symptoms. The VRF may mimic other conditions, commonly periodontal disease or failed root canal treatment. The tooth will have a history of root canal treatment and often is restored with a post; both create significant internal wedging forces. Some teeth have normal probing patterns; however, most have deep defects in narrow or rectangular patterns.[7] Radiographic evidence varies; only rarely will there be visible separation of the segments. Commonly, lesions are J-shaped and extend from apical to lateral surfaces. CBCT is not a good diagnostic tool for visualizing the fracture but will show the presence and shape of the bony lesion (Fig. 4.19). Signs, symptoms, tests, and probing patterns are not definitive in identifying a VRF. Flap reflection and visualization of the fracture, accompanied by a punched-out bony defect, has shown to be the best determinant.[64] Once identified, the tooth or the root must be removed.

Trauma

Traumatic injuries, including fractures of the crown and root, as well as luxation-type injuries and avulsions, require careful management. Pulpal and periapical pathosis will often develop related to the injuries. Evidence-based protocols related to the type and extent of injury exist.[65] These protocols are defined distinctly, in addition to the endodontic diagnosis. A detailed discussion of traumatic dental injuries and their management is in Chapter 11.

Resorption

Resorption of dental structures occurs due to lost unmineralized predentin or precementum, allowing for invasion of inflammation-mediated odontoclastic-type cells.[46] The presentation and effects of the varying types of resorption are heterogenous. Resorption occurs in a variety of forms, with multifaceted clinical and radiographic presentations, and even more varied management options (Fig. 4.20).

Internal Root Resorption

Inflammatory root resorption (IRR) is a combination of loss or damaged predentin along with adjacent pulpal inflammation. Usually, pulpal injury due to dental trauma, restorative dentistry without adequate coolant, pulp cap or pulpotomy occurs with resultant damage to the predentin, as well as localized coronal pulp necrosis. This damage leads to an inflammatory cascade in the adjacent pulp tissue, with resultant clastic activity to the surrounding chamber wall.[46,66] The resorption will arrest once complete pulp necrosis occurs.[67]

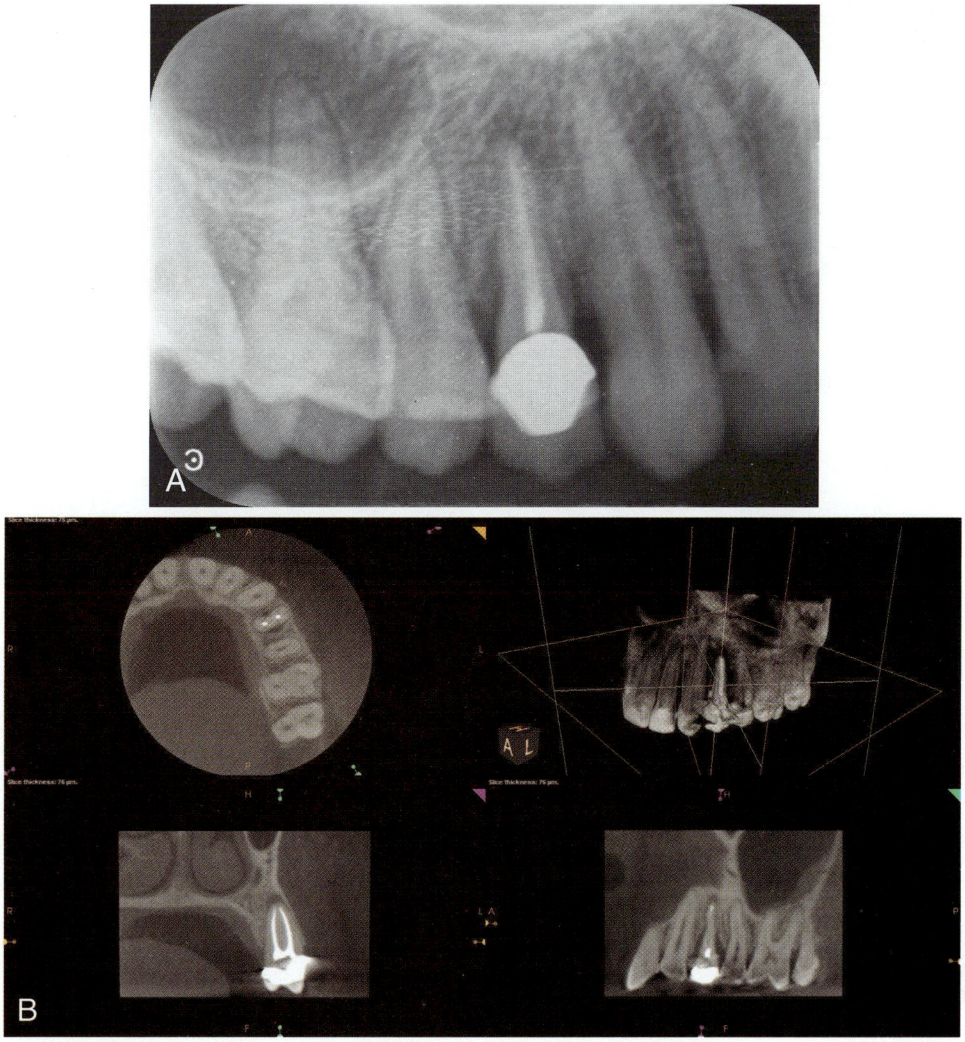

• **Fig. 4.19** The typical findings of a vertical root fracture seen on digital **(A)** and cone beam computed tomography (CBCT) **(B)** imaging.

IRR usually presents as a symmetric radiolucency continuous with the pulp space or a clinically enlarged pulp chamber.[67] Treatment of IRR involves removal of the pulp tissue to arrest the resorptive process. The prognosis for treatment is excellent if the lesions are nonperforating and is reduced when perforation is present.[68]

External Root Resorption

External root resorption involves loss or damage to the precementum with inflammation of the adjacent PDL.[46] It can present as external inflammatory root resorption (EIRR) either apically due to pulpally mediated periapical inflammation or laterally due to extensive luxation-type or avulsive traumatic dental injuries. The presentation includes a radiographically irregular or mottled appearance to the outside border of the root. Apical EIRR responds well to root canal therapy,[69] whereas the prognosis for lateral EIRR depends on the extent of root surface involved.[70] Extensive lateral EIRR can progress to replacement resorption, or ankylosis (fusion of dentin and bone) once bone directly contacts root surface, with progressive, irreversible loss of root structure.[70] Further discussion of lateral EIRR and replacement resorption secondary to traumatic dental injuries can be found in Chapter 11.

External root resorption may also take the form of pressure resorption. Pressure resorption occurs due to direct damage to the cementum by orthodontic tooth movement,[71] misaligned tooth eruption, or slow-growing jaw tumors or cysts.[46] Removal of the orthodontic forces or inciting adjacent pathology will result in immediate arrest of the process, though its damage to root structure is irreversible.

Invasive Cervical Root Resorption

Invasive cervical root resorption (ICRR) is a distinct type of resorption. It occurs due to either loss of precementum or a development gap between cementum and enamel, as well as inflamed junctional epithelium at the base of the periodontal sulcus.[72] Though no definitive causes have been established, several associated factors exist, including orthodontics, trauma, intracoronal restorations, nonvital bleaching, dentoalveolar surgery, periodontal therapy,[73] herpes viruses,[74] and potentially medications, including bisphosphonates.[75] ICRR is often found incidentally on radiographs as it is commonly asymptomatic, and its subgingival location renders clinical detection difficult. Because the predentin surrounding the pulp can act as a barrier for invasion of the resorptive process unless secondary caries develops, the pulp is usually unaffected

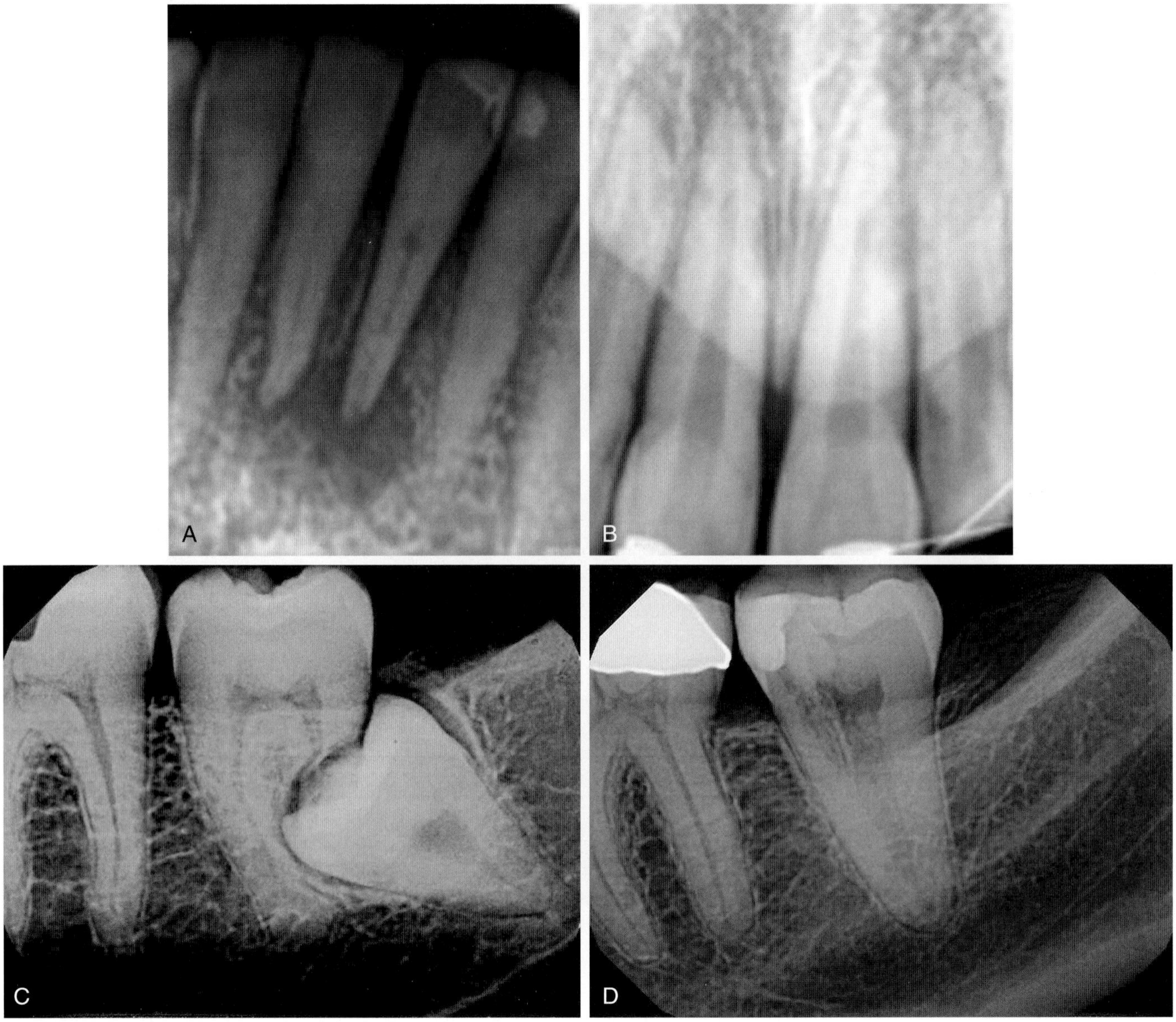

• **Fig. 4.20** The varying presentations of pathological root resorption, including internal **(A)**, apical external inflammatory root resorption **(B)**, pressure resorption **(C)**, and invasive cervical root resorption **(D)**.

until very late stages of disease.[72] Unless epithelial downgrowth occurs, a form of bony replacement can even occur, serving as a means of protection from periodontal pocketing and abscess formation.[76] Lesions are classified according to their size and extent[72] (Fig. 4.21). Class 1 lesions are small and localized to the cervical. Class 2 lesions are still localized but approach the pulp tissue. Class 3 lesions begin to invade into the coronal one third of the root. Class 4 lesions extend beyond the coronal one third of the root.

In early lesions, or when symptoms develop, treatment should involve surgical access, application of trichloroacetic acid to remove deep projections of vital resorbing tissue, and restoration, in addition to any additional endodontic and restorative treatment rendered necessary by the extension of the defect.[77] Extensive lesions involving root surface may be monitored as long as they are asymptomatic and not creating adjacent bony pathosis, though they may progress at any time to make treatment necessary.[72,76]

Endodontic–Periodontic Interrelationships

The pulp tissue and periodontium are connected through the apical foramen, lateral canals, and dentinal tubules. Pulpal diseases usually cause pathologic changes in the periodontium. Examination of pathogenesis of periapical lesions of pulpal origin and periodontitis shows that the mechanisms involved in both diseases are similar in nature.[78] The main differences between the two processes are their original source and the direction of their progression. Periapical lesions extend apically or coronally, whereas periodontal lesions tend to extend only apically. Because of their similarities, these lesions can mimic each other, and it is sometime difficult to make a proper diagnosis (Fig. 4.22). To arrive at the correct diagnosis and administer appropriate treatment, a systematic approach in obtaining information is required. Reliance on one test is a prelude to misdiagnosis and performing improper treatment. In general, periodontal disease is a chronic and generalized process that is associated with little or no significant pain. In contrast, pulpal and periapical lesions are localized conditions and are more likely to be associated with acute symptoms that require analgesics. However, chronic lesions of pulpal origin can cause periodontal defects that simulate periodontal disease.

Classification and Differential Diagnosis of Endodontic–Periodontic Lesions

Based on their origin, periodontal defects have been classified into three major categories.[79-81] These origins are either pulpal (endodontic) origin, periodontal origin, or endodontic–periodontic origin (true combined lesions) (Fig. 4.23). In very rare instances, long-standing primary defects of pulpal or periodontal origin can progress to secondary combined lesions.

Primary Periodontal Defects of Endodontic Origin

A periodontal defect of endodontic origin is usually associated with pulpal necrosis of at least one root (Fig. 4.24, *A*). The patient may or may not have any discomfort. Occasionally, there is a localized abscess with swelling. Radiographic examination reveals the presence of isolated periapical lesions. Pulp sensitivity tests show the absence of a response to thermal or electric stimuli. The involved tooth may or may not be sensitive to palpation or percussion sensitivity tests. Periodontal probing usually shows normal sulci around the tooth except in one area with a narrow defect. Placement of a gutta-percha cone or a periodontal probe in this sinus tract shows that the defect is deep, usually to the apex or possibly to the opening of a lateral canal. A periodontal defect of endodontic origin should be considered a coronally extended periapical lesion, which is initiated and perpetuated by the toxic materials in the root canal system (Fig. 4.24, *A*). This defect is not a true periodontal pocket, and adequate cleaning and shaping as well as obturation of the root canal system usually result in its complete resolution (Fig. 4.24, *B* and *C*). The defect does not usually require adjunctive periodontal treatment.[79-81]

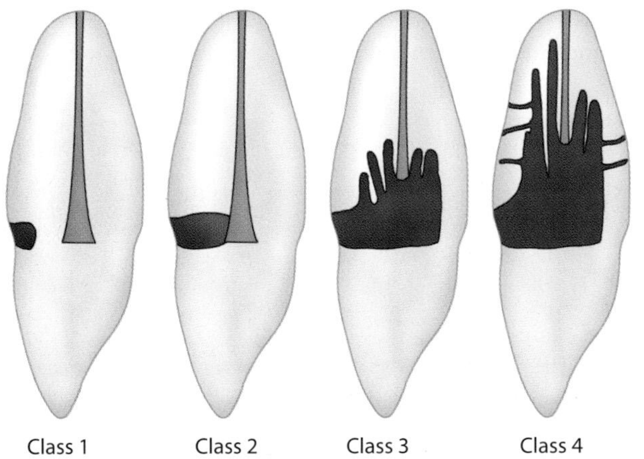

• **Fig. 4.21** Heithersay's classification of Invasive Cervical Root Resorption.[72] (Reprinted with permission from Blicher B, Lucier Pryles R, Lin J: *Endodontics review: a study guide*. Chicago, 2016, Quintessence.)

Primary Periodontal Defects

A periodontal defect of periodontal origin is usually associated with generalized gingivitis and/or periodontitis resulting from the accumulation of plaque and/or calculus formation. Except in cases of acute periodontal abscesses, patients usually have no significant symptoms. The affected tooth may or may not have extensive restorative procedures and is often associated with varying degrees of mobility. Radiographic examination of the involved tooth and its adjacent teeth shows the presence of generalized vertical and horizontal bone loss along the root surfaces (Fig. 4.25). Teeth with these defects respond within normal limits to pulp sensitivity testing. Unlike the lesions of pulpal origin, defects of periodontal origin are wide and V-shaped.[83] When probing, the crest is within normal limits. Then, in a "step-down" fashion, the probe reaches deeper. The pocket depth decreases in a "step-up" manner and reaches the normal depth on the other side of the pocket.[79] Because these defects are not of endodontic origin, root canal treatment will not result in their resolution. Only periodontal treatment is indicated.

Primary Periodontal Defects of Endodontic–Periodontic Origin (True Combined Lesions)

These defects have two concurrent components and occur less often than the previous two types. One component is an independent periapical lesion originating from a necrotic pulp. The other component is an independent periodontal lesion that has progressed apically toward the periapical lesion (Fig. 4.26, *A*). Depending on their stage of development, the lesions may or may not communicate with one another. A true combined defect is usually associated with clinical signs and symptoms of generalized

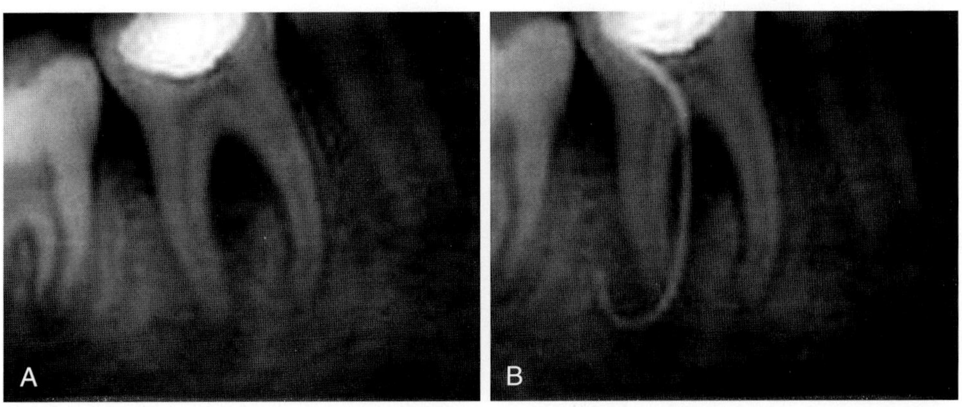

• **Fig. 4.22** **A**, Pulpal necrosis has caused development of a large lesion extending along the mesial aspect of the distal root and furcation of the first mandibular right molar. **B**, Sinus tract exploration using a gutta-percha cone shows that the lesion communicates with the oral cavity via a narrow defect on the buccal aspect of this tooth.

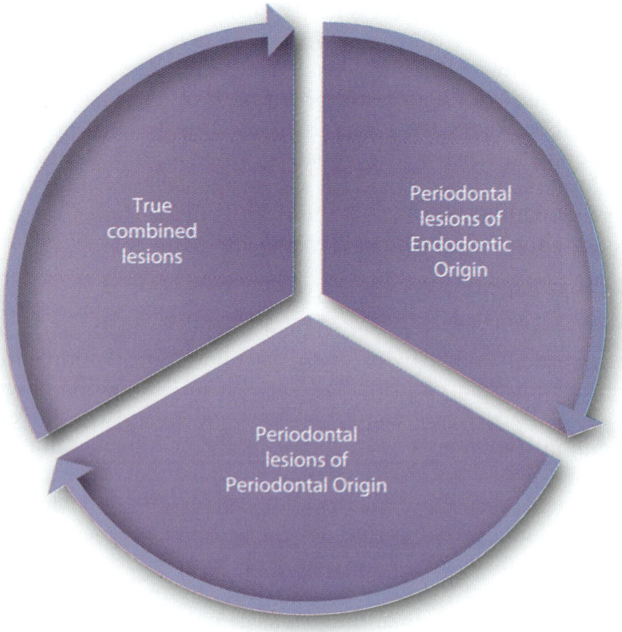

• **Fig. 4.23** Classifications of periodontal lesions by origin.

gingivitis and/or periodontitis with little or no discomfort. The affected tooth may or may not have had extensive operative procedures and is often mobile. Radiographically, the involved tooth and its adjacent teeth may show the presence of generalized vertical and horizontal bone loss along the root surfaces and periapical lesions isolated to that tooth. A tooth with true combined lesions is unresponsive to cold, heat, electric stimuli, or cavity tests. Periodontal examinations and probing of a tooth with a combined lesion reveal the presence of plaque, calculus, periodontitis, and wide and conical periodontal pockets characteristic of defects of periodontal disease origin. Treatment of true combined lesions consists of endodontic and periodontal treatments (Fig. 4.26, *B*). The overall prognosis of the affected tooth depends on the prognosis of each individual lesion. Generally, however, the prognosis of such advanced conditions is guarded.

Treatment Planning

Planning and delivery of care follow the definitive diagnosis of endodontic pathosis. As discussed, certain diagnoses will not require endodontic treatment. The diagnosis of reversible pulpitis should be addressed by whatever means will remove or reverse the inciting stimulus of inflammation, with expected resolution. Irreversible pulpitis, whether symptomatic or asymptomatic, and pulpal necrosis, should be considered for endodontic care. Previously initiated teeth will require definitive endodontic care or extraction, and previously endodontically treated teeth with associated

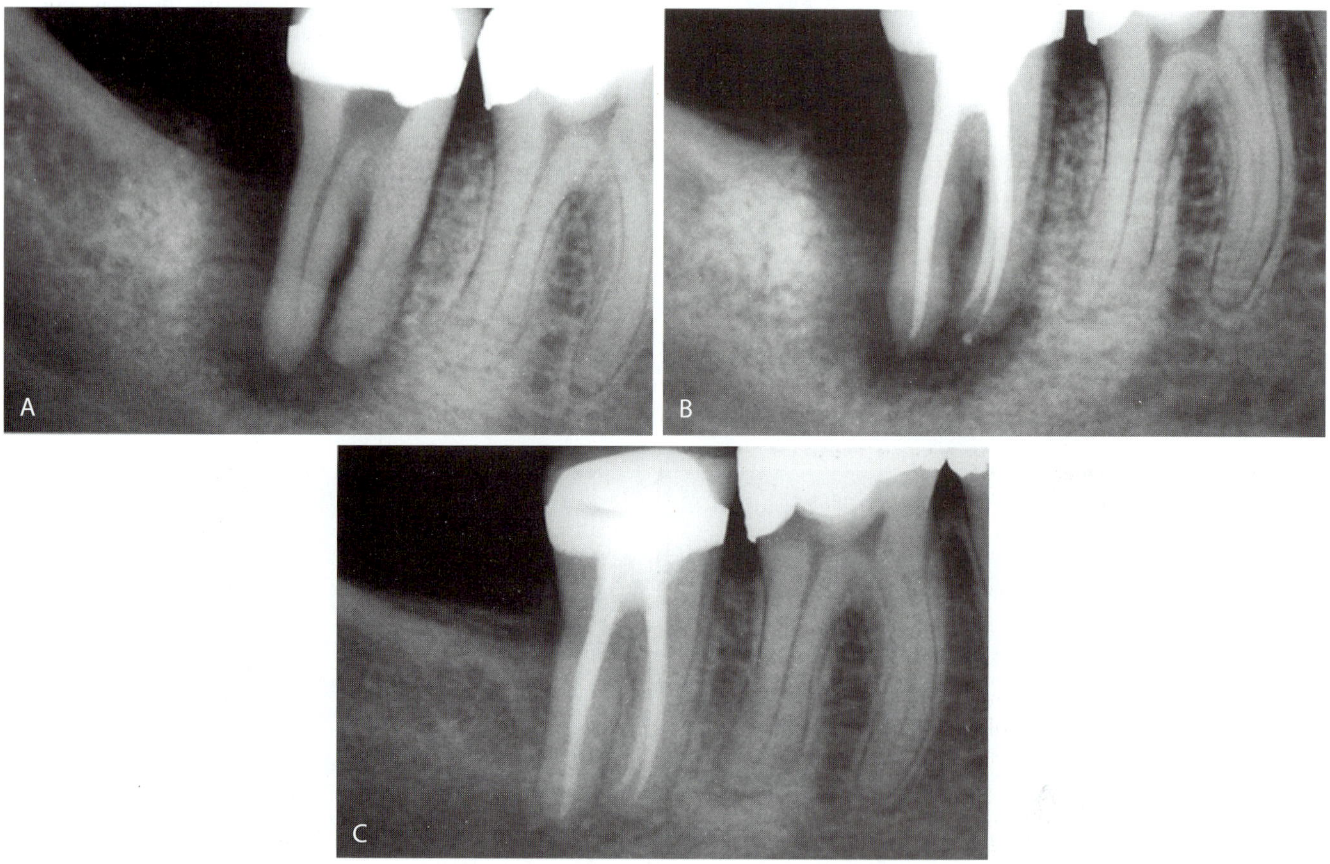

• **Fig. 4.24** **A,** Preoperative radiograph indicates bone loss from the crest of the ridge around the apices of the tooth. **B,** Root canal treatment completed. **C,** Four-year recall shows resolution of the radiolucency. (Reprinted from Harrington GW and Steiner DR, In Walton RE and Torabinejad M, *Principles and practice of endodontics,* ed 3, 2002:477.[82])

periapical pathosis require surgical or nonsurgical retreatment. Of course, all cases should be subject to a proper informed consent process, including discussions related to restorability, prognosis, treatment alternatives, and the strategic value of the tooth in the overall treatment plan.

Phasing Treatment

The diagnosis of endodontic pathosis can have a variety of presentations, and the urgency of treatment often follows. Patients presenting with pain and/or swelling require treatment sooner than those with incidental findings of endodontic disease.

Emergency Treatment

Endodontic emergencies are a special category and require skill in diagnosis, treatment planning, pharmacotherapeutics, anesthesia, and patient management (see Chapter 9).

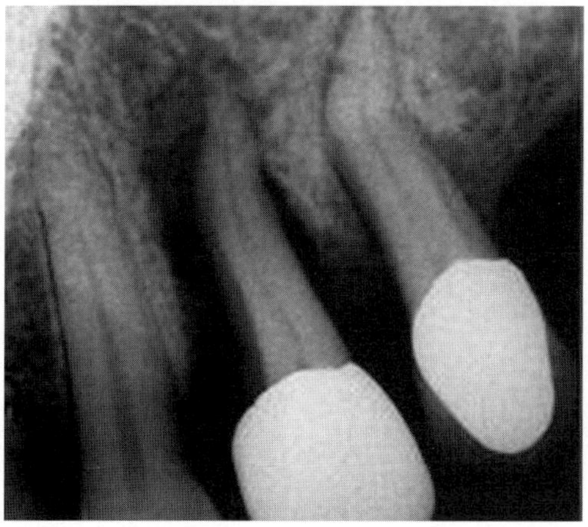

• **Fig. 4.25** Periapical radiograph of the maxillary premolar region reveals the presence of severe periodontal lesions in this area, with generalized vertical and horizontal bone loss along the root surfaces. This severe periodontal lesion indicates tooth extraction.

Definitive Treatment

Definitive treatment accompanies any provision for emergency care. Neither a pulpotomy nor pulpectomy, nor placement of any temporary restorative material, is expected to last long-term, and patient expectations should be set appropriately. Pursuit of definitive treatment of endodontic pathosis should involve options for nonsurgical root canal therapy, nonsurgical or surgical root canal retreatment, or extraction. Further details on the indications and contraindications for these treatments, as well as detailed descriptions of the endodontic procedures themselves can be found in Chapters 19 to 21.

Of course, the treatments explained in this section concern the management of mature teeth. Alternative treatments, including apexification and apexogenesis, can be considered when managing immature teeth, discussed in greater detail in Chapter 10.

The Comprehensive Treatment Plan

Consideration of the comprehensive treatment plan is included as part of the informed consent process. Even in cases of a severely painful pulpitis, local anesthesia can be administered so a patient can comfortably discuss his or her diagnosis, treatment options, and related factors with the provider before pursuit of definitive treatment.

Informed consent involves a discussion of the treatment advised and its expected prognosis, potential complications, as well as treatment alternatives. The discussion of treatment alternatives should always include the options for no treatment as well as extraction. Patients should be informed of the risks and benefits of each of these treatment alternatives, including expected short- and long-term effects. For example, in patients electing *not* to proceed with treatment, continued pain and other sequelae are expected (Fig. 4.27). In the long term, even if problems improve spontaneously or with analgesics, untreated endodontic pathosis can result in recurrent infections with a perhaps reduced prognosis for future treatment. Effects on neighboring bone and teeth may limit future implant options, as well as result in potentially serious sequelae like cellulitis or space infections.

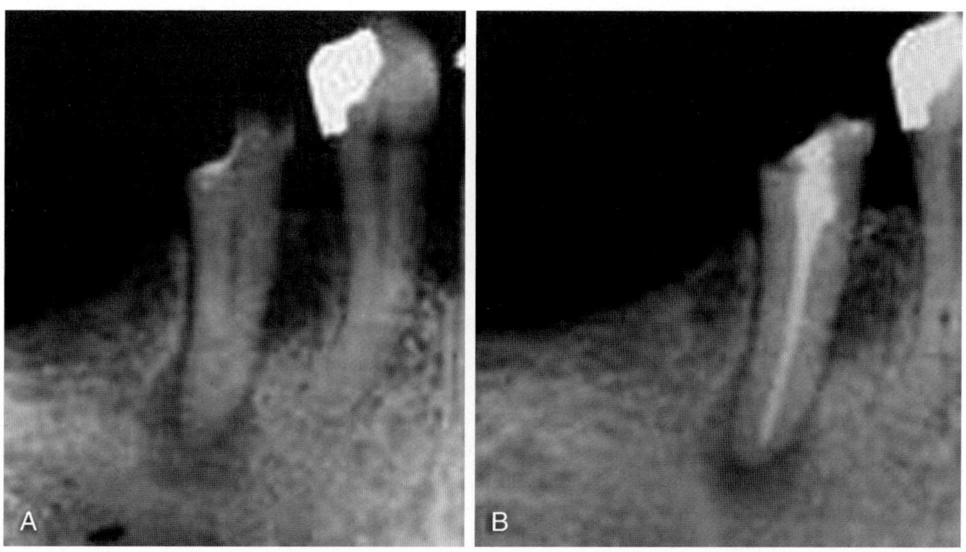

• **Fig. 4.26** **A**, A combined endodontic–periodontic lesion is observed in the second mandibular premolar. **B,** Endodontic and periodontal treatments of this tooth have resulted in the decrease of these lesions in 6 months.

In some cases, extraction is the only choice, due to coexisting periodontal disease, issues with restorability, cost-related factors, and a tooth's strategic value in the overall treatment plan. Reliable replacement options, including fixed partial dentures and implant-supported restorations, should be discussed, as well as the potential limitations of these treatment alternatives.

Patients should be advised of additional procedures that may be required after initiation of endodontic therapy. These include follow-up visits to complete treatment, restorative care, and when relevant, any adjunctive procedures, such as crown lengthening surgery or orthodontic extrusion.

All these considerations, including the patient's responses and preferences, must be recorded for possible further reference. Legal situations may arise by patients claiming they were never informed of adverse outcomes if the full, proposed treatment plan is not instituted.

Factors That May Alter the Treatment Plan

Beyond the factors already discussed, certain qualities may affect treatment planning or require consultation with a specialist or referral. They include systematic factors, physical limitations, tooth anatomy, and calcific metamorphosis. A detailed discussion of these factors may be found in Chapters 2, 6, 12, 19-22.

Study Questions

6. A tooth presenting with a carious pulpal exposure may present with which of the following pulpal diagnosis:
   a. Reversible pulpitis
   b. Asymptomatic irreversible pulpitis
   c. Symptomatic irreversible pulpitis
   d. Pulpal necrosis
   e. B, C, and D
7. A tooth presenting with pulpal necrosis can have which of the following corresponding periapical diagnosis:
   a. Normal periapical tissues
   b. Symptomatic apical periodontitis
   c. Asymptomatic apical periodontitis
   d. Acute apical abscess
   e. All of the above
8. VRF should be managed by…
   a. Root canal therapy
   b. Root-end surgery
   c. Extraction or root removal
   d. All of the above
   e. None of the above
9. Once pathological resorptive diseases are identified, endodontic therapy is required.
   a. True
   b. False
10. Teeth with primary periodontal defects of endodontic origin usually require…
    a. Endodontic treatment only
    b. Periodontal treatment only
    c. Endodontic treatment and periodontal treatment
    d. Extraction

ANSWERS

Answer Box 4

1 e. A, B, and C
2 c. Chronic apical abscess
3 b. Sometimes
4 b. False
5 b. False
6 e. B, C, and D
7 e. All of the above
8 c. Extraction or root removal
9 b. False
10 a. Endodontic treatment only

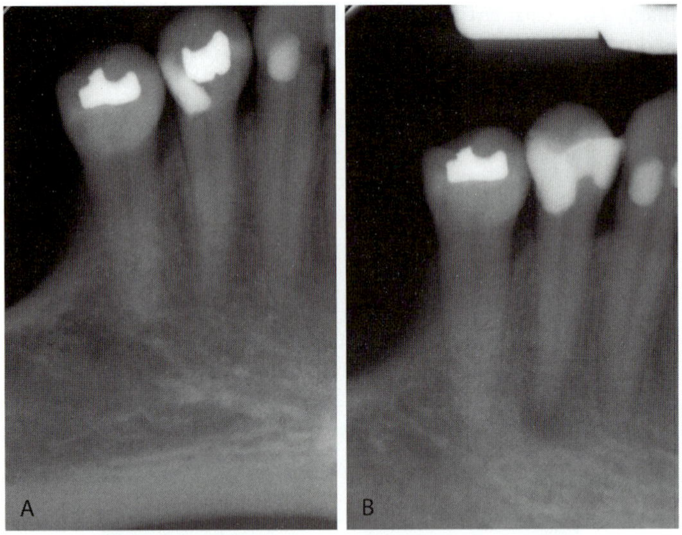

• **Fig. 4.27** **A**, Mandibular right first premolar was excavated and had a carious pulp exposure (diagnosis: asymptomatic irreversible pulpitis). The patient declined having endodontic treatment. **B**, Eight months later, the tooth had pulp necrosis and asymptomatic apical periodontitis, which has worse prognosis than the original diagnosis. (Courtesy Dr. Blythe Kaufman.)

References

1. Campanelli CA, Walton RE, Williamson AE, et al.: Vital signs of the emergency patient with pulpal necrosis and localized acute apical abscess, *J Endod* 34(3):264–267, 2008.
2. Baumgartner JC: *Antibiotics and the treatment of dental infections*, Endodontics, 2006, Colleagues for Excellence Newsletter. Summer.
3. Segura-Egea JJ, Gould K, Sen BH, et al.: European Society of Endodontology position statement: the use of antibiotics in endodontics, *Int Endod J* 51(1):20–25, 2018.
4. Bender IB: Pulpal pain diagnosis—a review, *J Endod* 26(3):175–179, 2000.
5. American Association of Oral and Maxillofacial Surgeons: *Medication-Related Osteonecrosis of the Jaw-2014 Update.* Position Paper 2014.
6. Kang SH, Kim BS, Kim Y: Cracked teeth: distribution, characteristics, and survival after root canal treatment, *J Endod* 42(4):557–562, 2016.
7. Tsesis I, Rosen E, Tamse A, et al.: Diagnosis of vertical root fractures in endodontically treated teeth based on clinical and radiographic indices: a systematic review, *J Endod* 36(9):1455–1458, 2010.

8. Kim SY, Kim SH, Cho SB, et al.: Different treatment protocols for different pulpal and periapical diagnoses of 72 cracked teeth, *J Endod* 39(4):449–452, 2013.
9. Seo DG, Yi YA, Shin SJ, Park JW: Analysis of factors associated with cracked teeth, *J Endod* 38(3):288–292, 2012.
10. Sasano T, Onodera D, Hashimoto K, et al.: Possible application of transmitted laser light for the assessment of human pulp vitality. Part 2. Increased laser power for enhanced detection of pulpal blood flow, *Dent Traumatol* 21(1):37–41, 2005.
11. Schnettler JM, Wallace JA: Pulse oximetry as a diagnostic tool of pulpal vitality, *J Endod* 17(10):488–490, 1991.
12. Emshoff R, Moschen I, Strobl H: Use of laser Doppler flowmetry to predict vitality of luxated or avulsed permanent teeth, *Oral Surg Oral Med Oral Pathol Oral Radiol Endod* 98(6):750–755, 2004.
13. Seltzer S, Bender IB, Ziontz M: The dynamics of pulp inflammation: correlations between diagnostic data and actual histologic findings in the pulp, *Oral Surg Oral Med Oral Pathol* 16:969–977, 1963.
14. Ricucci D, Loghin S, Siqueira Jr JF: Correlation between clinical and histologic pulp diagnoses, *J Endod* 40(12):1932–1939, 2014.
15. Weisleder R, Yamauchi S, Caplan DJ, et al.: The validity of pulp testing: a clinical study, *J Am Dent Assoc* 140(8):1013–1017, 2009.
16. Mainkar A, Kim SG: Diagnostic accuracy of 5 dental pulp tests: a systematic review and meta-analysis, *J Endod* 44(5):694–702, 2018.
17. Fulling HJ, Andreasen JO: Influence of maturation status and tooth type of permanent teeth upon electrometric and thermal pulp testing, *Scand J Dent Res* 84(5):286–290, 1976.
18. Jones VR, Rivera EM, Walton RE: Comparison of carbon dioxide versus refrigerant spray to determine pulpal responsiveness, *J Endod* 28(7):531–533, 2002.
19. White J, Cooley R: A quantitative evaluation of thermal pulp testing, *J Endod* 3(12):453–457, 1977.
20. Miller SO, Johnson JD, Allemang JD, Strother JM: Cold testing through full-coverage restorations, *J Endod* 30(10):695–700, 2004.
21. Trowbridge HO, Franks M, Korostoff E, Emling R: Sensory response to thermal stimulation in human teeth, *J Endod* 6(1):405–412, 1980.
22. Ketterl W: Age-induced changes in the teeth and their attachment apparatus, *Int Dent J* 33(3):262–271, 1983.
23. Rutsatz C, Baumhardt SG, Feldens CA, et al.: Response of pulp sensibility test is strongly influenced by periodontal attachment loss and gingival recession, *J Endod* 38(5):580–583, 2012.
24. Bierma MM, McClanahan S, Baisden MK, Bowles WR: Comparison of heat-testing methodology, *J Endod* 38(8):1106–1109, 2012.
25. Keir DM, Walker 3rd WA, Schindler WG, Dazey SE: Thermally induced pulpalgia in endodontically treated teeth, *J Endod* 17(1):38–40, 1991.
26. Bender IB, Landau MA, Fonsecca S, Trowbridge HO: The optimum placement-site of the electrode in electric pulp testing of the 12 anterior teeth, *J Am Dent Assoc* 118(3):305–310, 1989.
27. Petersson K, Söderström C, Kiani-Anaraki M, Levy G: Evaluation of the ability of thermal and electrical tests to register pulp vitality, *Endod Dent Traumatol* 15(3):127–131, 1999.
28. D'Souza JE, Walton RE, Peterson LC: Periodontal ligament injection: an evaluation of the extent of anesthesia and postinjection discomfort, *J Am Dent Assoc* 114(3):341–344, 1987.
29. Bender IB, Seltzer S: Roentgenographic and direct observation of experimental lesions in bone: II. 1961, *J Am Dent Assoc* 62:708–716, 1961.
30. Low KM, Dula K, Burgin W, von Arx T: Comparison of periapical radiography and limited cone-beam tomography in posterior maxillary teeth referred for apical surgery, *J Endod* 34(5):557–562, 2008.
31. Patel S, Dawood A, Mannocci F, et al.: Detection of periapical bone defects in human jaws using cone beam computed tomography and intraoral radiography, *Int Endod J* 42(6):507–515, 2009.
32. AAE/AAOMR: AAE and AAOMR Joint Position Statement: Use of cone beam computed tomography in endodontics 2015 update, *J Endod* 41(9):1393–1396, 2015.
33. Ricucci D, Mannocci F, Ford TR: A study of periapical lesions correlating the presence of a radiopaque lamina with histological findings, *Oral Surg Oral Med Oral Pathol Oral Radiol Endod* 101(3):389–394, 2006.
34. Shrout MK, Hall JM, Hildebolt CE: Differentiation of periapical granulomas and radicular cysts by digital radiometric analysis, *Oral Surg Oral Med Oral Pathol* 76(3):356–361, 1993.
35. Bender IB, Mori K: The radiopaque lesion: a diagnostic consideration, *Endod Dent Traumatol* 1(1):2–12, 1985.
36. Caliskan MK, Turkun M, Oztop F: Histological evaluation of a tooth with hyperplastic pulpitis and periapical osteosclerosis, *Int Endod J* 30(5):347–351, 1997.
37. Eversole LR, Stone CE, Strub D: Focal sclerosing osteomyelitis/focal periapical osteopetrosis: radiographic patterns, *Oral Surg Oral Med Oral Pathol* 58(4):456–460, 1984.
38. Marmary Y, Kutiner G: A radiographic survey of periapical jawbone lesions, *Oral Surg Oral Med Oral Pathol* 61(4):405–408, 1986.
39. Green TL, Walton RE, Clark JM, Maixner D: Histologic examination of condensing osteitis in cadaver specimens, *J Endod* 39(8):977–979, 2013.
40. McCabe PS, Dummer PM: Pulp canal obliteration: an endodontic diagnosis and treatment challenge, *Int Endod J* 45(2):177–197, 2012.
41. Edds AC, Walden JE, Scheetz JP, et al.: Pilot study of correlation of pulp stones with cardiovascular disease, *J Endod* 31(7):504–506, 2005.
42. Sayegh FS, Reed AJ: Calcification in the dental pulp, *Oral Surg Oral Med Oral Pathol* 25(6):873–882, 1968.
43. Pettiette MT, Wright JT, Trope M: Dentinogenesis imperfecta: endodontic implications. Case report, *Oral Surg Oral Med Oral Pathol Oral Radiol Endod* 86(6):733–737, 1998.
44. Pettiette MT, Zhong S, Moretti AJ, Khan AA: Potential correlation between statins and pulp chamber calcification, *J Endod* 39(9):1119–1123, 2013.
45. Gold SI: Root canal calcification associated with prednisone therapy: a case report, *J Am Dent Assoc* 119(4):523–525, 1989.
46. Tronstad L: Root resorption—etiology, terminology and clinical manifestations, *Endod Dent Traumatol* 4(6):241–252, 1988.
47. Walton RE, Leonard LA: Cracked tooth: an etiology for "idiopathic" internal resorption? *J Endod* 12(4):167–169, 1986.
48. Costa CP, Thomaz EB, Souza Sde F: Association between sickle cell anemia and pulp necrosis, *J Endod* 39(2):177–181, 2013.
49. Rauckhorst AJ, Baumgartner JC: Zebra. XIX. Part 2. Oral herpes zoster, *J Endod* 26(8):469–471, 2000.
50. Michaelson PL, Holland GR: Is pulpitis painful? *Int Endod J* 35(10):829–832, 2002.
51. Read JK, McClanahan SB, Khan AA, et al.: Effect of Ibuprofen on masking endodontic diagnosis, *J Endod* 40(8):1058–1062, 2014.
52. American Association of Endodontists. Glossary of Endodontics Terms. 2016. cited ed 9; ed ed 8. Available from http://www.nxtbook.com/nxtbooks/aae/endodonticglossary2016/index.php.

52a. Chevigny C, Dao TT, Basrani BR, et al.: Treatment outcomes in endodontics: The Toronto study—Phase 4: Initial treatment, *J Endod* 34:258–263, 2008.

53. Eliasson S, Halvarsson C, Ljungheimer C: Periapical condensing osteitis and endodontic treatment, *Oral Surg Oral Med Oral Path* 57(2):195–199, 1984.
54. Rivera E, Walton R: Longitudinal tooth cracks and fractures: an update and review, *Endod Topics* 33(1):14–42, 2015.
55. Alassaad SS: Incomplete cusp fractures: early diagnosis and communication with patients using fiber-optic transillumination and intraoral photography, *Gen Dent* 59(2):132–135, 2011.
56. Wright Jr HM, Loushine RJ, Weller RN, et al.: Identification of resected root-end dentinal cracks: a comparative study of transillumination and dyes, *J Endod* 30(10):712–715, 2004.
57. Rivera E, Walton R: Longitudinal tooth fractures. In Torabinejad M, Walton R, Fouad A, editors: *Endodontics: principles and practice*, ed 5, St. Louis, 2015, Elsevier, pp 121–141.

58. Abou-Rass M: Crack lines: the precursors of tooth fractures - their diagnosis and treatment, *Quintessence Int Dent Dig* 14(4):437–447, 1983.
59. Fennis WM, Kuijs RH, Kreulen CM, et al.: A survey of cusp fractures in a population of general dental practices, *Int J Prosthodont* 15(6):559–563, 2002.
60. Krell KV, Caplan DJ: 12-month success of cracked teeth treated with orthograde root canal treatment, *J Endod* 44(4):543–548, 2018.
61. Krell KV, Rivera EM: A six year evaluation of cracked teeth diagnosed with reversible pulpitis: treatment and prognosis, *J Endod* 33(12):1405–1407, 2007.
62. Tamse A, Tsesis I, Rosen E: *Vertical root fractures in dentistry*, Switzerland, 2015, Springer.
63. Walton RE, Michelich RJ, Smith GN: The histopathogenesis of vertical root fractures, *J Endod* 10(2):48–56, 1984.
64. Walton RE: Vertical root fracture: factors related to identification, *J Am Dent Assoc* 148(2):100–105, 2017.
65. American Association of Endodontists: The Recommended Guidelines of the American Association of Endodontists for the Treatment of Traumatic Dental Injuries, Revised 2013.
66. Wedenberg C, Lindskog S: Experimental internal resorption in monkey teeth, *Endod Dent Traumatol* 1(6):221–227, 1985.
67. Gartner AH, Mack T, Somerlott RG, Walsh LC: Differential diagnosis of internal and external root resorption, *J Endod* 2(11):329–334, 1976.
68. Caliskan MK, Turkun M: Prognosis of permanent teeth with internal resorption: a clinical review, *Endod Dent Traumatol* 13(2):75–81, 1997.
69. Vier FV, Figueiredo JA: Prevalence of different periapical lesions associated with human teeth and their correlation with the presence and extension of apical external root resorption, *Int Endod J* 35(8):710–719, 2002.
70. Andreasen JO, Kristerson L: The effect of limited drying or removal of the periodontal ligament. Periodontal healing after replantation of mature permanent incisors in monkeys, *Acta Odontol Scand* 39(1):1–13, 1981.
71. Zahrowski J, Jeske A: Apical root resorption is associated with comprehensive orthodontic treatment but not clearly dependent on prior tooth characteristics or orthodontic techniques, *J Am Dent Assoc* 142(1):66–68, 2011.
72. Heithersay GS: Clinical, radiologic, and histopathologic features of invasive cervical resorption, *Quintessence Int* 30(1):27–37, 1999.
73. Heithersay GS: Invasive cervical resorption: an analysis of potential predisposing factors, *Quintessence Int* 30(2):83–95, 1999.
74. von Arx T, Schawalder P, Ackermann M, Bosshardt DD: Human and feline invasive cervical resorptions: the missing link?—presentation of four cases, *J Endod* 35(6):904–913, 2009.
75. Gunst V, Huybrechts B, De Almeida Neves A, et al.: Playing wind instruments as a potential aetiologic cofactor in external cervical resorption: two case reports, *Int Endod J* 44(3):268–282, 2011.
76. Mavridou AM, Bergmans L, Barendregt D, Lambrechts P: Descriptive analysis of factors associated with external cervical resorption, *J Endod* 43(10):1602–1610, 2017.
77. Heithersay GS: Treatment of invasive cervical resorption: an analysis of results using topical application of trichloroacetic acid, curettage, and restoration, *Quintessence Int* 30(2):96–110, 1999.
78. Seymour GJ: Possible mechanisms involved in the immunoregulation of chronic inflammatory periodontal disease, *J Dent Res* 66(1):2–9, 1987.
79. Harrington GW: The perio-endo question: differential diagnosis, *Dent Clin North Am* 23(4):673–690, 1979.
80. Rotstein I, Simon JH: Diagnosis, prognosis and decision-making in the treatment of combined periodonta-endodontic lesions, *Periodontology* 34:165–203, 2000 2004.
81. Simon JH, Glick DH, Frank AL: The relationship of endodontic-periodontic lesions, *J Periodontol* 43(4):202–208, 1972.
82. Harrington GW, Steiner DR: Endodontic and periodontal interrelationship. In Walton R, Torabinejad M, editors: *Principles and practice of endodontics*, St. Louis, 2002, Elsevier.
83. Bergenholtz G: Interrelationship between periodontics and endodontics. In Lindhe J, editor: *Textbook of clinical periodontology*, Copenhagen, 1983, Munksgaard.

5

Differential Diagnosis of Pains and Radiolucencies of Nonpulpal Origin

BRADLEY ELI, NASSER SAID-AL-NAIEF, AND MAHMOUD TORABINEJAD

CHAPTER OUTLINE

LEARNING OBJECTIVES

After reading this chapter, the student should be able to:

1. Identify the personal and societal effect that orofacial pain conditions can have.
2. Understand the classification systems for common orofacial disorders that can cause tooth pain.
3. Understand both extracranial and intracranial conditions that can refer pain to the teeth.
4. Identify and manage confusing dental causes of tooth pain.
5. Identify and manage muscles, joint, neurovascular causes of tooth pain.
6. Understand head and neck structures that refer pain to the teeth.
7. Understand temporomandibular disorders (TMD) that can cause pain in the jaw, head, and neck.
8. Identify the radiographic features of normal anatomic structures and developmental entities and understand the clues on differentiating these entities from true pathologies of the maxillofacial region.
9. Identify the clinicopathologic and radiographic features of incisive canal cyst.
10. List the odontogenic and nonodontogenic tumors and cysts that involve the maxillofacial region.
11. Understand the key differentiating points when examining the odontogenic and nonodontogenic tumors and cysts that involve the maxillofacial region.
12. List different types of benign fibro-osseous lesions of the jaw and identify the clinicopathologic features of each.
13. Identify the clinicopathologic and radiographic features and etiopathogenesis of surgical ciliated cyst, traumatic bone cyst (TBC), and focal osteoporotic bone marrow defect, with a brief description of the histologic feature of each.
14. List and identify the clinicopathologic features of selective benign and malignant bone tumors.
15. Identify the spectrum of hematolymphoid disorders as well as plasma cell disorders and Langerhan cell disease (LCD).

Introduction

Several conditions of nonendodontic origin simulate clinical and the radiographic appearances of pulpal and/or periapical lesions. Determining the cause of these conditions is a critical first step in diagnosis and treatment planning. Without an accurate diagnosis, treatment is unlikely to be effective. Initially, the clinician must determine whether the cause of the problem is odontogenic (pulpal or periodontal) or nonodontogenic. Because of the similarities of clinical and radiographic appearance of many of these conditions, dentists must perform clinical tests in a systematic manner to arrive at an accurate diagnosis and avoid critical mistakes. Pulp vitality tests are the most important aids in differentiating most of these conditions. To avoid misdiagnosis and performing wrong treatment, all relevant patient history, clinical signs and symptoms, vitality tests, and radiographic examinations should be utilized. The purpose of this chapter is differentiating and treating (1) pains of nonpulpal origin from those of pulpal and or/periodontal origin, and (2) radiolucencies of nonpulpal origin from those of pulpal origin.

Pains of Nonpulpal Origin

Toothache of Nonpulpal Origin

Nonodontogenic pain can be extremely distressing to the patient and baffling to the clinician. For patients, this can result in years of misdiagnosis, mismanagement, and overtreatment, thus risking the development of chronic pain pathology. To further complicate the problem, patients will jump from one provider to another as treatment failures continue to mount. A history of unsuccessful treatment by numerous providers is a red flag for the endodontist to expand the differential diagnosis to include pain of a nonodontogenic origin. In this group of patients taking the time to complete a comprehensive history will avoid unneeded diagnostic tests and misdirected treatment.

All pain disorders have a negative effect on the patient and those around them. This is especially true when it comes to painful conditions in the facial region. These disorders have an especially high level of concern because this region is the center for both verbal and nonverbal communication as well as nourishment.

The face is also highly innervated by both sensory and special sensory nerves. The motor and special motor nerves respond to this afferent information. This cross talk of malfunctioning nerves can make specific diagnosis elusive for the provider and at the same time making the patient frantic for an explanation.

This combination is the perfect environment for unnecessary or unsupported treatment resulting in more failure and despair. Using a linear model of cause and treatment is not always successful. To address this issue further, the research diagnostic criteria of Dworkin and Leveche considered the psychosocial side of pain and that both physical conditions and psychologic conditions contribute to the suffering, pain behavior, and disability associated with a person's pain experience.[1]

Dentists are often the first clinicians involved in diagnosis and treatment of these conditions.[2,3]

To be successful in treating these patients, it is important to have a clear understanding of the many different ways in which the patient may experience nonodontogenic pain and how to avoid unnecessary treatment. In the dental field, the most useful pain consultants are (1) orofacial pain trained dentists, (2) endodontists, and (3) oral maxillofacial surgeons. These professionals are a resource for medically trained pain management providers as well as dentists. Referral to one of these specialists is preferable to sending a patient to an urgent care facility or an emergency room.

Incidence of Orofacial Pain

The frequency of continuing pain after endodontic treatment has been reported at 5%. Of these patients, 62% were found to be a pain of nonodontogenic origin.[4] The frequency of persistent pain after orthograde root canal treatment in one study subsequently identified as nonodontogenic pain was 53%. In this study myofascial pain was determined to be the source.[5] Another study found that 44% of patients with persistent pain had previously received endodontic treatment or tooth extractions in an attempt to resolve their pain.[6] Moreover, 23.5% of patients with headaches reported tooth pain referral as well.[7] The importance of comprehensive examination of the muscles in the head and neck is emphasized in a study that reported pain referral patterns to the teeth in 138 of 230 patients.[8]

In a survey of 827 randomly selected individuals from a general population group, 10% reported pain in the head, face, or neck.[9] Another group surveyed 1016 members of an HMO and found that 12% reported facial pain within the preceding 6 months and 26% reported headache.[10] Lipton et al. surveyed 45,711 households and found 22% had at least one of 5 types of orofacial pain in the preceding 6 months. Most common orofacial pains were toothache at 12.2%, temporomandibular (TM) joint pain at 5.3%, and face/cheek pain in 1.4%.[11]

To better understand disorders of the orofacial region, a study was undertaken titled "Orofacial Pain: Prospective Evaluation and Risk Assessment (OPPERA)."[12] This study provided improved insight into the number of people affected by pain in the orofacial region. Epidemiologic surveys in the United States, Canada, and the United Kingdom report the frequency of orofacial pain in the general adult population as ranging from 14% to 40%.

Basic Terminology in the Understanding and Diagnosis of Pain

Pain is defined as an unpleasant sensory and emotional experience associated with actual or potential tissue damage or described in terms of such damage.[13,14] Orofacial pain refers to oral pain, dental pain, and pain in the face above the neck, anterior to the ears, and below the orbitomeatal line.

Common Terms

Algesia – Any pain experience after a stimulus
Allodynia – Painful response to a nonpainful stimulus
Dysesthesia – An abnormal sensation that is unpleasant
Hyperalgesia – An increased pain response to a noxious stimulus
Hypoalgesia – A diminished pain response to a noxious stimulus
Hypoesthesia – A decreased sensitivity to stimulation similar to anesthesia
Neuroma – A mass of peripheral neurons formed by a healing damaged nerve
Neuropathic Pain – Aberrant sensation produced by a malfunctioning nerve
Nociception – Perception of pain arising from tissue damage or injury
Pain Threshold – The lowest level of stimulation perceived as painful
Pain Tolerance – The highest level of pain a subject is prepared (or able) to tolerate
Sensitization – The increased excitability of nerve terminals or neurons produced by trauma or inflammation of peripheral tissues

Diagnostic Process for Nondental Orofacial Pain

Due to the complexity of orofacial pain, many authors suggest classification or grouping of functional systems as the most direct method to evaluate these orofacial pain problems.[2,3,14] Effective diagnosis and treatment of these disorders require a working knowledge of functional neuroanatomy, peripheral nervous system (PNS) and central nervous system (CNS) pathways, descending pain-modulating systems, and their related structures. CNS changes may underlie persistent pain. The patient's emotional response to continuing pain is another factor that should be considered in the diagnostic process. To be an effective care provider, the clinician must have a solid understanding of the various categories in which persistent orofacial pain can be classified.

It is important to remember that directing and providing the most appropriate care may involve multiple clinicians. By taking a thorough medical history and carefully processing clinical characteristics, the clinician can begin to identify the unique characteristics of extracranial, intracranial, musculoskeletal, vascular, neurologic, and psychological symptoms. This assessment provides the most direct path to diagnosis, referral, or treatment.[2,3,5,16]

When a thorough assessment is completed, the clinician can confidently reassure the patient that his or her symptom will be appropriately managed. This proficiency is another critically important skill for the specialist to develop. Without confidence in the treatment provider, the patient's anxiety and worry can interfere with the diagnostic process and resulting care.

Localization of the Pain

1. Eyes, ears, nose, throat, sinuses, tongue, teeth, and glands are head and neck structures that may be a source of pain. The quality of pain in a region involving such a broad range of structures can range from mild aching to excruciating pain. As previously mentioned, the most common cause of pain in the orofacial region is dental pathology.
2. A diligent search for dental pathology should begin early and continue throughout diagnosis and treatment.
3. Pain of dental origin will often awaken a patient from sleep or prevent sleep. Patients may regard sleep disturbance as noncritical medical information.[2,3] Sleep disturbance is an important part of the differential diagnosis. It is important to ask very specific questions about the effect of pain on sleep patterns.
4. Pain of the pulpal tissues or periodontium is often very acute and easily localized on examination or by patient report. Affected teeth are typically painful to palpation or percussion. Use of percussion testing is extremely helpful in the diagnostic process.
5. Any tooth-related pain should be evaluated radiographically to exclude dental disease. Most computed tomography (CT) imaging and radiology reporting from a medical center do not provide an adequate evaluation of the dental structures. If imaging is completed, a dental provider should access the images and review them personally.
6. With nonodontogenic pain, the maxillary sinus and teeth are the areas that are most commonly affected by disease. Typical descriptors of sinus disease are "constant," "aching," "pressure," and "fullness." Pain will often include the teeth or ear. Fever, congestion, and/or discharge may also be present. Head position or movement can often exacerbate this symptomatology.[2,3]

Confusing Dental Pathology

Periodontal Ligament Pain

Caused by repetitive strain to the dental periodontal ligaments through clenching, gross occlusal prematurities, or trauma to the teeth, this type of pain is characterized by deep somatic musculoskeletal pain. Periodontal ligament pain is generally a dull, aching pain in and around the teeth and can affect multiple teeth. Inflammatory fluid accumulation from a periodontitis or an apical abscess may cause displacement of the tooth in its socket, with a resulting acute malocclusion and pain (Fig. 5.1). The most common sign is tenderness of the teeth to percussion in the absence of pulpitis or periapical/periodontal abscess. Treatment consists of using a splint to protect the teeth, reducing oral habits, and encouraging healing. The use of a transitional splint can help in diagnosing and treating these conditions.

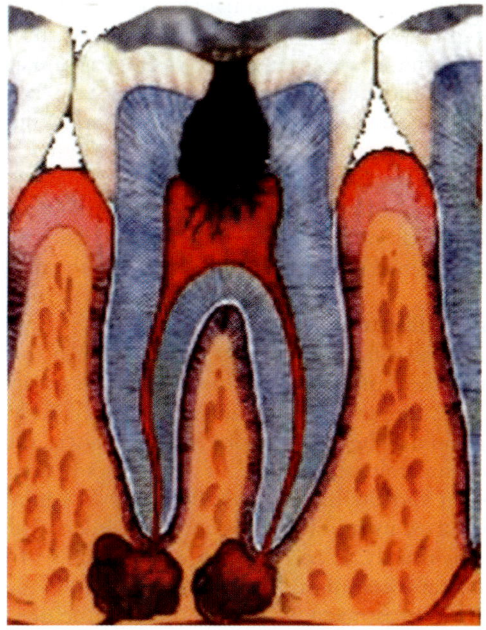

• **Fig. 5.1** Periodontal ligament pain is cause by inflammatory and fluid accumulation from either a periodontitis or an apical abscess. (Redrawn after Fricton J, Kroening R, Hathaway K: *TMJ and craniofacial pain: diagnosis and management*, St. Louis, 1988, Medico Dental Media International, Inc.)

Intracranial and Headache Pain

Although uncommon, neoplasm, hematoma, hemorrhage, edema, aneurysm, and infection of the CNS can result in facial pain. Space-occupying lesions are often associated with progressive pain complaints and associated neurologic deficit or signs. Patient descriptors, including the "worst" or "first," have been identified as specifically pathognomonic of more serious conditions.[2,3,15,16] These conditions can progress quickly and lead to permanent disability or even death. Prompt identification and referral for neurology consultation can be critical to successful diagnosis. The SNOOP acronym can be helpful to determine level of concern, as follows:

Systemic symptoms or disease: fever, weight loss, human immunodeficiency virus (HIV), systemic cancer
Neurologic signs or symptoms: confusion, clumsiness, weakness, aphasia, vision change
Onset sudden: thunderclap, progressive, positional
Onset after age 40 years: vascular (temporal arteritis), tumor, infection
Pattern change: any new or changed headache pattern or quality or increase in frequency or intensity

Some of the most difficult primary headache diagnoses involve the orofacial region. It is important to remember that headache disorders can and do occur anywhere in the trigeminal distribution and can be difficult to differentiate from disease. For example, midface migraine and sinus disease can look and act very similar in many ways to dental pathology. Careful history-taking is critical to diagnostic accuracy and treatment effectiveness. Recurrence and duration can often be helpful in differentiation of primary headache. In addition, with the introduction of the specific drug class triptans, a medication trial can help clarify the diagnosis.

Temporomandibular Disorders

Musculoskeletal conditions are the major cause of nonodontogenic pain in the orofacial region. Included in this group are cervical spine and temporomandibular joint disorders (TMD). Oral and facial pain may be the result of TMD, myofascial disorders, or systemic rheumatologic, collagen, or cervical spine disease. TMD refers to pain and dysfunction specific to the TM joint that frequently involves mandibular movement disorders. Palpation of the region is usually associated with exacerbations of pain, and functional pain is common.

The TM joint is made up of three major structures: the condyle, the disk, and the skull. The TM joint is a complex joint, capable of both rotational and translational movements. Rapid displacement of the joint can result in pressures that disrupt the disk–condyle relationship, resulting in lack of coordinated movement. On examination, this disorder can be identified as clicking or popping in the joint. Less subtle noises, such as crepitation, can occur with degenerative disease of the region and must be considered in the diagnostic process.

Mechanical disturbance of this joint is often associated with inflammatory events that often respond to antiinflammatory treatment.[2,15,16] Noise in the TM joint that presents without pain, catching, locking, or sudden and notable change in bite position is often simply a finding that requires no more than identification. Because of the TM joint's location in relation to the ear, patients' concerns about joint noise must be addressed and explained as present and being considered in the diagnostic process to avoid unnecessary treatment focused on the TM joint.

Trauma is thought to be the main cause of dysfunction in the region. Microtrauma resulting from tooth grinding or jaw clenching, or macrotrauma resulting from external forces such as a MVA or facial effect has been discussed in the literature as the etiology of such disorders.[2,3,15-17] Jaw joint and muscle strain and sprain (JAMSS) is another potential precedent to TMD and facial pain. Trauma may occur during dental treatment. Hyperextension of the mouth for extended time periods and excessive force placed on the jaw during a procedure or after local anesthetic injections may cause injury. More than 50% of patients with TMD associate initial onset of this problem with this type of trauma.[18]

Psychological Disturbances

Psychological disturbances have also been proposed as a cause of tooth pain. However, even though practitioners know factors such as stress, muscle tension, anxiety, and depression can contribute to an enhanced experience of pain, psychological factors have not been established as a cause of toothaches of nondental origin. Psychological disturbances are considered more of a contributing factor to periodontal ligament strain and muscle pain but not tooth pain. Psychological illness with reported pain complaints is common. Psychological illness requires the inclusionary criteria present for any other disease and should not be assumed. Once identified, treatment plans should be developed and presented as clearly and succinctly as those of the other pain etiologies discussed.

It is important to remember that many of the currently described pain disorders were, as recently as the 1990s, considered to be psychological illnesses. Therefore care should be exercised when allowing this diagnosis to be made by exclusion.[2,3] It is also important to remember that with extended time, multiple treatment failures, and constant pain, patients who present with depression, fear, and feelings of hopelessness and helplessness are actually showing signs of a "normal" response to a chronic condition.

Types of Pain

Musculoskeletal Pain

Myofascial pain is the most common muscle pain disorder of the orofacial region. Muscle splinting, muscle spasm, and myositis are the most common acute conditions and, based on duration, may precede myofascial pain in etiology.[17] Factors associated with aggravation of muscle pain include prolonged muscle tension, poor posture, parafunction, trauma, sleep disturbance, viral infection, metabolic disturbance, and specific joint pathology.[17] The most common examination finding associated with muscle problems involves pain with palpation, movement anomalies, and referred pain. Knowing the common referral patterns for the head and neck muscles will save hours of confounding findings and prevent failed treatments. The text by Travell and Simons is the best resource for information about this disorder.[17]

Joint Disorders

Joint disorders have been identified as a major cause of nondental pain in the orofacial region and are considered to be a subclassification of musculoskeletal disorders.[19]

Neurovascular Pain

Migraines, cluster headaches, and hemicrania continua are types of headaches that result from changes in the nerves and blood vessels of the head. In some cases, through referral patterns of the trigeminal nerve, these headaches can also be felt in the teeth, causing toothaches. The pain can be spontaneous, severe, and throbbing, and it can have periods of remission. Treatment is directed at the cause of the headache and often includes behavioral therapy and medications.

Neuropathic Pain

Neurologic or neuropathic pain is the result of abnormality in nociceptors. These receptors are activated by stimuli that threaten or damage the body's integrity. They respond to mechanical, thermal, and chemical stimuli. Both peripheral and central locations and mechanisms may be involved.

Decreased inhibition and/or increased peripheral activity result in two basic types of pain: paroxysmal and continuous neuralgias.[2,20,21]

Paroxysmal neuralgias are described as intense, sharp, stabbing, electric-like pains, usually of unilateral presentation involving a specific nerve.

The intensity of the pain is described as "the worst pain known to man." This type of pain can occur in short or extended-duration volleys.[20,21] Although the intensity of these types of pain is extreme, they do not often awaken the sleeping patient, which helps differentiate this pain from pulpal or periodontal pain.

Trigeminal neuralgia affects the fifth cranial nerve. It is usually unilateral and is more common in women over the age of 50.

Etiology includes idiopathic, demyelination, or vascular malformations.[2,3] Additional etiology theory includes pathologic (bone) cavities at the site of previous tooth extraction, periodontal lesions, and previous endodontic therapy.[3]

Because of the similarity between the symptoms of trigeminal neuralgia and dental etiology, it is common for patients to have consulted with an endodontist. The endodontic specialists must become very familiar with the unique features and provide the evaluation "to eliminate" toothache as the etiology.

The majority of patients describe the classic high-intensity, triggerable pain in association with such activities as eating and talking. Even simple things, such as a cold breeze, can trigger a pain episode.[20,21]

In addition to the paroxysmal nature of classic trigeminal neuralgia, a pretrigeminal neuralgia has also been described by Fromm.[22] This type of pain is of note due to its more constant, dull aching characteristics and is often described by patients as feeling "like a toothache." To further confound the pain provider, most neuralgias are disabled for 4 to 8 weeks by dental procedures such as endodontic treatment and oral surgery. When the pain returns, it is "transferred" to the next tooth in the same arch, which is then incorrectly treated. Patients can often undergo multiple endodontic procedures chasing this disorder.

Glossopharyngeal neuralgia and nervous intermedius neuralgia are more rare than trigeminal neuralgia and involve branches of the glossopharyngeal and vagus nerves.[20,21] Symptoms of pain often include the ear, throat, tonsillar pillar, and submandibular regions. Triggering mechanisms, including chewing, talking, and swallowing, are often the hallmark. Aggressive imaging of the region is recommended because of the high likelihood of regional lesion or pathology associated with this disorder.[3]

Deafferentation Syndromes

Partial or total loss of nerve supply to a region can result in a painful condition. This disorder can be a direct result of traumatic injury, surgery, or a breakdown of the neural structures.

Deafferentation-type pain is thought to involve the sympathetic nervous system, as blockade of this system may often eliminate or reduce the complaints of the patient. Characteristic descriptors used with this type of pain seem most commonly to include the words "burning," "stinging," "itching," and "crawling." Pain is not always present immediately at the time of injury or trauma and may be the result of a breakdown of the central inhibition.

Atypical Odontalgia

This term is used to describe a persistent, painful condition in the oral cavity that cannot be readily attributed to a known cause. The International Headache Society defines atypical odontalgia (AO) as a subgroup of persistent idiopathic facial pain that does not have the characteristic cranial neuralgias and is not attributed to another disorder."[23]

Phantom tooth pain, atypical facial neuralgia, and idiopathic toothache are terms that are used synonymously with AO.

Differential diagnosis includes these four findings:

- Duration longer than 4 months
- Normal radiographic examination
- No clinical observable cause
- Description as a toothache or tooth site pain

Words often used to describe this pain are "diffuse," "burning," "stabbing," or "throbbing."

It is generally thought that AO is a subset of neuropathic pain, i.e., "pain arising as a direct consequence of any lesion or disease affecting the somatosensory system."[24] In this instance, it is thought to result from injury to sensory fibers supplying the extirpated pulp or extracted tooth.

Dental procedures, testing, and diagnostic block of the somatic system are rarely conclusive. Confirmation is associated with positive sympathetic nerve block.[2,3,16]

Neuromas and Neuritis

Neuromas are a growth or tumor of nerve tissue and are often associated with trauma or a direct section of nerve tissue. Stimulation of the region is consistent for diagnostic purposes; however, treatment can be elusive due to recurrence. Neuritis as a systemic inflammatory response is often associated with herpes zoster viral infection. Aggressive and early identification and treatment can often decrease or eliminate the constant sequelae of a zoster episode.[20,21]

Referred Pain

Cervical Spine Pain

Disruption in spine position, structure, and movement can often refer pain into the orofacial region. Careful assessment, history, and clinical examination, including the cervical spine, are paramount to correct identification of etiology and exclusion of referred pain phenomena.[3,16,17]

These disorders can generally be subdivided into muscles or those from the cervical spine. These structures commonly refer to the face and should not be overlooked in cases wherein a diagnostic question exists.[25]

Pain Arising from Vascular Structures

Carotidynia and temporal arteritis are two such disorders that can present with pain in and around the teeth, jaws, and related structures. Palpation localized to their specific anatomic locations assist in the diagnostic process.[2,3,15,16]

Cardiac Toothache

Heart problems such as angina pectoris or acute myocardial infarction refer pain to the shoulder, arm, and even to the jaw. We know that these conditions can refer pain to teeth as well. Sometimes cardiac toothache is associated with chest pain, but occasionally it is not. When a toothache has a cardiac origin, it usually increases with exercise and decreases with medication specifically prescribed for the heart (such as nitroglycerin tablets). Treatment is directed to the underlying heart problem usually after a dentist has evaluated the tooth.

Sinus/Nasal Toothache

Problems in the maxillary sinuses and/or paranasal mucosa can refer pain to the upper teeth. The pain is usually felt in several teeth as dull aching or throbbing. Sometimes it is associated with pressure under the eyes, and it can increase with lowering the head (which puts pressure over the sinuses), coughing, or sneezing. Tests performed on the teeth, such as cold, chewing, and percussion, can increase the pain from sinus origin. A history of an upper respiratory infection, nasal congestion, or sinus problem should lead to suspicion of a "sinus toothache." Diagnostic tests such as visual nasal examination, sinus x-rays, or magnetic resonance imaging (MRI) will reveal this condition. Also, application of topical anesthesia to the offending area should eliminate the pain. Treatment with antihistamines, decongestants, and antibiotics will help (Fig. 5.2).

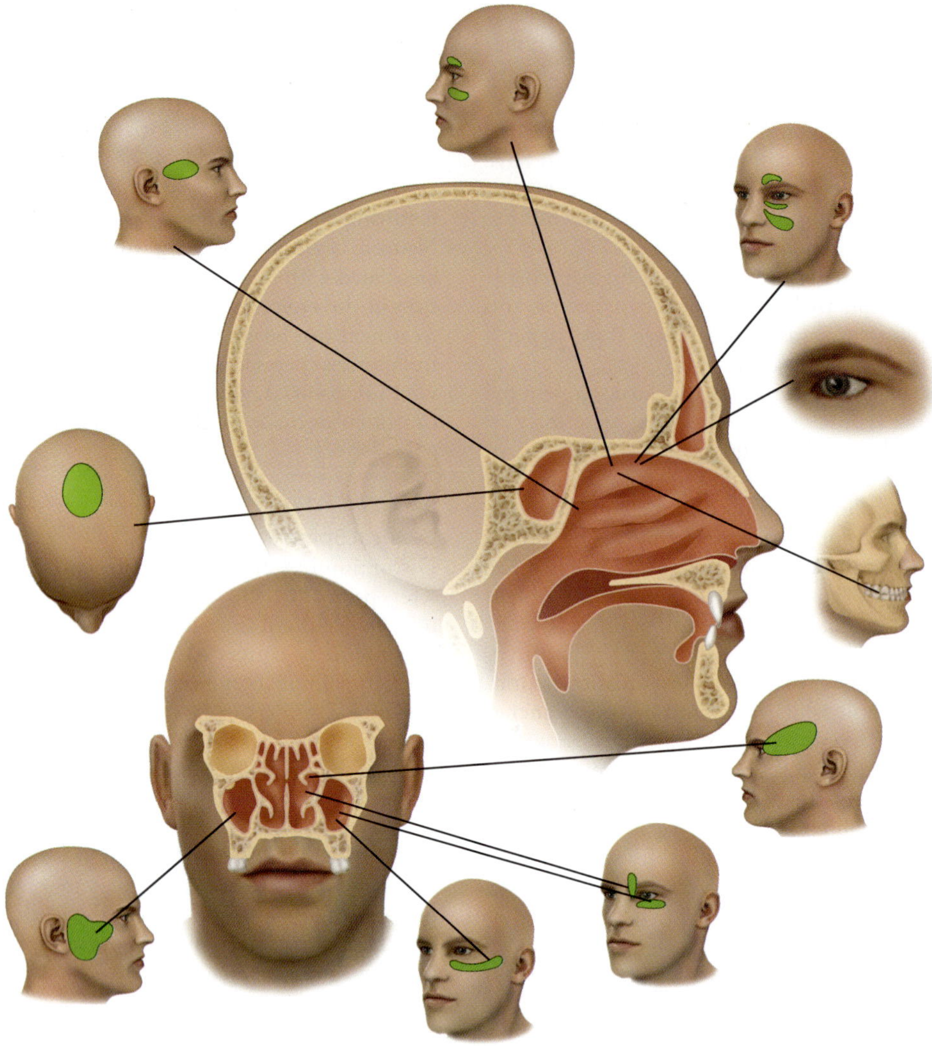

• **Fig. 5.2** Sinuses and Associated Structures. (Redrawn after Fricton J, Kroening R, Hathaway K: *TMJ and craniofacial pain: diagnosis and management*, St. Louis, 1988, Medico Dental Media International, Inc.)

Neoplasias and Other Lesions in the Head

Some tumors, aneurysms, and other intracranial disorders can cause pain in the mouth or teeth. The tooth symptoms are generally accompanied by other nerves malfunctioning or by systemic symptoms, such as weight loss, fatigue, and so on. These accompanying symptoms suggest more than a localized tooth problem is occurring. Tumors can also appear in the areas near the nerves of the teeth, which may cause the teeth to be loose or displaced. Proper imaging of the face, jaw, and head is important to evaluate for these problems. Although possible, these problems are very rare, and treatment needs to be directed to the specific problem.

Salivary Gland Dysfunction

Patients with salivary gland dysfunction can experience dental pain through different mechanisms. Pain may occur through referred pain from the glands to the teeth. It may also occur through compromising the health of the teeth and supporting structures and by the absence of the protective saliva. In such cases, a comprehensive evaluation of the salivary glands is needed (Fig. 5.3).

Treatment

Over the past three decades, significant progress has been made in understanding the pathophysiology of painful conditions.[26]

Treatment of painful conditions of the orofacial region involves identification of the specific illness and correction of the site. If there is no current curative understanding, a management strategy is employed, with the focus being on improving quality of life and decreasing unnecessary treatment and resulting suffering.

Management of painful conditions attempts to employ the most efficient medications and treatments with little or no negative experience, side effect, or misuse potential. This goal can be quite elusive and is the subject of another chapter in this book.

Radiolucencies of Nonpulpal Origin

The radiolucencies that simulate clinical and radiographic appearances of pulpal and/or periapical lesions include normal anatomic structures and developmental entities, odontogenic and nonodontogenic cysts and tumors, osseous pathology, as well as hematolymphoid conditions, malignancies, and related disorders.

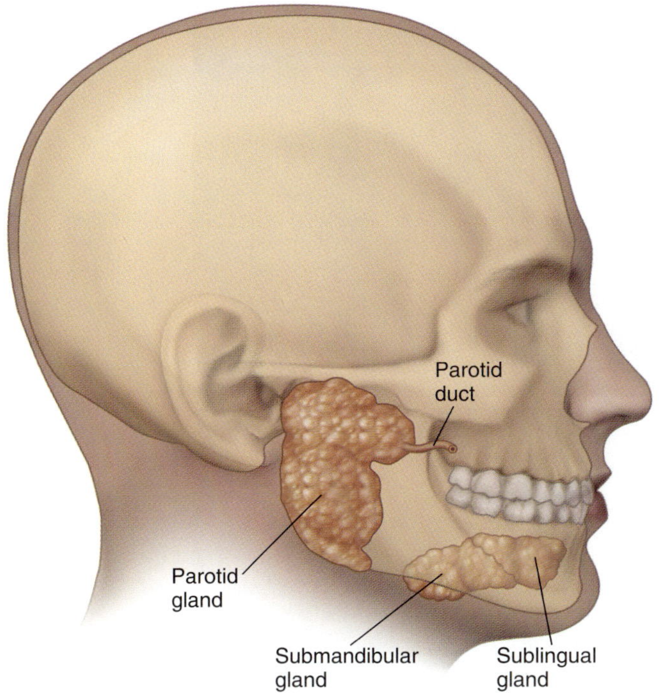

• **Fig. 5.3** Salivary Glands. (Redrawn after Fricton J, Kroening R, Hathaway K: *TMJ and craniofacial pain: diagnosis and management*, St. Louis, 1988, Medico Dental Media International, Inc.)

• BOX 5.1 Study Questions

1. Orofacial pain is present in what percent of the population:
   a. 5% to 9%
   b. 10% to 14%
   c. 15% to 40%
   d. More than 50%
2. Pain tolerance is best described by:
   a. The minimum amount of pain a person can perceive
   b. The average amount of discomfort a person reports
   c. The maximum a person will allow
   d. The maximum amount of energy a nerve can generate
3. Oral splints can be helpful in the diagnostic process of toothache:
   a. Only when a TM joint dysfunction is present
   b. When bruxism may be present
   c. When the patient has a history of "TMJ"
   d. When endodontic testing is resulting in inconsistent results
4. Clicking in the TM joint should be suspected:
   a. As always a contributing factor in endodontic diagnosis
   b. As present before endodontic therapy
   c. As likely the primary cause of toothache
   d. If directly associated with the onset of a person's chief complaint
5. "Classic" trigeminal neuralgia
   a. Involves V1
   b. Involves V2
   c. Involves V3
   d. All of the above
6. What does SNOOP refer to?
   a. Concerns regarding family members, opinions on what is wrong
   b. An animal-based contagious disorder
   c. A method to remember key risk factors in diagnosis
   d. Syndrome unrelated to the diagnostic process of facial pain

Normal Anatomic Structures and Developmental Entities

Several normal anatomic landmarks and developmental entities may be confused with true pathologic conditions.

The Mental Foramen

Clinical Features

This foramen bilaterally transmits the sensory and motor fibers of the mental nerve.

Radiographic Features

Despite the fact that the location and appearance of the mental foramen is well-characterized and described as asymmetric unilocular radiolucency between the roots of the premolar teeth, many variations in its position and number have been reported[27] and are best viewed on cone beam computed tomography (CBCT) imaging. Accessory foramina can sometimes appear as multiple, small, well-demarcated, or semi–well-defined radiolucencies, close to and/or juxtaposed to the mental foramen proper.[27,28] The foramen, which is typically located below the apices of the first and second premolars, may occasionally be confused with periapical pathology. Clinicians must use judgment during radiographic evaluation and account for age-related variation in the location of the foramen with respect to the width and height of the alveolar ridge and potential changes in respect to the ridge height (Fig. 5.4, *A* and *B*).

Histology

Histologic confirmation is not required, but it would demonstrate mature neural tissue with perineural sheath, representing the mental nerve. Tooth vitality testing and changing the angulation of radiographs can help in differentiating between the foramen and periapical lesions of pulpal origin.

Nasopalatine Duct Cyst

Also referred to as "incisive canal cyst" (Fig. 5.5), nasopalatine duct cyst (NPDC) is the most common developmental cyst of the maxillofacial region. It constitutes approximately 60% of all non-odontogenic cysts of this region and is derived from nasopalatine ductal epithelial lining remnants.

Clinical Features

The NPDC may be totally asymptomatic or may produce anterior maxillary palatal swelling, and occasionally a salty taste originating from the anterior palatal region may be experienced.

Radiographic Features

A well-circumscribed, round or heart-shaped radiolucency, identified slightly higher than the interradicular region of vital maxillary central incisors with intact lamina dura, is considered diagnostic of this cyst, which may be also potentially confused with periapical pathology of pulpal origin including a periapical cyst.[29-31]

Histology

Histomorphologic examination should easily distinguish NPDC from a periapical cyst. NPDC typically demonstrates a cystic cavity lined by pseudostratified columnar respiratory-type epithelium, an inflammatory cell infiltrate of variable intensity, and minor salivary gland lobules, compared with a

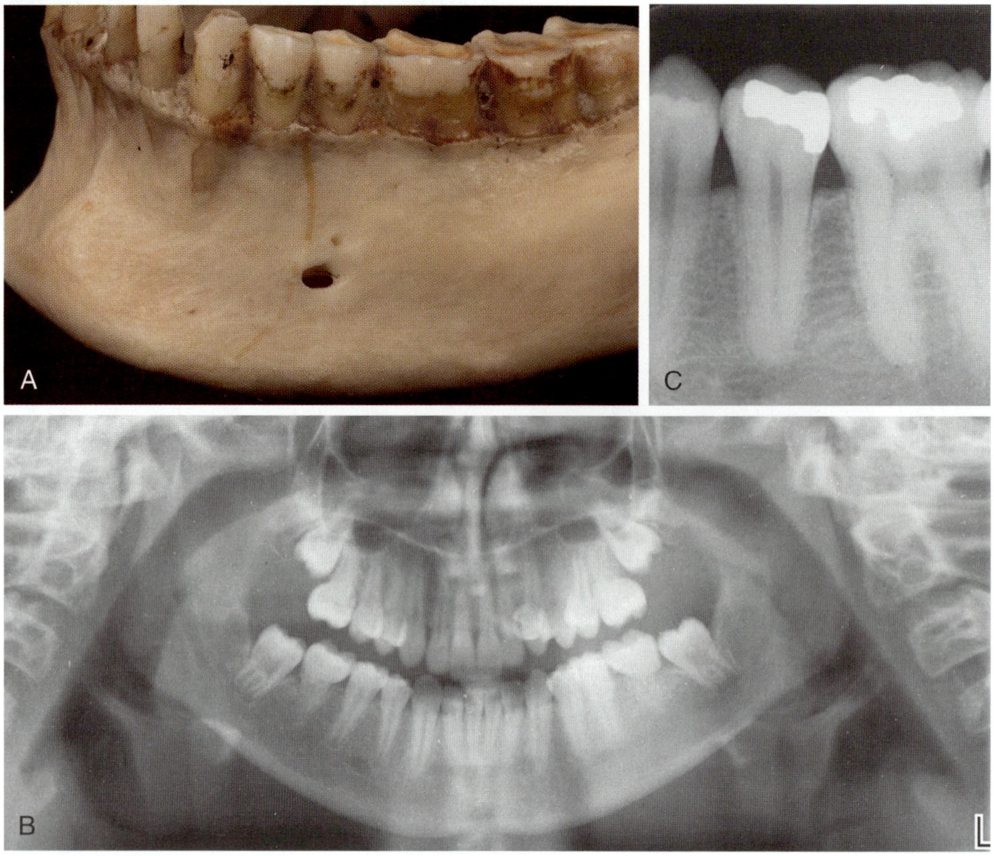

• **Fig. 5.4** **A**, A cadaver mandible, showing the typical location of the mental foramen between the roots of the mandibular premolars. **B**, The typical radiographic presentation of the mental foramen as a well demarcated radiolucency in the interradicular region of the mandibular premolars. **C**, The mental foramen appearing in close relationship to the mandibular second premolar, mimicking periapical pathosis. (**A** and **C**, Courtesy Dr. Dwight Rice, Loma Linda University; **B**, Courtesy Dr. Ying Wu, OHSU.)

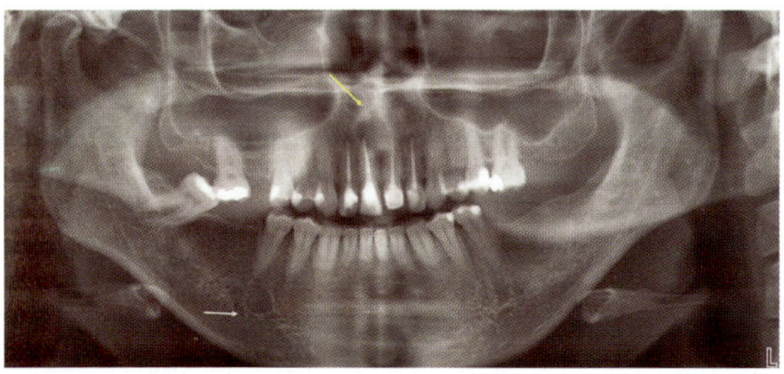

• **Fig. 5.5** Radiographic presentation of nasopalatine duct cyst, demonstrating a heart shaped radiolucency, situated above the roots of viable maxillary central incisors *(yellow arrow)*. The mental foramen could also be seen in the interproximal region of the mandible premolar teeth *(white arrow)*.

radicular cyst, which typically shows nonkeratinized stratified squamous epithelium that is intensely inflamed, hyperplastic, and edematous, and that often contains cholesterol clefts within the cyst wall.[29] A thorough pulp testing, confirming vitality status of the maxillary central incisors, should delineate NPDC from periapical pathosis. Changing the horizontal angulation of a periapical radiograph may further help differentiate NPDC from a radicular cyst, which, compared with NPDC, typically tends to maintain its position around the apex of the maxillary central incisor.

Incisive Foramen

Generally, the identification of an ill-defined 0.6-cm to 0.8-cm radiolucency in the interradicular area of maxillary central incisors should suggest the diagnosis of a normal but widened incisive foramen. The least-invasive technique to differentiate between a NPDC, radicular cyst, and an enlarged incisive foramen is a fine-needle aspiration and examination of the contents of the foramen.[31,32]

Stafne Defect

Stafne defect (SD), also called *Stafne bone cavity* and *static bone defect*, is a rare, asymptomatic developmental mandibular concavity.

Clinical Features

The condition is asymptomatic and is discovered during routine dental examination. It is overwhelmingly prevalent among males. A connection between the lower border of the lesion and inferior border of the mandible exists. This connection and lack of cortical bone leads to the herniation of the submandibular gland into the concavity that is often seen and best viewed on CBCT images.

Radiographic Features

Radiographic features present as a unilateral, homogeneous, well-circumscribed, unilocular radiolucency in the posterior part of the mandibular body, more commonly than in the anterior and ramus areas, below the inferior alveolar canal (Fig. 5.6). Documentation of stability in size with time is characteristic of this entity.

Histology

Fine-needle aspiration of the concavity may demonstrate salivary tissue within or may yield nothing. The stable size and pathognomonic radiographic presentation below the inferior alveolar canal can readily exclude other pathologies, including a residual cyst and aneurysmal bone cyst (ABC), among others.[33,34] Performing tooth vitality tests should also aid in differentiating between SD and true aforementioned pathologies.

Odontogenic and Nonodontogenic Cyst, Tumors, and Related Entities

Several odontogenic and nonodontogenic cysts and tumors can be included under this category of lesions. These include ameloblastoma (Am), calcifying odontogenic cyst (COC), calcifying epithelial odontogenic tumor (CEOT), odontogenic keratocyst (OKC), odontoma, ameloblastic fibro-odontoma (Amfo), ameloblastic fibroma (Amf), dentigerous cyst (DC), odontogenic myxoma, and adenomatoid odontogenic tumor (AOT).[34-39]

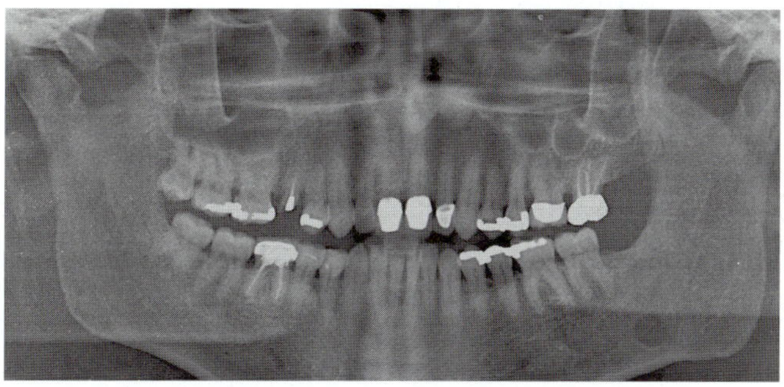

• **Fig. 5.6** Stafne bone defect appearing as a well-demarcated radiolucency below the inferior alveolar canal.

Ameloblastoma

Clinical Features

Am is the most common odontogenic tumor (aside from odontoma). It most commonly involves the posterior mandibular body and ramus regions, more than other gnathic areas, as an expansile asymptomatic mass with a potential for buccal and lingual cortical, as well as teeth root resorption. Am occurs in patients of a wide age range, from the third to seventh decades, with a mean age of 40 years old.

Radiographic Features and Differential Diagnosis

The majority of cases present as large, expansile, multilocular radiolucencies, more than unilocular radiolucencies, but may also present as a pericoronal, interradicular, or even a periapical lesion, mimicking radiolucencies of pulpal origin.[34-38] Differentiating Am from the latter from periapical pathology, which can be readily achieved by thorough tooth vitality testing and histologic examination, is of special significance, taking in consideration the locally aggressive nature of the tumor. The identification of a multilocular radiolucency in middle-aged patients, which involves the posterior mandibular area more than it does the maxilla or other gnathic regions, includes three entities in addition to the differential list: Am (Figs. 5.7 and 5.8), OKC, and odontogenic myxoma, whereas the detection of radiographic evidence of radiopacity within the same age spectrum favors CEOT and in a younger age favors the differential diagnosis of COC and Amfo.[40-44] Helpful clues in the diagnosis of odontogenic myxoma are the identification of fine bony trabeculation and septae that transect the radiolucency. Am characteristically does not demonstrate any evidence of hard tissue formation, histologically or radiographically reflecting the development of the tumor from the odontogenic epithelium of developing enamel organ before the processes of induction and cell differentiation taking place.

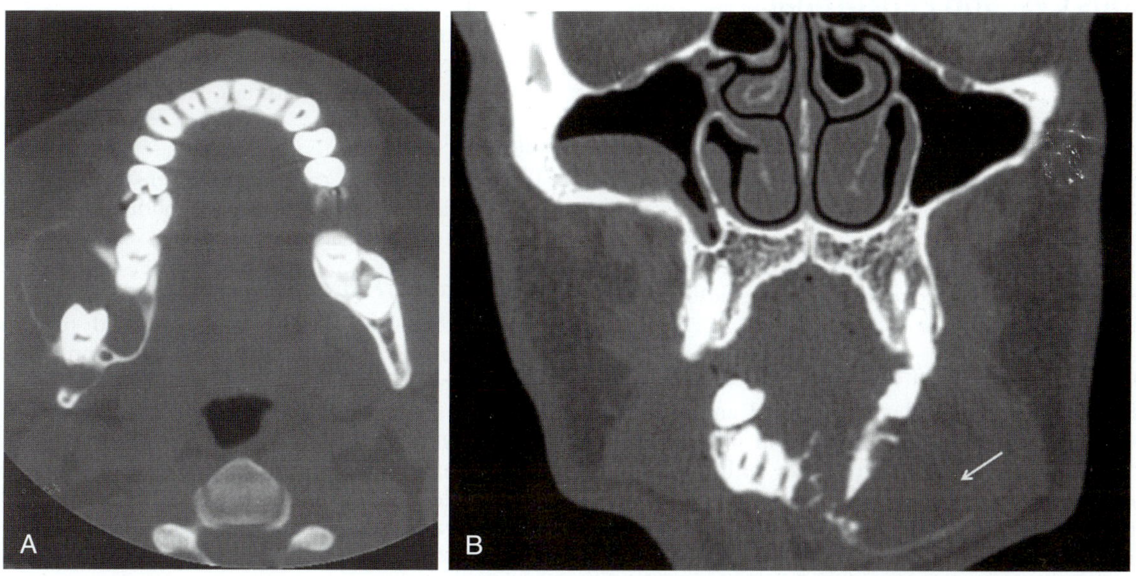

• **Fig. 5.7** **A**, A sagittal view of computed tomography (CT) scan demonstrating a large pericoronal radiolucency associated with impacted tooth #32. This was enucleated and demonstrated histologically dentigerous cyst. **B**, A large expansile radiolucency in the left mandibular body of a 45-year-old female, causing significant bone destruction, buccal cortical expansion and perforation. Biopsy revealed ameloblastoma. (Case courtesy Dr. Rui Fernandez, Jacksonville, FL.)

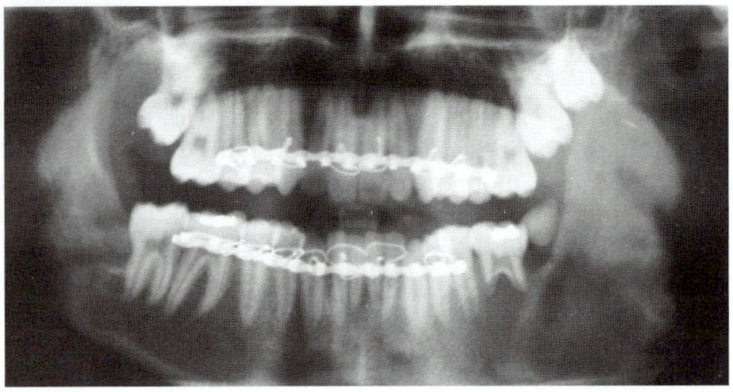

• **Fig. 5.8** A large multilocular radiolucency causing significant bone destruction in left mandibular angle and rams of a 50-year-old female. Biopsy showed ameloblastoma.

Histology

Am is characterized by islands, follicles, and cords of odontogenic epithelium showing reverse peripheral palisaded columnar cells and enclosing stellate reticulum-like tissue. The unicystic Am appears confined to cystic lining detected around an impacted tooth, compared with solid tumors where they show a diffuse infiltrative pattern. Variable histomormorphologic patterns have been reported, albeit with no significant prognostic differences. Nevertheless, in the desmoplastic type, a dense collagenous tissue background supports the ameloblastomatous islands, where the tumor displays a mixed radiolucent and opaque pattern and therefore is seldom diagnosed as Am but is rather easily confused for other osseous pathology. In CEOT, a monotonous benign epithelial tissue is seen, accompanied by concentric-type calcification (Liesegang rings) and also characteristically shows amyloid deposition, whereas in COC, ghost cells, many of which calcify, are characteristically seen. Odontogenic myxoma shows mildly vascular, loose, myxoid tissue that is gelatinous in nature due to high hyaluronic acid content and supports stellate-shaped nuclei with tapered ends.[38]

Dentigerous Cyst and Pericoronal Radiolucencies

Clinical Features

DC is the most common inflammatory odontogenic cyst of the gnathic region, and it may present with limited expansion but occasionally may also be associated with marked swelling, tooth displacement, and discomfort. The cyst occurs in a wide age range but most likely to be encountered in middle-aged adults and virtually around any impacted tooth, most specifically around impacted third molars.

Radiographic Features and Differential Diagnosis

DC appears as pericoronal radiolucency around any impacted teeth but is more commonly seen in association with impacted mandibular third molar teeth more often than with others. The differential diagnosis of pericoronal radiolucency in a middle identification of pericoronal radiolucency in adolescent- to middle-aged patients should include the differential diagnosis of DC, unicystic Am, OKC, and myxoma, whereas the detection of radiopacity in the same age range may favor CEOT. In comparison, similar lesions detected in young and adolescent patients may represent COC, Amf, and Amfo. AOT is another rare odontogenic tumor to be included in the differential of pericoronal radiolucencies when radiopacities are detected within. However, this tumor uniquely involves the anterior maxillary canine region more than other regions and is also typically seen in teenagers, 19 years old and under, with a slight female predilection. Thorough vitality teeth testing, coupled with a representative biopsy of the tumors discussed, should readily distinguish the aforementioned entities from periapical pathology of odontogenic origin.

Histology

A biopsy of a DC typically presents as a cystic cavity lined by hyperplastic inflamed and edematous stratified squamous epithelium, which often demonstrates variable histologic patterns, including the presence of cilia, mucous cell prosoplasia, and apocrine-type changes. Further, an inflamed cyst with bleeding may also depict cholesterol clefts with accompanying multinucleated foreign-body-type giant cell reaction. AOT demonstrates benign odontogenic epithelium, arranged in ducts and spherules and may or may not contain amyloid, and is diagnostic for AOT.[38] Occasionally, an apical displacement of DC or even an adenomatoid odontogenic tumor may also mimic periapical pathosis, and therefore vitality testing, in addition to a representative biopsy showing the histomorphologic features of DC and AOT, should confirm the diagnosis and exclude any periapical pathology present, avoiding any unnecessary root canal therapy and/or tooth extractions.

Differential Diagnosis of a Soft Tissue Mass, With or Without Opacity Obstructing the Eruption of a Permanent Tooth

In addition to what has been described in the previous section, the detection of a soft or mixed soft and hard tissue mass that is obstructing the eruption of a permanent tooth would most likely represent one of three entities, namely, an odontoma, Amf, or an Amfo.[34,37,38]

Odontoma

This tumor is considered the most common odontogenic tumor overall, despite the fact that some favor classifying the lesion as a hamartoma rather than a tumor.

Clinical Features

The majority of the cases are discovered incidentally during the investigation of lack of permanent tooth eruption, but rarely, jaw expansion has been also reported.

Radiographic Features

An odontoma may simulate miniature teeth or dense solid radiopaque pattern favoring compound and complex odontoma subtypes, respectively.

Histology

Odontomas basically recapitulate tooth formation, showing enamel, dentin, and cementum and odontogenic epithelial fragments arranged in teethlike figuration haphazardly, defining the compound and complex subtypes respectively.

Ameloblastic Fibroma

Clinical Features

Amf is typically detected in the posterior mandible discovered incidentally during the investigation of lack of the eruption of a permanent tooth in patients 20 years of age and under.

Radiographic Features

Almost half of the cases are associated with unerupted tooth; however, lesions may also demonstrate unilocular or multilocular well-defined radiolucent pattern.

Histology

Amf demonstrates cellular mesenchymal tissue-type proliferation with high resemblance to dental papilla tissue, supporting ameloblastic epithelium with inconspicuous stellate-reticulum component and also typically shows compressed and slender tumor islands.

Ameloblastic Fibro-odontoma

Clinical Features

This tumor is also most likely detected during the investigation of a soft and hard tissue mass that is preventing the eruption of a permanent tooth; however, similar to what has been described earlier, lesions may also cause painless expansion of the jaw.

Radiographic Features

The lesion most likely appears as a soft and hard tissue density overlying an impacted tooth, but it may also appear as a unilocular or a multilocular radiolucency with radiopacity within.

Histology

An identical feature to those described in Amf would be encountered in Amfo, albeit with the addition of an odontoma component, as described earlier,[34,37,38] although the aforementioned tumors are not easily confused with periapical pathosis and do not cause a challenge and diagnosis, especially after histologic confirmation and confirmation of the vitality status of the teeth should readily exclude the possibility of periapical pathology, especially when the soft tissue mass is apically or laterally displaced.

Odontogenic Keratocyst

Clinical Features

OKC is a rare, benign, locally aggressive developmental cyst that is more commonly encountered in the posterior mandibular body and ramus regions in adolescent and middle-aged adults, although it has also rarely been reported in wider age ranges. The cyst is also well-known for its high incidence of postsurgical recurrences.

Radiographic Features

OKC most commonly presents as a multilocular, pear-shaped, interradicular radiolucency, pericoronal radiolucency, or rarely as a periapical lesion associated with vital teeth, which is essential in distinguishing the lesion from periapical pathology, especially when taking into consideration its locally aggressive and destructive growth potential.

Histology

OKC demonstrates a stratified, squamous epithelium of uniform thickness, with a wavy parakeratinized surface, palisaded basal layer, and devoid of rete ridges. The latter feature is often associated with detachment of the cystic epithelium from the underlying connective tissue wall, which may significantly contribute to the recurrence to the characteristic high-recurrence potential. The differential diagnosis of an interradicular radiolucency of the jaw, identified within the context of tested and confirmed vital teeth, should include lateral periodontal cyst, Am, squamous odontogenic tumor (SOT), as well as OKC, among few other entities. It is also essential to differentiate a lateral radicular cyst, which occurs as a result of the lateral canal transmitting inflammation and bacteria to the periodontal ligament, from a true lateral periodontal cyst and OKCs, primarily to initiate appropriate treatment, as well as to avoid unnecessary endodontic treatment. An accurate pulp testing of vitality status should help the clinician exclude that possibility with confidence.

Squamous Odontogenic Tumor

Clinical Features

SOT is a benign, locally infiltrative odontogenic tumor, which arises within the periodontal ligament with a well-known familial transmission, and also shows equal tendency for maxillary and mandibular involvement. It is regarded by many to be a hamartomatous-type growth, rather than a true neoplasm because of its histologic features. The tumor may be asymptomatic or may produce mild painful gingival swelling.

Radiographic Features

SOT may appear as an interradicular radiolucency that pushes the roots of teeth apart or as a well- or an ill-defined radiolucency with or without sclerotic borders.

Histology

SOT demonstrates benign monotonous squamous epithelium that lacks atypia or abnormal morphology and may even produce keratinization, analogous to normal native epithelial tissue.[34,35,39]

Surgical Ciliated Cyst

Clinical Features

This is a true cyst of the maxillary sinus that develops iatrogenically secondary to surgical intervention with involvement of the sinus floor (Fig. 5.9).

Radiographic Features

The most common presentation is that of a well-demarcated unilocular radiolucency present in the sinus and is considered fairly nonspecific and should be excluded from other pathologies, including a residual cyst pushed into the sinus lining.

Histology

A cystic cavity lined by respiratory-type epithelium with the cystic wall contiguous with Schneiderian membrane is required to establish the diagnosis and exclude other sinonasal pathology, including those of pulpal origin; however, history of surgical intervention, coupled with the confirmation of vitality tests of the teeth in the region, and histomorphological confirmation can help arrive at the correct diagnosis.[40]

Other nonodontogenic entities, such as traumatic bone cyst (TBC), ABC, and central giant cell lesion (central giant cell granuloma [CGCG]), may be also included in this category of lesions.

Traumatic Bone Cyst

Clinical Features

TBC is a pseudocyst. The cyst is most likely discovered incidentally during radiographic examination of the patient's dentition during the second decade of life.

Radiographic Features

The presentation of an interradicular unilocular radiolucency, showing scalloping between the roots of teeth with the

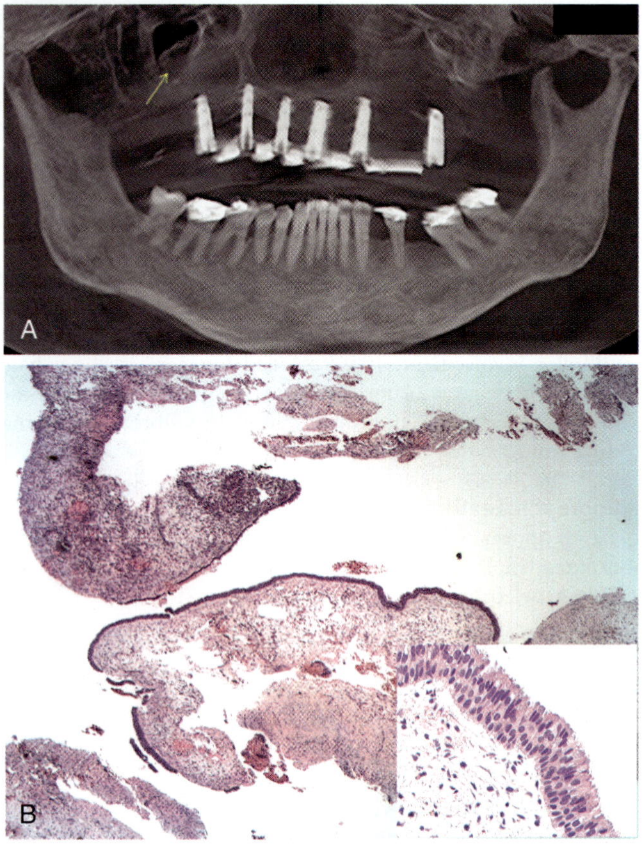

• **Fig. 5.9** Surgical Ciliated Cyst of the Maxillary Sinus. **A**, A Pantomogram generated from the cone beam computed tomography (CBCT) study, depicting a well-demarcated radiolucency detected within the R. maxillary sinuses *(yellow arrow)*. **B**, Histologic examination confirmed the diagnosis of surgical ciliated cyst, showing a cystic cavity, lined by respiratory type epithelium and inflamed Schneiderian membrane (hematoxylin and eosin stain, ×20, inset ×40.)

confirmation of the presence of an empty cavity upon surgical exploration is diagnostic and at the same time therapeutic for solitary bone cyst (also known as TBC or hemorrhagic bone cyst).[41] Complete bone repair is expected after surgical manipulation.[40,42]

Histology

Histology, TBC is usually noncontributory. Exploratory surgical manipulation reveals fragments of bony trabeculae, hemorrhage, and/or potential fragments of collagenous soft tissue.

Focal Osteoporotic Bone Marrow Defect

Clinical Features

This defect is a rare, reactive, nonneoplastic condition of the jaw, primarily affecting the posterior mandibular alveolar ridge and is discovered during routine dental examination in middle-aged females more than in others. It is often seen in the area of an extraction or surgical manipulation.

Radiographic Features

This defect most likely presents as an ill-defined radiolucency of variable dimensions, typically present above the inferior alveolar canal, and most often presents with fine lines/trabeculae within the radiolucency.

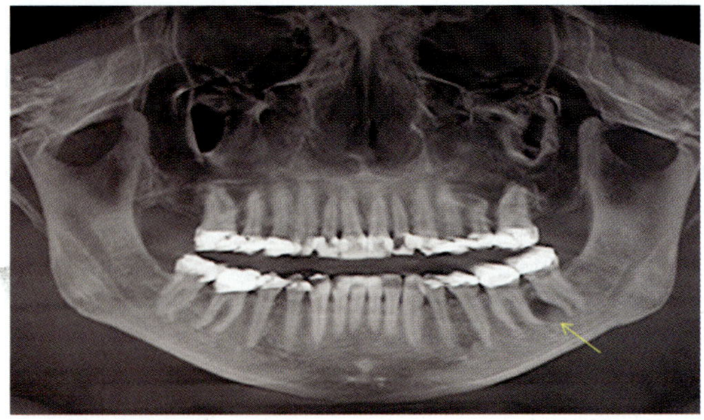

• **Fig. 5.10** Displaying a well-demarcated radiolucency located in the interradicular region of the posterior mandibular teeth. Histomorphological examination was consistent with aneurysmal bone cyst. (Courtesy Dr. Edwin Leung, Portland, OR.)

Histology

Although histology is very typical and diagnostic, showing red marrow elements, namely megakaryocytes and nucleated red blood cells (RBC), among other elements, histology is required for making the accurate diagnosis, especially because radiographic presentation may overlap with other odontogenic lesions such as Am, CGCG, ABC, as well as metastatic tumors. Further, it should be also distinguished from lesions of endodontic origin, and this clarification could be achieved tentatively with accurate teeth vitality testing and further confirmed with histologic examination.

ABC

Clinical Features

ABC of the maxillofacial region constitutes approximately 2% of all cases involving jaw bones. ABC may be self-limiting or may demonstrate an aggressive behavior with a tendency for marked expansion and post enucleation and curettage local recurrence[43] (Figs. 5.10 and 5.11). The etiopathogenesis of ABC is controversial and may be attributed to trauma, or nonneoplastic reactive malformation, with possible genetic predisposition, namely chromosome translocation t(16;17)(q22;p.13) abnormality.[43]

Radiographic Features

Variable presentations may be encountered, ranging from the well-demarcated unilocular radiolucency to a more common presentation as an expansile multilocular radiolucency that may also present with a lateral ballooning extension and extrusion from the alveolar ridge.

Histology

ABC demonstrates large blood-filled spaces, lacking true endothelial lining and often showing multinucleated giant cells in the vicinity of the blood-filled spaces.

Central Giant Cell Lesion

Clinical Features

CGCG (Figs. 5.12 and 5.13) is a reactive nonneoplastic entity that is somewhat unique to the gnathic–jaw region and tends to involve younger individuals, with a mean age of approximately 25 years old and with predilection for mandibular occurrence.

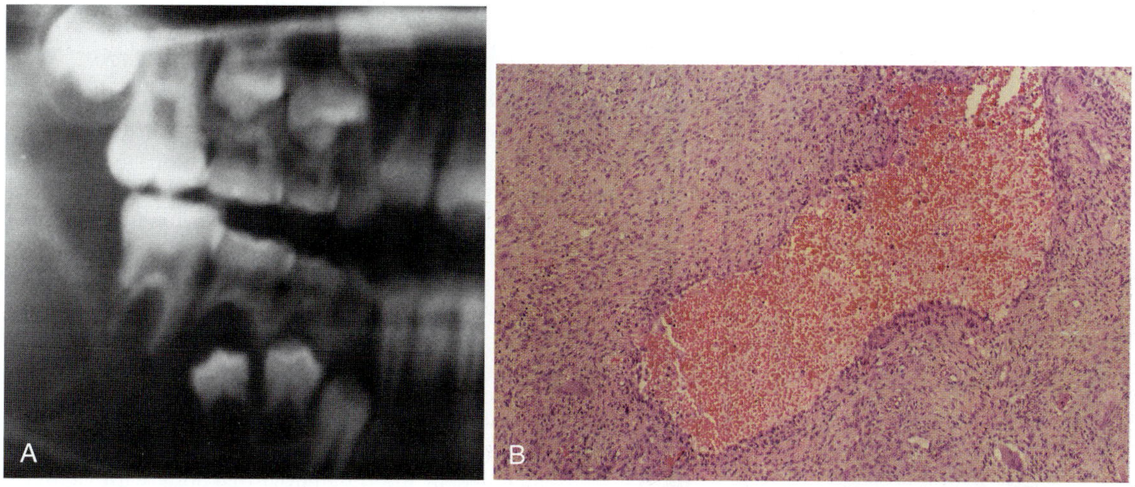

• **Fig. 5.11** **A**, Demonstrates a large multilocular radiolucency, occupying the entire mandibular ramus. **B,** Histomorphologic examination demonstrated large blood filled pseudocystic spaces, characteristically lacking endothelial lining, diagnostic of aneurysmal bone cyst. (Hematoxylin and eosin stain, original magnification ×20.)

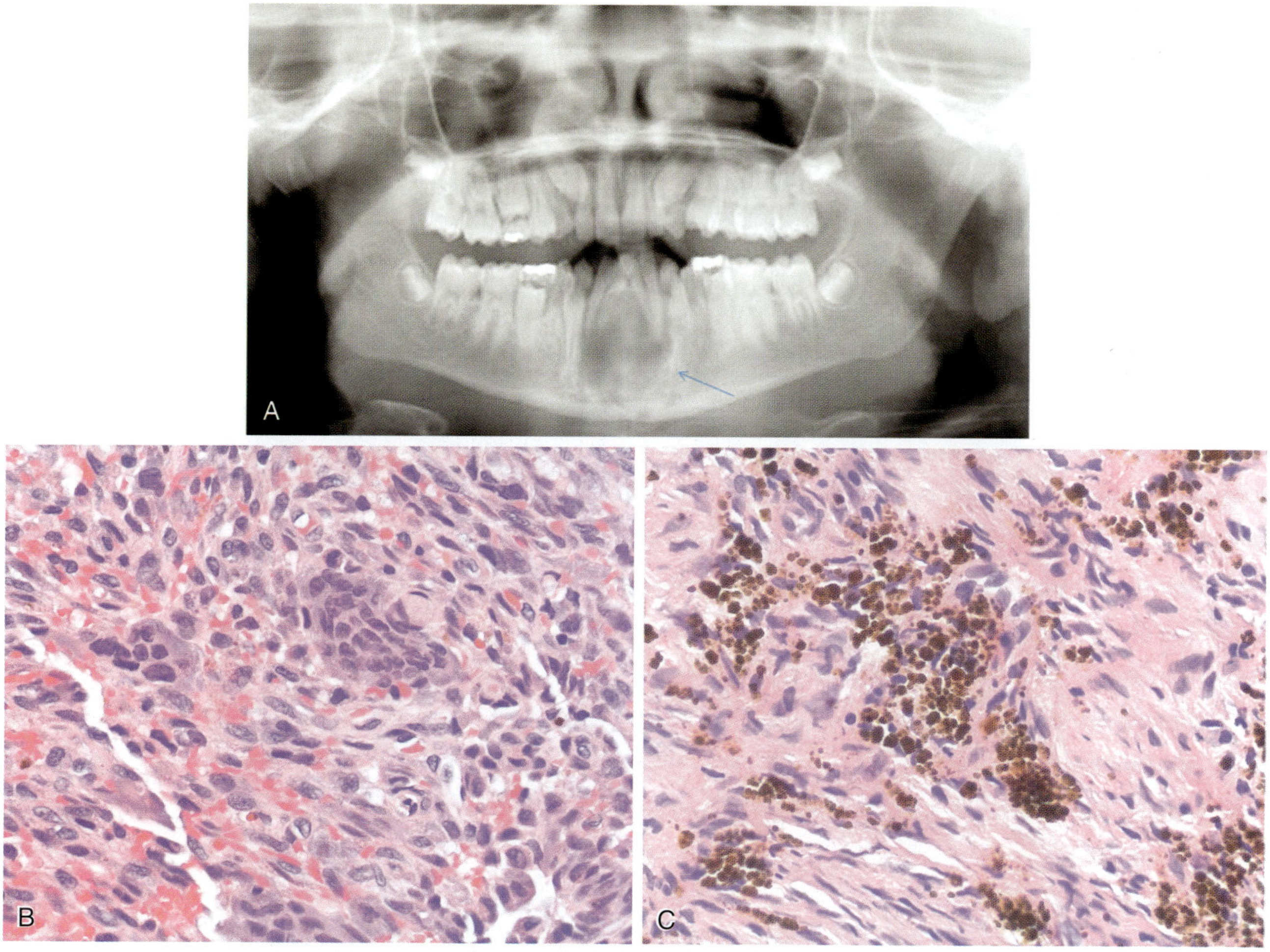

• **Fig. 5.12** **A**, A large expansile radiolucency of the anterior mandible in a 14-year-old male. **B,** Biopsy confirmed the diagnosis of recurrent central giant cell granuloma (CGCG), which was previously enucleated from the same region several months prior. **B**, The lesion demonstrated multinucleated osteoclasts type giant cells supported by a well vascularized cellular stroma. **C**, Hemorrhage with abundant hemosiderin pigment deposition is also evident (**A** and **B**, hematoxylin and eosin stain, original magnification ×40). (**A,** Courtesy Dr. Petrisor, OHSU.)

Radiographic Features

The most common radiologic presentation of central giant cell granuloma is a multilocular radiolucency; however, it may also be unilocular or may be also rarely seen in a periapical location, which may also constitute a diagnostic and management dilemma.[45] However, accurate pulpal status evaluation, coupled with thorough histomorphologic evaluation, should confidently distinguish CGCG and ABC from periapical radiolucencies of pulpal origin.

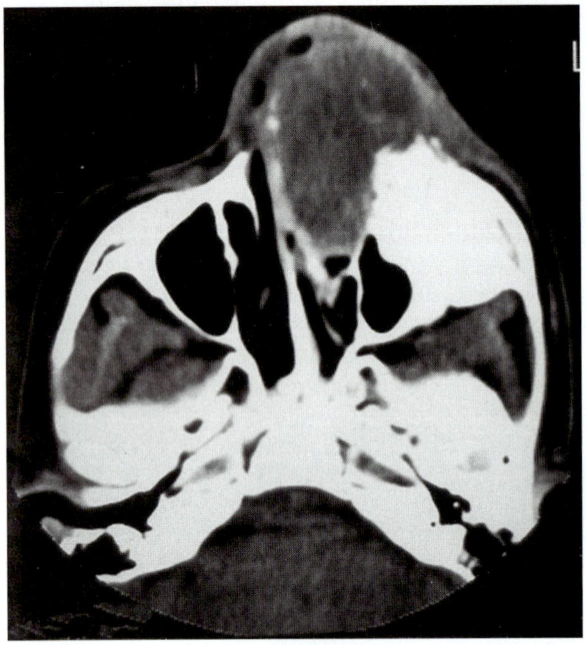

• **Fig. 5.13** Demonstrating large expansile radiolucency involving the maxillary sinus and left maxilla with considerable facial expansion. Biopsy revealed central giant cell granuloma (CGCG). (Courtesy Dr. Roman Carlos, Guatemala.)

Histology

Histologically, CGCG shows a highly vascularized collagenous stroma that is loaded with monotonous multinucleated osteoclast type giant cells observed. Fine-needle aspiration showing blood with hemosiderin pigmentation is highly suggestive of the diagnosis of ABC or CGCG but most significantly excludes other intraosseous true vascular lesions—specifically, high flow hemangiomas and arteriovenous malformation.[46]

Osseous Pathology

Bone pathology often presents with diverse radiographic manifestations, which in turn translate to a large list of entities to be included in the differential diagnosis with significant overlap in clinical and radiographic presentation.

Benign Fibro-osseous Lesions of the Maxillofacial and Gnathic Region

Clinical Features

Benign fibro-osseous lesions of the maxillofacial and gnathic region (BFOL) is a classic example of such diverse entities. They can be separated into one of three categories: (1) fibrous dysplasia (FD), which is considered by some to be a developmental type with neoplastic potential and by others to be a neoplastic condition from the very beginning, based on the identification of the *GNAS* gene mutation in these lesions and is characterized by a diffuse, ill-defined expansion of bone in younger individuals during adolescent years and constitutes less than 10% of all benign bone tumors; (2) ossifying fibroma (also known as *cementifying and ossifying fibroma*, or *CCOF*) (Fig. 5.14), which is a benign neoplastic

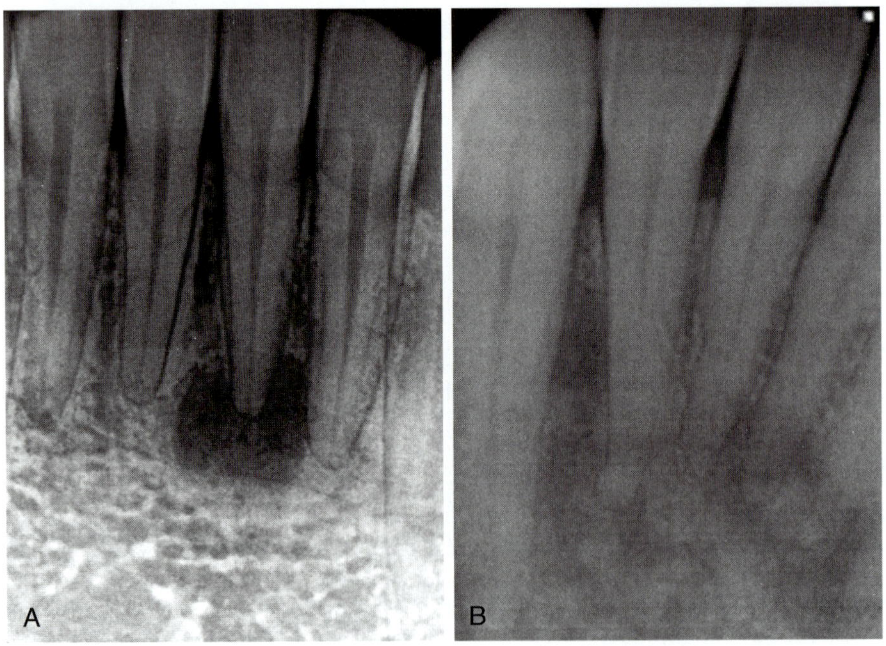

• **Fig. 5.14** **A**, A periapical radiograph which reveals the presence of an evolving periapical cementoosseous dysplasia, seen in association with vital mandibular central incisors. **B**, A mixed stage of periapical cemento-osseous dysplasia, with evidence of radiopacity, evolving at the edges of the radiolucent periapical lesion. (Courtesy Dr. Ying Wu, OHSU.)

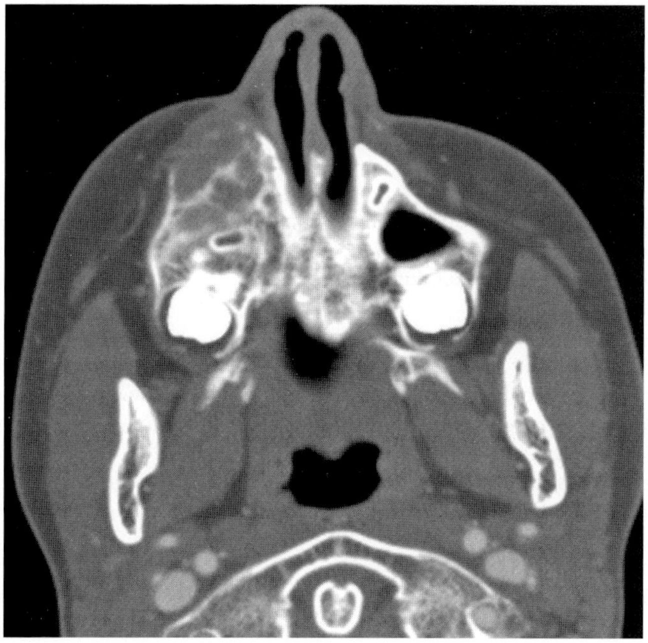

• **Fig. 5.15** Sagittal computed tomography (CT) scan demonstrating a large expansile mixed, radiolucent and radiopaque mass effacing the right maxillary sinus. Biopsy demonstrated central cementifying and ossifying fibroma. (Courtesy Dr. Patrick Louis, UAB.)

condition that is unique to the maxillofacial region. CCOF occurs in patients who are approximately10 years older than those seen with FD. It is also more common in females and also shows prevalence toward the posterior mandible; and (3) cemento-osseous dysplasias, representing a group of reactive nonneoplastic conditions. The last category, cemento-osseous dysplasia, is of special interest here because it is exclusive to the gnathic area and exists as focal cemento-osseous dysplasia, florid cemento-osseous dysplasia, and periapical cemento-osseous dysplasia, where the latter is of special significance because it could be easily confused with periapical pathology of endodontic origin.

Radiographic Features

FD typically presents as an ill-defined mixed radiolucent or radiolucent/radiopaque lesion which displays a ground-glass radiographic pattern which also demonstrates obliteration of the periodontal ligament spaces. In comparison, CCOF characteristically shows a well-defined radiolucent or a radiolucent/radiopaque mass that is also described to be easily shelled-out in one piece by the surgeon during its removal. Osseous dysplasia, on the other hand, presents initially with well-defined radiolucencies of the apical portion of vital mandibular central incisors with gradual production of radiopacities at the edges of the radiolucencies (Fig. 5.15). Furthermore, it typically involves the periapical region of vital mandibular central incisors and may therefore be mistaken for periapical pathology if pulpal vitality testing is not conducted, which leads to unnecessary endodontic treatment.[38,47-49] One exception to the well-demarcated routine presentation of CCOF is observed in the "juvenile cementifying-ossifying fibroma" subtype, which tends to be less well-demarcated radiographically, more aggressive clinically, and having higher tendency for local recurrence and a more cellular osteoblastic rimming with osteoid production on microscopic examination, which may be alarming to the untrained observer.[34,49]

Osteoblastoma

Clinical Features

Osteoblastoma (OB) is another rare benign bone tumor with known predilection for the maxillofacial and head and neck bones, especially the mandible.

Radiographic Features

OB may appear either as a well-defined or an ill-defined radiolucency, with or without radiopaque pattern, depending on the time the lesion is discovered. It may also rarely mimic lesions of endodontic origin but confirmation of the vital status of the adjacent teeth should easily delineate the lesion from periapical pathology.[50]

Histology

OB demonstrates osteoid and woven-bone production that also typically exhibits well-formed prominent and plump osteoblastic rimming, supported by dense well-vascularized fibrocollagenous background.[51]

Although rare, selective malignant entities may also be included here, specifically gnathic osteogenic and chondrogenic sarcomas.

Osteogenic Sarcoma

Clinical Features

Osteogenic sarcoma (OS) of the gnathic region accounts for 7% to 13% of all osteosarcomas with equal distribution between the maxilla and mandible. The tumor is slightly more commonly seen in males during the third and fourth decades of life. A painful swelling is typically seen and is often accompanied by paresthesia, loosening of teeth, as well as nasal obstruction and epistaxis in maxillary tumors.

Radiographic Features

OS is radiographically characterized by large destructive "moth-eaten" lytic or opaque lesions, accompanied by widening of the periodontal ligaments around the teeth in the involved region and a distinct sunray pattern, which is directly attributed to osteoblastic activity that is also often observed on the surfaces of these tumors.

Histology

Malignant osteoid, cartilage and/or fibrous tissue, or a combination of all of the aforementioned tissues may be detected. The bone is typically laid down in a lacelike pattern within this tumor.

Chondrogenic Sarcoma

Significant overlap in the clinical features and radiographic features between chondrogenic sarcoma (CS) and OS may be seen; however, CS of the maxillofacial and gnathic region is far rarer compared with OS. Additionally, pain is more characteristic of OS, whereas bone expansion, which may or may not be symptomatic, favors chondrosarcoma.

Radiographic Features

To reiterate, overlap in radiographic presentation of OS and CS may be seen, where both lesions can demonstrate widening of the periodontal ligament (PDL), spiky roots resorption, and lytic "moth-eaten" and destructive lesions. Further, chondrosarcoma may occasionally present as a multilocular lesion and thus would be potentially mistaken for an odontogenic tumor or cyst, or even other primary intraosseous pathology. Additionally, both entities may also rarely present as radiolucencies in the apical regions and thus may be also mistaken for periapical pathology. The presence of pain may further direct the clinician toward the diagnosis of periapical pathology of pulpal origin; however, accurate pulpal vitality assessment confirming vitality status of the teeth, coupled with histomorphologic examination confirmation of malignancies, can help the clinician reach an accurate diagnosis.

Histology

Lesions show malignant cartilaginous tissue with variation in histomorphology, including mesenchymal chondrosarcoma that demonstrates a small round cell tumor component within.

Ewing's Sarcoma

Ewing's sarcoma (ES) is a rare tumor of neuroectodermal origin that is considered rare in the head and neck region. Jaw involvement is extremely rare, less than 3% of cases seen involving this region; however, mandibular involvement is more common in comparison with involvement of maxilla. The tumor also shows prevalence for children and young adult Caucasian males.[45,52-54]

Clinical Features

The tumor typically exhibits an aggressive rapidly expanding and painful mass with high probability of metastasis, which is often discovered at the time of diagnosis.

Radiographic Features

The tumor exhibits a large destructive lytic lesion with buccal and/or lingual cortical erosion. Less commonly, lesions may also appear as a multilocular radiolucency and also have a tendency to periosteal reaction (onion skinning radiographic pattern). Although rare, reports of ES mimicking periapical pathology, including odontogenic infections, are also well-documented; however, a thorough vitality testing of the teeth coupled with representative histomorphologic confirmation should help clinicians arrive at the right diagnosis. Additionally, tumors involving the maxillary sinus and alveolar process may initially present with tooth pain and may even devitalize teeth, which results in undesirable delay in establishing the accurate diagnosis, as well as unnecessary endodontic treatment.[45] However, histomorphologic confirmation, the confirmation of tooth histology, and vitality status may allow clinicians to confidently exclude periapical pathosis. [45,52-54,]

Histology

ES demonstrates a cellular proliferation of small, round, blue cell with a well-demarcated nuclear contour and inconspicuous cytoplasm. A brisk mitotic activity and hyperproliferative index are often seen. The tumor cells demonstrate positive staining with vimentin, and desmin and a distinct membranous staining with anti-CD99. Other immunohistochemistry stains may also be performed to exclude other small round cell tumors including lymphoma. Chromosomal analysis, demonstrating t(11;22) gene rearrangement performed by FISH (fluorescence in situ hybridization) is also considered confirmatory and diagnostic.

Hematolymphoid Conditions, Malignancies, and Related Disorders

The involvement of the head and neck region with metabolic and neoplastic hematolymphoid conditions is well established.

Sickle Cell Anemia

Sickle cell anemia (SCA) is the most common inherited hemoglobinopathy worldwide, characterized by the production of abnormal hemoglobin (HgS),

Clinical Features

Patients characteristically have anemia, RBC deformity, and hemolysis; they also experience pain, including bone pain and necrosis, among other complications.

Radiographic Manifestations

SCA typically produces widening of the marrow spaces with course trabecular bone pattern, which may also be mistaken for periapical pathology, accentuated by the presence of pulpal necrosis that arises secondarily in these patients.[45,47-54,55-57] Detailed medical, social, and family history, as well as thorough laboratory and genetic workup, should definitely exclude lesions of endodontic origin.

Lymphoma

Lymphoma is a malignancy of the immune system cells, which could be roughly divided into Hodgkin's lymphoma, malignancy derived from B-cell lineage and non-Hodgkin's types, and those with T-, B-, or plasmablastic cell lineages. Approximately 40% of the non-Hodgkin's lymphomas are encountered in extranodal sites, and of these, approximately 2% to 3% involve the oral cavity and the gnathic bones with jaw bones representing the most common location of osseous lymphomas in the craniofacial skeleton.[58-61]

Clinical Features

Jaw involvement with this potentially aggressive and even deadly malignancy typically presents with marked bone destruction and expansion.

Radiographic Features

The majority of the cases present as large radiolucent lesions with significant bone resorption and destruction and are often accompanied by cervical lymphadenopathy; however, it may also rarely mimic periapical pathology.[60,61]

Histology

Although the majority of cases represent large B-cell lymphoma, the whole spectrum of hematolymphoid malignancies, including those of B-cell, T-cell, and plasmablastic cell lineage, may be seen. A diffuse atypical lymphoid infiltrate showing brisk mitotic activity and a variable amount of cytoplasm, depending on the tumor subtype and phenotype, may be observed. Subclassifying lymphomas requires a battery of immunohistochemistry staining in addition to other studies such as chromosomal analysis, flow cytometry, and others. Thorough vitality teeth testing, coupled with histomorphologic confirmation and immunohistochemistry staining, would aid in reaching an accurate diagnosis with definitive disease phenotyping.

Langerhan Cell Disease

Clinical Features

The vast majority of Langerhan cell disease (LCD) patients do not exceed 20 years of age, and the disease can be separated, in descending-age predilection, into three categories: eosinophilic granuloma (localized bone involvement); Hand–Schüller–Christian disease, characterized by the triad of exophthalmos, diabetes, and bone lesions of LCD; and Letterer–Siwe syndrome, characterized by cutaneous involvement with the disease.

Radiographic Features

Jaw involvement often presents with distinguished radiographic manifestations, displaying punched-out radiolucencies in the jaw, skull, and other bones, that lack sclerotic borders and may show the so-called "teeth floating in air" phenomenon mimicking an advanced periodontal disease.

Histology

LCD is characterized by an admixture of histiocytes that often exhibit grooved nuclei, a prominent number of eosinophils, and a distinct population of reactive plasma cells in the supporting connective tissue background. Positive immune-histochemical staining for anti S-100 protein, CD1a/Langerin are considered diagnostic and confirmatory of the diagnosis.[62] Although rare, LCD may also mimic periapical pathosis, and therefore a thorough tooth vitality testing in addition to histologic sampling showing features described previously may be required to confirm the diagnosis.

Multiple Myeloma

Multiple myeloma (MM) is an aggressive neoplasm of plasma cell origin characterized by proliferation of histologically atypical plasma cells that also characteristically display monoclonal plasma cell infiltrate.

Clinical Features

The disease is most often seen in adults, with age ranges between the sixth and seventh decades of life. It is also characterized by bone pain, most likely experienced in the spine, but could be also experienced with any bone involved, including the jaws. Additionally, patients with advanced disease may also suffer from bone fractures and repeated episodes of osteomyelitis.

Radiographic Features

In comparison with LCD, the identification of punched-out radiolucencies in the jaw or skull, which also may be accompanied by large lytic and destructive lesions of the jaw with a spiky pattern of teeth root resorption in older patients (age range is sixth to seventh decades),[34,62] is considered diagnostic of MM.[63-65] Generally, plasma cell dyscrasia may present as solitary jaw or sinus lesions or disseminated disease, and in the former, monoclonal and polyclonal plasma cell infiltrate may be detected.

Histology

A thorough histomorphologic examination, depicting an atypical plasma cell infiltrate, coupled with the immunohistochemistry assessment for kappa and lambda clonality studies should be confirmatory of the diagnosis. Rarely, the lytic lesions of MM may also mimic periapical pathosis, which may be further complicated by the fact that these lesions have been also found to devitalize teeth in long-term disease and which may further delay the diagnosis and lead to unnecessary endodontic treatment. However, the identification of malignant monoclonal plasma cell population in large painful lytic lesions of the jaw, spine, or skull is characteristic of MM. Additionally, patients also typically present with hypercalcemia and markedly elevated levels of monoclonal immunoglobulins (Bence Jones protein) and may also demonstrate the deposition of amyloid protein in the involved bones. The aforementioned features may collectively distinguish MM from periapical pathology of endodontic origin.[63-65] Despite the aggressive therapeutic regimens applied in its management, and the fact that up to 60% of patients may experience remission, the disease remains incurable, with a guarded prognosis and an overall median survival rate ranging from 13 to 31 months, depending on the overall underlying health status of the patient.[65]

Acknowledgment

The author acknowledges the help of Mrs. Carmelita Metz and Mrs. Debbi Schwarm administrative assistants, Oregon Health and Sciences University (OHSU), School of Dentistry for the help and support in the preparation of the manuscript.

• BOX 5.2 Study Questions

7. The mental foramen is typically situated between the first and second mandibular molars.
   a. True
   b. False
8. Nasopalatine duct cyst (NPDC) typically presents as heart-shaped radiolucency between the maxillary central incisors.
   a. True
   b. False
9. Am recapitulates the process of odontogenesis before epithelial/mesenchymal induction.
   a. True
   b. False
10. Which of the following is true regarding malignant myeloma (MM)?
    a. It is a disease of childhood.
    b. It is histologically characterized by eosinophils and histiocytes.
    c. Serologically, patients demonstrate high immunoglobulin production.
11. The majority of jaw lymphomas are of the large B-cell type.
    a. True
    b. False
12. What is the most common radiographic presentation of sickle cell anemia (SCA) in the mandible?
    a. Widened marrow spaces
    b. Sunray pattern
    c. Punched out radiolucencies
13. Which of the following does not typically present as a multilocular radiolucency?
    a. Ameloblastoma (Am)
    b. Odontogenic keratocyst (OKC)
    c. Traumatic bone cyst
14. Which of the following entities proves to be devoid of any content upon surgical exploration?
    a. Traumatic bone cyst (TBC)
    b. Odontogenic keratocyst (OKC)
    c. Surgical ciliated cyst
15. Of the following entities, which has a well-known familial transmission?
    a. Ameloblastoma (Am)
    b. Ameloblastic fibroma (Amf)
    c. Squamous odontogenic tumor (SOT)
16. All of the following are true regarding the radiographic features of Langerhan cell histiocytosis except one. Which is the exception?
    a. Often presents with teeth hanging in air pattern
    b. Often presents with punched-out radiolucencies
    c. Often present as multiple radiopaque jaw masses

ANSWERS

Answer Box 5

1 c. 15% to 40%
2 c. The maximum a person will allow
3 d. When endodontic testing is resulting in inconsistent results
4 d. If directly associated with the onset of a person's chief complaint
5 d. All of the above
6 c. A method to remember key risk factors in diagnosis
7 b. False
8 a. True
9 a. True
10 c. Serologically, patients demonstrate high immunoglobulin production.
11 a. True
12 a. Widened marrow spaces
13 c. Traumatic bone cyst
14 a. TBC.
15 c. SOT
16 c. Often present as multiple radiopaque jaw masses

References

1. Dworkin SF, LeResche L: Research diagnostic criteria for temporomandibular disorders: review, criteria, examinations and specifications, critique, *J Craniomandib Disord* 6:301–355. 1992.
2. Okeson JP, editor: *Orofacial pain: guidelines for assessment, classification, and management.* Carol Stream, IL, 1996, Quintessence.
3. Bell WE: *Orofacial pains: classification, diagnosis, management,* ed 4, Chicago, 1989, Year Book Medical Publishers.
4. Vena DA, Collie D, Wu H, et al: Prevalence of persistent pain 3 to 5 years post primary root canal therapy and its impact on oral health-related quality of life: PEARL network findings, *J Endod* 40(12):1917–1921, 2014.
5. Nixdorf DR, Law AS, John MT, et al: Differential diagnosis for persistent pain after root canal treatment: a study in the national dental practice-based research network, *J Endod* 41(4):457–463, 2015.
6. Linn J, Trantor I, Teo N, et al: The differential diagnosis of toothache from other orofacial pains in clinical practice, *Aust Dent J* 52(1 Suppl):S100–104, 2007.
7. Molina OF, Huber Simião BR, Yukio Hassumi M, et al: Headaches and pain referred to the teeth: frequency and potential neurophysiologic mechanisms, *Rev Sul-Brasileira Odontol (RSBO)* 12(2):151–159, 2015.
8. Wright EF: Referred craniofacial pain patterns in patients with temporomandibular disorder, *J Am Dent Assoc* 131(9):1307–1315, 2000.
9. Brattberg G, Thorslund M, Wikman A: The prevalence of pain in a general population. The results of a postal survey in a county of Sweden, *Pain* 37:215–222, 1989.
10. Von Koorff M, Dworkin SF, LeResche L, Kruger A: An epidemiologic comparison of pain complaints, *Pain* 32:173–183, 1988.
11. Lipton JA, Ship JA, Larach-Robinson D: Estimated prevalence and distribution of reported orofacial pain in the United States, *J Am Dent Assoc* 124:115–121, 1993.
12. Maixner W, Diatchenko L, Dubner R, et al: Orofacial pain prospective evaluation and risk assessment study – The OPPERA Study, *J Pain* 12(11 Suppl): T4–T11, 2011.
13. Merskey H, Bogduk N, editors: *Classification of chronic pain: descriptions of chronic pain syndrome and definitions of pain terms,* Seattle, 1994, IASP Press, pp 59–76.
14. de Leeuw R, Klasser G: *Orofacial pain guidelines for assessment, diagnosis and management,* ed 5, Quintessence, 2013.
15. Pertes RA, Heir GM: Temporomandibular disorders and orofacial pain, *Dent Clin North Am* 35:123–140, 1991.
16. Pertes RA, Gross SG, editors: *Clinical management of temporomandibular disorders and orofacial pain,* Carol Stream, IL, 1995, Quintessence.
17. Travell JG, Simon DG: *Myofascial pain and dysfunction: the trigger point manual,* Baltimore, 1999, Williams & Wilkins.
18. Fricton J, Eli B, Gupta A, Johnson N. Preventing chronic pain after acute jaw sprain or strain. *J Am Dent Assoc,* 147(12):979–986, 2016.
19. Okeson JP: Pains of muscle origin. In *Bell's orofacial pains,* ed 6, Chicago, 2005, Quintessence, pp. 287–328.
20. Long D: Contemporary diagnosis and management of pain, ed 2, Newtown, PA, 2001, Handbooks in Health Care.
21. Chapman CR, Syrjala KL: Measurement of pain. In Bonica JJ, editor: *The management of pain* (vol 1). ed 2, Philadelphia, 1990, Lea & Febiger, pp. 580–594.
22. Fromm GH, Graff-Radford SB, Terrence CF, Sweet WH: Pre-trigeminal neuralgia, *Neurology,* 40(10):1493–1495, 1990.
23. IHS Headache classification committee of the International Headache Society. *Classification and diagnosis criteria for headache disorders, cranial neuralgias and facial pain,* ed 2, *Cephalgia* (Suppl 1):1–160, 2004.
24. Treede, RD, et al: Neuropathic pain: redefinition and a grading system for clinical and research purposes, *Neurology* 70(18):1630–1635, 2008.
25. Piovesan EJ, Kowacs PA, Tatsui CE, et al: Referred pain after painful stimulation of the greater occipital nerve in humans: evidence of convergence of cervical afferences on trigeminal nuclei, *Cephalgia* 21:107–109, 2001.
26. American Pain Society Quality Assurance Standards for Relief of Acute Pain and Cancer Pain. In *Proceedings of the 6th World Congress on Pain,* New York, 1991, Elsevier.
27. Goyushov S, Tözüm MD, Tözüm TF: Accessory mental/buccal foramina: case report and review of literature, *Implant Dent* 26(5):796–801, 2017.
28. Rahpeyma A, Khajehahmadi S: Accessory mental foramen and maxillofacial surgery, *J Craniofac Surg* 1–2, 2017 (Volume publish ahead of print).
29. Barros CCDS, Santos HBP, Cavalcante IL, et al: Clinical and histopathological features of nasopalatine duct cyst: a 47-year retrospective study and review of current concepts, *J Craniomaxillofac Surg* 46:264–268, 2018.
30. Chapman MN, Nadgir RN, Akman AS, et al: Periapical lucency around the tooth: radiologic evaluation and differential diagnosis, *Radiographics* 33:15–32, 2013.
31. Abrams AM, Howell FV, Bullock WK: Nasopalatine cysts, *Oral Surg Oral Med Oral Pathol* 16:306–332, 1963.
32. Allard RH, van der Kwast WA, van der Waal I: Nasopalatine duct cyst. Review of the literature and report of 22 cases, *Int J Oral Surg* 10:447–461, 1981.
33. Assaf AT, Solaty M, Zrnc TA, et al: Prevalence of Stafne's bone cavity—retrospective analysis of 14,005 panoramic views, *In Vivo* 28:1159–1164, 2014.
34. Wright KR, Rice DD, Luo, Z: Chapter 1: Anatomical zones in endodontic surgery. In Torabinejad M, Rubinstein R, editors: *The art and science of contemporary surgical endodontics,* Philadelphia, 2016, Quintessence, pp. 1–17.
35. WHO: *World Health Organization classification of head and neck tumours,* ed 4, Lyon, 2017, IARC Press.
36. Dhanuthai K, Chantarangsu S, Rojanawatsirivej S, et al: Ameloblastoma: a multicentric study, *Oral Surg Oral Med Oral Pathol Oral Radiol* 13(6):782–788, 2012.
37. Zouhary KJ, Said-Al-Naief N, Waite PD: Ameloblastic fibro-odontoma: expansile mixed radiolucent lesion in the posterior maxilla: a case report, *Oral Surg Oral Med Oral Pathol Oral Radiol Endod* 106(4):15–21, 2008.
38. Said-Al-Naief N: Odontogenic tumors for general pathologists, *Review Adv Exp Med Biol* 563:148–164, 2005.
39. Chrcanovic BR, Gomez RS: Squamous odontogenic tumor and squamous odontogenic tumor-like proliferations in odontogenic cysts: an updated analysis of 170 cases reported in the literature, *J Craniomaxillofac Surg* 26(17):3045–3059, 2017.

40. Yamamoto S, Maeda K, Kouchi I, et al: Surgical ciliated cyst following maxillary sinus floor augmentation: a case report, *J Oral Implantol* 43:360–336, 2017.
41. Surej Kumar LK, Kurien N, Thaha KA: Traumatic bone cyst of mandible, *J Maxillofac Oral Surg* 14(2):466–469, 2015.
42. Hs CB, Rai BD, Nair MA, Astekar MS: Simple bone cyst of mandible mimicking periapical cyst, *Clin Pract* 2(3):59, 2012.
43. Urs AB, Augustine J, Chawla H, Aneurysmal bone cyst of the jaws: clinico-pathological study, *J Maxillofac Oral Surg* 13(4):458–463, 2014.
44. Regezi JA: Odontogenic cysts, odontogenic tumors, fibro-osseous and giant cell lesions of the jaws, *Mod Pathol* 15(3):331–341, 2002.
45. Bornstein MM, von Arx T, Altermatt HJ: Loss of pulp sensitivity and pain as the first symptoms of a Ewing's sarcoma in the right maxillary sinus and alveolar process: report of a case, *J Endod* 34(12):1549–1553, 2008.
46. Mohammedi H, Said-al-Naief N, Hafez LB: Arteriovenous malformation of the mandible: report of a case with a note on the differential diagnosis, *Oral Surg Oral Med Oral Pathol Oral Radiol Endod* 84(3):286–289, 1997.
47. Kontogiannis TG, Tosios KI, Kerezoudis NP, et al: Periapical lesions are not always a sequelae of pulpal necrosis: a retrospective study of 1521 biopsies, *Int Endod J* 48(1):68–73, 2015.
48. Daviet-Noual V, Ejeil AL, Gossiome C, et al: Differentiating early stage florid osseous dysplasia from periapical endodontic lesions: a radiological-based diagnostic algorithm, *BMC Oral Health* 17(1):161, 2017.
49. Spatafore CM, Griffin Jr JA, Keyes GG, et al: Periapical biopsy report: an analysis over a 10-year period, *J Endod* 16(5):239–241, 1990.
50. Ribera MJ: Osteoblastoma in the anterior maxilla mimicking periapical pathosis of odontogenic origin, *J Endod* 22(3):142–146, 1996.
51. Burić N, Jovanović G, Tijanić M: Endosteal (central) osteochondroma of the mandibular body, *Oral Surg Oral Med Oral Pathol Oral Radiol* 115(4):e20–22, 2013.
52. Bhadage CJ, Vaishampayan S, Kolhe S, Umarji H: Osteosarcoma of the mandible mimicking an odontogenic abscess: a case report and review of the literature, *Dent Update* 40(3):216–218 & 221, 2013.
53. Yamamoto-Silva FP, Silva BSF, Batista AC, et al: Chondroblastic osteosarcoma mimicking periapical abscess, *J Appl Oral Sci* 25(4):455–461, 2017.
54. Bueno MR, De Carvalhosa AA, De Souza Castro PH, et al: Mesenchymal chondrosarcoma mimicking apical periodontitis, *J Endod* 34(11):1415–1419, 2008.
55. Neville B, Damm DD, Allen C, Chi, A: *Oral and maxillofacial pathology*, ed 4, St. Louis, 2015, Elsevier.
56. Souza S, de Carvalho H, Costa C, Thomaz E: Association of sickle cell hemoglobinopathies with dental and jaw bone abnormalities, *Oral Dis* 20(3):393–403, 2018.
57. Andrews CH, England MC Jr, Kemp WB: Sickle cell anemia: an etiological factor in pulpal necrosis, *J Endod* 9(6):249–252, 1983.
58. Koivisto T, Bowles WR, Magajna WA, Rohrer M: Malignant lymphoma in maxilla with cystic involvement: a case report, *J Endod* 39(7):935–938, 2013.
59. Paes FM, Kalkanis DG, Sideras PA, et al: FDG PET/CT of extranodal involvement in non-Hodgkin lymphoma and Hodgkin disease, *Radiographics* 30:269–291, 2010.
60. Pereira DL, Fernandes DT, Santos-Silva AR, et al: Intraosseous non-Hodgkin lymphoma mimicking a periapical lesion, *J Endod* 10:1738–1742, 2015.
61. Wong GB, Spadafora S, Barbon N, Caputo M: Primary extranodal B-cell non-Hodgkin lymphoma mimicking an endodontic lesion: report of 2 cases, *J Can Dent Assoc* 79:d93, 2013.
62. Pinkus GS, Lones MA, Matsumura F, et al: Langerhans cell histiocytosis immunohistochemical expression of fascin, a dendritic cell marker, *Am J Clin Pathol* 118(3):335–343, 2002.
63. Dhanrajani PJ, Abdulkarim SA: Multiple myeloma presenting as a periapical lesion in the mandible, *Indian J Dent Res* 8(2):58–61, 1997.
64. Witt C, Borges AC, Klein K, Neumann HJ: Radiographic manifestations of multiple myeloma in the mandible: a retrospective study of 77 patients, *J Oral Maxillofac Surg* 55(5):450–453, 1997.
65. Tamura H, Zhonghua X, Ye X, Za Z: Immunopathogenesis and immunotherapy of multiple myeloma, *Int J Hematol* 107(3):27–285, 2018.

6

Endodontic Case Complexity and Working with the Specialist

BRADFORD JOHNSON, HAMID ABEDI, AND SHAHROKH SHABAHANG

CHAPTER OUTLINE

LEARNING OBJECTIVES

After reading this chapter, the student should be able to:

1. Evaluate the multiple factors that determine case difficulty and potential need for referral.
2. Identify the indications for referral to an endodontic specialist.
3. Explain the major differences in predoctoral training in endodontics and advanced specialty training in endodontics.
4. Describe differences in quantity and type of endodontic treatment performed by general dentists and endodontists in the United States.
5. Describe the optimal methods of communication between the general dentist and the endodontist.
6. Define the standards of care for endodontic treatment.
7. Identify the important elements of record keeping with respect to endodontic treatment.

Introduction

Dentistry is one of the most trusted professions in the United States, routinely ranked among the top five in surveys that ask the public to rate the honesty and ethical standards of people in different fields.[1] This high level of trust has been earned by generations of dentists who have consciously chosen to act in their patients' best interests. Perhaps nowhere else in the practice of endodontics is the responsibility to act in the patient's best interests more relevant than initial evaluation of case complexity and deciding whether to treat or refer to a specialist. The American Dental Association (ADA) Code of Ethics addresses the duty to refer, when indicated, by stating: "*The dentist's primary obligations include keeping knowledge and skills current, knowing one's own limitations and when to refer to a specialist or other professional...*".[2]

Although the definition of standard of care still varies somewhat by location, most states have moved away from a local, experience-based standard of care to acceptance of a national, evidence-based standard of care.[3] The standard of care for endodontic therapy is the same for specialists and general dentists; therefore, if case difficulty assessment determines that the procedure is beyond the level of skill and experience of the general dentist, referral to an endodontic specialist is indicated.[4] This chapter provides an overview of specialty training requirements, standard of care, communication between general dentists and specialists, and a more detailed review of evaluation of case complexity. The American Association of Endodontists (AAE) Endodontic Case Difficulty Assessment Form (Fig. 6.1) will be presented with guidance for clinical use.

AAE Endodontic Case Difficulty Assessment Form and Guidelines

PATIENT INFORMATION

Name______________________________

Address______________________________

City/State/Zip______________________________

Phone______________________________

DISPOSITION

Treat in Office: Yes ☐ No ☐

Refer Patient to:

____

Date:______________________________

Guidelines for Using the AAE Endodontic Case Difficulty Assessment Form

The AAE designed the Endodontic Case Difficulty Assessment Form for use in endodontic curricula. The Assessment Form makes case selection more efficient, more consistent and easier to document. Dentists may also choose to use the Assessment Form to help with referral decision making and record keeping.

Conditions listed in this form should be considered potential risk factors that may complicate treatment and adversely affect the outcome. Levels of difficulty are sets of conditions that may not be controllable by the dentist. Risk factors can influence the ability to provide care at a consistently predictable level and impact the appropriate provision of care and quality assurance.

The Assessment Form enables a practitioner to assign a level of difficulty to a particular case.

LEVELS OF DIFFICULTY

MINIMAL DIFFICULTY — Preoperative condition indicates routine complexity (uncomplicated). These types of cases would exhibit only those factors listed in the MINIMAL DIFFICULTY category. Achieving a predictable treatment outcome should be attainable by a competent practitioner with limited experience.

MODERATE DIFFICULTY — Preoperative condition is complicated, exhibiting one or more patient or treatment factors listed in the MODERATE DIFFICULTY category. Achieving a predictable treatment outcome will be challenging for a competent, experienced practitioner.

HIGH DIFFICULTY — Preoperative condition is exceptionally complicated, exhibiting several factors listed in the MODERATE DIFFICULTY category or at least one in the HIGH DIFFICULTY category. Achieving a predictable treatment outcome will be challenging for even the most experienced practitioner with an extensive history of favorable outcomes.

Review your assessment of each case to determine the level of difficulty. If the level of difficulty exceeds your experience and comfort, you might consider referral to an endodontist.

The contribution of the Canadian Academy of Endodontics and others to the development of this form is gratefully acknowledged.

AAE Endodontic Case Difficulty Assessment Form

Criteria and Subcriteria	Minimal Difficulty	Moderate Difficulty	High Difficulty
A. PATIENT CONSIDERATIONS			
Medical history	☐ No medical problem (ASA Class 1*)	☐ One or more medical problems (ASA Class 2*)	☐ Complex medical history/serious illness/disability (ASA Classes 3-5*)
Anesthesia	☐ No history of anesthesia problems	☐ Vasoconstrictor intolerance	☐ Difficulty achieving anesthesia
Patient disposition	☐ Cooperative and compliant	☐ Anxious but cooperative	☐ Uncooperative
Ability to open mouth	☐ No limitation	☐ Slight limitation in opening	☐ Significant limitation in opening
Gag reflex	☐ None	☐ Gags occasionally with radiographs/treatment	☐ Extreme gag reflex which has compromised past dental care
Emergency condition	☐ Minimum pain or swelling	☐ Moderate pain or swelling	☐ Severe pain or swelling
B. DIAGNOSTIC AND TREATMENT CONSIDERATIONS			
Diagnosis	☐ Signs and symptoms consistent with recognized pulpal and periapical conditions	☐ Extensive differential diagnosis of usual signs and symptoms required	☐ Confusing and complex signs and symptoms: difficult diagnosis ☐ History of chronic oral/facial pain
Radiographic difficulties	☐ Minimal difficulty obtaining/interpreting radiographs	☐ Moderate difficulty obtaining/interpreting radiographs (*e.g.*, high floor of mouth, narrow or low palatal vault, presence of tori)	☐ Extreme difficulty obtaining/interpreting radiographs (*e.g.*, superimposed anatomical structures)
Position in the arch	☐ Anterior/premolar ☐ Slight inclination (<10°) ☐ Slight rotation (<10°)	☐ 1st molar ☐ Moderate inclination (10-30°) ☐ Moderate rotation (10-30°)	☐ 2nd or 3rd molar ☐ Extreme inclination (>30°) ☐ Extreme rotation (>30°)
Tooth isolation	☐ Routine rubber dam placement	☐ Simple pretreatment modification required for rubber dam isolation	☐ Extensive pretreatment modification required for rubber dam isolation
Morphologic aberrations of crown	☐ Normal original crown morphology	☐ Full coverage restoration ☐ Porcelain restoration ☐ Bridge abutment ☐ Moderate deviation from normal tooth/root form (*e.g.*, taurodontism, microdens) ☐ Teeth with extensive coronal destruction	☐ Restoration does not reflect original anatomy/alignment ☐ Significant deviation from normal tooth/root form (*e.g.*, fusion, dens in dente)
Canal and root morphology	☐ Slight or no curvature (<10°) ☐ Closed apex (<1 mm in diameter)	☐ Moderate curvature (10-30°) ☐ Crown axis differs moderately from root axis. Apical opening 1-1.5 mm in diameter	☐ Extreme curvature (>30°) or S-shaped curve ☐ Mandibular premolar or anterior with 2 roots ☐ Maxillary premolar with 3 roots ☐ Canal divides in the middle or apical third ☐ Very long tooth (>25 mm) ☐ Open apex (>1.5 mm in diameter)
Radiographic appearance of canal(s)	☐ Canal(s) visible and not reduced in size	☐ Canal(s) and chamber visible but reduced in size ☐ Pulp stones	☐ Indistinct canal path ☐ Canal(s) not visible
Resorption	☐ No resorption evident	☐ Minimal apical resorption	☐ Extensive apical resorption ☐ Internal resorption ☐ External resorption
C. ADDITIONAL CONSIDERATIONS			
Trauma history	☐ Uncomplicated crown fracture of mature or immature teeth	☐ Complicated crown fracture of mature teeth ☐ Subluxation	☐ Complicated crown fracture of immature teeth ☐ Horizontal root fracture ☐ Alveolar fracture ☐ Intrusive, extrusive or lateral luxation ☐ Avulsion
Endodontic treatment history	☐ No previous treatment	☐ Previous access without complications	☐ Previous access with complications (*e.g.*, perforation, non-negotiated canal, ledge, separated instrument) ☐ Previous surgical or nonsurgical endodontic treatment completed
Periodontal-endodontic condition	☐ None or mild periodontal disease	☐ Concurrent moderate periodontal disease	☐ Concurrent severe periodontal disease ☐ Cracked teeth with periodontal complications ☐ Combined endodontic/periodontic lesion ☐ Root amputation prior to endodontic treatment

*American Society of Anesthesiologists (ASA) Classification System

Class 1: No systemic illness. Patient healthy.
Class 2: Patient with mild degree of systemic illness, but without functional restrictions, *e.g.*, well-controlled hypertension.
Class 3: Patient with severe degree of systemic illness which limits activities, but does not immobilize the patient.
Class 4: Patient with severe systemic illness that immobilizes and is sometimes life threatening.
Class 5: Patient will not survive more than 24 hours whether or not surgical intervention takes place.

www.asahq.org/clinical/physicalstatus.htm

• **Fig. 6.1** A and **B,** Case difficulty classification by the American Association of Endodontists. (Published with permission from the AAE.)

Advanced Dental Education Programs in Endodontics

Endodontics is one of the nine specialties recognized by the ADA. Specialty recognition is currently in a state of flux in the United States. To reduce potential bias and conflict of interest in the recognition process, the ADA recently supported the formation of an independent specialty recognition body, the National Commission on Recognition of Dental Specialties. Another independent specialty recognition board, the American Board of Dental Specialties, was also recently formed and recognizes four dental specialties that are not currently recognized by the ADA. Ultimately, it is under the purview of each individual state to determine which dental specialties to recognize.

Specialty recognition is separate from the actual accreditation of an advanced dental education training program. Advanced dental education programs in endodontics are accredited by the Commission on Dental Accreditation (CODA) and have specific and rigorous clinical, didactic, research, and teaching requirements. Programs are between 2 and 3 years in length, with a minimum of 24 months. Completion of a CODA-approved program in endodontics is required to announce specialty status in endodontics.

Communication Between Endodontists and General Dentists

According to the most recent ADA summary of dental services in 2005 to 2006,[5] there were 22.3 million endodontic procedures carried out, with general dentists performing 68.2% and endodontists accounting for 25.4% (the remainder carried out by other specialists). These trends are little changed from the ADA 1999[6] study, which reported 75.2% and 20.3%, respectively. Most endodontic procedures are performed by general dentists, and for optimal patient care it is important to have a good communication between the generalist and specialist. This partnership is essential in helping patients save their teeth.

Communication between general dentists and specialists takes place in the context of the referral of urgent or complex cases, discussion of an optimal treatment plan for a patient, and/or discussion of the latest evidence for a particular procedure or material used in endodontic treatment. Many endodontists also endeavor to speak at local study clubs or regional meetings to promote information on the latest technologies and practices in the field. Most interactions occur by printed forms or letters that are given to the patient (for subsequent delivery) or sent by mail. Phone communication is a common and secure means to efficiently exchange ideas and information about the patient. Electronic forms of communication have become very common. However, many popular methods of electronic communication, such as e-mail, text messages, and online portals, are not inherently secure. Some e-mail programs permit encryption, which must be used for communication related to patients. Some practice management software programs offer online sites where information can be uploaded and viewed in a secure manner. According to the Health Insurance Portability and Accountability Act (HIPAA), there are 19 information items that constitute protected health information (PHI), which can be used to potentially identify a patient. These include the name, birth date, contact information, and health record number, among other items, and they must be kept secure to comply with the law.

What Is Expected of a General Practitioner

Woodmansey and colleagues[7] found through an online survey of 40 predoctoral program directors at U.S. and Canadian dental schools that the average predoctoral student completed an average of 5.9 root canal procedures on live patients, and only 36% of the directors felt that their graduates were competent to perform molar root canals in private practice. By contrast most postgraduate endodontic programs in the United States run about 2 to 3 years. Gulabivala and coworkers (2010)[8] wrote a position paper published by the European Society of Endodontology stating that the minimal clinical requirement should be at 60% of the time, with a minimal number of 180 clinical cases completed.

Burry (2016)[9] looked at a very large database from insurance companies for up to 10 years for treatment completed by endodontists and general dentists, and the data indicated that there is no statistically significant difference in success and failure for incisors, canines, and premolars at 10 years. For molar teeth, however, the results were statistically significant at 10 years, with better outcomes for teeth in treatments performed by endodontists. This data is borne out in private practice as well, with studies showing that molars are the teeth most commonly referred to the endodontist.

Clearly this is a challenging gap and therein exists a potential opportunity for better relationships between the specialist and general dentist.

Abbott and colleagues[10] surveyed general dentists to assess their perceptions and understand the factors associated with referrals to endodontists. A total of 983 general dentists responded; 93% agreed that "endodontists are my partners for delivering quality dental care." In that study, the highest percentage of general dentists (96%) rated communications in the form of timely follow-up reports and images as the best ways to build relationships/partnerships, followed by referring the patient back for restorative treatment (94%) and patient scheduling accommodation (92%). Conversely only 38% mentioned that signs of appreciation, such as gifts, were an effective way to build a lasting relationship. This study reconfirms the importance of communications.

Explicit written instructions, pertinent findings, treatment history, and appropriate radiographs (original or duplicate) are mailed or sent via secure e-mail or website link to the endodontist. (Asking the patient to hand-carry these materials is discouraged.) These instructions should include how the tooth fits into the overall treatment plan, including the anticipated restoration.

What Is Expected of an Endodontist

Lin and colleagues[11] looked at the relationship between the endodontists and their referrals. They looked at many different factors related to the economics of endodontics and referral base. A total of 875 endodontists responded to the survey. In terms of marketing, the majority of participants reported providing gifts (77.8%), personally visiting general dentist offices (76.0%), having websites (66.8%), and organizing social activities (51.9%). Some participated in local study clubs (39.7%) or had their business in the Yellow Pages (29.9%) or on Facebook (19.4%). Seven percent of participants reported having mobile app presences. Also, of interest here was the fact that the most commonly referred tooth type was maxillary molar (60.2%), followed by mandibular molar (38.8%). Almost 10% of the referral cases were referred after a procedural mishap. Almost 50% of the endodontists had performed some form of regenerative procedure.

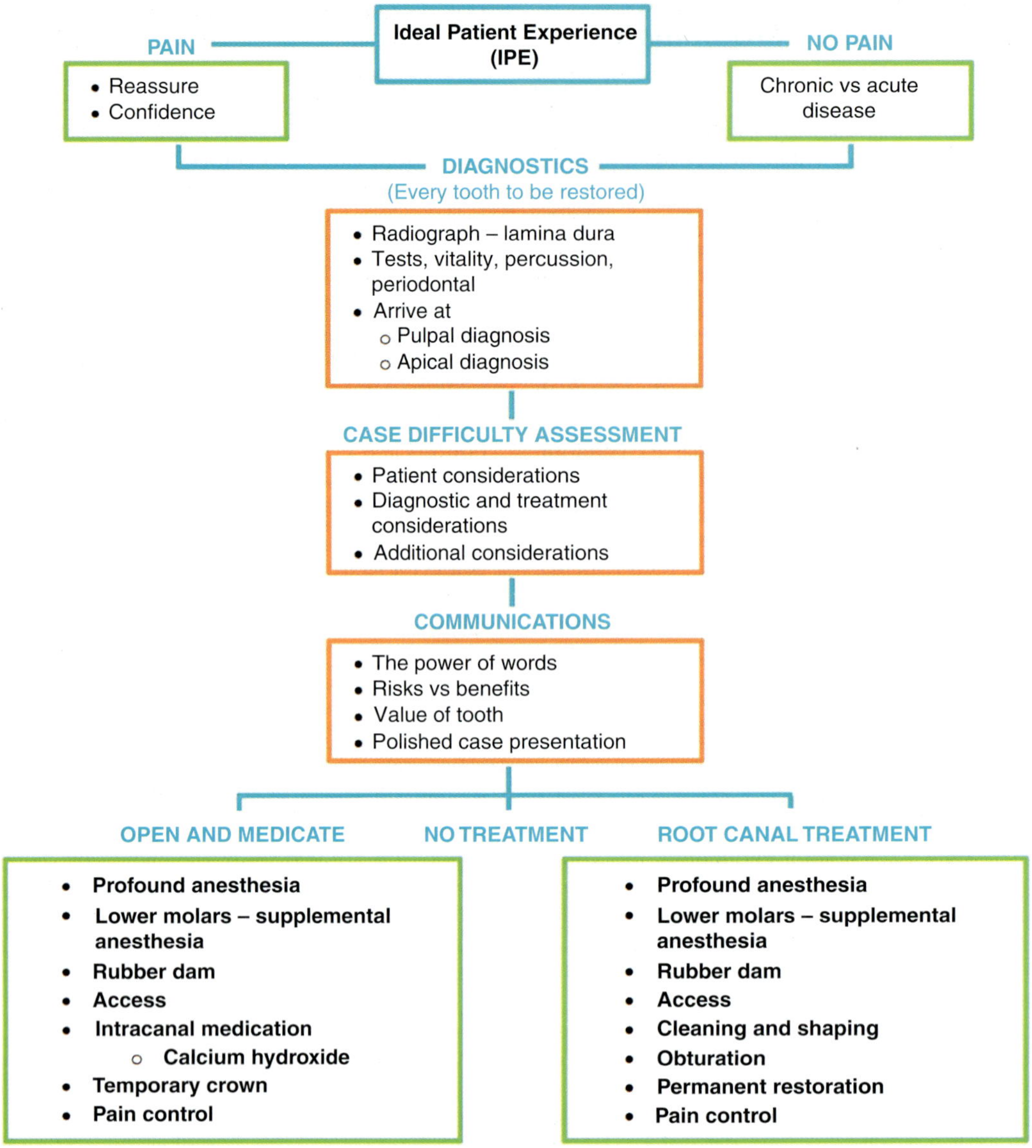

• **Fig. 6.2** Ideal steps in diagnosis, case difficulty assessment, communication with the patient, and treatment.

Specialists serve both the patient and referring dentist, and their responsibilities are to both. They should deliver appropriate treatment and communicate with the practitioner and the patient. When treatment is complete, the referring dentist should receive written confirmation from the endodontist that includes a radiograph of the obturation. A note is included about how the tooth was treated, anticipated recalls, the prognosis (both short term and long term), and unusual findings or circumstances. A suggestion regarding the definitive restoration is appropriate. Before and during treatment, the endodontist explains to the patient all the important aspects of the procedure and the anticipated outcome. After completion of treatment, the patient is informed of the prognosis, appropriate follow-up care, and any possible additional procedures in the future, as well as the need to return to the referring dentist for definitive restoration and continued care.[12]

Based on these findings, two main points become clear. First, there is a disparity in predoctoral dental education, and second, the general dentist has great confidence and belief in the partnership with the endodontist. As the pendulum shifts back to the maintenance of a healthy dentition related to our increased awareness of peri-implantitis, the generalist and specialist have a great opportunity to work together for the benefit of our patients.

Many endodontists are educators at heart, having taught in the undergraduate endodontic clinics, and are passionate about their craft. One of the best ways to nurture this relationship is through education and continuing education (CE) courses to develop the deep relationships that would strengthen and solidify these bridges and ultimately lead to a better patient experience. Fig. 6.2 shows the outline of a CE program that has worked well for one of the authors. There are many other topics, such as dental trauma, regenerative procedures, and cone beam computed tomography (CBCT), that are common areas of interest and will help with the synergistic relationship that will ultimately lead to better patient outcomes.

Standard of Care and Endodontic Case Documentation

Based on reports by the AAE, approximately 75% of nonsurgical root canal procedures are performed by general dentists, and 25% are performed by endodontists (endodontists perform 62% of molar root canals and the majority of retreatment root canal and endodontic microsurgery procedures).[13] Although case selection plays a significant role in these percentages, it is important to recognize that there is one uniform standard of care for providing endodontic treatment regardless of whether the procedures are performed by general dentists or endodontists. Case selection is made based on proper diagnosis, factors that affect long-term prognosis, and complexity of the case being considered. Each practitioner should be fully aware of his or her technical skills and levels of knowledge to determine which cases to treat and which to refer. The AAE has developed a Case Difficulty Assessment Form (see Fig. 6.1) that can be used to assist dentists in assessing the level of difficulty when treatment planning a tooth for endodontic procedures.

Once the decision is made to plan an endodontic procedure treatment of a tooth, the procedural steps and quality of services provided must adhere to the same standards, regardless of who provides the treatment. These steps include obtaining informed consent based on assessment of patient history, chief complaint, clinical and radiographic examination, diagnosis of pulpal and periapical status, and clear presentation of the treatment plan, which includes prognosis as well as risks, benefits, and alternatives. Accurate record keeping is paramount in documenting that the patient has been advised of his or her condition and understands the treatment recommended, including associated risks and costs. Accurate record keeping is also important to memorialize the examination procedures that were used, as well as specific materials employed during treatment. When performing the procedures, if a general dentist encounters challenges that could jeopardize the outcome or create procedural accidents, a consultation with a specialist is advisable.

Proper diagnosis and pretreatment assessment of long-term prognosis depend on accurate and complete gathering of relevant information. Diligent review of the patient's medical history and chief complaint provide an initial impression that can serve as guidance for next steps required to confirm a diagnosis. Even the best treatment based on the wrong diagnosis will predispose the clinician and patient to frustration and an unfavorable treatment outcome. In fact, no treatment is better than rendering the wrong treatment, regardless of how inclined the clinician is to perform services to help a patient in need. The next steps include employment of proper diagnostic tests and obtaining diagnostic radiographs.

The clinical tests currently available simply evaluate the response of an individual to a given stimulus. Thus control teeth are necessary to understand a normal response for the individual patient. For instance, some patients may have extreme sensitivity to cold with all dentition. Evaluation of a single tooth may yield a false impression of an elevated response indicating pulpitis. On the other hand, some individuals do not exhibit a response to stimulus from any teeth. In this case lack of response to a stimulus in the suspected tooth alone may falsely indicate pulpal necrosis. Inclusion of control teeth will help establish normal responses to pulp testing in unaffected teeth before testing the suspected tooth.

A complete radiographic evaluation requires multiple angulations when using intraoral radiographic images to 3-dimensionally visualize a single tooth with multiple roots, presence of severe dilacerations, or multiple canals in a single root. Further, more information can be gathered from multiple views. The radiographic image must capture the whole root and periapical structures, including the entire extent of an apical lesion when present. If apices are not clearly visible, additional images are required. All images obtained must be kept in the records regardless of quality because each angle can provide potentially beneficial information and because records must show all radiographs obtained. Bitewing radiographs allow visualization of bone levels in relation to existing restorations or caries, as well as visualization of the depth of the pulp chamber.[14] When challenges are encountered visualizing pathologic findings (e.g., incipient periapical lesions) to diagnose fractures or to determine proximity of certain anatomic structures, CBCT scans may be indicated.[15] Again, accurate documentation and recording of the preoperative test results are required for future reference.

The ultimate long-term prognosis of a tooth may be determined by other factors, such as periodontal status and restorability of the tooth in question. Measurement of periodontal attachment loss is critical in determining the correct diagnosis, which will ultimately dictate whether a tooth is likely to respond to endodontic treatment. Restorability may often require removal of existing restorations and caries to assess fully the remaining sound tooth structure. Patients must be informed of these considerations before initiation of treatment. Completion of endodontic treatment on an unrestorable tooth is as unethical as extraction of a sound tooth.[14]

Once a definitive diagnosis is made and the patient has consented to begin treatment, endodontic procedures performed must adhere to the accepted standard of care. These steps include the following:

Proper and profound anesthesia. Although this topic is covered in detail in Chapter 8, it is important to point out that most patients who express anxiety with regard to root canal therapy (RCT) have concerns about pain during the procedure. Profound anesthesia will provide a more pleasant experience for patient and clinician and will allow greater attention to performing the procedure properly.

Adequate rubber dam isolation. The primary goals of nonsurgical root canal treatment are to remove microbial contamination and to provide an adequate seal to prevent reinfection of the root canal system. To adhere to strict aseptic protocols, proper rubber dam isolation is necessary to prevent salivary contamination of the field of operation and to prevent aspiration of instruments, irrigants, or other materials. In short, tooth isolation using a rubber dam is standard of care and mandatory.[16]

Proper biomechanical débridement. Biomechanical débridement relies on the use of endodontic files to remove debris and to enlarge the canal space, allowing penetration of irrigating solution. Although canal enlargement should be adequate to allow passive insertion of a small-gauge needle, care must be taken not to overinstrument the canals at the expense of dentinal walls (no less than 1 mm). Proper working length determination early in the procedure is essential to minimize occurrences of overextension of material or creation of procedural mishaps, such as ledge formation or strip perforations.[13]

Use of approved materials. Mechanical instrumentation alone does not allow for optimum disinfection of the root canal system, and irrigation solutions with antimicrobial activity are required during canal débridement. Although sodium hypochlorite in various concentrations remains the most popular root canal irrigant, many new irrigation solutions have entered the market with various properties, including antimicrobial activity and/or smear layer removal activity. Because many of these irrigants can cause some degree of irritation to the periapical tissues, care must be taken to avoid inadvertent extrusion of the solution beyond the root apex, which may occur by locking the needle in the canal space.

Most obturation systems include a solid core used in conjunction with a sealer. Proper canal instrumentation and competency in techniques employed for placement of these materials is essential to prevent overextension of the materials beyond the root apex. Although relatively biocompatible, most root canal filling materials can cause irritation because the immune system in the periapical tissues may recognize these materials as foreign. Paste fillers generally are not recommended because they are more difficult to control during obturation. Further, paste fillers containing paraformaldehyde must be completely avoided.[17]

Adequate final restoration. After completion of endodontic treatment, proper coronal restoration is critical to prevent reinfection of the root canal system and protect the tooth. Studies have shown that properly instrumented and filled root canals can become rapidly contaminated if not properly restored and exposure of gutta-percha and sealer to saliva can cause rapid penetration of bacteria.[18-20] Provisional restorations placed after the completion of endodontic procedures serve as a temporary seal and must be planned for replacement with a permanent restoration, preferably within 30 days. Exposure of provisional access restorations to saliva can cause recontamination of the root canal system within 30 days.[21]

Proper postoperative care and instructions. Postoperative instructions should be provided before and after treatment to help patients know what to expect in the ensuing days. These instructions should be provided in written form because patients often forget verbal information. Additionally, adequate perioperative medications should be provided as needed. More specific information regarding medications will be provided in Chapter 9.

Study Questions

1. The ADA Code of Ethics position on duty to refer includes which of the following:
   a. Being current on knowledge and skill
   b. Knowing one's own limitations
   c. Recognizing when to refer
   d. All of the above
2. When performing root canal treatment, what is the difference in standard of care expected of a general dentist and an endodontist?
   a. General dentists are held to a higher standard of care than endodontists
   b. Endodontists are held to a higher standard of care than general dentists
   c. General dentists and endodontists are held to the same standard of care
   d. General dentists and endodontists are not held to a state but not national standard of care
3. How many years of additional training beyond dental school is required to become a specialist in endodontics?
   a. A minimum of 12 months
   b. A minimum of 22 months
   c. A minimum of 24 months
   d. A minimum of 36 months
4. To whom does the specialist have the primary responsibility?
   a. Patient
   b. Referring dentist
   c. Patient's financial guarantor
   d. No one
5. Who performs the majority of root canal procedures in the U.S.?
   a. Endodontists
   b. General dentists
   c. Oral surgeons
   d. Dental students

Case Difficulty Assessment—When to Treat and When to Refer

The AAE has developed a form to assist with assessment of case difficulty and potential need for referral to a specialist, *AAE Endodontic Case Difficulty Assessment Form and Guidelines* (see Fig. 6.1). The form is a free download available at https://www.aae.org/specialty/wp-content/uploads/sites/2/2019/02/19AAE_CaseDifficultyAssessmentForm.pdf The assessment form takes the user through a series of questions/conditions in three broad categories: patient considerations, diagnostic and treatment considerations, and additional considerations. Each of the three major categories is divided into subcategories.

The guidelines use the classifications titled minimal difficulty, moderate difficulty, and high difficulty to assist the practitioner in identifying the parameters of case difficulty and making a judgment as to whether the case is within his or her level of expertise. At first, the process may seem cumbersome. However, *repeated* usage and familiarity *reduces risk* for both patients and general dentists. This process should allow the dentist to provide optimum quality care. Referral can happen before, during, and after root canal treatment.

Patient Considerations

Medical History

Although some general dentists are well-trained in assessment and management of medically complex patients, especially clinicians who have completed a general practice residency (GPR) or Advanced Education in General Dentistry program (AEGD), a specialist is often better prepared to provide efficient RCT to a medically compromised patient. Frequently these patients are unable to stay in the dental chair for a long procedure, may require management under intravenous (IV) sedation or in the operating room, or require premedication and close monitoring during treatment. All these are factors that can complicate treatment, even if the technical aspects of the treatment do not appear to be complicated.

Anesthesia

Although true allergy to an amide local anesthetic is considered rare,[22] a patient's previous experiences with local anesthesia may nonetheless require some form of treatment modification. A thorough dental history should identify patients who have had previous problems with local anesthesia; most commonly reported problems are sensitivity to a vasoconstrictor or difficulty achieving profound anesthesia. Both of these situations, individually and collectively, will elevate the degree of difficulty and can usually be determined with a good dental history.

Patient Disposition

Anxious and uncooperative patients can present treatment challenges to both general dentists and specialists; however, the specialist's additional training and experience can often translate into a better patient experience or, at least, the ability to complete a procedure in a shorter period of time. Specialty training includes strategies for managing challenging patients.

Gag Reflex and Ability to Open Mouth

Patients with an active gag reflex present difficulties in acquiring diagnostic quality radiographs, especially for posterior teeth, as well as treatment. Alternatives such as a panoramic radiograph and/or CBCT imaging can often provide valuable additional information but should not be routinely used as a substitute for a high-quality periapical radiograph. Many patients with an active gag reflex often respond well to placement of a dental dam because the soft palate is then protected from stimulation, whereas other patients become claustrophobic and are not able to tolerate a dental dam. Oral anxiolytics or nitrous oxide/oxygen are sometimes useful, and there is a small subset of patients who will require general anesthesia for RCT. Because a dental dam is considered the standard of care for RCT, if it is not possible to place a dental dam, the patient is not a candidate for RCT.

Limited opening due to a variety of reasons can elevate the degree of difficulty from minimal to high.

Emergency Condition

Patients presenting in severe pain and/or with significant swelling require a high level of skill and experience to manage (Fig. 6.3). Profound anesthesia is often difficult to obtain in the presence of infection and for teeth with a diagnosis of symptomatic irreversible pulpitis, especially mandibular posterior teeth.

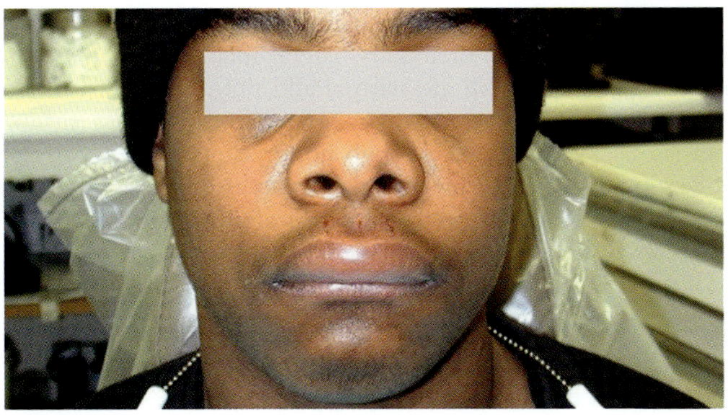

• **Fig. 6.3** A 17-year-old male presented on an emergency basis complaining of pain and swelling of the upper lip. The diagnosis was pulp necrosis with acute apical abscess and cellulitis. Obtaining profound local anesthesia in situations like this can be very difficult and painful for the patient due to the diffuse tissue edema.

Diagnostic and Treatment Considerations

Diagnosis

Appropriate treatment follows accurate diagnosis. Diagnostic difficulties include confusing test results, nonspecific or unusual patterns of pain from periradicular lesions of nonpulpal origin, endodontic or periodontal lesions, and resorption.

As noted in Chapter 4 the practitioner should be able to use the patient's signs and symptoms, the clinical and radiographic findings, and the results of clinical tests to establish a pulpal and periapical diagnosis and make treatment decisions accordingly. Applying these principles should allow the general practitioner to make an accurate diagnosis in most cases (Fig. 6.4). However, there are many cases in which the application of these basic principles is not sufficient, and the practitioner would need the expertise of a specialist to recognize and manage less common patient presentations or clinical conditions. These complex cases include situations in which diagnostic tests provide conflicting results or results that do not match the radiographic and clinical findings, traumatic injuries to teeth and their sequelae, diagnosis of symptomatic cases that were previously treated endodontically (Fig. 6.5), and/or orofacial pain or radiolucencies of nonendodontic origin that mimic endodontic pathosis.

Radiographic Difficulties

Radiographs are important tools for proper diagnosis and treatment planning. In cases in which obtaining and interpreting radiographs are difficult, the patient should be referred to an endodontist. This circumstance occurs with patients who have muscle trismus, have received radiation therapy to the orofacial musculature, have severe gagging issues, and/or have a small oral cavity.

Position in the Arch

Many dentists perform root canal treatment based on the location of the tooth in the arch. However, many other factors in addition to the location of the tooth in the arch make root canal treatment difficult. Depending on these factors, performing a root canal in a second molar in one patient may be easier than performing the procedure on a premolar in another patient.

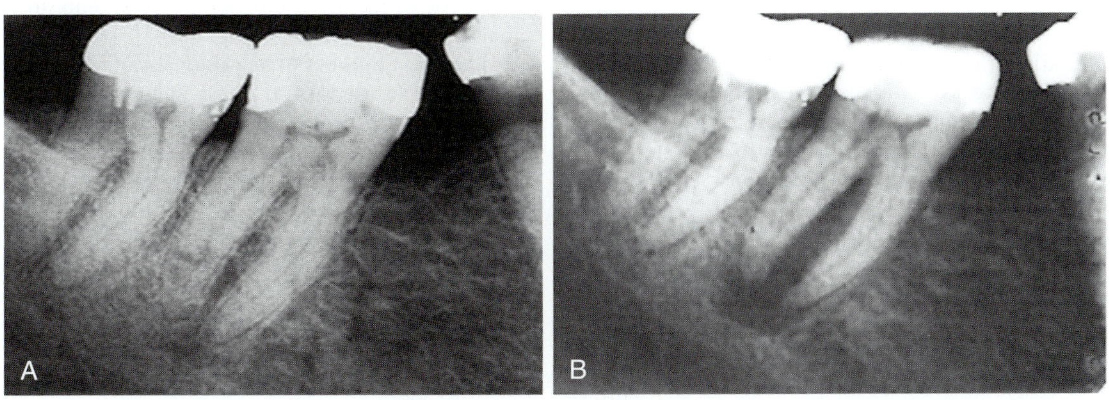

• **Fig. 6.4** An Example of Simple Diagnosis. Tooth #30 had caries and was not responsive to pulp testing. **A,** The dentist excavated the restoration and placed a temporary restoration because "the tooth did not have a pulp exposure." **B,** Three months later, a periapical lesion had developed. Endodontic treatment should have been initiated at the time of diagnosis for pulp necrosis.

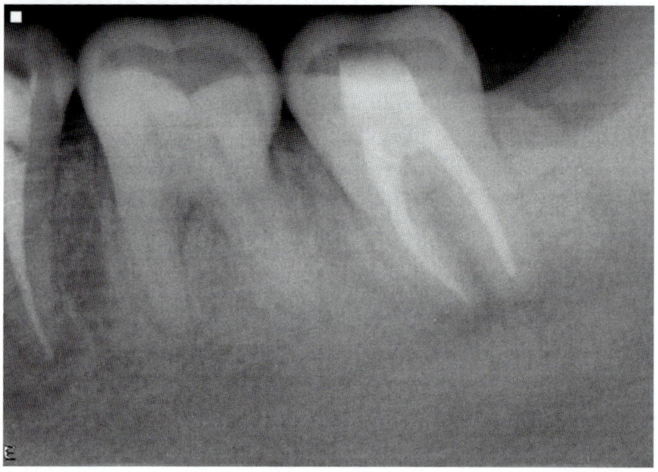

• **Fig. 6.5** An Example of Complex Diagnosis. The patient had a chronic, dull ache in the mandibular left quadrant. Endodontic treatment had been completed 2 years earlier by an endodontist, and the lesion appeared to be resolving. The chief complaint could not be reproduced, and the radiographic pattern of the bone suggested a possibility of bone pathosis. The case was diagnosed by an oral and maxillofacial surgeon as chronic sclerosing osteomyelitis.

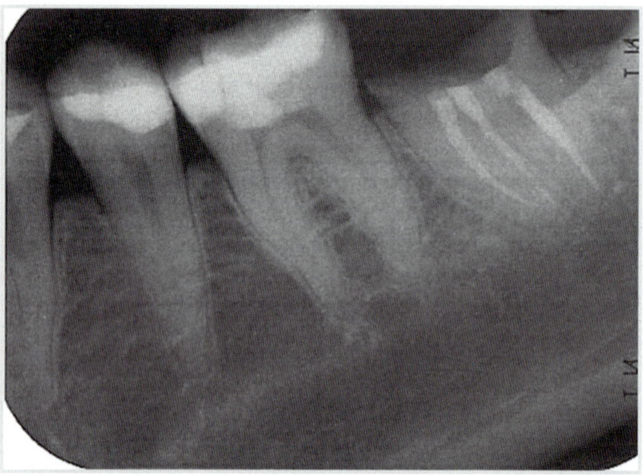

• **Fig. 6.6** In addition to the position of tooth #18 in the arch, this tooth will be challenging to isolate if retreatment root canal therapy (RCT) is indicated and has questionable restorability.

Tooth Isolation

Because of severe caries or crown fractures, a tooth may be too difficult to isolate or to restore; extraction may be the best alternative. In some instances, crown lengthening may be necessary to create biologic width before performing root canal treatment. Referral to a specialist for this type of treatment should be considered if such a problem exists (Fig. 6.6).

Crown Morphology

A number of anatomic factors should be considered in the treatment planning for a tooth intended for RCT. Many teeth that require root canal treatment have cast restorations. The restoration anatomy usually does not correspond to the original crown anatomy, and the pulp chamber can be difficult to locate. When a tooth that requires root canal treatment is part of a bridge, the angulation of the restoration to the original crown (Fig. 6.7), and its location in the arch must be examined carefully before an access preparation is made. These considerations are particularly important in maxillary first premolars, lateral incisors, and mandibular incisors. These teeth are narrow and prone to crown or root perforations during access cavity preparations. Access through gold is easier than access through nonprecious metals. Porcelain crowns are fragile and can break during access preparation. Newer zirconia-type crowns are very hard and often require special burs for access. When the pulp chamber and orifices to the root canals are not visible in the preoperative radiographs, referral to an endodontist should be considered (Fig. 6.8).

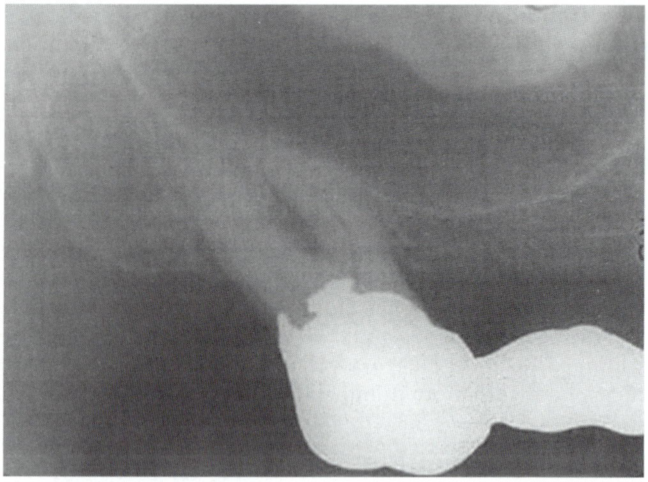

• **Fig. 6.7** This maxillary right second molar presents many challenges for endodontic therapy. It is mesially inclined about 45 degrees, has a full occlusal coverage restoration (abutment for a long-span fixed prosthesis), and moderately calcified canals. The degree of difficulty is high and would be even higher if the patient had limited ability to open.

Canal and Root Morphology

Several situations may limit access to the tooth in question, making it difficult to render routine treatment. These cases include limited mouth opening (particularly for the treatment of molars), tooth crowding, severe tilting or rotation, subgingival carious lesions necessitating crown lengthening or other procedures to ensure good isolation, and molars with very long working lengths. In the latter case, although the tooth may be accessible for routine restorative work, the use of long instruments to instrument the canals presents a challenge (Fig. 6.9).

There are a number of anatomic variations that may necessitate referral to an endodontist. These include teeth with an immature apex, teeth with severe canal curvature (Fig. 6.10, *A* and *B*), or teeth with a very calcified canal space. The general dentist should always be aware of the common anatomic variations of teeth and should rely on consultation or referral if he or she suspects additional canals that cannot be located, if the anatomic variation is unusual, or if the disease process persists despite treatment. Examples of circumstances in which the anatomic variations may render a case difficult to manage by the general dentist include mandibular premolars with more than one canal; maxillary premolars with more than two canals; radix entomolaris (extra roots in the mandibular molars); C-shaped canals (Fig. 6.11); dens invaginatus and evaginatus; fused and geminated teeth; teeth with palatal groove defects; and teeth with lateral or J-shaped lesions (which may have unusual canal branching).

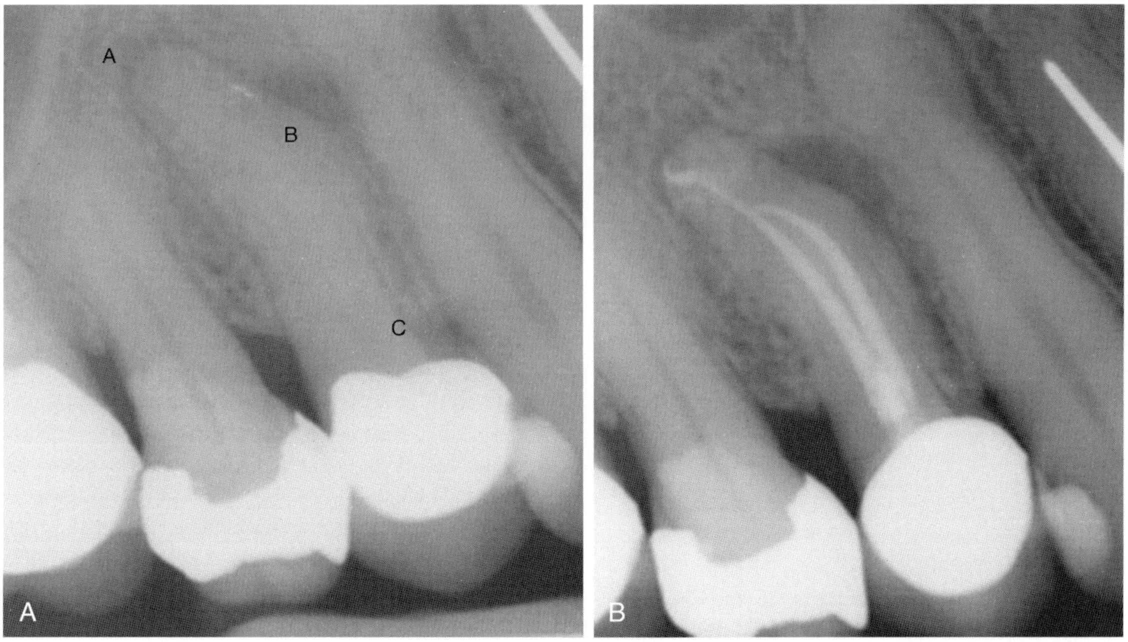

• **Fig. 6.8 A,** Periapical radiolucency *(A)* and mesial radiolucency in the apical third *(B)*. The canals are calcified, the root is narrow, and there is a hint of a significant mesial concavity in the coronal third *(C)*. The tooth is also crowned, thereby increasing access complexity. This case is considered a high risk. **B,** Post-operatively, the mesial radiolucency resulted from the buccal root exiting several millimeters shorter than the palatal root with a significant distal curvature. The practitioner must manage unexpected complications should problems arise during treatment.

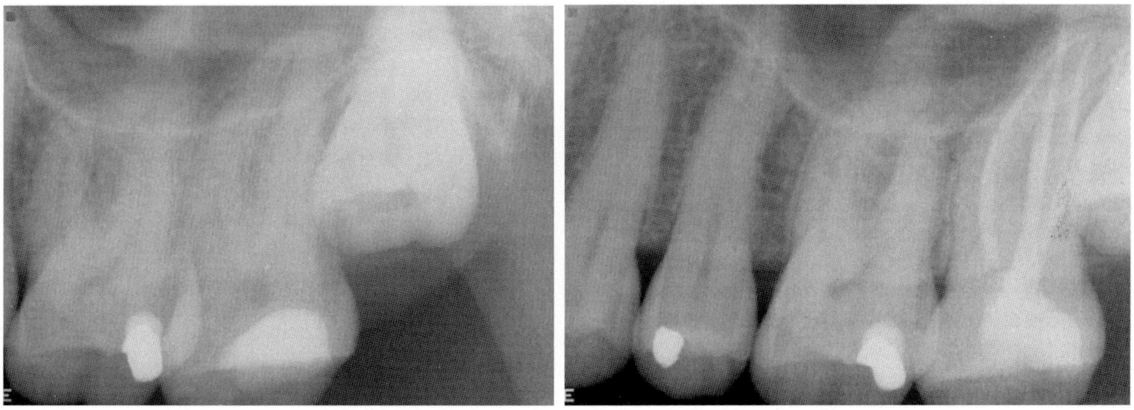

• **Fig. 6.9** Maxillary left second molar with working lengths that ranged from 26 to 28 mm.

Radiographic Appearance of Canal(s)

As a tooth ages, its pulp chamber and root canals calcify. Pulp chamber and root canal sizes, the presence of pulp stones, and the extent of calcifications in the root canal system must be considered before a decision is made regarding root canal treatment (Fig. 6.12). Management of these teeth is always challenging and typically requires use of a dental operating microscope and often CBCT imaging.

Resorption

Apical root resorption, common in necrotic teeth with long-standing apical periodontitis, requires careful determination and control of proper working length to help prevent overextension of root filling materials. Internal and external resorption (invasive cervical resorption) are two separate conditions, and both require a high level of diagnostic and treatment skill (Figs. 6.13, *A* and *B*).

Additional Considerations

Many of the cases that fall into the categories of traumatic injuries, retreatments, and surgeries are further described in the corresponding chapters (Chapters 11, 19, and 20, respectively); a general description of the interaction of the general dentist and the specialist is given here. Many cases of traumatic injuries are first seen by the patient's general dentist. The general dentist has an obligation to manage the emergency condition and triage the patient appropriately. The latest guidelines for management of traumatic injuries should be readily available and frequently reviewed. Diagnosis should include the pulpal and periapical

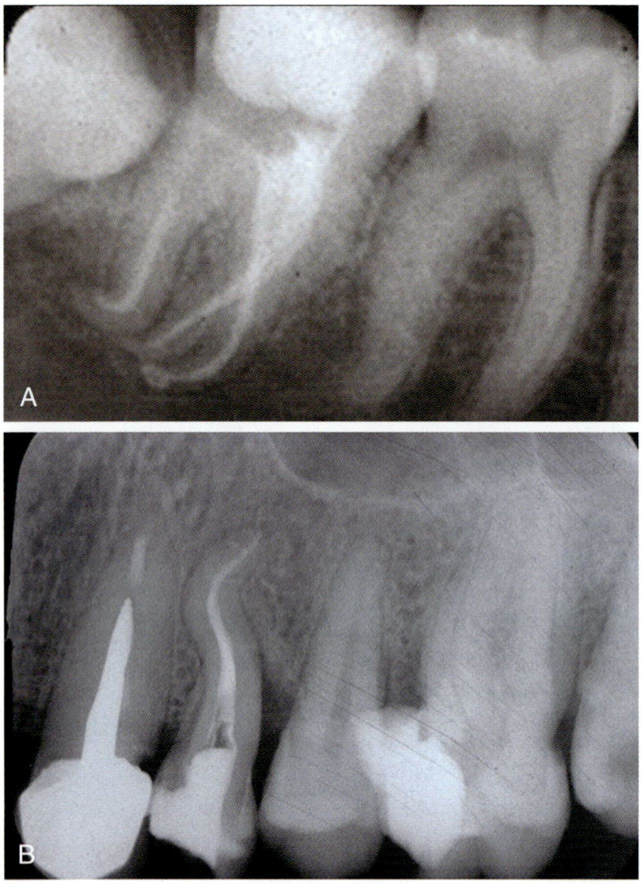

• **Fig. 6.10** **A,** This mandibular right second molar exhibited extreme root curvatures and presented access and isolation difficulties (Case courtesy Dr. Steve Weeks). **B,** Immediate postoperative radiograph of maxillary left second premolar demonstrating "S" curvature.

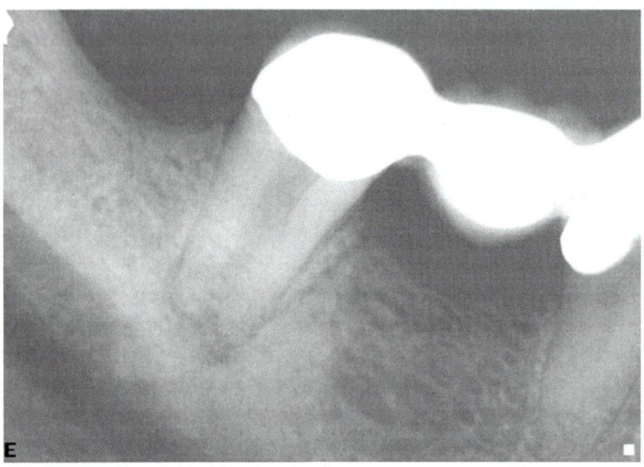

• **Fig. 6.11** Mandibular right second molar with suspected S-shaped canal space. The location in the arch, moderate mesial inclination, and presence of full occlusal coverage restoration would add to the complexity of treatment.

conditions of all the teeth in the area of trauma after the necessary examination and clinical testing has been performed. Management includes first aid for soft tissue injuries, repositioning of luxated teeth, and/or restoration of fractured teeth. The specialist should be involved in the diagnosis and management of

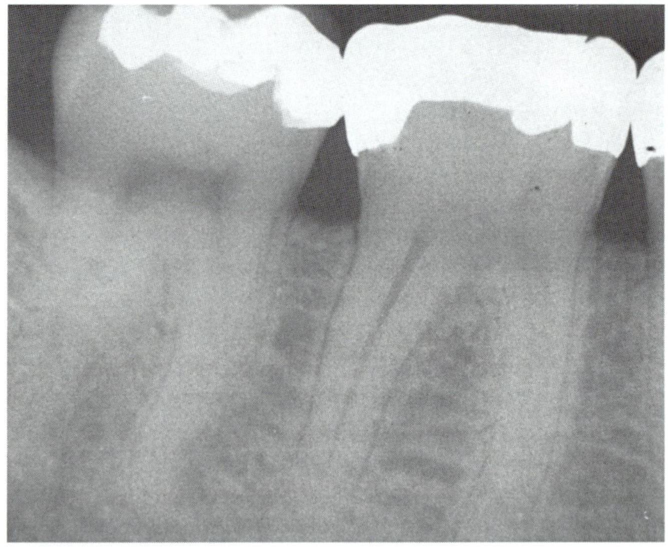

• **Fig. 6.12** Pulp chamber and root canals show calcific metamorphosis. This situation is rated as an extreme risk.

extensive injuries and complications, including luxations, fracture of the alveolar bone and obvious pulpal involvement, root fractures, root resorptions, teeth with immature apices, patients with behavioral or complex medical problems, and late complications of trauma.

The general dentist plays an important role as the gatekeeper of the patient's oral health in recognizing and referring cases with failure of previous endodontic treatment (Fig. 6.14, *A* and *B*) Many of these cases are asymptomatic; therefore recognizing them requires adequate clinical and radiographic examination of the patient (Fig. 6.15, *A* and *B*). The general dentist should be aware of the treatment procedures that are within the scope of endodontic practice and educate the patient accordingly. It is important that the general dentist present the patient with all the available treatment options before recommending that a tooth be extracted and replaced by an implant or prosthesis. There are many cases in which the general dentist recognizes that additional expertise in determining the prognosis and treatment options is needed and that consultation with an endodontist is warranted. In retrospect, many of the cases that are surgically or nonsurgically retreated by an endodontist should have been referred to the endodontist for primary treatment (Fig. 6.16). The prudent general dentist recognizes a case that is likely to be too complex and refers appropriately, rather than risk the development of treatment problems. There are many cases in which treatment appears to be routine, yet problems are encountered; referral to an endodontist can help ensure a good outcome.

Referral During Treatment

The timing and discussion of referral with the patient are important during treatment planning. It is poor practice to initiate treatment with the sense that problems will be encountered and that a referral will be made then. An initial referral prevents potential procedural accidents and improves the prognosis of difficult cases. Midtreatment referral may also result in misunderstanding and loss of confidence by the patient. Another issue is financial problems that may arise during midtreatment referrals. The

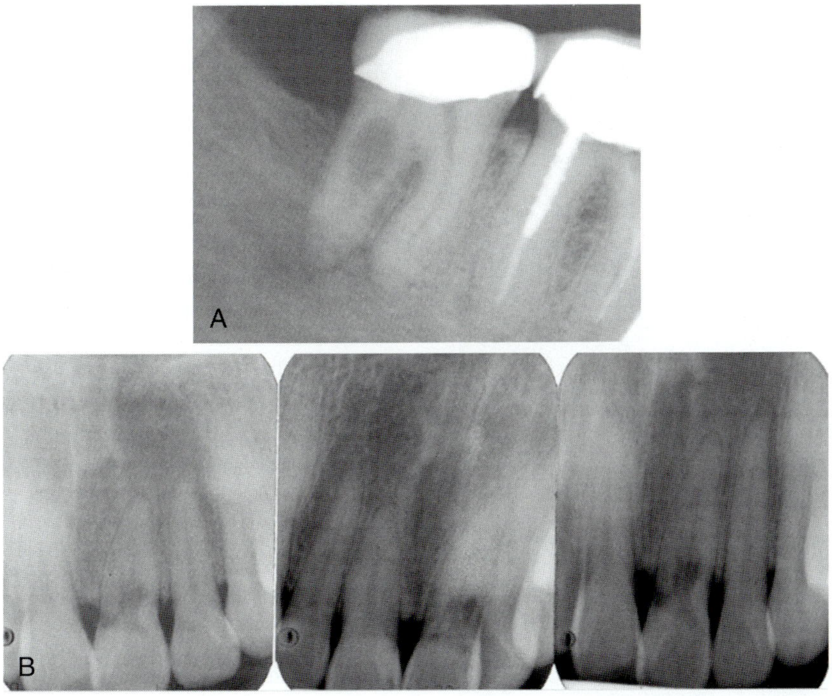

• **Fig. 6.13 A,** Large internal resorptive lesion observed in the distal root of the mandibular right second molar. **B,** Extensive invasive cervical resorption in maxillary left central incisor as seen in three angled radiographs. Cone beam computed tomography (CBCT) would be very useful to determine the extent of this lesion and develop a treatment plan.

endodontist is entitled to a full fee, and the patient should not be responsible for two fees for one tooth.

Despite all precautions and considerations, unanticipated problems may arise during treatments that require referral. A full explanation to the patient and a call to the endodontist are the necessary elements to prevent future problems. Reasons for referral during treatment include flare-ups (pain and/or swelling), procedural accidents, inability to achieve adequate anesthesia, and other factors that hinder completion of RCT.

Flare-ups

Usually most pain or swelling occurs before initial treatment. After emergency treatments, pain usually decreases significantly in most patients within 24 to 48 hours. Flare-ups are not common during root canal treatments.[23] However, some patients develop pain and/or swelling after initiation of root canal treatment. The general dentist may elect to treat such flare-ups with appropriate local procedures and systemic medications. If these measures prove inadequate, referral to an endodontist is in order.

Procedural Accidents

Procedural accidents during root canal treatment include ledge formation, creation of an artificial canal, root perforations, separated instruments, hypochlorite accidents, and underfilling and overfilling. (The causes, prevention, and prognosis of these mishaps are discussed in detail in Chapter 18) Consultation with an endodontist is advisable to handle these accidents nonsurgically or, in some cases, surgically (properly and expediently) with appropriate follow-up. Treatment approaches and long-term assessment of these cases are usually beyond the expertise of a general dentist.

Referral After Treatment

Persistent problems, such as pain, pathosis, and sinus tract after root canal treatment may indicate root canal failure and the need for further evaluation and treatment.

Pain

If pain and/or swelling persist or develop after treatment, the patient should be referred, or an endodontist should be consulted. These symptoms may be related to lack of débridement, inadequate obturation, missed canals, root fractures, or other causes. Surgical and/or nonsurgical retreatment procedures or extraction might be in order.

Persistent Pathosis

Persistent periapical lesions or the development of new lesions after root canal treatment is indicative of root canal failure. Surgical and/or nonsurgical retreatment procedures are needed to resolve the problem.

Sinus Tract

When a periodontal defect of pulpal origin or a sinus tract does not resolve after treatment, the patient should be referred to an endodontist. The presence of a new defect or sinus tract indicates treatment failure, and the patient must be referred for consultation or treatment by an endodontist.

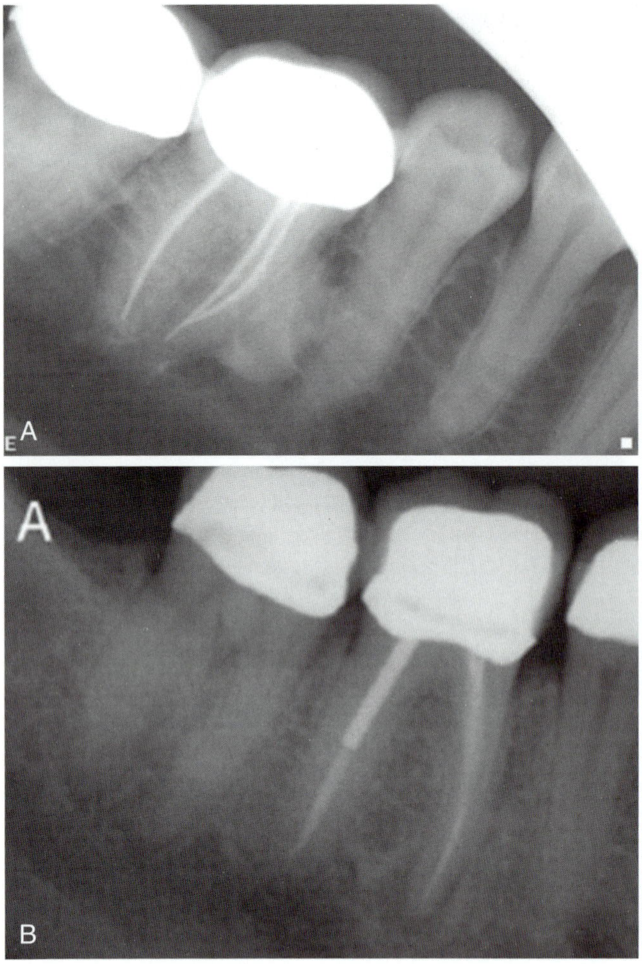

• **Fig. 6.14** These are examples of previously treated teeth that present a high level of difficulty. **(A)** is a previously treated mandibular right first molar with carrier-based filling material; **(B)** has a post in the distal canal. This tooth could be managed either with nonsurgical retreatment or endodontic microsurgery, and both options could lead to a predictable outcome when managed by a specialist.

Summary

Sometimes the most important treatment planning decision made by a general dentist is deciding when *not* to treat. Midtreatment referral to an endodontist to help manage a treatment complication creates unnecessary stress for all involved and can damage the patient–dentist relationship. A good endodontist will never disparage the work of a general dentist; however, most patients can sense when a general dentist has started treatment that might have been better managed by an initial referral to a specialist. Part of an endodontist's skill set is managing treatment complications, but every endodontist will tell you they would rather be the first clinician to initiate treatment on a difficult case rather than attempt corrective action.

Study Questions

6. Which of the following is a potential indication for referral to a specialist?
   a. A patient's report of difficulty with local anesthesia during previous dental procedures
   b. Severely calcified canal
   c. Challenges posed by location of a tooth in the arch
   d. Teeth with incomplete root development
   e. All of the above
7. Which of the following is the proper method of tooth isolation for endodontic therapy in patients with a severe gag reflex or claustrophobia?
   a. Cotton role and gauze
   b. Rubber dam
   c. Use of high-volume suction and mirror
   d. None of the above
8. The general dentist plays an important role in which of the following?
   a. Management of traumatic injuries
   b. Identifying failure of previous endodontic therapy
   c. Identifying complex cases, which may require referral to the appropriate specialist
   d. All of the above
9. What is the definition of a flare-up?
   a. Patient is upset about cost of treatment
   b. Pain to cold and heat
   c. A cracked tooth
   d. Pain and swelling after initiation of root canal therapy
10. Procedure accidents include all of the following except:
   a. Instrument separation during root canal therapy
   b. Perforation during access preparation
   c. Root fracture due to traumatic injury
   d. Hypochlorite accident

ANSWERS

Answer Box 6

1 One of dentist's primary obligations is knowing his or her own limitations and when to refer to a specialist.
2 No difference
3 2 or 3 years (minimum 24 months)
4 False. Specialists serve both the patient and the referring dentist.
5 False. General dentists perform approximately 75% of root canal procedures, although endodontists perform 62% of molar RCT.
6 True
7 False. Use of a dental dam is the standard of care for root canal treatment, primarily to protect the patient from aspiration or ingestion of endodontic instruments and also to maintain proper asepsis. Inability to place a dental dam is an absolute contraindication to performing root canal treatment.
8 False
9 True
10 False. There are many other factors in addition to the location of the tooth in the arch that make root canal treatment difficult.

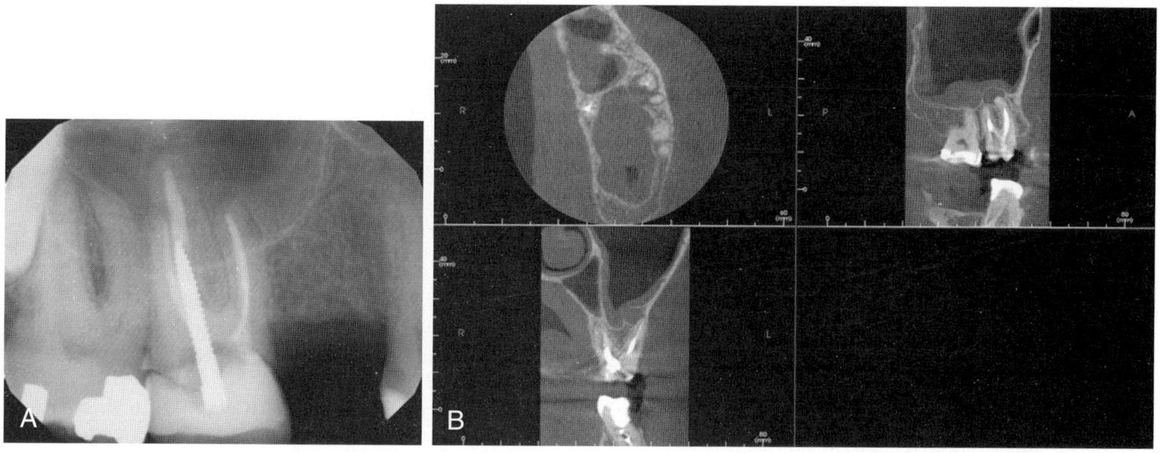

• **Fig. 6.15** This asymptomatic previously treated maxillary right first molar was referred to an endodontist to evaluate for possible retreatment or endodontic microsurgery before proceeding with a new crown. The standard two-dimensional image **(A)** was of limited value. However, cone beam computed tomography (CBCT) of the tooth demonstrated clear evidence of periapical pathosis and sinus mucositis secondary to persistent endodontic disease.

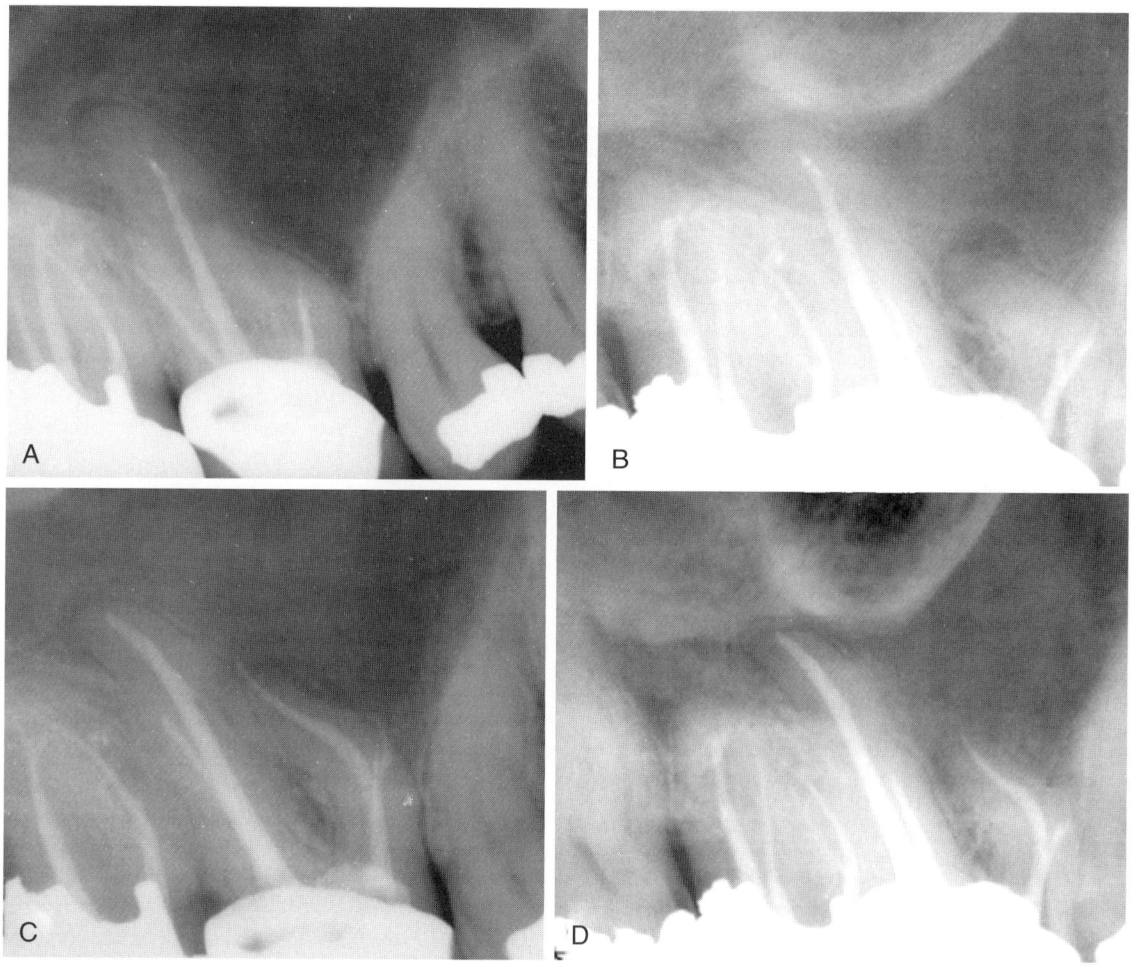

• **Fig. 6.16** Patient presented to the general dentist for root canal treatment of tooth #3. The tooth has severe curvature of mesial buccal (MB) root. The dentist performed root canal treatment and a crown for the tooth. **A,** Three months later, the patient was referred to the endodontist with continued pain. The straight radiograph shows that the MB canal could not be negotiated to length and had a possible perforation. There was blockage apically in the palatal (P) and distal buccal canals. The palatal root has a small radiolucency. **B,** Distal shift showing the perforation on the MB canal and the lesion related to this root. The root apex had apical root resorption. **C,** Retreatment was successful in negotiating the MB and P canals. Sealed the perforation with mineral trioxide aggregate (MTA). **D,** Six months follow-up showing healing of the lesions and absence of signs and symptoms of disease.

References

1. Americans Rate Healthcare Providers High on Honesty, Ethics. *Gallup.* December 19, 2016.
2. *Principles of Ethics and Code of Professional Conduct.* American Dental Association. Revised February 2018.
3. Niederman R, Richards D, Brands W: The changing standard of care, *J Am Dent Assoc* 143:434–437, 2012.
4. Zinman EJ: Endodontic records and legal responsibilities. In Hargreaves KM, Cohen S, Berman LH, editors: *Cohen's pathways of the pulp*, ed 10, St. Louis, 2011, Mosby, p 411.
5. ADA Health Policy Institute: 2005-06 *Survey of Dental Services Rendered.*
6. ADA Health Policy Institute: *Survey of Dental Services Rendered*, 1999.
7. Woodmansey K, Beck LG, Rodriguez TE: The landscape of predoctoral endodontic education in the United States and Canada: results of a survey, *J Dent Educ* 79:922–927, 2015.
8. Gulabivala K, Ahlquist M, Cunnington S, et al.: Accreditation of postgraduate speciality training programmes in endodontology. Minimum criteria for training specialists in endodontology within Europe, *Int Endod J* 43(9):725–737, 2010.
9. Burry JC, Stover S, Eichmiller F, Bhagavatula P: Outcomes of primary endodontic therapy provided by endodontic specialists compared with other providers, *J Endod* 42:702–705, 2016.
10. Abbott JA, Wolcott JF, Gordon G, Terlap HT: Survey of general dentists to identify characteristics associated with increased referrals to endodontists, *J Endod* 37:1191–1196, 2011.
11. Lin S, Sabbah W, Sedgley CM, Whitten B: A survey for endodontists in today's economy: exploring the current state of endodontics as a profession and the relationship between endodontists and their referral base, *J Endod* 41:325–332, 2015.
12. Kramer S: Communications regarding referrals, *Risk Manage Rep* I(IV):4, 1989.
13. *Treatment Standards*, pp 1–20. Available from www.aae.org, 2018.
14. *Endodontic competency in the diagnosis of endodontic treatment*, pp 1–11. Available from www.aae.org, 2017.
15. *AAE/AAOMR Joint Position Statement – Use of Cone Beam Computed Tomography in Endodontics*, pp 1–6. Available from www.aae.org, 2016.
16. *Dental Dams.* Available from www.aae.org, 2017.
17. Concerning Paraformaldehyde-Containing Endodontic Filling Materials and Sealers: *AAE Position Statement*, Reaffirmed, 2017, p 2017. Available from www.aae.org.
18. Torabinejad M, Ung B, Kettering JD: In vitro bacterial penetration of coronally unsealed endodontically treated teeth, *J Endod* 19:458–461, 1993.
19. Torabinejad M, Ung B, Kettering JD: In vitro bacterial penetration of coronally unsealed endodontically treated teeth, *J Endod* 16:566–569, 1990.
20. Khayat A, Lee SJ, Torabinejad M: Human saliva penetration of coronally unsealed obturated root canals, *J Endod* 19:458–461, 1993.
21. Magura ME, Kafrawy AH, Brown Jr CE, Newton CW: Human saliva coronal microleakage in obturated root canals: an in vitro study, *J Endod* 17:324–331, 1991.
22. Little JW, Miller CS, Rhodus NL, editors: *Little and Fallace's dental management of the medically compromised patient*, ed 9, St. Louis, 2018, Mosby, p 335.
23. Walton R, Fouad A: Endodontic interappointment flare-ups: a prospective study of incidence and related factors, *J Endod* 18:172, 1992.

7

Endodontic Armamentarium

ADHAM A. AZIM AND PHILIP MICHAELSON

CHAPTER OUTLINE

LEARNING OBJECTIVES

At the end of this chapter, the student should be able to:

1. Define the basic set of armamentarium appropriate for diagnosis, emergency treatment, canal preparation, obturation, and endodontic surgery.
2. Describe the general characteristics of endodontic armamentarium and show how these characteristics are related to their use.
3. Describe the importance of using magnification for proper endodontic treatment.
4. Present the advantages of three-dimensional (3D) versus two-dimensional (2D) radiographic imaging.
5. Explain the basis for sizing and taper of hand and rotary instruments.
6. Describe the basic design of the more common canal preparation instruments and their mode of use.
7. Describe the various adjunct tools needed to achieve adequate disinfection.
8. Identify the various temporary restorative materials used after endodontic treatment.
9. Describe the various adjunct tools used during endodontic surgery.

Introduction

The goals of nonsurgical root canal therapy (RCT) are to chemomechanically débride, disinfect, and shape the root canal spaces, followed by adequately sealing all portals of entry and exit.[1,2] To achieve these goals, multitudes of solutions and dental instruments have been specially designed and used. Historically, varied attempts at endodontic treatments have been documented since ancient times. In 1728 Pierre Fauchard wrote *The Surgeon Dentist*, which described the dental pulp space and the procedure to access this space to relieve abscess formation. Fauchard recommended leaving the access to the pulp space open for months and then filling the opening with lead foil. Advancing on this concept, Robert Woofendale in 1766 was credited with the first endodontic procedure in the United States. He would cauterize the dental pulp with a hot instrument and place cotton in the root canals. From this idea, the concept of pulp extirpation took hold. In 1838 Edwin Maynard fabricated the first endodontic instrument. He ground a watch spring into a broach, which he would then use to extirpate the dental pulp. Over the next several decades, endodontic instruments continued to evolve into the instruments and materials we use today. Over the past two decades, the endodontic armamentarium has undergone major renovations in nonsurgical and surgical treatment that have allowed endodontic treatment to become more successful.

This chapter provides an overview of basic and advanced endodontic armamentarium and describes their use in the clinical setting. Proper knowledge of the various instruments, materials, and equipment, together with their design, composition, and function, is critical to provide patients with proper diagnosis and treatment options. The field of endodontics is constantly evolving with improved armamentarium to assist clinicians with diagnosis and treatment. Clinicians should always consider using newer instruments, materials, and equipment to provide the best possible treatment for their patients. It will not be possible to include all armamentarium used in every endodontic procedure in this chapter. However, the most widely used instruments and materials will be covered in detail.

Examination and Diagnosis

Clinical Examination

The primary aim during endodontic diagnosis is to determine the vitality of the pulp and the status of the supporting periodontal structure. For that, clinicians use a basic examination kit, which is very similar to instruments used for restorative dentistry. It is composed of a mouth mirror, Shepherd's hook explorer, periodontal probe, and cotton pliers (Fig. 7.1). The vitality of the dental pulp is routinely examined using sensibility tests that aim to stimulate the pulp through temperature (cold or hot) or electric stimulation

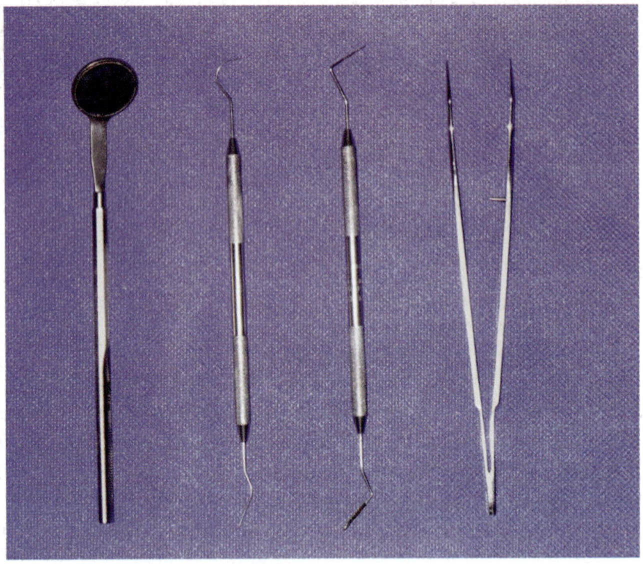

• **Fig. 7.1** Examination kit containing a mouth mirror, periodontal probe, dental probe, and cotton pliers.

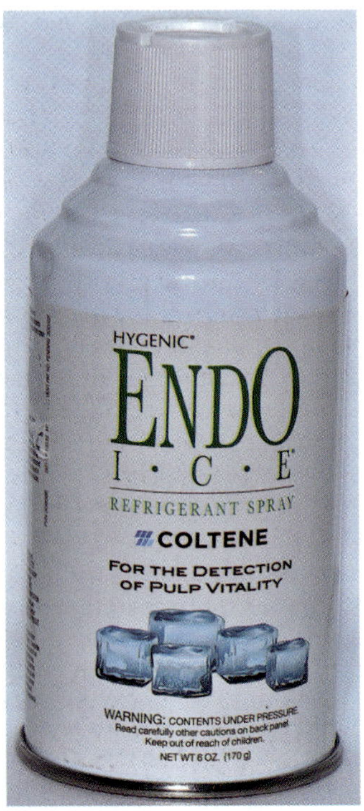

• **Fig. 7.2** EndoIce used for cold testing.

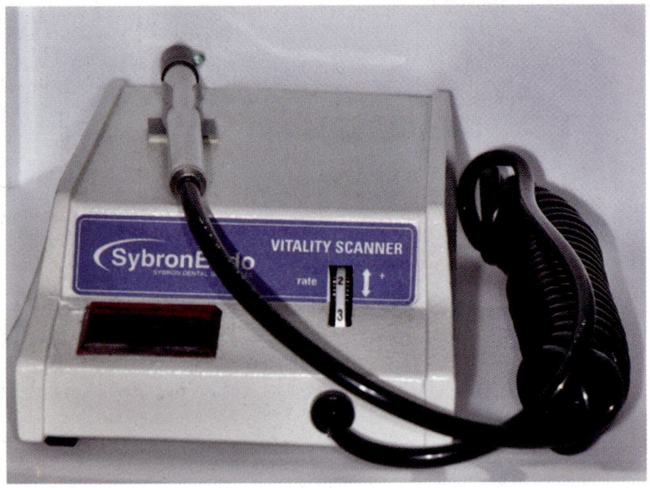

• **Fig. 7.3** Electric pulp testing used to determine pulp vitality.

(Figs. 7.2 and 7.3). The supporting periapical tissues can be examined with the back of the mirror (percussion), the index finger (palpation), and the periodontal probe. Other instruments can be used to determine the presence or absence of a coronal crack or a root fracture, such as a "Tooth Slooth," a transilluminator, methylene blue, or caries detection dye.

Radiographic Examination

Radiographic examination is the key diagnostic tool used to evaluate the periapex. Different types of radiographs can be used for endodontic diagnosis. Two-dimensional (2D) intraoral radiographs, periapical and bitewing, are used to evaluate the teeth, their supporting structures, and any existing restorations. Three-dimensional (3D) radiographs and cone beam computed tomography (CBCT) have become routinely used in endodontic diagnosis due to their ability to provide 3D images of the area of interest. In 2017 a survey sent to members of the American Association of Endodontists (AAE) showed that almost 50% of the endodontists in the United States have a CBCT machine in their offices.[3] CBCT use among endodontists is increasing because it can further assist clinicians in proper diagnosis and treatment planning.[4-8] Rodriguez et al.[7] investigated the influence of CBCT imaging on clinical decision-making choices of different specialists among cases with different levels of difficulty. The results showed that examiners altered their treatment plan after viewing the CBCT scan in 27.3% of the cases and up to 52.9% in high-difficulty-level cases. Although periapical radiographs are still used as the standard radiographic technique for endodontic diagnosis and treatment, there are several clinical situations in which 2D radiographs may not be able to properly assess the clinical condition. Periapical lesions have to reach a certain size and erode the inner cortical plates of the jaws to be visible on a periapical radiograph.[9,10] In addition, 2D radiographs have significant limitations in the detection, assessment, and treatment planning of external cervical root resorption compared with CBCT imaging.[6] In a joint statement by the AAE and the American Association of Oral and Maxillofacial Radiology (AAOMR),[11] they outlined several circumstances in which CBCT can be very useful for better clinical examination (see Chapter 3). These conditions include cases with external and internal resorptive defects, trauma and fracture cases, presurgical treatment planning, and vertical root fracture cases. In addition, they recommend using CBCT to evaluate the nonhealing

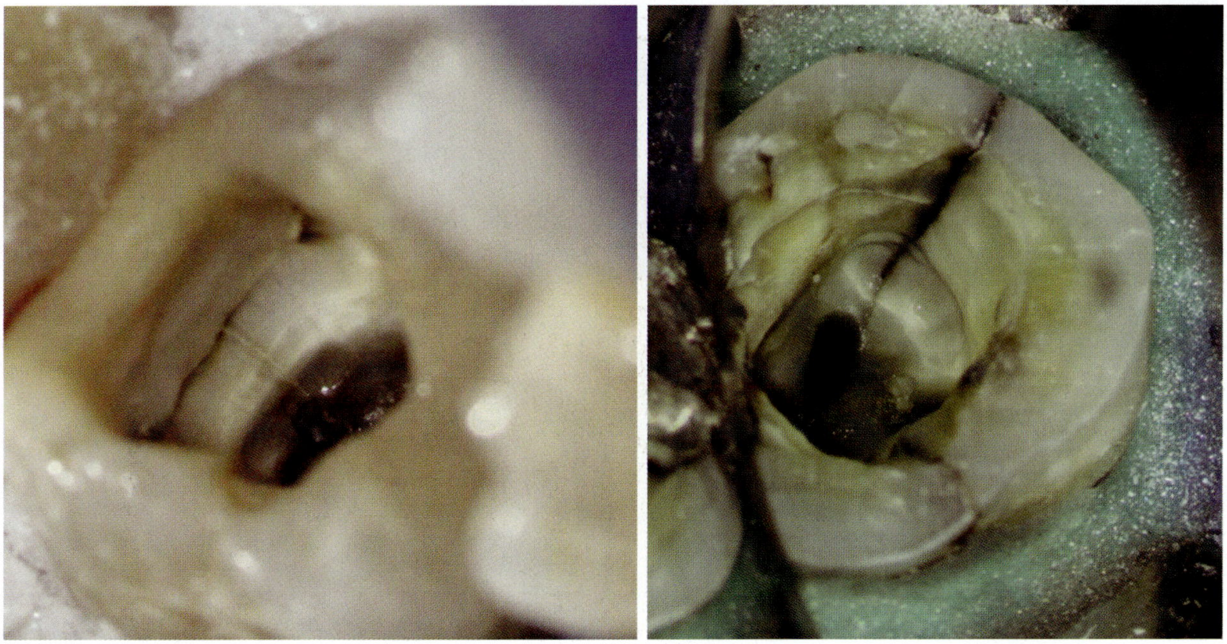

• **Fig. 7.4** Illustration of the use of the dental operating microscope to detect cracks within the crown and root. (Courtesy Dr. Hajar Albanian.)

of previous endodontic treatment, in intra-appointment identification and localization of calcified canals, for initial treatments with potential existence of extra canals and suspected complex morphology, and for the diagnosis of patients who present with contradictory or nonspecific clinical signs and symptoms associated with untreated or previously endodontically treated teeth. It should be noted, however, that the accuracy of CBCT relies to a great extent on the specifications and settings of the equipment used (field of view, voxel size, and artifact correction). Additionally, some lesions may not be accurately detected if they are smaller than 1.4 mm in diameter.[5]

Magnification

The dental operating microscope (DOM) is considered standard equipment in the endodontic office. Before the early 1990s, dental loops were used for magnification. The loops were limiting in two ways: first, only low-level magnification was possible; second, because the practitioner had to wear the loops, neck strain and postural problems often resulted. A web-based survey sent to AAE members in 2007[12] showed that 90% of endodontists were using a DOM during treatment in comparison with only 52% in 1999. The clinician can better visualize the root canal anatomy as a result of the magnification and illumination provided by the DOM. Khalighinejad et al. showed that maxillary first molars with nonhealed RCT in which DOM was not used were significantly more likely to have a missed MB2 canal in the affected MB root. This study indirectly shows the value of using the DOM on the outcome of nonsurgical root canal treatment, at least in this situation.[13] Other studies also showed that practitioners were better able to locate and negotiate canals when the DOM was used.[14,15] Although dental loops can be used during endodontic treatment, the DOM offers multiple advantages: a wider field of view, improved illumination, and less physical strain on the practitioner. DOM is also among the instruments and materials that have significantly improved the treatment outcome of endodontic surgery.[16,17] In addition to allowing excellent visualization, it is a great tool for documentation as well. Clinicians can easily take images and videos of the various procedures and use them for better patient communication and education (Fig. 7.4).

Isolation

In 1862 Dr. Sanford Barnum developed the rubber dam to allow a saliva-free field in the mouth. Later, Dr. G. A. Bowman improved the rubber dam by inventing the rubber dam clamp, which allowed the stabilization of the rubber dam to a tooth. The rubber dam is intended to isolate the tooth/teeth to be treated from the oral cavity to ensure no microbial contamination. In addition, it offers other kinds of benefits, such as enhancing visualization, providing a clean operative field, and preventing ingestion or aspiration of any instrument, material, or irrigant during treatment. The 2010 AAE Position Statement on Dental Dams indicated that "tooth isolation using the dental dam is ... integral and essential for any nonsurgical endodontic treatment." It is also considered the standard of care in today's practice.

An isolation kit is composed of (1) clamps that clasp the tooth and are available in different shapes and sizes, depending on the tooth to be isolated (Fig. 7.5); (2) rubber dam sheet, a physical barrier to isolate the tooth from the oral cavity; (3) rubber dam hole punch used to create a hole in the rubber dam sheet that allows for placement of the rubber dam clamp; and (4) a rubber dam frame used to hold the rubber dam sheet in place (Fig. 7.6). In some clinical cases, rubber dam placement alone may not sufficiently allow adequate isolation of the tooth before initiating treatment. Supplementary material such as OraSeal or OpalDam (Ultradent Products, Inc., South Jordan, Utah, USA) may be applied around the tooth/clamp junction to enhance tooth isolation (Fig. 7.7). In clinical cases in which an extensive amount of tooth structure is lost, restoration of the tooth to allow for proper isolation is recommended. This restoration can be achieved using glass ionomer or composite restorative materials (Fig. 7.8). If placing a clamp

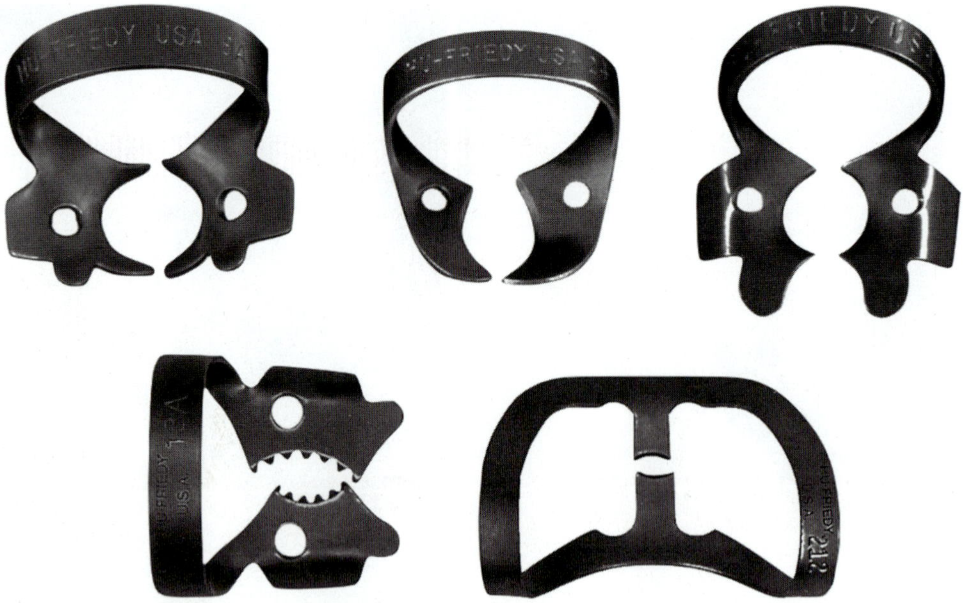

• **Fig. 7.5** Different types of clamps that can be used for rubber dam isolation, depending on the tooth morphology.

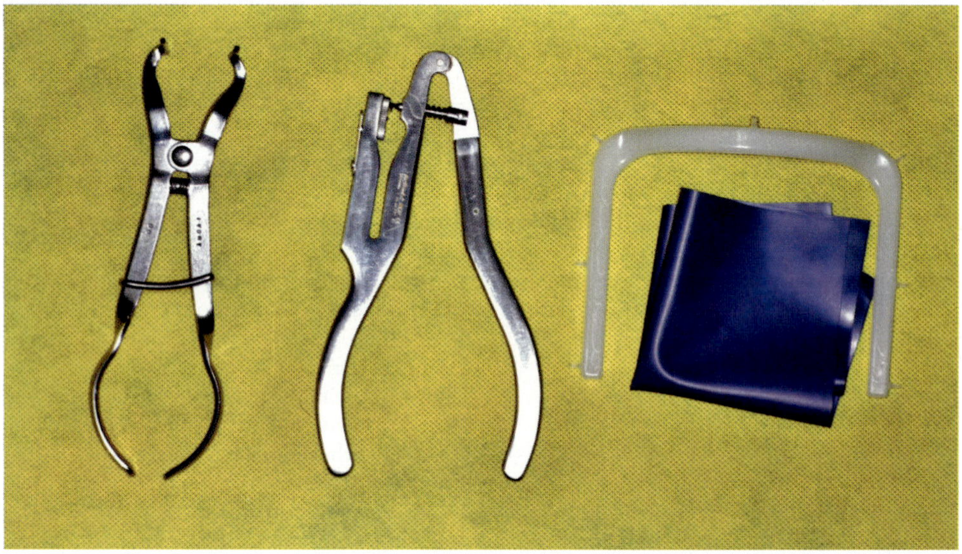

• **Fig. 7.6** Rubber dam kit composed of *(from left to right)* clamp holder, rubber dam punch, rubber dam frame *(white)*, and rubber dam sheet.

on the tooth might result in damage of an existing restoration, a dental dam stabilizing cord, such as Wedjets (Coltene/Whaledent GmbH), can be used to stabilize the rubber dam in place without the use of a clamp (Fig. 7.9).

Nonsurgical Root Canal Treatment

Nonsurgical Cassette

The nonsurgical treatment cassette includes all the instruments that are needed during RCT (Fig. 7.10). The cassette contains the instruments used in diagnosis in addition to other procedure-specific instruments, such as (1) local anesthesia syringe; (2) endodontic explorer (DG 16), an instrument that aids in the identification of root canal orifices; (3) a ruler used to measure the instruments for length control during the root canal procedure (Fig. 7.11); (4) endodontic spreaders, used for lateral condensation of gutta-percha; and (5) endodontic pluggers, used for vertical gutta-percha condensation during obturation. Endodontic spreaders and pluggers come in different sizes as well as both finger and handle design (Figs. 7.11 and 7.12). Finally, the cassette includes a metal or plastic instrument that is used to place the temporary filling into the pulp chamber.

Length Determination

To ensure proper length control during root canal treatment, electronic apex locators (EAL) have been used to determine the position of the apical foramen and/or constriction and thus the apical extent for root canal instrumentations. The first EAL was introduced in 1962 by Sunada.[18] Since their development, EAL have evolved to improve their accuracy and reliability in the

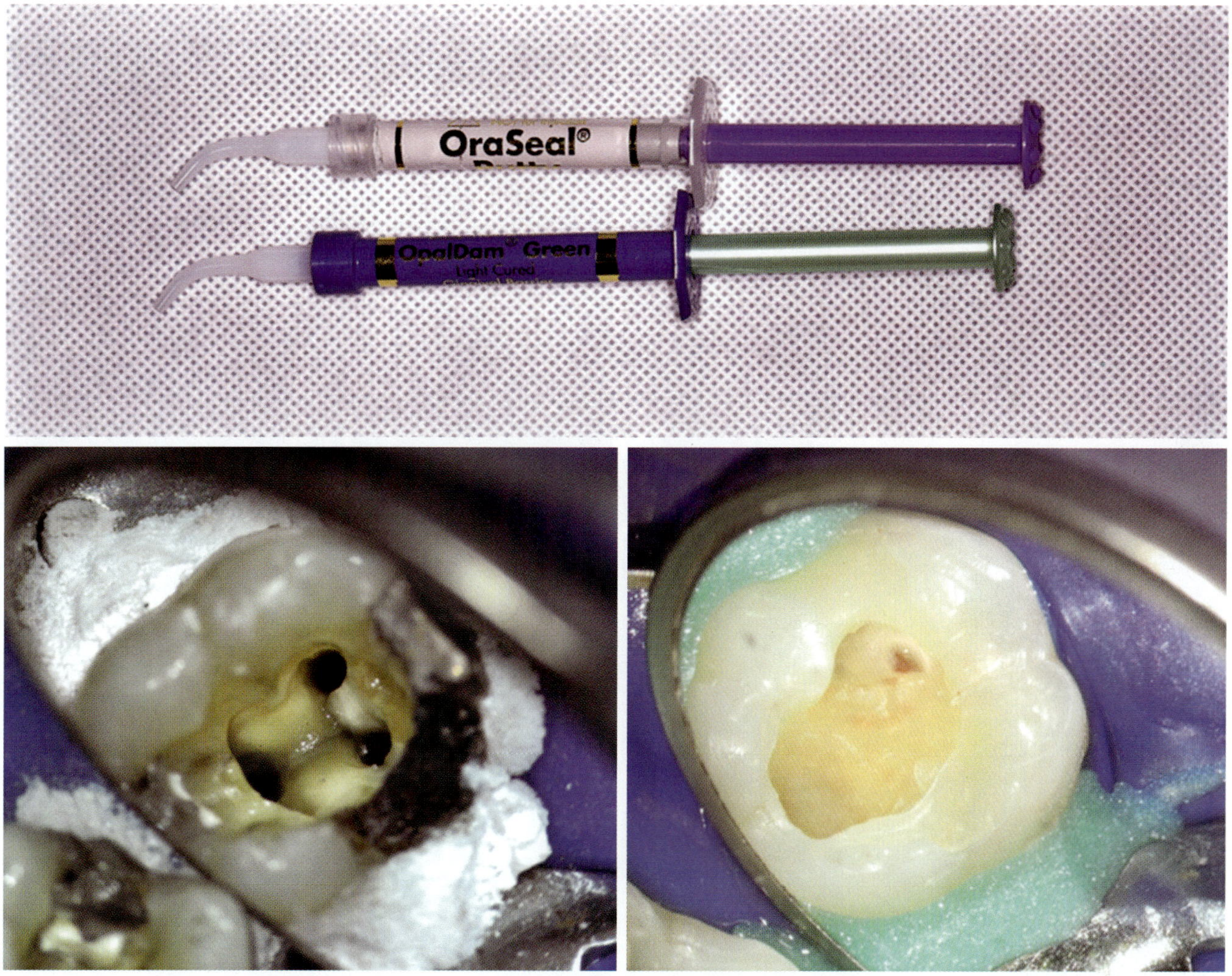

• **Fig. 7.7** Images illustrating the use of further isolation after rubber dam placement. Lower left: Isolation using OraSeal putty (Ultradent). Lower right: OpalDam (Ultradent).

various clinical conditions. Currently, EAL are consistently used by endodontists and widely used by general dentists.[19] EAL have been shown to be more accurate than standard 2D radiographs in working length determination.[20] When use of EAL is combined with a radiograph, clinicians can reduce the risk of over- or underinstrumentation during root canal treatment,[21] and thereby achieve more predictable results.[22,23]

Instrumentation Armamentarium

Endodontic Access

The endodontic access is the opening in the crown of the tooth that allows for localization of the root canal space. Classically, the outline form for the access has been governed by G. V. Black's principles of cavity preparation. However, the access for each tooth should be directed by the anatomy of both the pulp chamber and the curvature of the root. Existing restorations and decay can alter the outline form of the access. Due to the implementation of the DOM, modern endodontic accesses can be smaller and more precise in their location on the crown of the tooth. The access is prepared using a high-speed handpiece and burs with water coolant. The selection of burs for access depends on the material(s) in the crown of the tooth. Ceramic restorations and porcelain are best approached using diamonds burs. Carbide burs are acceptable for metal (amalgam, gold, crown undercasting) and composite restoration.[24] The typical armamentarium consists of sizes 2, 4, and 6 round diamond burs and size 4 round carbide or #1157 carbide burs. After achieving access to the pulp chamber, safe end burs (Endo Z) can be used to avoid any unnecessary damage to the floor of the pulp chamber.

Additional instruments are sometimes required to localize the root canal orifices/canals (Fig. 7.13). Root canal localization can be complicated by calcification in the form of pulp stones and dystrophic calcification of the root canal space. To remove these calcified structures, Munce burs, Mueller burs, or Swiss LN burs can be used. They are long shanked rotary burs that can be used for precise troughing to expose root canal orifices. These burs come in different sizes to facilitate drilling at different levels without the root canal space and are used without water coolant, which can generate a significant amount of debris. Specialized endodontic ultrasonic tips can also be used for root canal localization. The advantages of ultrasonic tips are that they can be used very precisely and, if desired, used with water irrigation. Irrigants, dyes, and light can also help in root canal localization. A drop of sodium hypochlorite (NaOCl) can be placed in the pulp chamber and viewed under the DOM. The solution will often bubble and "light

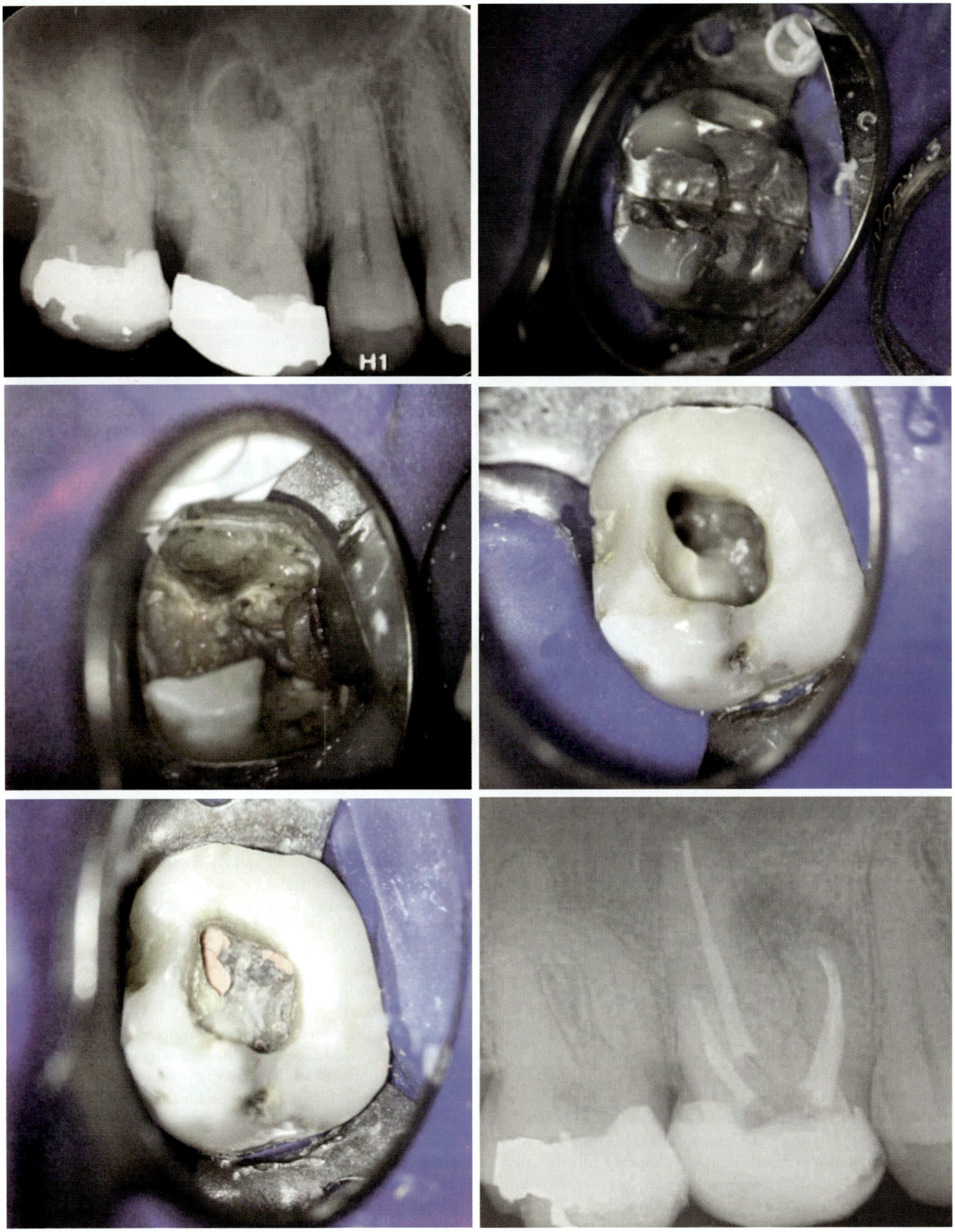

• **Fig. 7.8** Images illustrating the prebuildup using composite resin after removal of the old restoration and before initiating root canal treatment. (Courtesy Dr. Howard H Wang.)

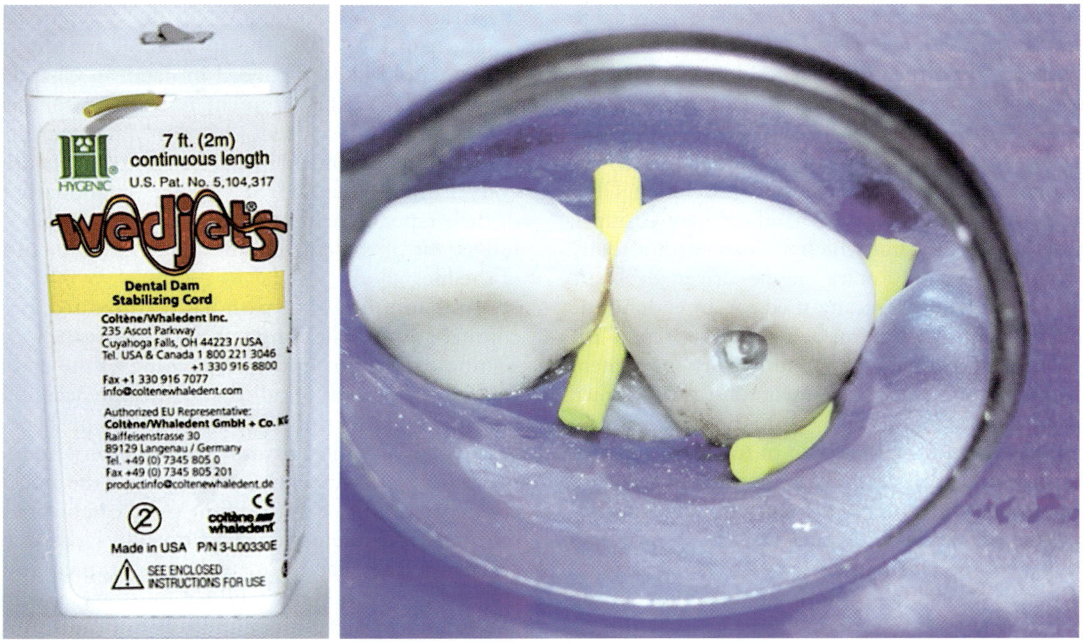

• **Fig. 7.9** Clampless rubber dam isolation using Wedjet in an upper anterior tooth with an all-ceramic crown. (Courtesy Dr. Elham Shadmehr.)

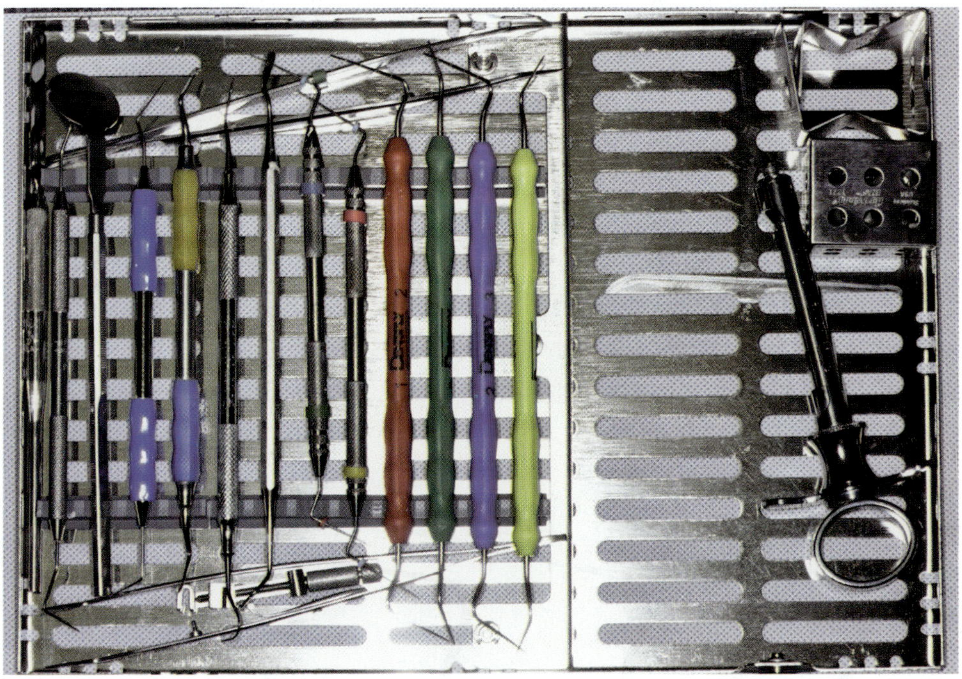

• **Fig. 7.10** Nonsurgical cassette used for endodontic treatment.

up" a canal orifice. Caries detection dye or other stains can also locate hard-to-find root canal orifices. Transillumination of the pulp chamber with a curing light has also been suggested to help locate root canal orifices. In summary, precise endodontic access is essential to a successful root canal treatment.

Cleaning and Shaping Instruments

Once access to the root canal system has been achieved, disinfection of the root canal space can be initiated. The goal of root canal disinfection is removing all pulp tissue and infected debris from the root canal system. Because achieving a sterile environment is currently impossible, the root canal space is then filled with a special filling material to "entomb" any remaining bacteria. Root canal disinfection is achieved through a step called "cleaning and shaping." Although the primary goal is only cleaning, the root canal space needs to be shaped by endodontic instruments to facilitate the cleaning process. It should be noted that the current disinfection process derives from the instruments and materials currently used. With the advancement in technology, noninstrumentation techniques may be used, and the need to further shape the canal to facilities cleaning may be no longer needed. Cleaning and shaping of the root canal space with the current endodontic armamentarium have two primary objectives: (1) the enlargement of the root canal space, and (2) creation of a space amenable to the filling "obturation" method being used. The instruments used for cleaning and shaping are classified by the ISO-Federation Dentaire Internationale. Instruments used by hand only are Group I. Instruments similar to Group I but which are used with a rotary engine or motor are Group II. Rotary engine–driven drills are Group III. All three groups are typically used for an endodontic procedure. Initially, small hand files can be inserted to "scout" the root canal space. After providing a glide path, rotary instrumentation can be commenced. Rotary instrumentation is performed using an endodontic electric motor (Fig. 7.14). The electric motor allows for more precise control of the speed of rotation than that allowed by an air-driven handpiece. Electric motors can also control the allowable torque, which can be set to maximize file performance and minimize file separation (breakage).

Hand and rotary files use standardized systems for sizing and identification. The size of a file is defined by 100 times the tip size. The taper of the file (the increase in diameter from the tip of the file to the handle) is based on 1/100th of a millimeter. The color-coded identification system is based on file size. With the exception of the three smallest file sizes (6, 8, and 10), the color pattern repeats to aid in file size identification (Fig. 7.15). Hand and rotary files come with different cross-sections and accordingly can be used in different motions and at different parts of the treatment. An illustration of the different hand instrument is shown in Fig. 7.16. The application and use of each of these instruments will be discussed in detail in Chapter 14. The taper for a standardized instrument is constant for the full length of the cutting flutes (typically 16 mm). The taper of the instrument refers to the incremental enlargement of the instrument diameter every 1 mm (Table 7.1). Some rotary endodontic files are variable in their taper, which means that the taper is not constant for the full extent of the cutting flutes and varies for different segments of the file.

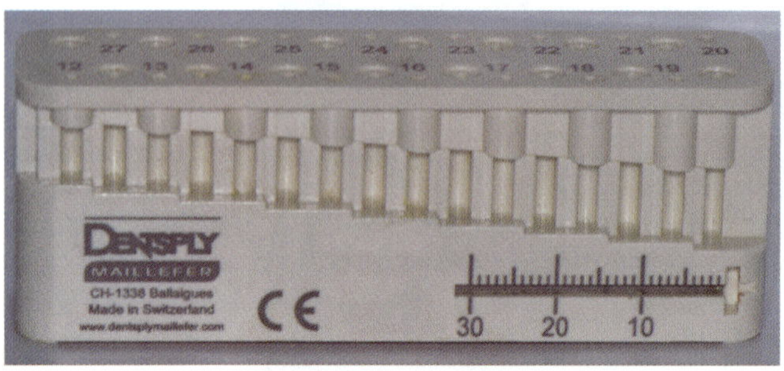

• **Fig. 7.11** Endodontic ruler.

After an initial glide path has been created, preparation of the coronal and middle thirds of the canal system can be started. A significant concept in the preparation of the coronal and middle thirds of the canal is called straight-line access. Root canal systems are typically similar to an hourglass in shape.[25] Straight-line access decreases the curvature in the coronal and middle thirds of the root canal, which favorably preserves the apical curvature. The coronal and middle thirds of the canal can be prepared with hand or rotary instrumentation. Traditionally, Hedstrom files were used to enlarge the space. Currently, the coronal and middle thirds are enlarged with Gates Glidden burs, Peeso reamers, specialized access burs, or nickel-titanium orifice openers. All can be effective in the coronal enlargement of the root canal system. Gates Glidden and Peeso reamers can also be used for the preparation of post space after completion of RCT (Fig. 7.17). Their use, however, should be restricted to the coronal and middle third of the canal. Both are available in various sizes (Table 7.2) and lengths. The apical third of the canal can be enlarged with hand or rotary files. The desired final size and taper of the root canal is determined by the width, curvature, and length of the root. Each root canal should be individually evaluated for maximum apical preparation size and taper. The physical attributes of the file (material and design) dictate its optimal use. The clinician should select the instrument type based on its mechanical properties and the desired goal needed to be achieved. Historically, files were made from carbon steel. Carbon steel had strength but was less flexible and degraded by sterilization. Stainless steel is used today and has the benefits of strength, improved flexibility compared with carbon steel, and heat tolerance. More recently, nickel titanium has been used for file fabrication. Nickel titanium allows for strength, flexibility, ability to withstand sterilization, and the ability to

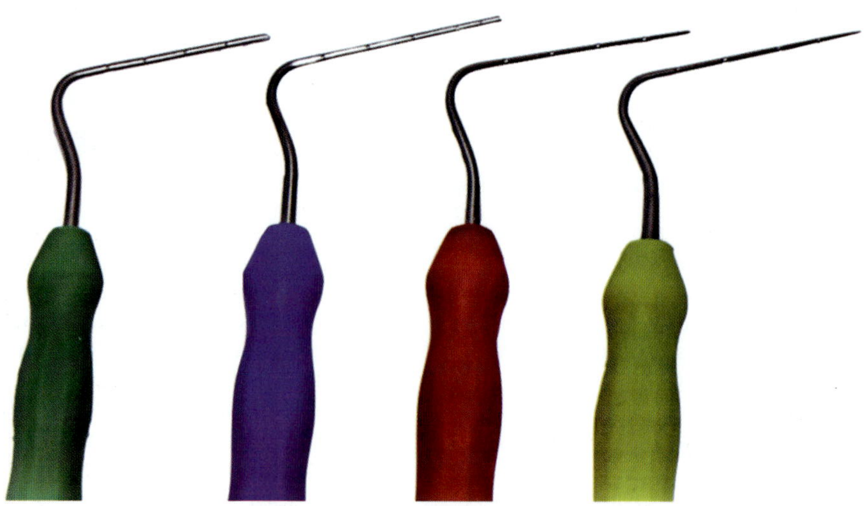

• **Fig. 7.12** Hand pluggers in different sizes.

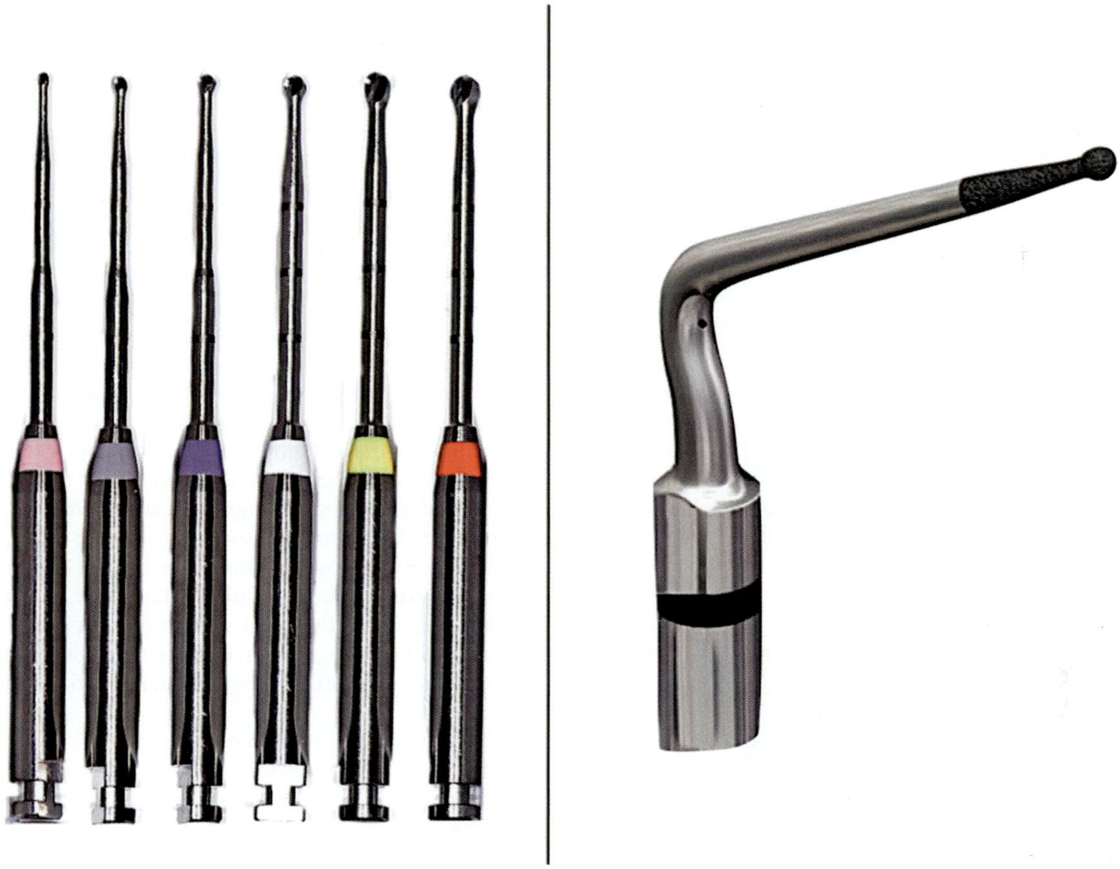

• **Fig. 7.13** Additional instruments used for canal localization. Long shank round burs in different sizes *(left)*. Ultrasonic tips with a round diamond tip *(right)*.

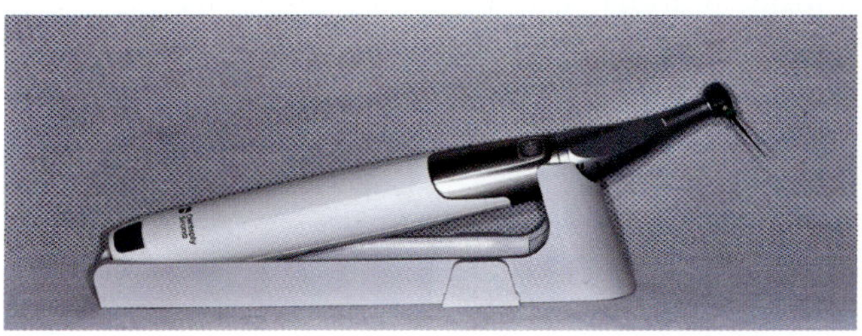

• **Fig. 7.14** Wireless endodontic motor used for endodontic rotary instruments.

tolerate engine-driven rotation. The combination of these characteristics allows nickel-titanium engine-driven files to produce a more consistent shape. Ultimately, the combined use of hand and engine-driven files is required due to the inherent limitations of each individual file. The ability to produce a consistent shape allows for more efficacious débridement, disinfection, and obturation of the root canal system.

Irrigants, Irrigation Devices, and Intracanal Medicaments

The use of hand and rotary instruments to adequately disinfect the root canal space should always be performed with an irrigant. From a conceptual point of view, the ultimate goal of irrigants is to provide a disinfected, tissue-free, and debris-free root canal space. Currently, there is no irrigant that can ultimately achieve all the required goals. As a result, numerous irrigants are used in modern endodontic treatment. The advantages and disadvantages of each irrigant should be considered during each step of endodontic treatment. Endodontic treatment should then be deconstructed into sections and the appropriate irrigant used for each step.

Numerous irrigants are used during endodontic therapy. NaOCl is the most commonly used irrigant in endodontics because it can dissolve pulp tissue and lubricate the root canals during treatment. In addition, NaOCl is bactericidal and can penetrate deep into the dentinal tubules.[26-30] Although 2% chlorhexidine (CHX) has antibacterial effects and is less caustic than NaOCl, CHX cannot dissolve organic tissue.[31-35] Ethylenediaminetetraacetic acid (EDTA or EDTAC) is used during endodontic treatment due to its ability to chelate inorganic molecules and remove the smear layer[36]; however, it lacks the degree of antibacterial or tissue dissolution properties of other irrigants.[34,37,38] Sterile saline has been used to irrigate root canals as well. Baker determined sterile saline to be an effective irrigant with sufficient volume.[39] However, its lack of disinfection and tissue dissolution are not ideal.[27] Sterile saline can be used as an intermediary solution between certain irrigants, such as NaOCl and CHX, to prevent any undesired chemical interactions.[40,41] Other disinfection solutions that contain a mixture of irrigants, such as MTAD and QMix (Dentsply Sirona, Inc., Tulsa, Oklahoma, USA) have been proposed to be used in endodontic treatment. Further discussion on these irrigants, their advantages, and drawbacks will be further discussed in Chapter 14.

In clinical practice, the practitioner must determine the proper combination of irrigants and the ultimate concentration needed

File #	D0 diameter (in mm)	Handle Color
06	0.06	
08	0.08	
10	0.10	
15	0.15	
20	0.20	
25	0.25	
30	0.30	
35	0.35	
40	0.40	
45	0.45	
50	0.50	
55	0.55	
60	0.60	
70	0.70	
80	0.80	
90	0.90	
100	1.00	
110	1.10	
120	1.20	
130	1.30	
140	1.40	

• **Fig. 7.15** Color-coding specifications for standardization of files and reamers.

for each irrigant on a case-by-case basis. Depending on the status of the pulp and the periapical tissue at the time of treatment, as well as the type of treatment being performed, the combination of different irrigants can improve the quality of canal débridement.[42] Irrigants are commonly delivered in the root canal space using an irrigation syringe and a small-gauge irrigation needle. Endodontic irrigation needles range between 25 to 31 gauge. Smaller-diameter (higher gauge) needles allow greater apical depth and irrigation delivery in the canal, and thus their use should be considered during root canal treatment (Fig. 7.18).[43-45] Endodontic needles have various tip designs. They can be open-ended, close-ended, or side-vented. A side-vented irrigation needle is recommended to minimize pressure buildup caused by an opened-ended needle and thus minimize irrigation extrusion into the periapical tissues.[46,47] Energetically augmenting an irrigant's effectiveness has also been determined to have a positive effect on root canal disinfection. Devices such as an Endoactivator (Fig. 7.19) can allow sonic activation of the irrigants through oscillating patterns of nodes and antinodes.[48,49] The use of a small endodontic file on an ultrasonic handpiece to freely oscillate inside the canal is another form of irrigation activation. The transmittal of acoustic energy generating a rapid movement of fluid in a circular motion (acoustic streaming) and cavitation through the irrigant can improve its effectiveness.[50] Several other methods of irrigation activation will be discussed in Chapter 14.

With the complete preparation and disinfection of the root canal system, the final component to nonsurgical endodontic treatment is obturation of the root canal space. However, in some clinical situations when treatment is not completed due to time constraints or inability to achieve a dry canal, intracanal medicaments can be placed between visits, which can also enhance root canal disinfection. Among the intracanal medicaments used in root canal treatment is calcium hydroxide [$Ca(OH)_2$]. It has antibacterial properties and can assist in dissolving remaining pulp tissue in the root canal space.[51,52] $Ca(OH)_2$ is available in different forms (powder + liquid or paste). Paste forms can be easily injected into the root canal space or inserted via lentulo spiral (Fig. 7.20) to allow adequate distribution on to the canal wall. Other medicaments, such as 2% CHX gel, can be also used as an intracanal medicament.

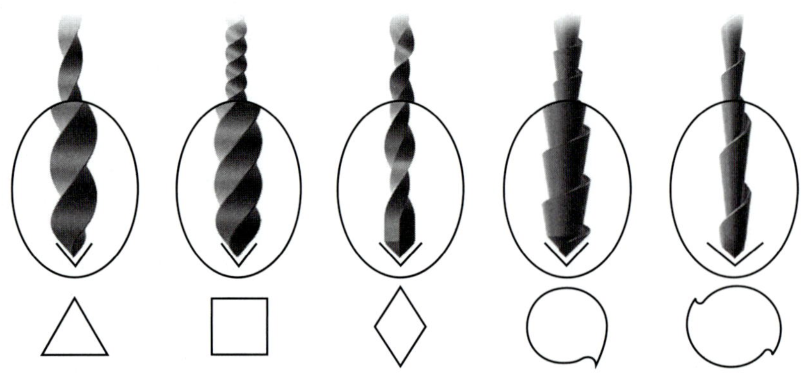

• **Fig. 7.16** Longitudinal and cross-sectional shapes of various hand-operated instruments. Note that small sizes of K-reamers, K-files, and the K-Flex have a different shape than the larger sizes.

TABLE 7.1 Hand Files Tip Size and Diameter Based on Different file Taper

File Size (Color)	Tip Size in mm	Diameter 3 mm from Tip with 02 Taper in mm	Diameter 3 mm from Tip with 04 Taper in mm	Diameter 3 mm from Tip with 06 Taper in mm
6 (Pink)	.06	.12	.18	.24
8 (Gray)	.08	.14	.20	.26
10 (Purple)	.10	.16	.22	.28
15 (White)*	.15	.21	.27	.33
20 (Yellow)*	.20	.26	.32	.38
25 (Red)*	.25	.31	.37	.43
30 (Blue)*	.30	.36	.42	.48
35 (Green)*	.35	.41	.47	.53
40 (Black)*	.40	.46	.52	.58

*Color code repeats starting at size 45 files. After size 60, files increase by 10 and not by 5.

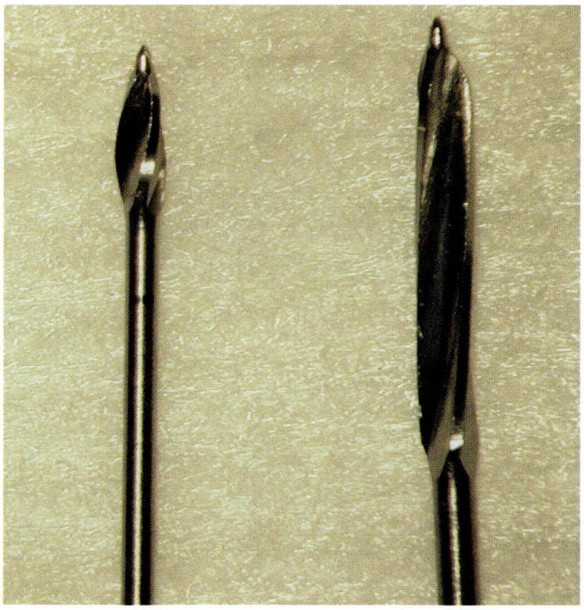

• **Fig. 7.17** *Left*, Gates Glidden drill. Note the noncutting tip and the elliptical shape. *Right*, Peeso reamer. Note the noncutting "safe" tip and parallel sides. These are stiffer and more aggressive than the Gates Glidden drill. Both are used for straight-line access preparation.

Obturation Armamentarium

Obturation of the root canal space is performed to seal the root canal space and prevent reinfection.[1] As mentioned earlier, Dr. Pierre Fauchard recommended obturating root canals with lead foil. During the past three centuries, numerous materials were promoted, including but not limited to, gold, plaster of Paris, rosin-chloroform, silver nitrate, formocresol, cotton, fiberglass, calcium hydroxide, silver cones, Hydron, and polyester. In 1867 Dr. G. A. Bowman introduced gutta-percha as a sole root canal obturation material. In 1925 U. G. Rickert suggested using a sealer in conjunction with gutta-percha to improve the obturation. This concept was later modified to allow for cold lateral condensation (compaction) of the primary gutta-percha cone and the subsequent placement of additional gutta-percha. In 1933 Dr. E. A. Jasper introduced silver cones as an obturation material.[53] The use of silver cones and cold lateral condensation of gutta-percha was the primary obturation methods for root canals until the 1960s. At that time, Dr. Herbert Schilder developed the warm vertical obturation method.[1] This technique included heating a gutta-percha mass and hydraulically compacting the molten material apically to obturate the pulp canal space. This method would create an apical seal, but the coronal and middle thirds of the canal would be devoid of material. The clinician would then continue obturating by inserting small pieces of gutta-percha into the root canal space, heating them, and condensing them, using endodontic pluggers until the entire root canal was obturated. Although silver cones are not used currently, cold lateral and warm vertical gutta-percha obturation techniques are still commonly used today.

TABLE 7.2 Rotary Flaring Instruments

Size	Gates Glidden Drills	Peeso Reamers
No. 1	0.4 mm	0.7 mm
No. 2	0.6 mm	0.9 mm
No. 3	0.8 mm	1.1 mm
No. 4	1.0 mm	1.3 mm
No. 5	1.2 mm	1.5 mm
No. 6	1.4 mm	1.7 mm

The armamentarium needed can vary depending on the obturation technique used and the complexity of each case. The following items are currently the most commonly used:

1. **Gutta-percha cones** are available in different sizes and tapers. Standardized gutta-percha cones correspond to the size and taper of endodontic files used during root canal instrumentation. They are also available in a nonstandardized form (fine,

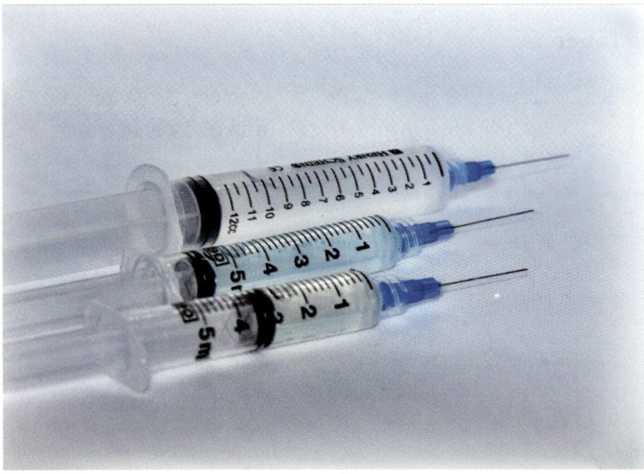

• **Fig. 7.18** Irrigation syringes containing different irrigation solutions that can be used during endodontic treatment. *From top to bottom*: (1) Sodium hypochlorite (NaOCl), (2) chlorhexidine (CHX), and (3) ethylenediaminetetraacetic acid (EDTA).

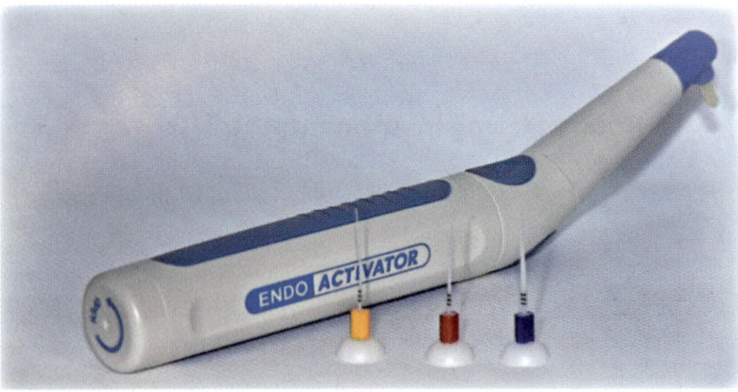

• **Fig. 7.19** EndoActivator used for irrigation activation.

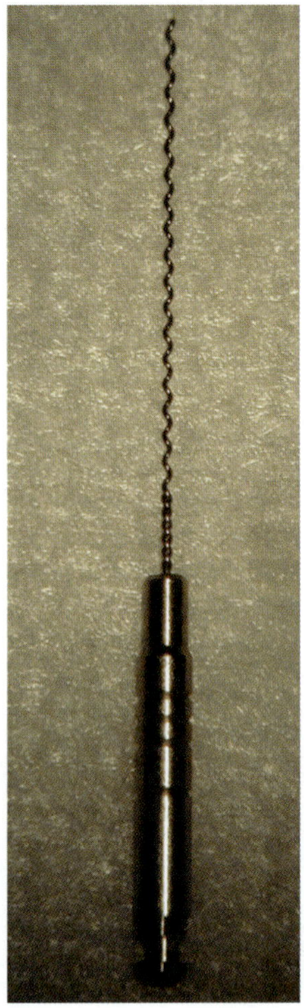

• **Fig. 7.20** The lentulo spiral drill is used to spin calcium hydroxide or sealer into canals.

fine medium, medium, medium fine, and coarse) that can be customized for every case.

2. **Paper points** are used to dry the root canal space before obturation. The rationale for drying the canal before obturation is that sealers tend to be hydrophobic,[54] preventing the flow of the sealer into the intricacies of the canal space. Moisture can also affect the setting property of sealers.[54] Like gutta-percha, paper points are available in different sizes in standardized and nonstandardized forms. Another method to dry the canal is the use of a surgical suction with a cannula within the canal to remove moisture before obturation.
3. **Sealer** is a cement applied inside the root canal space to adhere the obturation material to the root canal wall. The ideal properties for sealers were defined by Dr. Louis Grossman (Chapter 15). Sealers are available in different compositions. Zinc-oxide eugenol sealers have been traditionally used. However, modern sealers can be composed of epoxy resin or bioceramic materials (see Fig. 7.20). According to the type of sealer and the manufacturer, sealers can be supplied as either a powder and liquid, which are mixed at the time of use, or in a preprepared paste form. The obturation materials are classically placed on a glass slab before use. This placement allows for ease of visualization and a surface to mix the sealer (if required), and it can be used to form custom-made gutta-percha cones (if needed). The placement of the sealer into the canal can be performed by coating a gutta-percha cone or paper point and inserting it into the canal, or via rotary displacement of sealer with a lentulo engine-driven spiral (Fig. 7.21). Currently, several endodontic sealers are provided with an injection tip to facilitate direct application of the sealer in the root canal space.
4. **Spreaders** are used for lateral condensation of gutta-percha in the root canal space. Spreaders come in different shapes and sizes (standardized and nonstandardized). They can also be finger-held or hand-held (Fig. 7.22).
5. **Heat source** (e.g., System B) has the primary purpose of warming the gutta-percha, allowing it to flow under pressure. A heat source can also remove gutta-percha at any level within the root canal space.
6. Thermoplasticized gutta-percha dispensers (e.g., Obtura [Obtura Spartan, Algonquin, IL, USA] and Calamus [Dentsply Sirona, Tulsa, Oklahoma, USA]) are devices that preheat gutta-percha in a chamber, changing its physical properties from a beta phase to an alpha phase, thereby making it softer and easy to pack using endodontic pluggers. The gutta-percha can then be injected in the root canal space and compacted. Once the gutta-percha cools within the root canal space, it changes back to its beta phase, which is more stable. Some devices, such as Dual Calamus (Dentsply Sirona, Tulsa, Oklahoma, USA) can have both, a heat source and a thermoplasticized gutta-percha dispenser, in the same device (Fig. 7.23). Additional details are provided in Chapter 15 regarding the various obturation techniques and armamentarium that can be used to manage various clinical cases.

Study Questions

1. All of the following are normally included in an examination kit EXCEPT:
   a. Mouth mirror
   b. Periodontal probe
   c. Cotton pliers
   d. Periosteal elevator
   e. Dental explorer
2. Which of the following is not found in a typical nonsurgical treatment cassette?
   a. DG16 explorer
   b. Anesthetic syringe
   c. Retro-pluggers
   d. Cotton pliers
   e. Plastic instrument
3. A CBCT scan is recommended for examining all the following conditions EXCEPT:
   a. Dental caries detection
   b. Internal resorption
   c. External resorption
   d. Traumatic injuries
   e. Treatment planning for apical surgery
4. Rubber dam isolation…
   a. Provides a clean operation field
   b. Improves visualization of the tooth to be treated
   c. Prevents aspiration of dental instruments
   d. Limits the visibility to the floor of the mouth
   e. All of the above
5. All of the following irrigants are used for nonsurgical root canal treatment EXCEPT:
   a. NaOCl
   b. EDTA
   c. formocresol
   d. Chlorhexidine
   e. Sterile saline

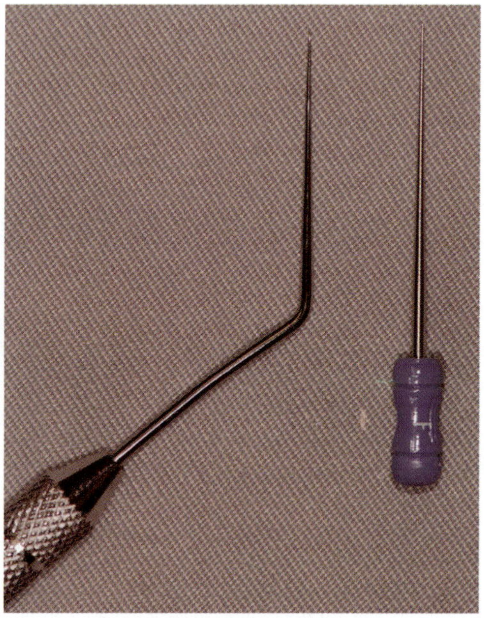

• **Fig. 7.22** D11 handled spreader *(left)* and a fine finger spreader *(right)*. Both are designed for lateral condensation.

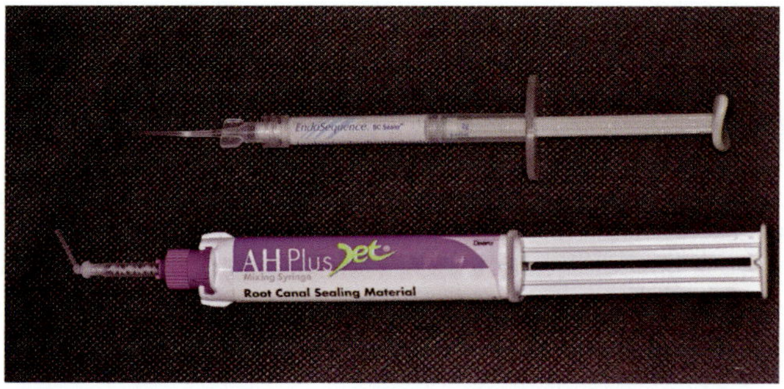

• **Fig. 7.21** Different types of endodontic sealers. *Top*: Bioceramic sealer (Brassler, Augusta, GA, USA). *Bottom*: AH plus sealer (Dentsply Sirona, Tulsa, OK, USA).

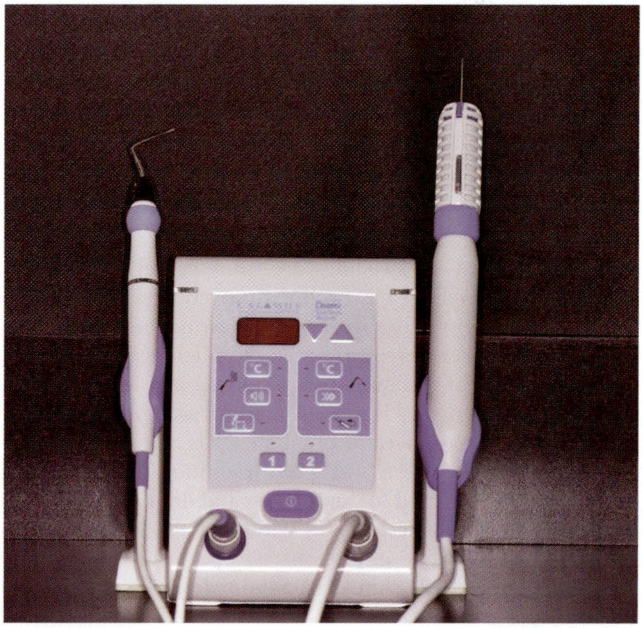

• **Fig. 7.23** Dual Calamus obturation device. On the left side is the heat system; on the right side is a thermoplasticized gutta-percha dispenser.

Coronal Seal

After completion of RCT, the access opening in the tooth must be restored. Although some treatments can allow for the placement of a permanent restoration at the time of treatment, the tooth after root canal treatment is often sealed with a temporary material. The pulp chamber is cleaned of all sealer and gutta-percha with a solvent. This process is typically performed using isopropyl alcohol on a cotton pellet or microbrush. Once complete, a piece of sterile cotton or sponge is placed in the pulp chamber. The access is then sealed with a temporary material. Numerous temporary materials have been used historically. Most materials were eugenol-based, such as zinc oxide eugenol (ZOE) or intermediate restorative material (IRM). Noneugenol based materials, such as Cavit or glass ionomer are more commonly used today due to their improved mechanical properties.[55-58] A plastic instrument is then used to adapt the temporary filling material to the access cavity. It should be noted that the success of endodontic treatment is significantly affected by the quality of the final restoration.[59,60] In a systematic review by Gillen et al., researchers showed that the quality of the coronal restoration is as important as the quality of the root canal filling for the success of the endodontic treatment.[59] Thus nonsurgical endodontic treatment is fully completed only with a proper permanent restoration in place.

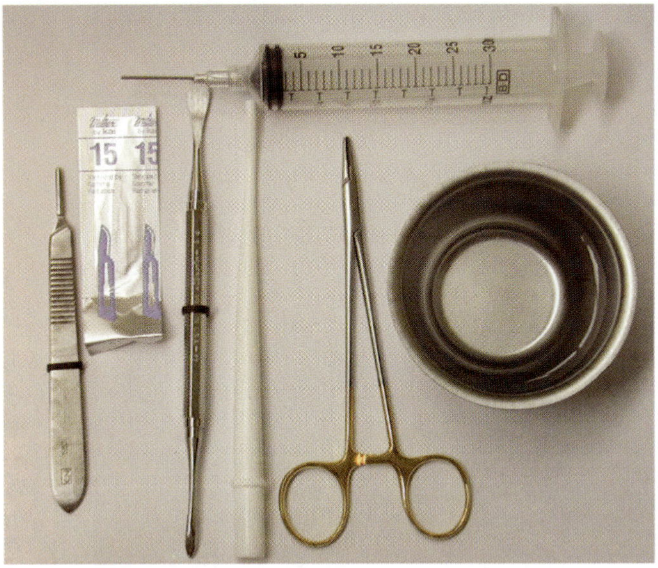

• **Fig. 7.24** Basic emergency kit for an incision for drainage includes (1) scalpel handle, (2) blade, (3) periosteal elevator, (4) suction tip, (5) needle holder, (6) irrigating syringe with an 18-gauge needle, and (7) sterile saline. A rubber dam drain is a frequent addition.

Surgical Armamentarium

Incision and Drainage Armamentarium

Patients can present with swelling before or after endodontic therapy. The swelling can be defined as indurated (cellulitis) or fluctuant (abscess). The swelling can be confined to one fascial space or spread to multiple spaces. The practitioner should always remember that not all swellings are from dental (endodontic) cause. After the swelling has been definitively determined to be of endodontic origin and a thorough review of the patient's past medical history does not contraindicate patient treatment, incision and drainage of the swelling is required. Incision and drainage for endodontic issues is not a solitary treatment. Endodontic therapy in addition to incision and drainage is required to remove the source of the infection and speed resolution of the swelling. The armamentarium used for an incision and drainage is relatively basic and includes (1) scalpel, (2) periosteal elevator, (3) hemostat and (4) sterile saline in a plastic syringe, and (5) drain (Fig. 7.24). Proper anesthesia should be administered before any incision. A scalpel is used to make an incision in the dependent base of the swelling. Number 12 and 15 blades are the most commonly used blades for this procedure. The type of blade used, however, may vary depending on the location and accessibility of the most fluctuant part of the swelling. The incision should not simply cut the gingiva but extend to the cortical bone. Whether the incision should be vertical or horizontal in origin is debatable. Classically, the incision is made in a horizontal direction. Care should be exercised to avoid important anatomic landmarks (e.g., the mental foramen) where transient or permanent injury to the underlying tissues can occur. After making the incision, a periosteal elevator is then placed in the incision to perform blunt dissection. If the swelling is fluctuant, this procedure should provide laudable pus and exudate drainage. In some cases, a curved hemostat may be needed to drain and decompress the swelling. The hemostat is inserted and bluntly forced into the swelling to lyse any loculations. The incision should then be copiously irrigated with sterile saline. After drainage, the clinician must decide whether to place a physical drain. Most swellings of endodontic origin that comprise one fascial space do not require the placement of a physical drain. The incision site will heal and close after treatment. However, the site is still weakened and therefore remains the path of least resistance for future swelling, should it occur. If a physical drain would appear to be beneficial, a piece of rubber dam cut with a dovetail can be inserted into the incision. The dovetail should prevent dislodgement. A suture can also be placed to stabilize the drain if needed. For more extensive swellings, a Penrose drain can be inserted and sutured in place. The steps and techniques of drain placement will be further covered in Chapter 9.

Root End Surgery (Apicoectomy) Armamentarium

Endodontic treatment is usually initiated by cleaning and sealing the root canal space through the crown portion of the tooth. In certain clinical situations or when a previously root canal–treated tooth fails, cleaning and sealing the root canal space may require further treatment using a surgical approach in an attempt to address the canals from the apical end (root end side). For that, a completely different set of instruments and materials are used to allow reflection of the soft tissue and bone, removal of the granulomatous tissue, resection of the apical portion of the root, preparation, and filling of the root end portion from an apical approach. This process can be followed by guided tissue regeneration, if needed, and suturing the soft tissue back to its place. The surgical cassette (Fig. 7.25) consists of (1) scalpel, (2) periosteal elevator, (3) retractors, (4) bone curettes, (5) periodontal curettes, (6) micromirrors, (7) retro pluggers, and (9) needle holders. Also, other instruments and materials are needed in combination with the surgical cassette, such as (1) blades, (2) Impact Air handpiece (see later section), (3) burs, (4) retro-preparation ultrasonic tips, (5) hemostatic agents, (6) dye, (7) retro-filling material, and (8) suture material. The armamentarium used for root end surgery has been modified in the past two decades to allow better management of the soft tissue, bone structure, and root end portion of the tooth. The term used for these instruments in today's practice is "microsurgical armamentarium," and hence the procedure today is termed "microapical surgery," rather than just traditional "apical surgery." The success rate of microsurgery is very high, in the 90% range,[61-64] and has been shown to be superior to traditional endodontic surgery.[17,65] Thus the use of the appropriate armamentarium (and filling material) can play a major role in the success of the treatment provided. The blades used in microsurgery, such as microblades or #15 C, are smaller and more precise to cut soft tissue, compared with traditional surgery that often involved a #15 blade (Fig. 7.26). If microblades are to be used, a microscalpel will be needed. Using the appropriate blade together with proper flap design will result in less recession of the soft tissue after treatment. Periosteal elevators or mold curettes are used to reflect the soft tissue away from the bone. They usually come in different shapes and sizes (Fig. 7.27). Selection of the appropriate size will prevent laceration of the soft tissue during reflection. Unlike nonsurgical treatment, the Impact Air surgical handpiece is designed with a 45-degree angled head to allow for better visibility while cutting the bone (Fig. 7.28). It also does not release any air into the surgical site to avoid the possibility of surgical emphysema. The flap is retracted using the appropriate retractor. A classical retractor often used is the Minnesota retractor. Other retractors have been developed to facilitate easier retraction in the

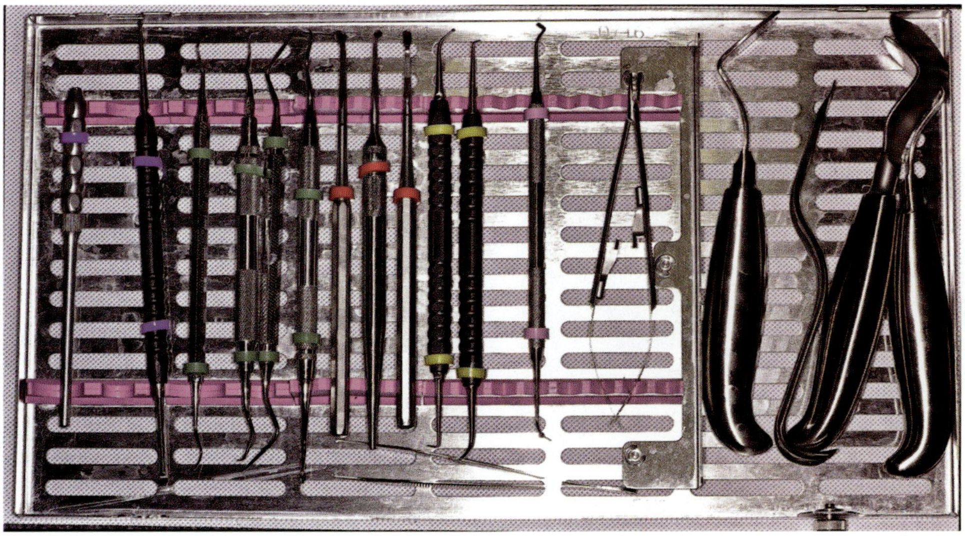

• **Fig. 7.25** Surgical cassette for root end surgery.

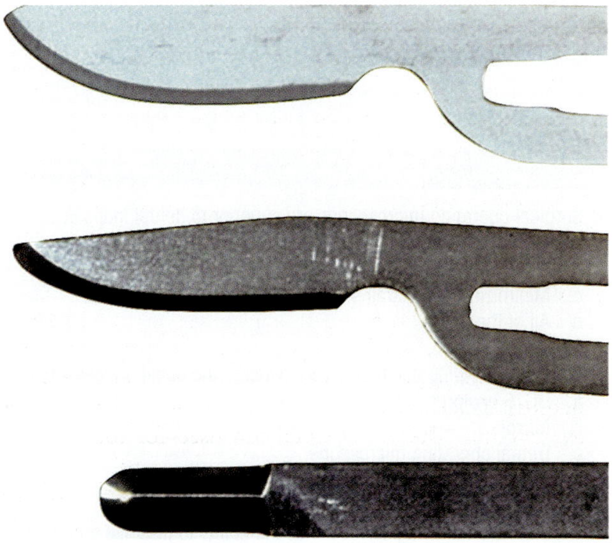

• **Fig. 7.26** Different types of blades, *from top to bottom*: (1) standard 15 blade, (2) 15 C blade, and (3) microblade.

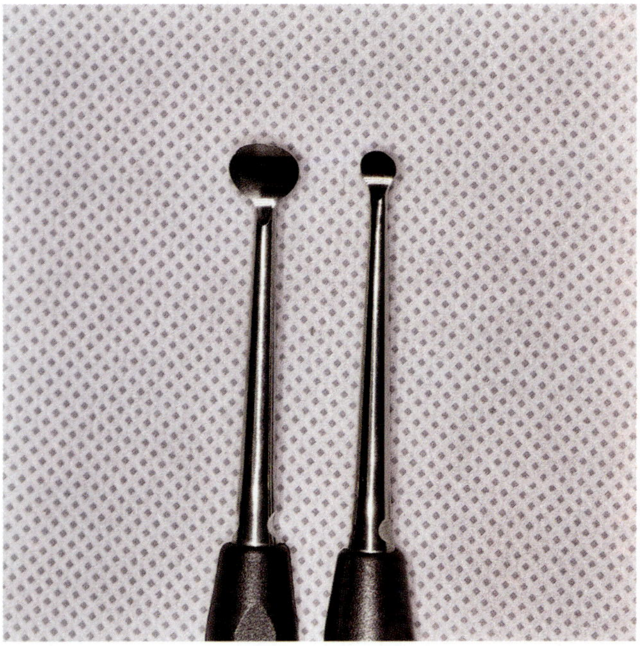

• **Fig. 7.27** Mold curettes used to reflect the flap off the bone and elevate the periosteum.

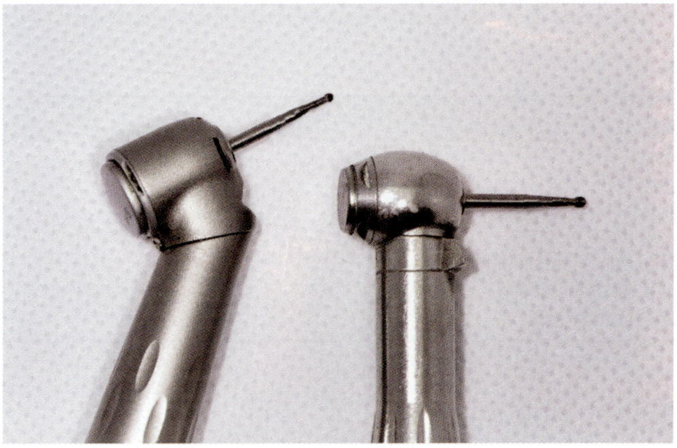

• **Fig. 7.28** Surgical handpiece with a 45-degree angled head *(left)*. Non-surgical handpiece for standard dental work.

anterior and posterior area (Fig. 7.29). Surgical burs are used to remove bone, create the osteotomy, and cut the root end portion of the tooth. After the osteotomy, bone curettes are needed to remove the granulation tissue from the bony crypt. They also come in different sizes to accommodate for the size of the bony crypt (Fig. 7.30). The granulation tissue is often attached to the root; thus periodontal curettes are used to release the granulation tissue from the root surface (Fig. 7.31). Retro preparation is then initiated using specially designed ultrasonic tips (retro-preparation tips), which come in different angulations and sizes to accommodate the different roots (anterior or posterior) (Fig. 7.32). They are also available in different lengths (3 mm, 6 mm, and 9 mm). Although 3 mm retro preparation tips are the most commonly used, 6 mm and 9 mm tips can be often used to allow further cleaning of the root canal space from an apical direction in special clinical cases. Micromirrors are used to visualize the root end portion of the tooth after retro preparation to ensure that no cracks are present (Fig. 7.33). This technique can be combined with the use of dyes to stain the apical end of the root as well

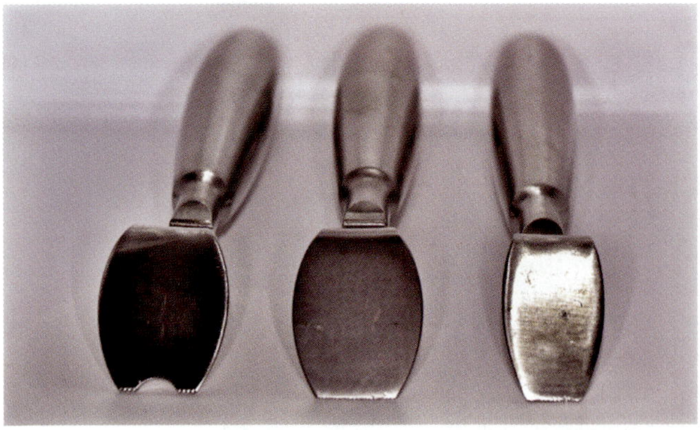

• **Fig. 7.29** Surgical retractors with different tip design for retraction at various locations.

as transillumination to visualize any apical defects[66] (Fig. 7.34). Adequate bleeding control is required for proper visualization and placement of the root end filling. For that, hemostatic agents such as epinephrine pellets, ferric sulfate, or resorbable collagen can be used to control bleeding. The retro-filling material is then placed, using carriers or hand instruments, into the retro cavity. Different categories of retro-filling materials have been used in endodontic surgery. Traditionally, amalgam has been used as a retro-filling material. Due to its moisture sensitivity, it did not provide an adequate seal in the apical area,[67,68] and as a result, the outcome of apical surgery was affected.[17] Over the years, several other retro-filling materials have been introduced, such as IRM, glass ionomer, and resin-based retro-filling material. The most recently introduced and commonly used material in today's microsurgery armamentarium are calcium silicate–based materials such as mineral trioxide aggregate (MTA; Dentsply Sirona, Tulsa, Oklahoma, USA) or Bioceramic putty (Brassler, Augusta, Georgia, USA). These materials have shown superiority in their sealing ability as well as stimulation of hard tissue repair.[68,69] Depending on the crypt size and bone structure, bone substitutes and resorbable membranes can be placed into the bony crypt to enhance and/or restore the integrity of the supporting structure.[70,71] Finally, sutures are used to place the flap back in position. Sutures also come in different sizes, starting 1-0 to 10-0. Usually, 5-0 or 6-0 sutures are used to approximate the flap back to its place. For that process, specially designed needle holders would be used to allow adequate manipulation of the small threads (Fig. 7.35). More details regarding the use of all these instruments are discussed in Chapter 21.

Study Questions

6. Endodontic surgery "apicoectomy" includes:
   a. Resection of an entire root
   b. The placement of a retro-filling material to seal the root canal apically
   c. The use of NaOCl to disinfect the osteotomy site
   d. Stimulation of bleeding to improve visualization and placement of a retro-filling material
7. Dental operating microscopes are beneficial for:
   a. The prevention of carpal tunnel syndrome in the operator
   b. Decreased illumination of the surgical field
   c. Location and negotiation of root canals
   d. Low level magnification
   e. Nonsurgical treatment only
8. Which of the following radiographic methods is not commonly used in endodontic diagnosis?
   a. Periapical radiographs
   b. Bitewings
   c. CBCT
   d. Panoramic x-ray
9. Surgical operating microscopes are superior to dental loops in
   a. Provides higher magnification
   b. Allowing minimal illumination
   c. Minimizing neck strains
   d. All of the above
   e. Only a and c
10. All of the following can be utilized to locate the canal orifices EXCEPT:
    a. DG16 explorer
    b. Mirror
    c. Dental operating microscope
    d. Apex locator
    e. Caries detection dye
11. Which of the following irrigants has the ability to dissolve pulp tissue and disinfect the root canal system?
    a. NaOCl
    b. $Ca(OH)_2$
    c. EDTA
    d. Chlorhexidine
    e. Formocresol

ANSWERS

Answer Box 7

1 d. Periosteal elevator
2 c. Retro pluggers
3 a. Dental caries detection
4 e. All of the above
5 c. formocresol
6 b. The placement of a retro-filling material to seal the root canal apically
7 c. Location and negotiation of root canals
8 d. Panoramic x-ray
9 e. Only A & C
10 d. Apex locator

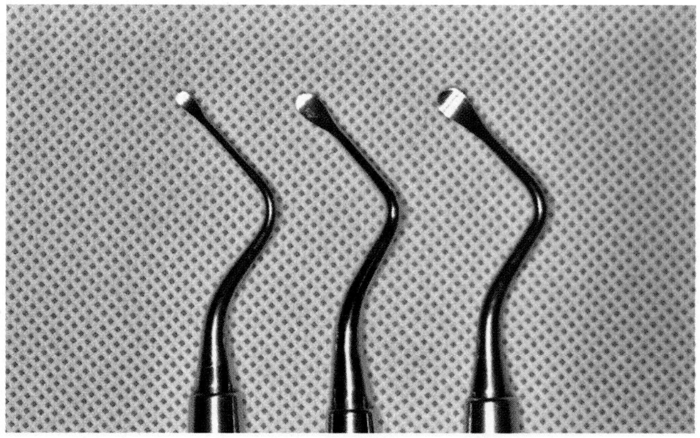

• **Fig. 7.30** Angulated bone curettes to facilitate removal of granulation tissue from the periapical lesion.

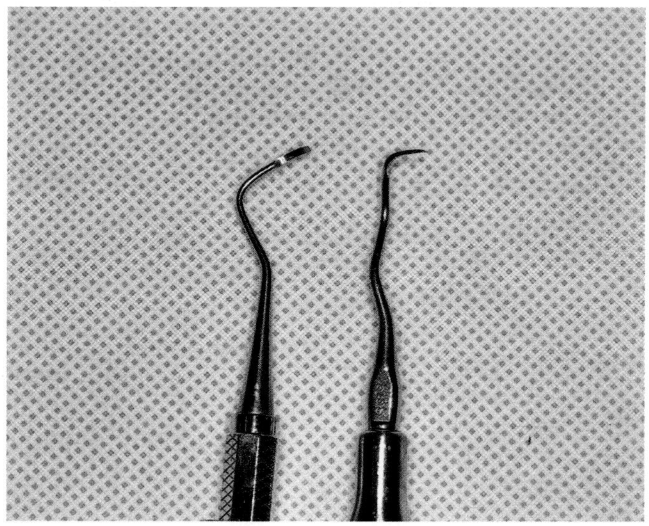

• **Fig. 7.31** Periodontal curette to scale the root surface after apical resection and removal of granulation tissue.

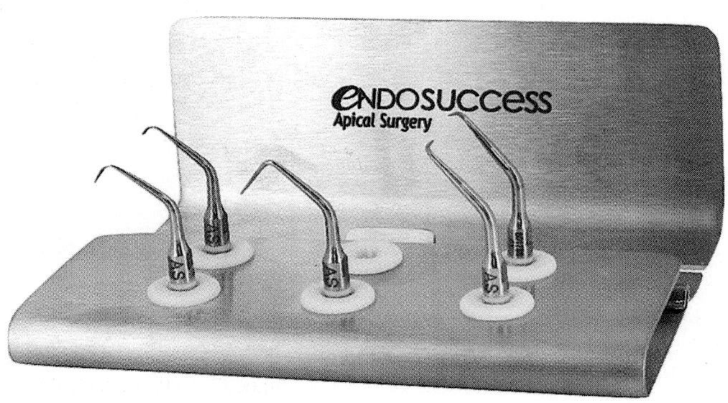

• **Fig. 7.32** Ultrasonic set showing the different ultrasonic tip designs that can be used for root end preparation in the anterior and posterior roots.

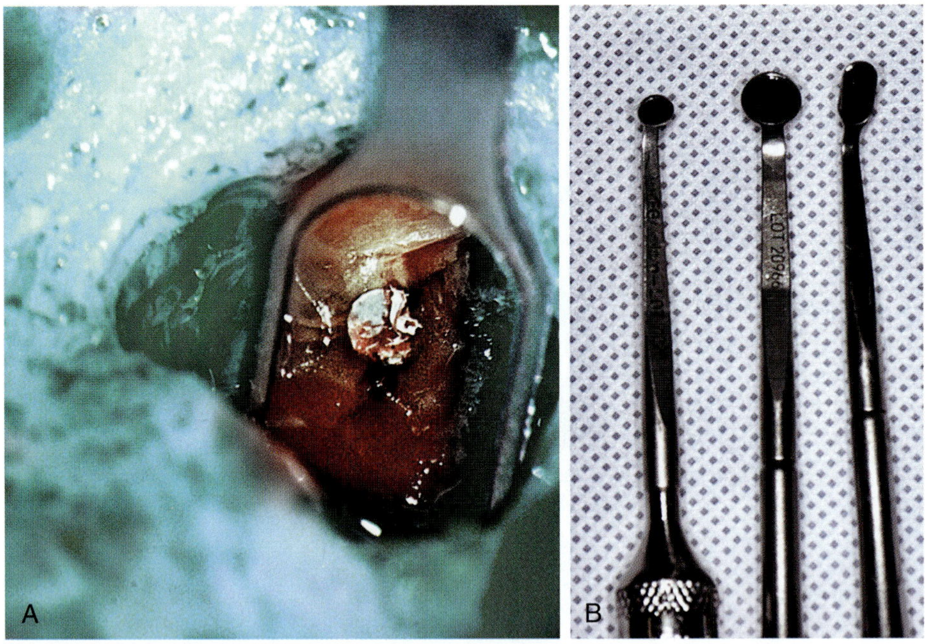

• **Fig. 7.33** Micromirrors used during endodontic surgery *(right)*. Illustration of the use of a micromirror to visualize an apical crack *(left)*.

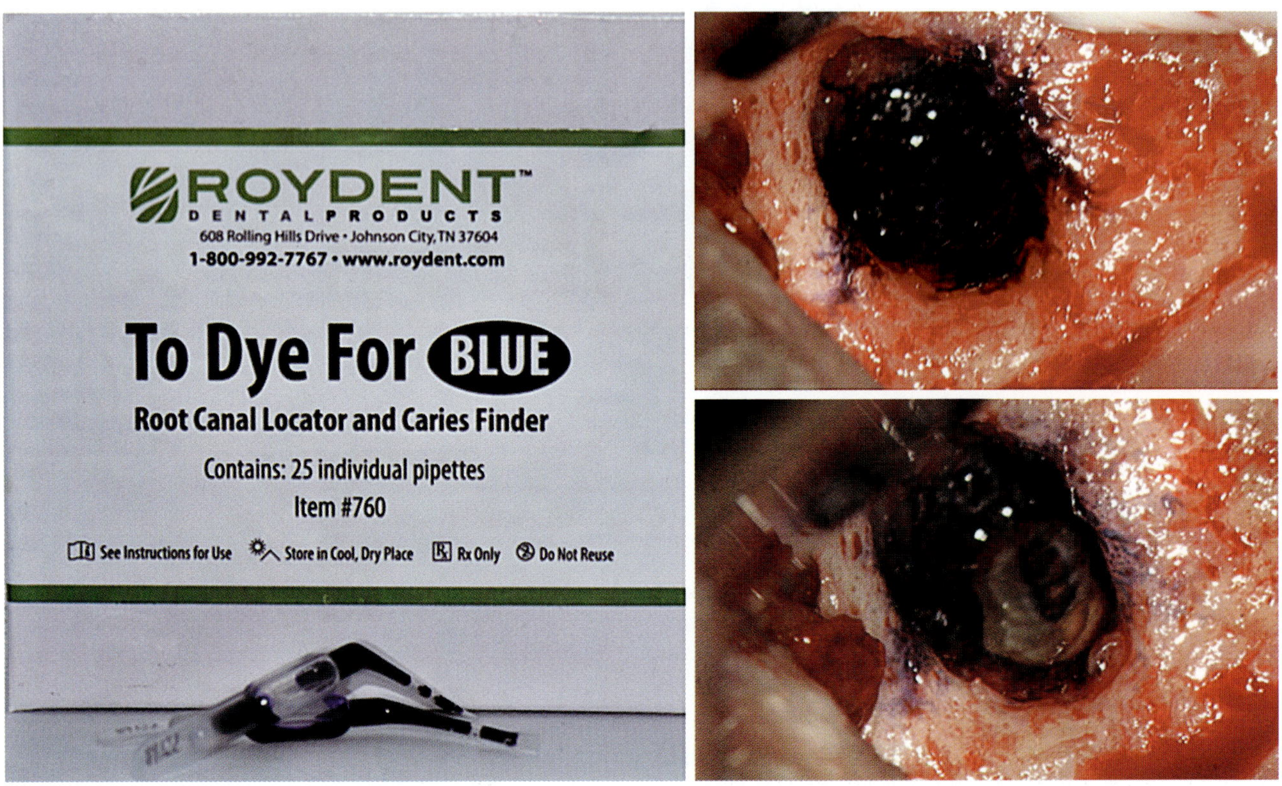

• **Fig. 7.34** The product called "To Dye For," used to stain the root surface *(left)*. Illustration of the staining process in root end surgery (*top* and *bottom right*).

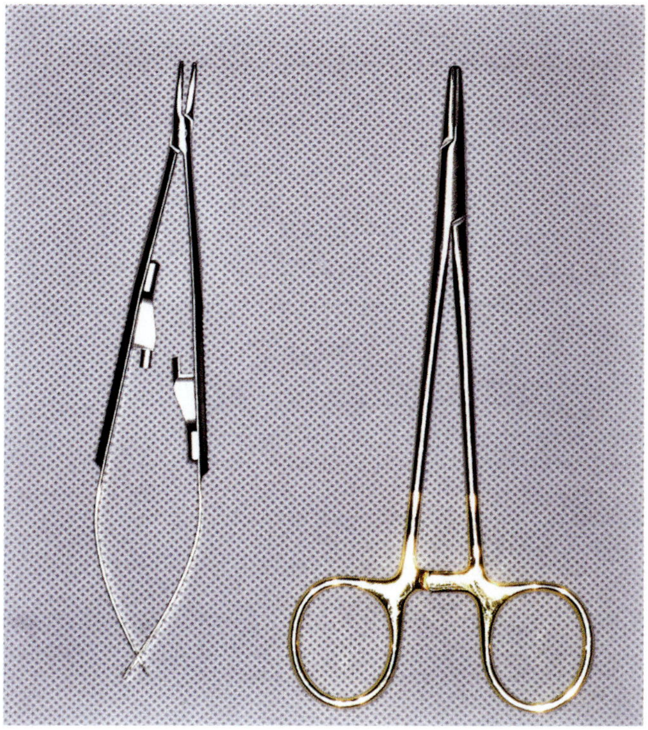

• **Fig. 7.35** Standard needle holder *(left)* and Castroviejo needle holder *(right)*.

References

1. Schilder H: Filling root canals in three dimensions, *Dent Clin North Am* 723–744, 1967.
2. Schilder H: Cleaning and shaping the root canal, *Dent Clin North Am* 18(2):269–296, 1974.
3. Setzer FC, Hinckley N, Kohli MR, Karabucak B: A survey of cone-beam computed tomographic use among endodontic practitioners in the United States, *J Endod* 43(5):699–704, 2017.
4. Mota de Almeida FJ, Knutsson K, Flygare L: The impact of cone beam computed tomography on the choice of endodontic diagnosis, *Int Endod J* 48(6):564–572, 2015.
5. Tsai P, Torabinejad M, Rice D, Azevedo B: Accuracy of cone-beam computed tomography and periapical radiography in detecting small periapical lesions, *J Endod* 38(7):965–970, 2012.
6. Patel K, Mannocci F, Patel S: The assessment and management of external cervical resorption with periapical radiographs and cone-beam computed tomography: a clinical study, *J Endod* 42(10):1435–1440, 2016.
7. Rodriguez G, Abella F, Duran-Sindreu F, Patel S, Roig M: Influence of cone-beam computed tomography in clinical decision making among specialists, *J Endod* 43(2):194–199, 2017.
8. Edlund M, Nair MK, Nair UP: Detection of vertical root fractures by using cone-beam computed tomography: a clinical study, *J Endod* 37(6):768–772, 2011.
9. Bender IB, Seltzer S: Roentgenographic and direct observation of experimental lesions in bone: I. 1961, *J Endod* 29(11):702–706, 2003; discussion 701.
10. Bender IB, Seltzer S: Roentgenographic and direct observation of experimental lesions in bone: II. 1961, *J Endod* 29(11):707–712, 2003; discussion 701.
11. AAE and AAOMR Joint Position Statement: Use of cone beam computed tomography in endodontics 2015 update, *J Endod* 41(9):1393–1396, 2015.
12. Kersten DD, Mines P, Sweet M: Use of the microscope in endodontics: results of a questionnaire, *J Endod* 34(7):804–807, 2008.
13. Khalighinejad N, Aminoshariae A, Kulild JC, et al.: The effect of the dental operating microscope on the outcome of nonsurgical root canal treatment: a retrospective case-control study, *J Endod* 43(5):728–732, 2017.
14. Azim AA, Deutsch AS, Solomon CS: Prevalence of middle mesial canals in mandibular molars after guided troughing under high magnification: an in vivo investigation, *J Endod* 41(2):164–168, 2015.
15. Stropko JJ: Canal morphology of maxillary molars: clinical observations of canal configurations, *J Endod* 25(6):446–450, 1999.
16. Setzer FC, Kohli MR, Shah SB, et al.: Outcome of endodontic surgery: a meta-analysis of the literature—Part 2: Comparison of endodontic microsurgical techniques with and without the use of higher magnification, *J Endod* 38(1):1–10, 2012.
17. Tsesis I, Rosen E, Taschieri S, et al.: Outcomes of surgical endodontic treatment performed by a modern technique: an updated meta-analysis of the literature, *J Endod* 39(3):332–339, 2013.
18. Sunada: New method for measuring the length of the root canal, *J Dent Res* 41(2):1, 1962.
19. Savani GM, Sabbah W, Sedgley CM, Whitten B: Current trends in endodontic treatment by general dental practitioners: report of a United States national survey, *J Endod* 40(5):618–624, 2014.
20. Piasecki L, Carneiro E, da Silva Neto UX, et al.: The use of micro-computed tomography to determine the accuracy of 2 electronic apex locators and anatomic variations affecting their precision, *J Endod* 42(8):1263–1267, 2016.
21. Martins JN, Marques D, Mata A, Carames J: Clinical efficacy of electronic apex locators: systematic review, *J Endod* 40(6):759–777, 2014.
22. Azim AA, Griggs JA, Huang GT: The Tennessee study: factors affecting treatment outcome and healing time following nonsurgical root canal treatment, *Int Endod J* 49(1):6–16, 2016.
23. Ng YL, Mann V, Gulabivala K: A prospective study of the factors affecting outcomes of nonsurgical root canal treatment: Part 1: periapical health, *Int Endod J* 44(7):583–609, 2011.
24. Stokes AN, Tidmarsh BG: A comparison of diamond and tungsten carbide burs for preparing endodontic access cavities through crowns, *J Endod* 14(11):550–553, 1988.
25. Leeb J: Canal orifice enlargement as related to biomechanical preparation, *J Endod* 9(11):463–470, 1983.
26. Baumgartner JC, Cuenin PR: Efficacy of several concentrations of sodium hypochlorite for root canal irrigation, *J Endod* 18(12):605–612, 1992.
27. Gordon TM, Damato D, Christner P: Solvent effect of various dilutions of sodium hypochlorite on vital and necrotic tissue, *J Endod* 7(10):466–469, 1981.
28. Rosenfeld EF, James GA, Burch BS: Vital pulp tissue response to sodium hypochlorite, *J Endod* 4(5):140–146, 1978.
29. Siqueira Jr JF: Rocas IN, Favieri A, Lima KC: Chemomechanical reduction of the bacterial population in the root canal after instrumentation and irrigation with 1%, 2.5%, and 5.25% sodium hypochlorite, *J Endod* 26(6):331–334, 2000.
30. Zou L, Shen Y, Li W, Haapasalo M: Penetration of sodium hypochlorite into dentin, *J Endod* 36(5):793–796, 2010.
31. Jeansonne MJ, White RR: A comparison of 2.0% chlorhexidine gluconate and 5.25% sodium hypochlorite as antimicrobial endodontic irrigants, *J Endod* 20(6):276–278, 1994.
32. Khademi A, Usefian E, Feizianfard M: Tissue dissolving ability of several endodontic irrigants on bovine pulp tissue, *Iran Endod J* 2(2):65–68, 2007.
33. Naenni N, Thoma K, Zehnder M: Soft tissue dissolution capacity of currently used and potential endodontic irrigants, *J Endod* 30(11):785–787, 2004.
34. Ohara P, Torabinejad M, Kettering JD: Antibacterial effects of various endodontic irrigants on selected anaerobic bacteria, *Endod Dent Traumatol* 9(3):95–100, 1993.
35. Okino LA, Siqueira EL, Santos M, et al.: Dissolution of pulp tissue by aqueous solution of chlorhexidine digluconate and chlorhexidine digluconate gel, *Int Endod J* 37(1):38–41, 2004.

36. Yamada RS, Armas A, Goldman M, Lin PS: A scanning electron microscopic comparison of a high volume final flush with several irrigating solutions: part 3, *J Endod* 9(4):137–142, 1983.
37. Bystrom A, Sundqvist G: The antibacterial action of sodium hypochlorite and EDTA in 60 cases of endodontic therapy, *Int Endod J* 18(1):35–40, 1985.
38. Nygaard-Ostby B. Chelation in root canal therapy: ethylenediaminetetraacetic acid for cleansing and widening of root canals. *Odontol Tidskr* 65:3–11, 1957.
39. Baker NA, Eleazer PD, Averbach RE, Seltzer S: Scanning electron microscopic study of the efficacy of various irrigating solutions, *J Endod* 1(4):127–135, 1975.
40. Basrani BR, Manek S, Sodhi RN, et al.: Interaction between sodium hypochlorite and chlorhexidine gluconate, *J Endod* 33(8):966–969, 2007.
41. Bui TB, Baumgartner JC, Mitchell JC: Evaluation of the interaction between sodium hypochlorite and chlorhexidine gluconate and its effect on root dentin, *J Endod* 34(2):181–185, 2008.
42. Baumgartner JC, Mader CL: A scanning electron microscopic evaluation of four root canal irrigation regimens, *J Endod* 13(4):147–157, 1987.
43. Chow TW: Mechanical effectiveness of root canal irrigation, *J Endod* 9(11):475–479, 1983.
44. Psimma Z, Boutsioukis C, Kastrinakis E, Vasiliadis L: Effect of needle insertion depth and root canal curvature on irrigant extrusion ex vivo, *J Endod* 39(4):521–524, 2013.
45. Boutsioukis C, Lambrianidis T, Verhaagen B, et al.: The effect of needle-insertion depth on the irrigant flow in the root canal: evaluation using an unsteady computational fluid dynamics model, *J Endod* 36(10):1664–1668, 2010.
46. Gao Y, Haapasalo M, Shen Y, et al.: Development and validation of a three-dimensional computational fluid dynamics model of root canal irrigation, *J Endod* 35(9):1282–1287, 2009.
47. Boutsioukis C, Verhaagen B, Versluis M, et al.: Evaluation of irrigant flow in the root canal using different needle types by an unsteady computational fluid dynamics model, *J Endod* 36(5):875–879, 2010.
48. Caron G, Nham K, Bronnec F, Machtou P: Effectiveness of different final irrigant activation protocols on smear layer removal in curved canals, *J Endod* 36(8):1361–1366, 2010.
49. Desai P, Himel V: Comparative safety of various intracanal irrigation systems, *J Endod* 35(4):545–549, 2009.
50. van der Sluis LW, Versluis M, Wu MK, Wesselink PR: Passive ultrasonic irrigation of the root canal: a review of the literature, *Int Endod J* 40(6):415–426, 2007.
51. Hasselgren G, Olsson B, Cvek M: Effects of calcium hydroxide and sodium hypochlorite on the dissolution of necrotic porcine muscle tissue, *J Endod* 14(3):125–127, 1988.
52. Law A, Messer H: An evidence-based analysis of the antibacterial effectiveness of intracanal medicaments, *J Endod* 30(10):689–694, 2004.
53. Jasper E: Root canal therapy in modern dentistry, *Dental Cosmos* 75:823–829, 1933.
54. Whitworth J: Sealer selection: a considered approach, *Endod Prac* 2(3):31–38, 1999.
55. Anderson RW, Powell BJ, Pashley DH: Microleakage of temporary restorations in complex endodontic access preparations, *J Endod* 15(11):526–529, 1989.
56. Kazemi RB, Safavi KE, Spangberg LS: Assessment of marginal stability and permeability of an interim restorative endodontic material, *Oral Surg Oral Med Oral Pathol* 78(6):788–796, 1994.
57. Webber RT, del Rio CE, Brady JM, Segall RO: Sealing quality of a temporary filling material, *Oral Surg Oral Med Oral Pathol* 46(1):123–130, 1978.
58. Bobotis HG, Anderson RW, Pashley DH, Pantera Jr EA: A microleakage study of temporary restorative materials used in endodontics, *J Endod* 15(12):569–572, 1989.
59. Gillen BM, Looney SW, Gu LS, et al.: Impact of the quality of coronal restoration versus the quality of root canal fillings on success of root canal treatment: a systematic review and meta-analysis, *J Endod* 37(7):895–902, 2011.
60. Ray HA, Trope M: Periapical status of endodontically treated teeth in relation to the technical quality of the root filling and the coronal restoration, *Int Endod J* 28(1):12–18, 1995.
61. Rubinstein RA, Kim S: Long-term follow-up of cases considered healed one year after apical microsurgery, *J Endod* 28(5):378–383, 2002.
62. Shinbori N, Grama AM, Patel Y, et al.: Clinical outcome of endodontic microsurgery that uses EndoSequence BC root repair material as the root-end filling material, *J Endod* 41(5):607–612, 2015.
63. Kim S, Song M, Shin SJ, Kim E: A randomized controlled study of mineral trioxide aggregate and super ethoxybenzoic acid as root-end filling materials in endodontic microsurgery: long-term outcomes, *J Endod* 42(7):997–1002, 2016.
64. Chong BS, Pitt Ford TR, Hudson MB: A prospective clinical study of mineral trioxide aggregate and IRM when used as root-end filling materials in endodontic surgery, *Int Endod J* 36(8):520–526, 2003.
65. Setzer FC, Shah SB, Kohli MR, et al.: Outcome of endodontic surgery: a meta-analysis of the literature—part 1: comparison of traditional root-end surgery and endodontic microsurgery, *J Endod* 36(11):1757–1765, 2010.
66. Tawil PZ, Saraiya VM, Galicia JC, Duggan DJ: Periapical microsurgery: the effect of root dentinal defects on short- and long-term outcome, *J Endod* 41(1):22–27, 2015.
67. Torabinejad M, Lee SJ, Hong CU: Apical marginal adaptation of orthograde and retrograde root end fillings: a dye leakage and scanning electron microscopic study, *J Endod* 20(8):402–407, 1994.
68. Torabinejad M, Higa RK, McKendry DJ, Pitt Ford TR: Dye leakage of four root end filling materials: effects of blood contamination, *J Endod* 20(4):159–163, 1994.
69. Baek SH, Plenk Jr H, Kim S: Periapical tissue responses and cementum regeneration with amalgam, SuperEBA, and MTA as root-end filling materials, *J Endod* 31(6):444–449, 2005.
70. Taschieri S, Corbella S, Tsesis I, et al.: Effect of guided tissue regeneration on the outcome of surgical endodontic treatment of through-and-through lesions: a retrospective study at 4-year follow-up, *Oral Maxillofac Surg* 15(3):153–159, 2011.
71. Tsesis I, Rosen E, Tamse A, et al.: Effect of guided tissue regeneration on the outcome of surgical endodontic treatment: a systematic review and meta-analysis, *J Endod* 37(8):1039–1045, 2011.

8

Local Anesthesia

AL READER, JOHN M. NUSSTEIN, AND MELISSA DRUM

CHAPTER OUTLINE

LEARNING OBJECTIVES

After reading this chapter, the student should be able to:

1. Explain why apprehension and anxiety, fatigue, and tissue inflammation create difficulties in obtaining profound anesthesia.
2. Define the pain threshold and the factors affecting it.
3. Describe patient management techniques that facilitate obtaining adequate anesthesia.
4. List techniques that are helpful in reducing the pain of injections.
5. Describe the "routine" approach to conventional local anesthesia: when and how to anesthetize.
6. Describe circumstances that create difficulties in obtaining profound anesthesia using conventional techniques.
7. Describe when to use supplemental methods of obtaining pulpal anesthesia if standard block or infiltration methods fail.
8. Review techniques of infiltration, intraosseous, periodontal ligament, and intraseptal and intrapulpal injections.
9. Discuss how to obtain anesthesia for specific pulpal and periapical pathoses: symptomatic irreversible pulpitis, symptomatic teeth with pulpal necrosis, asymptomatic teeth with pulpal necrosis, and surgical procedures.

Factors Affecting Endodontic Anesthesia

Emotional considerations, in addition to tissue changes, impair the effectiveness of local anesthesia.[1] A patient who is psychologically distraught and has an inflamed pulp or periapex has a lower pain threshold (i.e., less stimulus is required to produce pain).[2]

Apprehension and Anxiety

Many endodontic patients have heard horror stories about root canal treatment. The cause may not be the treatment but the experience of a painful or "infected" tooth. They vividly recall the pain, swelling, and sleepless nights associated with the tooth before treatment. The procedure itself is generally less threatening; a survey of endodontic patients completing therapy indicated that 96% would agree to have future root canal treatment.[3] Therefore because they fear the unknown and have heard unfavorable stories, patients are apprehensive or anxious. This emotion plays a role in their perceptions and affects how they react to pain. Many patients can effectively mask this apprehension!

Fatigue

Over a course of days, many patients with a toothache have not slept well, have not eaten properly, or otherwise have not functioned normally. In addition, many are apprehensive or anxious about the appointment. The result is a patient with a decreased ability to manage stress and less tolerance for pain.

Tissue Inflammation

Inflamed tissues have a lower threshold of pain perception[4]; this phenomenon is called *allodynia.* In other words, a tissue that is inflamed is much more sensitive and reactive to a mild stimulus.[4] Therefore an inflamed tissue responds painfully to a stimulus that otherwise would be unnoticed or perceived only mildly. Because root canal treatment procedures generally involve inflamed pulpal or periapical tissues, this phenomenon has obvious importance. A related complication is that inflamed tissues are more difficult to anesthetize.[5]

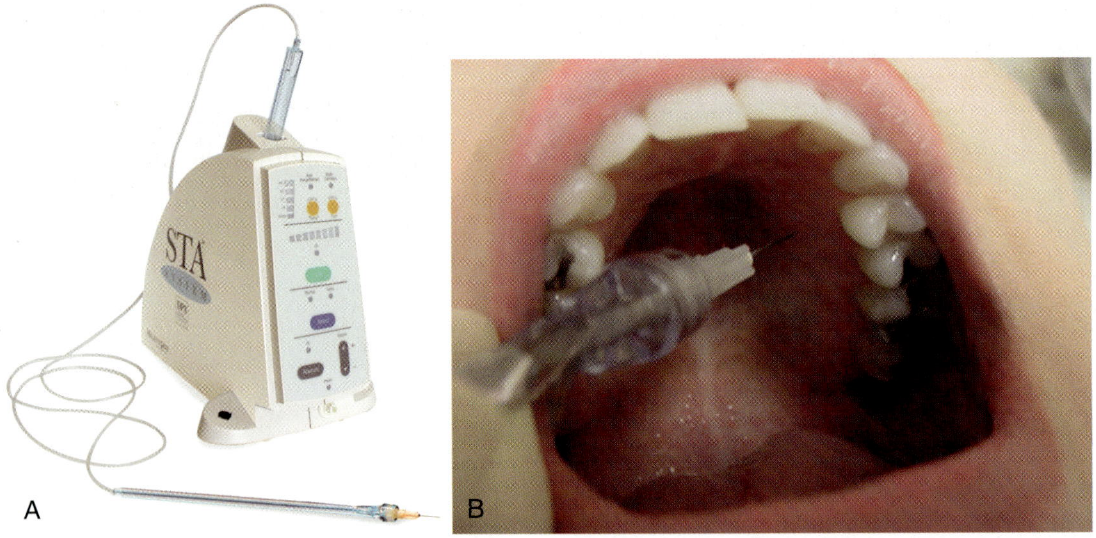

• **Fig. 8.1** **A,** Computer-controlled injection device. Note the handpiece assembly and microtubing. **B,** The specialized handpiece and needle may be used in most situations. (A, courtesy Milestone Scientific, Inc., Livingston, NJ, USA.)

A good example of the allodynia is sunburn. Exposed tissues that have been sunburned are irritated and inflamed. The skin has now become quite sensitive (lower pain threshold) to contact and is painful. The same principle applies to inflamed pulpal and periapical tissues.[6]

Previous Unsuccessful Anesthesia

Unfortunately, profound pulpal anesthesia is not always obtained with conventional techniques. Previous difficulty with teeth becoming anesthetized is associated with a likelihood of subsequent unsuccessful anesthesia.[7] These patients are likely to be apprehensive (lower pain threshold) and generally identify themselves by comments such as, "Novocain never seems to work very well on me" or "A lot of shots are always necessary to deaden my teeth." The practitioner should anticipate difficulties in obtaining anesthesia in such patients. Often, psychological management and supplemental local anesthesia techniques are required.

Initial Management

The early phase of treatment is most important. If the patient is managed properly and anesthetic techniques are performed smoothly, the pain threshold elevates. The result is more predictable anesthesia and a less apprehensive, more cooperative patient.

Psychological Approach

The psychological approach involves the four Cs: control, communication, concern, and confidence. *Control* is important and is achieved by obtaining and maintaining the upper hand. *Communication* is accomplished by listening to the patient and explaining what is to be done and what the patient should expect. *Concern* is shown by verbalizing awareness of the patient's apprehensions. *Confidence* is expressed in body language and in a professional approach and communication style, giving the patient confidence in the management, diagnostic, and treatment skills of the dentist. Management of the four Cs effectively calms and reassures the patient, thereby raising the pain threshold.

Topics Related to Injection Pain

Obtaining the Patient's Confidence

Obtaining the patient's confidence is critical. Before any injection is given, establishing communication, exhibiting empathy, and informing patients of an awareness of their apprehension in addition to their dental problem markedly increases the patient's confidence levels.[8] Most important, having the patient's confidence gives control of the situation to the dentist; this is a requisite!

Topical Anesthetic

Use of a topical anesthetic is popular as an adjunct to oral injections. Some investigators have shown topical anesthetics to be effective,[9-11] whereas others have not.[12,13] The most important aspect of using topical anesthesia is not primarily the actual decrease in mucosal sensitivity, but rather the demonstrated concern that everything possible is being done to prevent pain. Another aspect is the power of suggestion that the topical anesthetic will reduce the pain of injection.[13] When a topical anesthetic gel is used, a small amount on a cotton-tipped applicator is placed on the dried mucosa for 1 minute before the injection.[14]

Needle Insertion

Initially, the needle is inserted *gently* into the mucosal tissue.

Small-Gauge Needles

A common misconception is that smaller needles cause less pain; this is not true for dental needles. Patients cannot differentiate between 25-, 27-, and 30-gauge needles during injections.[15-17] These sizes have similar deflection patterns and resistance to breakage.[17,18] However, to prevent broken needles when administering inferior alveolar nerve blocks, do not use 30-gauge needles, bury the needle to the hub, or bend needles at the hub.[19] As a recommendation, a 27-gauge needle is suitable for most conventional dental injections.

Slow Injection

A slow injection decreases both pressure and the patient's discomfort.[20] A slow inferior alveolar nerve block is more comfortable than a rapid injection.[20,21] A technique for slow injection is to use a computer-controlled anesthetic delivery system (CCLAD) (Fig. 8.1, *A* and *B*).

Most studies on CCLADs compared the pain of injection with delivery systems and pain with standard syringe injections,[22-28] generally with favorable results.[24-28] Therefore although the CCLAD reduces the pain of the injection, the system does not produce a painless injection.[22-28]

Two-Stage Injection

A two-stage injection consists of initial, very slow administration of approximately a quarter-cartridge of anesthetic just under the mucosal surface. After regional numbness has been obtained, the remainder of the cartridge is deposited to the full depth at the target site. The two-stage injection decreases the pain of needle placement for females in the inferior alveolar nerve block.[29] This injection technique is indicated for apprehensive and anxious patients or pediatric patients, but it may be used on anyone. It is also effective for any injection, including the inferior alveolar nerve block.

Gender Differences in Pain

Women try to avoid pain more than men, accept it less, and fear it more.[30,31] Anxiety may also modulate differences in pain responses between males and females.[31] Women react differently to pain and are more likely to present anesthetic challenges.

When to Anesthetize

Preferably, anesthesia should be given at each appointment. A common belief is that instruments may be used in canals with necrotic pulps and periapical lesions painlessly without anesthesia. Occasionally there may be ingrowth of vital tissue in the apical few millimeters of the canal.[32] This inflamed tissue contains nerves and is sensitive. Not only is this vital tissue contacted during instrumentation, but also pressure is created. These factors may cause discomfort if the patient is not anesthetized.

There is an antiquated notion that canal length can be determined in a nonanesthetized patient by passing an instrument into a necrotic canal until the patient shows an "eye-blink response." Unfortunately, patient perceptions and responses are too variable for accuracy. Pain may be felt when the instrument is far short of the apex, or some patients may have no sensation even when the instrument is several millimeters beyond the apex. Not using anesthesia to aid in length determination cannot replace radiographs or an electronic apex locator for accuracy. Another misconception is that after the canals have been cleaned and shaped, it is not necessary to anesthetize the patient at the obturation appointment. Unfortunately, during obturation, pressure is created, and small amounts of sealer may be extruded beyond the apex. This occurrence may be quite uncomfortable for the patient. Many patients (and the dentist) are more at ease if regional hard and soft tissue anesthesia is present.

Adjunctive Pharmacologic Therapy

Anxious patients may benefit from sedation (oral, inhalation, intravenous). However, even with conscious sedation, profound local anesthesia is required to eliminate pain during dental treatment.[33-35] Nitrous oxide administration helps reduce pain during treatment in patients presenting with symptomatic irreversible pulpitis.[34,36] A discussion of agents that control anxiety is included in Chapter 9.

Conventional Pulpal Anesthesia for Restorative Dentistry

Success of local anesthesia is variable. Two surveys of patients and dentists indicated that inadequate anesthesia was common during restorative treatment.[7,37] Several factors affect anesthesia, such as

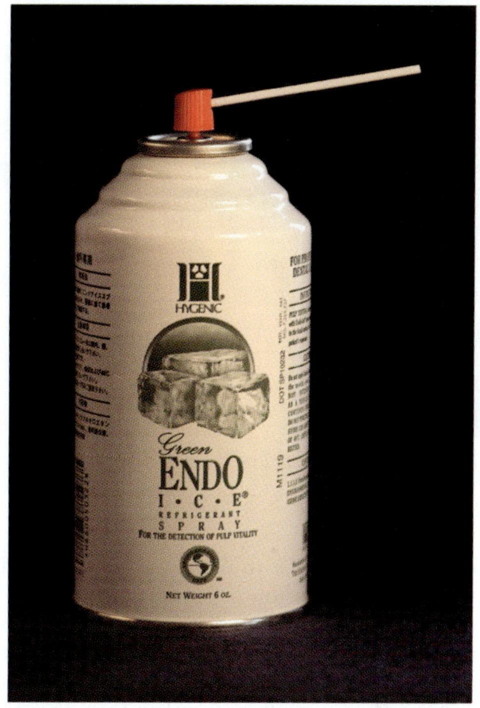

• **Fig. 8.2** A cold refrigerant may be used to test for pulpal anesthesia before the start of a clinical procedure. (Courtesy Coltene/Whaledent, Cuyahoga Falls, OH, USA.)

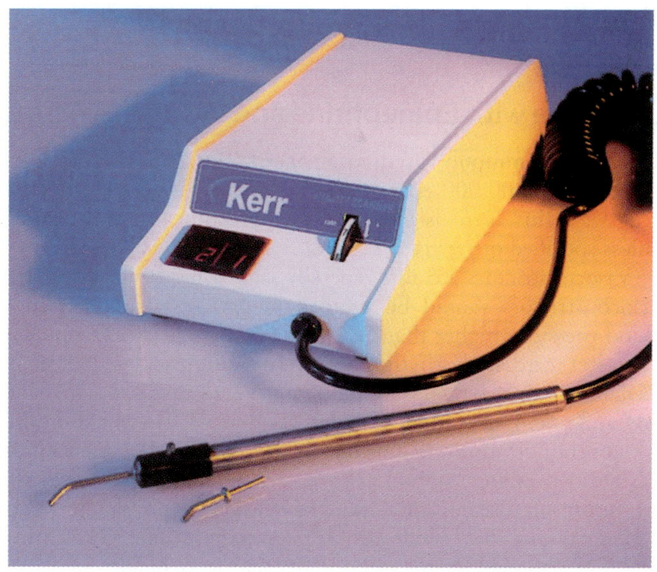

• **Fig. 8.3** An electrical pulp tester (EPT) also may be used to test for pulpal anesthesia before a clinical procedure is started. (Courtesy SybronEndo, Glendora, CA, USA.)

the type of procedure (endodontic, extraction, restorative, periodontal, implant placement, etc.), arch location (maxillary or mandibular), the patient's anxiety level, and the presence of inflamed tissue. This chapter emphasizes the evidence-based requirements for pulpal anesthesia, which differ from those for oral surgery, implant dentistry, periodontics, and pediatric dentistry.

Many clinical studies have objectively evaluated local anesthetic agents and techniques. A measurement of pulpal anesthesia before beginning a clinical procedure is obtained with a cold spray refrigerant (Fig. 8.2) or electric pulp tester (Fig. 8.3). The cold

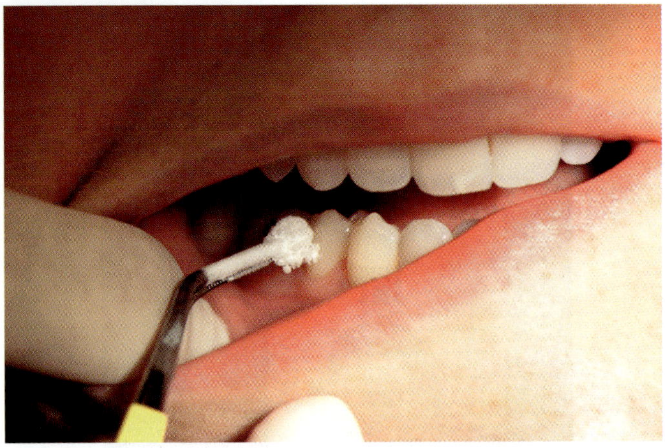

• **Fig. 8.4** The pellet with the cold refrigerant is applied to the surface of the tooth.

spray refrigerant is the easiest to use clinically. The cold refrigerant is sprayed on a large cotton pellet held with cotton tweezers. The cold pellet is then placed on the tooth (Fig. 8.4). No pulpal response to the stimuli after administration of anesthetic means probable profound pulpal anesthesia in asymptomatic teeth with vital pulps.[38,39] Experimental studies that have investigated the use of local anesthesia are discussed in the following sections. Conventional injection techniques are detailed in other textbooks.

Mandibular Anesthesia for Restorative Dentistry

Lidocaine with Epinephrine and Vasoconstrictors

The most commonly used local anesthetic agent is 2% lidocaine with 1:100,000 epinephrine, which is a safe and effective drug.[14,40] This agent is indicated for procedures in this chapter unless specified otherwise.

Vasoconstrictors are also generally safe. It has been stated that vasoconstrictors should be avoided in patients who have high blood pressure (higher than 200 mm Hg systolic or 115 mm Hg diastolic), cardiac dysrhythmias, severe cardiovascular disease, or unstable angina, or who are less than 6 months past a myocardial infarction or cerebrovascular accident.[14] These conditions are contraindications to routine dental treatment. Patients taking antidepressants, nonselective beta-blocking agents, medicine for Parkinson disease, and cocaine are at risk for problems.[14,40] In patients taking these medications, plain mepivacaine (3% Carbocaine) can be used for the inferior alveolar nerve block.

Anesthetic Factors Associated with the Inferior Alveolar Nerve Block

Although the most common method of mandibular anesthesia is the inferior alveolar nerve block, this injection also has the greatest number of failures.[40] The following sections discuss the expected signs of successful (and unsuccessful) anesthesia after administration of one cartridge of 2% lidocaine with 1:100,000 epinephrine.

Lip Numbness

Lip numbness usually occurs in 4 to 6 minutes after injection.[40-47] Lip numbness indicates only that the injection blocked the nerves to the soft tissues of the lip, not necessarily that pulpal anesthesia has been obtained.[40-50] If lip numbness is not obtained, the block has been "missed." This circumstance occurs approximately 4% to 6% of the time in asymptomatic patients and 2% to 8% in patients with irreversible pulpitis.[51] Fowler et al. also found that administration of a two-cartridge volume was significantly better than a one-cartridge volume in both asymptomatic subjects and emergency patients presenting with irreversible pulpitis.[51] If missed blocks occur frequently, the injection technique should be reviewed.

Soft Tissue Anesthesia

Lack of mucosal or gingival response to a sharp explorer does not indicate pulpal anesthesia.[40-50]

Onset of Pulpal Anesthesia

Pulpal anesthesia usually occurs in 5 to 9 minutes in the molars and premolars and 14 to 19 minutes in the anterior teeth.[40-50] In some patients, onset occurs sooner, and in others it is delayed.[40-50]

Duration

The duration of pulpal anesthesia in the mandible is very good.[40-50] Therefore if successful anesthesia usually (but not always) persists for approximately 2½ hours.[48]

Success

The incidence of successful mandibular pulpal anesthesia tends to be higher in molars and premolars and lower in anterior teeth.[40-50] Pulpal anesthesia is not achieved in all patients after what appears to be a clinically successful inferior alveolar nerve block (i.e., numb lip and chin). In such cases, other approaches are required.

Alternative Attempts to Increase Anesthetic Success

Increasing the Volume

Increasing the volume of anesthetic from one to two cartridges does not increase the success rate for obtaining pulpal anesthesia with the inferior alveolar nerve block.[40,41,49,50]

Increasing the Epinephrine Concentration

There is no improvement in pulpal anesthesia with a higher concentration (1:50,000) of epinephrine in an inferior alveolar nerve block.[50,52]

Alternative Solutions

2% Mepivacaine with 1:20,000 Levonordefrin, 4% Prilocaine with 1:200,000 Epinephrine, and Plain Solutions (3% Mepivacaine and 4% Prilocaine)

As alternative solutions, 2% mepivacaine with 1:20,000 levonordefrin; 4% prilocaine with 1:200,000 epinephrine; and plain solutions (3% mepivacaine and 4% prilocaine) are equivalent to 2% lidocaine with 1:100,000 epinephrine in providing pulpal anesthesia for approximately 1 hour after an inferior alveolar nerve block.[44,47]

4% Articaine with Epinephrine for Inferior Alveolar Nerve Blocks

Articaine is a safe and effective local anesthetic agent.[53-62] Anecdotally, articaine has been see to have an improved local anesthetic

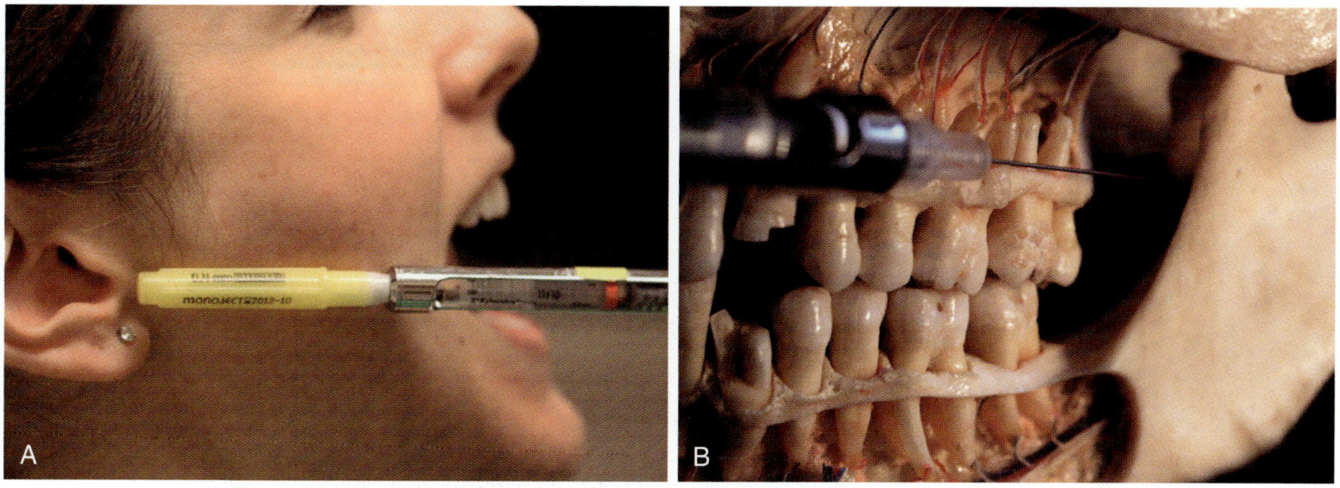

• **Fig. 8.5** **A,** Extraoral landmark for the Gow-Gates technique: the lower border of the tragus of the ear and the corner of the mouth. The intraoral target site for the Gow Gates technique is the neck of the mandibular condyle. **B,** Vazirani-Akinosi technique. This closed-mouth technique has the landmark for needle insertion online with the mucogingival junction of the maxillary second molar.

effect.[63] However, clinical trials have failed to detect any superiority of articaine over lidocaine in inferior alveolar nerve block anesthesia.[58,61]

Articaine, like prilocaine, has the potential to cause neuropathies.[64] Some authors have found the incidence of paresthesia (involving the lip and/or tongue) associated with articaine and prilocaine to be higher than that found with either lidocaine or mepivacaine.[64-66] Other authors have not found a higher incidence when using articaine.[67] However, because there is no difference in success of pulpal anesthesia between articaine and lidocaine for inferior alveolar nerve blocks, and some attorneys are aware of the proposed association of articaine to paresthesia, it seems reasonable to use articaine for infiltrations but not for nerve blocks.

Long-Acting Agents

Clinical trials of bupivacaine and etidocaine have been conducted in oral surgery, endodontics, and periodontics.[68-71] These agents provide a prolonged analgesic period and are indicated when postoperative pain is anticipated. However, not all patients want prolonged lip numbness.[69] For those patients, analgesics may be prescribed. Compared with lidocaine, bupivacaine has a somewhat slower onset but almost double the duration of pulpal anesthesia in the mandible (approximately 4 hours).[48]

Buffered Lidocaine

Buffering lidocaine with sodium bicarbonate raises the pH of the anesthetic solution. In medicine there is evidence that buffering lidocaine results in less pain during the injection.[72,73] In dentistry, some studies[74-77] found that buffered lidocaine produced less pain on injection and a faster onset of anesthesia. A number of recent studies[78-84] failed to establish a significant reduction in injection pain, a faster onset, or better success with buffered anesthetic solutions.

Alternative Injections and Locations

Gow-Gates and Vizarani-Akinosi Techniques (Fig. 8.5)

Neither the Gow-Gates[85] nor the Vizarani-Akinosi[86] technique is superior to the standard inferior alveolar nerve block injection.[87-92] These techniques are not replacements for the inferior alveolar nerve block, and both require a two-cartridge volume. The Vizarani-Akinosi is a closed-mouth technique and is useful for patients presenting with trismus. However, patients with trismus should be referred to an endodontist because patient management is complicated.

Neither the Gow-Gates nor the Vazirani-Akinosi technique provides adequate pulpal anesthesia for mandibular posterior teeth in patients presenting with symptomatic irreversible pulpitis.[93] Both injections would require supplemental anesthesia.

Incisive Nerve Block/Infiltration at the Mental Foramen

The incisive nerve block is successful 80% to 83% of the time in anesthetizing the premolar teeth for about 20 to 30 minutes.[46,94-96] It is not effective for the central and lateral incisors.[46]

Lidocaine Infiltration Injections

Labial or lingual infiltrations of a lidocaine solution alone are not effective for pulpal anesthesia in the mandible.[97-99]

Articaine Infiltration Injections

Articaine is significantly better than lidocaine for buccal infiltration of the mandibular first molar.[100-103] However, articaine alone does not predictably provide pulpal anesthesia of the first molar. There is no difference between 4% articaine with 1:100,000 and 1:200,000 epinephrine for buccal infiltration.[104]

In anterior teeth, buccal and lingual infiltrations of articaine provide initial pulpal anesthesia, but anesthesia declines over the course of 60 minutes from the time the injection was given.[105,106]

Evaluating Mechanisms of Failure with the Inferior Alveolar Nerve Block

Accuracy of Needle Placement

Accurate anatomic positioning of the needle is no guarantee of a successful block.[107,108] It is interesting to note that even locating the inferior alveolar nerve with ultrasound or with a peripheral nerve stimulator before the injection did not improve success.[109,110] The anesthetic solution may not completely diffuse into the nerve trunk (Fig. 8.6) to reach and block all nerves, even if deposited at the correct site, thus resulting in failure.[111]

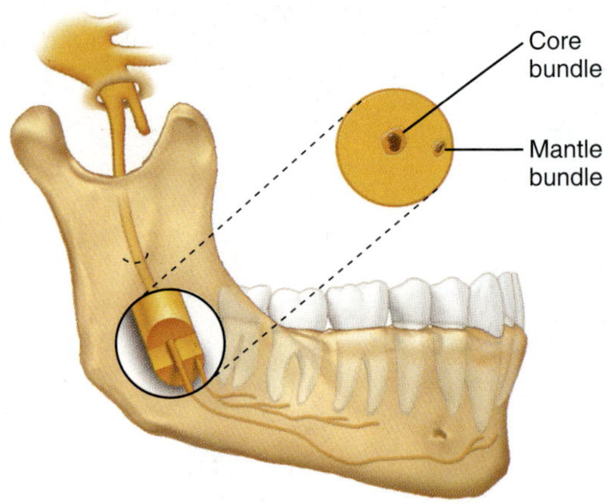

• **Fig. 8.6** Central Core Theory. The large diameter and density of the bundle may inhibit diffusion of a sufficient quantity of anesthetic to provide profound pulpal anesthesia.

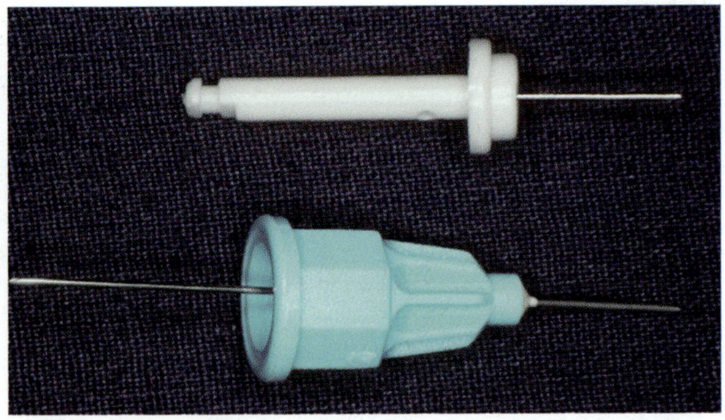

• **Fig. 8.7** Components of an Intraosseous Injection System. The perforator *(top)* is a small, sharp, latch-type drill used to make an opening through soft tissue and bone. The needle *(bottom)* is short and of small gauge to allow insertion and injection directly through the opening.

Needle Deflection and Needle Bevel

Needle deflection has been theorized to be a cause of failure of the inferior alveolar nerve block.[18,112-115] However, two studies have shown that needle bevel orientation (away or toward the mandibular foramen or ramus) does not affect the success of the inferior alveolar nerve block.[116,117]

Accessory Innervation

Anatomic evidence suggests that accessory innervation exists from branches of the mylohyoid nerve.[118] A study using a mylohyoid injection lingual and inferior to the retromolar fossa, in addition to an inferior alveolar nerve block, showed no enhancement of pulpal anesthesia.[119] Therefore, the mylohyoid nerve is not a major factor in failure of the inferior alveolar nerve block.

Cross-Innervation

Cross-innervation from the contralateral inferior alveolar nerve has been implicated in failure to achieve anesthesia in anterior teeth after an inferior alveolar nerve block injection. Cross-innervation does occur in incisors, but it is the failure of the initial inferior alveolar nerve block that accounts for failure of pulpal anesthesia in anterior teeth.[120]

Red Hair

In medicine, red-haired females have shown reduced subcutaneous efficacy of lidocaine and increased requirements for desflurane.[121] However, in dentistry, red hair was unrelated to success rates for the inferior alveolar nerve block. Red hair was associated with higher levels of dental anxiety.[121] Because of this higher dental anxiety, red-haired women may be more likely to report nonpainful sensations (pressure, vibration, etc.) as painful during treatment. This circumstance would cause clinicians to mistake a difference in anxiety for a difference in quality of anesthesia.

Patient Position for an Inferior Alveolar Nerve Block

It has been recommended to place patients in an upright position after administration of an inferior alveolar nerve block, theoretically allowing the anesthetic to diffuse in an inferior direction and resulting in better pulpal anesthesia. When an upright and a supine position were compared after an inferior alveolar nerve block, a study found the two positions were equally successful in the molars.[122] However, clinically, neither position for administration of the inferior alveolar nerve block would provide complete pulpal anesthesia.

Another study evaluated the effect of the head tilted in the direction of the block versus the head tilted to the opposite side in patients with symptomatic irreversible pulpitis. The study found no significant difference in the same side position and the opposite side position. [123]

Methods to Increase Success of the Inferior Alveolar Nerve Block

Infiltrations of Articaine After an Inferior Alveolar Nerve Block

A very important clinical finding is that a supplemental, buccal articaine infiltration of the first molar, premolars, and labial infiltration of anterior teeth after an inferior alveolar nerve block should provide pulpal anesthesia for approximately 1 hour.[105,124,125] The second molar may require a supplemental intraosseous (IO) or periodontal ligament (PDL) injection to achieve success.

Intraosseous Anesthesia After an Inferior Alveolar Nerve Block

Supplemental IO injections of lidocaine and mepivacaine with vasoconstrictors allow quick onset and increase the success of the inferior alveolar nerve block for approximately 60 minutes.[126,127] Using 3% mepivacaine plain results in pulpal anesthesia for approximately 30 minutes.[128] (Figs. 8.7 to 8.11)

Periodontal Ligament Anesthesia After an Inferior Alveolar Nerve Block

Supplemental PDL injections of 2% lidocaine with 1:100,000 epinephrine increase the success of the inferior alveolar nerve block, but the duration is approximately 23 minutes.[129]

Injection Speed and Success

A slow inferior alveolar nerve block increases success over a fast injection[20] but not for patients diagnosed with irreversible pulpitis.[21]

Pain and Inflammation

Most studies have evaluated anesthesia in the absence of symptoms and inflammation; results differ if these conditions are

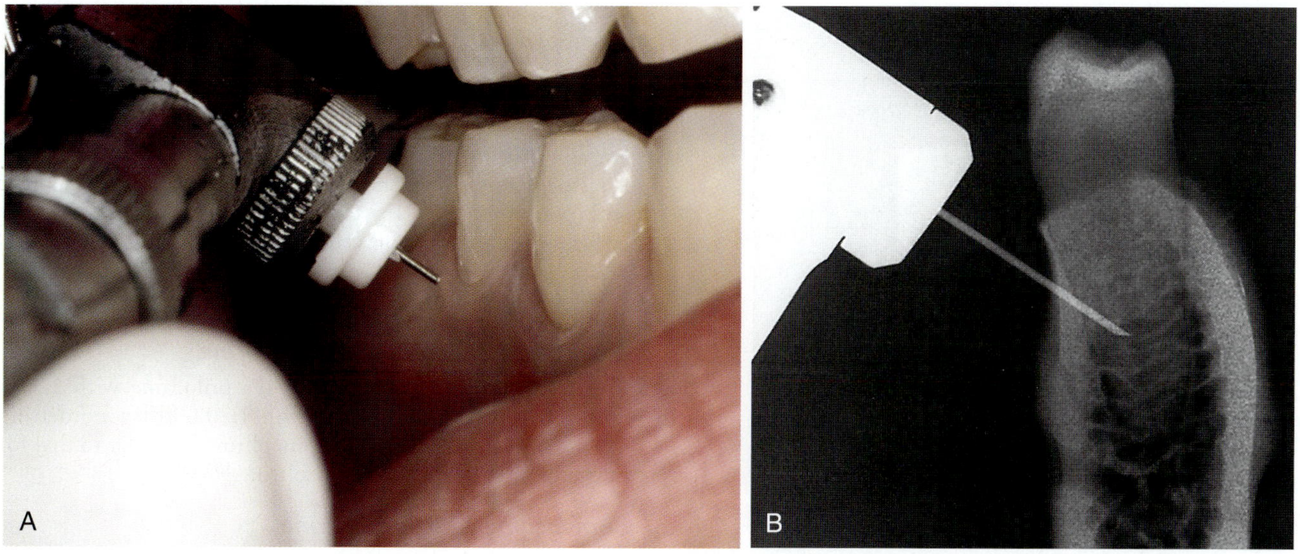

• **Fig. 8.8** Intraosseous Injection Technique. **A,** Location and angulation of the perforator. **B,** The perforator "breaks through" cortical bone into the medullary space.

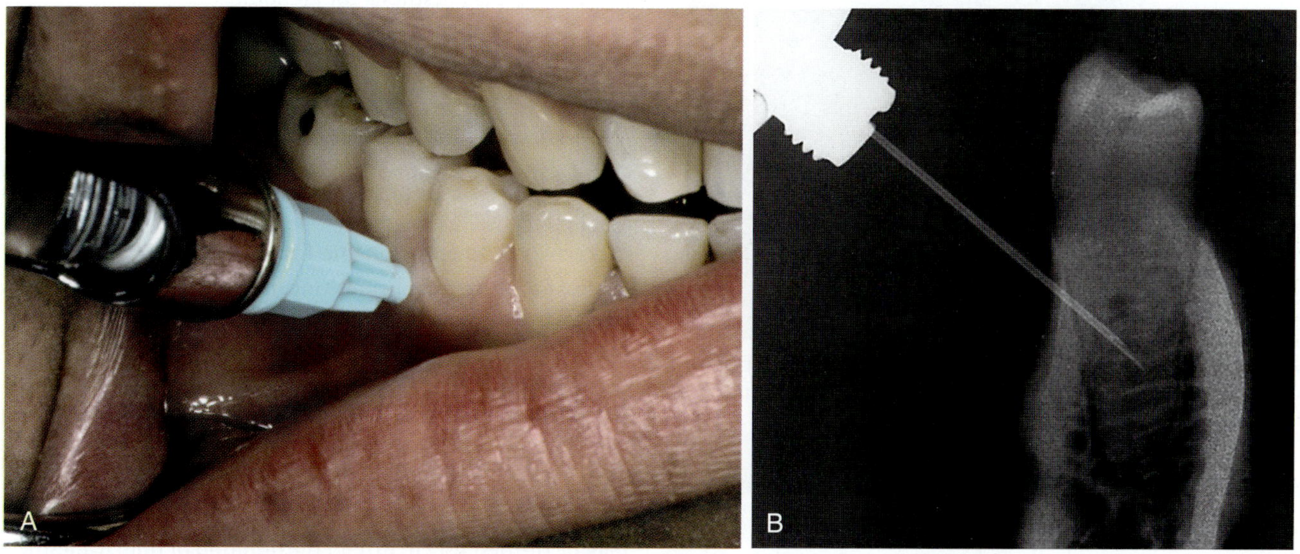

• **Fig. 8.9** **A,** The needle is inserted directly into the opening. **B,** Anesthetic is injected into medullary bone, where it diffuses widely to block dental nerves.

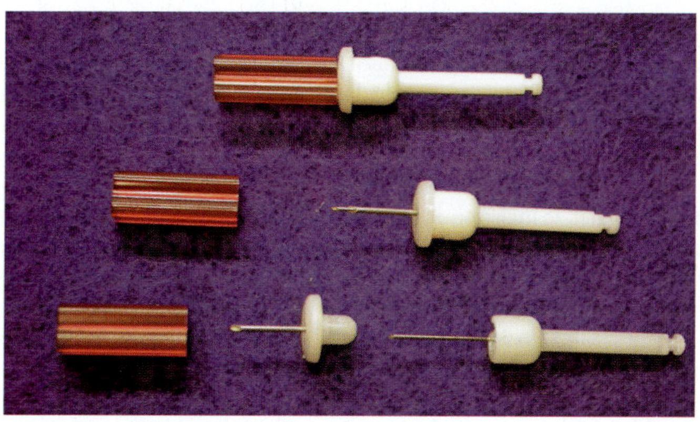

• **Fig. 8.10** Components of another approach to intraosseous injection: the drill and guide sleeve and cover *(top).* The drill (a special hollow needle) leads the guide sleeve through the cortical plate *(middle),* in which it is separated and withdrawn *(bottom).* The remaining guide sleeve is designed to accept a 27-gauge needle that injects the anesthetic solution.

present.[5,40,130] As discussed later, patients who have symptomatic pulpal or periapical pathosis (and/or who are anxious) present significant anesthesia problems.

Maxillary Anesthesia for Restorative Dentistry

Unless otherwise specified, the conventional solution used is 2% lidocaine with 1:100,000 epinephrine.

Anesthesia-Related Factors

Anesthesia is more successful in the maxilla than in the mandible.[40] The most common injection for the maxillary teeth is infiltration. Several events can be expected with this technique when one cartridge of anesthetic is used.

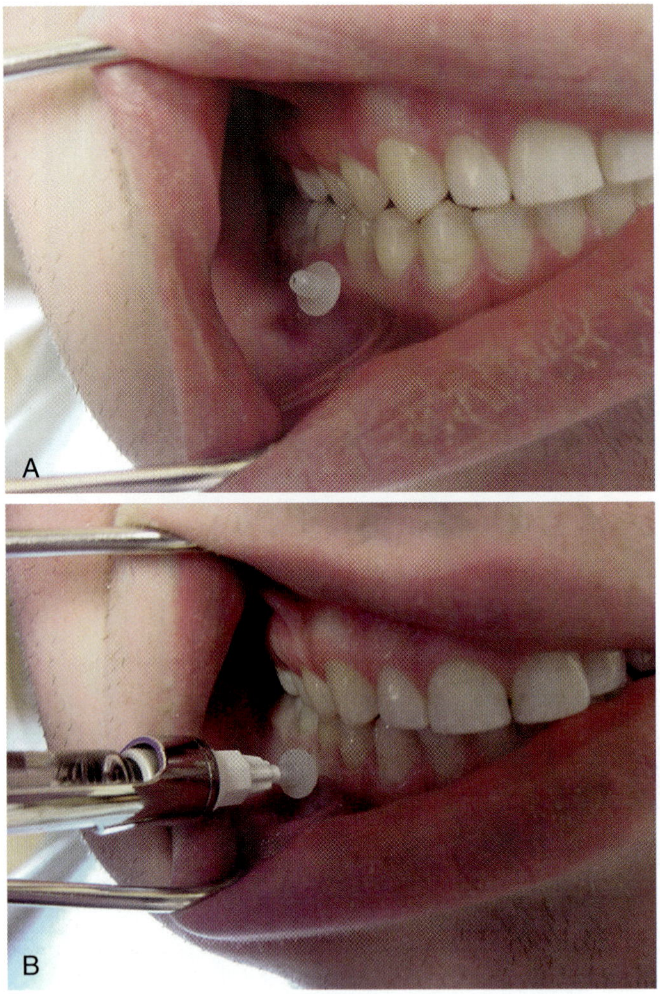

• **Fig. 8.11** **A,** The tissue and bone have been perforated, and the perforator now serves as a guide sleeve. **B,** The anesthetic needle is in place in the guide sleeve.

Lip/Cheek Numbness or Dead Feeling of the Teeth

Lip/cheek numbness usually occurs within a few minutes. Lip or cheek numbness or a dead feeling when tapping the teeth together does not always indicate pulpal anesthesia. Additionally, lip or cheek numbness does not correspond to the duration of pulpal anesthesia, because the pulp does not remain anesthetized as long as the soft tissues do.[40,131-139]

Success

Infiltration results in a fairly high incidence of successful pulpal anesthesia (around 87% to 92%).[11,40,131-139] However, some patients may not be anesthetized due to individual variations in response to the drug administered, operator differences, and variations of anatomy, in addition to tooth position.

Onset of Pulpal Anesthesia

Pulpal anesthesia usually occurs in 3 to 5 minutes.[40,131-139]

Duration of Pulpal Anesthesia

A problem with maxillary infiltration is the duration of pulpal anesthesia.[40,131-139] Pulpal anesthesia of the anterior teeth declines after about 30 minutes, with most losing anesthesia by 60 minutes.[40,131-139] In premolars and first molars, pulpal anesthesia is effective until about 40 to 45 minutes, and then it starts to decline.[40,131-139] Additional local anesthetic must be administered, depending on the duration of the procedure and the tooth group affected.

Alternative Anesthetic Solutions

Plain Solutions of Mepivacaine and Prilocaine

Anesthesia duration is shorter with plain solutions of mepivacaine and prilocaine.[137,138] Therefore these anesthetics are used for procedures of short duration (10 to 15 minutes).

4% Prilocaine with 1:200,000 Epinephrine, 2% Mepivacaine with 1:20,000 Levonordefrin, and 4% Articaine with 1:100,000 Epinephrine

The duration of anesthesia with 4% prilocaine with 1:200,000 epinephrine; 2% mepivacaine with 1:20,000 levonordefrin; and 4% articaine with 1:100,000 epinephrine is similar to that for 2% lidocaine with 1:100,000 epinephrine.[134,138,139]

Bupivacaine with Epinephrine

Bupivacaine has a lower success rate than a lidocaine formulation in anterior teeth.[132,140] There is no difference between success rates of the two formulations in the first molar.[132] Neither agent provides pulpal anesthesia for an hour.[132,140]

Increasing the Duration of Pulpal Anesthesia

Increasing the Volume of Solution

A two-cartridge volume of 2% lidocaine with epinephrine extends the duration of pulpal anesthesia but not for 60 minutes.[133]

Increasing the Epinephrine Concentration

Increasing the epinephrine concentration to 1:50,000 epinephrine increases duration for the lateral incisor but not for the first molar.[137] Neither tooth achieved a duration of 60 minutes.[137]

Repeating an Infiltration After 30 or 45 Minutes

Adding a cartridge of 2% lidocaine with epinephrine at 30 minutes in anterior teeth and 45 minutes in posterior teeth significantly improves the duration of pulpal anesthesia and may be the best way to extend the duration of pulpal anesthesia.[136]

Alternative Injection Techniques

The *posterior superior alveolar (PSA) nerve block* anesthetizes the second molars and about 80% of first molars.[141,142] An additional mesial infiltration injection may be necessary to anesthetize the first molar. Generally, the PSA block injection is not advocated for routine restorative procedures. An infiltration of the molars is preferred.

The *infraorbital block* results in lip numbness but does not predictably anesthetize incisor pulps.[143,144] It usually anesthetizes the canines and premolars, but duration is less than 1 hour.[143,144] Generally, the infraorbital injection is not advocated for routine restorative procedures. An infiltration of the individual teeth is preferred.

The *second division block* usually anesthetizes pulps of molars and some second premolars but does not predictably anesthetize first premolars, canines, or lateral and central incisors.[145,146] The high tuberosity technique is preferred to the greater palatine approach, because it is easier and less painful.[145] Generally, the second division nerve block is not advocated for routine restorative procedures. An infiltration of the individual teeth is preferred.

The *palatal anterior superior alveolar (P-ASA) nerve block* has been advocated for anesthetizing all the maxillary incisors with a single palatal injection into the incisive canal.[147] However, this injection technique does not provide predictable pulpal anesthesia for the incisors and canines[148] and is often painful.[26]

The *anterior middle superior alveolar (AMSA) nerve block* has been advocated for unilaterally anesthetizing the maxillary central and lateral incisors, canines, and first and second premolars with a single palatal injection in the premolar region.[149] However, this injection technique does not provide predictable pulpal anesthesia for these maxillary teeth[150] and is often painful.[27]

Pain, Inflammation, and Anxiety

As mentioned, results differ from normal when an anesthetic is given to patients with either pain or inflammation (or both) or to those with anxiety.

Supplemental Anesthesia for Restorative Dentistry in the Mandible and Maxilla

Indications

A supplemental injection is used if the standard injection is not effective. It is useful to repeat an initial injection only if the patient is not exhibiting the "classic" signs of soft tissue anesthesia. Generally, if the classic signs are present, reinjection is not very effective.[151] For example, after the inferior alveolar nerve block, the patient develops lip, chin, and tongue numbness and quadrant "deadness" of the teeth. A useful procedure is to test the pulp of the tooth with cold (cold refrigerant) or an electric pulp tester before the cavity preparation is begun.[38,39] If the patient feels pain to cold, a supplemental injection is indicated. Assuming that reinjection using the inferior alveolar nerve block approach will be successful is wishful thinking; failure the first time is usually followed by failure on the second attempt. The dentist should go directly to a supplemental technique. Four such injections are the (1) *infiltration injection,* (2) *IO injection,* (3) *PDL injection,* and (4) *intraseptal injection.*

Infiltration

Additional Infiltration of Lidocaine in the Maxilla

Because the duration of pulpal anesthesia for infiltration in the maxilla is less than 60 minutes, adding a cartridge of 2% lidocaine with epinephrine at 30 minutes in the anterior teeth and at about 45 minutes in premolar and molar teeth significantly improves the duration of pulpal anesthesia and may be the best way to extend the duration of pulpal anesthesia in maxillary teeth.[136] That is, if the patient experiences pain during the later stages of a dental appointment, an additional infiltration will be helpful.

Infiltration of Articaine in the Mandible

An important clinical finding is that a supplemental, buccal articaine infiltration of the first molar and premolars and a labial infiltration of the anterior teeth, after an inferior alveolar nerve block, should provide pulpal anesthesia for approximately 1 hour.[105,124,125] The second molar may require a supplemental IO or PDL injection.

Intraosseous Anesthesia (Figs 8.7–8.11)

The IO injection has been shown to be effective by substantial research and clinical use. It is particularly useful in conjunction with a conventional injection when it is likely that supplemental anesthesia will be necessary (e.g., in mandibular second molar teeth).[126-128] The IO injection allows placement of a local anesthetic directly into the cancellous bone adjacent to the tooth. There is an IO system with two components (Stabident; Fairfax Dental, Miami, Florida, USA). One part is a slow-speed handpiece–driven perforator, which drills a small hole through the cortical plate. The anesthetic solution is delivered into cancellous bone through a matching 27-gauge, ultrashort injector needle. Another IO system uses a guide sleeve (X-tip; Dentsply Maillefer Tulsa, Oklahoma, USA) that remains in the perforation. This sleeve serves as a guide for the needle, and it may remain in place throughout the procedure in case reinjection is necessary. The perforation may be made in attached gingiva or alveolar mucosa with this system.[152]

Technique for the Stabident System

The area of perforation and injection is on a horizontal line of the buccal gingival margins of the adjacent teeth and a vertical line that passes through the interdental papilla distal to the tooth to be injected. A point approximately 2 mm below the intersection of these lines is selected as the perforation site. This site must be in attached gingiva. The soft tissue is first anesthetized by infiltration. The perforator is placed through the gingiva perpendicular or a 45-degree angle to the cortical plate. With the point gently resting against bone, the clinician activates the handpiece at full speed while pushing the perforator, with light pressure, against bone and then slightly withdrawing the perforator and pushing it again against the bone (i.e., a pecking motion). This action is continued until a "breakthrough" into the cancellous bone is achieved (this process takes approximately 2 to 5 seconds).[152]

The standard syringe is held in a "pen-gripping" fashion, and the needle is precisely aligned with and inserted into the perforation. A full cartridge of anesthetic solution is *slowly* delivered over 1 to 2 minutes with light pressure. If back-pressure is encountered, the needle is rotated approximately a quarter turn, and deposition is reattempted. If this attempt is unsuccessful, the needle should be removed and checked for blockage. If the needle is not blocked, it is reinserted or the site is opened with a new perforator and the injection is repeated.[152]

Perforator "Breakage"

Rarely, the metal perforator "separates" from the plastic hub. If this separation occurs, the perforator is easily removed with a hemostat; there are no reports of a perforator breaking into parts.[126-128,152-154]

Injection Discomfort

When the IO injection is used as a primary injection, pain is experienced about one-fourth of the time.[153-155] When the IO injection is used as a supplemental injection, fewer patients experience pain.[126-128,156,157]

Selection of Perforation Site

With IO injections, a distal perforation site results in the best anesthesia.[126-128,152-154,156,157] The second molars are an exception; in those teeth, a mesial site is prefer red.[126-128,152-154,156,157]

Anesthetic Agents

When the IO injection is used as a supplemental injection after the inferior alveolar nerve block in patients without pain, excellent success has been reported for 2% lidocaine with 1:100,000 epinephrine and 2% mepivacaine with 1:20,000 levonordefrin.[126,127] However, because of the adverse cardiovascular reactions with a long-acting anesthetic (0.5% bupivacaine with 1:200,000 epinephrine)[158] and the lack of a prolonged duration of pulpal anesthesia, this agent does not offer any advantage over lidocaine. Furthermore, 3% mepivacaine plain is successful, but the duration of pulpal anesthesia is shorter.[128]

Onset of Anesthesia

Onset of anesthesia is rapid with the IO injection.[126-128,152-154,156,157] There is no waiting period for anesthesia.

Success

When the IO injection is used as a supplemental injection after an inferior alveolar nerve block in pain-free patients, success rates are very good.[126,127]

Failure

If the anesthetic solution squirts out of the perforation (backflow) with an IO injection, anesthesia will not be obtained.[152] Reperforation or choosing another perforation site is then necessary.

Duration

With a primary IO injection, the duration of pulpal anesthesia declines steadily over 1 hour.[153,154] There is an even shorter duration with 3% mepivacaine, compared with 2% lidocaine with 1:100,000 epinephrine.[154] With a supplemental IO injection of lidocaine with 1:100,000 epinephrine after the inferior alveolar nerve block in patients without pain, the duration of pulpal anesthesia is very good for 1 hour.[126,127] A solution of 3% mepivacaine, when used as a supplemental IO injection, results in a shorter anesthetic duration.[128]

Postoperative Pain and Problems

With primary and supplemental IO injection techniques, the majority of patients report no pain or mild pain postoperatively.[126-128,152-154,156,157] Fewer than 5% develop exudate and/or localized swelling at the perforation site, possibly from overheating of the bone during perforation.[126-128,152-154,156,157]

Systemic Effects

With both primary and supplemental IO injection techniques using anesthetics with a vasoconstrictor (epinephrine or levonordefrin), most patients perceive an increased heart rate.[153,154,156,157,159] When these agents are used, patients should be informed *before the injection* of this tachycardia to lessen their anxiety. No significant heart rate increase occurs with 3% mepivacaine plain.[154,160] The venous plasma levels of lidocaine are the same for an IO injection as for infiltration injection.[161] Therefore the same precautions for the maximum amount of lidocaine given for an infiltration injection also apply to an IO injection.[161]

Medical Contraindications

Patients taking antidepressants, nonselective beta-blocking agents, medicine for Parkinson disease, and cocaine should not receive IO injections of solutions containing epinephrine or levonordefrin[40]; 3% mepivacaine plain is preferred.

Precautions

An IO injection should not be used with painful necrotic teeth with periapical radiolucencies or with teeth exhibiting cellulitis or abscess formation. This injection would be very painful and would likely not provide profound anesthesia.

Periodontal Ligament Injection

The PDL injection is also a useful technique if a conventional injection is unsuccessful.[162,163] The technique is clinically less effective than the IO injection technique because more anesthetic solution can be delivered to the cancellous bone.[151]

Technique

The procedure for a PDL injection (Fig. 8.12, *A–D*) is not difficult but does require practice and familiarity. A standard syringe or pressure syringe is equipped with a 30-gauge, ultrashort needle or a 27- or 25-gauge short needle. The needle is inserted into the mesial gingival sulcus at a 30-degree angle to the long axis of the tooth. The needle is supported by the fingers or a hemostat and is positioned with maximum penetration (wedged between the root and crestal bone). Heavy pressure is *slowly* applied on the syringe handle for approximately 10 to 20 seconds (conventional syringe), or the trigger is *slowly* squeezed once or twice with resistance (pressure syringe). *Back-pressure is important.* If there is no back-pressure (resistance)—that is, if the anesthetic readily flows out of the sulcus—the needle is repositioned, and the technique is repeated until back-pressure is attained. The injection is then repeated on the distal surface. Only a small volume of anesthetic (approximately 0.2 mL) is deposited on each surface.

Mechanism of Action

The PDL injection forces anesthetic solution through the cribriform plate (Fig. 8.13) into the marrow spaces and into the vasculature in and around the tooth (Figs. 8.14 and 8.15).[162-165] The primary route is not the PDL; the mechanism of action is not related to direct pressure on the nerves.[166,167]

Injection Discomfort in Asymptomatic Patients

When the PDL injection is the primary injection, needle insertion and injection may be painful about one third of the time.[166-168] In maxillary anterior teeth, the PDL injection may be quite painful[168] and should not be used. An infiltration is preferred. As a supplemental injection after an inferior alveolar nerve block, the PDL injection has a low potential to be painful.[129]

Onset of Anesthesia

The onset of anesthesia is rapid with a PDL injection; there is no waiting period to begin the clinical procedure.[166-168] If anesthesia is still not adequate, reinjection is necessary.

Success in Asymptomatic Teeth

Success rates for the PDL injection, when used as a primary injection, have been reported to be about 75% in mandibular and maxillary posterior teeth, with a duration of pulpal anesthesia of 10 to 15 minutes.[167,168] Success rates have been low in anterior teeth.[167-169] Anesthetic solutions without vasoconstrictors (3% mepivacaine) or with reduced vasoconstrictor concentrations (bupivacaine with 1:200,000 epinephrine) are not very effective.[167,170-172] Articaine is equivalent to lidocaine.[60]

When the PDL injection is used as a supplemental injection (standard techniques have failed to provide adequate anesthesia), good success rates are achieved, but the duration of pulpal anesthesia is approximately 23 minutes.[129]

Duration in Asymptomatic Teeth

The duration of profound pulpal anesthesia (either primary or supplemental) with PDL injections is approximately 10 to 15 minutes.[60,129,166-168]

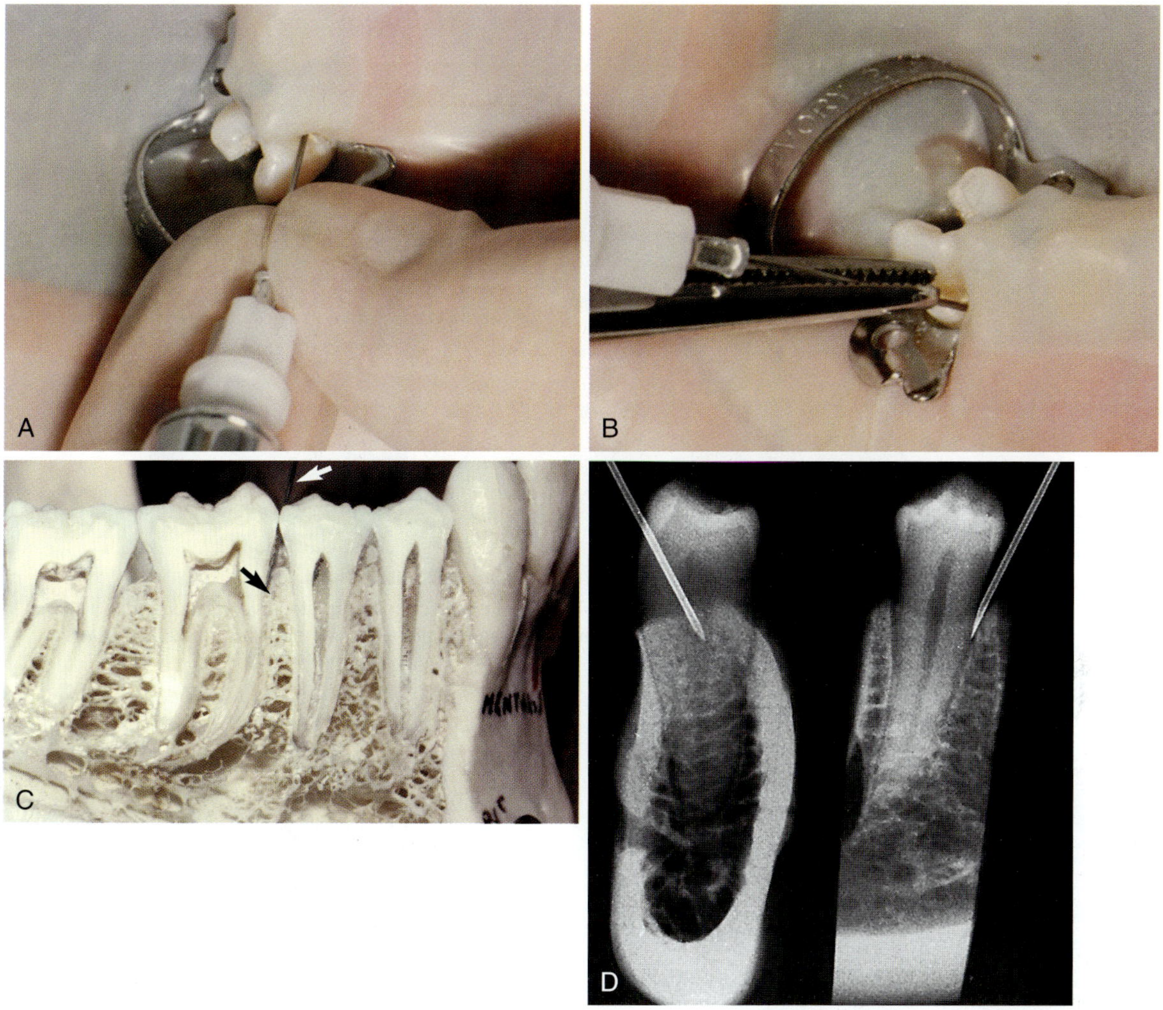

• **Fig. 8.12** Intraligamentary Injection. **A,** Needle insertion using the fingers to prevent needle buckling. **B,** A hemostat may be substituted for the fingers to support and direct the needle. The injection may be given with or without the rubber dam in place. **C,** Note the direction and position of the needle *(arrows).* The tip of the needle will be wedged between the crestal bone and the root surface. **D,** Angle of the needle relative to the long axis of the tooth *(left).* With approximately a 30-degree orientation, the needle tip will be positioned close to the midline of the root.

Postoperative Discomfort in Asymptomatic Teeth

When the PDL injection is used as a primary technique, postoperative pain occurs in one-third to three-fourths of patients, with a duration of 14 hours to 3 days.[60,129,166-168,173,174] There is no difference between articaine and lidocaine.[60] The discomfort is related to damage from needle insertion rather than to the pressure of depositing the solution.[173] About one-third of patients report that their tooth feels "high."[167,168]

Selective Anesthesia

It has been suggested that a PDL injection may be used in the differential diagnosis of poorly localized, painful irreversible pulpitis.[175] However, adjacent teeth are often anesthetized with PDL injection of a single tooth.[166-168] Therefore this injection is *not* useful for differential diagnosis.

Systemic Effects

Although some authors[176] have found that the PDL injection raises the heart rate, human studies have shown that these injections do not cause significant changes in heart rate.[174,177]

Other Factors

Different needle gauges (25-, 27-, or 30-gauge) are equally effective for PDL injections.[178] Special pressure syringes have been marketed (Fig. 8.16) but have not proved to be more effective than a standard syringe.[167,168,178]

Damage to the Periodontium

Clinical and animal studies have demonstrated the relative safety of the PDL injection.[166-169,174,178-184] Minor local damage is limited to the site of needle penetration (Fig. 8.17); this damage subsequently undergoes repair.[179] In some instances, periodontal infections have occurred.[167,168] The clinician should be aware that this may happen. Histologic areas of root resorption after PDL injections have also been reported, but they heal with time.[183,184] Damaging effects from injecting into an area of periodontal disease are unlikely.[185]

Damage to the Pulp

Clinical and animal studies have shown no adverse effects on the pulp after PDL injections.[166-168,186,187] However, physiologic

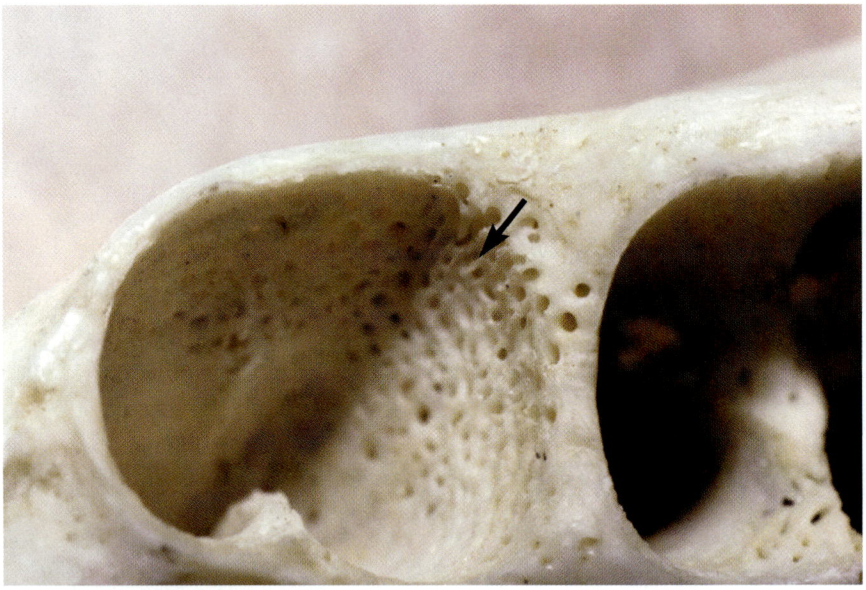

• **Fig. 8.13** Extraction Socket of a Second Molar. The bone of the cribriform plate is very porous, particularly in the cervical region *(arrow)*. During the intraligamentary injection, this is the region of passage of most anesthetic solution into the medullary space.

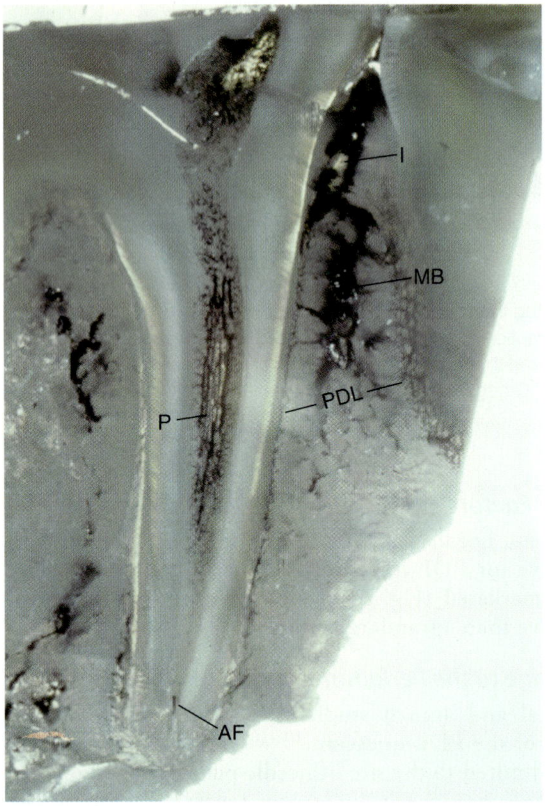

• **Fig. 8.14** A single intraligamentary injection of carbon dye adjacent to a dog's tooth demonstrates the distribution of dye particles. Particles are concentrated at the injection site *(I)* and in the medullary bone *(MB)*, the apical foramen *(AF)*, and the pulp *(P)* of the injected tooth. Dye particles have spread through the periodontal ligament *(PDL)* of both the injected and adjacent teeth.

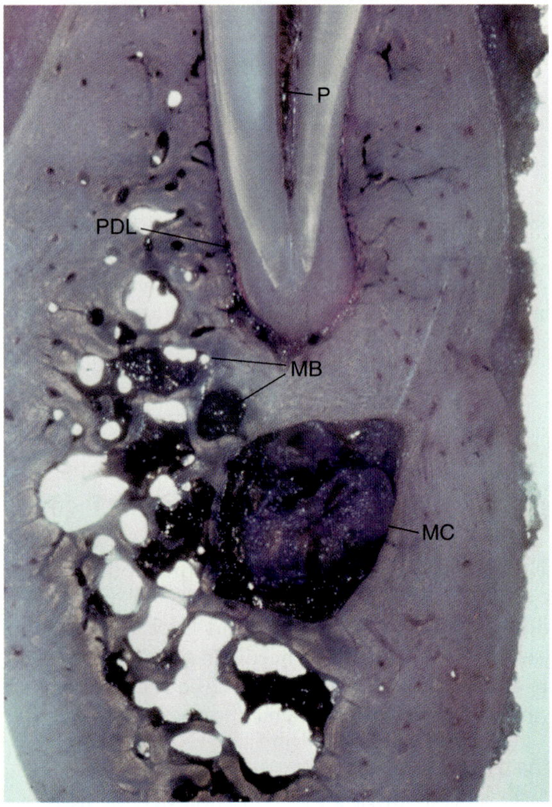

• **Fig. 8.15** A single injection of dye was made in the distal periodontal ligament. This frontal section, including the tooth apex and surrounding structures, shows that dye distributes to the pulp *(P)*, periodontal ligament space *(PDL)*, medullary bone space *(MB)*, and mandibular canal *(MC)*. The widespread distribution of solutions from the intraligamentary injection may anesthetize the adjacent teeth.

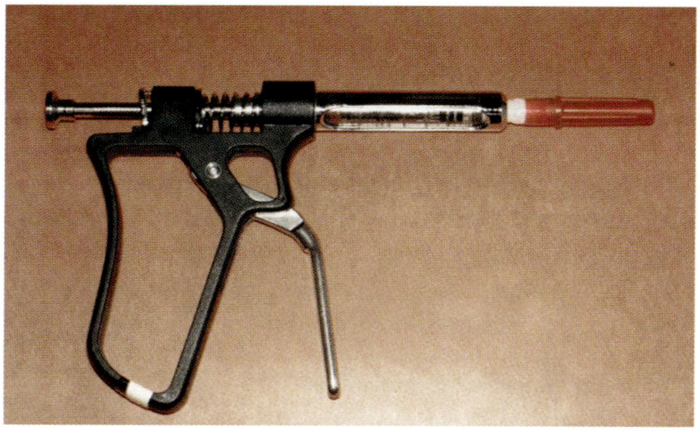

• **Fig. 8.16** Example of a special syringe used for the intraligamentary injection. Although these devices are capable of injecting with more pressure, they have not been shown to be superior to the standard syringe.

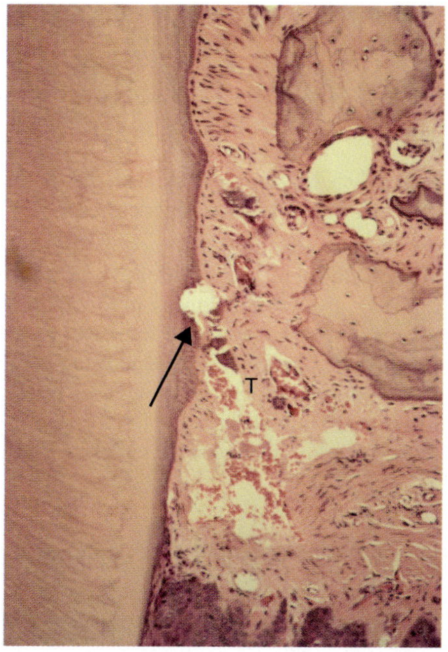

• **Fig. 8.17** The Injection Site at the Time of Injection. The needle tract *(T),* which ends in a gouge in cementum *(arrow),* is apparent in the connective tissue. No tissue changes are evident outside the penetration site, including the more apical tissues.

changes in the pulp do occur, including a rapid and prolonged marked decrease in blood flow caused by epinephrine.[188] This vascular impairment has no demonstrated damaging effect, even in conjunction with restorative procedures.[189] The PDL injection probably would not result in severe pulpal injury, although this event has not been studied with extensive (crown) preparations or in teeth with significant caries.

Damage to Primary Teeth

Minor enamel hypoplasia of succedaneous teeth has been seen after PDL injections in primary teeth.[190] However, this effect was caused by the cytotoxicity of the local anesthetic rather than by the actual injection. Therefore this injection may be used for anesthetizing primary teeth.

Precautions

The PDL injection should not be used with necrotic pulps and periapical pathosis or with cellulitis or abscess formation. This would be very painful and likely would not provide profound anesthesia.

Anesthesia Difficulties in Endodontics

The following is a classic scenario: The diagnosis is irreversible pulpitis. The dentist administers the standard inferior alveolar nerve block. The patient reports classic signs of anesthesia (lip numbness and a dull feeling of the tooth or quadrant). After isolation, access preparation is begun. When the bur is in enamel, the patient feels nothing. Once the bur enters dentin or possibly not until the pulp is exposed, the patient feels sharp pain. Obviously, pulpal anesthesia is not profound and additional anesthetic is required. The following are some of the theories as to why this problem occurs.

1. The anesthetic solution may not completely penetrate to the sensory nerves that innervate the pulp, especially in the mandible.
2. The *central core theory* states that nerves on the outside of the nerve bundle supply molar teeth, whereas nerves on the inside supply anterior teeth (see Fig. 8.6). The anesthetic solution may not diffuse into the nerve trunk to reach all nerves to produce an adequate block, even if deposited at the correct site. This theory would explain the higher experimental failure rates in anterior teeth with the inferior alveolar nerve block.[40-50,52]
3. *Local tissues change* because of inflammation. This popular theory states that the lowered pH of inflamed tissue reduces the amount of the base form of the anesthetic available to penetrate the nerve membrane.[14] Consequently, there is less of the ionized form within the nerve to achieve anesthesia. Although this theory may have some validity for regions with swelling, it does not relate to anesthesia difficulties in the mandible.[40] It does not explain the major problem, which is the mandibular molar with pulpitis that is not anesthetized by an inferior alveolar injection. The injection site is distant from the area of inflammation; changes in tissue pH would be unrelated to the anesthesia problem.
4. *Hyperalgesia.* Change in nociceptor (pain receptor) pathways is a more plausible explanation. This theory states that the nerves arising in inflamed tissue have altered resting potentials and decreased excitability thresholds. These changes are not restricted to the inflamed pulp itself but rather affect the entire neuronal membrane, extending to the central nervous system.[5,6] Local anesthetic agents are not sufficient to prevent impulse transmission, owing to these lowered excitability thresholds.[5]
5. *Apprehension.* Patients in pain often are anxious, which lowers the pain threshold. A vicious cycle may be established in which initial apprehension leads to a decreased pain threshold, which leads to anesthesia difficulties, which lead to increased apprehension, which results in loss of control and confidence, and so on. Therefore, if this cycle becomes evident, the practitioner should stop treatment immediately and regain control, schedule another appointment, or consider referral to an endodontist. Most patients will endure some pain during the initial stages of root canal treatment if they have confidence in the dentist. However, they will not tolerate being hurt repeatedly!

6. *Insufficient time allowed after injection.* The dentist may not allow adequate time for the anesthetic to diffuse and to block the sensory nerves. Onset may be very slow, particularly with the inferior alveolar block.

Success of the Inferior Alveolar Nerve Block with Symptomatic Irreversible Pulpitis

Fowler and coauthors determined the success of the inferior alveolar nerve block in first and second molars and premolars using 2% lidocaine with 1:100,000 epinephrine in emergency patients presenting with symptomatic irreversible pulpitis.[191] They found success (no or mild pain upon endodontic access or instrumentation) was 28% for the first molars, 25% for the second molars, and 39% for the premolars. These success rates for the inferior alveolar nerve block of the molars and premolars would not be high enough to ensure profound pulpal anesthesia.

For patients presenting with irreversible pulpitis, success was not significantly different between a 3.6 mL volume and 1.8 mL volume of 2% lidocaine with 1:100,000 epinephrine.[51] The success rates (28% to 39%) with either volume were not high enough to ensure complete pulpal anesthesia.[192]

Gow-Gates and Vizarani-Akinosi Techniques

Neither the Gow-Gates[85] (see Fig, 8.5) nor the Vizarani-Akinosi[86] (see Fig. 8.5) technique is superior to the standard inferior alveolar nerve block injection.[87-92] These techniques are not replacements for the inferior alveolar nerve block, and both require a two-cartridge volume. The Vizarani-Akinosi is a closed-mouth technique and is useful for patients presenting with trismus. However, patients with trismus should be referred to an endodontist because patient management is complicated.

Neither the Gow-Gates nor Vazirani-Akinosi technique provides adequate pulpal anesthesia for mandibular posterior teeth in patients presenting with symptomatic irreversible pulpitis.[93] Both injections would require supplemental anesthesia.

Do Buffered Lidocaine Formulations Increase the Success of the Inferior Alveolar Nerve Block in Patients with Symptomatic Irreversible Pulpitis?

Two systems are commercially available to buffer local anesthetics. Onset (Onpharma, Los Gatos, California, USA) buffers a local anesthetic solution using a unique dispensing system. The other system is Anutra (Anutra Medical Inc., Morrisville, North Carolina, USA), which consists of a dispenser, a 5-mL multiple-dose syringe, and cassette.

Two studies evaluated a buffered 2% lidocaine with 1:80,000 epinephrine formulation, or buffered 4% lidocaine with 1:100,000 epinephrine formulation for inferior alveolar nerve blocks in patients presenting with symptomatic irreversible pulpitis.[79,83] Both studies concluded that buffering did not statistically improve the success of the inferior alveolar nerve block or decrease injection pain.

Effect of Preemptive Nitrous Oxide in Irreversible Pulpitis

Nitrous oxide is the most commonly used inhalation anesthetic in dentistry.[34] It has an impressive safety record and is excellent for providing conscious sedation for dental patients. Moreover, nitrous oxide provides a mild analgesic effect. The most common estimate of analgesic efficacy suggests 30% nitrous oxide is equivalent to 10 to 15 mg morphine.[34] Nitrous oxide has significant benefits because of its sedation and analgesic effects.

Two studies have found administration of 30% to 50% nitrous oxide resulted in a statistically significant increase in the success of the inferior alveolar nerve block in patients presenting with symptomatic irreversible pulpitis.[34,36]

Success of Maxillary Molar Infiltration with Irreversible Pulpitis

Clinical studies of maxillary posterior buccal infiltrations in patients presenting with irreversible pulpitis reported successful infiltration 54% to 85% of the time with an average rate of 64%.[193-195] There does not appear to be a difference between articaine and lidocaine formulations.[196,197]

Asymptomatic Irreversible Pulpitis Versus Symptomatic Irreversible Pulpitis

Patients who have spontaneous pain (symptomatic irreversible pulpitis) have less successful anesthesia after an inferior alveolar nerve block than patients who do not have spontaneous pain or who have pain only when the tooth is stimulated by the application of cold (asymptomatic irreversible pulpitis).[198] It is important to distinguish between these patients when evaluating clinical success, because the success rates differ.

Use of Preoperative Analgesic Medications to Increase the Success of the Inferior Alveolar Nerve Block

Many studies have used analgesic medications (for example, ibuprofen, acetaminophen, hydrocodone, and combinations of these medications) given 60 minutes before administering an inferior alveolar nerve block to try to increase the success of the inferior alveolar nerve block. There are varying results but, currently, it appears that preoperative analgesic medications may not show a significant advantage.[199-201] If any increase in success is seen, it is not enough to prevent the use of supplemental anesthesia.

Adjunctive Pharmacologic Therapy

Anxious patients may benefit from sedation (oral, inhalation, intravenous). However, even with conscious sedation, profound local anesthesia is required to eliminate pain during dental treatment.[33-35] Nitrous oxide administration helps reduce pain during treatment in patients presenting with symptomatic irreversible pulpitis.[34,36] A discussion on agents that control anxiety is included in Chapter 9.

Reversing Soft-Tissue Numbness

Patients may feel that residual soft-tissue numbness interferes with their normal daily activities in three specific areas: perceptual (perception of altered physical appearance); sensory (lack of sensation); and functional (diminished ability to speak, smile, drink, and control drooling). Patients often do not want to have lip and tongue numbness for hours after the appointment. Phentolamine mesylate (0.4 mg in a 1.7 mL cartridge, OraVerse; Septodont, Lancaster, Pennsylvania, USA) is an agent that shortens the duration of soft tissue anesthesia.

Fowler and coauthors studied the use of OraVerse for reversal of soft-tissue anesthesia in asymptomatic endodontic patients.[202] They found it shortened mandibular and maxillary soft tissue sensations. Postoperative pain and complications were minimal. Many patients may benefit from the use of a reversal agent when they have speaking engagements or important meetings or perform in musical or theatrical events.

Supplemental Techniques for Mandibular Teeth in Endodontics

Supplemental Buccal Infiltration of Articaine After an Inferior Alveolar Nerve Block in Patients Presenting with Symptomatic Irreversible Pulpitis

Fowler and coauthors determined the anesthetic success of a supplemental, articaine buccal infiltration after a failed inferior alveolar nerve block, in premolars and first and second molars, in emergency patients presenting with symptomatic irreversible pulpitis.[191] Success was defined as the ability to access and instrument the tooth with mild to no pain. They found success was 42% for the first molars, 48% for the second molars, and 73% for the premolars. Therefore supplemental anesthesia should be considered.

This result should be compared with the finding in asymptomatic (nonpainful) teeth where the buccal infiltration of a cartridge of 4% articaine with 1:100,000 epinephrine after an inferior alveolar nerve block was successful 88% of the time.[124]

Supplemental Intraosseous Injections

For use as a supplemental injection with irreversible pulpitis, high success rates (about 90%) have been reported for IO injections.[193,199,203,204] There is no difference between lidocaine and articaine.[204] Three percent mepivacaine has an 80% success rate, which increases to 98% with a second IO injection of 3% mepivacaine.[205]

Although some studies[206,207] have suggested that an IO injection alone can successfully anesthetize patients presenting with irreversible pulpitis, it is doubtful that this would be successful.[193,199-201,208]

Supplemental Periodontal Ligament Injections

Supplemental PDL injections are not as successful as supplemental IO injections.[151,209] For example, in patients with irreversible pulpitis, use of a computer-controlled local anesthetic delivery system (see Fig. 8.1) for supplemental PDL injections was successful in about half of patients with irreversible pulpitis.[209] Others have reported success in about three-quarters to half of patients.[151,210] Reinjection increases the success rate.[178,210]

Supplemental Intraseptal Injection

Intraseptal anesthesia is the deposition of the anesthetic solution directly into the interdental septum, allowing solution to flow through the porous crestal alveolar bone and hence into the medullary bone surrounding the tooth.[211]

A study in endodontics determined the anesthetic efficacy of the supplemental intraseptal technique in mandibular posterior teeth diagnosed with symptomatic irreversible pulpitis when the conventional inferior alveolar nerve block failed.[212] Success was defined as the ability to perform endodontic access and instrumentation with mild to no pain. The supplemental intraseptal injection provided success in 29% of patients and would not provide a predictable level of anesthesia.

Supplemental Intrapulpal Injection

Besides the supplemental infiltration, IO, and PDL injections discussed previously, the intrapulpal (IP) injection is used when other methods fail.

Indications

After the inferior alveolar nerve block, on occasion IO and PDL injections do not produce profound anesthesia, even when repeated, and pain persists when the pulp is entered. This occurrence is an indication for an IP injection. However, the IP injection should not be given without first administering an inferior alveolar block plus an IO or PDL injection. The IP injection is very painful without some other form of supplemental anesthesia.

Advantages and Disadvantages

Although the IP injection is somewhat popular, it has disadvantages as well as advantages, making it the last supplemental injection of choice. The major drawback is that the needle is inserted directly into a vital and very sensitive pulp; thus the injection may be exquisitely painful. Also, the effects of the injection are unpredictable if it is not given under pressure. Once anesthesia has been obtained, the duration is short (5 to 15 minutes). Therefore the bulk of the pulp must be removed quickly and at the correct working length to prevent recurrence of pain during instrumentation. Another disadvantage is that the pulp must be exposed to permit direct injection; often problems with anesthesia occur before pulpal exposure.

The advantage is the predictability of profound anesthesia if the IP injection is given under back-pressure. The onset of anesthesia is immediate, and no special syringes or needles are required, although different approaches may be necessary to attain the desired back-pressure.

Mechanism of Action

Strong back-pressure has been shown to be the major factor in producing anesthesia.[212,213] Depositing anesthetic passively into the pulp chamber is not adequate; the solution will not diffuse throughout the pulp. Therefore the anesthetic agent is not solely responsible for IP anesthesia; it also depends on pressure.

Technique

The patient must be informed that a "little extra" anesthetic will ensure comfort and that there will be "a sharp sensation" as the injection is given.

One technique creates back-pressure by stoppering the access with a cotton pellet to prevent backflow of anesthetic (Fig. 8.18).[213,214] Other stoppers, such as gutta-percha, waxes, or pieces of rubber, have been used. If possible, the roof of the pulp chamber should be penetrated by a half-round bur, which allows the needle to fit snugly in the bur hole.

Another approach is an injection into each canal after the chamber has been unroofed. A standard syringe is usually equipped with a bent short needle. With fingers supporting the needle shaft to prevent buckling, the needle is positioned in the access opening and then moved down the canal, as the anesthetic is slowly expressed, to the point of wedging. Maximum pressure is then applied slowly on the syringe handle for 5 to 10 seconds. If there is no back-pressure, anesthetic flows out of the access opening. The needle is then wedged deeper or withdrawn and replaced with a larger diameter needle (or stoppered with a cotton pellet), and the injection is repeated. This procedure may be necessary in each canal.

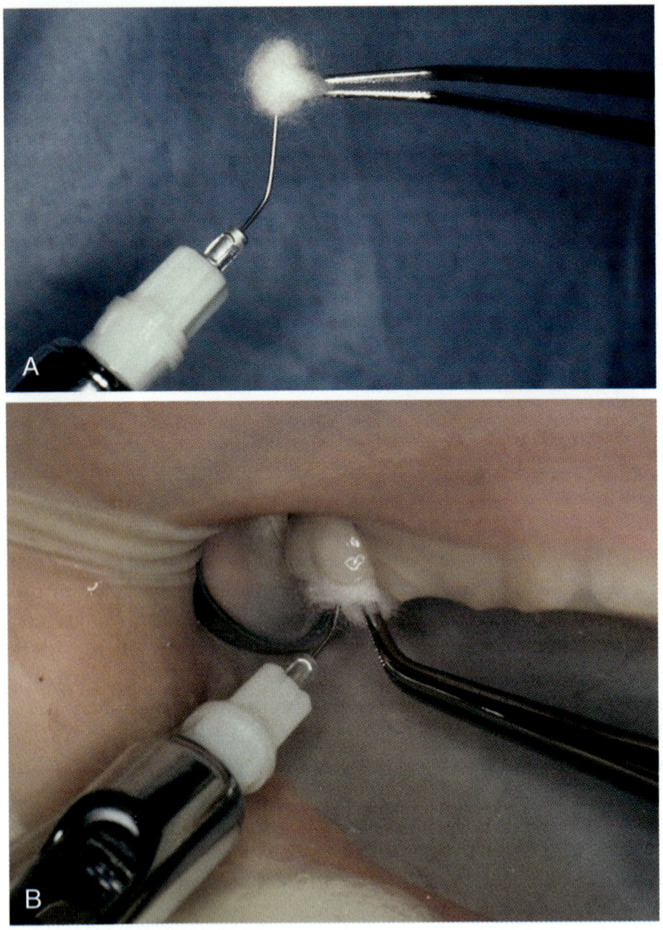

• **Fig. 8.18** Intrapulpal Injection Technique. **A,** A 45-degree bend is placed on the needle. To stopper the injection site, a cotton pellet is pulled over the needle and the needle is placed in the opening in the pulp (the patient is forewarned of discomfort!). **B,** The cotton pellet is packed *tightly* and held in the access opening, and the syringe handle is pushed *slowly.* The patient often feels sharp pain with resistance on the syringe handle; this resistance usually indicates successful anesthesia.

What Is the Effect of No Endodontic Débridement on Postoperative Pain for Symptomatic Teeth with Pulpal Necrosis?

Patients without a dentist or access to care often present to hospital emergency departments with painful teeth. These patients are typically prescribed pain medication and an antibiotic. If they do not seek immediate dental treatment, what postoperative pain do they experience?

Sebastian and coauthors compared the effect of complete endodontic débridement (cleaning and shaping of the root canal system) versus no endodontic débridement on postoperative pain in emergency patients with symptomatic teeth, a pulpal diagnosis of necrosis, and a periapical radiolucency.[215] Success was defined as mild or no postoperative pain and no use of narcotic medication. Patients receiving débridement or no débridement had a decrease in postoperative pain over the 5 days. However, débridement resulted in a statistically higher success rate than no débridement.

Therefore an important consideration is that if there is not time or ability to perform complete débridement, an option is to refer the patient to an endodontist or defer treatment until the patient is asymptomatic.

Anesthetic Management of Pulpal or Periapical Pathoses

Symptomatic Irreversible Pulpitis

With irreversible pulpitis, the teeth most difficult to anesthetize are the mandibular molars, followed in order by the mandibular and maxillary premolars, maxillary molars, mandibular anterior teeth, and maxillary anterior teeth. The vital inflamed pulp must be instrumented and removed. Also, pulpal tissue has a very concentrated sensory nerve supply, particularly in the pulp chamber. These factors, combined with others related to inflammatory effects on sensory nerves and failures that occur with conventional techniques, make anesthetizing patients with painful irreversible pulpitis a challenge.

Different clinical situations present surprises. In some cases, inflamed vital tissue exists only in the apical canals, and the tissue in the chamber is necrotic and does not respond to the cold refrigerant or electric pulp testing. Obviously, in this situation the chamber is entered with no problem, but when the operator attempts to place a file to length, severe pain results. IO or PDL injections are helpful, and an IP injection may be used. However, irreversible pulpitis must be differentiated from a symptomatic necrotic tooth with a distinct radiographic apical abscess, because IO, PDL, and IP injections are contraindicated in the latter condition.

General Considerations

A conventional anesthetic using primary techniques is administered to the patient, and after signs of soft tissue anesthesia occur, the pain abates and the patient relaxes. Frequently, however, on access opening or when the pulp is entered, pain results because not all sensory nerves have been blocked. A useful procedure is to test the pulp of the tooth with cold (cold refrigerant) before the access is begun.[193,209] If the patient responds, an IO or PDL injection is given. However, no response does not ensure complete anesthesia.[193,209] The patient is always informed that the procedure will be immediately discontinued if pain is experienced during treatment or if there is a "premonition" of impending pain. Appropriate supplementary injections are then used. Occasionally, all attempts fail, and in that case, it is best to place a temporary restoration and refer the patient to an endodontist.

Mandibular Posterior Teeth

For mandibular posterior teeth, a conventional inferior alveolar nerve block is administered, usually in conjunction with a long buccal injection for the molars. The tooth is tested with cold refrigerant. If the result is negative, the clinician may proceed with access; if the result is positive, an IO or PDL injection is administered before access is begun. Before the supplemental IO injection, buccal infiltration of a cartridge of 4% articaine with 1:100,000 epinephrine is given over the tooth to reduce the pain of the injection. If pain is felt during access, the IO or PDL injection may be repeated, or an IP injection is given if the pulp is exposed. Usually, once the pulp has been removed, further pain is minimal, owing to the longer duration of mandibular anesthesia.[43-48,193]

Mandibular Anterior Teeth

For mandibular anterior teeth, an inferior alveolar injection is given. The tooth is tested with cold refrigerant. If the result is negative, the clinician may proceed with access; if the result is positive, an IO injection is administered before access is begun (the PDL injection does not work well in mandibular anterior teeth). Before the supplemental IO injection, labial infiltration of a cartridge of 4% articaine with

1:100,000 epinephrine is given over the tooth to reduce the pain of the IO injection. If pain is felt upon access, the IO injection is repeated. If this is unsuccessful, an IP injection is added.

Maxillary Posterior Teeth

The approaches for maxillary posterior teeth are the same as those outlined under "General Considerations" *except* that the initial dose of 2% lidocaine with 1:100,000 epinephrine is doubled (3.6 mL) for buccal infiltration, and a palatal infiltration is given for the rubber dam retainer. The tooth is tested with cold refrigerant. If the result is negative, the clinician may proceed with access; if the result is positive, an IO or PDL injection is administered before access is begun. If pain is felt during access, the IO or PDL injection is repeated. In some cases, an IP injection may be needed.

The duration of anesthesia in the maxilla is less than in the mandible.[131-139] Therefore if pain is experienced during instrumentation or obturation, additional primary and/or supplemental injections are necessary.

Maxillary Anterior Teeth

In the maxillary anterior teeth, anesthetic is administered initially as a labial infiltration and occasionally as a palatal infiltration for the rubber dam retainer. The tooth is tested with cold refrigerant. If the result is negative, the clinician may proceed with access; if the result is positive, an IO injection is administered before access is begun (the PDL injection is not effective[168]). Rarely is an IO injection needed. The duration of anesthesia may be less than 1 hour, requiring additional infiltration.[131-139]

Symptomatic Pulp Necrosis

A diagnosis of symptomatic pulp necrosis indicates pain and/or swelling and therefore periapical inflammation. Because the pulp is necrotic and apical tissues are inflamed, anesthesia problems are different. These teeth may be painful when manipulated during treatment.

For the mandible, an inferior alveolar nerve block and a long buccal injection (for the molars) are administered. For maxillary teeth, if no swelling is present, the anesthetic is given with a conventional infiltration. If soft-tissue swelling is present (cellulitis or abscess), infiltration is administered on either side of the swelling. Occasionally a regional block may be necessary. Access is begun *slowly*. Usually the pulp chamber is entered without discomfort if the tooth is not torqued excessively during use of the high-speed handpiece. File placement and débridement also can be performed without much pain if instruments are used gently.

Occasionally, conventional injections do not provide adequate anesthesia. IO, PDL, and IP injections are *contraindicated.* Although effective for vital pulps, these injections are painful and ineffective with apical pathosis. Rather, the patient should be informed that profound anesthesia is not present, owing to inflammation in the bone. Therefore an important consideration is that if the pain is too severe to perform complete débridement, an option is to refer the patient to an endodontist or defer treatment until the patient is asymptomatic.

In patients with severe preoperative pain without drainage from the tooth (or when no swelling can be incised), a long-acting anesthetic (e.g., bupivacaine) may help control postoperative pain in mandibular teeth; however, this is not very successful in maxillary teeth.[132,140] The duration of analgesia in the mandible is usually not so long as to preclude the prescription of oral analgesics.[48]

Asymptomatic Pulp Necrosis

Asymptomatic teeth are the easiest to anesthetize. Although it may be tempting to proceed without anesthesia, vital sensitive tissue (ingrowth of periapical tissue into canal) may be encountered in the apical portion of canals, or placement of files may cause pressure and extrusion of fluid periapically.

The conventional injections are usually administered: inferior alveolar nerve block and long buccal injection (molars) for mandibular teeth and infiltration in the maxilla. Usually the patient remains comfortable. Rarely, there may be some sensitivity during canal preparation that requires an IO or IL injection. IP injection is not indicated, because bacteria and debris may be forced periapically. In the maxilla, an additional infiltration may be necessary during longer procedures.

Anesthesia for Surgical Procedures

Incision for Drainage

Patients tolerate the procedure better when adequate anesthesia is present before incision and drainage (I&D) of a swelling. However, obtaining profound anesthesia is difficult, which should be explained to the patient. In the mandible, an inferior alveolar nerve block plus a long buccal injection (for molars) and an inferior alveolar nerve block plus labial infiltration away from the swelling (for premolars and anterior teeth) are administered. In the maxilla, infiltration is given mesial and distal to the swelling. For palatal swellings, a small volume of anesthetic is infiltrated over the greater palatine foramen (for posterior teeth) or over the nasopalatine foramen (for anterior teeth). With swelling over either foramen, lateral infiltration is indicated.

Injection directly into a swelling is contraindicated. These inflamed tissues are hyperalgesic and difficult to anesthetize. Traditionally it has been believed that the anesthetic solution may be affected by the lower pH of these tissues and rendered less effective and that direct injection "spreads the infection," although neither belief has been proved. Nevertheless, reasons for avoiding injection into a swelling are the pain from the injection pressure and the ineffectiveness of this technique. Theoretically, the area of swelling has an increased blood supply; therefore the anesthetic is transported quickly into the systemic circulation, diminishing its effect. Also, edema and purulence may dilute the solution.

Incision and Drainage—Buffered Anesthetics

In dentistry, I&D of an odontogenic facial swelling is an emergency procedure. Adequate pain control during the I&D procedure is difficult. Buffered local anesthetics have been purported to reduce pain particularly during painful procedures such as I&D. The reasoning behind buffering of local anesthetics is logical according to the Henderson-Hasselbalch equation: if a local anesthetic solution is buffered to a pH that is closer to its pKa, more of the free base form will be available upon injection to enter the nerve sheath. The most common method for buffering local anesthetics is by the addition of sodium bicarbonate.

Two investigations studied the pain of local anesthetic infiltration (mesial and distal to the swelling) and the pain of the I&D procedure of a buffered versus a nonbuffered formulation in symptomatic emergency patients presenting with a diagnosis of pulpal necrosis, associated periapical area, and an acute clinical swelling.[81,84] Moderate to severe pain was experienced in a large number of patients with both the infiltrations and during the I&D procedure. Buffering did not significantly decrease the pain of infiltrations or significantly decrease the pain of the I&D procedure.

Although the theory of buffering local anesthetics is logical, in reality the presence of a buffer in the local anesthetic may not be enough to overcome the lowered excitability thresholds and peripheral sensitization associated with such significant inflammatory and infectious conditions of a patient with pulpal necrosis and associated acute swelling.[84]

Outcome of an Incision and Drainage Procedure

Endodontic textbooks recommend I&D to treat swollen endodontic patients. The rationale is that I&D prevents further spread of the infection, relieves pressure and pain, and allows introduction of oxygen, which may aid in reducing the number of anaerobic bacteria. However, there is no evidence-based research to support that the outcome of an endodontic I&D procedure is related to these factors.

One recent study found there was more postoperative pain when an I&D procedure was performed.[216] This result may have been related to tissue damage caused by the surgical wounding of the infected and inflamed tissue by the incision and dissection of the swelling.[216] The authors also found that whether an I&D was performed or not, patients had a decrease in postoperative pain and medication use over the 4 days.

Regardless, patients with facial swelling should be closely monitored and possibly referred to an endodontist because clinical management of these patients requires special care.[216]

Periapical Surgery

Most periapical surgery should be performed by an endodontist, because these practitioners have received advanced training in surgical procedures, the periapical bone anatomy of the mandible and maxilla, the use of magnification technologies, the complex canal anatomy, and advanced microsurgical techniques for retrograde preparation and filling.

Additional considerations in periapical surgery involve anesthesia of both soft tissue and bone. Also, inflammation is usually present. In the mandible the inferior alveolar injection is reasonably effective. Additional infiltration injections in the vestibule are useful to achieve vasoconstriction, particularly in the mandibular anterior region. In the maxilla, infiltration and block injections are generally effective, and larger volumes usually are necessary to provide anesthesia over the surgical field.

If the area of operation is inflamed or the patient is apprehensive, anesthesia may not be totally successful. Additionally, the effectiveness of surgical anesthesia is decreased by half compared with anesthesia for nonsurgical procedures. With flap reflection and opening into bone, the anesthetic solution is diluted by bleeding and removed by irrigation.[217]

Use of a long-acting anesthetic has been advocated.[14,69,218] In the mandible, use of a long-acting anesthetic is reasonably effective. In the maxilla, long-acting agents have decreased epinephrine concentrations, which result in more bleeding during surgery.[219] After periapical surgery, administration of a long-acting anesthetic has been suggested.[14] However, postsurgical pain is usually not severe and can be managed by analgesics.[219]

Acknowledgement

The authors would like to thank Dr. Richard Walton for authoring the first chapter of Local Anesthesia and the continued support through the years in helping to write the many excellent chapters.

Study Questions

1. Giving a thorough explanation of the procedure and how to converse if there is any discomfort is an example of exercising which of the 4 Cs?
   a. Control
   b. Communication
   c. Concern
   d. Confidence
2. Why do we use topical anesthesia?
   a. Decreases pain of depositing the anesthetic solution for the IAN block
   b. Decreases pain of depositing the anesthetic solution for infiltrations
   c. Provides an increase in pulpal anesthesia
   d. Demonstrates to the patient that the doctor is doing everything possible to prevent pain
3. Which of the following statements is true?
   a. One way to determine working length is by not administering anesthesia.
   b. Anesthesia is not necessary for teeth with pulpal necrosis.
   c. Anesthesia is not necessary for obturation appointments.
   d. The "eye-blink response" should not be used as an assessment of working length.
4. Which of the following has been shown to increase the success of the inferior alveolar nerve block in asymptomatic patients?
   a. Slow injection
   b. Buffered anesthetic
   c. Increased epinephrine concentration
   d. Increased volume (1.8 mL versus 3.6 mL)
5. Articaine is best used for which type of injection?
   a. Inferior alveolar nerve block
   b. Mandibular infiltration after an IANB
   c. PDL injection after an IANB
   d. Intraosseous injection after an IANB
6. If a patient's lower lip is numb but she or he feels pain when their mandibular tooth is prepared, the next step is to administer
   a. Another inferior alveolar nerve block
   b. A solution with more epinephrine
   c. A mylohyoid nerve injection
   d. Supplemental anesthesia
7. Which type of maxillary anesthesia is preferred for endodontic treatment of maxillary canines?
   a. Infiltration of the tooth
   b. Second division nerve block
   c. Palatal–anterior superior alveolar nerve block
   d. Infraorbital nerve block
8. Which of the following statements is true?
   a. After infiltration anesthesia, performing an incision & drainage procedure is painless.
   b. Cold testing for anesthesia should be done before beginning endodontic therapy.
   c. A repeat inferior alveolar nerve block should be used when patients have pain during endodontic treatment.
   d. Infiltrations should be given directly into a swelling to have the best anesthesia for an incision & drainage procedure.
9. Which of the following should be used for an intraosseous injection:
   a. Both lidocaine and mepivacaine
   b. Only mepivacaine
   b. Only lidocaine
   d. Only bupivacaine
10. A supplemental intraosseous injection is more successful than a supplemental PDL injection because it is administered
    a. In a more apical site
    b. With more anesthetic
    c. More slowly
    d. In the cancellous bone

ANSWERS

Answer Box 8

1 b. Communication
2 d. Demonstrates to the patient that the doctor is doing everything possible to prevent pain
3 d. The "eye-blink response" should not be used as an assessment of working length.
4 a. Slow injection
5 b. Mandibular infiltration after an IANB
6 d. Supplemental anesthesia
7 a. Infiltration of the tooth
8 b. Cold testing for anesthesia should be done before beginning endodontic therapy.
9 a. Both lidocaine and mepivacaine
10 b. With more anesthetic

References

1. Walton R, Torabinejad M: Managing local anesthesia problems in the endodontic patient, *J Am Dent Assoc* 123:97, 1992.
2. Walton R: Managing endodontic anaesthesia problems, *Endod Pract* 1:15, 1998.
3. LeClaire A, Skidmore A, Griffin Jr J, et al.: Endodontic fear survey, *J Endod* 14:560, 1988.
4. Rood J, Pateromichelakis S: Inflammation and peripheral nerve sensitization, *Br J Oral Surg* 19:67, 1981.
5. Wallace J, Michanowicz A, Mundell R, et al.: A pilot study of the clinical problem of regionally anesthetizing the pulp of an acutely inflamed mandibular molar, *Oral Surg Oral Med Oral Pathol* 59:517, 1985.
6. Byers M, Taylor P, Khayat B, et al.: Effects of injury and inflammation on pulpal and periapical nerves, *J Endod* 16:78, 1990.
7. Weinstein P, Milgrom P, Kaufman E, et al.: Patient perceptions of failure to achieve optimal local anesthesia, *Gen Dent* 33:218, 1985.
8. Fiset L, Milgrom P, Weinstein P: Psychophysiological responses to dental injections, *J Am Dent Assoc* 11:4, 1985.
9. Meechan J: Intra-oral topical anaesthetics: a review, *J Dent* 28:3, 2000.
10. Rosivack R, Koenigsberg S, Maxwell K: An analysis of the effectiveness of two topical anesthetics, *Anesth Prog* 37:290, 1990.
11. Nusstein J, Beck M: Effectiveness of 20% benzocaine as a topical anesthetic for intraoral injections, *Anesth Prog* 50:159, 2003.
12. Parirokh M, Sadeghi A, Nakhaee N, et al.: Effect of topical anesthesia on pain during infiltration injection and success of anesthesia for maxillary central incisors, *J Endod* 38:1553, 2012.
13. Martin M, Ramsay D, Whitney C, et al.: Topical anesthesia: differentiating the pharmacological and psychological contributions to efficacy, *Anesth Prog* 41:40, 1994.
14. Malamed S: *Handbook of local anesthesia*, ed 6, St. Louis, 2013, Elsevier/Mosby.
15. Flanagan T, Wahl MJ, Schmitt MM, et al.: Size doesn't matter: needle gauge and injection pain, *Gen Dent* 55:216, 2007.
16. Fuller N, Menke R, Meyers W: Perception of pain to intraoral penetration of three needles, *J Am Dent Assoc* 99:822, 1979.
17. Cooley R, Robison S: Comparative evaluation of the 30-gauge dental needle, *Oral Surg Oral Med Oral Pathol* 48:400, 1979.
18. Robison S, Mayhew R, Cowan R, et al.: Comparative study of deflection characteristics and fragility of 25-, 27-, and 30-gauge short dental needles, *J Am Dent Assoc* 109:920, 1984.
19. Pogrel MA: Broken local anesthetic needles: a case series of 16 patients, with recommendations, *J Am Dent Assoc* 140:1517, 2009.
20. Kanaa H, Meechan J, Corbett P, et al.: Speed of injection influences efficacy of inferior alveolar nerve blocks: a double-blind randomized controlled trial in volunteers, *J Endod* 32:919, 2006.
21. Aggarwal V, Singla M, Miglani S, et al.: A prospective, randomized single-blind evaluation of effect of injection speed on anesthetic efficacy of inferior alveolar nerve block in patients with symptomatic irreversible pulpitis, *J Endod* 38:1578, 2012.
22. Saloum FS, Baumgartner JC, Marshall G, et al.: A clinical comparison of pain perception to the Wand and a traditional syringe, *Oral Surg Oral Med Oral Pathol Oral Radiol Endod* 86:691, 2000.
23. Goodell GG, Gallagher FJ, Nicoll BK: Comparison of a controlled injection pressure system with a conventional technique, *Oral Surg Oral Med Oral Pathol Oral Radiol Endod* 90:88, 2000.
24. Nicholson JW, Berry TG, Summitt JB, et al.: Pain perception and utility: a comparison of the syringe and computerized local injection techniques, *Gen Dent* 249:167, 2001.
25. Primosch RE, Brooks R: Influence of anesthetic flow rate delivered by the wand local anesthetic system on pain response to palatal injections, *Am J Dent* 15:15, 2002.
26. Nusstein J, Burns Y, Reader A, et al.: Injection pain and postinjection pain of the palatal anterior superior alveolar injection, administered with the wand plus system, comparing 2% lidocaine with 1:100,000 epinephrine to 3% mepivacaine, *Oral Surg Oral Med Oral Pathol Oral Radiol Endodon* 97:164, 2004.
27. Nusstein J, Lee S, Reader A, et al.: Injection pain and postinjection pain of the anterior middle superior alveolar injection administered with the wand or conventional syringe, *Oral Surg Oral Med Oral Pathol Oral Radiol Endod* 98:124, 2004.
28. Palm AM, Kirkegaard U, Poulsen S: The wand versus traditional injection for mandibular nerve block in children and adolescents: perceived pain and time of onset, *Pediatr Dent* 26:481, 2004.
29. Nusstein J, Steinkruger G, Reader A, et al.: The effects of a two-stage injection technique on inferior alveolar nerve block injection pain, *Anesth Prog* 53:126, 2006.
30. Liddell A, Locker D: Gender and age differences in attitudes to dental pain and dental control, *Community Dent Oral Epidemiol* 25:314, 1997.
31. Fillingim R, Edwards R, Powell T: The relationship of sex and clinical pain to experimental pain responses, *Pain* 83:419, 1999.
32. Lin L, Shovlin F, Skribner J, et al.: Pulp biopsies from the teeth associated with periapical radiolucency, *J Endod* 10:436, 1984.
33. Lindemann M, Reader A, Nusstein J, et al.: Effect of sublingual triazolam on the success of inferior alveolar nerve block in patients with irreversible pulpitis, *J Endod* 34:1167, 2008.
34. Stanley W, Drum M, Nusstein J, et al.: Effect of nitrous oxide on the efficacy of the inferior alveolar nerve block in patients with irreversible pulpitis, *J Endod* 38:565, 2012.
35. Khademi AA, Saatchi M, Minaiyan M, et al.: Effect of preoperative alprazolam on the success of inferior alveolar nerve block for teeth with irreversible pulpitis, *J Endod* 38:1337, 2012.
36. Stentz D, Drum M, Reader A, et al.: Effect of a combination of intranasal ketorolac and nitrous oxide on the success of the inferior alveolar nerve block in patients with symptomatic irreversible pulpitis: a prospective, randomized, double-blind study, *J Endod* 44:9, 2018.
37. Kaufman E, Weinstein P, Milgrom P: Difficulties in achieving local anesthesia, *J Am Dent Assoc* 108:205, 1984.
38. Dreven L, Reader A, Beck M, et al.: An evaluation of an electric pulp tester as a measure of analgesia in human vital teeth, *J Endod* 13:233, 1987.
39. Certosimo A, Archer R: A clinical evaluation of the electric pulp tester as an indicator of local anesthesia, *Oper Dent* 21:25, 1996.
40. Reader A, Nusstein J, Drum M: *Successful local anesthesia for restorative dentistry and endodontics*, ed 2, Hanover Park, IL, 2017, Quintessence.
41. Nusstein J, Reader A, Beck M: Anesthetic efficacy of different volumes of lidocaine with epinephrine for inferior alveolar nerve blocks, *Gen Dent* 50:372, 2002.
42. Ågren E, Danielsson K: Conduction block analgesia in the mandible, *Swed Dent J* 5:81, 1981.

43. Vreeland D, Reader A, Beck M, et al.: An evaluation of volumes and concentrations of lidocaine in human inferior alveolar nerve block, *J Endod* 15:6, 1989.
44. Hinkley S, Reader A, Beck M, et al.: An evaluation of 4% prilocaine with 1:200,000 epinephrine and 2% mepivacaine with 1:20,000 levonordefrin compared with 2% lidocaine with 1:100,000 epinephrine for inferior alveolar nerve block, *Anesth Prog* 38:84, 1991.
45. Chaney M, Kerby R, Reader A, et al.: An evaluation of lidocaine hydrocarbonate compared with lidocaine hydrochloride for inferior alveolar nerve block, *Anesth Prog* 38:212, 1992.
46. Nist R, Reader A, Beck M, et al.: An evaluation of the incisive nerve block and combination inferior alveolar and incisive nerve blocks in mandibular anesthesia, *J Endod* 18:455, 1992.
47. McLean C, Reader A, Beck M, et al.: An evaluation of 4% prilocaine and 3% mepivacaine compared with 2% lidocaine (1:100,000 epinephrine) for inferior alveolar nerve block, *J Endod* 19:146, 1993.
48. Fernandez C, Reader A, Beck M, et al.: A prospective, randomized, double-blind comparison of bupivacaine and lidocaine for inferior alveolar nerve blocks, *J Endod* 31:499, 2005.
49. Yared GM, Dagher BF: Evaluation of lidocaine in human inferior alveolar nerve block, *J Endod* 23:575, 1997.
50. Wali M, Drum M, Reader A, et al.: Prospective, randomized single-blind study of the anesthetic efficacy of 1.8 and 3.6 milliliters of 2% lidocaine with 1:50,000 epinephrine for inferior alveolar nerve blocks, *J Endod* 36:1459, 2010.
51. Fowler S, Reader A, Beck M: Incidence of missed inferior alveolar nerve blocks in vital asymptomatic subjects and in patients with symptomatic irreversible pulpitis, *J Endod* 41:637, 2015.
52. Dagher FB, Yared GM, Machtou P: An evaluation of 2% lidocaine with different concentrations of epinephrine for inferior alveolar nerve block, *J Endod* 23:178, 1997.
53. Malamed SF, Gagnon S, LeBlanc D: Articaine hydrochloride: a study of the safety of a new amide local anesthetic, *J Am Dent Assoc* 132:177, 2001.
54. Oertel R, Rahn R, Kirch W: Clinical pharmacokinetics of articaine, *Clin Pharmacokinet* 33:417, 1997.
55. Malamed SF, Gagnon S, Leblanc D: A comparison between articaine HCl and lidocaine HCl in pediatric dental patients, *Pediatr Dent* 22:307, 2000.
56. Malamed SF, Gagnon S, Leblanc D: Efficacy of articaine: a new amide local anesthetic, *J Am Dent Assoc* 131:635, 2000.
57. Haas DA, Harper DG, Saso MA, et al.: Comparison of articaine and prilocaine anesthesia by infiltration in maxillary and mandibular arches, *Anesth Prog* 37:230, 1990.
58. Claffey E, Reader A, Nusstein J, et al.: Anesthetic efficacy of articaine for inferior alveolar nerve blocks in patients with irreversible pulpitis, *J Endod* 30:568, 2004.
59. Vahatalo K, Antila H, Lehtinen R: Articaine and lidocaine for maxillary infiltration anesthesia, *Anesth Prog* 40:114, 1993.
60. Berlin J, Nusstein J, Reader A, et al.: Efficacy of articaine and lidocaine in a primary intraligamentary injection administered with a computer-controlled local anesthetic delivery system, *Oral Surg Oral Med Oral Pathol Oral Radiol Endod* 99:361, 2005.
61. Mikesell P, Nusstein J, Reader A, et al.: A comparison of articaine and lidocaine for inferior alveolar nerve blocks, *J Endod* 31:265, 2005.
62. Moore PA, Boynes SG, Hersh EV, et al.: The anesthetic efficacy of 4 percent articaine 1:200,000 epinephrine: two controlled clinical trials, *J Am Dent Assoc* 137:1572, 2006.
63. Schertzer ER, Malamed SF: Articaine vs lidocaine, *J Am Dent Assoc* 131:1248, 2000.
64. Haas DA, Lennon D: A 21-year retrospective study of reports of paresthesia following local anesthetic administration, *J Can Dent Assoc* 61:319, 1995.
65. Gaffen AS, Haas DA: Retrospective review of voluntary reports of nonsurgical paresthesia in dentistry, *J Can Dent Assoc* 75:579, 2009.
66. Garisto GA, Gaffen AS, Lawrence HP, et al.: Occurrence of paresthesia after dental local anesthetic administration in the United States, *J Am Dent Assoc* 141:836, 2010.
67. Pogrel M: Permanent nerve damage from inferior alveolar nerve blocks: an update to include articaine, *J Calif Dent Assoc* 35:271, 2007.
68. Davis W, Oakley J, Smith E: Comparison of the effectiveness of etidocaine and lidocaine as local anesthetic agents during oral surgery, *Anesth Prog* 31:159, 1984.
69. Rosenquist J, Rosenquist K, Lee P: Comparison between lidocaine and bupivacaine as local anesthetics with diflunisal for postoperative pain control after lower third molar surgery, *Anesth Prog* 35:1, 1988.
70. Dunsky J, Moore P: Long-acting local anesthetics: a comparison of bupivacaine and etidocaine in endodontics, *J Endod* 10:6, 1984.
71. Crout R, Koraido G, Moore P: A clinical trial of long-acting local anesthetics for periodontal surgery, *Anesth Prog* 37:194, 1990.
72. Cepeda MS, Tzortzopoulou A, Thackrey M, et al.: Adjusting the pH of lidocaine for reducing pain on injection (review), *Cochrane Database Syst Rev*, 2010.
73. Hanna MN, Elhassan A, Veloso PM, et al.: Efficacy of bicarbonate in decreasing pain on intradermal injection of local anesthetics: a meta-analysis, *Reg Anesth Pain Med* 34:122, 2009.
74. Bowles WH, Frysh H, Emmons R: Clinical evaluation of buffered local anesthetic, *Gen Dent* 43:182, 1995.
75. Kashyap VM, Desai R, Reddy PB, et al.: Effect of alkalinisation of lignocaine for intraoral nerve block on pain during injection, and speed of onset of anaesthesia, *Br J Oral Maxillofac Surg* 49:e72, 2011.
76. Al-Sultan AF: Effectiveness of pH adjusted lidocaine versus commercial lidocaine for maxillary infiltration anesthesia, *Al-Rafidain Dent J* 4:34, 2004.
77. Al-Sultan AF, Fathie WK, Hamid RS: A clinical evaluation on the alkalization of local anesthetic solution in periapical surgery, *Al-Rafidain Dent J* 6:71, 2006.
78. Whitcomb M, Drum M, Reader A, et al.: A prospective, randomized double-blind study of the anesthetic efficacy of sodium bicarbonate buffered 2% lidocaine with 1:100,000 epinephrine in inferior alveolar nerve blocks, *Anesth Prog* 57:59, 2010.
79. Saatchi M, Farhad AR, Shenasa N, et al.: Effect of sodium bicarbonate buccal infiltration on the success of inferior alveolar nerve block in mandibular first molars with symptomatic irreversible pulpitis: a prospective, randomized double-blind study, *J Endod* 42:1458, 2016.
80. Hobeich P, Simon S, Schneiderman E, et al.: A prospective, randomized, double-blind comparison of the injection pain and anesthetic onset of 2% lidocaine with 1:100,000 epinephrine buffered with 5% and 10% sodium bicarbonate in maxillary infiltrations, *J Endod* 39:597, 2013.
81. Harreld TK, Fowler S, Drum M, et al.: Efficacy of a buffered 4% lidocaine formulation for incision and drainage: a prospective, randomized, double-blind study, *J Endod* 41:1583, 2015.
82. Shurtz R, Nusstein J, Reader A, et al.: Buffered 4% articaine as a primary buccal infiltration of the mandibular first molar: a prospective, randomized, double-blind study, *J Endod* 41:1403, 2015.
83. Schellenberg J, Drum M, Reader A, et al.: Effect of buffered 4% lidocaine on the success of the inferior alveolar nerve block in patients with symptomatic irreversible pulpitis: a prospective, randomized, double-blind study, *J Endod* 41:791, 2015.
84. Balasco M, Drum M, Reader A, et al.: Buffered lidocaine for incision and drainage: a prospective, randomized double-blind study, *J Endod* 39:1329, 2013.
85. Gow-Gates G: Mandibular conduction anesthesia: a new technique using extra-oral landmarks, *Oral Surg Oral Med Oral Pathol* 36:321, 1973.
86. Akinosi J: A new approach to the mandibular nerve block, *Br J Oral Surg* 15:83, 1977.
87. Todorovic L, Stajcic Z, Petrovic V: Mandibular versus inferior alveolar dental anaesthesia: clinical assessment of 3 different techniques, *Int J Oral Maxillofac Surg* 15:733, 1986.
88. Goldberg S, Reader A, Drum M, et al.: Comparison of the anesthetic efficacy of the conventional inferior alveolar, Gow-Gates, and Vazirani-Akinosi techniques, *J Endod* 34:1306, 2008.

89. Montagnese T, Reader A, Melfi R: A comparative study of the Gow-Gates technique and a standard technique for mandibular anesthesia, *J Endod* 10:158, 1984.
90. Sisk AL: Evaluation of the Akinosi mandibular block technique in oral surgery, *Oral Maxillofac Surg* 44:113, 1986.
91. Yucel E, Hutchison IL: A comparative evaluation of the conventional and closed mouth technique for inferior alveolar nerve block, *Aust Dent J* 40:15, 1995.
92. Martinez GJM, Benito PB, Fernandez CF, et al.: A comparative study of direct mandibular nerve block and the Akinosi technique, *Med Oral* 8:143, 2003.
93. Click V, Drum M, Reader A, et al.: Evaluation of the Gow-Gates and Vazirani-Akinosi techniques in patients with symptomatic irreversible pulpitis: a prospective randomized study, *J Endod* 41:16, 2015.
94. Joyce AP, Donnelly JC: Evaluation of the effectiveness and comfort of incisive nerve anesthesia given inside or outside the mental foramen, *J Endod* 19:409, 1993.
95. Whitworth JM, Kanaa MD, Corbett IP, et al.: Influence of injection speed on the effectiveness of incisive/mental nerve block: a randomized, controlled, double-blind study in adult volunteers, *J Endod* 33:1149, 2007.
96. Batista da Silva C, Berto LA, Volpato MC, et al.: Anesthetic efficacy of articaine and lidocaine for incisive/mental nerve block, *J Endod* 36:438, 2010.
97. Yonchak T, Reader A, Beck M, et al.: Anesthetic efficacy of infiltrations in mandibular anterior teeth, *Anes Prog* 48:55, 2001.
98. Meechan JG, Ledvinka JI: Pulpal anesthesia for mandibular central incisor teeth: a comparison of infiltration and intraligamentary injections, *Int Endod J* 35:629, 2002.
99. Meechan JG, Kanaa MD, Corbett IP, et al.: Pulpal anesthesia for permanent first molar teeth: a double-blind randomized cross-over trial comparing buccal and buccal plus lingual infiltration injections in volunteers, *Int Endod J* 39:764, 2006.
100. Kanaa MD, Whitworth JM, Corbett IP, et al.: Articaine and lidocaine mandibular buccal infiltration anesthesia: a prospective randomized double-blind cross-over study, *J Endod* 32:296, 2006.
101. Jung Y, Kim JH, Kim ES, et al.: An evaluation of buccal infiltrations and inferior alveolar nerve blocks in pulpal anesthesia for mandibular first molars, *J Endod* 34:11, 2008.
102. Corbett IP, Kanaa MD, Whitworth JM, et al.: Articaine infiltration for anesthesia of mandibular first molars, *J Endod* 34:514, 2008.
103. Robertson D, Nusstein J, Reader A, et al.: The anesthetic efficacy of articaine in buccal infiltration of mandibular posterior teeth, *J Am Dent Assoc* 138:1104, 2007.
104. McEntire M, Nusstein J, Drum M, et al.: Anesthetic efficacy of 4% articaine with 1:100,000 epinephrine versus 4% articaine with 1:200,000 epinephrine as a primary buccal infiltration in the mandibular first molar, *J Endod* 37:450, 2011.
105. Nuzum FM, Drum M, Nusstein J, et al.: Anesthetic efficacy of articaine for combination labial plus lingual infiltrations versus labial infiltration in the mandibular lateral incisor, *J Endod* 36:952, 2010.
106. Jaber A, Whitworth JM, Corbett IP, et al.: The efficacy of infiltration anaesthesia for adult mandibular incisors: a randomized double-blind cross-over trial comparing articaine and lidocaine buccal and buccal plus lingual infiltrations, *Br Dent J* 209:e16, 2010.
107. Berns J, Sadove M: Mandibular block injection: a method of study using an injected radiopaque material, *J Am Dent Assoc* 65:735, 1962.
108. Galbreath J: Tracing the course of the mandibular block injection, *Oral Surg Oral Med Oral Pathol* 30:571, 1970.
109. Hannan L, Reader A, Nist R, et al.: The use of ultrasound for guiding needle placement for inferior alveolar nerve blocks, *Oral Surg Oral Med Oral Pathol Oral Radiol Endod* 87:658, 1999.
110. Simon F, Reader A, Drum M, et al.: A prospective, randomized single-blind study of the anesthetic efficacy of the inferior alveolar nerve block administered with a peripheral nerve stimulator, *J Endod* 36:429, 2010.
111. Strichartz G: Molecular mechanisms of nerve block by local anesthetics, *Anesthesiology* 45:421, 1976.
112. Cooley R, Robison S: Comparative evaluation of the 30-gauge dental needle, *Oral Surg Oral Med Oral Pathol* 48:400, 1979.
113. Davidson M: Bevel-oriented mandibular injections: needle deflection can be beneficial, *Gen Dent* 37:410, 1989.
114. Hochman MN, Friedman MJ: In vitro study of needle deflection: a linear insertion technique versus a bidirectional rotation insertion technique, *Quintessence Int* 31:33, 2000.
115. Aldous J: Needle deflection: a factor in the administration of local anesthetics, *J Am Dent Assoc* 77:602, 1968.
116. Kennedy S, Reader A, Nusstein J, et al.: The significance of needle deflection in success of the inferior alveolar nerve block in patients with irreversible pulpitis, *J Endod* 29:630, 2003.
117. Steinkruger G, Nusstein J, Reader A, et al.: The significance of needle bevel orientation in achieving a successful inferior alveolar nerve block, *J Am Dent Assoc* 137:1685, 2006.
118. Wilson S, Johns P, Fuller P: The inferior and mylohyoid nerves: an anatomic study and relationship to local anesthesia of the anterior mandibular teeth, *J Am Dent Assoc* 108:350, 1984.
119. Clark S, Reader A, Beck M, et al.: Anesthetic efficacy of the mylohyoid nerve block and combination inferior alveolar nerve block/mylohyoid nerve block, *Oral Surg Oral Med Oral Pathol Oral Radiol Endod* 87:557, 1999.
120. Yonchak T, Reader A, Beck M, et al.: Anesthetic efficacy of unilateral and bilateral inferior alveolar nerve blocks to determine cross innervation in anterior teeth, *Oral Surg Oral Med Oral Pathol Oral Radiol Endod* 92:132, 2001.
121. Droll B, Drum M, Nusstein J, et al.: Anesthetic efficacy of the inferior alveolar nerve block in red-haired women, *J Endod* 38:1564, 2012.
122. Crowley C, Drum M, Reader A, et al.: Anesthetic efficacy of supine and upright positions for the inferior alveolar nerve block: a prospective, randomized study, *J Endod* 44:202, 2018.
123. Aggarwal V, Singla M, Miglani S: Effect of relative head position on the anesthetic efficacy of inferior alveolar nerve block during endodontic treatment of patients with irreversible pulpitis, *J Dent Anesth Pain Med* 18:41, 2018.
124. Haase A, Reader A, Nusstein J, et al.: Comparing anesthetic efficacy of articaine versus lidocaine as a supplemental buccal infiltration of the mandibular first molar after an inferior alveolar nerve block, *J Am Dent Assoc* 139:1228, 2008.
125. Kanaa MD, Whitworth JM, Corbett IP, et al.: Articaine buccal infiltration enhances the effectiveness of lidocaine inferior alveolar nerve block, *Int Endod J* 42:238, 2009.
126. Dunbar D, Reader A, Nist R, et al.: Anesthetic efficacy of the intraosseous injection after an inferior alveolar nerve block, *J Endod* 22:481, 1996.
127. Guglielmo A, Reader A, Nist R, et al.: Anesthetic efficacy and heart rate effects of the supplemental intraosseous injection of 2% mepivacaine with 1:20,000 levonordefrin, *Oral Surg Oral Med Oral Pathol Oral Radiol Endod* 87:284, 1999.
128. Gallatin E, Stabile P, Reader A, et al.: Anesthetic efficacy and heart rate effects of the intraosseous injection of 3% mepivacaine after an inferior alveolar nerve block, *Oral Surg Oral Med Oral Pathol Oral Radiol Endod* 89:83, 2000.
129. Childers M, Reader A, Nist R, et al.: Anesthetic efficacy of the periodontal ligament injection after an inferior alveolar nerve block, *J Endod* 22:317, 1996.
130. Bunczak-Reeh M, Hargreaves K: Effect of inflammation on the delivery of drugs to dental pulp, *J Endod* 24:822, 1998.
131. Nusstein J, Wood M, Reader A, et al.: Comparison of the degree of pulpal anesthesia achieved with the intraosseous injection and infiltration injection using 2% lidocaine with 1:100,000 epinephrine, *Gen Dent* 53:50, 2005.
132. Gross R, McCartney M, Reader A, et al.: A prospective, randomized, double-blind comparison of bupivacaine and lidocaine for maxillary infiltrations, *J Endod* 33:1021, 2007.

133. Mikesell A, Drum M, Reader A, et al.: Anesthetic efficacy of 1.8 mL and 3.6 mL of 2% lidocaine with 1:100,000 epinephrine for maxillary infiltrations, *J Endod* 34:121, 2008.
134. Evans G, Nusstein J, Drum M, et al.: A prospective, randomized double-blind comparison of articaine and lidocaine for maxillary infiltrations, *J Endod* 34:389, 2008.
135. Brunetto PC, Ranali J, Ambrosano GMB, et al.: Anesthetic efficacy of 3 volumes of lidocaine with epinephrine in maxillary infiltration anesthesia, *Anesth Prog* 55:29, 2008.
136. Scott J, Drum M, Reader A, et al.: The efficacy of a repeated infiltration in prolonging duration of pulpal anesthesia in maxillary lateral incisors, *J Am Dent Assoc* 140:318, 2009.
137. Mason R, Drum M, Reader A, et al.: A prospective, randomized, double-blind comparison of 2% lidocaine with 1:100,000 and 1:50,000 epinephrine and 3% mepivacaine for maxillary infiltrations, *J Endod* 35:1173, 2009.
138. Katz S, Drum M, Reader A, et al.: A prospective, randomized, double-blind comparison of 2% lidocaine with 1:100,000 epinephrine, 4% prilocaine with 1:200,000 epinephrine and 4% prilocaine for maxillary infiltrations, *Anesth Prog* 57:45, 2010.
139. Lawaty I, Drum M, Reader A, et al.: A prospective, randomized, double-blind comparison of 2% mepivacaine with 1:20,000 levonordefrin versus 2% lidocaine with 1:100,000 epinephrine for maxillary infiltrations, *Anesth Prog* 57:139, 2010.
140. Danielsson K, Evers H, Nordenram A: Long-acting local anesthetics in oral surgery: an experimental evaluation of bupivacaine and etidocaine for oral infiltration anesthesia, *Anesth Prog* 32:65, 1985.
141. Loetscher C, Melton D, Walton R: Injection regimen for anesthesia of the maxillary first molar, *J Am Dent Assoc* 117:337, 1988.
142. Pfeil L, Drum M, Reader A, et al.: Anesthetic efficacy of 1.8 milliters and 3.6 milliters of 2% lidocaine with 1:100,000 epinephrine for posterior superior alveolar nerve blocks, *J Endod* 36:598, 2010.
143. Berberich G, Reader A, Drum M, et al.: A prospective, randomized, double-blind comparison of the anesthetic efficacy of 2% lidocaine with 1:100,000 and 1:50,000 epinephrine and 3% mepivacaine in the intraoral, infraorbital nerve block, *J Endod* 35:1498, 2009.
144. Karkut B, Reader A, Drum M, et al.: A comparison of the local anesthetic efficacy of the extraoral versus the intraoral infraorbital nerve block, *J Am Dent Assoc* 141:185, 2010.
145. Broering R, Reader A, Drum M, et al.: A prospective, randomized comparison of the anesthetic efficacy of the greater palatine and high tuberosity second division nerve blocks, *J Endod* 35:1337, 2009.
146. Forloine A, Drum M, Reader A, et al.: A prospective, randomized, double-blind comparison of the anesthetic efficacy of two percent lidocaine with 1:100,000 epinephrine and three percent mepivacaine in the maxillary high tuberosity second division nerve block, *J Endod* 36:1770, 2010.
147. Friedman M, Hochman M: P-ASA block injection: a new palatal technique to anesthetize maxillary anterior teeth, *J Esthet Dent* 11:63, 1999.
148. Burns Y, Reader A, Nusstein J, et al.: Anesthetic efficacy of the palatal anterior superior alveolar injection, *J Am Dent Assoc* 135:1269, 2004.
149. Friedman M, Hochman M: Using AMSA and P-ASA nerve blocks for esthetic restorative dentistry, *Gen Dent* 5:506, 2001.
150. Lee S, Reader A, Nusstein J, et al.: Anesthetic efficacy of the anterior middle superior alveolar (AMSA) injection, *Anesth Prog* 51:80, 2004.
151. Kanaa MD, Whitworth JM, Meechan JG: A prospective trial of different supplementary local anesthetic techniques after failure of inferior alveolar nerve block in patients with irreversible pulpitis in mandibular teeth, *J Endod* 38:421, 2012.
152. Gallatin J, Reader A, Nusstein J, et al.: A comparison of two intraosseous anesthetic techniques in mandibular posterior teeth, *J Am Dent Assoc* 134:1476, 2003.
153. Coggins R, Reader A, Nist R, et al.: Anesthetic efficacy of the intraosseous injection in maxillary and mandibular teeth, *Oral Surg Oral Med Oral Pathol Oral Radiol Endod* 81:634, 1996.
154. Replogle K, Reader A, Nist R, et al.: Anesthetic efficacy of the intraosseous injection of 2% lidocaine (1:100,000 epinephrine) and 3% mepivacaine in mandibular first molars, *Oral Surg Oral Med Oral Pathol Oral Radiol Endod* 83:30, 1997.
155. Gallatin J, Nusstein J, Reader A, et al.: A comparison of injection pain and postoperative pain of two intraosseous anesthetic techniques, *Anesth Prog* 50:111, 2003.
156. Reitz J, Reader A, Nist R, et al.: Anesthetic efficacy of the intraosseous injection of 0.9 mL of 2% lidocaine (1:100,000 epinephrine) to augment an inferior alveolar nerve block, *Oral Surg Oral Med Oral Pathol Oral Radiol Endod* 86:516, 1998.
157. Stabile P, Reader A, Gallatin E, et al.: Anesthetic efficacy and heart rate effects of the intraosseous injection of 1.5% etidocaine (1:200,000 epinephrine) after an inferior alveolar nerve block, *Oral Surg Oral Med Oral Pathol Oral Radiol Endod* 89:407, 2000.
158. Bacsik CJ, Swift JQ, Hargreaves KM: Toxic systemic reactions of bupivacaine and etidocaine hydrochloride, *Oral Surg Oral Med Oral Pathol Oral Radiol Endod* 79:18, 1995.
159. Chamberlain TM, Davis RD, Murchison DF, et al.: Systemic effects of an intraosseous injection of 2% lidocaine with 1:100,000 epinephrine, *Gen Dent* 48:299, 2000.
160. Gallatin E, Stabile P, Reader A, et al.: Anesthetic efficacy and heart rate effects of the intraosseous injection of 3% mepivacaine after an inferior alveolar nerve block, *Oral Surg Oral Med Oral Pathol Oral Radiol Endod* 89:83, 2000.
161. Wood M, Reader A, Nusstein JM, et al.: Comparison of intraosseous and infiltration injections for venous lidocaine blood concentrations and heart rate changes after injection of 2% lidocaine with 1:100,000 epinephrine, *J Endod* 31:435, 2005.
162. Smith G, Walton R, Abbott B: Clinical evaluation of periodontal ligament anesthesia using a pressure syringe, *J Am Dent Assoc* 107:953, 1983.
163. Eriksen H, Aamdal H, Kerekes K: Periodontal anesthesia: a clinical evaluation, *Endod Dent Traumatol* 2:267, 1986.
164. Dreyer W, van Heerden J, Joubert J: The route of periodontal ligament injection of local anesthetic solution, *J Endod* 9:471, 1983.
165. Tagger M, Tagger E, Sarnat H: Periodontal ligament injection: spread of solution in the dog, *J Endod* 20:283, 1994.
166. Moore K, Reader A, Meyers W, et al.: A comparison of the periodontal ligament injection using 2% lidocaine with 1:100,000 epinephrine and saline in human mandibular premolars, *Anesth Prog* 34:181, 1987.
167. Schleder J, Reader A, Beck M, et al.: The periodontal ligament injection: a comparison of 2% lidocaine, 3% mepivacaine, and 1:100,000 epinephrine to 2% lidocaine with 1:100,000 epinephrine in human mandibular premolars, *J Endod* 14:397, 1988.
168. White J, Reader A, Beck M, et al.: The periodontal ligament injection: a comparison of the efficacy in human maxillary and mandibular teeth, *J Endod* 14:508, 1988.
169. Meechan JG, Ledvinka JI: Pulpal anesthesia for mandibular central incisor teeth: a comparison of infiltration and intraligamentary injections, *Int Endod J* 35:629, 2002.
170. Johnson G, Hlava G, Kalkwarf K: A comparison of periodontal intraligamental anesthesia using etidocaine HCl and lidocaine HCl, *Anesth Prog* 32:202, 1985.
171. Gray R, Lomax A, Rood J: Periodontal ligament injection: alternative solutions, *Anesth Prog* 37:293, 1990.
172. Meechan JG: A comparison of ropivacaine and lidocaine with epinephrine for intraligamentary anesthesia, *Oral Surg Oral Med Oral Pathol Oral Radiol Endod* 93:469, 2002.
173. D'Souza J, Walton R, Peterson L: Periodontal ligament injection: an evaluation of extent of anesthesia and postinjection discomfort, *J Am Dent Assoc* 114:341, 1987.
174. Nusstein J, Berlin J, Reader A, et al.: Comparison of injection pain, heart rate increase and post-injection pain of articaine and lidocaine in a primary intraligamentary injection administered with a computer-controlled local anesthetic delivery system, *Anesth Prog* 51:126, 2004.

175. Simon D, Jacobs L, Senia S, et al.: Intraligamentary anesthesia as an aid in endodontic diagnosis, *Oral Surg Oral Med Oral Pathol* 54:77, 1982.
176. Pashley D: Systemic effects of intraligamental injections, *J Endod* 12:501, 1986.
177. Cannell H, Kerwala C, Webster K, et al.: Are intraligamentary injections intravascular? *Br Dent J* 175:281, 1993.
178. Walton R, Abbott B: Periodontal ligament injection: a clinical evaluation, *J Am Dent Assoc* 103:103, 1981.
179. Walton R, Garnick J: The periodontal ligament injection: histologic effects on the periodontium in monkeys, *J Endod* 8:22, 1981.
180. List G, Meister Jr F, Nery E, et al.: Gingival crevicular fluid response to various solutions using the intraligamentary injection, *Quintessence Int* 19:559, 1988.
181. Brannström M, Nordenvall K, Hedstrom K: Periodontal tissue changes after intraligamentary anesthesia, *J Dent Child* 11:417, 1982.
182. Galili D, Kaufman E, Garfunkel A, et al.: Intraligamental anesthesia: a histological study, *Int J Oral Surg* 13:511, 1984.
183. Roahen J, Marshall J: The effects of periodontal ligament injection on pulpal and periodontal tissues, *J Endod* 16:28, 1990.
184. Pertot W, Dejou J: Bone and root resorption: effects of the force developed during periodontal ligament injections in dogs, *Oral Surg Oral Med Oral Pathol* 74:357, 1992.
185. Cromley NL, Adams DF: The effect of intraligamentary injections on diseased periodontiums in dogs, *Gen Dent* 39:33, 1991.
186. Peurach J: Pulpal response to intraligamentary injection in cynomolgus monkey, *Anesth Prog* 32:73, 1985.
187. Torabinejad M, Peters D, Peckham N, et al.: Electron microscopic changes in human pulps after intraligamental injection, *Oral Surg Oral Med Oral Pathol* 76:219, 1993.
188. Kim S: Ligamental injection: a physiological explanation of its efficacy, *J Endod* 12:486, 1986.
189. Plamondon T, Walton R, Graham G, et al.: Pulp response to the combined effects of cavity preparation and periodontal ligament injection, *Oper Dent* 15:86, 1990.
190. Brannström M, Lindsko S, Nordenvall K: Enamel hypoplasia in permanent teeth induced by periodontal ligament anesthesia of primary teeth, *J Am Dent Assoc* 109:735, 1984.
191. Fowler S, Drum M, Reader A, et al.: Anesthetic success of an inferior alveolar nerve block and supplemental articaine buccal infiltration for molars and premolars in patients with symptomatic irreversible pulpitis, *J Endod* 42:390, 2016.
192. Fowler S, Reader A: Is a volume of 3.6 mL better than 1.8 mL for inferior alveolar nerve blocks in patients with symptomatic irreversible pulpitis? *J Endod* 39:970, 2013.
193. Nusstein J, Reader A, Nist R, et al.: Anesthetic efficacy of the supplemental intraosseous injection of 2% lidocaine with 1:100,000 epinephrine in irreversible pulpitis, *J Endod* 24:487, 1998.
194. Aggarwal V, Singla M, Miglani S, et al.: A prospective, randomized, single-blind comparative evaluation of anesthetic efficacy of posterior alveolar nerve blocks, buccal infiltrations, and buccal plus palatal infiltrations in patients with irreversible pulpitis, *J Endod* 37:1491, 2011.
195. Kanaa MD, Whitworth JM, Meechan JG: A comparison of the efficacy of 4% articaine with 1:100,000 epinephrine and 2% lidocaine with 1:80,000 epinephrine in achieving pulpal anesthesia in maxillary teeth with irreversible pulpitis, *J Endod* 38:279, 2012.
196. Brandt RG, Anderson PF, McDonald NJ, et al.: The pulpal anesthetic efficacy of articaine versus lidocaine in dentistry: a meta-analysis, *J Am Dent Assoc* 142:493, 2011.
197. Kung J, McDonagh M, Sedgley CM: Does articaine provide an advantage over lidocaine in patients with symptomatic irreversible pulpitis? A systematic review and meta-analysis, *J Endod* 41:1784, 2015.
198. Argueta-Figueroa L, Arzate-Sosa G, Mendieta-Zeron H: Anesthetic efficacy of articaine for inferior alveolar nerve blocks in patients with symptomatic versus asymptomatic irreversible pulpitis, *Gen Dent* 60:e39, 2012.
199. Oleson M, Drum M, Reader A, et al.: Effect of preoperative ibuprofen on the success of the inferior alveolar nerve block in patients with irreversible pulpitis, *J Endod* 36:379, 2010.
200. Simpson M, Drum M, Reader A, et al.: Effect of preoperative ibuprofen/acetaminophen on the success of the inferior alveolar nerve block in patients with symptomatic irreversible pulpitis, *J Endod* 37:593, 2011.
201. Fullmer S, Drum M, Reader A, et al.: Effect of preoperative acetaminophen/hydrocodone on the efficacy of the inferior alveolar nerve block in patients with symptomatic irreversible pulpitis: a prospective, randomized, double-blind, placebo-controlled study, *J Endod* 40:1, 2014.
202. Fowler S, Nusstein J, Drum M, et al.: Reversal of soft-tissue anesthesia in asymptomatic endodontic patients: a preliminary, prospective, randomized, single-blind study, *J Endod* 37:1353, 2011.
203. Matthews R, Drum M, Reader A, et al.: Articaine for supplemental, buccal mandibular infiltration anesthesia in patients with irreversible pulpitis when the inferior alveolar nerve block fails, *J Endod* 35:343, 2009.
204. Bigby J, Reader A, Nusstein J, et al.: Articaine for supplemental intraosseous anesthesia in patients with irreversible pulpitis, *J Endod* 32:1044, 2006.
205. Reisman D, Reader A, Nist R, et al.: Anesthetic efficacy of the supplemental intraosseous injection of 3% mepivacaine in irreversible pulpitis, *Oral Surg Oral Med Oral Pathol Oral Radiol Endod* 84:676, 1997.
206. Reemers T, Glickman G, Spears R, et al.: The efficacy of the IntraFlow intraosseous injection as a primary anesthesia technique, *J Endod* 34:280, 2008.
207. Pereira LA, Groppo FC, Bergamaschi CD, et al.: Articaine (4%) with epinephrine (1:100,000 or 1:200,000) in intraosseous injections in symptomatic irreversible pulpitis of mandibular molars: anesthetic efficacy and cardiovascular effects, *Oral Surg Oral Med Oral Pathol Oral Radiol Endod* 116:e85, 2013.
208. Zarei M, Ghoddusi J, Sharifi E, et al.: Comparison of the anesthetic efficacy of and heart rate changes after periodontal ligament or intraosseous X-tip injection in mandibular molars: a randomized controlled clinical trial, *Int Endod J* 45:921, 2012.
209. Nusstein J, Claffey E, Reader A, et al.: Anesthetic effectiveness of the supplemental intraligamentary injection, administered with a computer-controlled local anesthetic delivery system, in patients with irreversible pulpitis, *J Endod* 31:354, 2005.
210. Cohen H, Cha B, Spangberg L: Endodontic anesthesia in mandibular molars: a clinical study, *J Endod* 19:370, 1993.
211. Bonar T, Nusstein J, Reader A, et al.: Anesthetic efficacy of articaine and lidocaine in a primary intraseptal injection: a prospective, randomized double-blind study, *Anesth Prog* 64:203, 2017.
212. Webster Jr S, Drum M, Reader A, et al.: How effective is supplemental intraseptal anesthesia in patients with symptomatic irreversible pulpitis? *J Endod* 42:1453, 2016.
213. Birchfield J, Rosenberg P: Role of the anesthetic solution in intrapulpal anesthesia, *J Endod* 1:26, 1975.
214. VanGheluwe J, Walton R: Intrapulpal injection: factors related to effectiveness, *Oral Surg Oral Med Oral Pathol Oral Radiol Endod* 83:38, 1997.
215. Sebastian R, Drum M, Reader A, et al.: What is the effect of no endodontic debridement on postoperative pain for symptomatic teeth with pulpal necrosis? *J Endod* 42:378, 2016.
216. Beus H, Fowler S, Drum M, et al.: What is the outcome of an incision and drainage procedure in endodontic patients? A prospective, randomized, single-blind study, *J Endod* 44:193, 2018.
217. Yamazaki S, Seino H, Ozawa S, et al.: Elevation of a periosteal flap with irrigation of the bone for minor oral surgery reduces the duration of action of infiltration anesthesia, *Anes Prog* 53:8, 2006.
218. Davis W, Oakley J, Smith E: Comparison of the effectiveness of etidocaine and lidocaine as local anesthetic agents during oral surgery, *Anesth Prog* 31:159, 1984.
219. Meechan J, Blair G: The effect of two different local anaesthetic solutions on pain experience following apicoectomy, *Br Dent J* 175:410, 1993.

9

Endodontic Emergencies and Therapeutics

RICHARD WALTON AND NIKITA B. RUPAREL

CHAPTER OUTLINE

LEARNING OBJECTIVES

After reading this chapter, the student should be able to:

1. Identify causes of emergencies as they occur before treatment, between appointments, and after obturation, differentiating urgency from a true emergency.
2. Identify patients who are at greater risk for experiencing pain after endodontic procedures.
3. Describe the psychological and physiologic factors that affect pain perception and pain reaction and how these are managed.
4. Define the flare-up and describe its management.
5. List the factors that relate to greater frequency of interappointment or postobturation flare-ups.
6. Describe and outline a sequential approach to endodontic emergencies:
   a. Determine the source of pain (pulpal or periapical)
   b. Establish a pulpal and periapical diagnosis
   c. Identify the etiologic factor of the pathosis
   d. Design an emergency (short-term) treatment plan
   e. Design a long-term treatment plan
7. Outline a system of subjective and objective examinations and radiographic findings to identify the source of pain and the pulpal or periapical diagnosis.
8. Describe when pretreatment emergencies might occur and how to manage these emergencies.
9. Outline the steps involved in treatment of painful, irreversible pulpitis.
10. Describe the steps involved in treatment of necrotic pulp with acute apical periodontitis.
11. Describe treatment of acute apical abscess and include the indications and procedure for incision and drainage.
12. Detail pharmacologic supportive therapy (analgesics, anxiolytics, antibiotics, and antiinflammatory agents) used in emergencies and its role in controlling pain and infection.

Introduction

Endodontic emergencies constitute approximately two-thirds of all dental emergencies,[1,2] with many patients seeking emergency care for a painful tooth.[1-3] There are a very large number of hospital emergency room visits for mouth abscess/facial cellulitis.[4] These painful and infectious emergencies pose significant challenges to patients and dental providers. Pain and/or swelling occur in patients before (pretreatment), during (interappointment), and after (postobturation) root canal treatment.[5-10] Understanding the causes of such emergencies results in appropriate diagnosis and treatment protocols for resolution of signs and symptoms.

Classical studies by Stanley, Fitzgerald, and Kakehashi[11] as well as the preponderance of endodontic literature point to a bacterial etiology as the initial causative factor for pulpal pathosis. Both primary and secondary endodontic infections are polymicrobial in nature with an average of 10 to 20 microorganisms in primary[12] and 1 to 3 microbial species in secondary infections.[13] Examples of endodontic pathogens include gram positive (*Enterococcus* species) and gram-negative (*Porphyromonas, Prevotella, Bacteroides* species) bacteria as well as members of the spirochete family (*Treponema* species). Other pathogens include viruses and fungi. Bacterial byproducts from such a mixed flora therefore constitute a soup of toxins that breakdown host tissues and initiate an inflammatory response. An untimely management attenuating such a response can lead to spread of the inflammatory mediators into the periapical regions, posing greater risks, such as facial abscesses and cellulitis (see Chapter 1).

Bacterial toxins fall into two categories: exotoxins and endotoxins. Exotoxins are secreted and released by the microorganism to degrade host tissues such as the extracellular matrix. Many of these function via enzymatic tissue breakdown and include enzymes belonging to the family of collagenases, proteases, lipases, chondroitinases, hyaluronidases, and cysteine and serine proteinases, among others. On the other hand, endotoxins are typically cell membrane/wall components such as lipoteichoic acid (LTA) and lipopolysaccharide (LPS). Still other specialized toxins include hemolysins and flagellins. Endotoxins play a crucial role in mediating pulpal pain. Because pain is the #1 reason why patients seek dental care, an in-depth understanding of pain detection and transmission is critical for management of a painful emergency.

LPS from a known endodontic pathogen, *Porphyromonas gingivalis,* has been shown in recent years to activate and sensitize trigeminal sensory neurons via Toll-like receptor-4 (TLR-4) expressed on sensory neurons.[14,15] On the other hand, non-TLR mechanisms have also been demonstrated for other bacterial species such as *Staphylococcus aureus* and *Escherichia coli.*[16-18] Moreover, these studies suggest that bacterium-induced pain does not depend on tissue edema or immune cell activation.[18] Collectively, these studies demonstrate that the concentration of the bacterial load dictates hyperalgesic conditions rather than local tissue inflammation (see Chapter 1).

Nonbacterial etiologies can also contribute to pulpal inflammation and emergency situations. These emergency situations include pulpal inflammation caused at the time of caries removal or crown preparations performed without adequate coolant, characteristics of the cavity preparation most importantly, remaining dentin thickness over the pulp, and type of restorative material.[19] It is well known that certain restorative materials promote marginal breakdown due to polymerization shrinkage and promote bacterial microleakage, whereas others release chemical agents such as resin monomers namely, BisGMA, urethane dimethacrylate (UDMA), and triethylene glycol dimethacrylate (TEGDMA), among others. These along with monomers present in dentin bonding agents such as hydroxyethyl methacrylate (HEMA) can be toxic to the underlying pulp if not polymerized fully.[19-22] Biomaterial studies indicate that the hydrophobicity of nonpolymerized monomers displaces dentinal fluid, thereby diffusing through the tubules and into the pulp.[20,23] Collectively, factors that do not directly point to a microbial etiology must be considered in emergencies and appropriate diagnosis must be determined to deliver a suitable treatment.

Both microbial and nonmicrobial etiologies culminate in an immunologic response. Patients with emergencies often report symptoms of spontaneous pain, pain to swallow, referred pain, pain that wakes them up, and pain that lingers after a stimulus. These symptoms are often mediated by an immunologic response and by (1) inflammatory mediators and (2) fluid pressure. Management of such a painful episode cannot be efficiently achieved by pharmacologic means alone.[24-26] Peripheral nerve sprouting,[27-31] increased expression of tetrodotoxin resistant (TTX-R) sodium channels,[32] as well as increased expression of transient receptor potential (TRP) channels,[33,34] all culminate in dramatic reduction of peripheral nerve thresholds of Aδ and C-fibers. Clinical studies consistently implicate preoperative pain as a strong predictor of postoperative pain.[35] Therefore emergency protocols must make every effort to attenuate preoperative pain to minimize development of chronic odontogenic pain conditions.

Endodontic emergencies are therefore a challenge for both diagnosis and management. Knowledge and skill in several aspects of endodontics are required; failure to apply these can result in serious consequences. Incorrect diagnosis and/or treatment can shift an acute condition to a chronic pain or infection-induced life-threatening condition. The clinician must have knowledge of pain mechanisms, patient management, diagnosis, anesthesia, therapeutics, and appropriate treatment measures for both hard and soft tissues. This chapter discusses approaches to the diagnosis and treatment of various categories of emergencies. It includes a review of etiologic factors and details of a systematic approach to identifying and diagnosing the offending cause; then appropriate treatment, including pharmacotherapy, is described.

Definition

By definition, endodontic emergencies are usually associated with pain and/or swelling and require immediate diagnosis and treatment. These emergencies are caused by pathoses in the pulp or periradicular tissues. They also include severe traumatic injuries that result in luxation, avulsion, or fractures of the hard tissues. Management of emergencies related to trauma will not be included in this chapter (see Chapter 11).

Categories

Pretreatment Emergency

These are situations in which the patient is seen initially with severe pain and/or swelling. Problems occur with both diagnosis and treatment.

Interappointment and Postobturation Emergency

Also referred to as a "flare-up," an interappointment and postobturation emergency problem occurs after an endodontic appointment. Although an upsetting event, this problem is easier to manage because the offending tooth has already been identified and a diagnosis has been previously established. Also, the clinician has knowledge of the prior procedure and will be better able to correct the problem.

The Challenge

It is satisfying and rewarding to successfully manage a distraught patient who has an emergency (Fig. 9.1). In contrast, it is very distressing to have a patient with a flare-up after root canal treatment in a previously asymptomatic tooth. The aim is to increase occurrences in the first category and decrease those in the second.

Differentiation of Emergency and Urgency

Whether a pretreatment, interappointment, or postobturation problem, it is important to differentiate between a *true emergency* and the less critical *urgency.* A *true emergency* is a condition requiring an unscheduled office visit with diagnosis and treatment. The

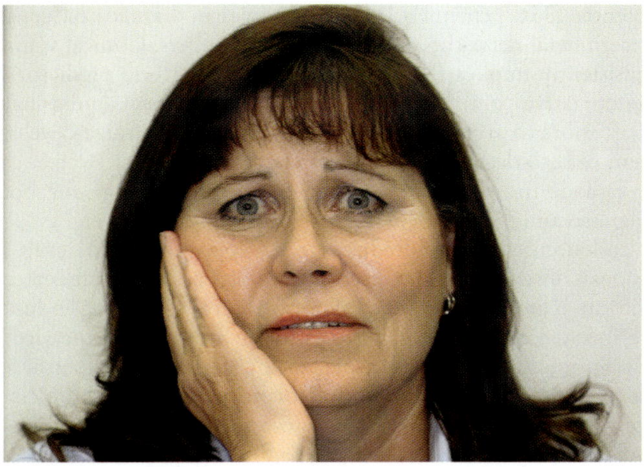

• **Fig. 9.1** Patient is distraught from severe pain of irreversible pulpitis. This patient will be a challenge to diagnose and treat.

visit cannot be rescheduled because of the severity of the problem. *Urgency* indicates a less severe problem; a visit may be scheduled for mutual convenience of the patient and the dentist. Key questions, which may be asked by telephone, to determine severity include the following:

1. Does the problem disturb your sleeping, eating, working, concentrating, or other daily activities? (A true emergency disrupts the patient's activities or quality of life.)
2. How long has this problem been bothering you? (A true emergency has rarely been severe for more than a few hours to 2 days.)
3. Have you taken any pain medication? Was the medication ineffective? (Analgesics do not relieve the pain of a true emergency.)

Affirmative answers to these questions require an immediate office visit for management and constitute a true emergency. Obviously, the patient's emotional and mental status must also be determined. To some patients, even a minor problem has major proportions and is disruptive.

Development of a System

Because a misdiagnosis will probably result in improper treatment and an exacerbation of the problem, a systematic approach is mandatory. The emotional status of the patient, pressures of time, and stress on dentist and staff should not affect such an orderly approach.

Pain Perception and Pain Reaction

Pain is a complex physiologic and psychological phenomenon. Pain perception levels are not constant; pain thresholds as well as reactions to pain change significantly in various circumstances.[36] Psychological components of pain perception and pain reaction comprise cognitive, emotional, and symbolic factors. The pain reaction threshold is significantly altered by past experiences and by present anxiety levels and emotional status. Anxiety decreases levels of both pain perception and pain reaction.[37]

To reduce anxiety and consequently obtain reliable information about the chief complaint and to receive cooperation during treatment, the clinician should (1) establish and maintain control of the situation, (2) gain the confidence of the patient, (3) provide attention and sympathy, and (4) treat the patient as an important individual.[38] Providing positive written information about pain control during root canal therapy can also reduce the fear associated with an emergency endodontic procedure.[39] By managing these pain components, pain perception and reaction thresholds are raised significantly, greatly facilitating the procedure. Psychological management of the patient is the most important factor in emergency treatment!

Adjunctive pharmacotherapy may also be required in the management of patient anxiety during emergency treatment.[36] Reducing anxiety at this stage will not only reduce the response to potentially painful stimuli during treatment, but also will decrease the tendency for the patient to recall the endodontic procedure as unpleasant.[37] Mild anxiety may be managed with nitrous oxide[40]; however, the apparatus may be a bit cumbersome when obtaining treatment radiographs. Oral benzodiazepines can be very effective in managing more significant anxiety. Triazolam has a fast onset and a relatively short half-life and, because of its lipophilic nature, can be administered sublingually for rapid absorption.[41] Thus this anxiolytic medication is quite convenient for sedation in the dental office. One quarter of a milligram of oral triazolam has been shown to be as effective as intravenous diazepam.[42] Of course, patients who have taken or are given an oral sedative in the dental office must have transportation provided. Importantly, the potential drug interactions with other centrally acting agents must also be considered.

System of Diagnosis

Patients in pain often provide information and responses that are exaggerated and inaccurate. They tend to be confused as well as apprehensive. Clinicians may find it easy (and tempting) to rush through the diagnosis to institute treatment for a suffering patient. After pertinent information regarding the medical and dental histories is obtained, both subjective questioning and an objective examination are performed carefully and completely (See Box 9.1).[43,44]

A rule of the true emergency is that *one tooth is the offender,* that is, the source of pain. In the excitement of the moment, the patient might believe that the severe pain is emanating from more than a single tooth. The clinician may become convinced also, leading to overtreatment.

Medical and Dental Histories

Medical and dental histories should be reviewed first. If the patient is the dentist's own patient, the medical history is briefly reviewed and updated. If the patient is new, a standard, complete history is obtained. An important medical complication may be easily overlooked in an emergency situation. Certainly, the need for antibiotic prophylaxis must be determined even before initiating any portion of the oral examination that might induce a bacteremia, such as periodontal probing. Either a short or a complete dental history is recorded. This process includes recollection of dental procedures, recording a chronology of symptoms, or discussing an earlier relevant comment by a dentist.

Subjective Examination

When the patient is in pain, the subjective examination comprises careful questioning and is the most important aspect of diagnosis. Questions relate to the history, location, severity, duration, character, and eliciting stimuli of pain. Questions relating to the cause or stimulus that elicits or relieves the pain help select appropriate objective tests to arrive at a final diagnosis.

Pain that is elicited by thermal stimuli and/or pain that is referred is likely to originate from the pulp. Pain that occurs on mastication or tooth contact and is well localized is probably apical.

The three important factors constituting the quality and magnitude of pain are its spontaneity, intensity, and duration. If the patient reports any of these symptoms (and assuming that the patient is not exaggerating), significant pathosis is likely to be present. Careful questioning provides important information about the source of the pain and whether it is pulpal or periradicular. In fact, a perceptive, clever clinician should be able to arrive at a tentative diagnosis by means of a thorough subjective examination; objective tests and radiographic findings are then used for confirmation. For example, a reported complaint of severe, continuous (lingering) pain when the patient drinks cold beverages and marked tenderness on mastication indicates irreversible pulpitis and symptomatic apical periodontitis. These stimuli are then repeated in an objective examination to confirm the patient's response.

Objective Examination

An endodontic diagnosis consists of two parts: pulpal and periapical diagnoses. Therefore objective examination is a comprehensive evaluation of the health of the pulp and periapical tissues. The clinician's first clue to identifying the offending tooth is to carefully listen to the patient's chief complaint and reproduce it using all the available tools. Objective examination includes the following clinical tests.

Physical Condition/Extraoral Examination

It is imperative to not miss signs of an infectious spread systemically. Signs include extraoral swelling (unilateral or bilateral), facial cellulitis, lymphadenopathy, trismus, and eye shut. Such signs are commonly also involved with elevated temperature. In addition to the emotional factors that complicate the diagnosis of endodontic emergencies, physical conditions induced as a result of these situations also contribute to the problems. Pain or swelling may limit mouth opening, thereby hampering diagnostic procedures as well as treatment (Fig. 9.2, *A–D*). In addition, hypersensitivity to thermal stimuli or pressure influences diagnosis and treatment. Therefore the most severe aspect of the emergency is treated first to facilitate diagnosis.

Intraoral Examination

Included under this examination is observation for intraoral swelling or sinus tracts, as well as mirror and explorer examination to note the presence of defective restorations, discolored crowns, recurrent caries, and fractures.

Pulp Vitality Tests

Pulp vitality tests are the most commonly used objective tests for diagnosing a painful or offending tooth. Although cold, hot, and electric pulp tests (EPTs) truly test only the function of nerves rather than pulpal inflammation or vitality, they are the most convenient tests available. Among these assessments, cold testing is the most accurate test[45] and a combination of cold with EPT increases accuracy.

Again, it is important in identifying the offending tooth to repeat tests that mimic what the patient reports subjectively. In other words, the best test is to repeat the stimulus that reportedly causes the pain. This is especially true for pulpal disease that has not extended to the periradicular tissues (e.g., irreversible pulpitis with asymptomatic apical periodontitis). It is often difficult for the patient to localize the pain to a particular tooth due to the paucity of proprioceptive neurons in the dental pulp. As in the previous example, applying cold should reproduce pain of basically the same type and magnitude as that related by the patient. If similar subjective symptoms are not reproduced, this situation may not be a true emergency; the patient may be "overreporting" (exaggerating the problem), or the pain may be referred from a source other than that perceived by the patient.

Periapical Tests

Periapical inflammation occurs as early as 1 to 3 days after pulp exposure.[46-48] Conceivably, periapical symptoms such as tenderness to biting, chewing, and pain to palpation or pressure can ensue shortly after.[49,50] These symptoms often occur despite absence of periapical bone resorption on radiographic examination, and therefore clinical tests that can localize pain to the offending tooth are essential tools for diagnosis of the periapical inflammatory status. These include (1) palpation over the apex; (2) digital pressure on, or wiggling of, teeth (preferred if the patient reports severe pain on mastication); (3) light percussion with the end of the mirror handle; and (4) selective biting on an object such as a cotton swab or Tooth Slooth.

Periodontal Examination

A periodontal examination is always necessary. Probing helps in differentiating endodontic from periodontal disease. For example, a periodontal abscess can simulate an acute apical abscess (Fig. 9.3); however, with a localized periodontal abscess, the pulp is usually vital (see Chapter 7). In contrast, an acute apical abscess is related to an unresponsive (necrotic) pulp. These abscesses occasionally communicate with the sulcus and have a deep probing defect. In addition to these tests, when the differential diagnosis is difficult, a test cavity may identify the pulp status and isolate the offending tooth. A narrow-walled, isolated probing defect may also indicate a coronal fracture that has extended beyond the level of sulcular attachment, or a vertical root fracture (see Chapter 8).

Radiographic Examination

Radiographic examination is a crucial tool in diagnosing the offending tooth. As stated before, patients often have difficulty localizing pulpal pain. Additionally, studies have demonstrated that approximately half the teeth with periapical pathosis are asymptomatic to periapical tests.[3] Vitality tests certainly aid in narrowing down the source of pain to one to two teeth. When vitality tests cannot confirm the true diagnosis due to presence of crowns, multiple teeth involvement, an anxious patient, or a patient with heightened responses to clinical tests, radiographic examination can provide several key clues that point to the offender. Recurrent caries, possible pulpal exposure, internal or external resorption, unusual appearance of the lamina dura, periapical pathosis, and traceable sinus tracts are some very important identifiers that help confirm diagnosis.

Both periapical and bitewing radiographs must be exposed during initial evaluation, as clinicians must never miss an opportunity to determine restorability of a tooth in addition to identifying the cause of the emergency. Additionally, three-dimensional

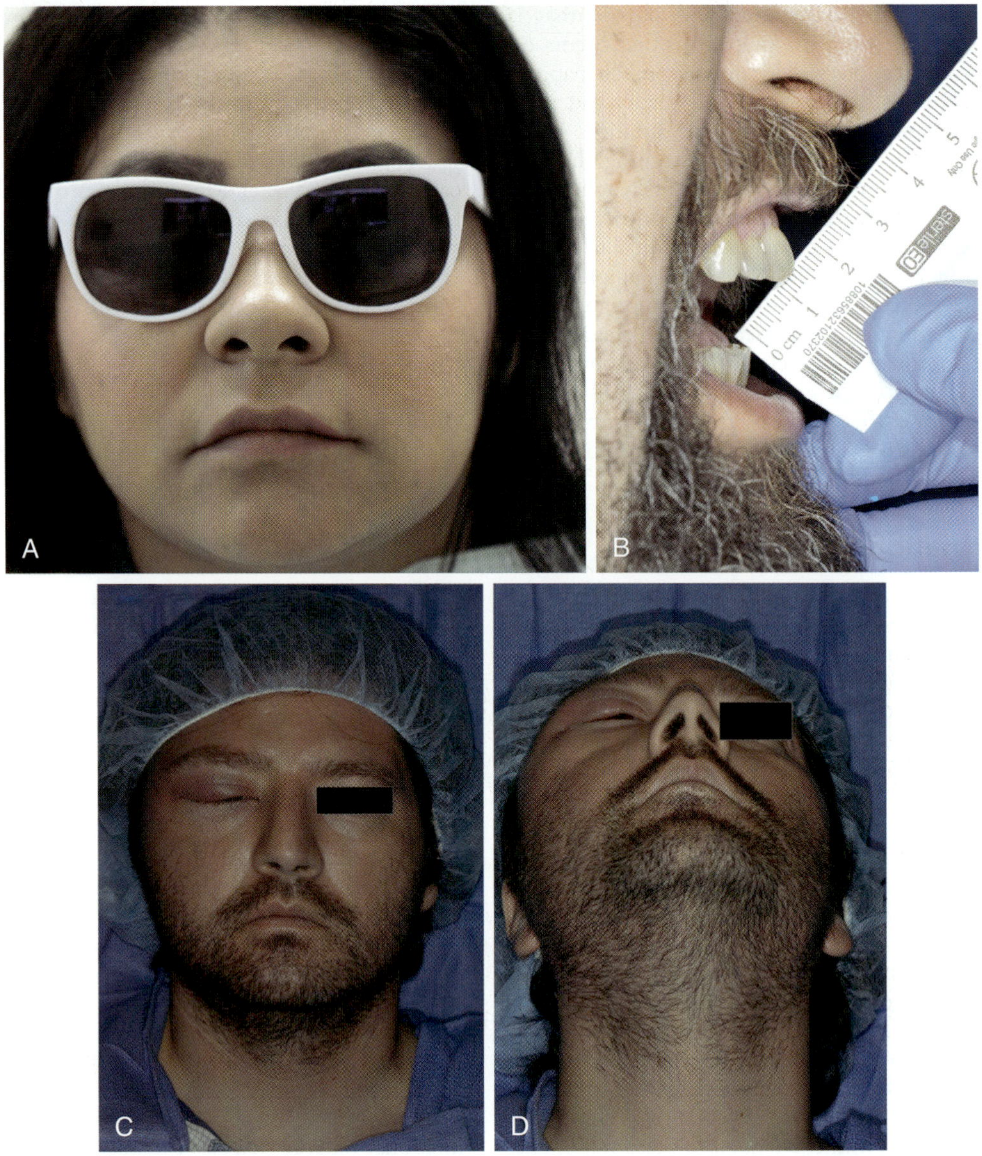

• **Fig. 9.2** Examples of **A,** mandibular swelling; **B**, trismus; **C** and **D**, eye shut. (Courtesy Dr. Daniel Perez, UTHSCSA, San Antonio, TX, USA.)

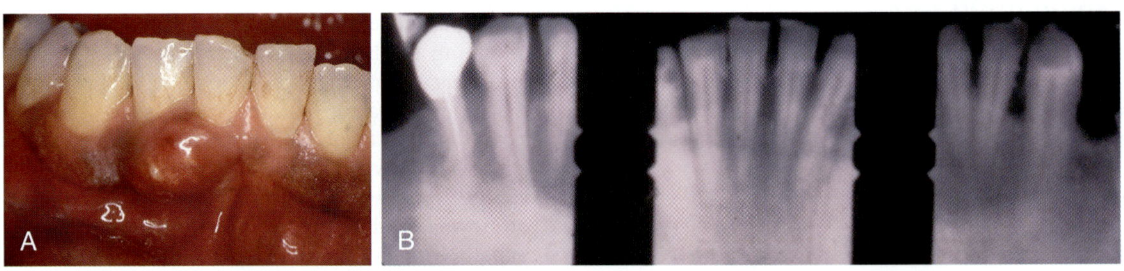

• **Fig. 9.3** Periodontal abscess with vital mandibular anterior teeth. **A,** Clinical photo obuccal swelling; and **B,** Periapical radiograph of periodontal bone loss. (Courtesy Dr. Brian Mealey, UTHSCSA, San Antonio.)

(3D) cone beam computed tomography (CBCT) renders diagnosis more predictable than two-dimensional (2D) imaging alone. Some of the most diagnostically challenging cases are ones with tooth fractures. A recent meta-analysis suggests that CBCT has greater accuracy in confirming tooth fractures in teeth with clinically suspected but periapical-radiography–undetected tooth fractures.[51] CBCT imaging therefore not only elevates a clinician's ability to accurately diagnose, but also to appropriately treat an emergency case. To this end, knowing the offending tooth's anatomy, the 3D relationship of critical anatomic structures such

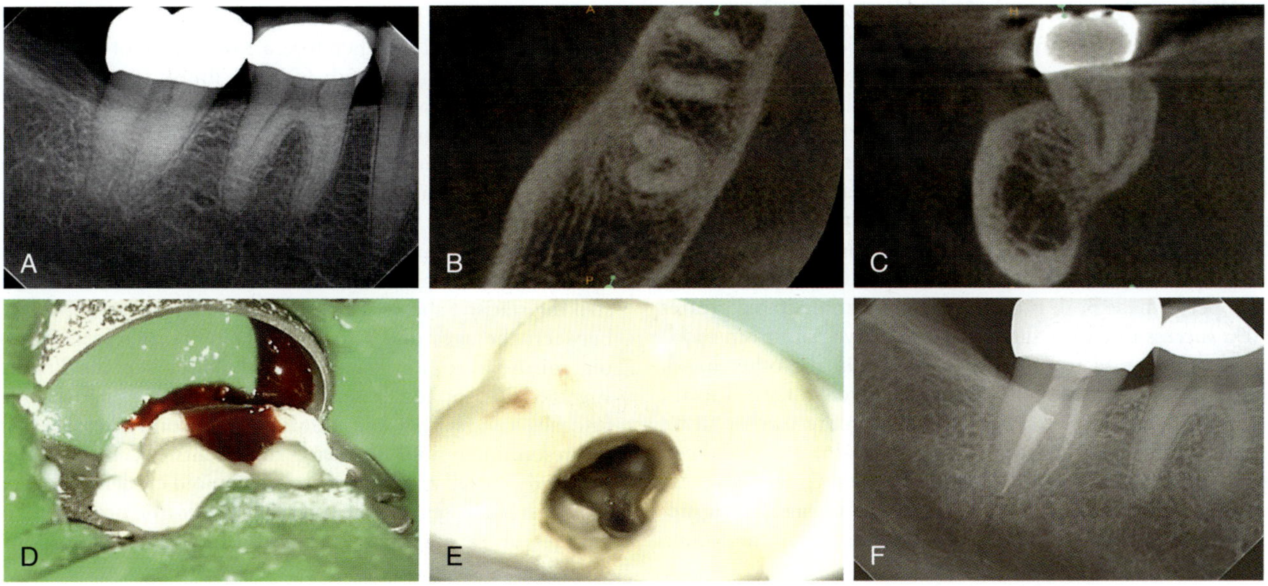

• **Fig. 9.4** A difficult management case of symptomatic irreversible pulpitis with symptomatic apical periodontitis for a 60-year-old female patient with pain at 10/10 on visual analog scale (VAS). **A**, Preoperative radiograph of #31. **B**, Axial view of #31 showing mesiobuccal (MB) canal and C-shaped canal. **C,** Sagittal view of #31 showing anatomy of the C-shaped canal. **D**, Photograph of #31 with profuse hemorrhage upon access. **E**, MB and C-shaped canal anatomy at orifice level. **F**, Postoperative radiograph of completed obturation and access restoration at second visit. (Courtesy Dr. Anibal Diogenes, UTHSCSA San Antonio, TX, USA.)

as the inferior alveolar nerve (IAN), and the extent of resorptive defects, are some unique advantages of 3D imaging.[52]

Collectively, a systematic approach to diagnosis must be followed, and a combination of subjective and objective findings are carefully collected before attempting treatment. More specifics of diagnosis are included in Chapter 4.

Diagnostic Outcome

After carefully working through the sequence described in the previous sections, the offending tooth and the tissue (pulpal or periapical) that is the source of pain should have been identified and a pulpal and periradicular diagnosis recorded. For many reasons, all or none of these conclusions may be clear. This circumstance may not be a true emergency, or the problem may be beyond the capability of the general dentist, and the patient should be referred (Fig. 9.4). However, if the diagnosis is clear, treatment planning follows.

Treatment Planning

As previously discussed, inflammation and its consequences, i.e., increased tissue pressure and release of chemical mediators in the inflamed pulp or periapical tissues, are the major causes of painful dental emergencies.[53] Therefore reducing the irritant, reduction of pressure, or removal of the inflamed pulp or periapical tissue should be the immediate goal; this approach usually results in pain relief. Of the two, pressure release is the most effective.

Pretreatment Emergencies

These emergencies require a diagnosis and treatment sequencing. Each of these steps is important: (1) categorizing the problem, (2) taking a medical history, (3) identifying the source, (4) making the diagnosis, (5) planning the treatment, and (6) treating the patient.

Patient Management

Patient management is always the most critical factor. The frightened patient in pain must have confidence that his or her problem is being properly managed.

Profound Anesthesia

Obtaining profound anesthesia of inflamed painful tissues is a challenge. Adequate anesthesia, however, will instill confidence and cooperation and influence the patient's desire to save the offending tooth. Maxillary anesthesia is usually obtained by infiltration, or block injections in the buccal and palatal regions. With mandibular teeth, in addition to an IAN block with lidocaine, a long buccal injection for soft tissue anesthesia as well as infiltration of articaine on the facial may be necessary. Often (particularly with mandibular molars), although all "classic" signs of profound anesthesia are present (such as lip numbness), access into the dentin or pulp is painful, presumably due to sensitized pulpal nociceptors. It is therefore prudent to retest the tooth with a cold stimulus to assess pulpal anesthesia before initiating access into the pulp space. For those patients who still respond with pain, periodontal, intrapulpal, or intraosseous injection techniques are indicated.[54,55] These supplemental injections are often administered prophylactically, particularly with painful irreversible pulpitis.[54] Other conditions (for example, acute apical abscess) require other approaches. Chapter 8 contains details.

Management of Symptomatic Irreversible Pulpitis

Because pain is the result of inflammation, primarily in the coronal pulp, removal of the inflamed tissue will usually reduce the pain.

With or Without Symptomatic Apical Periodontitis

Teeth with caries, large restorations, cracked teeth, or trauma are some etiologies of symptomatic irreversible pulpitis. Complete cleaning and shaping of the root canals are the preferred treatments if time permits. Access to contemporary aids such as the electronic apex locator (EAL), surgical operating microscope (SOM), ultrasonic instruments, and CBCT facilitates complete instrumentation. However, during times when time- or patient-related factors prevent complete instrumentation, pulpotomy or a partial pulpectomy on the largest canals (palatal or distal root of molars) is performed. Both procedures have demonstrated greater than 90% success rate in reducing postoperative pain from moderate to severe to mild to no pain.[25,35,56-59] On the other hand, partial pulpectomy, but not pulpotomy of severely inflamed teeth, upregulates inflammatory mediators that promote further nerve sprouting, leading to greater postoperative pain, and has been strongly discouraged.[56,60] When there is a vital, inflamed pulp, other procedures such as trephination (artificial fistulation) by creating an opening through mucosa and bone are not useful and are contraindicated.[59,61]

An old but still popular idea is that chemical medicaments sealed in chambers help control or prevent additional pain; this idea is not true. A dry cotton pellet alone is as effective in relieving pain as a pellet moistened with camphorated monochlorophenol (CMCP), formocresol, Cresatin, eugenol, or saline.[58,62] Therefore after irrigation of the chamber or canals with sodium hypochlorite (NaOCl), a dry cotton pellet is placed, and the access is sealed temporarily. These cases can be completed in a single visit; however, results of a recent meta-analysis suggest that cases completed in one visit are more likely to have postoperative pain medication consumption.[63] Moreover, as stated before, preoperative pain is a strong predictor of postoperative pain. Additionally, calcium hydroxide [$Ca(OH)_2$] has been shown to significantly reduce inflammatory mediators such as cytokines and neuropeptides[64] commonly known to activate and sensitize nociceptors.[65,66] Therefore allowing further reduction in the inflammatory load with intracanal medicament placement may reduce the probability of postoperative pain associated with one-visit cases. Lastly, reducing the occlusion to eliminate contact has been shown to aid in relief of symptoms[67] but does not prevent symptoms.[68]

Postoperative Pharmacologic Management

Pain Management: Recent systematic reviews and meta-analysis demonstrate that 600 mg ibuprofen or 600 mg ibuprofen with N-acetyl-p-aminophenol (APAP) 1000 mg is most effective in attenuating postoperative endodontic pain.[69,70] To prevent the build-up of the arachidonic acid metabolites that contribute a large portion of the inflammatory pain stimulus, the patient should take the first dose before the loss of local anesthesia and then take the nonsteroidal antiinflammatory drug (NSAID) "by the clock," rather than "as needed" (PRN). Administering ibuprofen to the patient while in the chair has been shown to reduce initial postoperative pain.[71] Moreover, a newer ibuprofen formulation, ibuprofen sodium dihydrate at a 512-mg dose has been shown to have a faster onset of action than ibuprofen acid producing a greater reduction in spontaneous pain and mechanical allodynia.[26] It is noteworthy that the U.S. Food and Drug Administration (FDA)-recommended maximum daily dose of APAP is 4 gm per day, owing to the increasing evidence of APAP-induced hepatoxicity.[72-74] However, it is well known that patients often underreport their use of over-the-counter (OTC) medications, such as NyQuil, Theraflu, and so on, that contain as high as 500 to 1000 mg APAP.[75] Therefore a lower dose of 325 to 500 mg APAP in combination with 600 mg ibuprofen will have a safer drug profile compared with 1000 mg APAP, and will avoid "therapeutic misadventures."

For patients with severe postoperative pain, other drug classes such as opioids maybe considered. However, the clinician must be fully aware of the recent opioid crisis that prevails; opioid overdose-related deaths have increased five-fold since 1999 (https://www.cdc.gov/drugoverdose/epidemic/index.html). An even more striking statistic shows that prescription opioid use by adolescents between the ages of 19 to 23 has a 33% increased risk of opioid misuse at a later stage in life.[76] Moreover, the Practitioners Engaged in Applied Research and Learning (PEARL) Network findings suggest that endodontists are second after oral surgeons in prescribing opioid-like drugs to patients.[77] Clinicians must significantly curtail contributing to the opioid epidemic. For patients with persistent, severe pain after an endodontic procedure, opioids with less abuse potential must be considered. Tramadol, a mu-opioid agonist, at varying doses has shown to have fewer opioid-like central effects compared with morphine[78] (RA, 2018 #924); however, it is not devoid of addiction and abuse potential and must be used judiciously for severe postoperative pain. Ultracet (325 mg APAP, 37.5 mg tramadol) is a combination drug, which is a viable option for patients with severe postoperative pain. See Fig. 9.5 for a flexible analgesic strategy.

Postoperative pain is attributed in large part to a process called *central sensitization.* Constant input from primary afferent nerve fibers can increase activity in the second-order neuron located in the trigeminal nucleus and cause signal amplification. Randomized clinical trials have elegantly demonstrated that administration of 0.5% bupivacaine with 1:200,000 epinephrine preoperatively significantly reduces postoperative pain at 6 and 12 hours compared with 2% lidocaine with 1:80,000 epinephrine after treatment of teeth with symptomatic irreversible pulpitis.[79,80]

Other pharmacologic drugs targeted at minimizing postendodontic pain include corticosteroids. Steroids inhibit phospholipase A2 enzyme upon membrane release of arachidonic acid, thereby inhibiting effects mediated by both lipoxygenases and cyclooxygenases. Several studies have evaluated the effects of corticosteroids in the prevention of postoperative endodontic pain and have demonstrated that drugs such as prednisolone and dexamethasone significantly attenuate the incidence of pain at 6, 12, and 24 hours posttreatment.[81,82] Collectively, several strategies are available to the clinician to reduce postoperative pain in patients with symptomatic irreversible pulpitis.

Use of Antibiotics: The irreversibly inflamed pulp is still vital and immunocompetent, with the ability to resist bacterial infection. Antibiotics, therefore, are definitely not indicated in cases of irreversible pulpitis without swelling.[83] Moreover, antibiotics are not analgesics and have no role in inhibition of nociceptors.[5,35] Unfortunately, old habits die hard, and there are still practitioners who prescribe antibiotics inappropriately, as in the case of irreversible pulpitis.[84] Antibiotic administration has the potential to result in at least two very serious sequelae: adverse reaction to the antibiotic, as well as increasing antibiotic-resistant microbial strains. The former is a local problem in which injudicious use of an antibiotic could lead to a life-threatening situation for an allergic patient. The latter is a global problem. Resistant microbial strains are emerging faster than pharmaceutical companies

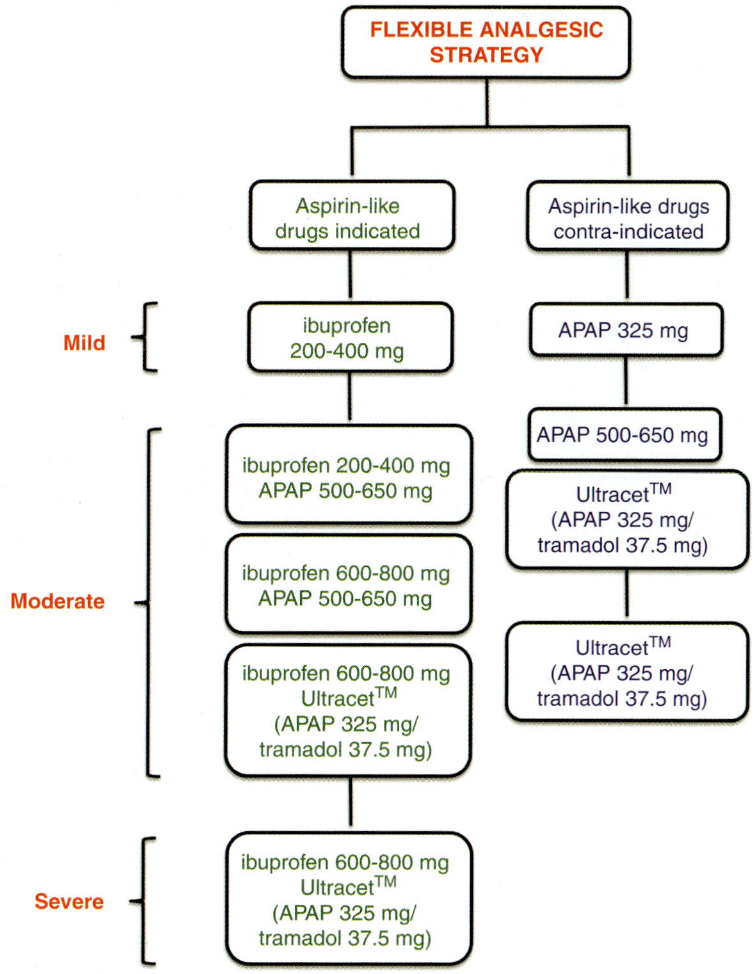

• **Fig. 9.5** Simplified analgesic strategy to guide drug selection based on patient history and level of present or anticipated posttreatment pain.

are developing new antibiotics; therefore it is critical that health care providers practice good stewardship with existing antibiotics.[85] Otherwise, in the near future there may not be a pharmacologic option in treating severe odontogenic or systemic infections.

Management of Pulp Necrosis with Apical Pathosis

The pain is related to periradicular inflammation, which results from potent irritants in the necrotic tissue in the pulp space. Treatment now is biphasic: (1) remove or reduce the pulp irritants and (2) relieve the apical fluid pressure (when possible). Therefore with pulp necrosis and pain from periradicular tissues there may be (1) symptomatic apical periodontitis without swelling, (2) acute apical abscess with localized intraoral swelling, or (3) acute apical abscess with diffuse extraoral swelling. Each circumstance is managed differently.

Pulp Necrosis/Symptomatic Apical Periodontitis Without Swelling

The microbiota is much more developed and stable compared with severely inflamed pulps. These teeth harbor not just planktonic bacteria but also well-established biofilms that release their toxins and byproducts into the canal system as well as into the periapical tissues. An inflammatory response consisting of activation of innate and adaptive immune cells and release of inflammatory mediators such as interleukin-1 (IL-1), prostaglandin E2 (PGE2), and tumor necrosis factor-α (TNF-α)[53,86] activate osteoclasts, leading to bone resorption. Some of these lesions expand and form an abscess that is confined to bone. These abscesses are often painful, primarily because of fluid pressure in a noncompliant environment. The two-fold aim is to reduce the canal irritants and to try to encourage some drainage through the tooth. Complete canal débridement, after determining the correct working length, is the treatment of choice. If time is limited, partial débridement at the estimated working length is performed with light instrumentation with a passive step-back or crown-down technique to reduce or remove irritating debris. Canals are not enlarged without knowledge of the working length. During cleaning, canals are flooded and flushed with copious amounts of full-strength NaOCl (6% or 8%). Finally, canals are irrigated with 17% ethylene diaminetetraacetic acid (17% ethylenediaminetetraacetic acid [EDTA]) followed by NaOCl, dried with paper points, filled with $Ca(OH)_2$ paste (if the preparation is large enough), and sealed with a dry cotton pellet and a temporary restoration. The access must never be left open for drainage.

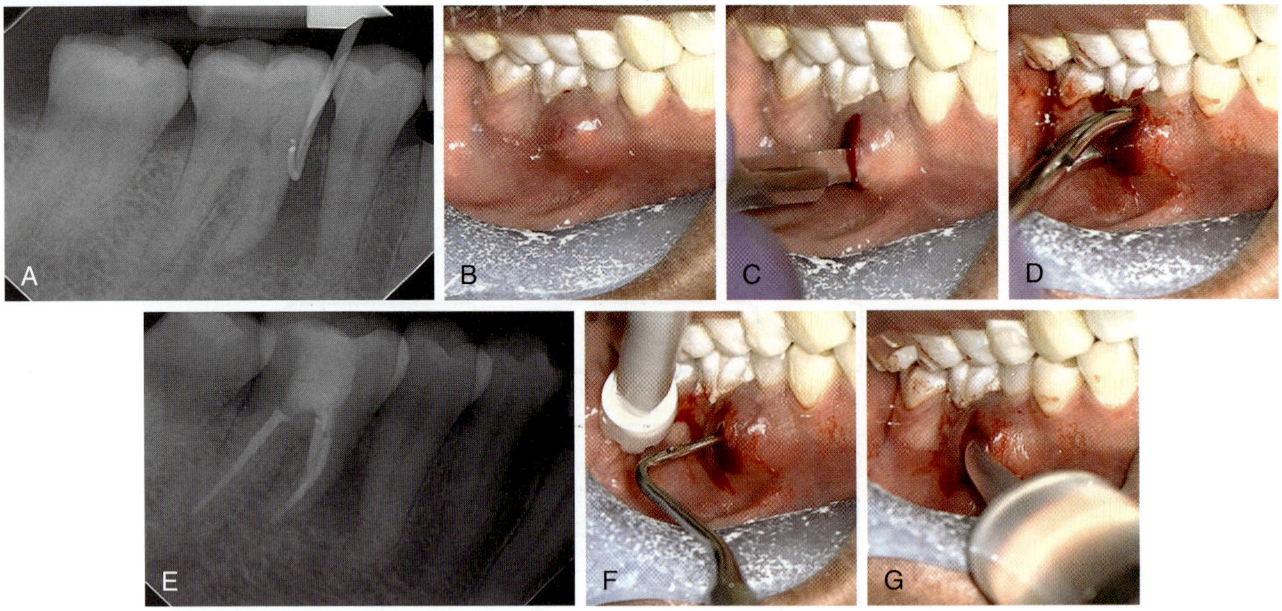

• **Fig. 9.6** Management of pulp necrosis with acute apical abscess with localized intraoral swelling for a 60-year-old female patient with pain at 5/5 on visual analog scale (VAS). **A,** Preoperative radiograph of #30 with sulcular sinus tract. **B,** Preoperative photograph of intraoral swelling. **C,** Photograph of incision. **D,** Blunt dissection. **E,** Postoperative radiograph of completed obturation and access restoration at second visit. **F,** Curettage. **G,** Sterile saline irrigation. (Courtesy Dr. Saeed Bayat, UTHSCSA, San Antonio, TX, USA.)

Postoperative Pharmacologic Management

Pain Management: Pain-management protocols follow guidelines similar to those stated previously. Antibiotics are not indicated due to lack of systemic involvement.[87] The patient is informed that there will still be some pain (the inflamed, sensitive periapical tissues are still present), but that the pain usually subsides during the next 2 or 3 days, as the inflammation decreases.

Management of Infections: These patients seldom have elevated temperatures or other systemic signs.[88] Therefore in acute apical abscess with localized swelling, the use of systemic antibiotics is not necessary, having been shown to be of no benefit.[87,89,90]

Pulp Necrosis/Acute Apical Abscess with Localized Intraoral Swelling

In these situations, an abscess has invaded regional soft tissues, and, at times, there is purulent exudate in the canal. Radiographic findings range from no periapical change (seldom) to a large radiolucency. Again, treatment is biphasic. *First and most important* is débridement (complete cleaning and shaping if time permits) of the canal or canals. *Second in urgency* is drainage. Localized swelling (whether fluctuant or nonfluctuant) should be incised (Fig. 9.6). Drainage accomplishes three things: (1) relief of pressure and pain, (2) removal of potent irritants (purulence and inflammatory mediators), and (3) prevention of the spread of infection to fascial spaces.

In teeth that drain readily after opening, instrumentation should be confined to the root canal system (Fig. 9.7). In patients with a periapical abscess but no drainage through the canal, penetration of the apical foramen with small files (up to #25) may initiate drainage and release of pressure. This release often does not occur because the abscess cavity does not communicate directly with the apical foramen. Copious irrigation with NaOCl reduces amounts of necrotic tissue and bacteria. The canals are then dried with paper points and filled with $Ca(OH)_2$ paste. Occasionally, purulence will continue to fill the canal during the preparation (the so-called "weeping" canal). If this occurs, the patient should sit for some time. Usually, the flow will cease, and the access may be closed. After placement of a dry cotton pellet, the access is sealed temporarily. These teeth should not be left open to drain. A canal exposed to the oral cavity is a potential home for introduced bacteria, food debris, and even viruses and leads to increased exacerbation from an activated immune response.[91]

After débridement, an incision and drainage (I&D) procedure must be performed in cases with more than one abscess (see Fig. 9.7): one that communicates with the apex when another separate abscess is found in the vestibule. Because they do not communicate, drainage must occur through both the tooth and a mucosal incision. Steps of an I&D procedure typically involve a vertical incision followed by blunt dissection of the incised area, thorough curettage and copious irrigation with sterile saline and/or 0.12% chlorhexidine (see Fig. 9.7). A drain maybe placed if cessation of drainage does not occur during the appointment. Postoperative pain may be associated with the I&D procedure; however, this pain typically resolves within 2 to 3 days.[92]

Postoperative Pharmacologic Management

Pain Management: An analgesic regimen appropriate for mild to moderate pain should be followed as described previously; relief of pressure is most important in pain control for these patients.

Management of Infections: These patients seldom experience an elevated temperature or other systemic signs. Therefore in acute apical abscess with localized swelling, the use of systemic antibiotics is not necessary, having been shown to be of no benefit.[88]

Pulp Necrosis with Diffuse Swelling

Endodontic abscesses that perforate through the cortical bone can spread to nearby fascial spaces; these occurrences are also referred to as cellulitis. The muscle attachment and arrangement

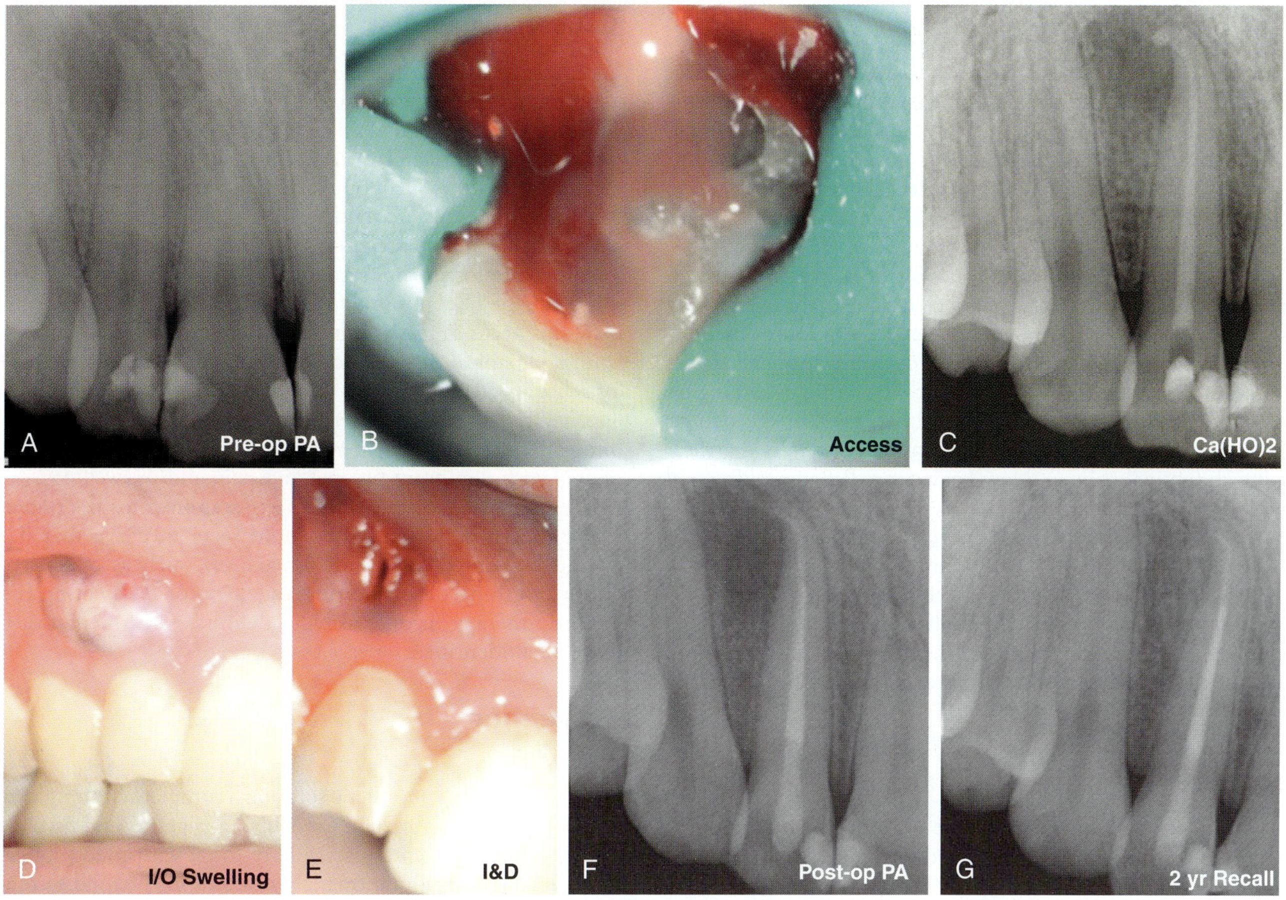

• **Fig. 9.7** Management of pulp necrosis with acute apical abscess with localized intraoral swelling for a 60-year-old female patient with pain at 5/5 on visual analog scale (VAS). **A,** Preoperative radiograph of #7. **B**, Drainage through tooth upon access. **C**, Radiograph of #7 with calcium hydroxide [$Ca(OH)_2$]. **D**, Preoperative photograph of intraoral swelling. **E**, Photograph post–incision and drainage. **F**, Postoperative radiograph of completed obturation and access restoration at second visit. **G**, Postoperative radiograph at 2 years post treatment. (Courtesy Dr. Obadah Austah, UTHSCSA, San Antonio, TX, USA.)

of fasciae will determine the pathway of spread and the possible site of localization. These rapidly progressive and spreading swellings are not localized and may have dissected into the fascial spaces (Fig. 9.2A-D). Limited opening, pain and difficulty in swallowing, and occasionally bilateral spread may also occur. Fortunately, these serious infections seldom occur. There may be elevated temperature or other systemic signs indicating a potentially serious infection. These patients should be referred to an oral surgeon for extraoral drainage, intravenous antibiotics, and pain management. Often, the patient is hospitalized for this aggressive treatment.

Once stable, the patient may return for initiation of canal débridement. Most important is removal of the irritant by canal débridement (cleaning and shaping is completed, if possible) or by extraction. The apical foramen may be gently penetrated with a file to permit any possible flow of exudate, although drainage often does not occur. After placing $Ca(OH)_2$ paste and a dry pellet, the access is closed with a temporary restoration.

Postoperative Pharmacologic Management

Pain Management: An analgesic regimen appropriate for moderate-severe pain should be followed as described previously; resolution of extraoral swelling will provide for maximum pain relief for these patients.

Management of Infections: Systemic antibiotics are indicated for diffuse, rapidly spreading swelling (cellulitis).[93] Culturing and molecular identification techniques used to study odontogenic abscesses reveal a polymicrobial infection, with anaerobic species predominating.[94-96] Antibiotic sensitivity testing confirms that the majority of isolates are susceptible to penicillin VK (Pen VK).[95] However, its bactericidal efficacy is significantly lower than that of other drugs such as amoxicillin due to inferior penetration and absorption properties. Moreover, it is associated with gastrointestinal side effects due to depletion of gut commensal flora.[93] Amoxicillin with clavulanic acid has shown a 100% efficacy against pathogens found in endodontic abscesses followed by amoxicillin with metronidazole at 99%. Amoxicillin achieves higher serum levels, maintained over a longer period of time than Pen VK. A loading dose of amoxicillin 1-g load followed by 500 mg every 6 hours for 2 to 3 days must be prescribed.

For patients with penicillin allergy, clindamycin is an alternative that demonstrates 96% antibacterial efficacy in vitro. It has superior oral absorption with excellent distribution in bone. It has both bacteriostatic and bactericidal effects and is effective against gram-positive aerobes and gram-positive and negative anaerobes, thereby satisfying a broad spectrum of microbes. A loading dose of 300 to 600 mg followed by 150 to 300 mg every 6 hours for 2 to 3 days must be prescribed. Note: Shorter prescription duration has been recommended based on emerging evidence and recommendations. Recent evidence suggests that shorter prescription duration of 2 to 3 days until resolution of symptoms is equally efficacious as longer prescription duration of 7 to 10 days. Moreover, the longer the commensal microbes in our bodies are exposed to antibiotics, the greater their ability to select for resistance. Therefore our threat increases more from the commensal bacteria than from pathogenic bacteria.[93,97-100]

Because of the reduction in normal gut flora, patients on oral antibiotics occasionally develop signs of colitis due to the overgrowth of *Clostridium difficile* and a potentially fatal condition of pseudomembranous colitis. This problem can occur with nearly all classes of antibiotics, especially clindamycin, which has an eight-fold higher risk of *C. difficile* infection compared with penicillin; the patient should be warned to watch for the development of watery diarrhea, cramping abdominal pain, and low-grade fever. Patients taking oral contraceptives for whom antibiotics are prescribed should also be warned to use alternative methods during, and for 1 week after, the course of antibiotic therapy. There is some clinical, albeit empirical, evidence that probiotics may minimize the superinfections.

Speed of recovery (whether the swelling is localized or diffuse) depends primarily on canal débridement and drainage. Because edema (fluid) has spread through the tissues, diffuse swelling decreases slowly over several days.

Postoperative Instructions

With all emergencies, patients must be informed of their responsibilities and of what to expect. Pain and swelling will take time to resolve. Proper nutrition and adequate intake of fluids are important, and medications must be taken as prescribed. The problem may recur or worsen (flare-up), requiring another emergency visit.[5] Communication is very important; calling the patient the day after the appointment reduces pain perception and analgesic needs[101] and allows for closer monitoring of progress.

Interappointment Emergencies

The interappointment flare-up is a true emergency that occurs after an endodontic appointment and is so severe that an unscheduled patient visit and treatment are required. Despite judicious and careful treatment procedures, complications such as pain, swelling, or both may occur. Regional temporary paresthesia has even been reported.[57] As with emergencies occurring before root canal therapy, these flare-ups are undesirable and disruptive events and must be resolved quickly. Occasionally flare-ups are unexpected, although they can often be better predicted according to certain patient presenting factors.

Incidence

The reported incidence of flare-ups in endodontics varies widely due to variations in study parameters. Properly controlled prospective studies show an incidence of approximately 3%.[5,102,103] Even though the occurrence is low, interappointment flare-ups represent such a stressful situation to the patient (most postoperative discomfort is in the mild to moderate range), that it behooves the prudent clinician to consider the likely related factors and to try to prepare the patient for the possibility of such an event. It is especially distressing for the patient who had minimal preoperative discomfort to experience pain and/or swelling after treatment.

Causative Factors

Assessing causality is difficult when reviewing the literature on flare-ups; however, certain risk factors have emerged. These factors generally can be categorized as related to the patient (including pulpal or periapical diagnosis). Treatment procedures are unrelated to flare-ups, although this is a popular belief. Patient factors include gender (more flare-ups are reported to occur in females, although this circumstance may represent a greater tendency for females to seek medical care for painful symptoms)[104] and preoperative diagnosis. Flare-ups are uncommon in teeth with vital pulps.[5,105] More often, flare-ups occur in teeth with necrotic pulps, and especially in those with a periapical diagnosis of symptomatic periapical periodontitis or acute apical abscess.[5,102,105,106] The presence of a periapical radiolucency has also been shown to be a risk factor.[5,102,103,107] Clearly, the patient who experiences a flare-up is more likely to have presented with significant preoperative pain and/or swelling.

Treatment factors have also been examined for the potential to cause flare-ups. Although it would seem intuitive that flare-ups would be related to certain procedures, such as overinstrumentation, pushing debris beyond the apex, or completing the endodontic therapy in one visit, no definitive treatment risk factors have been identified.

Prevention

Procedures

Use of long-acting anesthetic solutions, complete cleaning and shaping of the root canal system (possibly), analgesics, and psychological preparation of patients (particularly those with preoperative pain) will decrease interappointment symptoms in the mild to moderate levels.[35] There are, however, no demonstrated treatment or therapeutic measures that will reduce the number of interappointment flare-ups. In other words, no particular relationship has been shown between flare-ups and specific treatment procedures.

Verbal Instructions

Most important is the preparation of patients for what to expect after the appointment. They should be told that discomfort ("soreness") is likely; the discomfort should subside within a day or two. Increases in pain, noticeable swelling, or other adverse signs necessitate a call and sometimes a visit. This explanation reduces the number of calls from unnecessarily concerned patients.

Therapeutic Prophylaxis

A popular preventive approach has been the prescribing of antibiotics to minimize postoperative symptoms. This practice has been demonstrated to be not useful and needlessly exposes the patient to expensive, potentially dangerous drugs, as described previously.[108-110] In contrast, certain NSAIDs have been shown to reduce postendodontic treatment pain.[71,111] For patients at risk for a flare-up, 400-600 mg of ibuprofen should be given while the patient is in the chair, and then taken by the clock for the first 24 to 48 hours postoperatively. Although this medication will reduce postoperative symptoms, it is uncertain whether it will reduce the incidence of flare-ups.

Diagnosis

The same basic procedure is followed as outlined earlier in this chapter for pretreatment emergencies, although with modifications. The problem has already been diagnosed initially; the clinician has an advantage. However, a step-by-step approach to diagnosing the existing condition reduces confusion and error; most important, it calms a patient who has been frightened by the episode of pain or swelling. After the underlying complications are identified, treatment is initiated.

Treatment of Flare-Ups

Reassurance (the "Big R") is the most important aspect of treatment. The patient is generally frightened and upset and may even assume that extraction is necessary. The explanation is that the flare-up is neither unusual nor irrevocable and will be managed. Next in importance are restoring the patient's comfort and breaking the pain cycle. For extended anesthesia and analgesia, administration of bupivacaine hydrochloride is recommended.[112]

Interappointment emergencies are divided into patients with an initial diagnosis of a vital or a necrotic pulp, and patients with or without swelling.

Previously Vital Pulps with Complete Débridement

If complete removal of the inflamed vital pulp tissues was accomplished at the first visit, this situation is unlikely to be a true flare-up, and patient reassurance and the prescription of a mild to moderate analgesic (9.5) often will suffice. Generally, nothing is to be gained by opening these teeth; the pain will usually regress spontaneously, but it is important to check that the temporary restoration is not in traumatic occlusion. Placing corticosteroids in the canal or administering an intraoral or intramuscular injection of these medications after cleaning and shaping reduces inflammation and somewhat lowers the level of moderate pain.[113-115] Flare-ups, however, have not been shown to be prevented by steroids, whether administered intracanal or systemically.[116]

Previously Vital Pulps with Incomplete Débridement

In previously vital pulps with incomplete débridement, it is likely that tissue remnants have become inflamed and have become a major irritant. The working length should be rechecked, and the canal(s) should be carefully cleaned with copious irrigation with NaOCl. A dry cotton pellet is then placed, followed by a temporary restoration, and a mild to moderate analgesic is prescribed (see Fig. 9.5). Occasionally, a previously vital pulp (with or without complete débridement) will develop into an acute apical abscess. This problem will occur sometime after the appointment and indicates that pulpal remnants have become necrotic and are invaded by bacteria.

Previously Necrotic Pulps with No Swelling

Occasionally teeth with previously necrotic pulps but no swelling develop an acute apical abscess (flare-up) after the appointment (1). The abscess is confined to bone and can be very painful. The tooth is opened, and the canal is gently recleaned and irrigated with NaOCl. Drainage should be established if possible (see Fig. 9.7). If there is active drainage from the tooth after opening, the canal should be recleaned (or débridement completed) and irrigated with NaOCl. The rubber dam is left in place after the tooth is opened; the patient is allowed to rest pain-free for at least 30 minutes or until drainage stops. Then, the canals are dried, $Ca(OH)_2$ paste is placed, and the access is sealed. The tooth should not be left open! If there is no drainage, the tooth should also be lightly instrumented and gently irrigated, medicated with $Ca(OH)_2$ paste, and then closed. The symptoms usually subside but do so more slowly than if drainage were present. Again, patient education and reassurance are critical. A long-acting anesthetic and an analgesic regimen for moderate to severe pain are helpful; antibiotics are not indicated.[87,89]

Previously Necrotic Pulps with Swelling

These cases are best managed with I&D (see Fig. 9.6). In addition, it is most important that the canals have been débrided. If not, they should be opened and débrided, medicated with $Ca(OH)_2$ paste, and sealed. Then I&D with placement of a drain (if there is continuous drainage) are completed. Occasionally, but rarely, a flare-up or a presenting acute apical abscess may be serious or even life-threatening (Fig. 9.8). These situations may require hospitalization and aggressive therapy with the cooperation of an oral surgeon.

Follow-Up Care

With flare-ups, the patient should be contacted daily until the symptoms abate. Communication may be made by telephone; patients with more serious problems or those that are not resolving (many may not and require additional measures) should return to the dentist for treatment as described previously, depending on findings. When symptoms recur or cannot be controlled, these patients should be considered for referral. Ultimate treatment by a specialist may include extra measures, such as apical surgery, or even hospitalization.

Postobturation Emergencies

True emergencies (flare-ups) postobturation are infrequent, although pain at the mild level is common. Therefore active intervention is seldom necessary; usually symptoms will resolve spontaneously.

Causative Factors

Little is known about the etiologic factors involved in postoperative pain after obturation. Reports of the incidence of postobturation pain vary; however, most reports show that the pain tends to occur in the first 24 hours.[35,117] A correlation has been found between the level of obturation and pain incidence, with overextension associated with the highest incidence of discomfort.[35,117] Postobturation pain also relates to preobturation pain; levels of pain reported after obturation tend to correlate to levels of pain before the appointment.[117,118]

Treatment

Information about possible discomfort for the first few days (especially in patients who had higher levels of preoperative pain), reassurance about the availability of emergency services, and administration of analgesics for mild pain (see Fig. 9.5) significantly control the patient's anxiety and prevent overreaction. This support, in turn, decreases the incidence of postobturation frantic telephone calls or "emergency" visits. Some patients, however, do develop serious complications and require follow-up treatment.

Retreatment is indicated when prior treatment obviously has been inadequate. Apical surgery is often required when an acute apical abscess develops, and there is uncorrectable, inadequate root canal treatment. If root canal treatment was acceptable, I&D of swelling after obturation (an occasional occurrence) should be performed; usually the swelling resolves without further treatment. At times, the patient reports severe pain, but there is no evidence of acute apical abscess, and the root canal treatment has been well done. These patients are treated with reassurance and appropriate analgesics (see Fig. 9.5); again, the symptoms usually subside spontaneously.

Patients with postobturation emergencies that do not respond to therapy should be referred to an endodontist for other treatment modalities, such as surgery.

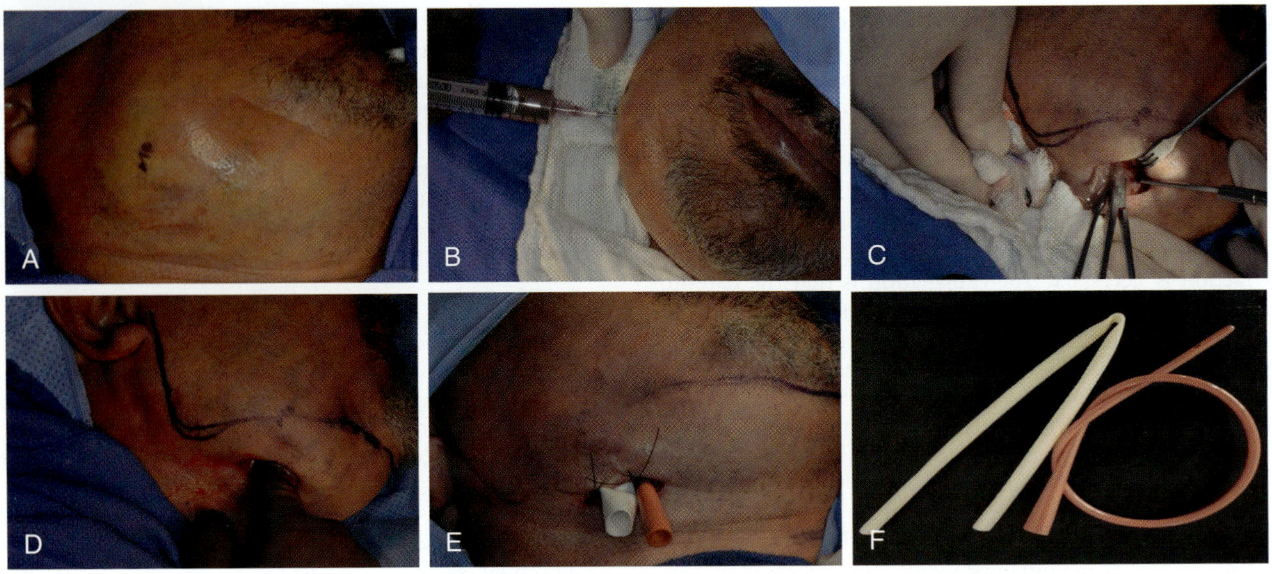

• **Fig. 9.8** Management of pulp necrosis with acute apical abscess with diffused extraoral swelling for a 43-year-old male patient hospitalized for aggressive therapy with nasal intubation. Pain at 5/5 on visual analog scale (VAS). **A**, Preoperative photograph of extraoral swelling. **B**, Photograph of syringe aspiration. **C** and **D**, Drainage. **E**, Postoperative photograph of two drains placed and sutured. **F**, Types of extraoral drains: Covidien Dover Rob-Nel Urethral Catheter and Penrose drain. (Courtesy Dr. Daniel Perez, UTHSCSA, San Antonio, TX, USA.)

Study Questions

1. What effect does anxiety have on pain threshold levels?
   a. Increases
   b. Decreases
   c. No effect
2. The most important aspect of diagnosis is
   a. Subjective examination
   b. Pulp testing with cold
   c. Pulp testing with electrical pulp test device
   d. Percussion test
   e. Radiographic examination
3. Anesthesia of mandibular teeth is enhanced by
   a. Infiltration of articaine on the facial
   b. Injecting buffers in the region of the mandibular foramen
   c. Increasing the concentration of epinephrine
   d. Repeating the injection while itipositioning the patient upright
   e. Injecting on the lingual to block the mylohyoid nerve
4. Most important in managing symptomatic irreversible pulpitis is:
   a. Selecting the appropriate intracanal medicament
   b. Removing the inflamed tissue
   c. Reducing the occlusion
   d. Prescribing opiate/NSAID combinations
   e. Prescribing the appropriate antibiotic
5. Antibiotic administration is recommended for:
   a. Prophylaxis to minimize flare-ups
   b. Severe pain with symptomatic irreversible pulpitis
   c. Localized swelling with a large radiolucency
   d. Retreatment of a failed root canal treatment
   e. Cellulitis
   f. None of the above
6. An analgesic choice for severe pain is
   a. Ibuprofen 400 to 600 mg
   b. Combination: Ibuprofen 200 to 400 mg and APAP 500 mg
   c. Combination: Ibuprofen 200 to 400 mg and APAP 325 mg/tramadol 37.5 mg
   d. Combination: Ibuprofen 600 to 800 mg and APAP/tramadol 37.5 mg
   e. Combination: APAP 325 mg and tramadol 37.5 mg
7. The incidence of flare-ups is
   a. Approximately 3%
   b. Approximately 15%
   c. Decreased with prophylactic antibiotics
   d. Higher in inflamed versus necrotic pulps
   e. Higher in preoperative asymptomatic versus symptomatic conditions
8. Most important for resolution of pulp necrosis/acute apical abscess is
   a. Administering appropriate medications (antibiotics and analgesics)
   b. Obtaining drainage through the tooth
   c. Removing irritants from the canal space
   d. Modifying the immune response with regional steroid injections
9. In an emergency situation, the most important objective test is
   a. Cold
   b. Heat
   c. Test cavity
   d. Percussion
   e. The test that reproduces the painful stimulus
10. The best way to differentiate an endodontic from a periodontal abscess swelling is
    a. Endodontic is over the apex, periodontal is more cervical
    b. Endodontic swelling is more painful
    c. Periodontal swelling is associated with probing defects
    d. Periodontal swelling is associated with cervical bone loss
    e. Determining pulp status; endodontic swelling results from pulp necrosis

• BOX 9.1

Diagnosis Sequence

1. Obtain pertinent information about the patient's medical and dental histories.
2. Ask pointed subjective questions about the patient's pain: history, location, severity, duration, character, and eliciting stimuli.
3. Perform an extraoral examination.
4. Perform an intraoral examination.
5. Perform pulp testing as appropriate.
6. Use palpation and percussion sensitivity tests to determine periapical status.
7. Interpret appropriate radiographs.
8. Identify the offending tooth and tissue (pulp or periapex).
9. Establish a pulpal and periapical diagnosis.
10. Design a treatment plan (both emergency and definitive).

References

1. Estrela C, Guedes OA, Silva JA, et al.: Diagnostic and clinical factors associated with pulpal and periapical pain, *Braz Dent J* 22(4):306–311, 2011.
2. Rechenberg DK, Held U, Burgstaller JM, et al.: Pain levels and typical symptoms of acute endodontic infections: a prospective, observational study, *BMC Oral Health* 16(1):61, 2016.
3. Owatz CB, Khan AA, Schindler WG, et al.: The incidence of mechanical allodynia in patients with irreversible pulpitis, *J Endod* 33(5):552–556, 2007.
4. Kim MK, Allareddy V, Nalliah RP, et al.: Burden of facial cellulitis: estimates from the Nationwide Emergency Department Sample, *Oral Surg Oral Med Oral Pathol Oral Radiol* 114(3):312–317, 2012.
5. Walton R, Fouad A: Endodontic interappointment flare-ups: a prospective study of incidence and related factors, *J Endod* 18(4):172–177, 1992.
6. Mor C, Rotstein I, Friedman S: Incidence of interappointment emergency associated with endodontic therapy, *J Endod* 18(10):509–511, 1992.
7. Marshall JG, Liesinger AW: Factors associated with endodontic posttreatment pain, *J Endod* 19(11):573–575, 1993.
8. Albashaireh ZS, Alnegrish AS: Postobturation pain after single- and multiple-visit endodontic therapy. A prospective study, *J Dent* 26(3):227–232, 1998.
9. Glennon JP, Ng YL, Setchell DJ, Gulabivala K: Prevalence of and factors affecting postpreparation pain in patients undergoing two-visit root canal treatment, *Int Endod J* 37(1):29–37, 2004.
10. Ng YL, Glennon JP, Setchell DJ, Gulabivala K: Prevalence of and factors affecting post-obturation pain in patients undergoing root canal treatment, *Int Endod J* 37(6):381–391, 2004.
11. Kakehashi S, Stanley HR, Fitzgerald RJ: The effects of surgical exposures of dental pulps in germ-free and conventional laboratory rats, *Oral Surg Oral Med Oral Pathol* 20:340–349, 1965.
12. Siqueira Jr JF, Rôças IN: Distinctive features of the microbiota associated with different forms of apical periodontitis, *J Oral Microbiol* 1, 2009.
13. Sundqvist G, Figdor D, Persson S, Sjogren U: Microbiologic analysis of teeth with failed endodontic treatment and the outcome of conservative re-treatment, *Oral Surg Oral Med Oral Pathol Oral Radiol Endod* 85(1):86–93, 1998.
14. Diogenes A, Ferraz CC, Akopian AN, et al.: LPS sensitizes TRPV1 via activation of TLR4 in trigeminal sensory neurons, *J Dent Res* 90(6):759–764, 2011.
15. Ferraz CC, Henry MA, Hargreaves KM, Diogenes A: Lipopolysaccharide from *Porphyromonas gingivalis* sensitizes capsaicin-sensitive nociceptors, *J Endod* 37(1):45–48, 2011.
16. Chiu IM, Pinho-Ribeiro FA, Woolf CJ: Pain and infection: pathogen detection by nociceptors, *Pain* 157(6):1192–1193, 2016.
17. Meseguer V, Alpizar YA, Luis E, et al.: TRPA1 channels mediate acute neurogenic inflammation and pain produced by bacterial endotoxins, *Nat Commun* 5:3125, 2014.
18. Chiu IM, Heesters BA, Ghasemlou N, et al.: Bacteria activate sensory neurons that modulate pain and inflammation, *Nature* 501(7465):52–57, 2013.
19. Murray PE, Windsor LJ, Smyth TW, et al.: Analysis of pulpal reactions to restorative procedures, materials, pulp capping, and future therapies, *Crit Rev Oral Biol Med* 13(6):509–520, 2002.
20. Bouillaguet S: Biological risks of resin-based materials to the dentin-pulp complex, *Crit Rev Oral Biol Med* 15(1):47–60, 2004.
21. Asmussen E: Factors affecting the quantity of remaining double bonds in restorative resin polymers, *Scand J. Dent. Res* 90(6):490–496, 1982.
22. Imazato S, McCabe JF, Tarumi H, et al.: Degree of conversion of composites measured by DTA and FTIR, *Dent Mater* 17(2):178–183, 2001.
23. Hume WR, Gerzina TM: Bioavailability of components of resin-based materials which are applied to teeth, *Crit Rev Oral Biol Med* 7(2):172–179, 1996.
24. Curtis Jr P, Gartman LA, Green DB: Utilization of ketorolac tromethamine for control of severe odontogenic pain, *J Endod* 20(9):457–459, 1994.
25. Penniston SG, Hargreaves KM: Evaluation of periapical injection of Ketorolac for management of endodontic pain, *J Endod* 22(2):55–59, 1996.
26. Taggar T, Wu D, Khan AA: A randomized clinical trial comparing 2 ibuprofen formulations in patients with acute odontogenic pain, *J Endod* 43(5):674–678, 2017.
27. Byers MR: Dynamic plasticity of dental sensory nerve structure and cytochemistry, *Arch Oral Biol* 39(Suppl):13S–21S, 1994.
28. Byers MR: Sensory innervation of periodontal ligament of rat molars consists of unencapsulated Ruffini-like mechanoreceptors and free nerve endings, *J Comp Neurol* 231(4):500–518, 1985.
29. Byers MR, Narhi MV: Dental injury models: experimental tools for understanding neuroinflammatory interactions and polymodal nociceptor functions, *Crit Rev Oral Biol Med* 10(1):4–39, 1999.
30. Byers MR, Suzuki H, Maeda T: Dental neuroplasticity, neuro-pulpal interactions, and nerve regeneration, *Microsc Res Tech* 60(5):503–515, 2003.
31. Byers MR, Taylor PE: Effect of sensory denervation on the response of rat molar pulp to exposure injury, *J Dent Res* 72(3):613–618, 1993.
32. Henry MA, Luo S, Foley BD, et al.: Sodium channel expression and localization at demyelinated sites in painful human dental pulp, *J Pain* 10(7):750–758, 2009.
33. Fehrenbacher JC, Sun XX, Locke EE, et al.: Capsaicin-evoked iCGRP release from human dental pulp: a model system for the study of peripheral neuropeptide secretion in normal healthy tissue, *Pain* 144(3):253–261, 2009.
34. El Karim IA, Linden GJ, Curtis TM, et al.: Human dental pulp fibroblasts express the "cold-sensing" transient receptor potential channels TRPA1 and TRPM8, *J Endod* 37(4):473–478, 2011.
35. Torabinejad M, Cymerman JJ, Frankson M, et al.: Effectiveness of various medications on postoperative pain following complete instrumentation, *J Endod* 20(7):345–354, 1994.
36. Hansen GR, Streltzer J: The psychology of pain, *Emerg Med Clin North Am* 23(2):339–348, 2005.
37. Gedney JJ, Logan H, Baron RS: Predictors of short-term and long-term memory of sensory and affective dimensions of pain, *J Pain* 4(2):47–55, 2003.
38. Wepman BJ: Psychological components of pain perception, *Dent Clin North Am* 22(1):101–113, 1978.

39. van Wijk AJ, Hoogstraten J: Reducing fear of pain associated with endodontic therapy, *Int Endod J* 39(5):384–388, 2006.
40. Saxen MA, Newton CW: Managing the endodontic patient with disabling anxiety or phobia, *J Indiana Dent Assoc* 78(4):21–23, 1999.
41. Berthold CW, Dionne RA, Corey SE: Comparison of sublingually and orally administered triazolam for premedication before oral surgery, *Oral Surg Oral Med Oral Pathol Oral Radiol Endod* 84(2):119–124, 1997.
42. Kaufman E, Hargreaves KM, Dionne RA: Comparison of oral triazolam and nitrous oxide with placebo and intravenous diazepam for outpatient premedication, *Oral Surg Oral Med Oral Pathol* 75(2):156–164, 1993.
43. Torabinejad M, Walton RE: Managing endodontic emergencies, *J Am Dent Assoc* 122(5), 1991. 99, 101, 103.
44. Hargreaves KM, Keiser K: Development of new pain management strategies, *J Dent Educ* 66(1):113–121, 2002.
45. Weisleder R, Yamauchi S, Caplan DJ, et al.: The validity of pulp testing: a clinical study, *J Am Dent Assoc* 140(8):1013–1017, 2009.
46. Graunaite I, Lodiene G, Maciulskiene V: Pathogenesis of apical periodontitis: a literature review, *J Oral Maxillofac Res* 2(4):e1, 2012.
47. Akamine A, Hashiguchi I, Toriya Y, Maeda K: Immunohistochemical examination on the localization of macrophages and plasma cells in induced rat periapical lesions, *Endod Dent Traumatol* 10(3):121–128, 1994.
48. Okiji T, Kawashima N, Kosaka T, et al.: Distribution of Ia antigen-expressing nonlymphoid cells in various stages of induced periapical lesions in rat molars, *J Endod* 20(1):27–31, 1994.
49. Khan AA, McCreary B, Owatz CB, et al.: The development of a diagnostic instrument for the measurement of mechanical allodynia, *J Endod* 33(6):663–666, 2007.
50. Khan AA, Owatz CB, Schindler WG, et al.: Measurement of mechanical allodynia and local anesthetic efficacy in patients with irreversible pulpitis and acute periradicular periodontitis, *J Endod* 33(7):796–799, 2007.
51. Long H, Zhou Y, Ye N, et al.: Diagnostic accuracy of CBCT for tooth fractures: a meta-analysis, *J Dent* 42(3):240–248, 2014.
52. AAE AAMOR: AAE and AAOMR Joint Position Statement: Use of Cone Beam Computed Tomography in Endodontics 2015 Update, *Oral Surg Oral Med Oral Pathol Oral Radiol* 120(4):508–512, 2015.
53. Stashenko P, Teles R, D'Souza R: Periapical inflammatory responses and their modulation, *Crit Rev Oral Biol Med* 9(4):498–521, 1998.
54. Reisman D, Reader A, Nist R, Beck M, Weaver J: Anesthetic efficacy of the supplemental intraosseous injection of 3% mepivacaine in irreversible pulpitis, *Oral Surg Oral Med Oral Pathol Oral Radiol Endod* 84(6):676–682, 1997.
55. Smith GN, Walton RE: Periodontal ligament injection: distribution of injected solutions, *Oral Surg Oral Med Oral Pathol* 55(3):232–238, 1983.
56. Oguntebi BR, DeSchepper EJ, Taylor TS, et al.: Postoperative pain incidence related to the type of emergency treatment of symptomatic pulpitis, *Oral Surg Oral Med Oral Pathol* 73(4):479–483, 1992.
57. Nyerere JW, Matee MI, Simon EN: Emergency pulpotomy in relieving acute dental pain among Tanzanian patients, *BMC Oral Health* 6(1), 2006.
58. Hasselgren G, Reit C: Emergency pulpotomy: pain relieving effect with and without the use of sedative dressings, *J Endod* 15(6):254–256, 1989.
59. Moos HL, Bramwell JD, Roahen JO: A comparison of pulpectomy alone versus pulpectomy with trephination for the relief of pain, *J Endod* 22(8):422–425, 1996.
60. Hildebrand C, Fried K, Tuisku F, Johansson CS: Teeth and tooth nerves, *Prog Neurobiol* 45(3):165–222, 1995.
61. Nist E, Reader A, Beck M: Effect of apical trephination on postoperative pain and swelling in symptomatic necrotic teeth, *J Endod* 27(6):415–420, 2001.
62. Maddox DL, Walton RE, Davis CO: Incidence of posttreatment endodontic pain related to medicaments and other factors, *J Endod* 3(12):447–457, 1977.
63. Figini L, Lodi G, Gorni F, Gagliani M: Single versus multiple visits for endodontic treatment of permanent teeth: a Cochrane systematic review, *J Endod* 34(9):1041–1047, 2008.
64. Khan AA, Sun X, Hargreaves KM: Effect of calcium hydroxide on proinflammatory cytokines and neuropeptides, *J Endod* 34(11):1360–1363, 2008.
65. Khan AA, Diogenes A, Jeske NA, et al.: Tumor necrosis factor alpha enhances the sensitivity of rat trigeminal neurons to capsaicin, *Neuroscience* 155(2):503–509, 2008.
66. Binshtok AM, Wang H, Zimmermann K, et al.: Nociceptors are interleukin-1beta sensors, *J Neurosci* 28(52):14062–14073, 2008.
67. Rosenberg PA, Babick PJ, Schertzer L, Leung A: The effect of occlusal reduction on pain after endodontic instrumentation, *J Endod* 24(7):492–496, 1998.
68. Creech 3rd JL, Walton RE, Kaltenbach R: Effect of occlusal relief on endodontic pain, *J Am Dent Assoc* 109(1):64–67, 1984.
69. Smith EA, Marshall JG, Selph SS, et al.: Nonsteroidal anti-inflammatory drugs for managing postoperative endodontic pain in patients who present with preoperative pain: a systematic review and meta-analysis, *J Endod* 43(1):7–15, 2017.
70. Elzaki WM, Abubakr NH, Ziada HM, Ibrahim YE: Double-blind randomized placebo-controlled clinical trial of efficiency of nonsteroidal anti-inflammatory drugs in the control of post-endodontic pain, *J Endod* 42(6):835–842, 2016.
71. Menke ER, Jackson CR, Bagby MD, Tracy TS: The effectiveness of prophylactic etodolac on postendodontic pain, *J Endod* 26(12):712–715, 2000.
72. Yoon E, Babar A, Choudhary M, et al.: Acetaminophen-induced hepatotoxicity: a comprehensive update, *J Clin Transl Hepatol* 4(2):131–142, 2016.
73. Blieden M, Paramore LC, Shah D, Ben-Joseph R: A perspective on the epidemiology of acetaminophen exposure and toxicity in the United States, *Expert Rev Clin Pharmacol* 7(3):341–348, 2014.
74. Bunchorntavakul C, Reddy KR: Acetaminophen-related hepatotoxicity, *Clin Liver Dis* 17(4):587–607, 2013. viii.
75. Fontana RJ, Adams PC: "Unintentional" acetaminophen overdose on the rise: who is responsible? *Can J Gastroenterol* 20(5):319–324, 2006.
76. Miech R, Johnston L, O'Malley PM, et al.: Prescription opioids in adolescence and future opioid misuse, *Pediatrics* 136(5):e1169–1177, 2015.
77. Wong YJ, Keenan J, Hudson K, et al.: Opioid, NSAID, and OTC analgesic medications for dental procedures: PEARL Network Findings, *Compendium of Continuing Education in Dentistry, Jamesburg, NJ* 37(10):710–718, 1995. 2016.
78. Preston KL, Jasinski DR, Testa M: Abuse potential and pharmacological comparison of tramadol and morphine, *Drug Alcohol Depend* 27(1):7–17, 1991.
79. Al-Kahtani A: Effect of long acting local anesthetic on postoperative pain in teeth with irreversible pulpitis: randomized clinical trial, *Saudi Pharm J* 22(1):39–42, 2014.
80. Parirokh M, Yosefi MH, Nakhaee N, et al.: Effect of bupivacaine on postoperative pain for inferior alveolar nerve block anesthesia after single-visit root canal treatment in teeth with irreversible pulpitis, *J Endod* 38(8):1035–1039, 2012.
81. Nogueira BML, Silva LG, Mesquita CRM, et al.: Is the use of dexamethasone effective in controlling pain associated with symptomatic irreversible pulpitis? a systematic review, *J Endod* 44(5):703–710, 2018.
82. Shamszadeh S, Shirvani A, Eghbal MJ, Asgary S: Efficacy of corticosteroids on postoperative endodontic pain: a systematic review and meta-analysis, *J Endod* 44(7):1057–1065, 2018.
83. Keenan JV, Farman AG, Fedorowicz Z, Newton JT: Antibiotic use for irreversible pulpitis, *Cochrane Database Syst Rev*(2)CD004969, 2005.

84. Yingling NM, Byrne BE, Hartwell GR: Antibiotic use by members of the American Association of Endodontists in the year 2000: report of a national survey, *J Endod* 28(5):396–404, 2002.
85. Fishman N: Antimicrobial stewardship, *Am J Infect Control* 34(5 Suppl 1):S55–63; discussion S64–73, 2006.
86. Stashenko P, Wang CY: Characterization of bone resorptive mediators in active periapical lesions, *Proceedings of the Finnish Dental Society, Suom Hammaslaak Toim* 88(Suppl 1):427–432, 1992.
87. Fouad AF, Rivera EM, Walton RE: Penicillin as a supplement in resolving the localized acute apical abscess, *Oral Surg Oral Med Oral Pathol Oral Radiol Endod* 81(5):590–595, 1996.
88. Campanelli CA, Walton RE, Williamson AE, et al.: Vital signs of the emergency patient with pulpal necrosis and localized acute apical abscess, *J Endod* 34(3):264–267, 2008.
89. Henry M, Reader A, Beck M: Effect of penicillin on postoperative endodontic pain and swelling in symptomatic necrotic teeth, *J Endod* 27(2):117–123, 2001.
90. Canadian Collaboration on Clinical Practice Guidelines in D: Clinical practice guideline on treatment of acute apical abscess (AAA) in adults, *Evid Based Dent* 5(1):8, 2004.
91. Weine FS, Healey HJ, Theiss EP: Endodontic emergency dilemma: leave tooth open or keep it closed? *Oral Surg Oral Med Oral Pathol* 40(4):531–536, 1975.
92. Beus H, Fowler S, Drum M, et al.: What is the outcome of an incision and drainage procedure in endodontic patients? a prospective, randomized, single-blind study, *J Endod* 44(2):193–201, 2018.
93. AAE. AAE: Position Statement: AAE Guidance on the Use of Systemic Antibiotics in Endodontics, *J Endod* 43(9):1409–1413, 2017.
94. Khemaleelakul S, Baumgartner JC, Pruksakorn S: Identification of bacteria in acute endodontic infections and their antimicrobial susceptibility, *Oral Surg Oral Med Oral Pathol Oral Radiol Endod* 94(6):746–755, 2002.
95. Siqueira Jr JF, Rôças IN: Exploiting molecular methods to explore endodontic infections: part 2—Redefining the endodontic microbiota, *J Endod* 31(7):488–498, 2005.
96. Baumgartner JC, Xia T: Antibiotic susceptibility of bacteria associated with endodontic abscesses, *J Endod* 29(1):44–47, 2003.
97. Llewelyn MJ, Fitzpatrick JM, Darwin E, et al.: The antibiotic course has had its day, *BMJ (Clinical research ed.)* 358:j3418, 2017.
98. Martin MV, Longman LP, Hill JB, Hardy P: Acute dentoalveolar infections: an investigation of the duration of antibiotic therapy, *Br Dent J* 183(4):135–137, 1997.
99. Lewis MA, McGowan DA, MacFarlane TW: Short-course high-dosage amoxycillin in the treatment of acute dentoalveolar abscess, *Br Dent J* 162(5):175, 1987.
100. Singh N, Rogers P, Atwood CW, et al.: Short-course empiric antibiotic therapy for patients with pulmonary infiltrates in the intensive care unit. A proposed solution for indiscriminate antibiotic prescription, *Am J Respir Crit Care Med* 162(2 Pt 1):505–511, 2000.
101. Touyz LZ, Marchand S: The influence of postoperative telephone calls on pain perception: a study of 118 periodontal surgical procedures, *J Orofac Pain* 12(3):219–225, 1998.
102. Imura N, Zuolo ML: Factors associated with endodontic flare-ups: a prospective study, *Int Endod J* 28(5):261–265, 1995.
103. Trope M: Flare-up rate of single-visit endodontics, *Int Endod J* 24(1):24–26, 1991.
104. Dao TT, LeResche L: Gender differences in pain, *J Orofac Pain* 14(3):169–184; discussion 184–195, 2000.
105. Sim CK: Endodontic interappointment emergencies in a Singapore private practice setting: a retrospective study of incidence and cause-related factors, *Singapore Dent J* 22(1):22–27, 1997.
106. Torabinejad M, Kettering JD, McGraw JC, et al.: Factors associated with endodontic interappointment emergencies of teeth with necrotic pulps, *J Endod* 14(5):261–266, 1988.
107. Genet JM, Hart AA, Wesselink PR, Thoden van Velzen SK: Preoperative and operative factors associated with pain after the first endodontic visit, *Int Endod J* 20(2):53–64, 1987.
108. Eleazer PD, Eleazer KR: Flare-up rate in pulpally necrotic molars in one-visit versus two-visit endodontic treatment, *J Endod* 24(9):614–616, 1998.
109. Walton RE, Chiappinelli J: Prophylactic penicillin: effect on posttreatment symptoms following root canal treatment of asymptomatic periapical pathosis, *J Endod* 19(9):466–470, 1993.
110. Pickenpaugh L, Reader A, Beck M, et al.: Effect of prophylactic amoxicillin on endodontic flare-up in asymptomatic, necrotic teeth, *J Endod* 27(1):53–56, 2001.
111. Gopikrishna V, Parameswaran A: Effectiveness of prophylactic use of rofecoxib in comparison with ibuprofen on postendodontic pain, *J Endod* 29(1):62–64, 2003.
112. Gordon SM, Dionne RA, Brahim J, et al.: Blockade of peripheral neuronal barrage reduces postoperative pain, *Pain* 70(2-3):209–215, 1997.
113. Calderon A: Prevention of apical periodontal ligament pain: a preliminary report of 100 vital pulp cases, *J Endod* 19(5):247–249, 1993.
114. Liesinger A, Marshall FJ, Marshall JG: Effect of variable doses of dexamethasone on posttreatment endodontic pain, *J Endod* 19(1):35–39, 1993.
115. Marshall JG, Walton RE: The effect of intramuscular injection of steroid on posttreatment endodontic pain, *J Endod* 10(12):584–588, 1984.
116. Trope M: Relationship of intracanal medicaments to endodontic flare-ups, *Endod Dent Traumatol* 6(5):226–229, 1990.
117. Harrison JW, Baumgartner JC, Svec TA: Incidence of pain associated with clinical factors during and after root canal therapy. Part 2. Postobturation pain, *J Endod* 9(10):434–438, 1983.
118. Gesi A, Hakeberg M, Warfvinge J, Bergenholtz G: Incidence of periapical lesions and clinical symptoms after pulpectomy—a clinical and radiographic evaluation of 1- versus 2-session treatment, *Oral Surg Oral Med Oral Pathol Oral Radiol Endod* 101(3):379–388, 2006.

10

Management of the Vital Pulp and of Immature Teeth

ANIBAL DIOGENES, TATIANA BOTERO, AND MO KANG

CHAPTER OUTLINE

LEARNING OBJECTIVES

After reading this chapter, the student should be able to:

1. Understand the special physiologic and structural characteristics of the dentin-pulp complex and how they affect the pulpal response to injury.
2. Discuss the effects of pulpal injury in teeth with developing roots.
3. Differentiate reparative and reactionary dentin.
4. Recognize the indications, contraindications, and expected outcomes of the vital pulp therapy protocols.
5. Describe diagnosis and case assessment of immature teeth with pulp injury.
6. Determine the techniques for vital pulp therapy and prognosis.
7. Indicate the treatment options for immature teeth with pulp necrosis.
8. Describe apexification procedures and prognosis.
9. Explain the technique and the goals of regenerative endodontic therapy.
10. Recognize the tissue engineering techniques used to regenerating the dentin-pulp complex.
11. Indicate the stem cells present in dental tissues and their potential to regenerate the dentin-pulp complex.

The Dentin-Pulp Complex

Pulp Defense Mechanisms

The dental pulp is a highly specialized and complex loose connective tissue encased by mineralized tissues, namely enamel, dentin, and cementum. The dental pulp has close anatomic and functional relationship with the dentin, often referred as dentin-pulp complex (Fig. 10.1). Although the dental pulp is protected by a mineralized case, it is not impervious to irritation. Dental caries, trauma, anatomic defects, and iatrogenic mishaps can lead to inflammation and possibly pulp necrosis. However, the dentin-pulp complex has elaborate defense mechanisms.

Invading microorganisms reaching the dentin will encounter an outward flow of dentinal fluid. This positive pressure maintained by the dental pulp acts to "push" out the ingression of microorganisms, and it increases if pulpal inflammation and edema occur. A notable aspect is that this fluid will carry important molecules released from cells of the innate and adaptive immune response such as cytokines, immunoglobulins, and complement proteins.[1] These molecules are able to initiate the pulpal defense before these organisms reach the pulpal cells. In addition, bacteria-mediated demineralization of dentin releases key noncollagenous proteins (NCPs) that mediate reparative responses.[2] Thus dentin is no longer thought to be an inert tissue but instead comprises myriad growth factors, morphogens, and neurotrophins that have shown to be "fossilized" within the dentinal matrix and that can be released upon demineralization and mediate processes of angiogenesis, neurogenesis, and dentinogenesis.[3] These processes are part of an elaborate response of the dentin-pulp complex to increase vascularity, overhauling the immune response and the metabolic demand of an injured area undergoing remodeling, repair, and possibly regeneration.[4] In addition, inflammatory foci within the dental pulp have increased innervation density due to robust neuronal sprouting in the area. These neuronal fibers, mainly nociceptors, play their best recognized role of surveillance by providing nociceptive signals but also participate in the

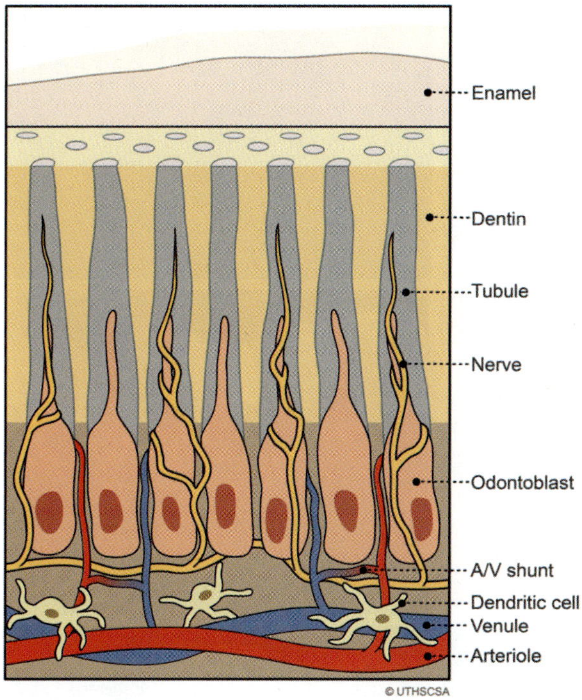

• **Fig. 10.1** Illustration of the dentin-pulp interphase in normal conditions. The fluid-filled dentinal tubules are occupied by odontoblastic processes and free nerve endings that might extend farther than odontoblasts toward the enamel junction. The subodontoblastic complex is composed of a rich capillary bed and innervation network. The pulp capillaries are equipped with arteriole/venule (A/V) shunts that may open upon injury, diverting the circulation to uninjured areas. Dendritic cells are the main antigen presenting cells in the dental pulp that are usually located in the subodontoblastic process in normal conditions of homeostasis.

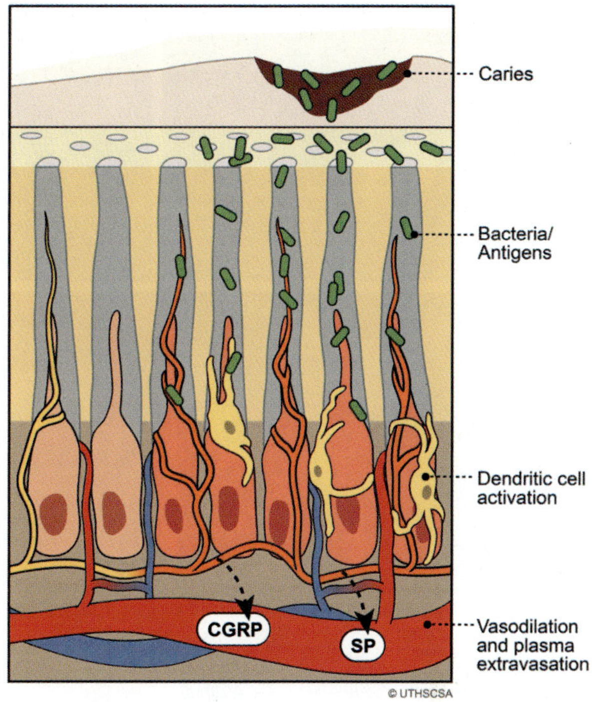

• **Fig. 10.2** Illustration of early events of microbial insult to the dentin-pulp complex. Microbes and their antigens diffuse through dentinal tubules reaching the free nerve endings of the trigeminal ganglia. These neuronal fibers express microbial recognition receptors (i.e., Toll-like receptors) and are activated and sensitized, resulting in the neuronal release of vasoactive peptides (i.e., calcitonin gene–related peptide [CGRP] and substance P [SP]) that, in turn, promote vasodilation and plasma extravasation, also known as neurogenic inflammation. Odontoblasts also express Toll-like receptors that upon recognition of microbial presence, trigger the release of chemokines, attracting dendritic cells to the dentinal tubules. These dendritic cells engulf and digest microbial antigens into epitopes and present these to cells of the adaptive immune cells (i.e., T cells). Subsequent events of pulp inflammation include the exuberant accumulation of polymorphonuclear (PMN) and adaptive immune response cells.

inflammatory process known as *neurogenic inflammation* by the release of vasoactive peptides such as calcitonin gene–related peptide (CGRP) and substance P, which are responsible for promoting vasodilation and plasma extravasation, respectively, as well as modulation of immune cell function (Fig. 10.2).[5]

The progressive ingress of antigen and microorganisms into the dentin first reaches the cells positioned with the dentinal tubules (see Fig. 10.2). These cells include nociceptive primary afferent neuronal terminals that have been shown to extend up to 200 μm into the dentinal tubules and odontoblastic processes (see Figs. 10.1 and 10.2).[6] Interestingly, pulpal neuronal afferent fibers are mainly nociceptors but have also been shown to have a role in directly detecting microorganisms.[7] This characteristic is particularly interesting because the dentin-pulp complex is one of the most densely innervated tissues in the human body with nociceptors. These neuronal fibers within the dental pulp, regardless their degree of myelination, have been shown to mediate only nociceptive signals. Thus teeth are constantly under surveillance of this neuronal network dedicated to detecting injury or potential injury. These neurons have been shown to express the Toll-like receptor 4 (TLR4) that recognizes liposaccharides or endotoxins from gram-negative bacteria.[7,8] The activation of TLR4 in neurons results in sensitization of these fibers, lowering their activation threshold and increasing the response magnitude.[7,8] This increased response, in turn, leads to secretion of vasoactive peptides such as CGRP and substance P (see Fig. 10.2). The action of these peptides results in vasodilation and plasma extravasation (i.e., edema) at the site of injury, a process called *neurogenic inflammation*. The vasodilation and plasma extravasation allow for greater vascularity in the area with increased immune cellular presence and greater outward fluid flow, decelerating the ingress of microorganisms (see Fig. 10.2). This unique neuronal–bacterial communication is a sophisticated mechanism for sensory neurons to detect, alert the breach of the biological barrier, and initiate a process of neurogenic inflammation that will be immediately integrated with the immune-driven inflammation. An interesting aspect is that the early symptoms of a carious lesion can be manifested as painful responses to low-intensity stimuli and exaggerated responses to noxious stimuli in reversible pulpitis, matching the previously described neurophysiology.

Odontoblasts are highly specialized cells that serve the primary role of secreting dentin. As with other cell types within the dentin-pulp complex, these cells also have other functions that extend beyond their best-recognized role as secretory cells. Odontoblasts have also been shown to act as "sentinels" because these cells express many subtypes of TLRs and thus can detect the presence of gram-negative and gram-positive viruses and fungi within the dentinal tubules.[9,10] Activation of these TLRs have been shown to result in upregulation of expression and release of key chemokines and cytokines.[9,11] These factors are crucial for the recruitment of dendritic cells from the subodontoblastic plexus area to the areas

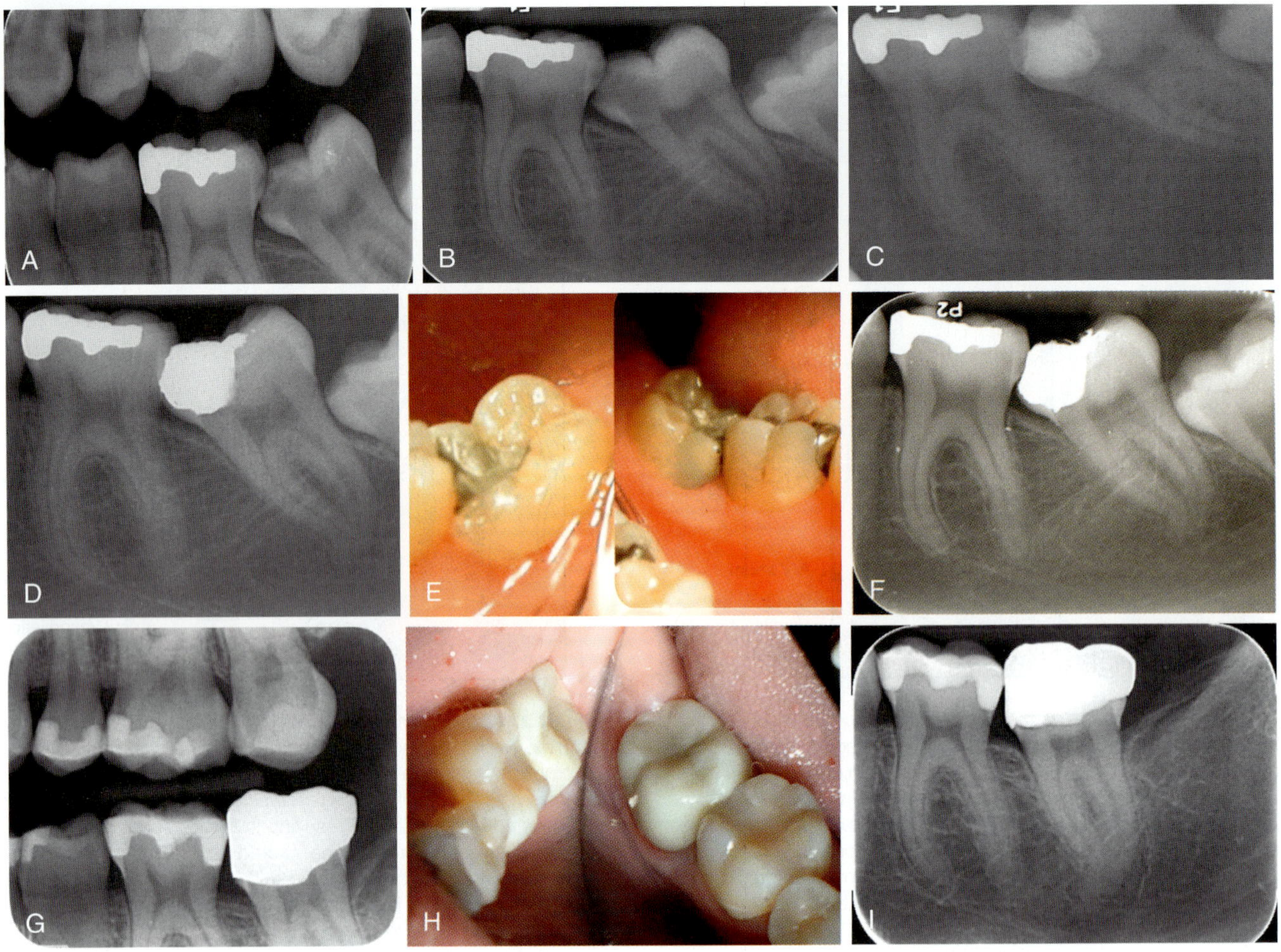

• **Fig. 10.3** Indirect pulp capping. A 14-year-old female patient consulting with symptoms of reversible pulpitis and symptomatic apical periodontitis on tooth #18 (**A** and **B**). Extensive decay and infected dentin were removed, exposed, and sealed with WMTA-ketac silver glass ionomer under rubber dam isolation **(C)**. Final obturation was performed 1 month later with amalgam (**D** and **E**). At 1-year follow-up, the patient was asymptomatic, and tooth #18 responded normal to clinic tests and radiographic evaluation (**F**). At 5.5-year follow-up, tooth #17 had been extracted and tooth #18 had a received a full-cuspal coverage crown. The patient was asymptomatic, and tooth #18 had normal response to clinicals test (**G**, **H**, and **I**). (Courtesy Dr. Tatiana M. Botero, faculty dental practice, University of Michigan, Ann Arbor, MI, USA.)

of insult (see Fig. 10.2). These cells represent the major form of antigen-presenting cells in the dental pulp and are analogous to Langerhans cells in the skin.[12] They are equipped to engulf, process, and present the antigens to other cells of the immune response system. In addition, dendritic cells will release additional chemokines and cytokines that in conjunction with odontoblast-derived factors and neurogenic inflammation will recruit additional cells of the innate and eventually adaptive immune response, resulting in the amplification of the inflammatory process. It is noteworthy that inflammation is a normal homeostatic response and is essential for containing the invasion of microorganisms. If successful, tertiary dentin is deposited in the area of insult in the form of either reactionary or reparative dentin, providing an additional mineralized barrier. Last, the presence of arteriole/venule (A/V) shunts (see Figs. 10.1 and 10.2) that open upon injury[13] allows for the compartmentalization of microabscess regions within the dental pulp that are surrounded by vascularized dental pulp. The careful removal of the infected tissue, allowing the surrounding tissue to promote repair, represents the biologic basis for pulpotomy procedures (Fig. 10.3).

Tertiary Dentinogenesis

The process of dentin mineralization occurs prenatally for most teeth and throughout the life of a tooth as long as the pulp is vital. The primary dentin is formed during tooth development, whereas secondary dentin is deposited at a slower rate, after tooth maturation, resulting in the gradual deposition of dentin throughout the entire extent of the pulp canal spaces and pulp chamber.[14] The most superficial layer of dentin in contact with the dental pulp is the predentin that is formed by the unmineralized matrix secreted by the odontoblasts. It is the mineralization of the predentin that forms the mature primary and secondary dentin that are composed roughly by 70% hydroxyapatite crystals, 20% organic matrix, and 10% water.[15] Thus primary dentin and secondary dentin are deposited in response to normal physiologic conditions. Tertiary dentin, on the other hand, is secreted in response to any injury to the dentin-pulp complex.

A mild injury to the pulp that can provide sufficient inflammatory stimuli for odontoblasts, increasing the secretion of tertiary dentin at a higher rate, promotes "reactionary" dentinogenesis (Fig. 10.4). This reaction of the surviving odontoblasts results

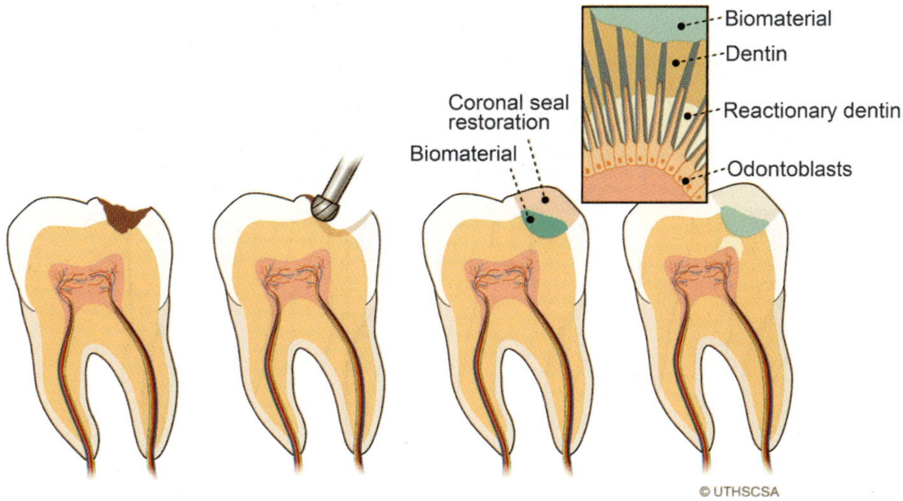

• **Fig. 10.4** Reactionary dentin formation as result of an indirect pulp capping procedure. Upon the removal of infected dentin, the cavity is layered with a biomaterial that stimulates surviving odontoblasts to secrete dentin at a faster rate, creating a localized accumulation of dentin, distancing the pulp from the area of mild injury.

in localized increased thickness of the dentinal layer as it maintains the overall architecture of the dentin odontoblast interphase. Odontoblast death could occur with more intense stimuli for a period of time sufficient to lead to the loss of odontoblasts in the area of injury. If the surrounding pulp remains vital and there is a favorable balance between inflammation and repair, progenitor cells are recruited to the site of injury,[16] possibly by chemotactic factors released from the demineralized dentin matrix and neighboring cells. These progenitor cells differentiate into mineralizing cells often referred as "odontoblast-like cells." Although these cells differ in morphology from native odontoblasts, they also secrete a matrix that upon mineralization forms a "mineralized bridge" over the area of injury called *reparative dentin* (Fig. 10.5). This dentin is typically atubular and, due to its rapid secretion, often traps the mineralizing cells within its matrix resembling osteocytes; it is often referred to as "osteodentin." This nontubular dentin bridge, if formed uniformly without tubular defects, can provide a biological barrier with fluid permeability seen with tubular dentin.[17] This inherent reparative and regenerative capacity of the dental pulp forms the basis for contemporary vital pulp therapies.

Pulp Necrosis and Root Development

Despite the advanced defense and reparative mechanisms already described in this chapter and in Chapter 1, the dental pulp may succumb to infections. The progressive process of liquefaction pulp necrosis results in complete loss of homeostatic functions. An important factor is that the loss of odontoblasts in the radicular pulp results in arrested tooth development in teeth still undergoing development. Indeed, root development is known to continue 2 to 3 years after the eruption of a permanent tooth in the oral cavity.[18,19] This process of root formation and maturation requires the complex interaction of the epithelial root sheath and mesenchymal cells located in the dental apical papilla.[20] Pulp necrosis and/or trauma can severely disrupt this interaction, resulting in interruption of normal development in addition to the development and maintenance of apical periodontitis. Thus all efforts must be directed toward avoiding complete pulp necrosis through vital pulp therapies. Nonetheless, vital pulp therapy as a treatment alternative depends on the initial clinical presentation and the often-challenging assessment of the degree of inflammation.

Etiologic Factors of the Dentin-Pulp Complex Injury

Preserving the vitality of the dentin-pulp complex tissue is the principal goal when treating teeth that have been damaged by trauma, caries, dental anomalies, or iatrogenic factors. Each of the etiologic factors will cause an initial inflammatory reaction: pulpitis. If not treated, this reaction will progress to irreversible pulpitis, leading finally to necrosis. Recognition of these factors will contribute to the preventive therapeutic approaches and preservation of the pulp vitality. Maintenance of pulp vitality requires a good understanding of the interplay of biologic factors influencing regenerative events such as the infection and the inflammation occurring. Vital pulp therapies may not be suitable for all cases, especially those showing deep pulpal inflammation and involving the periapical tissues. The correlation of clinical symptoms with the pathophysiologic status of the dental pulp remains a significant diagnostic challenge before attempting a regenerative procedure, for example.

Trauma

When patients present with traumatic dental emergencies, management is crucial for the prognosis of the tooth. It is important to perform an extensive evaluation and diagnosis of the case as well as schedule adequate follow-up visits to detect possible complications such as pulp necrosis and resorptions. The incidence of dental trauma is higher among boys than among girls, and the anterior maxillary teeth are the most commonly affected teeth,[21,22] particularly in patients with increased overjet and active participation in sports.[23-27] The incidence of dental trauma has overall (all ages) a frequency of 5%, but in 0- to 6-year-old patients it is 17%.[28] Traumatic injuries are more common in permanent (58%) than in primary teeth (36%).[29,30] The maxillary central incisor is more frequently affected (66%) than is the lateral incisor (17%). Uncomplicated crown fractures (without pulp exposure) are the

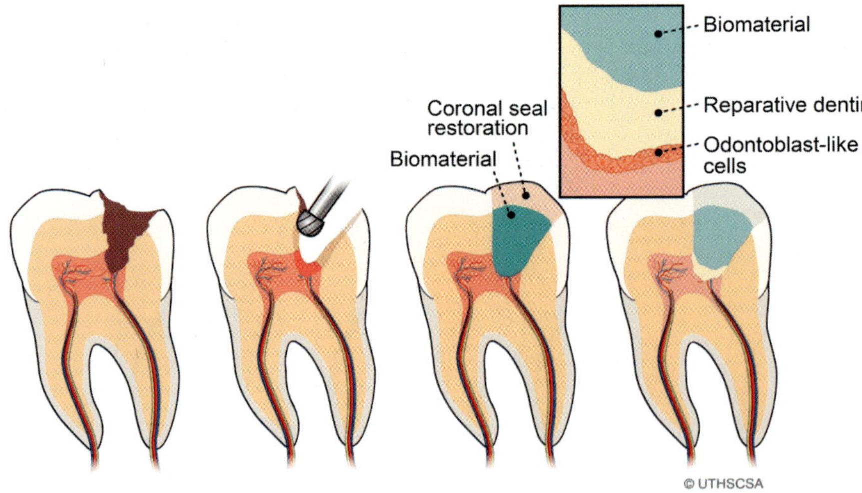

• **Fig. 10.5** Reparative dentin formation as result of a direct pulp capping or partial pulpotomy. Upon the removal of infected dentin and part of the injured pulp, the cavity is layered with a biomaterial that stimulates migration of pulp progenitor cells (such as a tricalcium silicate material) and the differentiation into mineralizing cells in the area of injury. These cells secrete a mineralized bridge called reparative dentin in the attempt to create a biologic seal between the injured area and the underlying dental pulp.

most common traumatic lesions (41% to 68%).[23,24,26] Pulpitis and necrosis can also occur as a result of dentinal exposure to bacteria and bacterial byproducts in uncomplicated (nonpulp-exposed) or complicated (pulp-exposed) crown or crown-root fractures. The incidence of pulp necrosis after uncomplicated crown fractures is low (2% to 5%), but when there is a concomitant injury such as a luxation the chances of necrosis increases, especially in cases with a close apex (55% to 65%) compared with open apex teeth (3.5% to 11%). The traumatized dental pulp in immature or open apex teeth will have greater chances to heal and survive.[31-33]

Trauma to the periradicular tissues can disrupt the neurovascular supply of the dental pulp, leading to necrosis. Severe traumatic incidents such as intrusions, lateral luxations, and avulsions result in greater incidence of pulp necrosis and resorptions. Indeed, depending on the type of luxation injury, an immature permanent tooth would become necrotic 14% to 67% of the time.[31] If an immature permanent tooth is avulsed and replanted, the risk of pulp necrosis is as high as 77%.[34] Therefore dental trauma is a major cause of interruption of tooth development because the dental pulp is readily infected and becomes necrotic in immature permanent teeth.

Caries

Dental caries is one of the most common infectious diseases in children and young adults, with high prevalence in the United States.[35,36] The National Health and Nutrition Examination Survey (NHANES) showed a decrease in its overall incidence, although 21% of children (6 to 11 years old) continue to have dental caries on permanent teeth, with 8% of children having untreated decay. Approximately 59% of adolescents (12 to 19 years old) and 92% of adults (20 to 64 years old) have dental caries in their permanent teeth. Untreated decay affects 20% of adolescents and 26% of adults.[37-39] The incidence and rate of progression of dental caries are multifactorial, depending on genetics, diet, and oral hygiene habits.[35] The lack of prompt treatment for carious lesions and/or the resulting microleakage from defective restorations leads to pulpitis, which can eventually progress to pulp necrosis, periapical lesions, infection dissemination, and systemic involvement, with eventual tooth loss. Therefore early treatment is crucial to maintain the vitality of the pulp, especially in young patients with immature teeth undergoing development. In active caries lesions, it is important to differentiate the infected from affected dentin. As discusses previously, indirect or direct pulp capping procedures can be employed after adequate caries excavation, allowing for remineralization of affected dentin or formation of a new mineralized bridge.[40-43]

Dental Anomalies

Dental anomalies such as dens evaginatus, dens invaginatus, or radicular lingual or palato-gingival groove are less frequent etiologic factors but can also cause pulpal necrosis. In these conditions, bacteria will have a direct access to the pulp through the malformations. Dens evaginatus, which is an occlusal tubercle formed during development by folding of inner enamel epithelium into the stellate reticulum, is most commonly found in mandibular secondary premolars.[44] Dens evaginatus has been reported to be prevalent in 1% to 4% of Asian populations and up to 15% in Alaskan Yupik and Inupiat people and North American Indian population.[44-47] Dens invaginatus, on the other hand, is formed from in-folding of the inner enamel epithelium and odontoblast layer into the pulp. The highest incidence of dens invaginatus is observed in maxillary lateral incisors, and the overall prevalence has been reported as 1% to 10%.[45,48,49] Oehlers has classified this anomaly by the degree of invagination affecting either the periodontium, pulp canal space, or both.[50] The pulp is exposed, in the most severe cases, when the communication passes directly to the apical papilla, communicating with the apical third of the canal and giving a direct entrance for bacteria. The radicular lingual grooves, similarly to dens invaginatus, are mostly found in lateral incisors and less common in central incisors.[48,50]

Iatrogenic Factors

Cavity Preparation Aspects and Remaining Dentin

The blood flow to the pulp is reduced to less than half its normal rate when local anesthetics containing vasoconstrictors are used in restorative dentistry.[51] In procedures on teeth with pulps that are already compromised, this reduction may be an additional stressor. A healthy pulp may survive episodes of ischemia lasting for 1 hour or longer.[52] An already ischemic pulp subjected to severe injury may hemorrhage (blush) when subjected to trauma such as that associated with full crown preparation without the use of coolant.[53] Any intervention that extends to the dentin during cavity preparation may result in some degree of injury to the odontoblasts and their processes. However, dentin matrix demineralization during the carious process of cutting and etching of the dentin during cavity preparation can lead to release of important bioactive molecules, with the consequent stimulation of reparative cellular responses in the pulp.[54,55] Dentin is an effective insulator; for this reason, careful cutting with adequate cooling is less likely to damage the pulp unless the thickness of the dentin between preparation and pulp is less than 1 mm.[56] Even then, the inflammatory response may be mild (Fig. 10.6). The greatest amount of frictional heat is generated during crown preparations when the pulp is particularly at risk of injury. The heat generated may also have a desiccating effect by "boiling" away dentinal tubule fluid at the dentin surface. The "blushing" of dentin during cavity or crown preparation is thought to be due to frictional heat, resulting in vascular injury (hemorrhage) in the pulp.[57] Dentin may take on an underlying pinkish hue soon after a operative procedure, reflecting significant vascular changes that could result in the development of pulpitis. Thus crown preparation must be performed with adequate use of profuse water spray with new sharp burs and minimizing the pressure of the instrument on the tooth and the time of contact. In addition, it is imperative to establish the preoperative and postoperative pulp status through vitality testing.

Dentin permeability increases exponentially with increasing cavity depth, because both the diameter and density of dentinal tubules also increase with cavity depth (Fig. 10.7).[58,59] Thus the deeper the cavity, the greater the tubular surface area into which potentially toxic substances can penetrate and diffuse to the pulp. The length of the dentinal tubules beneath the cavity is also important. The farther substances diffuse, the more they are diluted and buffered by the dentinal fluid. Deeper cavity preparations sever the odontoblast processes in their region of greater length.

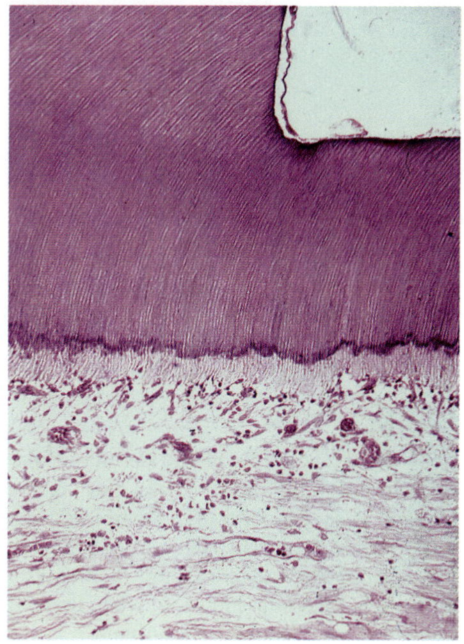

• **Fig. 10.6** Mild inflammation beneath a deep cavity preparation with adequate coolant. (Courtesy Dr. H.O. Trowbridge.).

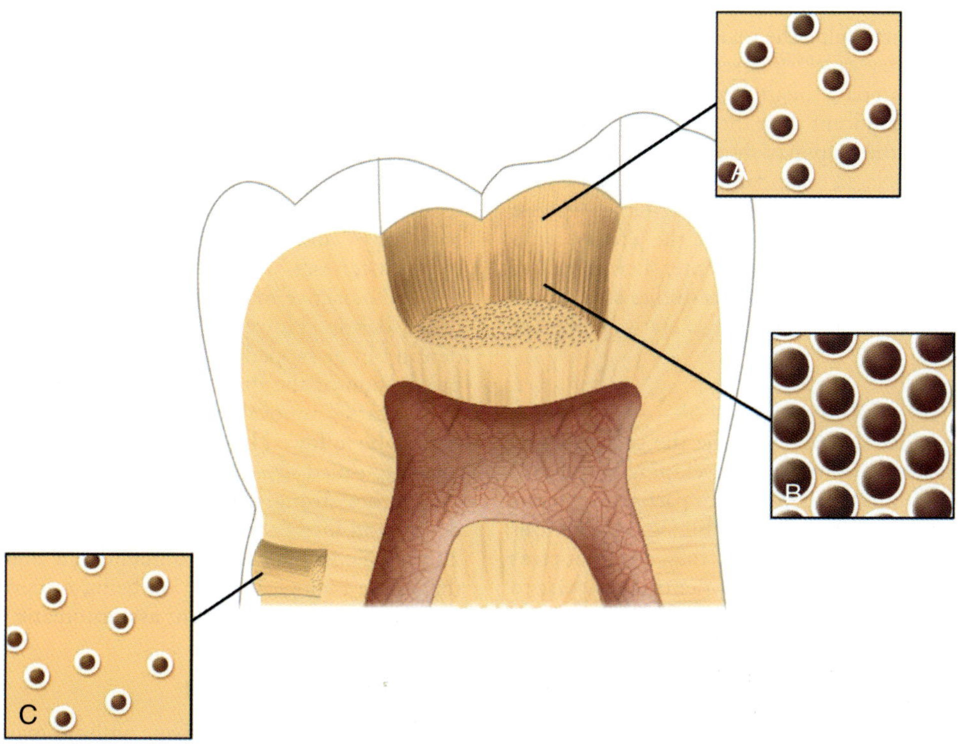

• **Fig. 10.7** Difference in size and number of tubules in the dentinal floor of a shallow **(A)**, deep **(B)** and cervical **(C)** cavity preparations. (From Trowbridge HO: Dentistry today, *Dentistry* 82:22, 1982.)

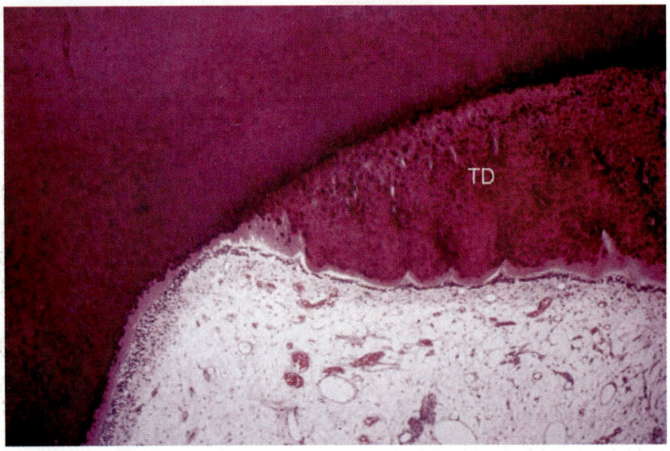

• **Fig. 10.8** Tertiary dentin (TD) formed under a deep preparation and irritating material. (Courtesy Dr. H.O. Trowbridge.)

This severing negatively affects the cell's attempts to restore its membrane integrity and increases the risk of a cell leaking its contents.

Dental Materials

The most important characteristic of any restorative material on its effect on the pulp is its ability to form a seal that prevents the leakage of bacteria and their products onto dentin and the pulp.[60-63] Cytotoxicity is another important factor to evaluate in the restorative materials, because they are composed of chemicals that have the potential to irritate the pulp. However, when these materials are placed in a cavity, the intervening dentin usually neutralizes or prevents leachable ingredients from reaching the pulp in a high enough concentration to cause injury. Materials are more toxic when they are placed directly on an exposed pulp. Cytotoxicity tests carried out on materials in vitro or in soft tissues may not predict the effect of these materials on the dental pulp. The toxicity of the individual components of a material may vary.[64,65] A set material may differ in toxicity from an unset material. The immediate pulpal response to a material is much less significant than the long-term response. A few days after placement, the pulp may show a strong inflammatory response. A few months later, the inflammatory response may subside, and repair occurs. A good measure of long-term response is the thickness of tertiary dentin laid down by the affected pulp (Fig. 10.8). As discussed previously in this chapter, new bioactive silicate materials have been found by numerous studies to promote healing of the injured pulp by reparative and regenerative processes.

Vital Pulp Therapy

Maintenance of pulp vitality should always be the goal in treatment planning, and considerable interest is developing in the concept of regenerative endodontics for complete or partial pulp tissue regeneration. This interest in maintaining the biological functions of the dental pulp and the recognition that they are important for the longevity and overall health of the patients dates back to 1756 with the original attempts of pulp capping.[66] The introduction of calcium hydroxide[67] and more recently, the widespread use of hydraulic tricalcium silicates such as mineral trioxide aggregate (MTA; Dentsply, York, Pennsylvania, USA), Biodentine™ (Septodont, Saint-Maur-des-Fossés, France) and Endosequence® RRM™ (Root Repair Material) (Brasseler, USA) among others[68,69] have all emphasized the central role for biologically based therapies in endodontics. In general, vital pulp therapies can be classified in two broad categories: capping procedures and pulpotomies. These procedures differ in degrees of invasiveness and largely depend on the clinician's assessment of the extent of contamination and pulpal inflammation. This subjective assessment is performed chairside and relies on accurate clinical testing and diagnosis based on the signs and symptoms of disease and direct inspection of residual dentin and/or pulpal tissue under high-power magnification and illumination. Once vitality has been confirmed clinically by pulp sensitivity tests such as the application of cold or electrical pulp testing (EPT), careful inspection of the residual healthy tissue must be performed. Hemorrhage or lack thereof is often used as an indicator of the level of inflammation in the dental pulp. Continued bleeding despite application of mild pressure by an operator is interpreted as pulp that is too severely inflamed to be directly capped. Instead, more of the pulp tissue must be removed until its healthy appearance is observed and hemostasis is achieved. Although there have been attempts to develop methods to determine the level of inflammation of the residual pulp tissue based on biomarkers,[70] these methods have not yet been fully validated and are not immediately available for clinicians. Thus clinicians still rely on their expertise and subjective assessment when determining which vital pulp therapy is most suited for each particular case.

Capping Procedures

Indirect Pulp Capping

A clinician must always first identify the etiology of the insult and reach an accurate diagnosis. In the case of caries or uncomplicated crown fractures (without pulp exposure), excavation of infected dentin and cavity disinfection must be first achieved. If possible, the pulp tissue should not be violated. This goal can be achieved by progressive removal, using caries indicator to detect contaminated dentinal tissue. It has been shown that cavity preparations with residual dentin thickness of at least 0.5 mm from the pulp could be successfully capped with a bioactive material, resulting in the desirable formation of reactionary dentin, particularly in young patients.[71] This capping approach is called *indirect pulp capping* because the bioactive material does not directly contact the pulp tissue. Yet its bioactive components and high pH can neutralize bacteria[72,73] and their antigens and directly stimulate odontoblasts to produce reactionary tertiary dentin in the site of injury.[74] Ideally, the bioactive materials are placed over residual healthy, uninfected dentin. However, there is evidence that residual softened dentin can be capped, still resulting in tertiary dentin and arrested progression of the disease with the use of these materials.[74] This partial caries removal approach can be accomplished in one visit or may be followed by additional visits for excavation followed by capping, called *step-wise caries excavation*.[75,76] These conservative approaches strongly rely on the remineralization of the residual dentin and further formation of tertiary dentin by a healthy pulp. Therefore clinicians need to maintain a close follow-up to ensure that these biological goals are being achieved and that the pulp remains vital and the patient asymptomatic (Fig. 10.9).

Direct Pulp Capping

The exposure of the pulp tissue without major contamination can happen upon mechanical exposure of the dental pulp by trauma or during cavity preparation. In this instance the pulp may be

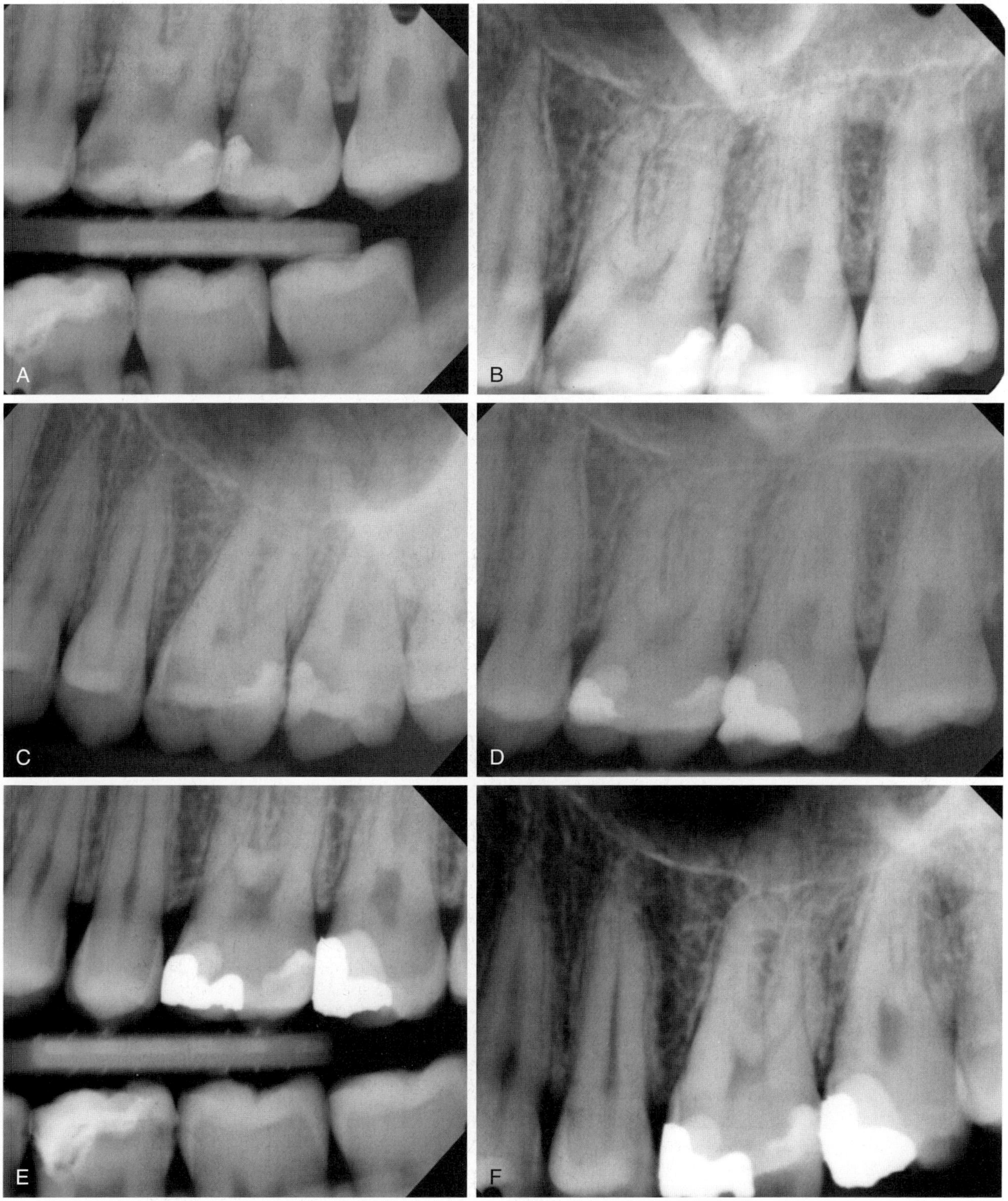

• **Fig. 10.9** An 18-year-old male patient with asymptomatic deep caries lesions on #14 and #15 and diagnosed with reversible pulpitis and normal periapical tissues diagnosed (**A**, **B**, and **C**). Caries were removed and indirect pulp capping performed on both teeth under rubber dam isolation with Biodentine™ (Septodont, Saint-Maur-des-Fossés, France) and coronal seal with Fuji IILC (GC America), followed by an amalgam final coronal restoration (**D**). At 1-year follow-up, tooth was asymptomatic and was diagnosed with normal pulp and normal periradicular tissues (**E** and **F**). (Case courtesy Dr. Tatiana M. Botero, private practice, Alsip, Illinois, USA.)

protected and its vitality maintained by immediately covering it (pulp capping) with a bioactive material and placing a restoration, thereby avoiding root canal treatment. This approach has been shown to have an excellent prognosis in incompletely formed teeth but has also been shown successful in permanent teeth with fully formed roots. However, in cases of long-standing carious exposure of the pulp, lower success rates are expected when a direct pulp-capping procedure is performed.[77] Recently, new data on the regenerative potential of the dental pulp and the development of newer bioactive materials have broadened the effectiveness of direct pulp-capping procedures.

Pulpotomies

If the exposure is large or seriously contaminated, it may require the removal of the superficial layer of the diseased pulp (partial pulpotomy) or the entire coronal pulp to the level of the root canal orifice (pulp chamber pulpotomy). As with direct pulp capping, close follow-up is recommended to ensure that, if needed, appropriate further treatment is provided in a timely fashion (Fig. 10.10).

Partial pulpotomies (also known as *Cvek pulpotomies*)[78] rely on the removal of the superficial most layer of infected or irreversibly injured pulp, followed by the direct capping of the residual healthy pulp. This technique relies on the subjective clinical assessment of inflammation upon direct visualization of the tissues. This assessment is best achieved with the use of the operating microscope that facilitates the visualization of hemorrhagic parts of the dental pulp. Typically, a pulp is considered irreversibly inflamed if it bleeds profusely despite local hemostasis measures. In these instances, the clinician may elect to remove more of the pulp or the complete removal of the pulp in the chamber to the level of the canal orifices (pulp chamber pulpotomy). In brief, the affected tooth is adequately isolated with the dental dam, and the infected

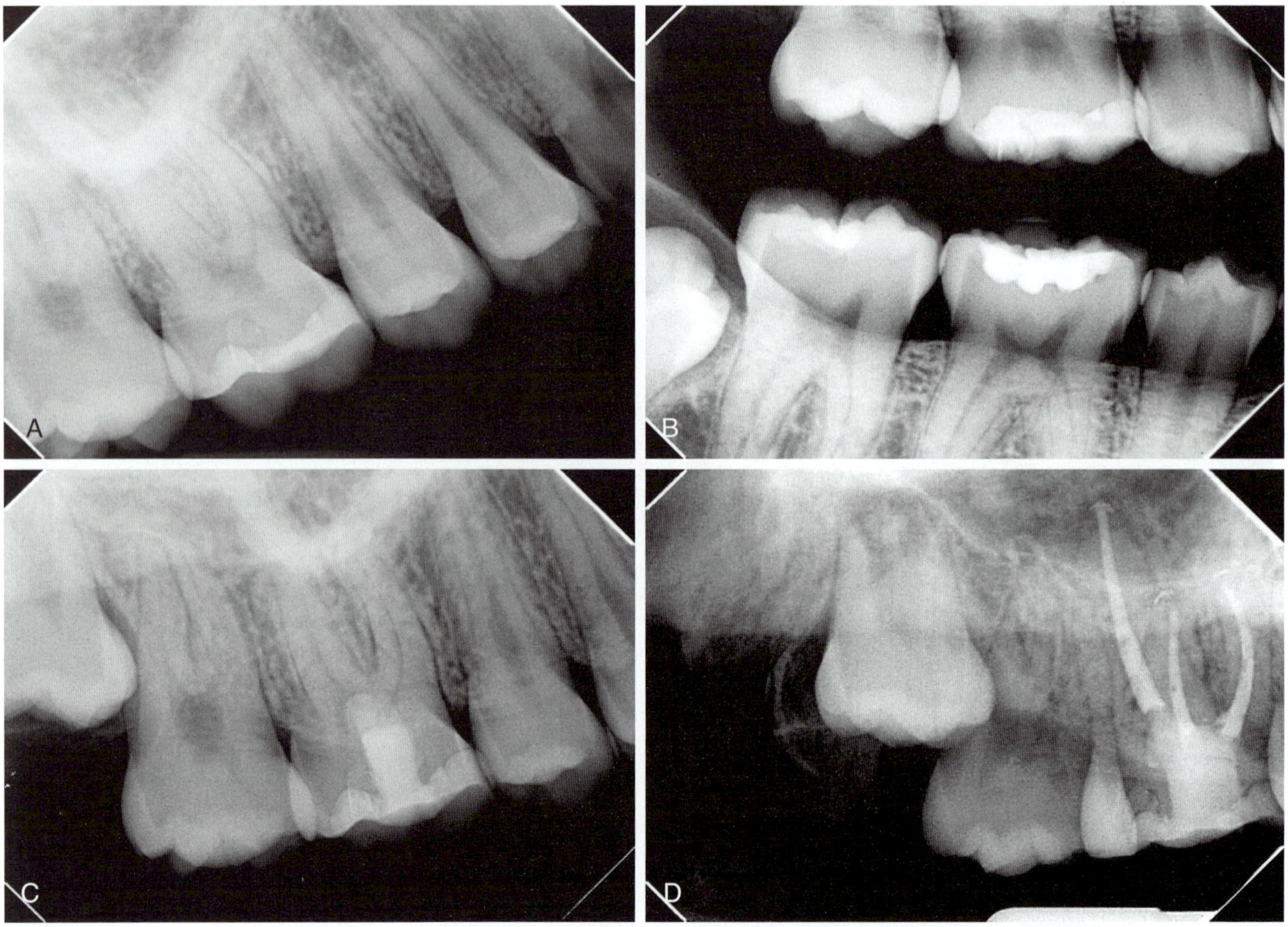

• **Fig. 10.10** A 16-year-old female presents to clinic with a chief complaint of pain in the upper right tooth. Tooth #3 was restored 4 months before with an occlusal composite restoration. Patient reported pain triggered by hot, cold, and chewing but she was not experiencing spontaneous pain or pain that woke her up at night (**A** and **B**). Vital pulp therapy was completed under rubber dam isolation. The pulp chamber was accessed, coronal pulp tissue removed, and hemostasis achieved with less than 5 minutes of a sodium hypochlorite (NaOCl)-soaked cotton pellet pressure. Biodentine™ was placed in the pulp chamber, and restoration completed with Fuji II LC and composite core build-up material **(C)**. Patient returned 4 weeks later with throbbing pain triggered by hot and chewing, which had started 2 weeks earlier. Nonsurgical root canal treatment was completed under rubber dam isolation, obturation completed with gutta-perch and Roth's sealer. Tooth was restored with glass ionomer and core build-up material **(D)**. Patient was asymptomatic 2 months post-non-surgical root canal therapy (NSRCT). (Case courtesy Dr. Sukhpreet Sandhu, Advanced Program in Endodontics at the University of Texas Health at San Antonio, San Antonio, TX, USA.)

dentin and damaged pulp is removed with water-cooled diamond bur at high speed. Next, a cotton pellet soaked in sodium hypochlorite is placed over the pulp with gentle pressure, followed by 17% ethylenediaminetetraacetic acid (EDTA). After the cavity is dried, a tricalcium silicate material is placed over the pulp/dentin, followed by a final coronal sealing restoration. Partial pulpotomies, when performed with good aseptic techniques and using bioactive silicate materials, demonstrate excellent success rates, allowing root maturation (maturogenesis) and normal physiologic responses[79] (Figs. 10.11 and 10.12).

A complete pulp chamber pulpotomy is often required when the coronal pulp is heavily inflamed or with a questionable vitality status. Once the pulp in the chamber is removed under rubber dam isolation with a diamond bur at high speed with plenty of sterile water as coolant, a cotton pellet soaked in sodium hypochlorite is placed over the pulp stump(s) and gentle pressure is applied for 2 to 5 minutes. This technique allows for disinfection and hemostasis (if not irreversibly inflamed), which should result in pulp stumps with minimal to no bleeding. Next, the chamber is quickly rinsed with 17% EDTA and gently air dried, and a layer of >4 mm of a bioactive tricalcium silicate material is placed over the pulp stumps. Finally, the tooth is sealed with a definitive restoration (e.g., composite restoration). Patients should be reevaluated at 6 and 12 months, followed by annual evaluations for the first 4 years. This procedure has been shown to have excellent clinical results, promoting the maintenance of vitality, continued root development, and the lack of symptoms, and it may be considered definitive treatment in certain cases[80] (Figs. 10.13 and 10.14).

It is important to recognize, however, that pulp inflammation is a progressive disease, and the use of regenerative approaches to maintain pulp vitality requires a good understanding of the interplay of biologic factors influencing regenerative events, in addition to appropriate case selection. Such approaches may not be suitable for all cases, especially those showing deep pulp inflammation involving the radicular tissue, and the correlation of clinical symptoms with the pathophysiologic status of the dental pulp remains a significant challenge. In addition, there are no studies evaluating the long-term outcomes of these procedures in large patient populations,[15] and patients should be evaluated closely to ensure that the biologic outcome of continued root development and vitality are being achieved, and conventional root canal therapies should always be considered if vital pulp therapies fail to achieve their biologic goals.

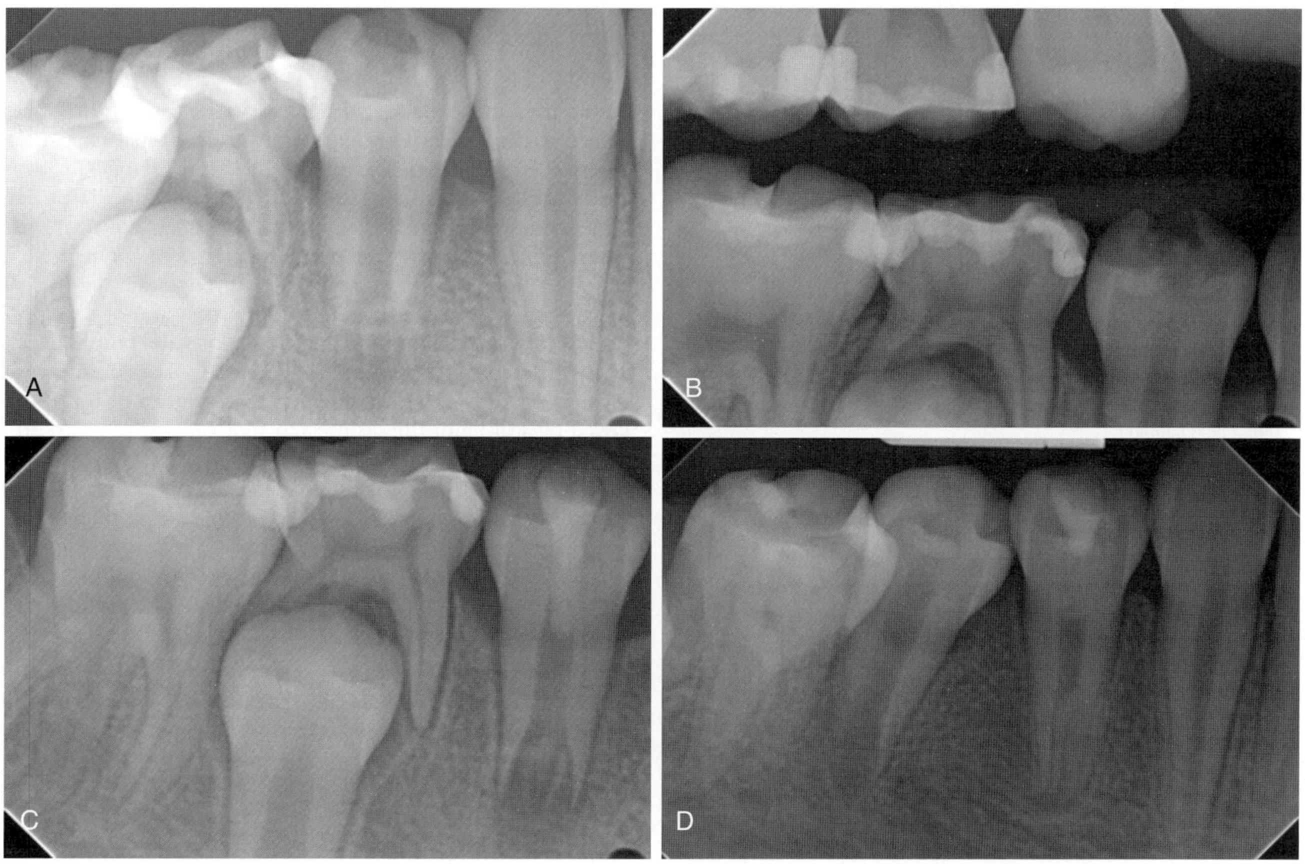

• **Fig. 10.11** A 10-year-old female patient was evaluated for pain upon mastication on tooth #28 for approximately 2 weeks. The tooth had occlusal caries and immature, partially formed root, and it was diagnosed as reversible pulpitis with normal periradicular tissues (**A** and **B**). A partial pulpotomy was performed under rubber dam isolation with Biodentine™ being placed over the vital pulp, followed by a glass ionomer and composite restoration **(C)**. At 1-year recall, the patient was asymptomatic, responded normally to vitality testing, and demonstrated the completion of development of a bifurcated root and normal periapical tissues **(D)**. (Case courtesy Dr. Saeed Bayat Movahed, Graduate Endodontics Program. University of Texas Health at San Antonio, San Antonio, TX, USA.)

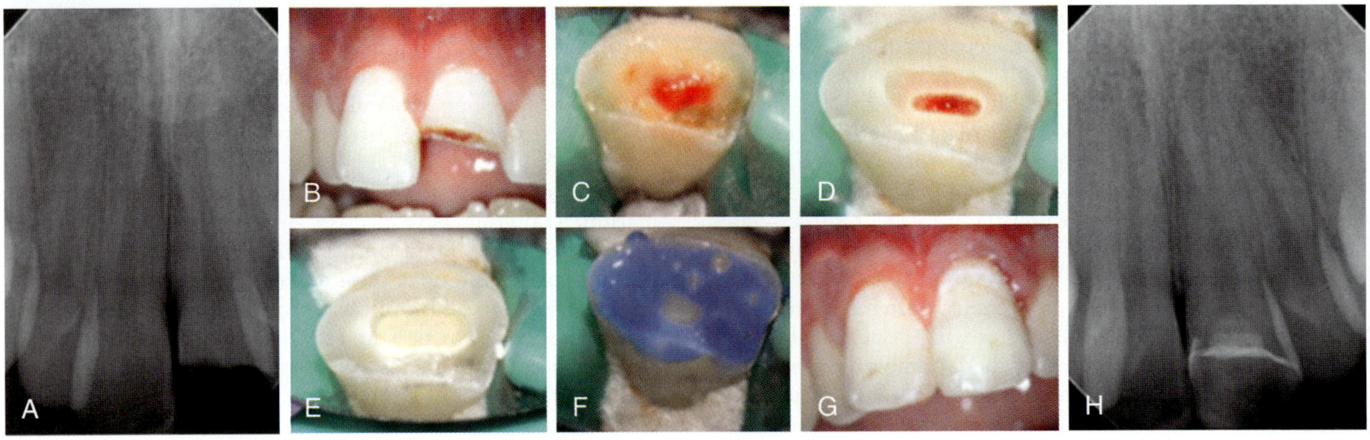

• **Fig. 10.12** A 17-year-old male patient presented with a complicated crown fracture after trauma of tooth #9 approximately 24 hours before the appointment. A preoperative periapical radiograph **(A)** and clinical examination **(B)** confirmed the presence of a frank pulp exposure **(C)**. The tooth responded to vitality testing with an exaggerated but nonlingering response to cold test, and it was diagnosed as reversible pulpitis. Approximately 2 mm of the affected coronal pulp was removed under rubber dam isolation and hemostasis was achieved with topical application of 2.5% sodium hypochlorite (NaOCl) followed by 17% ethylenediaminetetraacetic acid (EDTA) **(D)**. A 3-mm-thick layer of Biodentine™ (Septodont, Saint-Maur-des-Fossés, France) was placed over the vital pulp **(E)**. The tooth was etched **(F)** and the fractured fragment kept by the patient was bonded and restored with composite **(G)**. A postoperative periapical radiograph revealed adequate coronal seal and adaptation of the fractured segment **(H)**. The patient has remained asymptomatic since the treatment. (Case courtesy Dr. Koyo Takimoto, Advanced Program in Endodontics at the University of Texas Health at San Antonio, San Antonio, TX, USA.)

Study Questions

1. The following are defense mechanisms of the dental pulp:
   a. Outward fluid flow
   b. Neurogenic inflammation
   c. Arteriole/venule (A/V) shunt
   d. Tertiary dentinogenesis
   e. All of the above
2. The following is NOT an example of vital pulp therapy:
   a. Partial pulpotomy
   b. Full chamber pulpotomy
   c. Pulpectomy
   d. Direct pulp capping
   e. Indirect pulp capping
3. The following is true regarding partial or complete pulp chamber pulpotomies:
   a. Use of bioactive dental materials is advocated.
   b. They are considered only temporary therapies.
   c. They have considerably lower success rates compared with nonvital therapies.
   d. Teeth diagnosed with pulp necrosis can benefit from these procedures.
4. What are the most common teeth affected by traumatic injuries?
   a. Anterior maxillary
   b. Anterior mandibular
   c. Posterior maxillary
   d. Posterior mandibular

Treatment of Immature Teeth with Pulp Necrosis

Immature teeth with pulpal necrosis present clinical challenges due to persistent infection in the root canal system, often associated with periradicular bone loss and inability to effectively disinfect the root canals and seal the root canal space. These cases are exemplified in premolars with dens evaginatus, a form of enamel defect at the occlusal surface resulting in pulpal exposure after abrasion of the occlusal enamel.[46] Necrotic changes in the pulp after exposure in dens evaginatus often occurs in pediatric patients with incomplete root development and open apices.[81] Alternatively, pulpal necrosis can occur in any permanent teeth from carious lesions that have penetrated through the dentinal layers to cause the root canal infection at any stage of root development. Endodontic treatment of immature teeth with pulpal necrosis is vastly different from vital pulp therapies. In cases of infection, the focus is on root canal débridement and control of infection, followed by sealing of the disinfected root canal space with artificial material, or an attempt to regenerate vital tissue. On the contrary, vital pulp therapies are primarily focused on preservation of the remaining vital pulp tissues, as seen in the cases of direct pulp capping or pulpotomies as described previously in this chapter. Thus this section of the chapter will discuss our treatment strategies for immature teeth with pulpal necrosis, which mainly include apexification and regenerative endodontic therapies.

Apexification—Indications, Approach, and Limitations

For immature teeth with pulp necrosis, root canal débridement can be accomplished with mechanical instrumentation and copious irrigation with antimicrobial irrigating solutions. Obturation of the root canal space is necessary to avoid remaining bacteria or microbial biofilm growth after the clinician's attempt to disinfect the root canal space. In particular, teeth with pulpal necrosis are generally considered infected with bacteria within the complexities of root canal space, including dentinal tubules, especially when radiographic lesions are visible. It has been shown that tubular infection with bacteria occurs rapidly after dentinal inoculation with the microorganisms and that the depth of tubular penetration

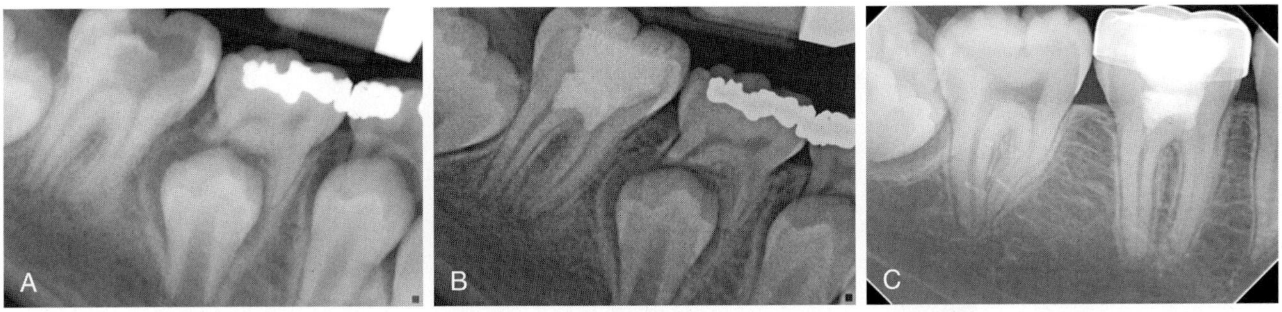

• **Fig. 10.13** An 11-year-old male with large carious lesion and diagnosis of reversible pulpitis **(A)** was treated with full pulp chamber pulpotomy performed with white mineral trioxide aggregate (MTA) (Dentsply, York, PA, USA) and a composite restoration **(B)** followed by a stainless-steel crown. At 7-year recall, the tooth is asymptomatic, responds normally to vitality testing and displays completion of root development and normal periradicular tissues **(C)**. (Case courtesy Dr. Tyler Lovelace, Advanced Program in Endodontics at the University of Texas Health at San Antonio, San Antonio, TX, USA.)

occurs in a time-dependent manner.[82] Hence in cases in which the apical constriction has not yet been formed, the obturation of the root canal system can be accomplished by a procedure called *apexification*. In these procedures, a calcific barrier is formed after long-term calcium hydroxide medicament or immediately with the use of an MTA or other tricalcium silicate as an apical plug.

Apexification is different from apexogenesis, which is accomplished with vital pulp therapies. In apexification, no vital pulp tissue is preserved because root canal obturation will occur to the most apical extent of the root, regardless of the size of the apical opening. Thus no further root development is anticipated in teeth treated by apexification, whereas apical closure and further root development is anticipated in those treated by apexogenesis. Studies have clearly demonstrated that immature teeth treated by apexification do not undergo changes in the root dimension, such as lengthening or thickening of the root dentin.[83-87] Conceptually, apexification has as its primary goal apical closure, which can be accomplished by an indirect approach using $Ca(OH_2$ as intracanal medicament or directly by placement of MTA or other hydraulic silicate cement to the apical extent of the root canal space. The $Ca(OH)_2$-mediated apical closure formation is an indirect approach because it relies on the establishment of a hard tissue apical barrier, which often requires an extended period of $Ca(OH)_2$ medicament and multiple appointments.[88] Typically, $Ca(OH)_2$-mediated apical plug formation requires 3- to 9-month period of treatment, during which time the $Ca(OH)_2$ medicament needs to be replaced periodically, thereby requiring multiple patient visits. In addition, there is increasing evidence that long-term calcium hydroxide treatment can weaken dentin,[89,90] resulting in increased susceptibility to fractures.[91] These aspects are the major shortcomings of apexification with $Ca(OH)_2$ intracanal medicament. On the contrary, MTA (or other tricalcium silicate cements) apexification is a direct approach that does not require prior hard tissue formation induction; instead, an apical barrier as collagen plug followed by a bioactive cement will provide immediate apical barrier without the need for prolonged $Ca(OH)_2$ (Fig. 10.15). For this reason, apexification can be accomplished in a single visit (known as *one-step apexification*) without having to wait for the calcific barrier formation when the apical plug is established using MTA with same expected clinical success rate.[92,93]

Apexification has been the treatment of choice for many decades for immature teeth with pulpal necrosis since the 1970s. A retrospective study involving 98 teeth treated with apexification showed greater than 90% success in terms of resolution of apical periodontitis over long-term follow-up period.[94] Other studies also demonstrated close to 100% success in resolution of apical periodontitis by apexification for teeth with open apices.[95,96] However, one of the main limitations of apexification is arrest of root development posttreatment, when the treatment is rendered in immature teeth with large open apex, underdeveloped root structures with thin and short root dentin. Consequently, there is increased probability of root fracture in immature teeth treated by apexification. When teeth with immature root development were treated and maintained after root canal filling, the incidence of cervical root fracture was significantly higher than those of mature-root filled teeth and depended on the stage of root development.[91] Thus cervical root fracture remains a plausible risk factor for those immature teeth treated by apexification, primarily because of absence of root dentin development despite resolution of apical periodontitis.

Apexification—Clinical Protocols

The clinical procedure for apexification varies among clinicians but may be accentuated as following, as previously described by Kang and Bogen.[97] Under profound local anesthesia, access is made using a #2 long-shank round bur, and root canals are débrided with hand instrumentation with larger K-files, primarily by circumferential filing due to enlarged lumen of the root canals. Passive irrigation of root canals may proceed with 1.5% sodium hypochlorite (NaOCl) for 15 to 20 minutes while performing the canal instrumentation. For patients that present with soft tissue swelling around the buccal gingiva or with draining through the sinus tract, intracanal medicament using $Ca(OH)_2$ is necessary with temporization with a cotton pellet and temporary restoration. Subsequently, after confirming the resolution of the soft tissue lesions, placement of MTA into the root canal apex may proceed, with drying the canals using extra-coarse paper points. In certain cases, a collagen membrane (e.g., CollaPlug™ or CollaTape™, Zimmer Dental Inc, Warsaw, Indiana,USA) can be placed in contact with the periradicular tissues at the apex to serve as internal matrix to prevent or minimize the extrusion of MTA into the periradicular tissues. Apical condensation of MTA using the back end of paper points or gutta-percha points may be necessary to ensure the material adaptation to the most apical extent of the divergent root canal apices. Radiographs should be taken to confirm the adequate placement of the apical MTA plug to assess the density and thickness of the apical plug. After at least 5 mm of apical plug is established, ensuring adequate apical seal, the coronal root canal space may be filled with either MTA or flowable gutta-percha, depending on the clinical

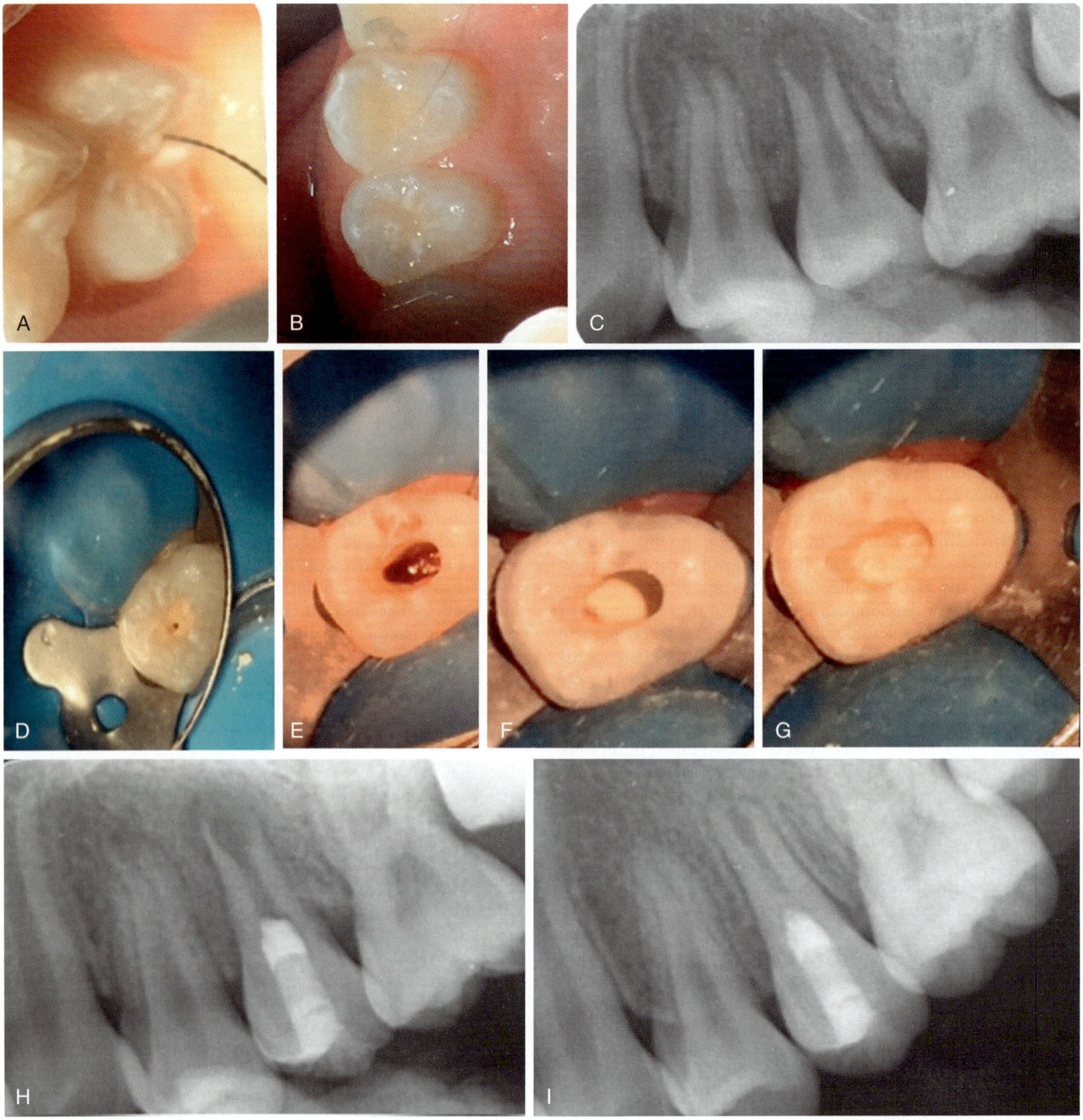

• **Fig. 10.14** An 11-year-old female patient with tooth #13 diagnosed with pulp necrosis and history of swelling. **(A)** A file could be placed in the communication between the pulp and the oral environment created by the dens evaginatus. **(B)** The opening of the tubercle is seen on the occlusal surface of tooth #13 *(black arrow)*. **(C)** Periapical radiograph revealed the presence of an immature root with thin dentinal walls and open apex. **(D)** Upon accessing through the dens communication, a vital pulp was seen under high magnification. **(E–G)** A full pulpotomy was performed with placement of Biodentine™, glass ionomer, and a composite coronal seal **(G, H)**. **(I)** At 1-year follow-up, the patient was asymptomatic, and radiographic examination revealed a mineralized bridge formation under the Biodentine™ and evidence of further root maturation with closure of the apex and normal periradicular tissues. (Courtesy of Dr. Tatiana M. Botero and Dr. Anna DeGraft-Johnson, Graduate Endodontic Program, University of Michigan, Ann Arbor, MI, USA.)

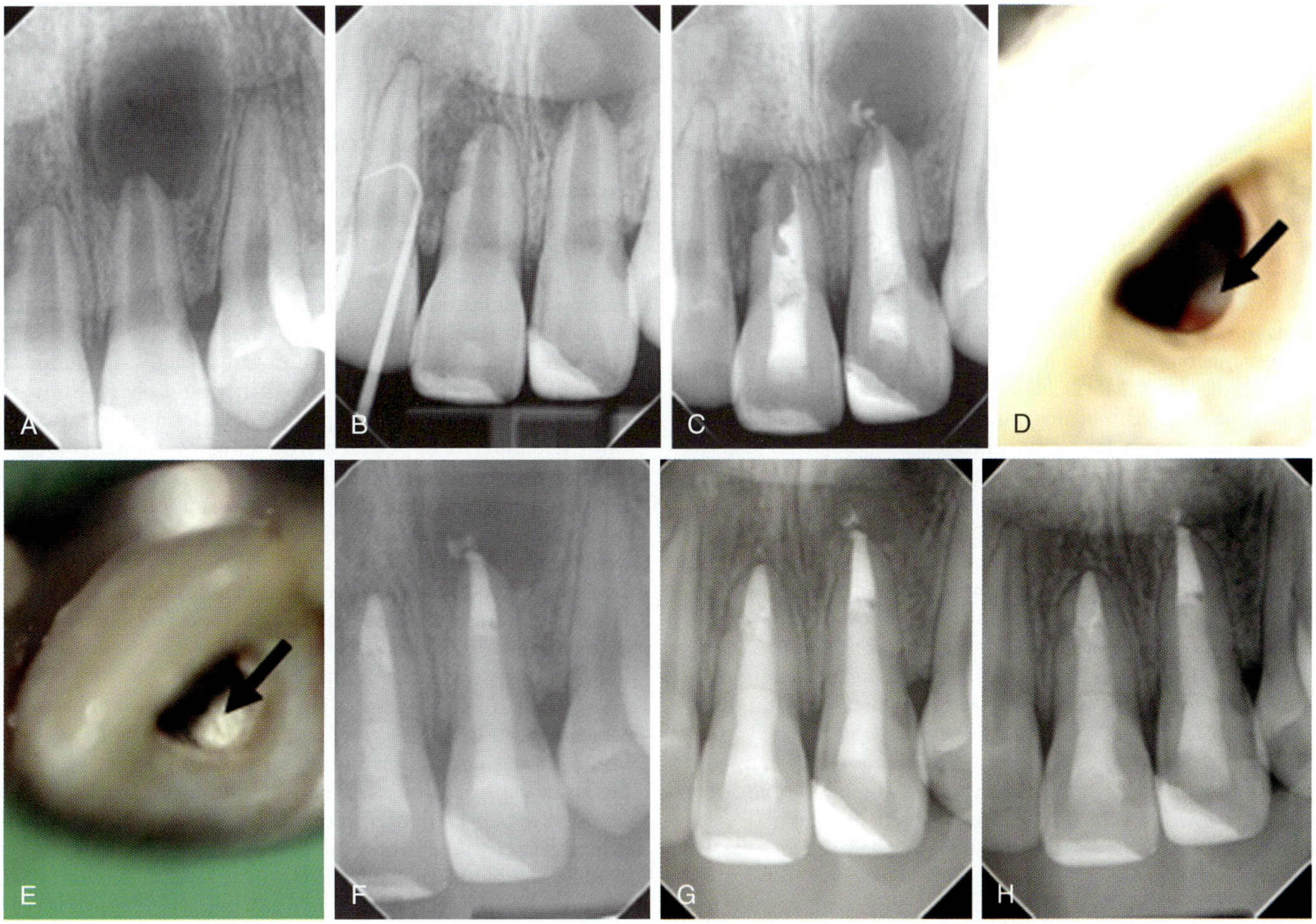

• **Fig. 10.15** A 16-year-old male patient with history of trauma to the anterior teeth due to a car accident 9 years prior has the chief complaint of intermittent pain, swelling, and intraoral drainage **(A)**. Intraoral examination revealed a sinus tract that was traced with a gutta-percha cone to tooth #8, which was diagnosed with pulp necrosis and chronic apical abscess; periradicular inflammatory root resorption is also observed on the periapical radiograph (**A** and **B**). Tooth #9 was diagnosed with pulp necrosis and symptomatic apical periodontitis due to lack of responses to vitality testing and the extreme tenderness to percussion and the large periapical radiolucency (**A** and **B**). On first visit, both teeth were accessed, and canals were débrided with Hedstrom files and irrigation with 6% sodium hypochlorite (NaOCl) and 17% ethylenediaminetetraacetic acid (EDTA), followed by placement of calcium hydroxide medicament for 1 month and access seal with Fuji Triage glass ionomer **(C)**. On the second visit (1 month later), the sinus tract had closed, and the patient was asymptomatic. Teeth were reaccessed, and canals were irrigated as in first visit. Next, a collagen membrane was placed at the apical foramen to prevent mineral trioxide aggregate (MTA) extrusion (*black arrow*; **D**). Next, white MTA was placed at apical one-third of each tooth (*black arrow*; **E**), and the canals were backfilled with thermoplasticized gutta-percha and accesses sealed a composite restoration **(F)**. At both 1-year **(G)** and 2-year recall **(H)**, both teeth were asymptomatic without swelling or sinus tract history with radiographic evidence of complete healing and arrestment of the resorptive process in tooth #8. (Case courtesy Dr. Anibal Diogenes, Endodontic Faculty Practice, University of Texas Health at San Antonio, San Antonio, TX, USA.)

needs and restorative plan for the tooth. Coronal restoration may be finalized using bonded composite material. Radiographic follow-up examination should be scheduled to assess resolution of apical periodontitis and absence of complications after 6 and 12 months postoperatively.

Regenerative Endodontic Procedures (REPs)—Indications, Approach, and Limitations

In 2000 reports of isolation and characterization of multipotent adult stem cells from the dental pulp, namely dental pulp stem cells (DPSCs), had been published[98] followed by the identification of stem cells of the apical papilla (SCAP).[99] Shortly after, a case report demonstrated successful treatment of immature teeth with periapical abscess via regenerative approaches, which led to resolution of apical periodontitis and apical closure.[100] Those two findings have fueled the explosion of interest and research endeavors in regenerative endodontics, which led at least to an alternative treatment protocol for necrotic immature teeth through development of regenerative endodontic procedure (REP), also known as *pulp revascularization* or *pulp revitalization*. At present, REP is considered a viable treatment option for immature teeth with pulpal necrosis. This protocol presents critical advantages over apexification in that teeth undergo dimensional changes posttreatment that result in increased root dentin thickness and length.[83,87] Consequently, REP is expected to address the major shortcomings of apexification, which are the arrest of root development and the permanent loss of pulp vitality.

The basic premise of REP is to allow indigenous mesenchymal stem cells (MSCs) around the periapex to continue the root development in the immature teeth by débriding the infected root canal space. The typical REP procedure involves disinfection of the root canal space by minimal instrumentation with antimicrobial irrigation and placement of medicaments (e.g., $Ca[OH]_2$ or triple antibiotic paste [TAP]), which includes metronidazole, ciprofloxacin, and minocycline, follow by coronal seal. In a second appointment, typically 2 to 4 weeks after the placement of medicament, indigenous MSCs from periapical tissues are recruited by means of induced bleeding into the root canal space[101,102] or placement of growth factor–enriched scaffold, such as platelet-rich plasma (PRP) or plate-rich fibrin (PRF), followed by capping material (MTA or other tricalcium silicate) and coronal restoration. Recent studies demonstrate successful REP through various clinical protocols.[96,103-106] The success/survival rate of REP in the literature is surprisingly high, nearing 100%, and successful outcome is defined by resolution of apical periodontitis.[96,104,105,107] Thus it is important to note that the success of REP in resolving apical periodontitis does not seem to depend on the variations of treatment protocols but is determined largely by successful disinfection of the root canal space, recruitment of MSCs, and biocompatibility of the coronal restoration. Whether the root canals were disinfected by $Ca(OH)_2$ medicament or mixture of antibiotics or whether the MSCs were recruited by induced bleeding[101,102] or placement of PRP/PRF,[108] no difference in the outcome has yet been seen.[109]

Although REP has clearly revolutionized how clinicians treat immature teeth with pulp necrosis, it falls short on de novo regeneration of the dentin-pulp complex with currently used techniques. Histologic studies on teeth treated by REP have revealed the absence of organized pulp tissues, such as a palisading odontoblast layer juxtaposed with the dentinal surface, and occurrence of ectopic tissue formation inside the lumen of root canals, which included bone, cementum, and fibrous tissues.[110] These findings were corroborated with large animal studies, which also revealed ectopic tissue formation in the root canal space after REP, in lieu of dentin-pulp regeneration.[111] Thus REP may represent "tissue repair" rather than de novo regeneration of functional dental pulp, although the procedure demonstrates efficacy in the resolution of apical periodontitis. These procedures have also been called "guided endodontic repair" (GER),[112] acknowledging the role of each clinical step of these procedures favoring formation of a vital tissue resembling the pulp as being a connective tissue with rich vascularity[113] and innervation,[114] but lacking the organization of the native dental pulp. The ectopic mineralization in the root canals after REP may manifest as rampant calcifications visible on the follow-up radiographs (Fig. 10.16). Song et al. recently reported the clinical outcome of 29 REP cases with varying clinical parameters and treatment protocols with 1- to 6-year recall period.[115] This longitudinal retrospective study also showed very high proportion of treatment success, with 80% of apical closures for those with open apices. Researchers were surprised to find that intracanal calcification was evident in 62% of REP cases to varying degrees, some with complete canal obliteration; REP cases that were followed at multiple time points revealed progressive increases in the level of canal calcifications. Hence, the so-called REP-associated intracanal calcification (RAIC) is a very common treatment complication and illustrates the major limitation of this treatment approach because RAIC could impede restoration of functional dental pulp after REP.

REP—Clinical Protocols

There are many variants of REP protocols that lead to successful treatment outcome. The American Association of Endodontists (AAE) has developed Clinical Considerations for Regenerative Procedures(https://www.aae.org/specialty/clinical-resources/regenerative-endodontics/), which outlines detailed protocols to be employed for REP. In addition, these treatment recommendations closely resemble those of the European Society of Endodontology (ESE).[116] In essence, the cases that would benefit from REP include immature teeth with pulp necrosis and adequate coronal tooth structure to be restored with direct restoration. Débridement of the root canal space may proceed with minimal instrumentation and irrigation with low concentration (1.5%) NaOCl, followed by intracanal $Ca(OH)_2$ or TAP dressing to resolve periradicular inflammation. The tooth is then temporarily restored until the second appointment. After confirming the absence of gross periradicular inflammation, such as resolution of soft tissue swelling or draining sinus tract, the tooth is ready for the second phase of REP, which involves recruitment of MSCs into the root canal space. The patient is anesthetized with a local anesthetic without vasoconstrictor, e.g., 3% mepivacaine, and the tooth is isolated with a rubber dam. After intracanal irrigation with 17% EDTA and visual confirmation of absence of draining exudate or necrotic debris, bleeding is induced into the root canal space by agitation of periapical tissues beyond the root apex, using small #10 K-files to allow the blood clot formation to the level of cementoenamel junction (CEJ). Collagen matrix, e.g., CollaPlug™ or CollaTape™, may be placed over the blood clot to provide a barrier onto which MTA or other tricalcium silicate can be placed as coronal capping material. In the final visit, the patient should be recalled for a 1-week postoperative check to confirm the absence of periradicular infection and resolution of the patient's symptoms. The tooth can then be restored with direct restoration (e.g., composite resin over MTA or other tricalcium silicate) (Fig. 10.17) and be followed up with a 6-month check, followed by yearly recall visits. Importantly, clinicians must become more familiar with this new treatment alternative and realize that the radiographic presentation of teeth treated with this treatment modality will appear as if endodontic the "filling" or obturation is missing. Therefore adequate treatment history and current vitality testing must be performed when history of this kind of treatment is suspected to prevent unnecessary re-treatment and the violation of a newly formed reparative vital tissue.

Tissue Engineering Approaches

Although efficacious, REP presents limitations that involve ectopic tissue formation and calcification of the canal space, which may impede functional pulp regeneration. To circumvent these issues, pulp tissue engineering approaches have been developed and involve isolation, expansion, and transplantation of autologous pulpal MSCs. An earlier animal study revealed that de novo regeneration of the dentin-pulp complex requires transplantation of pulpal MSCs, whereas transplantation of scaffold alone led to ingrowth of fibrous tissues with no pulp tissue regeneration.[117] Likewise, a large animal study involving pulpectomy model in dogs showed successful

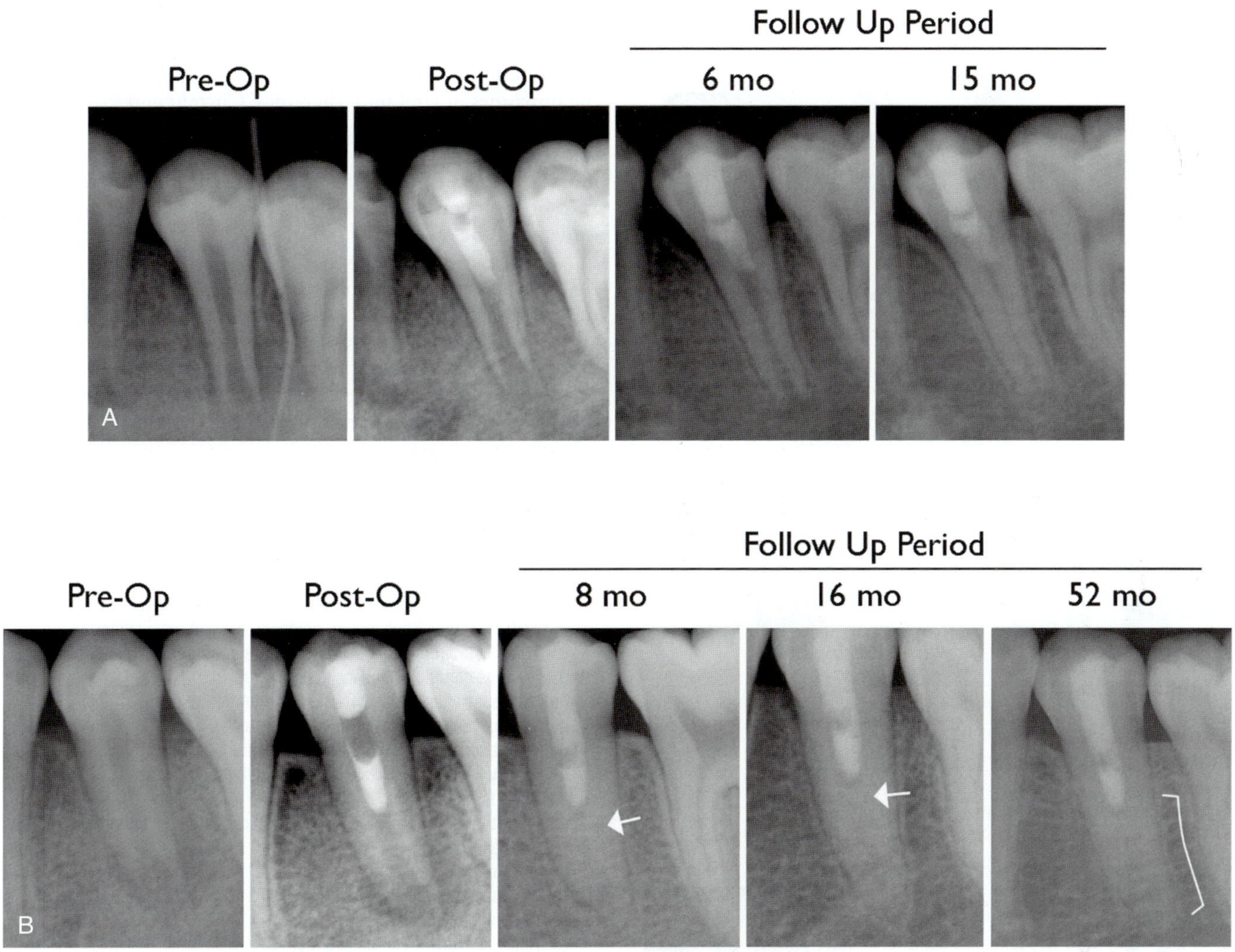

• **Fig. 10.16** Regenerative endodontic procedures (REPs) are efficacious in resolving apical periodontitis but with frequent occurrence of intracanal calcification. Tooth #20 is shown with large periapical radiolucency and gutta-percha tracing of sinus tract **(A)**. Due to open apex, regenerative endodontic therapy was performed, followed by coronal restoration with mineral trioxide aggregate (MTA). When the patient was recalled for 6-month follow-up, apical periodontitis had been completely resolved, and the tooth demonstrated complete closure of the apex. Also visible on the 6- and 15-month follow-up radiograph was lengthening and thickening of root dentin without evidence of intracanal calcification. **(B)** In a similar clinical scenario, tooth #20 presented with periapical radiolucency with open apex and was treated by REP and coronal MTA placement. In this case, REP successfully resolved apical periodontitis, but there is appearance of intracanal calcification at 8-, 16-, and 52-month follow-up, with progressive increase in the level of calcification with time after completion of REP (*arrows* and *bracket*). (Figures were modified from Martin G, Ricucci D, Gibbs JL, Lin LM: Histological findings of revascularized/revitalized immature permanent molar with apical periodontitis using platelet-rich plasma, *J Endod* 39(1):138–144, 2013.)

regeneration of whole pulp by transplantation of pulpal MSCs enriched with CD105+ immunophenotyped.[118] These animal studies demonstrated that functional pulp regeneration requires pulpal MSC transplantation, supporting the concept of cell-based approaches for endodontic regeneration. Recently a phase I clinical trial of MSC transplantation was performed successfully in patients presenting with symptomatic irreversible pulpitis.[119] This study tested the efficacy and safety of cell-based therapy, by which the investigators débrided coronal caries lesions, shaped the root canals, and transplanted autologous pulp MSCs into the root canal space mixed with a collagen scaffold. At successive evaluations, the investigators documented the resolution of patient symptoms, restoration of vitality and sensibility of pulp tissues, and absence of canal calcification in patients who received MSC transplantation in the root canal space. Hence, the cell-based tissue engineering strategy is feasible for endodontic regeneration and may circumvent the limitations of REP. Further research endeavors will focus on practicalities of cell-based endodontic regeneration to bring the technology chairside to benefit the public.

Conclusions

The dental pulp has elaborate defense mechanisms designed to minimize damage from microbial insults and trauma. Early intervention with minimally invasive procedures addressing the

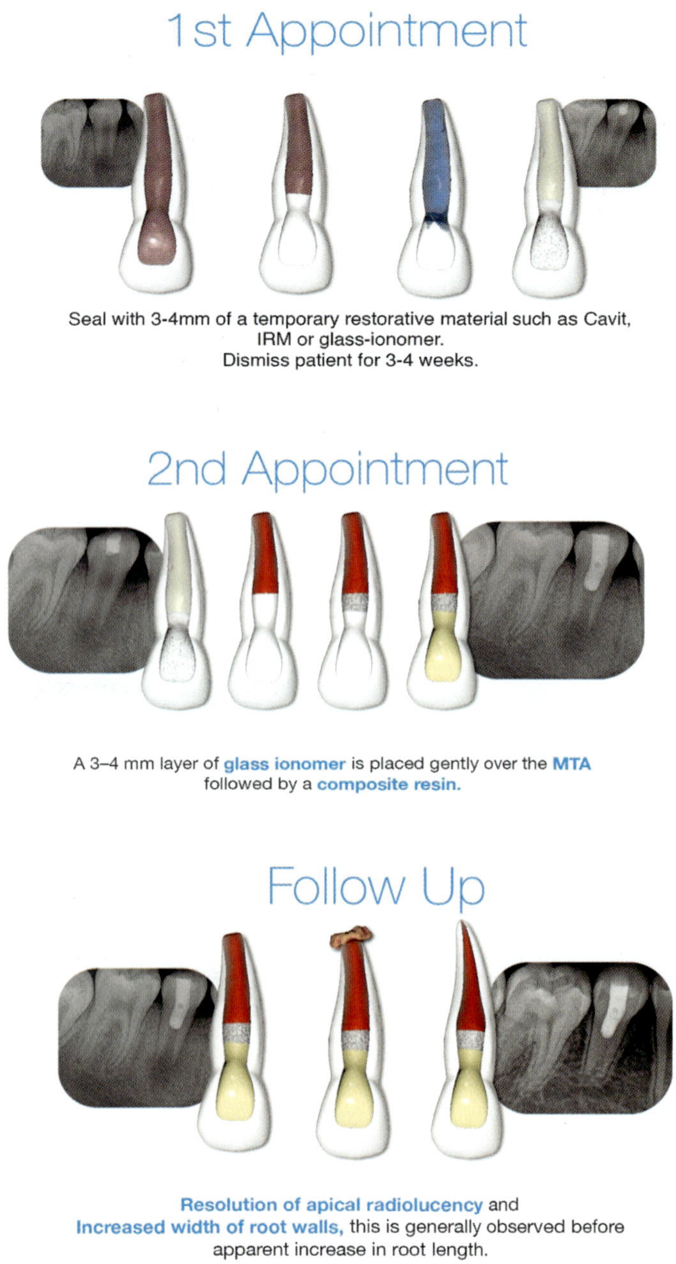
1st Appointment
Seal with 3-4mm of a temporary restorative material such as Cavit, IRM or glass-ionomer.
Dismiss patient for 3-4 weeks.
2nd Appointment
A 3–4 mm layer of glass ionomer is placed gently over the MTA followed by a composite resin.
Follow Up
Resolution of apical radiolucency and Increased width of root walls, this is generally observed before apparent increase in root length.

• **Fig. 10.17** Regenerative endodontic procedure (REP) treatment protocol as recommended by the American Association of Endodontists (AAE) and European Society of Endodontology (ESE). At first appointment, after access and disinfection, the intracanal medication is placed and left for several weeks, rendering the root canal progressively more disinfected *(seen as color change in the illustration)*. At second appointment, the medication is removed, and bleeding is induced from periapical tissues. Blood clot is formed and capped with a collagen membrane and a tricalcium silicate cement (e.g., white mineral trioxide aggregate [MTA]; Dentsply, York, PA, USA or Biodentine™; Septodont, Saint-Maur-des-Fossés, France). Follow-up for 6, 12, and 24 months after treatment completion. Clinical case of an immature premolar with dens evaginatus and pulp necrosis at a 2-year follow-up. (Case courtesy Dr. Viraj Vora, private practice, Toronto, Canada. Graphics by Dr. Diogo Guerreiro, University of Michigan Ann Arbor, MI.) Figure was modified from Botero-D TM, Vodopyanov D, Degraft-Johnson A., Guerreiro D., "Procedures endodontiques regeneratives" Revue d'odonto stomatology. Tome 47, No 4, Dec 2018; 338-349.

etiology of the disease has the potential to favor regeneration and repair with excellent clinical prognosis. Advances in pulp biology and dental materials have played a fundamental role in improving outcomes of vital pulp therapies. Current and further knowledge gained on molecular markers of inflammation could result in better diagnosis and even more predictable outcomes. For the most severe cases of insult that resulted in pulp necrosis, the field of regenerative endodontics has made significant strides in understanding the role of stem cells, dentin growth factors, and biocompatible disinfection in the reestablishment of a vital tissue that fosters continued root development and acceptable clinical outcomes. Further efforts focused on better control of the regenerative process will improve the predictability and acceptance of regenerative endodontic therapies. In conclusion, clinicians must be ready to provide early biocompatible interventions to preserve pulp vitality, accepting their role as "facilitators" of the inherent great regenerative potential of human dental pulp.

Study Questions

5. When the patient presents a dental anomaly such as dens invaginatus or dens evaginatus, the dental pulp can become infected because:
   a. The enamel is less mineralized and prompt to decay.
   b. These patients have higher incidence of cariogenic bacteria.
   c. There is a direct access to bacteria though the malformation.
   d. There is generic predisposition to necrosis.
6. Select the iatrogenic factor that affects the dental pulp.
   a. Coronal leakage from inadequate restorations
   b. The vasoconstriction provoked by dental anesthetics
   c. The lack or cooling while drilling with high-speed burs
   d. All of the above
7. Which of the following is the limitation of regenerative endodontic procedures (REP)?
   a. Resolution of apical periodontitis
   b. Increased stability of the root
   c. Intracanal calcification
   d. Apical closure for immature teeth
8. Which of the following tissue type(s) have been shown to be present in the newly formed tissue after REP?
   a. Bone
   b. Cementum
   c. Fibrous tissues
   d. All of the above
9. Which of the following is NOT a requirement for successful REP?
   a. Bioactive, biocompatible material
   b. Control of inflammation and infection
   c. Presence or recruitment of mesenchymal stem cells
   d. Biomechanical instrumentation of canals

ANSWERS

Answer Box 10

1 e. All of the above
2 c. Pulpectomy
3 a. Use of bioactive dental materials is advocated.
4 a. Anterior maxillary
5 c. There is a direct access to bacteria through the malformation.
6 d. All of the above
7 c. Intracanal calcification
8 d. All of the above
9 d. Biomechanical instrumentation of canals

References

1. Hahn CL, Liewehr FR: Innate immune responses of the dental pulp to caries, *J Endod* 33(6):643–651, 2007.
2. Smith AJ, Tobias RS, Plant CG, et al.: In vivo morphogenetic activity of dentine matrix proteins, *J Biol Buccale* 18(2):123–129, 1990.
3. Smith AJ, Duncan HF, Diogenes A, et al.: Exploiting the bioactive properties of the dentin-pulp complex in regenerative endodontics, *J Endod* 42(1):47–56, 2016.
4. Cooper PR, Holder MJ, Smith AJ: Inflammation and regeneration in the dentin-pulp complex: a double-edged sword, *J Endod* 40(Suppl 4):S46–51, 2014.
5. Caviedes-Bucheli J, Munoz HR, Azuero-Holguin MM, Ulate E: Neuropeptides in dental pulp: the silent protagonists, *J Endod* 34(7):773–788, 2008.
6. Carda C, Peydro A: Ultrastructural patterns of human dentinal tubules, odontoblasts processes and nerve fibres, *Tissue & Cell* 38(2):141–150, 2006.
7. Diogenes A, Ferraz CC, Akopian AN, et al.: LPS sensitizes TRPV1 via activation of TLR4 in trigeminal sensory neurons, *J Dent Res* 90(6):759–764, 2011.
8. Ferraz CC, Henry MA, Hargreaves KM, Diogenes A: Lipopolysaccharide from *Porphyromonas gingivalis* sensitizes capsaicin-sensitive nociceptors, *J Endod* 37(1):45–48, 2011.
9. Farges JC, Keller JF, Carrouel F, et al.: Odontoblasts in the dental pulp immune response, *J Exp Zool B Mol Dev Evol* 312B(5):425–436, 2009.
10. Botero TM, Shelburne CE, Holland GR, et al.: TLR4 mediates LPS-induced VEGF expression in odontoblasts, *J Endod* 32(10):951–955, 2006.
11. Farges JC, Carrouel F, Keller JF, et al.: Cytokine production by human odontoblast-like cells upon Toll-like receptor-2 engagement, *Immunobiology* 216(4):513–517, 2011.
12. Yang G, Kawashima N, Kaneko T, Suzuki N, Okiji T, Suda H: Kinetic study of immunohistochemical colocalization of antigen-presenting cells and nerve fibers in rat periapical lesions, *J Endod* 33(2):132–136, 2007.
13. Kim S: Regulation of pulpal blood flow, *J Dent Res* 64:590–596, 1985.
14. Hammarstrom L: Enamel matrix, cementum development and regeneration, *J Clin Periodontol* 24(9 Pt 2):658–668, 1997.
15. Bergenholtz G, Axelsson S, Davidson T, et al.: Treatment of pulps in teeth affected by deep caries - a systematic review of the literature, *Singapore Dent J* 34(1):1–12, 2013.
16. Heys DR, Fitzgerald M, Heys RJ, Chiego Jr DJ: Healing of primate dental pulps capped with Teflon, *Oral Surg Oral Med Oral Pathol* 69(2):227–237, 1990.
17. Nair PN, Duncan HF, Pitt Ford TR, Luder HU: Histological, ultrastructural and quantitative investigations on the response of healthy human pulps to experimental capping with mineral trioxide aggregate: a randomized controlled trial, *Int Endod J* 41(2):128–150, 2008.
18. Moorrees CF, Kent Jr RL: Interrelations in the timing of root formation and tooth emergence, *Proceedings of the Finnish Dental Society, Suom Hammaslaak Toim* 77(1-3):113–117, 1981.
19. Moorrees CF, Gron AM, Lebret LM, et al.: Growth studies of the dentition: a review, *Am J Orthod* 55(6):600–616, 1969.
20. Xu L, Tang L, Jin F, et al.: The apical region of developing tooth root constitutes a complex and maintains the ability to generate root and periodontium-like tissues, *J Periodont Res* 44(2):275–282, 2009.
21. Altun C, Ozen B, Esenlik E, et al.: Traumatic injuries to permanent teeth in Turkish children, Ankara, *Dent Traumatol* 25(3):309–313, 2009.
22. Navabazam A, Farahani SS: Prevalence of traumatic injuries to maxillary permanent teeth in 9- to 14-year-old school children in Yazd, Iran, *Dent Traumatol* 26(2):154–157, 2010.
23. Fakhruddin KS, Lawrence HP, Kenny DJ, Locker D: Etiology and environment of dental injuries in 12- to 14-year-old Ontario schoolchildren, *Dent Traumatol* 24(3):305–308, 2008.
24. Kumar A, Bansal V, Veeresha KL, Sogi GM: Prevalence of traumatic dental injuries among 12- to 15-year-old schoolchildren in Ambala district, Haryana, India, *Oral Health Prev Dent* 9(3):301–305, 2011.
25. Soriano EP, Caldas Ade Jr F, Diniz De Carvalho MV, Amorim Filho Hde A: Prevalence and risk factors related to traumatic dental injuries in Brazilian schoolchildren, *Dent Traumatol* 23(4):232–240, 2007.
26. Taiwo OO, Jalo HP: Dental injuries in 12-year old Nigerian students, *Dent Traumatol* 27(3):230–234, 2011.
27. Gupta S, Kumar-Jindal S, Bansal M, Singla A: Prevalence of traumatic dental injuries and role of incisal overjet and inadequate lip coverage as risk factors among 4–15 years old government school children in Baddi-Barotiwala Area, Himachal Pradesh, India, *Med Oral Patol Oral Cir Bucal* e960–e965, 2011.
28. Petersson EE, Andersson L, Sorensen S: Traumatic oral vs non-oral injuries, *Swed Dent J* 21(1-2):55–68, 1997.
29. Granville-Garcia AF, de Menezes VA, de Lira PI: Dental trauma and associated factors in Brazilian preschoolers, *Dent Traumatol* 22(6):318–322, 2006.
30. Marcenes W, al Beiruti N, Tayfour D, Issa S: Epidemiology of traumatic injuries to the permanent incisors of 9-12-year-old schoolchildren in Damascus, Syria, *Endod Dent Traumatol* 15(3):117–123, 1999.
31. Lauridsen E, Hermann NV, Gerds TA, et al.: Combination injuries 3. The risk of pulp necrosis in permanent teeth with extrusion or lateral luxation and concomitant crown fractures without pulp exposure, *Dent Traumatol* 28(5):379–385, 2012.
32. Lauridsen E, Hermann NV, Gerds TA, et al.: Combination injuries 1. The risk of pulp necrosis in permanent teeth with concussion injuries and concomitant crown fractures, *Dent Traumatol* 28(5):364–370, 2012.
33. Lauridsen E, Hermann NV, Gerds TA, et al.: Combination injuries 2. The risk of pulp necrosis in permanent teeth with subluxation injuries and concomitant crown fractures, *Dent Traumatol* 28(5):371–378, 2012.
34. Hecova H, Tzigkounakis V, Merglova V, Netolicky J: A retrospective study of 889 injured permanent teeth, *Dent Traumatol* 26(6):466–475, 2010.
35. Selwitz RH, Ismail AI, Pitts NB: Dental caries, *Lancet* 369(9555):51–59, 2007.
36. JH S: Causes and control of dental caries, *N Engl J Med* 31(16):996–1004, 1987.
37. Dye BA, Thornton-Evans G, Li X, Iafolla TJ: Dental caries and sealant prevalence in children and adolescents in the United States, 2011-2012, *NCHS Data Brief*(191)1–8, 2015.
38. Naaman R, El-Housseiny AA, Alamoudi N: The use of pit and fissure sealants-a literature review, *Dent J (Basel)* 5(4), 2017.
39. Macek MD, Beltran-Aguilar ED, Lockwood SA, Malvitz DM: Updated comparison of the caries susceptibility of various morphological types of permanent teeth, *J Public Health Dent* 63(3):174–182, 2003.
40. Banerjee A, Watson TF, Kidd EA: Dentine caries: take it or leave it? *Dental update* 27(6):272–276, 2000.
41. Maltz M, de Oliveira EF, Fontanella V, Bianchi R: A clinical, microbiologic, and radiographic study of deep caries lesions after incomplete caries removal, *Quintessence Int* 33(2):151–159, 2002.
42. Maltz M, Oliveira EF, Fontanella V, Carminatti G: Deep caries lesions after incomplete dentine caries removal: 40-month follow-up study, *Caries Res* 41(6):493–496, 2007.
43. Schwendicke F, Frencken JE, Bjorndal L, et al.: Managing carious lesions: consensus recommendations on carious tissue removal, *Adv Dent Res* 28(2):58–67, 2016.
44. Merrill RG: Occlusal anomalous tubercles on premolars of Alaskan Eskimos and Indians, *Oral Surg Oral Med Oral Pathol* 17:484–496, 1964.
45. Naseri M, Ahangari Z, Shahbazi Moghadam M, Mohammadian M: Coronal sealing ability of three temporary filling materials, *Iran Endod J* 7(1):20–24, 2012.

46. Levitan ME, Himel VT: Dens evaginatus: literature review, pathophysiology, and comprehensive treatment regimen, *J Endod* 32(1):1–9, 2006.
47. Rao YG, Guo LY, Tao HT: Multiple dens evaginatus of premolars and molars in Chinese dentition: a case report and literature review, *Int J Oral Sci* 2(3):177–180, 2010.
48. Alani A, Bishop K: Dens invaginatus. Part 1: classification, prevalence and aetiology, *Int Endod J* 41(12):1123–1136, 2008.
49. Hulsmann M: Dens invaginatus: aetiology, classification, prevalence, diagnosis, and treatment considerations, *Int Endod J* 30(2):79–90, 1997.
50. Oehlers FA: Dens invaginatus (dilated composite odontome). I. Variations of the invagination process and associated anterior crown forms, *Oral Surg Oral Med Oral Pathol* 10(11):1204–1218, 1957. contd.
51. Ahn J, Pogrel MA: The effects of 2% lidocaine with 1:100,000 epinephrine on pulpal and gingival blood flow, *Oral Surg Oral Med Oral Pathol Oral Radiol Endod* 85(2):197–202, 1998.
52. Pitt Ford TR, Seare MA, McDonald F: Action of adrenaline on the effect of dental local anaesthetic solutions, *Endod Dent Traumatol* 9(1):31–35, 1993.
53. Nyborg H, Brannstrom M: Pulp reaction to heat, *J Prosthet Dent* 19(6):605–612, 1968.
54. Mjor IA, Odont D: Pulp-dentin biology in restorative dentistry. Part 2: initial reactions to preparation of teeth for restorative procedures, *Quintessence Int* 32(7):537–551, 2001.
55. Smith AJ, Scheven BA, Takahashi Y, et al.: Dentine as a bioactive extracellular matrix, *Arch Oral Biol* 57(2):109–121, 2012.
56. Murray PE, Lumley PJ, Smith AJ: Preserving the vital pulp in operative dentistry: 3. Thickness of remaining cavity dentine as a key mediator of pulpal injury and repair responses, *Dent Update* 29(4):172–178, 2002.
57. Mullaney TP, Laswell HR: Iatrogenic blushing of dentin following full crown preparation, *J Prosthet Dent* 22(3):354–359, 1969.
58. Pashley DH, Pashley EL: Dentin permeability and restorative dentistry: a status report for the American Journal of Dentistry, *Am J Dent* 4(1):5–9, 1991.
59. Murray PE, About I, Lumley PJ, et al.: Cavity remaining dentin thickness and pulpal activity, *Am J Dent* 15(1):41–46, 2002.
60. Bergenholtz G: Effect of bacterial products on inflammatory reactions in the dental pulp, *Scand J Dent Res* 85(2):122–129, 1977.
61. Bergenholtz G: Evidence for bacterial causation of adverse pulpal responses in resin-based dental restorations, *Crit Rev Oral Biol Med* 11(4):467–480, 2000.
62. Bergenholtz G, Cox CF, Loesche WJ, Syed SA: Bacterial leakage around dental restorations: its effect on the dental pulp, *J Oral Pathol* 11(6):439–450, 1982.
63. Camps J, Dejou J, Remusat M, About I: Factors influencing pulpal response to cavity restorations, *Dent Mater* 16(6):432–440, 2000.
64. Al-Hiyasat AS, Darmani H, Milhem MM: Cytotoxicity evaluation of dental resin composites and their flowable derivatives, *Clin Oral Investig* 9(1):21–25, 2005.
65. Lonnroth EC, Dahl JE: Cytotoxicity of liquids and powders of chemically different dental materials evaluated using dimethylthiazol diphenyltetrazolium and neutral red tests, *Acta Odontol Scand* 61(1):52–56, 2003.
66. Dammaschke T: The history of direct pulp capping, *J Hist Dent* 56(1):9–23, 2008.
67. Hermann BW: On the reaction of the dental pulp to vital amputation and calxyl capping, *Dtsch Zahnaztl Z* 7:1446, 1952.
68. Torabinejad M, Chivian N: Clinical applications of mineral trioxide aggregate, *J Endod* 25(3):197–205, 1999.
69. Zanini M, Sautier JM, Berdal A, Simon S: Biodentine induces immortalized murine pulp cell differentiation into odontoblast-like cells and stimulates biomineralization, *J Endod* 38(9):1220–1226, 2012.
70. Zehnder M, Wegehaupt FJ, Attin T: A first study on the usefulness of matrix metalloproteinase 9 from dentinal fluid to indicate pulp inflammation, *J Endod* 37(1):17–20, 2011.
71. Murray PE, About I, Lumley PJ, Smith G, Franquin JC, Smith AJ: Postoperative pulpal and repair responses, *J Am Dent Assoc* 131(3):321–329, 2000.
72. Bjorndal L, Larsen T: Changes in the cultivable flora in deep carious lesions following a stepwise excavation procedure, *Caries Res* 34(6):502–508, 2000.
73. Maltz M, Henz SL, de Oliveira EF, Jardim JJ: Conventional caries removal and sealed caries in permanent teeth: a microbiological evaluation, *J Dent* 40(9):776–782, 2012.
74. Bjorndal L, Demant S, Dabelsteen S: Depth and activity of carious lesions as indicators for the regenerative potential of dental pulp after intervention, *J Endod* 40(Suppl 4):S76–81, 2014.
75. Bjorndal L, Reit C, Bruun G, et al.: Treatment of deep caries lesions in adults: randomized clinical trials comparing stepwise vs. direct complete excavation, and direct pulp capping vs. partial pulpotomy, *Eur J Oral Sci* 118(3):290–297, 2010.
76. Maltz M, Garcia R, Jardim JJ, et al.: Randomized trial of partial vs. stepwise caries removal: 3-year follow-up, *J Dent Res* 91(11):1026–1031, 2012.
77. Barthel CR, Rosenkranz B, Leuenberg A, Roulet JF: Pulp capping of carious exposures: treatment outcome after 5 and 10 years: a retrospective study, *J Endod* 26(9):525–528, 2000.
78. Mejare I, Cvek M: Partial pulpotomy in young permanent teeth with deep carious lesions, *Endod Dent Traumatol* 9(6):238–242, 1993.
79. Taha NA, Khazali MA: Partial pulpotomy in mature permanent teeth with clinical signs indicative of irreversible pulpitis: a randomized clinical trial, *J Endod* 43(9):1417–1421, 2017.
80. Simon S, Perard M, Zanini M, et al.: Should pulp chamber pulpotomy be seen as a permanent treatment? Some preliminary thoughts, *Int Endod J* 46(1):79–87, 2013.
81. Sobhi MB, Rana MJ, Ibrahim M, et al.: Frequency of dens evaginatus of permanent anterior teeth, *J Coll Physicians Surg Pak* 14(2):88–90, 2004.
82. Perez F, Calas P, de Falguerolles A, Maurette A: Migration of a Streptococcus sanguis strain through the root dentinal tubules, *J Endod* 19(6):297–301, 1993.
83. Bose R, Nummikoski P, Hargreaves K: A retrospective evaluation of radiographic outcomes in immature teeth with necrotic root canal systems treated with regenerative endodontic procedures, *J Endod* 35(10):1343–1349, 2009.
84. Nagy MM, Tawfik HE, Hashem AA, Abu-Seida AM: Regenerative potential of immature permanent teeth with necrotic pulps after different regenerative protocols, *J Endod* 40(2):192–198, 2014.
85. Saoud TM, Zaazou A, Nabil A, et al.: Clinical and radiographic outcomes of traumatized immature permanent necrotic teeth after revascularization/revitalization therapy, *J Endod* 40(12):1946–1952, 2014.
86. Flake NM, Gibbs JL, Diogenes A, et al.: A standardized novel method to measure radiographic root changes after endodontic therapy in immature teeth, *J Endod* 40(1):46–50, 2014.
87. Jeeruphan T, Jantarat J, Yanpiset K, et al.: Mahidol study 1: comparison of radiographic and survival outcomes of immature teeth treated with either regenerative endodontic or apexification methods: a retrospective study, *J Endod* 38(10):1330–1336, 2012.
88. Frank AL: Therapy for the divergent pulpless tooth by continued apical formation, *J Am Dent Assoc* 72(1):87–93, 1966.
89. Andreasen JO, Munksgaard EC, Bakland LK: Comparison of fracture resistance in root canals of immature sheep teeth after filling with calcium hydroxide or MTA, *Dent Traumatol* 22(3):154–156, 2006.
90. Yassen GH, Vail MM, Chu TG, Platt JA: The effect of medicaments used in endodontic regeneration on root fracture and microhardness of radicular dentine, *Int Endod J* 46(7):688–695, 2013.
91. Cvek M: Prognosis of luxated non-vital maxillary incisors treated with calcium hydroxide and filled with gutta-percha. A retrospective clinical study, *Endod Dent Traumatol* 8(2):45–55, 1992.
92. Witherspoon DE, Small JC, Regan JD, Nunn M: Retrospective analysis of open apex teeth obturated with mineral trioxide aggregate, *J Endod* 34(10):1171–1176, 2008.

93. Ree MH, Schwartz RS: Long-term success of nonvital, immature permanent incisors treated with a mineral trioxide aggregate plug and adhesive restorations: a case series from a private endodontic practice, *J Endod* 43(8):1370–1377, 2017.
94. Bucher K, Meier F, Diegritz C, et al.: Long-term outcome of MTA apexification in teeth with open apices, *Quintessence Int* 47(6):473–482, 2016.
95. Alobaid AS, Cortes LM, Lo J, et al.: Radiographic and clinical outcomes of the treatment of immature permanent teeth by revascularization or apexification: a pilot retrospective cohort study, *J Endod* 40(8):1063–1070, 2014.
96. Jeeruphan T, Jantarat J, Yanpiset K, et al.: Mahidol study 1: comparison of radiographic and survival outcomes of immature teeth treated with either regenerative endodontic or apexification methods: a retrospective study, *J Endod* 38(10):1330–1336, 2012.
97. Kang MK, Bogen G: Regenerative approaches in endodontic therapies of immature teeth. In Chugal N, Lin LM, editors: *Endodontic prognosis*, Los Angeles, 2018, Springer, pp 65–86.
98. Gronthos S, Mankani M, Brahim J, et al.: Postnatal human dental pulp stem cells (DPSCs) in vitro and in vivo, *Proc Natl Acad Sci USA* 97(25):13625–13630, 2000.
99. Sonoyama W, Liu Y, Yamaza T, et al.: Characterization of the apical papilla and its residing stem cells from human immature permanent teeth: a pilot study, *J Endod* 34(2):166–171, 2008.
100. Banchs F, Trope M: Revascularization of immature permanent teeth with apical periodontitis: new treatment protocol? *J Endod* 30(4):196–200, 2004.
101. Lovelace TW, Henry MA, Hargreaves KM, Diogenes A: Evaluation of the delivery of mesenchymal stem cells into the root canal space of necrotic immature teeth after clinical regenerative endodontic procedure, *J Endod* 37(2):133–138, 2011.
102. Chrepa V, Henry MA, Daniel BJ, Diogenes A: Delivery of apical mesenchymal stem cells into root canals of mature teeth, *J Dent Res* 94(12):1653–1659, 2015.
103. Cehreli ZC, Isbitiren B, Sara S, Erbas G: Regenerative endodontic treatment (revascularization) of immature necrotic molars medicated with calcium hydroxide: a case series, *J Endod* 37(9):1327–1330, 2011.
104. Chen MY, Chen KL, Chen CA, et al.: Responses of immature permanent teeth with infected necrotic pulp tissue and apical periodontitis/abscess to revascularization procedures, *Int Endod J* 45(3):294–305, 2012.
105. Shah N, Logani A, Bhaskar U, Aggarwal V: Efficacy of revascularization to induce apexification/apexogensis in infected, nonvital, immature teeth: a pilot clinical study, *J Endod* 34(8):919–925, 2008; Discussion 1157.
106. Wang Y, Zhu X, Zhang C: Pulp revascularization on permanent teeth with open apices in a middle-aged patient, *J Endod* 41(9):1571–1575, 2015.
107. Bukhari S, Kohli MR, Setzer F, Karabucak B: Outcome of revascularization procedure: a retrospective case series, *J Endod* 42(12):1752–1759, 2016.
108. Kontakiotis EG, Filippatos CG, Tzanetakis GN, Agrafioti A: Regenerative endodontic therapy: a data analysis of clinical protocols, *J Endod* 41(2):146–154, 2015.
109. Torabinejad M, Nosrat A, Verma P, Udochukwu O: Regenerative endodontic treatment or mineral trioxide aggregate apical plug in teeth with necrotic pulps and open apices: a systematic review and meta-analysis, *J Endod* 43(11):1806–1820, 2017.
110. Martin G, Ricucci D, Gibbs JL, Lin LM: Histological findings of revascularized/revitalized immature permanent molar with apical periodontitis using platelet-rich plasma, *J Endod* 39(1):138–144, 2013.
111. Wang X, Thibodeau B, Trope M, et al.: Histologic characterization of regenerated tissues in canal space after the revitalization/revascularization procedure of immature dog teeth with apical periodontitis, *J Endod* 36(1):56–63, 2010.
112. Diogenes A, Ruparel NB, Shiloah Y, Hargreaves KM: Regenerative endodontics: a way forward, *J Am Dent Assoc* 147(5):372–380, 2016.
113. Shimizu E, Jong G, Partridge N, et al.: Histologic observation of a human immature permanent tooth with irreversible pulpitis after revascularization/regeneration procedure, *J Endod* 38(9):1293–1297, 2012.
114. Lei L, Chen Y, Zhou R, et al.: Histologic and Immunohistochemical findings of a human immature permanent tooth with apical periodontitis after regenerative endodontic treatment, *J Endod* 41(7):1172–1179, 2015.
115. Song M, Cao Y, Shin SJ, et al.: Revascularization-associated intracanal calcification: assessment of prevalence and contributing factors, *J Endod* 43(12):2025–2033, 2017.
116. Galler KM, Krastl G, Simon S, et al.: European Society of Endodontology position statement: revitalization procedures, *Int Endod J* 49(8):717–723, 2016.
117. Huang GT, Yamaza T, Shea LD, et al.: Stem/progenitor cell-mediated de novo regeneration of dental pulp with newly deposited continuous layer of dentin in an in vivo model, *Tissue Eng Part A* 16(2):605–615, 2010.
118. Iohara K, Imabayashi K, Ishizaka R, et al.: Complete pulp regeneration after pulpectomy by transplantation of CD105+ stem cells with stromal cell-derived factor-1, *Tissue Eng Part A* 17(15-16):1911–1920, 2011.
119. Nakashima M, Iohara K, Murakami M, et al.: Pulp regeneration by transplantation of dental pulp stem cells in pulpitis: a pilot clinical study, *Stem Cell Res Ther* 8(1):61, 2017.

11

Management of Traumatic Dental Injuries

AVINA PARANJPE AND CRAIG NOBLETT

CHAPTER OUTLINE

LEARNING OBJECTIVES

After reading this chapter, the student should be able to:

1. Describe the clinical and radiographic features of enamel fractures, uncomplicated crown fractures, complicated crown fractures, crown-root fractures, root fractures, concussion, subluxation, luxations (lateral, extrusive, and intrusive), avulsions, and alveolar fractures.
2. Describe possible short- and long-term responses of pulp, periradicular tissues, and hard tissues to the injuries listed previously.
3. List pertinent information needed when examining patients with dental injuries (health history, nature of injury, and symptoms).
4. Describe the diagnostic tests, radiographic imaging, and procedures needed in examining patients with dental injuries and interpret the findings.
5. Describe the importance of cone beam computed tomography (CBCT) imaging in patients with dental trauma.
6. Describe appropriate treatment strategies (immediate and long-term) for various types of traumatic injuries.
7. Recognize outcomes of traumatic dental injuries.
8. Recognize pulp space obliteration and describe management considerations.
9. Recognize surface resorption, inflammatory (infection-related) resorption, replacement (ankylosis-related) resorption, and cervical resorption and describe their respective prevention/treatment strategies.
10. Describe the preventive measures and treatment strategies for traumatic dental injuries in primary and permanent dentition.

Examination and Diagnosis

Patients who have suffered impact trauma to the head often present with dental injuries that may be their chief concern. These types of incidents often result in injuries to other tissues ranging from soft tissue lacerations to bone fractures and even brain injury. For this reason, a complete history and examination are always indicated, even though the dentist may not be the first provider encounter for the patient. The urgency often associated with an accident or injury can easily result in important signs or symptoms being overlooked, so repetitive examinations can help ensure that all injuries are identified and addressed. For dentists, it is easy to focus solely on injuries to the teeth and the oral cavity, but a basic knowledge of extraoral examination procedures in these scenarios is critical to the overall care of the patient.[1]

Mental Status

The first step in examining a patient who has suffered a head injury is to assess his or her mental status. A reliable and true history can only come from someone whose mental status is unimpaired. This step can be accomplished with just a few basic questions about the patient's name, age, the current date, and current general location.[2] If the patient can answer these questions without hesitation or confusion, the assumption that his or her mental state is unaffected can be made, and the practitioner can proceed with taking a history and performing the necessary examinations.

History

The patient history typically starts with the chief complaint, which normally involves a statement in the patient's own words regarding the current problem that has caused him or her to seek care. In the case of trauma, for example, that might be: "I fell and broke my tooth," or "I got an elbow to the mouth playing basketball, and now my teeth feel loose."

Next, the history of the present illness should be explored. The details regarding how the injury occurred can help direct the subsequent physical examination. Important questions to ask include:

When and how did the injury occur? Date and time should be recorded as well as the nature of the injury, such as a fall, a fight, a sports injury, or an auto or bicycle accident. It is also critical to ask the patient if he or she lost consciousness. This information can alert the practitioner to the possibility of a concussion or possible brain injury and might indicate that a neurologist referral is appropriate. Reports of headache, dizziness, and blurred or double vision would also indicate the need for a referral and should be the topic of inquiries as well.

Have you experienced other injuries to your mouth or teeth in the past? Repeated injuries, particularly of similar patterns, might indicate physical abuse, particularly in children. They can also result from sports injuries or other high-risk behaviors or occupations.[1] Previous injuries may have resulted in previously undetected crown or root fractures, or even osseous fractures. Repeated injuries in the same anatomic region may affect the healing capacity of the tissues due to scarring and changes in the vascular anatomy.

What problems are you currently having with your mouth? Pain, mobility, bleeding, and occlusal interferences are common symptoms. The patient's description of symptoms can aid in diagnosis.

Medical History

The patient's medical history must also be obtained because there may be significant findings that could affect treatment decisions. Medications taken and medication allergies should be recorded. A review of systems should also be completed to determine whether any systemic conditions are present. The patient's tetanus immunization status should also be determined because a booster might be necessary in the presence of injuries that carry the potential for contamination, such as an avulsion or penetrating lip and soft tissue injuries.[3]

Clinical Examination

Examination of the patient should begin with extraoral structures to determine the extent of any injuries. A cranial nerve examination is appropriate and should be completed. Sense of smell, visual acuity, and perception of sound are subjective and will depend on patient response, but movement of facial muscles, eyes, tongue, and the ability to "tense" the neck are clinically observable and will provide an objective assessment of cranial nerve function.[2]

• BOX 11.1 Selected Symptoms of Concussion

Affective/Emotional Symptoms

- Anxiety/nervousness
- Clinginess
- Depression
- Emotional distress
- Irritability*
- Personality changes
- Sadness

Cognitive Symptoms

- Amnesia
- Confusion
- Delayed verbal and other responses
- Difficulty concentrating*
- Difficulty remembering*
- Disorientation*
- Feeling "foggy"*
- Feeling "slowed down"*
- Feeling stunned
- Inability to focus
- Loss of consciousness
- Slurred speech
- Vacant stare

Sleep

- Decreased sleep
- Difficulty falling asleep
- Drowsiness*
- Increased sleep*

Somatic/Physical symptoms

- Blurred vision
- Convulsions
- Dizziness/poor balance
- Fatigue
- Headache
- Lightheadedness
- Light sensitivity
- Nausea
- Noise sensitivity
- Numbness/tingling
- Tinnitus
- Vomiting

*Common in self-report symptoms checklists.
From Scorza, KA, Raleigh, MF, O'Connor, FG. Current concepts in concussion: evaluation and management, *Am Fam Physician*, 85: 123–132, 2012.

Cognitive function is also important. As previously mentioned, loss of consciousness, headache, dizziness, and visual disturbances can indicate a brain injury.[4] Clinically, speech difficulties, inability to focus, or displaying a "vacant stare" may also alert the practitioner to the possibility of a concussion or other brain injury (Box 11.1).

Soft Tissue Examination

The extraoral soft tissues should be examined to determine the extent of any lacerations or soft tissue injuries. The presence of ecchymosis should also be noted. Postauricular ecchymosis is a cardinal sign of a LeFort III fracture, which is often otherwise asymptomatic. Any foreign bodies or material should also be identified and removed from injured soft tissues. This requirement is particularly true in the instance of crown fractures paired with

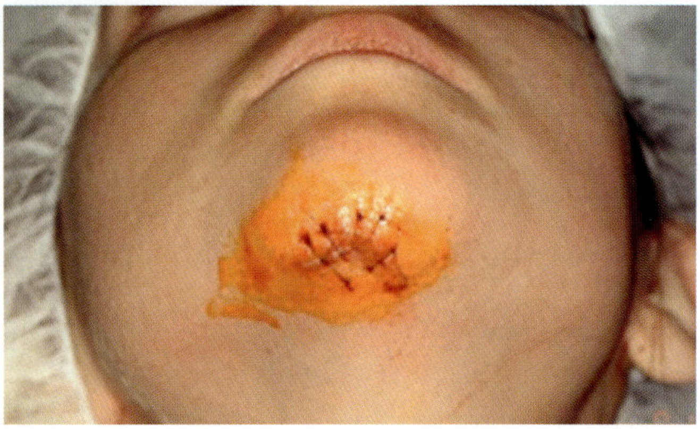

• **Fig. 11.1** Laceration of soft tissues requiring sutures.

lip lacerations. Radiographic confirmation as to the presence or absence of tooth fragments in the lip or perioral tissues is important. Severe lacerations could require suturing for adequate healing (Fig. 11.1).

Facial Skeleton

The facial skeleton should be examined for potential fractures. Extraorally, this is accomplished largely through palpation, but the presence of ecchymosis can provide a clue as to a possible fracture. A "step" in the borders of the orbit, abnormal mobility of the nose, or depression and mobility of the zygomatic arch are all indications of fractures. Intraorally, abnormal mobility of segments of the dentition can indicate a cortical plate fracture or, more extensively, an alveolar fracture. A marked change in alignment or displacement of the teeth as a block may indicate a fracture of the maxilla or mandible. The posttreatment significance of these fractures is that teeth involved in the plane of fracture are at risk of developing pulp necrosis.[5,6]

Teeth and Supporting Structures

Examination of the teeth and supporting structures will provide the information necessary to assess the extent of damage to the hard tissues, potential pulpal injury, and periodontal damage. A methodical approach to this examination will ensure a thorough evaluation of all injuries.

Mobility

Teeth should be examined gently for mobility, noting whether adjacent teeth move with the same degree of mobility. In the presence of an alveolar fracture, when one tooth is tested for mobility, the adjacent teeth involved in the fracture will move in unison. The degree of horizontal mobility should be recorded: 0 for physiologic mobility, 1 for slight mobility (up to 1 mm), 2 for significant mobility (1 to 2 mm), and 3 for severe mobility (greater than 2 mm), both horizontally and vertically. If no mobility is detected, the teeth should be percussed to detect any sign of intrusion or ankylosis, which would present as a "metallic" sound relative to other teeth.

Displacement

Displacement of teeth from their normal position should be noted. This type of injury is referred to as a *luxation* (discussed later in this chapter).

Periodontal Damage

Injury to the supporting structures of the teeth can result in a spectrum of clinical signs, including swelling, bleeding, ecchymosis, and lacerations. Visual inspection of the soft tissues for signs of injury should be the first step, followed by gentle palpation of the periodontium and alveolar processes. Palpation can reveal signs of cortical plate or alveolar fractures that may not have been noted during mobility testing. Injury to the periodontal ligament (PDL) can often result in edema and bleeding in the ligament, which may not be visible to the clinician. In this instance the teeth will likely be sensitive to percussion, which is a useful test for the identification of periodontal injury. This testing method should be performed as gently as possible, because injured teeth/periodontium are likely to exhibit a much lower threshold for pain. It is preferable to test unaffected teeth first to establish a baseline response and to gain the patient's confidence and understanding of the procedure. It is always important to test several adjacent teeth away from the site of injury, as well as opposing teeth. This additional test permits recognition of other dental injuries of which the patient may not have been aware and which might not have been obvious on visual examination. This test also provides baseline information in the event that future complications arise.

Pulpal Injury

The ideal pulpal response to an impact injury would be complete recovery after a traumatic incident. Two other potential outcomes may occur, however. One outcome would be calcific metamorphosis in which the pulp is gradually replaced by calcified tissue. This result can be recognized clinically by a yellow discoloration of the crown and radiographically by a narrowing or even disappearance of the pulp space. The other potential outcome is pulp necrosis, which can be caused by apical displacement that disrupts the pulpal blood supply.[7] Pulp necrosis can lead to external inflammatory root resorption if not treated in a timely manner. Typically, resorption occurs without clinical symptoms, so continued follow-up is vitally important in ensuring optimal treatment.

The status of the pulp tissue may be determined by symptoms, history, and clinical testing. The most commonly employed and reliable tests are electrical pulp testing (EPT) and the cold test. These modalities test the neural response of the pulp tissue and depend on the patient's subjective response. Fulling and Andreasen demonstrated that the late differentiation of the Aδ nerve fibers in the dental pulp explain the lack of reliable and predictable responses to pulp testing in erupting, developing teeth.[8] In young patients, cold testing is the most reliable subjective test to assess pulp status. Ideally, an objective assessment of the pulpal blood supply would provide a better diagnostic test in determining pulp vitality. Current evidence demonstrates that pulpal blood circulation can be accurately assessed with laser Doppler flowmetry and with pulse oximetry (Fig. 11.2).[9-15] In a study by Gopikrishna and colleagues, pulse oximetry was shown to provide a more constant indication of pulp vitality compared with EPT or cold testing after an impact injury, although with time, the EPT and cold tests would often return to normal responses.[16] The overriding principle regarding the necessity of endodontic treatment in the case of impact injury is the development of pulp necrosis; accurate assessment of the pulp status is critical, so the ability to detect pulpal blood circulation would represent the definitive test in making this determination.

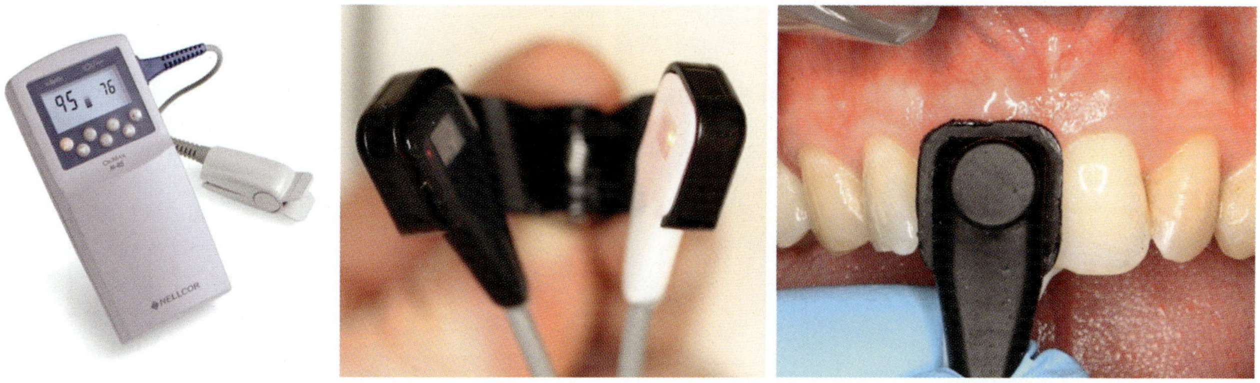

• **Fig. 11.2** Pulse oximetry unit with a commercially available sensor that fits dental tissues. (Courtesy Covidien.)

TABLE 11.1 Radiographic Classification of Odontogenic Development

Classification	Description
0	No crypt
1	Presence of a crypt
2	Initial calcification
3	One-third crown completed
4	Two-thirds crown completed
5	Crown almost completed
6	Crown completed
7	One-third root completed
8	Two-thirds root competed
9	Root almost open (open apex)
10	Root apex completed

Radiographic Examination

Radiographs can assist in revealing fractures of the bone and teeth as well as the stage of root development in children. Knowledge of the developmental stages of permanent teeth is essential for clinical practice in several dental specialties, because it may influence diagnosis, treatment planning, and outcomes. In 1960 Nolla published a classification system for odontogenic development based on radiographic interpretation (Table 11.1). This system has been widely used,[17] and it is particularly important for appropriate diagnosis and treatment of traumatized teeth. Luxation injuries and horizontal root fractures are often overlooked on routine radiographic examination, so multiple angles of exposure are indicated to increase the predictability of identifying these entities, making assessment and diagnosis as complete as possible (Fig. 11.3).[18,19] Crown fractures are more likely to be detected by conventional radiographs and clinical examination, but root fractures depend on the angulation of two-dimensional (2D) radiographs for detection and diagnosis. Recent advances in three-dimensional (3D) imaging (cone beam computed tomography [CBCT]) allow evaluation in three dimensions to detect fractures of the roots and alveolar bone (Fig. 11.4).[20]

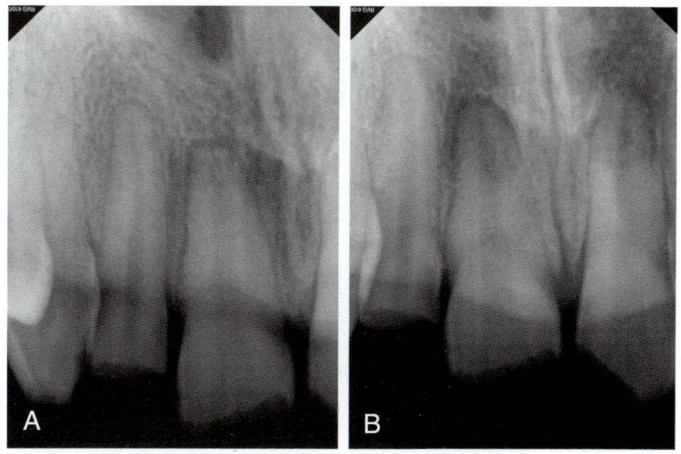

• **Fig. 11.3** Complicated crown fracture of the maxillary right central and lateral incisors and maxillary left central incisor. **A** and **B,** Periapical radiographs at different horizontal angles.

Importance of Cone Beam Computed Tomographic Analysis in Trauma

Traumatic dental injuries are complex and could involve several tissues. Furthermore, they can be challenging when discussing diagnosis and treatment planning. As stated in the previous section, radiographic examination is important in identifying the type and the extent of traumatic injuries to the dental tissues and the periodontium. The guidelines provided by the International Association of Dental Traumatology (IADT) outline the number and types of 2D radiographs that would be helpful in diagnosis of dental traumatic injuries.[21] However, 2D imaging has its limitations in serving as a diagnostic tool in trauma due to its limitation to two dimensions, superimposition of other structures, projection geometry, and so on.[22] Hence, there may be incidences where some types of trauma may go undiagnosed and therefore untreated.

3D imaging includes various imaging modalities that include computed tomography (CT), magnetic resonance imaging (MRI), and CBCT.[23] CBCT produces images in three dimensions with less radiation exposure than a traditional CT.[24,25] CBCT units can be classified according to the imaged volume or field of view (FOV) as large FOV (6- to 12-inch or 15- to 30.5-cm) or limited FOV systems (1.6- to 3.1-inch or 4- to 8-cm).[26]

The use of CBCT in dental trauma was first described in 2007. Several studies have reported the use of CBCT and digital

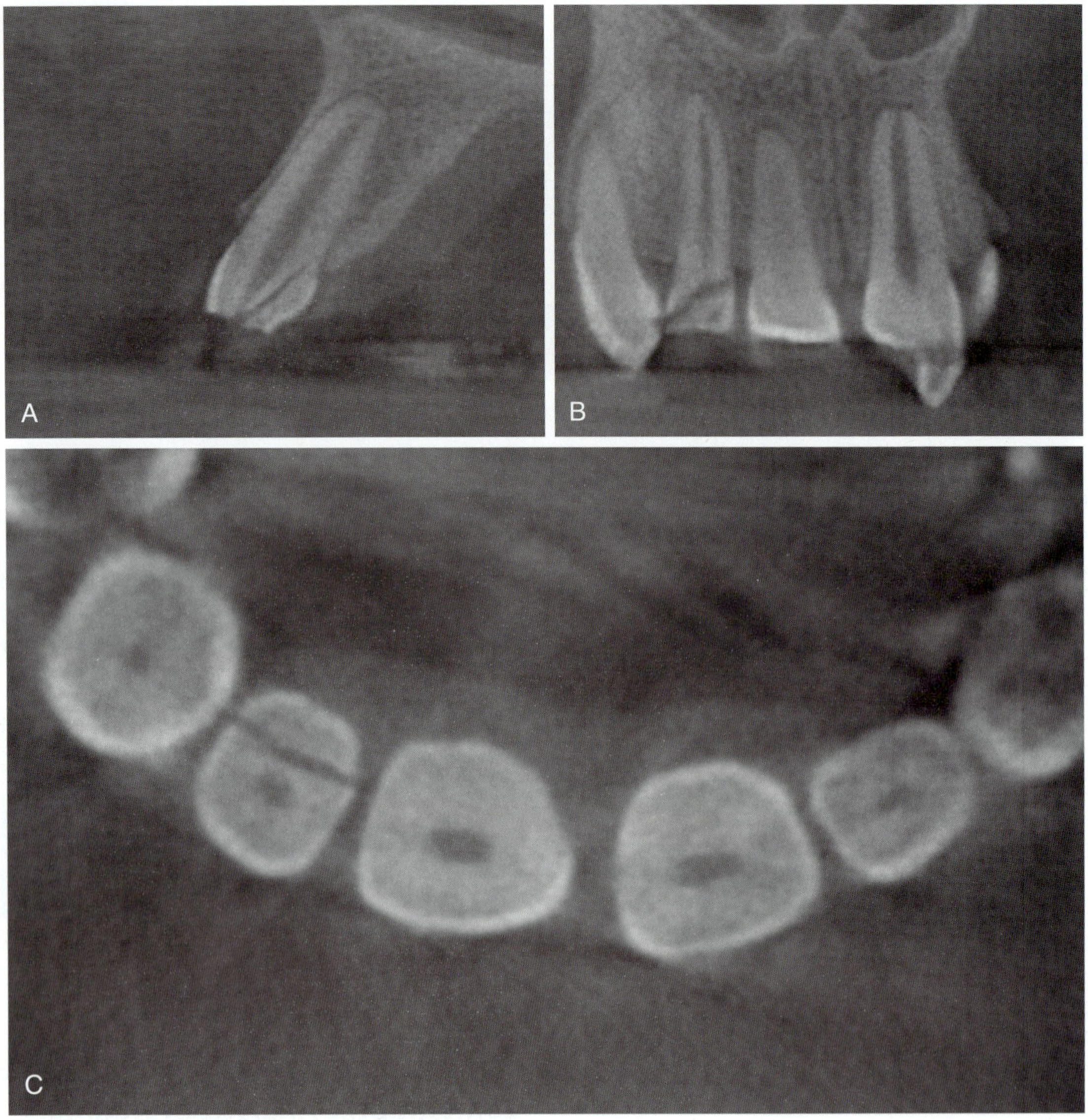

• **Fig. 11.4** Complicated crown fracture of the maxillary right central and lateral incisors and maxillary left central incisor – as seen in the saggital **(A),** coronal **(B)** and axial **(C)** sections of this CBCT image. (same case as in Fig. 11.7).

radiography for differential diagnosis,[27-29] assessment of treatment outcomes[30,31] endodontics,[32] oral and maxillofacial surgery,[26] implantology,[33] and orthodontics, with reliable measurements for reconstruction and imaging of dental and maxillofacial structures.[34,35] CBCTs provide a 3D image of a 3D structure in three orthogonal planes (axial, sagittal, and coronal).[36,37]

In 2016 the American Academy of Oral and Maxillofacial Radiology/American Association of Endodontists (AAOMR/AAE) joint position statement gave multiple recommendations for the use of limited FOV CBCT. Recommendation #11 states, "Limited FOV CBCT should be considered the imaging modality of choice for diagnosis and management of limited dento-alveolar trauma, root fractures, luxation, and/or displacement of teeth and localized alveolar fractures, in the absence of other maxillofacial or soft tissue injury that may require other advanced imaging modalities."

CBCT overcomes several limitations of 2D radiographs. CBCT provides a considerable amount of information and can differentiate between many types of airspaces and structures such as bones, airways, sinuses, and so on.[22] CBCT imaging also enables the clinician to view teeth in three dimensions, and often cases that appear to be straightforward on a periapical radiograph may have a completely different presentation when viewed in three dimensions (Figs. 11.5 and 11.6).

Injuries to the Hard Dental Tissues and the Pulp

Enamel Fractures

Chips or cracks that are confined to the enamel do not directly constitute a threat to the pulp tissue. However, when those cracks or chips are the result of an impact injury, they may also cause a slight luxation injury that can damage blood vessels that supply the pulp. A clinical sign that this injury may have occurred is tenderness to percussion of the affected tooth. If this injury is indeed a finding on examination, the practitioner should follow the recommended guidelines according to the type of trauma (discussed later in the chapter). Simply smoothing any rough edges or restoring missing structure may be all that is necessary to address the chips or cracks noted.

Uncomplicated Crown Fractures

Uncomplicated crown fractures involve the dentin as well as the enamel but do not result in a pulp exposure. This type of injury is not often severely painful but may present more of a cosmetic concern to the patient. This situation does not require urgent care in most instances, and generally prognosis for pulp survival is favorable unless there is a concurrent luxation injury.[18] If there is no observable displacement, a luxation injury might be suspected in cases where tenderness to percussion or bleeding from the sulcus is present.

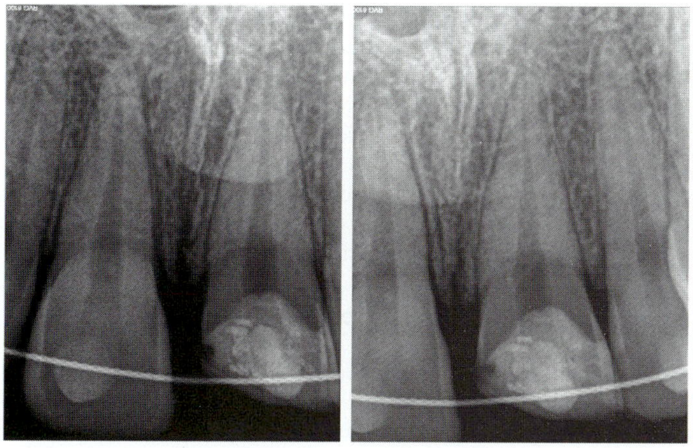

• **Fig. 11.5** Preoperative radiograph of the maxillary left central incisor that was diagnosed with a complicated crown fracture. The fractured segment was removed, a partial pulpotomy was completed and the tooth was restored with a composite restoration.

Treatment of uncomplicated crown fractures normally involves the restoration of the missing tooth structure, typically by employing an acid etch composite resin technique (Fig. 11.7). This conservative approach generally will not present a significant risk of pulp pathosis. An even more conservative approach would be to bond the tooth fragment back into place if it was salvaged. Both clinical studies and in vitro bonding experiments have demonstrated that reattachment of dentin-enamel crown fragments is an acceptable restorative procedure.[38] Employing this technique restores the dental anatomy with normal tooth structure, so esthetics and wear will match the adjacent teeth, and the status of the pulp can be reliably monitored.

Complicated Crown Fractures

Complicated crown fractures involve the enamel and dentin in a location that results in an exposure of the pulp tissue. The extent of the fracture, stage of root development, and time since the injury occurred should be recorded because these parameters will influence treatment decisions.

Considering the extent of the fracture will help determine the treatment of the pulp and what restorative needs exist. A smaller fracture that appears amenable to an acid-etch restoration may be a good candidate for vital pulp therapy, whereas an extensive fracture that will require a foundation and crown to restore would be a candidate for conventional endodontic treatment (Fig. 11.8). The final treatment plan will of course depend on the age of the patient.

The stage of root development is an important factor to consider when choosing between vital pulp therapy and conventional endodontic treatment. Teeth with incomplete root formation often have thin dentin walls, so every effort should be made to preserve the pulp so that continued dentin deposition can proceed, and root

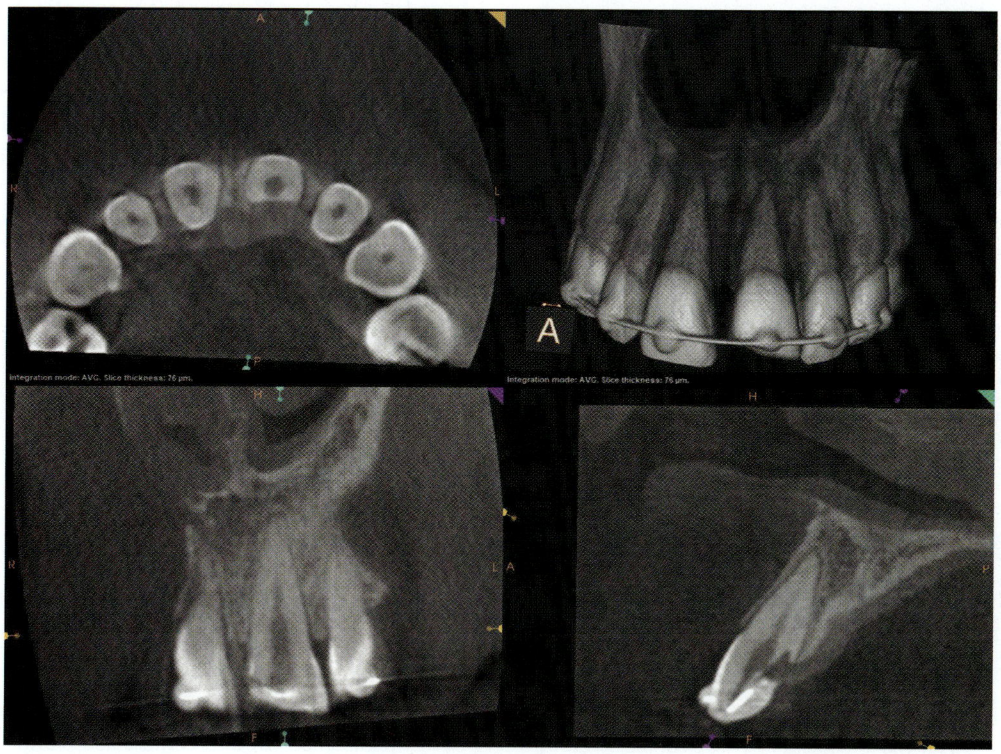

• **Fig. 11.6** Cone beam computed tomography (CBCT) (same case as Fig. 11.5). Sagittal section demonstrates the palatal aspect of the maxillary left central incisor, which was not restored adequately. This problem could not be visualized clinically or with the PA radiograph (Fig. 11.5) taken before the CBCT. The PA (Fig. 11.5) showed an intact restoration on tooth #9 and the palatal aspect could not be visualized on the PA.

development can continue to completion. The most accepted technique to accomplish this goal is a shallow pulpotomy followed by an acid-etch composite restoration or reattachment of the enamel-dentin fragment. Depending on the amount of tooth loss and restorative needs, this treatment plan can also be appropriate for fully formed teeth in adults. However, if there is structure loss that requires a crown to restore the tooth, endodontic treatment is recommended.[39]

Treatment of Crown Fractures

Teeth with crown fractures that expose the pulp tissue can be treated by pulp capping or a shallow pulpotomy, both of which constitute vital pulp therapy, or by conventional endodontic treatment. If vital pulp therapy is planned, the prognosis will be maximized if the time between the injury and treatment is minimal, although successful pulpotomy procedures after several weeks of exposure have been reported.[40-42]

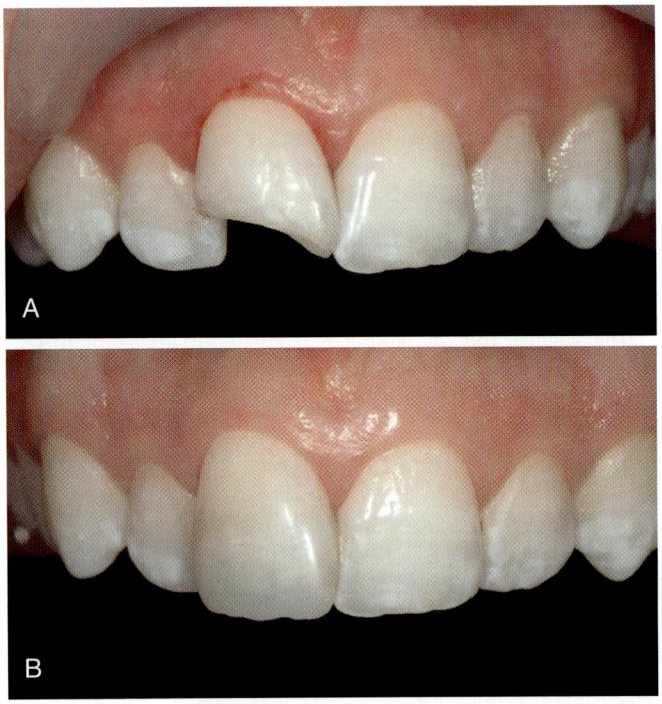

• **Fig. 11.7** Uncomplicated crown fracture of the maxillary right central incisor. Preoperative **(A)** and postoperative **(B)** views of restoration with composite resins. (Courtesy Dr. Gabriela Ibarra.)

Vital Pulp Therapy

The primary reason for considering vital pulp therapy is to preserve the pulp tissue. As previously mentioned, this therapy is of paramount importance in teeth with incomplete root formation. Continued root development will result in increased dentin thickness, which will translate to increased strength and fracture resistance. In the classic literature, pulpotomy is described as removal of the pulp tissue to a point just apical to the cementoenamel junction (CEJ). If the cervical dentin has not reached optimum thickness, performing a pulpotomy in this fashion will prevent any further dentin formation in this critical area of the tooth. Subsequently, a more conservative approach to pulp removal has been popularized by Cvek, which involves removing a minimal amount of tissue to a point where hemostasis can be obtained.[40] This technique will not only preserve the radicular pulp but will also likely preserve the majority of the coronal pulp, allowing the opportunity for greater hard tissue formation.

Case Selection for Vital Pulp Therapy

Both immature and mature teeth that can subsequently be restored with an acid-etch composite are candidates for the shallow pulpotomy technique. In general, this procedure is more important in those immature teeth in which root formation is not yet completed.

Technique

The shallow pulpotomy procedure (Fig. 11.9) requires anesthesia and rubber dam isolation. Once isolated, the dentin surface should be cleaned to remove any foreign matter and any loose fragments that might remain. Extruding granulation tissue at the pulp exposure site can be removed by a spoon excavator so that the actual size of the exposure can be observed. Next, the pulp tissue is removed to a depth of approximately 2 mm below the exposure. This is a relatively small volume of tissue but helps ensure removal of contaminated pulp. This stage of pulp removal is accomplished using a water-cooled, round diamond bur in a high-speed handpiece. After removing the pulp

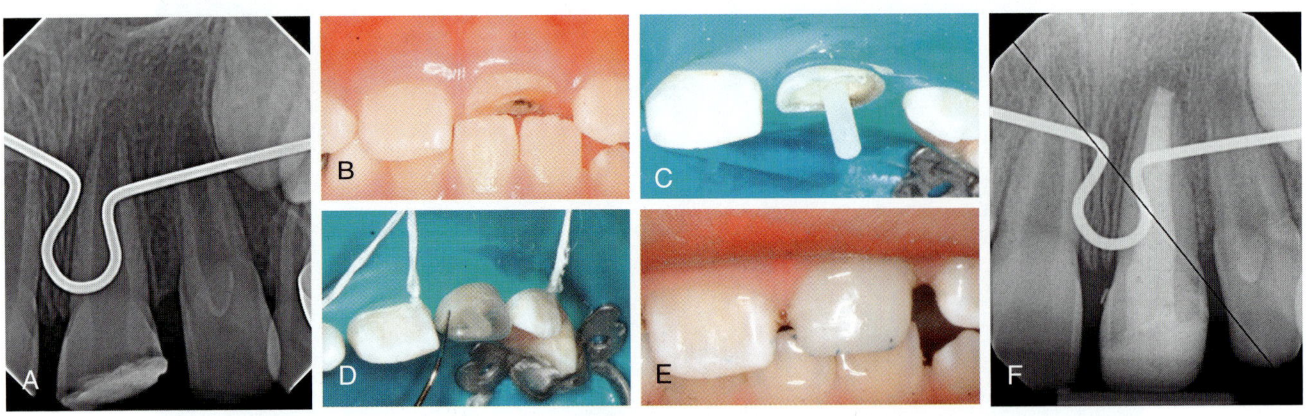

• **Fig. 11.8** Preoperative periapical radiograph **(A)** and clinical photograph **(B)** of a complicated crown fracture of the maxillary left central incisor. **C** and **D,** Upon completion of the endodontic therapy, a fiber post was placed, followed by the coronal restoration. The results are shown in a postoperative clinical photograph **(E)** and a final periapical radiograph **(F)**.

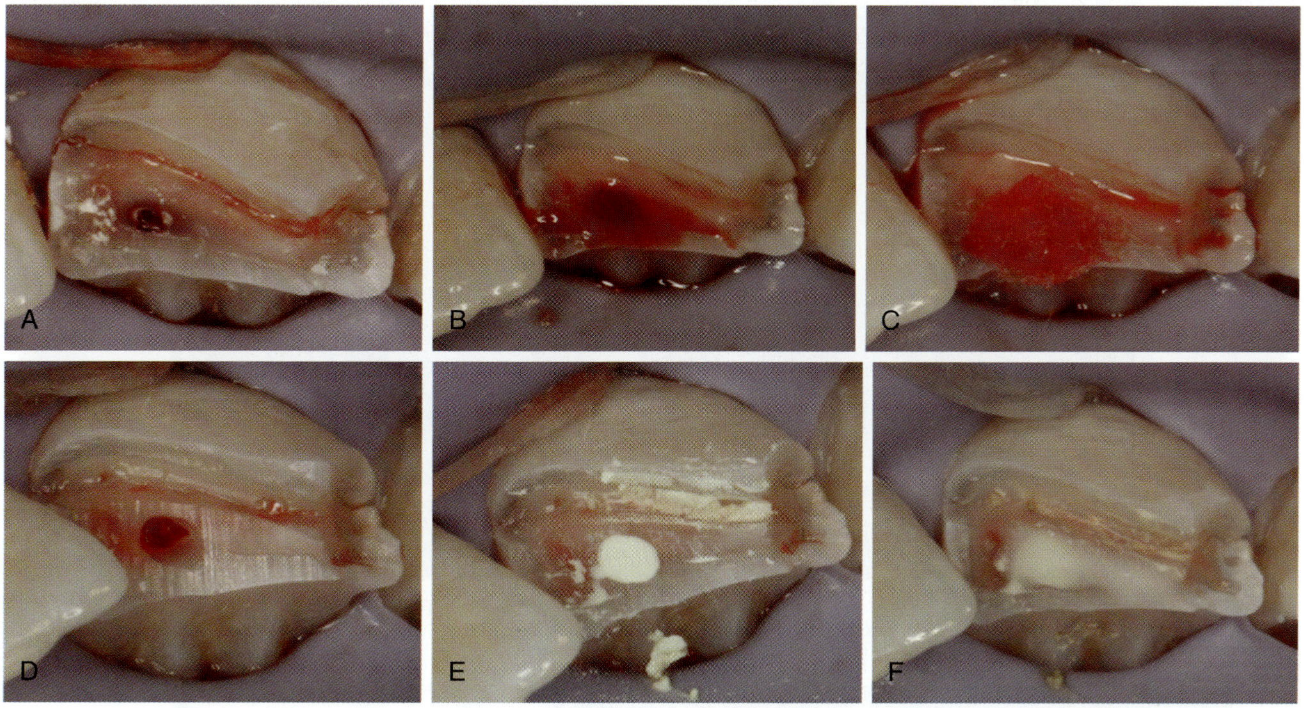

• **Fig. 11.9** Complicated crown fracture of the maxillary right central incisor. The partial pulpotomy procedure is clinically illustrated in the following steps: **A,** Pulp is exposed; **B,** pulpal tissue is excised 2 mm below the exposure; **C,** bleeding is controlled by pressure only (cotton pellet moistened with saline); **D,** hemostasis is obtained; **E,** white mineral trioxide aggregate (MTA) seal is applied; **F,** protection of the MTA is achieved using a layer of glass ionomer lining.

to the desired depth, the area can be irrigated with saline and hemostasis obtained, which may occasionally require some gentle compression. Typically, hemostasis will be obtained within 5 minutes, at which time the exposure site should be sealed with either a bioceramic putty or mineral trioxide aggregate (MTA). Care should be taken to avoid forcing the material into the pulp space. If MTA is used, it is preferable to confirm that it has set completely, which would necessitate that the patient return the next day. With a high viscosity bioceramic putty, the tooth can be restored immediately. Once the exposure site is sealed, the tooth is then restored with an acid-etch composite to replicate the contour, or the enamel-dentin fragment is bonded back into place.[43] This step completes the treatment, but follow-up to monitor pulp status is indicated.

Treatment Evaluation

Treatment outcome should be assessed after 6 months and then annually. This examination should include evaluation of pulp responsiveness to either cold or EPT, or both. Radiographic evidence of continued root formation is a strong indication of treatment success. If the pulp remains responsive and if continued root formation is observed, the vital pulp therapy procedure would be considered definitive treatment, which should have a favorable long-term prognosis (Fig. 11.10).[42,44]

Endodontic Treatment

Teeth with complete root formation can be treated either by vital pulp therapy or by conventional endodontic treatment. In cases where restorative needs dictate that a crown, or particularly a post and crown, are necessary, conventional root canal treatment is necessary.

Crown-Root Fractures

These fractures typically present in an oblique orientation, often splitting the crown in a diagonal direction and extending onto the root surface, which makes it a more serious injury. A less common variation of this type of fracture is one in which the crown appears to have shattered (Fig. 11.11). The pieces are held in place only by the part of a fractured segment that remains attached to the PDL. In these fractures, the pulp is usually exposed.

In contrast to the previously described impact injuries in which posterior teeth are rarely involved, crown-root fractures are often seen in premolars and molars as well. Cusp fractures that extend subgingivally are common. Diagnostically, however, they may be difficult to identify in the earlier stages of development and might require transillumination or a dye technique to detect at this point. Similar difficulties are encountered in detecting vertical fractures along the long axis of the root.

Crown-root fractures of the posterior teeth are not always associated with a single impact of a traumatic event. If that is the case, however, bicycle or motor vehicle accidents are often the culprits. The risk of this type of fracture is also increased with a sharp blow to the chin, which can cause the teeth to slam together. Skin abrasions under the chin may be an extraoral sign of such an injury.

Until recently, removal of all loose fragments was recommended as part of the examination to determine the extent of the injury and determine restorability of the tooth or teeth. This practice may still be necessary in some instances, but with the current

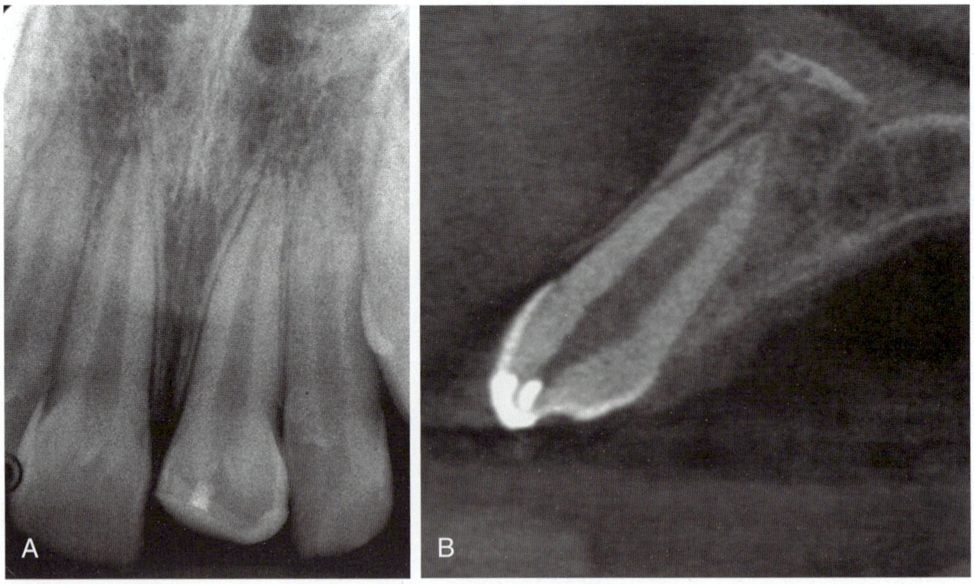

• **Fig. 11.10** Six-month follow-up after partial pulpotomy. Periapical radiograph **(A)** and sagittal view **(B)** obtained with cone beam computed tomography (CBCT).

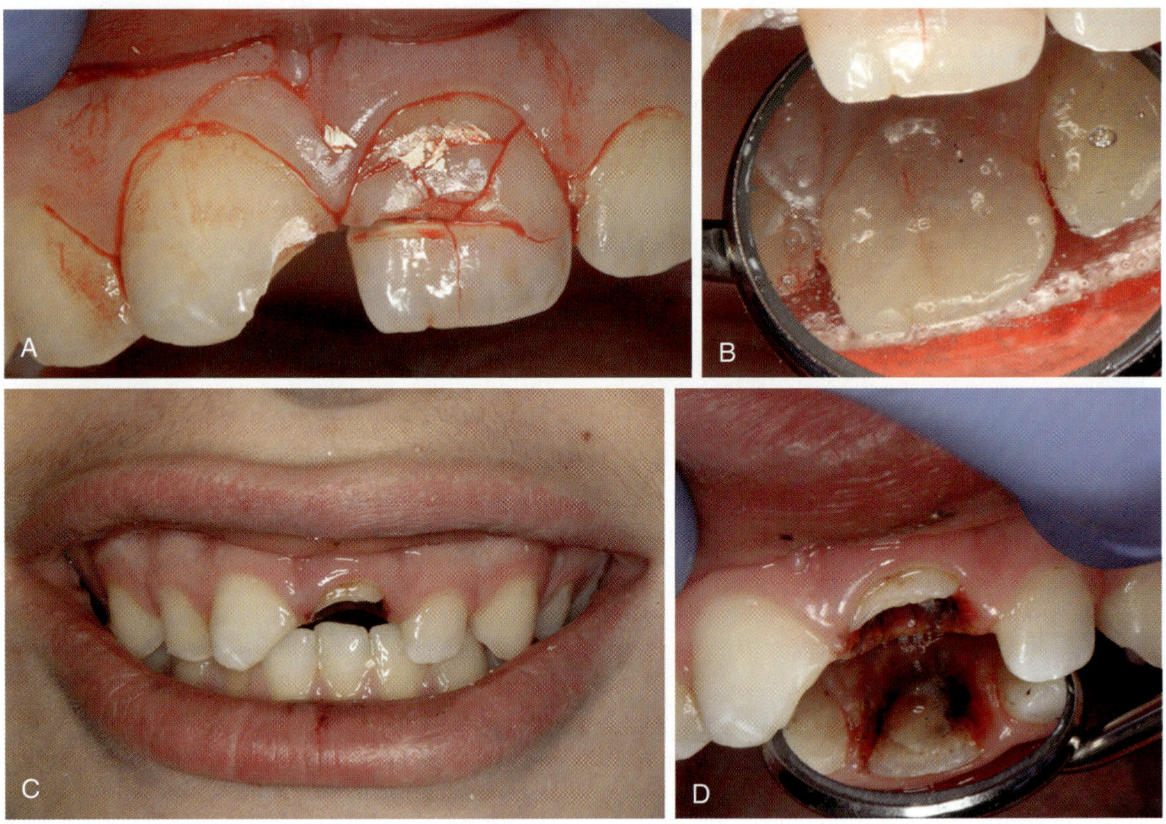

• **Fig. 11.11** A and **B,** Buccal and lingual photographs of a crown and root fracture immediately upon presentation. **C** and **D,** Images after removal of the fractured segments.

restorative options in adhesive dentistry, repair of these injuries can be more predictable than in the past. Current recommendations are to attempt bonding loose fragments together, particularly if root development is not yet complete.[39]

Teeth that present with a "shattered" appearance often have extension of the cracks onto the root surface. Additional imaging studies such as angled radiographs and CBCT may assist in identifying radicular as well as osseous fracture lines (Fig. 11.12).[19,45]

Emergency Care and Treatment Planning

Teeth exhibiting crown-root fractures often present with significant symptoms of pain and discomfort, particularly if there is a

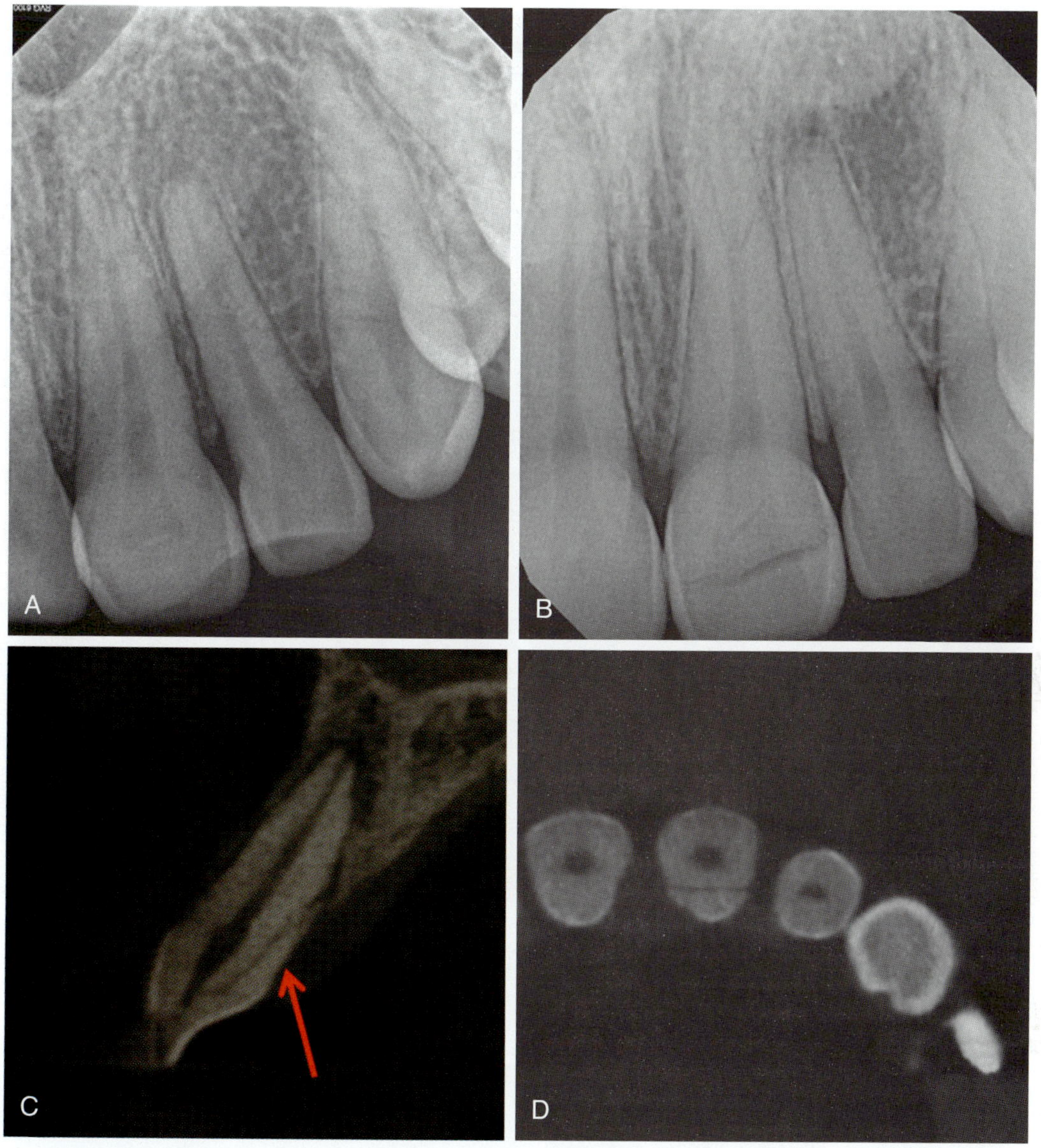

• **Fig. 11.12** A and **B,** Periapical radiographs demonstrating a crown fracture line. **C** and **D,** Sagittal and axial slides confirming the presence and extension of the fractures lines *(arrow).*

mobile fragment that moves easily with speaking or other functional movements. Injuries such as these require urgent care to alleviate the patient's symptoms and stabilize the teeth. This care may consist of simply bonding loose tooth fragments but often includes the initiation of pulpal treatment as well (Fig. 11.13). In teeth with incomplete root formation, a shallow pulpotomy would be preferable to a pulpectomy so that root formation might continue. Pulpectomy is the treatment of choice if the root formation is complete and fully developed (Fig. 11.14). Definitive treatment is best postponed until the overall endodontic/restorative treatment plan has been finalized.[39]

Crown-root fractures are often complicated by pulp exposures and extensive loss of tooth structure. In developing a definitive treatment plan, several aspects must be considered:

- Will pulpotomy or pulpectomy be the better choice for treating a particular tooth?
- After removal of all loose fragments, will the tooth still be restorable? In the event that fragments are bonded together to allow root formation to continue, will this last long enough for root formation to be complete or to allow the alveolus to develop adequately for the placement of an implant?
- Is the subgingival fracture margin at a level that would allow placement of a restoration margin, or will extrusion or periodontal surgery be necessary?
- Should the tooth be extracted and replaced with a bridge or implant? Alternately, if the tooth is extracted, could the space be closed with orthodontic treatment?

These are a few critical considerations that must be included in making treatment decisions. Because of the complexity involved in these cases, a team approach involving specialists in pediatric dentistry, endodontics, periodontics, orthodontics, oral and maxillofacial surgery, and prosthodontics is beneficial in developing a treatment plan to optimize the outcome for the patient.

Root Fractures

Root fractures that do not involve the crown of the tooth have also been termed *intra-alvelor root fractures, horizontal root fractures,*

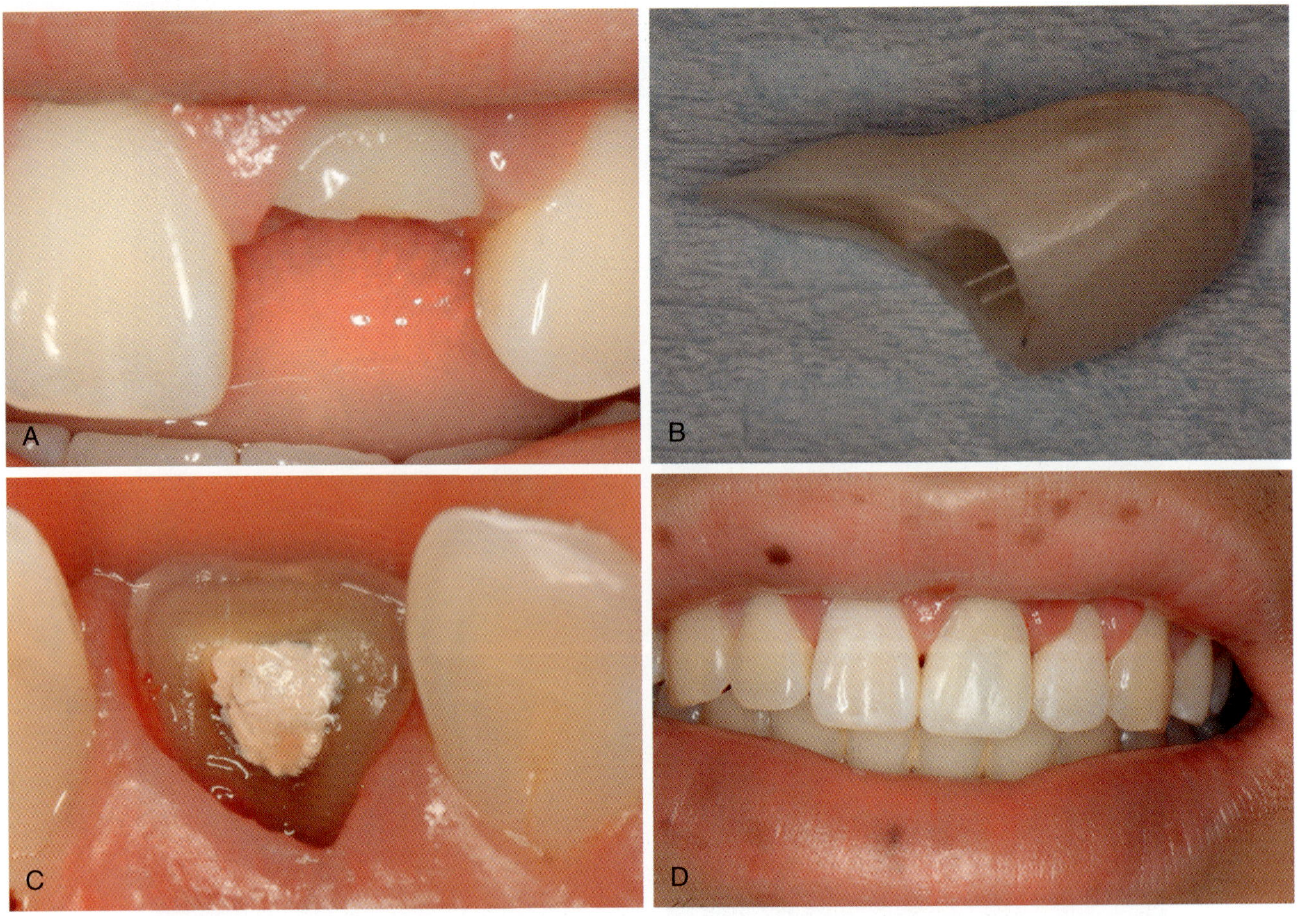

• **Fig. 11.13** **A–D,** Crown-root fracture of the maxillary left central incisor. Emergency procedure for stabilization of the coronal fragment using acid etch/resin applied to the remaining tooth structure.

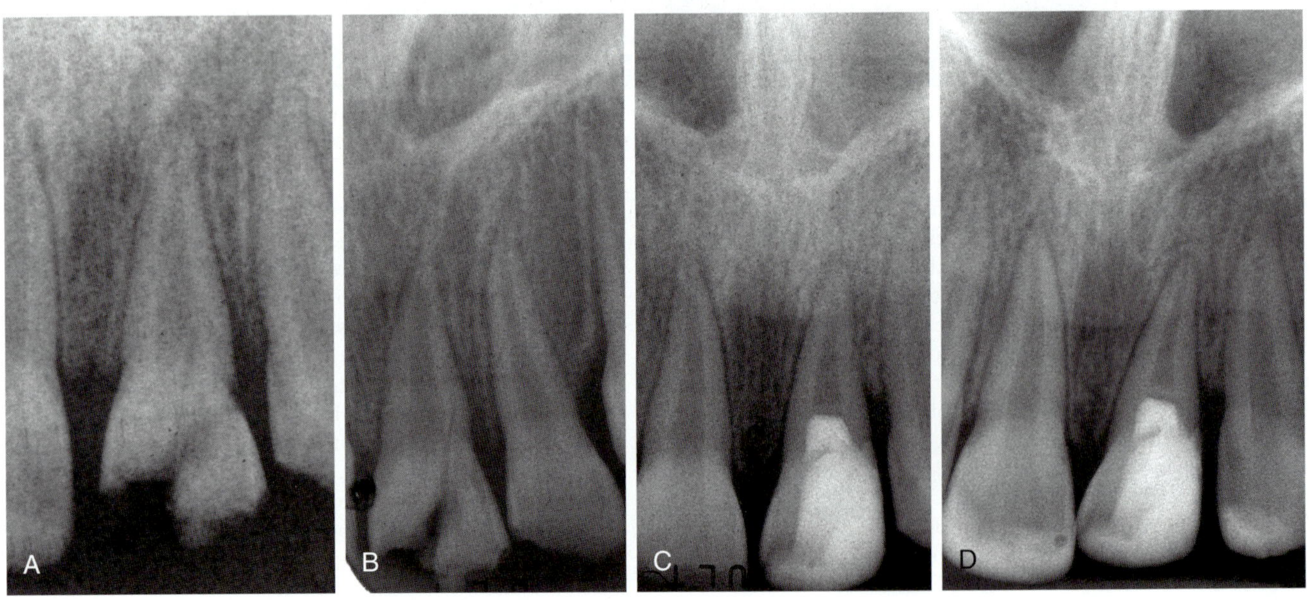

• **Fig. 11.14** Crown-root fracture of the maxillary left central incisor treated with cervical pulpotomy. **A** and **B,** Periapical radiographs at different horizontal angles. **C,** Two-month follow-up. **D,** Six-month follow-up.

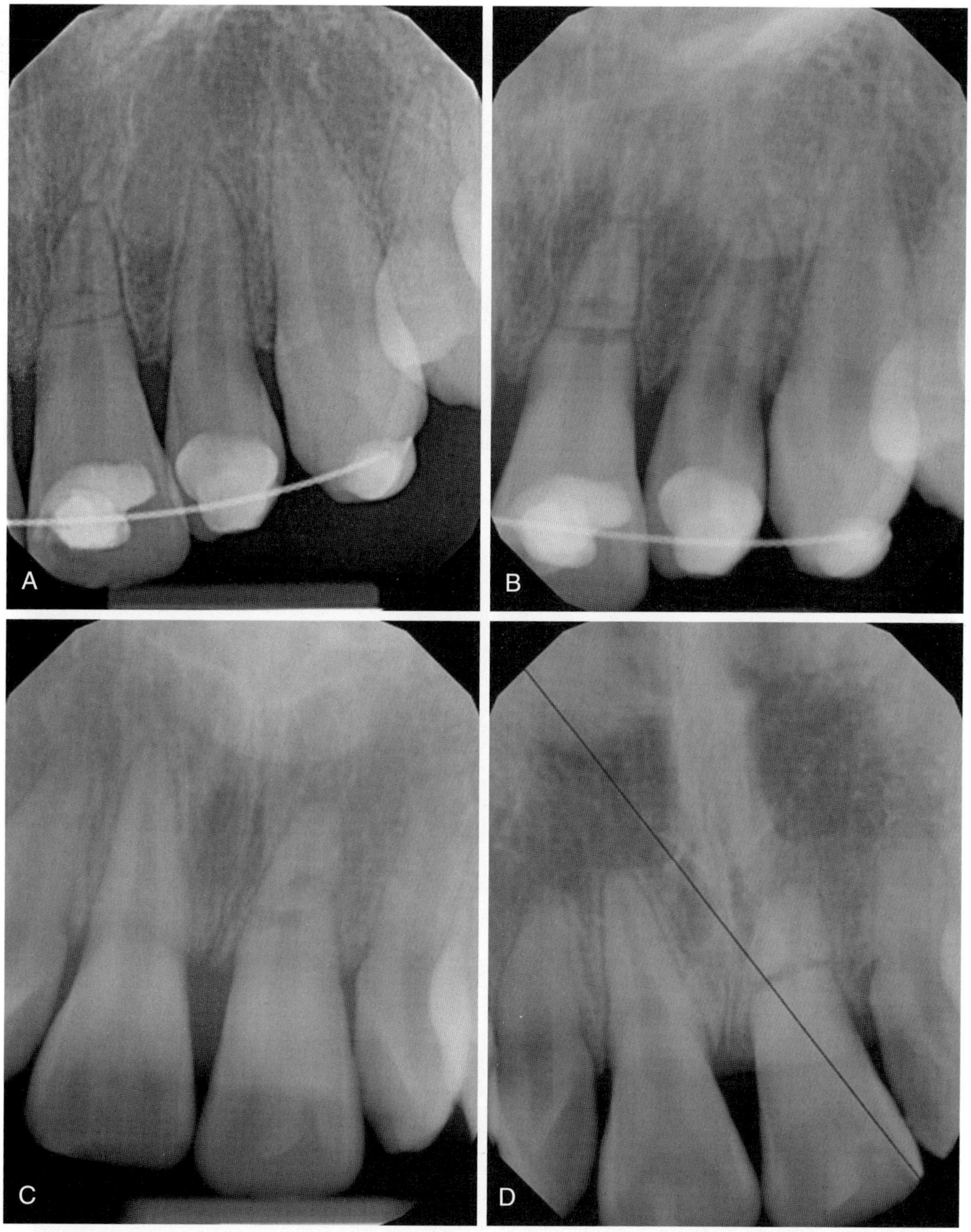

• **Fig. 11.15** Root fracture of the maxillary left central incisor. **A** and **B,** Immediate postoperative radiographs after reduction and splinting. **C,** Six-month follow-up. **D,** Follow-up at 18 months.

and *transverse root fractures*, depending on location and orientation relative to the long axis of the tooth. These types of fractures do not occur often and may be difficult to detect and diagnose.[1,19,46,47]

Radiographically, a root fracture is visualized only if the beam passes through the fracture line. Because these fractures are often oblique in orientation, they may be missed by a radiograph exposed by conventional paralleling technique. For this reason, it is recommended to obtain an additional exposure at a steep vertical angle whenever a root fracture is suspected. This additional angle (approximately 45 degrees) allows detection of many fractures, particularly in the apical area (Fig. 11.15).[46,48] Recently May and colleagues demonstrated that CBCT is most useful in cases in which conventional radiography yields inconclusive results or shows a fracture in the middle third of the root.[49] In such cases, CBCT may rule out or confirm the presence and allow evaluation of the course of the fracture through the root structure in a labiolingual direction (Fig. 11.16).

Clinically, root fractures may present as mobile or displaced teeth with pain upon biting and possible occlusal interference. Symptoms are typically mild, and if there is no mobility or displacement of the coronal segment, the patient may not be aware of any problem and may not seek treatment.[50] In general terms, the more cervical (or coronal) the location of the fracture, the greater the chance and degree of mobility and displacement of the coronal segment and the greater the likelihood of pulp necrosis of this segment if it is not promptly repositioned. Splinting is indicated for fractures occurring in the cervical or middle thirds of the root.[39,51,52] Root fractures

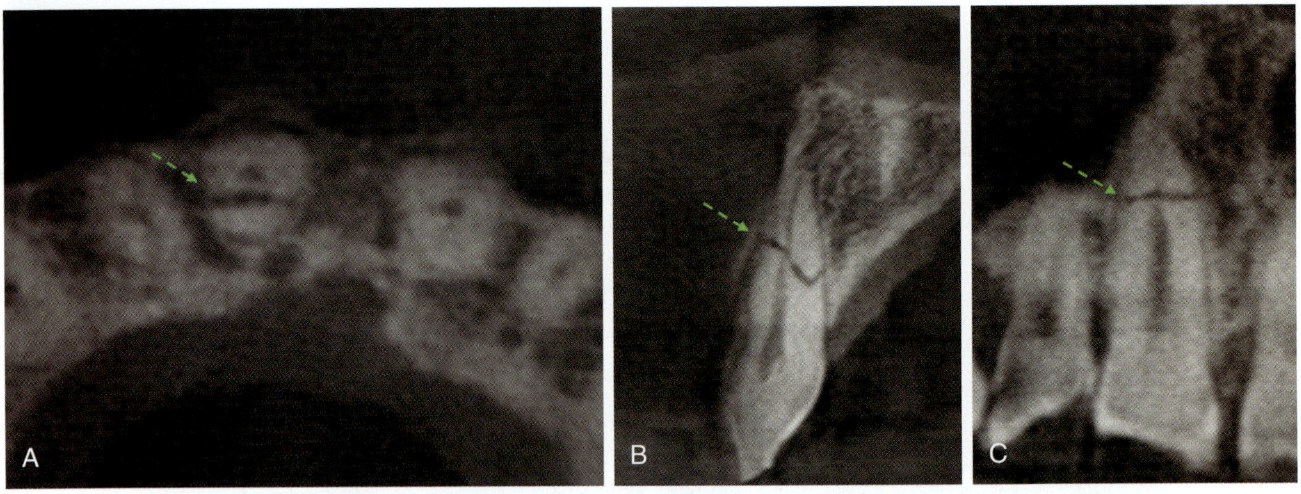

• **Fig. 11.16** Root fracture of the maxillary left central incisor. Cone beam computed tomography demonstrates the fracture in all three planes: axial **(A)**, sagittal **(B)**, and coronal **(C)**.

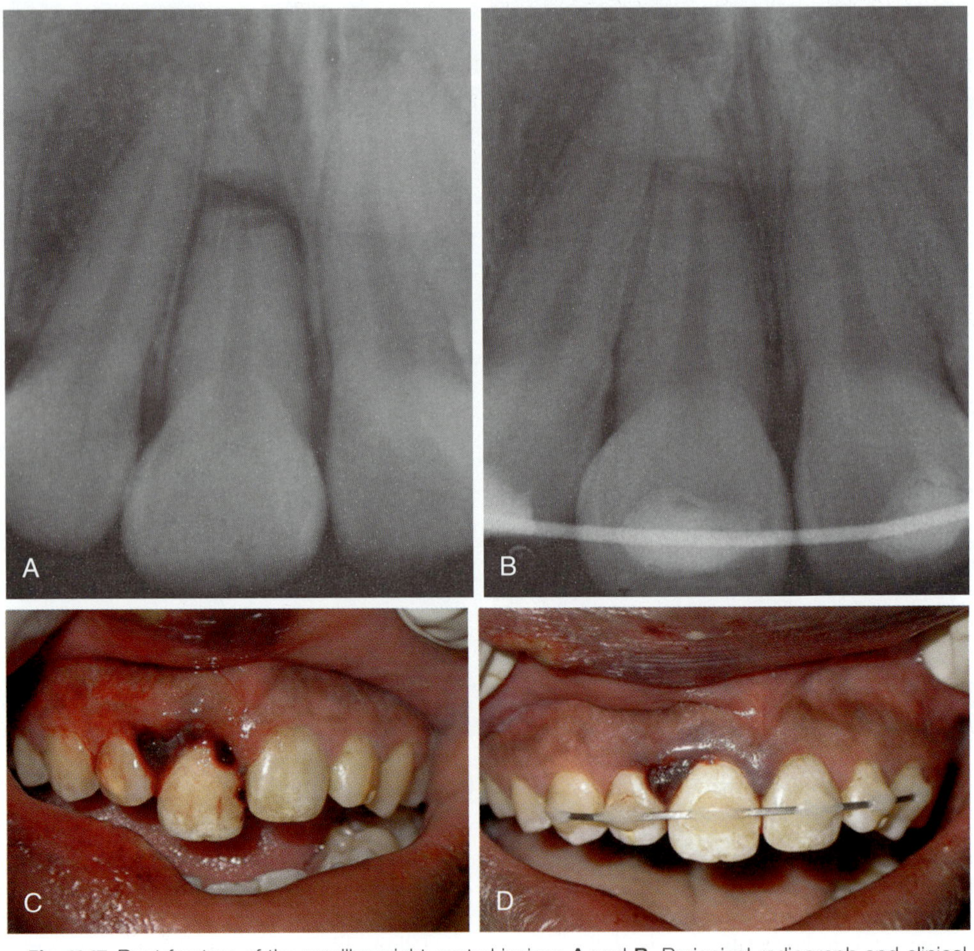

• **Fig. 11.17** Root fracture of the maxillary right central incisor. **A** and **B,** Periapical radiograph and clinical photograph of the tooth when the patient arrived at the emergency department. **C** and **D,** Reduction, repositioning, and splinting.

that occur in the apical third typically do not require any immediate treatment, but long-term observation is indicated.[51]

Emergency care for root fractures: specifically repositioning and stabilization should be completed without delay for the most favorable outcome (Fig. 11.17). Repositioning of the displaced coronal tooth segments is easier if completed soon after the injury because healing will not have started. Delayed repositioning may require orthodontic intervention to allow movement of the coronal segment into optimal position. After the repositioning, the coronal segment must be splinted to stabilize its position and

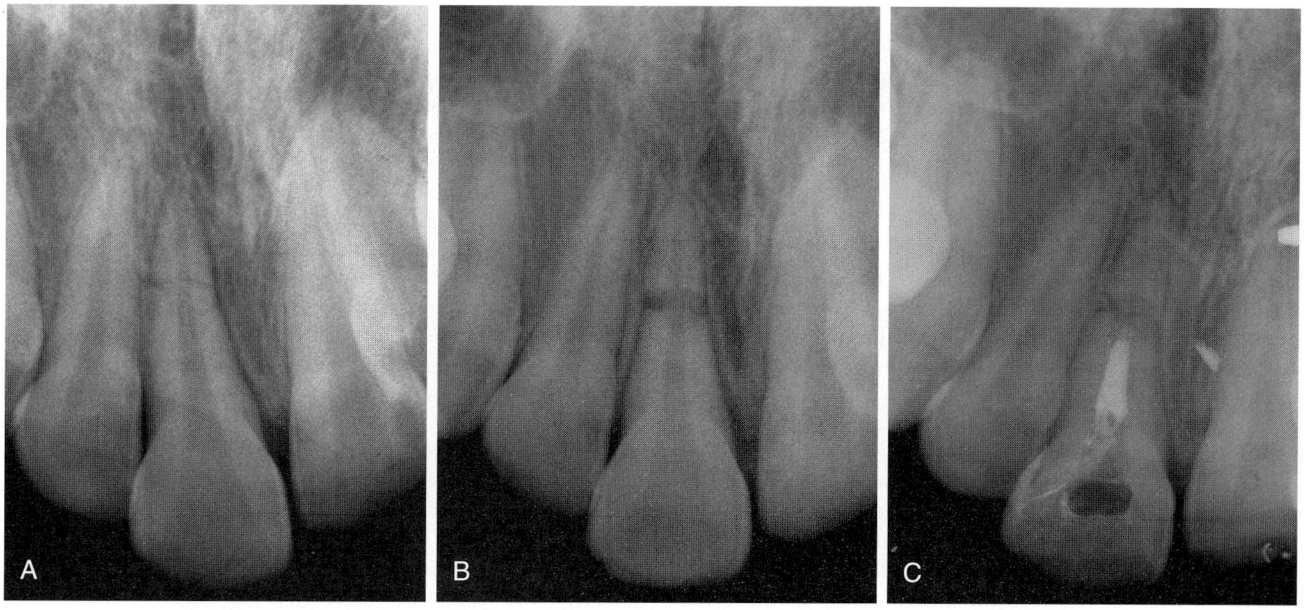

• **Fig. 11.18** Root fracture of the maxillary right central incisor. **A,** Preoperative periapical radiograph. **B,** One month later after removal of the splint. Note the separation of the coronal and apical fragments. Endodontic therapy of the coronal fragment was initiated. **C,** Two-year follow-up.

allow repair of the periodontal tissues and alveolar bone (see Fig. 11.17). Four to 6 weeks of stabilization is normally sufficient, although fractures located close to the crest of the alveolar bone may require longer periods of stabilization.[51] The outcome of this treatment should be evaluated periodically.

Sequelae of Root Fractures

Calcific metamorphosis is a common occurrence after a root fracture, usually in the coronal segment, but occasionally both coronal and apical segments can be affected. In this event, EPT may be of limited value in evaluating pulp status. In the absence of other signs of pulp necrosis, such as a radiolucency, either apical or adjacent to the fracture, lack of response to EPT alone does not necessarily indicate the necessity for root canal treatment. Frequently, the apical pulp will remain vital, even if pulp necrosis develops in the coronal segment (see Fig. 11.15).[53-56]

The healing of root fractures will occur either through hard tissue healing or connective tissue healing, or there can be a lack of healing. Hard tissue healing occurs with the deposition of calcified tissue originating from the apical pulp and PDL and is most likely to occur when little or no displacement of the coronal segment occurred during the injury. Connective tissue healing is more likely to occur with a greater degree of displacement and would be characterized by a fracture line that remains visible radiographically, but the lamina dura of the socket wall appears to be intact. Lack of healing after a root fracture typically occurs in the presence of bacterial contamination and pulp necrosis. This circumstance may present with apical symptoms such as tenderness to percussion, and the lamina dura of the socket may be disrupted on radiographic examination[46,54,57,58]

Root Canal Treatment

Root canal treatment is indicated when pulp pathosis develops subsequent to a root fracture. Normally this pathosis will be due to pulp necrosis in the coronal segment that will subsequently lead to inflammatory changes in the adjacent supporting tissues, resulting in radiolucencies adjacent to the fracture (Fig. 11.18).[54] When necessary, endodontic treatment in these cases can be complex, and referral to a specialist should be strongly considered. When treatment is indicated for teeth with horizontal root fractures, it is normally limited to the coronal segment as the pulp in the apical segment usually remains vital.[53-56]

Study Questions

1. Which of the following is a pulpal response after a traumatic incident?
   A. Calcific metamorphosis
   B. Discoloration of the crown
   C. Pulpal necrosis
   D. All of the above.
2. The unreliable responses to pulp testing in erupting, developing teeth has been attributed to the
   A. Lack of nerve fibers.
   B. Late differentiation of the Ad fibers.
   C. Late differentiation of the C fibers.
   D. Late differentiation of the Ab fibers.
3. Treatment of uncomplicated crown fractures involves
   A. Restoration of the missing tooth Structure.
   B. Pulpotomy.
   C. Root canal therapy.
   D. Extraction of the tooth.
4. Which of the following statements best describes a Cvek pulpotomy?
   A. Removal of minimal amount of the coronal pulp.
   B. Removal of the entire coronal pulp.
   C. Removal of the entire coronal pulp and part of the radicular pulp.
   D. No removal of any pulp tissue.
5. Which of the following is a sequelae of root fractures?
   A. Calcific metamorphosis.
   B. Healing of the root fracture with hard tissue.
   C. Healing of the root fracture with connective tissue.
   D. All of the above.

Injuries to the Periodontium

Injuries to the periodontium involve trauma to the supporting structures of teeth and often affect the neurovascular supply to the pulp. These injuries include:

- Concussion
- Subluxations
- Luxations (extrusive, lateral, intrusive)
- Avulsions

In general, the more severe the degree of displacement of the tooth from the socket, the greater the damage to the periodontium and to the dental pulp. Injuries to the periodontium could range from mild to severe and treatments for each of them may differ, depending on the type of injury.

The clinical descriptions of these injuries should be sufficient to make the initial diagnosis However, the pulpal status must be continually monitored until a definitive diagnosis can be made, which in some cases may require several months or years. Dichlorodifluoromethane (DDM) and EPT are used in monitoring pulpal status.[59] Table 11.2 provides a summary of the typical clinical findings associated with different types of injuries to the periodontium.

Examination, Diagnosis, and Pulp Testing

A good clinical examination followed by sensitivity tests, which include cold (DDM) and EPT, should be used to evaluate the sensory response of teeth that have been injured. Several adjacent and opposing teeth should be included in the test. An initial lack of response is not unusual, nor is a high reading on the pulp tester.[60] In these cases, the sensibility tests are repeated in 4 to 6 weeks, and the results are recorded and compared with the initial responses. If the pulp responds in both instances, the prognosis for pulp survival is good. A pulp response that is absent initially and present at the second visit indicates a probable recovery of vitality, although cases of subsequent reversals have been noted.[61] If the pulp fails to respond both times, the prognosis is questionable, and the pulp status uncertain. In the absence of other findings indicating pulp necrosis, the tooth is retested in 3 to 4 months. Continued lack of response may indicate pulp necrosis, but lack of response may not be enough evidence to make a diagnosis of pulp necrosis; that is, the pulp may permanently lose sensory nerve supply but retain its blood supply. After some time, the pulp often responds to testing if it recovers.[62]

Concussion injuries generally respond to pulp testing. Because the injury is less severe, the pulpal blood supply is more likely to return to normal.

Teeth in the *subluxation* injury group also tend to retain or recover pulpal responsiveness but less predictably than teeth with concussion injuries.

Extrusive, *lateral*, and *intrusive luxation* injuries involve displacement of the teeth and therefore more damage to apical vessels and nerves. Pulp responses in teeth with extrusive, lateral, or intrusive luxations are often absent. These pulps often do not recover even if the pulp is vital (has blood supply) because sensory nerves may be permanently damaged. Exceptions are immature teeth with wide-open apices; these teeth often regain or retain pulp vitality (responsiveness to sensitivity tests) even after severe injuries.[62]

Monitoring of pulpal status with pulp testing and radiographic evaluations is essential for a long enough period to permit determination of the outcome with a degree of certainty (this process may take 2 years or longer). Pulpal status is best monitored with pulp testing, radiographic findings, and observation for developing symptoms and for crown color changes.[62,63]

TABLE 11.2 Differential Diagnosis for the Most Common Injuries to the Periodontium

	Sensitivity Percussion	Mobility	Displacement
Concussion	Yes	No	No
Subluxation	Yes	Yes	No
Luxation	Yes	Yes	Yes

Radiographic Evaluation

The initial radiograph taken after the injury will not disclose the pulpal condition. However, it is important for evaluation of the general injury to the tooth and alveolus and serves as a basis for comparison for subsequent radiographs. Additionally, as stated in the earlier section, CBCT is important in trauma cases, especially in luxation and avulsion injuries, when a concomitant alveolar fracture is suspected (Figs. 11.19 and 11.20). 3D imaging allows for better

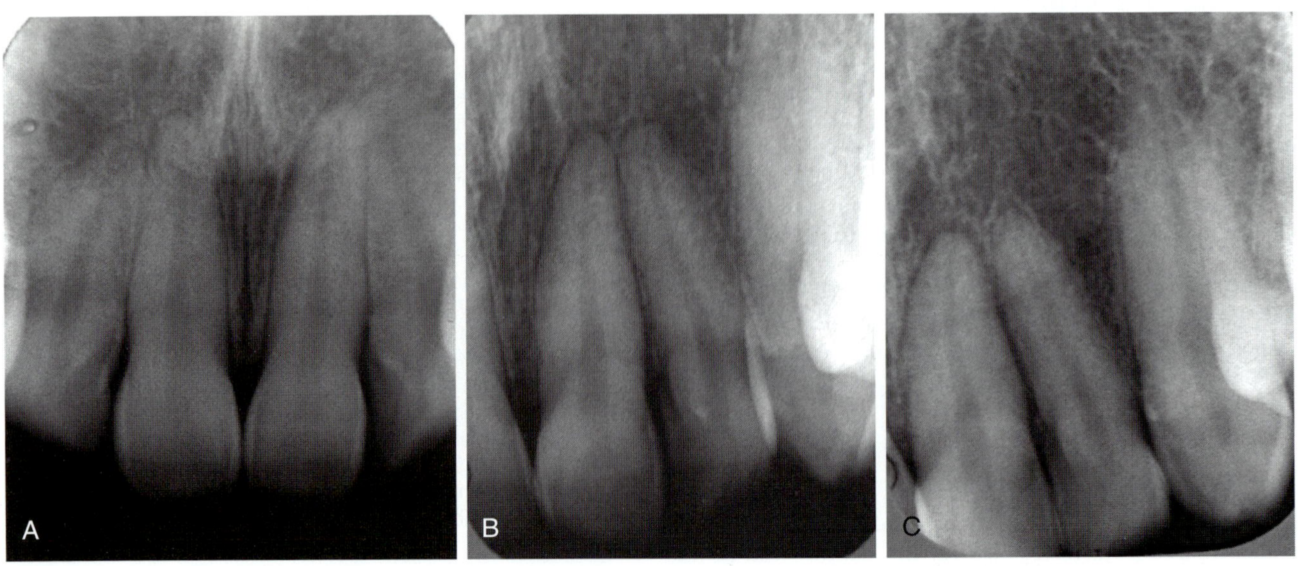

• **Fig. 11.19 A–C,** Periapical radiographs failed to reveal the position of the tooth in relation to its alveolus.

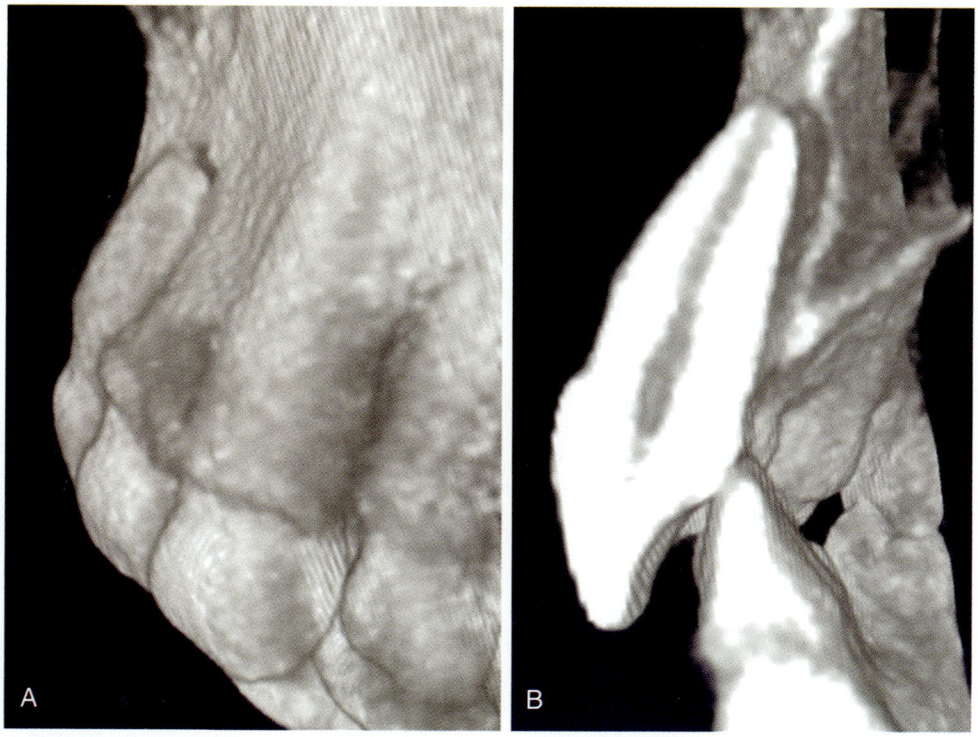

• **Fig. 11.20** Cone beam computed tomography. Transaxial volumetric reconstruction **(A)** and sagittal plane view **(B)** demonstrating lateral luxation of the maxillary left central incisor with a concomitant alveolar fracture.

diagnosis of alveolar fractures and confirms the correct position of the tooth in the socket, as stated previously in this chapter.

Radiographs are also indicated for early diagnosis and treatment of external resorptions and periradicular bony changes. Resorptive changes, particularly external changes, may occur soon after injury; if no attempt is made to arrest the destructive process, much of the root may be rapidly lost. Inflammatory (infection-related) resorption can be intercepted by timely endodontic intervention.[64]

Periodic radiographs show whether the root of a developing tooth is continuing to grow (a positive sign indicating recovery of the pulp). Another finding may be pulp space calcification or obliteration, a common finding after luxation injuries in immature teeth.[65] Also called *calcific metamorphosis*, this canal obliteration may be partial or nearly complete (after several years) and does not indicate a need for root canal treatment, except when other signs and symptoms suggest pulp necrosis.[65]

Crown Color Changes

Pulpal injury may cause discoloration, even after only a few days. Initial changes tend to be pink. Subsequently, if the pulp does not recover and becomes necrotic, there may be a grayish darkening of the crown, often accompanied by a loss in translucency (Fig. 11.21). In addition, color changes may take place as a result of calcific metamorphosis of the pulp. Such color changes are likely to be yellow to brown and do not indicate pulp pathosis. Other signs, findings, or symptoms are necessary to diagnose pulp necrosis.[62,65]

Discoloration could be reversed. This reversal usually happens relatively soon after the injury and indicates that the pulp is vital. Because of unpredictable changes associated with traumatized teeth, long-term evaluation is recommended.[62]

The next part of this chapter describes the injuries and the recommended treatment for each type.

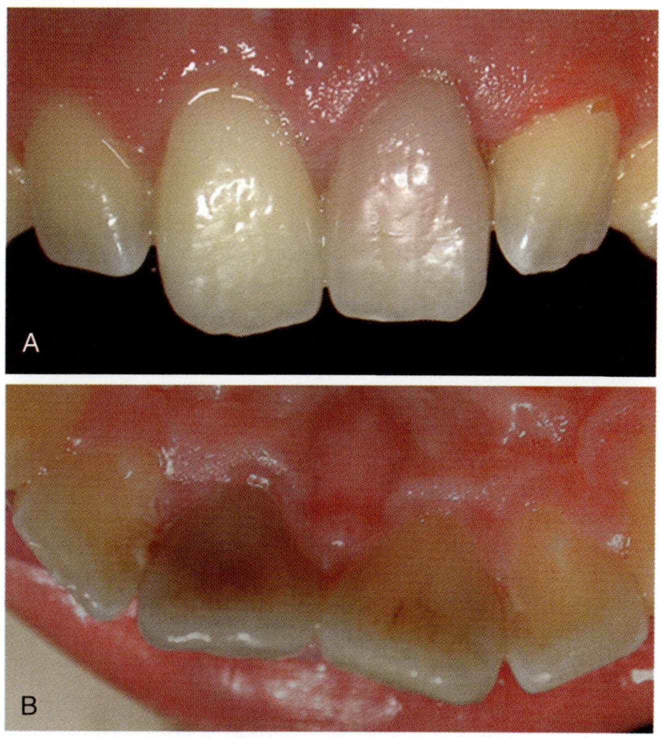

• **Fig. 11.21** Crown color changes as a result of pulpal injury after a luxation injury: buccal view **(A)** and lingual view **(B)**.

Concussion

This is an injury to the tooth-supporting structures *without increased mobility or displacement* of the tooth *but with pain on percussion.* Concussion injuries generally respond to pulp testing because the injury is less severe; the pulpal blood supply is more likely to return to normal. No radiographic changes are found.[66]

Treatment:
1. Note that no treatment is usually necessary.
2. Prescribe a soft diet for 14 days.
3. Prescribe chlorhexidine rinses.
4. Follow up.

Subluxation

Subluxation is an injury to the tooth-supporting structures resulting *in increased mobility* but *without displacement of the tooth.* Although sulcular bleeding might be present, this clinical finding does not provide a diagnosis.

Teeth with subluxation injuries are sensitive to percussion. The teeth are not displaced, and the pulp may respond normally to testing, sometimes after initially failing to respond. No radiographic changes are noted.[66]

Treatment:
1. Note that no treatment is usually necessary.
2. Relieve the occlusion.
3. Prescribe a soft diet.
4. Apply a splint only in case of marked loosening for up to 2 weeks.[67]
5. Prescribe chlorhexidine rinses.
6. Follow up and monitor pulpal status.

Luxation

Luxation is an injury to the tooth-supporting structures resulting *in increased mobility, with displacement of the tooth.*[66] The injury may displace the tooth in three possible directions: extrusive, lateral, or intrusive.

Extrusive Luxation

With extrusive luxation, teeth are partially displaced from the socket along the long axis. Extruded teeth have greatly increased mobility, and radiographs show displacement. The pulp usually does not respond to testing.[59,66]

Lateral Luxation

Teeth may be displaced in any direction besides axially. These teeth could be displaced lingually, buccally, mesially, or distally (i.e., away from their normal position in a horizontal direction).[66] However, this type of luxation injury is usually accompanied by comminution or fracture of either the labial or the palatal/lingual alveolar bone. This consequence is because of the impact, which usually comes from the facial aspect that causes the crown to be displaced lingually and the apex buccally, creating a subsequent alveolar fracture. If the apex has been severely displaced, the pulp may permanently lose sensory nerve supply but retain its blood supply. A metallic sound on percussion might indicate that the root tip has been forced into the alveolar bone.

Treatment for extrusive and lateral luxations:
1. Reposition and splint. Extrusive and lateral luxation injuries require repositioning and splinting. The duration of splinting varies with the severity of injury. Extrusions may need only 2 weeks, whereas lateral luxations that involve bony fractures need 4 weeks.[66]
2. Prescribe a soft diet.
3. Prescribe chlorhexidine rinses.
4. Treat with root canal therapy. Root canal treatment is indicated for teeth with a diagnosis of irreversible pulpitis or pulp necrosis. Such a diagnosis often requires a combination of signs and symptoms, such as discoloration of the crown, lack of pulp response to pulp testing, and a periradicular lesion seen radiographically.[66]
5. Monitor for possible endodontic treatment. Severe cases of either extrusive or lateral luxation of mature teeth may require endodontic therapy within the first 2 weeks to prevent the onset of resorption (Fig. 11.22).

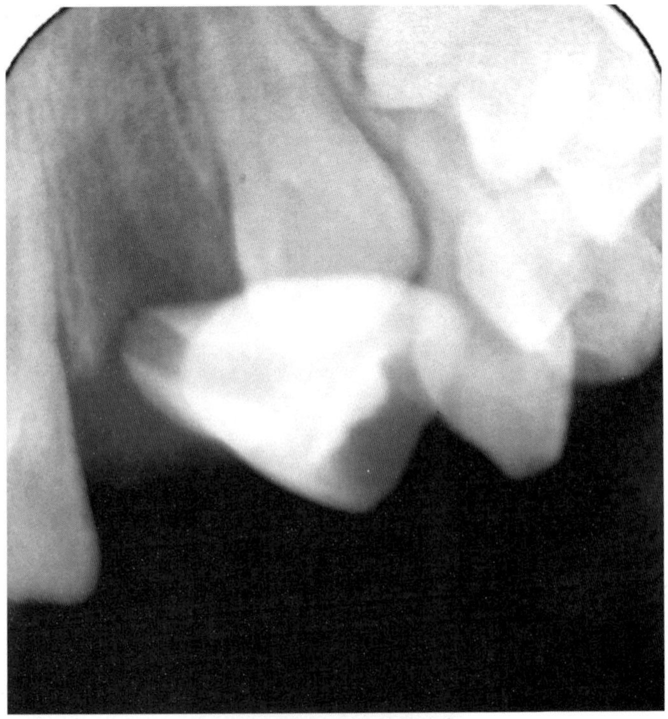

• **Fig. 11.22** Severe extrusive luxation. The tooth was retained only by soft tissue.

Intrusive Luxation

In this type of injury, the teeth are forced into the sockets in an axial (apical) direction, at times to the point of not being clinically visible. They have no mobility, resembling ankyloses (Fig. 11.23).[68,69]

Treatment for Intrusive Luxation

This treatment differs slightly from the extrusive and lateral luxation cases and depends on stage of root maturity.[68-70]

Open Apex

If the root is incompletely formed with an open apex, it may reposition spontaneously. A clinical study revealed that in young patients 12 to 17 years of age who have complete root formation, spontaneous reeruption is possible and was found to be the best treatment with regard to marginal periodontal healing.[68]

In teeth with immature roots, the pulp may revascularize.[68,71] However, the patient must be monitored carefully, because complications that include pulp necrosis along with lack of continued root development could arise. Root canal treatment should be performed in these cases.

Closed Apex

In older patients (i.e., older than 17 years of age) with complete root formation, either surgical or orthodontic extrusion should be attempted. Intrusively luxated teeth undergo pulp necrosis approximately 85% to 100% of the time.[68,69,71,72] Hence, root

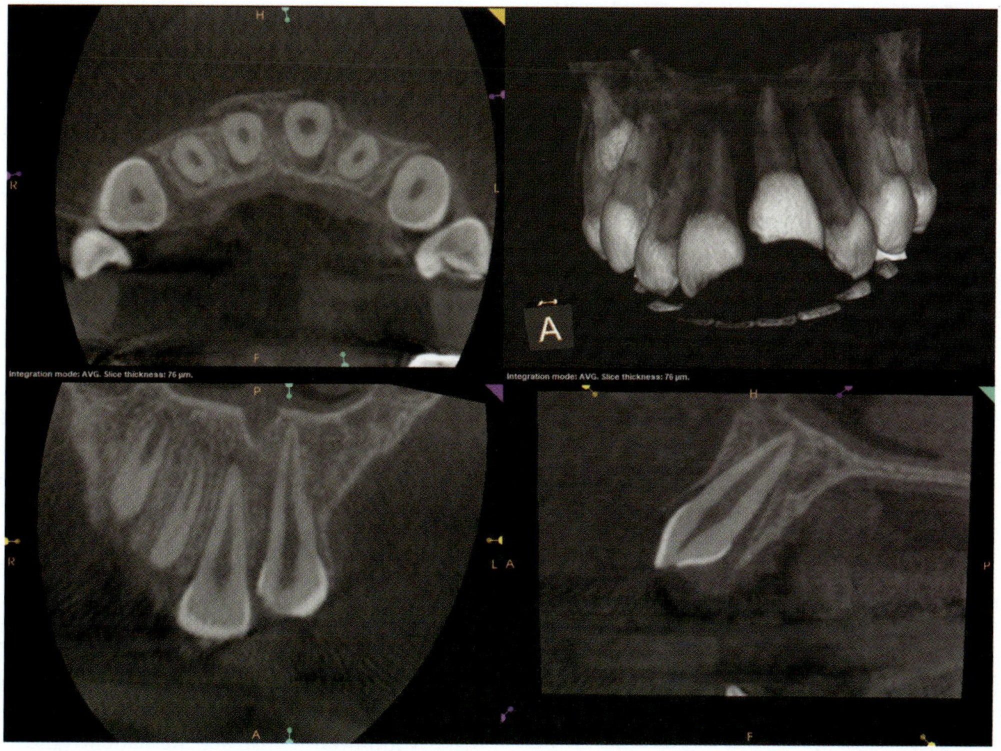

• **Fig. 11.23** Severe intrusive luxation: Cone beam computed tomographic imaging shows the extent of intrusion of the maxillary left central incisor.

canal therapy is indicated for these teeth within the first 2 weeks to prevent the onset of resorption.

Avulsion

This circumstance could be described as the complete separation of a tooth from its alveolus by traumatic injury. This separation can lead to extensive damage to the pulp and the periodontal tissues. The prognosis of the teeth depends entirely on the *extraoral dry time/period* and the *storage media*. The storage media is important to preserve the PDL cells and the fibers attached to the root surface.[73]

Treatment

Three situations involving avulsions may arise: (1) the tooth has already been replanted; (2) the extraoral dry time has been less than 60 minutes; or (3) the tooth has been out for *longer* than 60 minutes and has not been kept in a storage medium.

Immediate Replantation

The prognosis is improved by replantation immediately after avulsion and should always be encouraged.[74-76]

- Leave the tooth in place.
- Clean the area with water spray, saline, or chlorhexidine.
- Verify normal position of the replanted tooth both clinically and radiographically.
- Apply a flexible splint for up to 2 weeks.
- Administer systemic antibiotics.
- If the avulsed tooth has been in contact with soil, and if tetanus coverage is uncertain, refer to a physician for a tetanus booster.
- Initiate root canal treatment within 7 to 10 days after replantation and before splint removal.

Replantation Within 60 Minutes of Avulsion—Tooth with a Closed Apex

If replantation is not feasible at the place of injury, the tooth should be brought to the dental office in media to keep it moist and prolong the vitality of the PDL cells.[77,78] The most common storage medium is Hanks Balanced Salt Solution (HBSS), which is commercially available as a kit (Save-A-Tooth; Phoenix-Lazerus, Pottstown, Pennsylvania, USA). However, if not available, milk is an excellent alternative.[79-84]

When the patient arrives, the following steps are recommended:

1. Place the tooth in a cup of physiologic saline while preparing for replantation.
2. Take radiographs of the area of injury to look for evidence of alveolar fracture. Consider the use of CBCT, if indicated.
3. Administer local anesthetic.
4. Examine the avulsion site carefully for any loose bone fragments that may be removed. If the alveolus is collapsed, spread it open gently with an instrument.
5. Clean the root surface and apical foramen with a stream of saline and soak the tooth in saline, thereby removing contamination and dead cells from the root surface.
6. Irrigate the socket gently with saline to remove contaminated coagulum.
7. Grasp the crown of the tooth and avoid handling the root and replant the tooth with slight digital pressure to accomplish complete seating.
8. Check for proper alignment and correct any hyperocclusion. Soft tissue lacerations should be tightly sutured, particularly cervically.
9. Stabilize the tooth for 2 weeks with a flexible splint; nylon, stainless steel, or nickel-titanium wires up to 0.016 inch (0.4 mm) in diameter are significantly more flexible.[85]

Replantation Within 60 Minutes of Avulsion—Tooth with an Open Apex

When the patient arrives, the following steps are recommended:

1. Place the tooth in a cup of physiologic saline while preparing for replantation.
2. Administer a local anesthetic.
3. Examine the alveolar socket, looking for fracture of the socket wall.
4. If available, cover the root surface topically with a tetracycline-based antibiotic before replanting the tooth.[86-88]
5. Replant the tooth with slight digital pressure.
6. Suture gingival lacerations, especially in the cervical area.
7. Verify normal position of the replanted tooth.
8. Apply a flexible splint for 2 weeks.
9. If the avulsed tooth has been in contact with soil and if tetanus coverage is uncertain or if the previous one was administered more than 10 years earlier, refer to a physician for a tetanus booster.
10. Administer systemic antibiotics. Unlike mature teeth for which endodontic therapy should be initiated within a week, immature teeth with open apices may revascularize, but they must be evaluated at regular intervals of 2, 6, and 12 months after replantation. If subsequent evaluations indicate pulp necrosis, lack of root development, and apical closure, root canal treatment, probably including apexification, is indicated.[89]

Replantation with Dry Time Longer Than 60 Minutes—Tooth with a Closed Apex

If a tooth has been out of the alveolar socket for longer than 60 minutes (and has not been kept moist in a suitable medium), PDL cells and fibers will not survive, regardless of the stage of root development.[73,79] Replacement root resorption (characterized by ankylosis) is likely to be the eventual sequela of replantation. Therefore treatment efforts before replantation include treating the root surface with fluoride to slow the resorptive process.[73]

When the patient arrives, the following steps are recommended:

1. Examine the area of tooth avulsion and examine the radiographs for evidence of alveolar fractures.
2. Remove attached nonviable soft tissue/PDL carefully with gauze.
3. Root canal treatment can be performed before replantation, or it can be done within 2 weeks.
4. Administer local anesthesia.
5. Irrigate the socket with saline.
6. Replant the tooth slowly with slight digital pressure.
7. Verify normal position of the replanted tooth clinically and radiographically.
8. Stabilize the tooth for 4 weeks using a flexible splint.
9. Administer systemic antibiotics.
10. If the avulsed tooth has been in contact with soil, and if tetanus coverage is uncertain, refer to a physician for a tetanus booster.

Soaking the tooth in a 2.4% solution of sodium fluoride (acidulated to a pH of 5.5) for 20 minutes has been suggested to slow down osseous replacement, but this approach is not an absolute recommendation.[90]

Replantation with Dry Time Longer Than 60 Minutes—Tooth with an Open Apex

The management of these teeth is similar to those with a closed apex.

1. Remove attached nonviable soft tissue carefully with gauze.
2. Root canal treatment can be performed before replantation, or it can be done 7 to 10 days later.
3. Administer local anesthesia
4. Irrigate the socket with saline.
5. Examine the alveolar socket.
6. Replant the tooth slowly with slight digital pressure.
7. Verify normal position of the replanted tooth clinically and radiographically.
8. Stabilize the tooth for 4 weeks using a flexible splint.
9. Administer systemic antibiotics.
10. If the avulsed tooth has been in contact with soil, and if tetanus coverage is uncertain, refer to a physician for a tetanus booster.

Patient Instructions

Antibiotics are recommended for patients with replanted avulsed teeth.[91,92]

- For children under the age of 12 years, penicillin V 25-50 mg/kg of body weight in divided doses every 6 hours for 7 days can be prescribed.
- In patients 12 years of age or older, doxycycline 100 mg two times per day for 7 days is the current recommendation. Amoxicillin in an appropriate dose for age and weight, can also be given as alternative to tetracycline.

A tetanus booster injection is recommended if the previous one had been administered more than 10 years earlier.[93] Supportive care is important. Instruct the patient (and parents) to maintain a soft diet for up to 2 weeks, to brush with a soft toothbrush after every meal, and to use a chlorhexidine mouth rinse (0.12%) twice a day for a week.

Sequelae of Dental Trauma

Pulp Necrosis

When the pulp is diagnosed as necrotic, the main factor to be considered is the stage of root development. If the root is fully matured, root canal therapy is the treatment of choice as stated in the next section. In immature teeth with open apices, treatment options include apexification or, more recently, regenerative endodontic treatment.

Teeth with Open Apices

1. *Calcium hydroxide apexification:* Apexification could be done in the traditional manner, which incorporates long-term use of calcium hydroxide for up to 18 months. This method was first introduced by Kaiser in 1964 and made popular by Frank in 1966.[94,95] Many studies have described the successful formation of an apical barrier with the long-term use of calcium hydroxide.[96,97] However, such long-term treatment processes may result in decreased fracture resistance of these teeth.[98-100]
2. *MTA apexification:* In 2001 Witherspoon and Ham reported using MTA for single-visit apexification treatment of immature teeth with necrotic pulps.[101] This study demonstrated that the use of an MTA apical plug provided a scaffolding for the formation of a hard tissue barrier and subsequently a better apical seal. Furthermore, MTA apical plug has shown to increase the fracture resistance of immature teeth.[102,103]
3. *Regenerative endodontics:* Regenerative endodontic procedures (REPs) for the treatment of immature teeth with necrotic pulps and apical periodontitis have gained much attention in recent years.[104,105] Studies have shown that although the outcomes of these procedures are somewhat unpredictable, in successful cases there is increased thickness of the canal wall and length of the root, which makes these teeth less prone to fractures.[104-107]

Teeth with Closed Apices

Root Canal Treatment

An avulsion injury causes the neurovascular supply to be severely compromised along with loss of vascularization to the pulp, thereby causing necrosis.[75,108] In the mature replanted tooth, root canal treatment is indicated and should be started 7 to 10 days after replantation.[21] The use of calcium hydroxide as an antimicrobial intracanal interappointment medicament may be helpful.[92,109] It is particularly beneficial if the root canal is infected, a condition that would be likely to occur when root canal treatment is delayed more than a few weeks after replantation. However, as discussed in the previous section, long-term calcium hydroxide therapy could significantly decrease fracture strength.[98-100]

The procedure consists of cleaning and shaping, followed by calcium hydroxide placement for a minimum of 1 to 2 weeks.[109] The root canal is then obturated with gutta-percha and sealer. Long-term evaluation is necessary to monitor for possible resorption.

Restoration of the coronal access opening is necessary once the root canal treatment is completed. This step is important to prevent bacterial leakage into the root canal system.[110,111]

Pulp Canal Obliteration (Calcific Metamorphosis)

The complete or partial calcification of the root canal space is a common finding after luxation injuries in immature teeth with a well-vascularized pulp.[65,112] Canal obliteration may be partial or nearly complete (after several years) and does not indicate a need for root canal treatment except when other signs and symptoms suggest pulp necrosis.[65]

Root Resorption

External root resorption is a frequent occurrence in replanted avulsed teeth.[113] Three types have been identified and studied extensively: surface, inflammatory, and replacement.[114,115]

Surface Resorption

Also called "repair-related resorption," surface resorption is transient and shows as lacunae of resorption in the cementum of replanted teeth. They are not usually visible on radiographs. If resorption does not continue, the lacunae are repaired by deposition of new cementum.

Inflammatory Resorption

Inflammatory resorption occurs as a response to the presence of infected necrotic pulp tissue in conjunction with injury to the PDL (Fig. 11.24). It occurs with replanted teeth in addition to other types of luxation injuries. Inflammatory resorption is characterized by loss of tooth structure and adjacent alveolar bone. Resorption usually subsides after removal of the necrotic, infected pulp, so the prognosis is good. Hence, root canal treatment is recommended routinely for replanted teeth with closed apices to prevent the occurrence of inflammatory resorption.

External Replacement (PDL-Related) Resorption

In replacement resorption, the tooth structure is resorbed and replaced by bone, resulting in ankylosis in which bone fuses directly to the root surface (Fig. 11.25). The characteristics of ankylosis are lack of physiologic mobility, failure of the tooth to erupt along with adjacent teeth (leading to infraocclusion in young individuals), and a "solid" metallic sound on percussion. Currently no treatment is available for replacement resorption, which tends to be progressive until the root is completely replaced by bone.[114-116] In teeth that have had long extraoral dry periods, the resorptive process may be slowed (but not halted) by immersing the tooth in fluoride before replantation.[117-119] Research is ongoing to delineate the mechanism of replacement resorption and find various methods to slow or halt the process.[117]

Alveolar Fractures

Pulp necrosis and luxation injuries are often associated with alveolar fractures, which may in turn be associated with other major facial injuries (Fig. 11.26).[120] It is important to diagnose the presence of the fracture, which would dictate the treatment options and management, consisting of reduction and splinting of the segment to the adjacent teeth. The use of CBCT is highly recommended (as mentioned earlier in the chapter). When the patient is able to have the teeth examined, those in the line of fracture and adjacent teeth are evaluated. Lack of response to pulp testing, if not reversed within 3 to 6 months, may indicate pulp necrosis, but the presence of other indicators (apical radiolucency or symptoms) is necessary before root canal treatment is recommended.[121] Major facial injuries are usually managed by oral and maxillofacial surgeons who would also manage the related dental trauma.

Management of Traumatic Injuries in the Primary Dentition

Young children are often difficult to examine and treat primarily due to the sustained traumatic experience and fear. In some instances, the treatment of traumatic injuries to the primary dentition may mirror those of the permanent dentition; however, the clinician should be aware that the root of the injured primary tooth may be in close proximity to the permanent successor (Fig. 11.27). Treatment involves a thorough clinical and radiographic examination, followed by a diagnosis and necessary treatment, keeping in mind that these injuries may or may not have significant effects on the permanent successors.[122-124] Multiple studies have reported the possible sequelae to the permanent teeth after trauma to the primary teeth. These mainly included discoloration, tooth malformation, and enamel hypoplasia.[122,125] After diagnosis and an explanation of the treatment options to the parents or guardians, the clinician along with the parent or guardian should decide the treatment option that would benefit the patient.

Primary teeth could sustain various types of trauma; however, luxation injuries are the most common and most of these injuries will heal spontaneously.[126-129] Some other injuries, like complicated crown fractures (with pulp exposure), root fractures, alveolar fractures, extrusive and lateral luxations, require urgent treatment (Fig. 11.28). Treatment options depend on the proximity of the apex of the primary tooth and its developing permanent successor and on the degree of root resorption of the primary tooth. Hence, treatment should be aimed at minimizing additional trauma or damage to the permanent successors.

The following are some of the guidelines for treating traumatized primary teeth.[127,128]

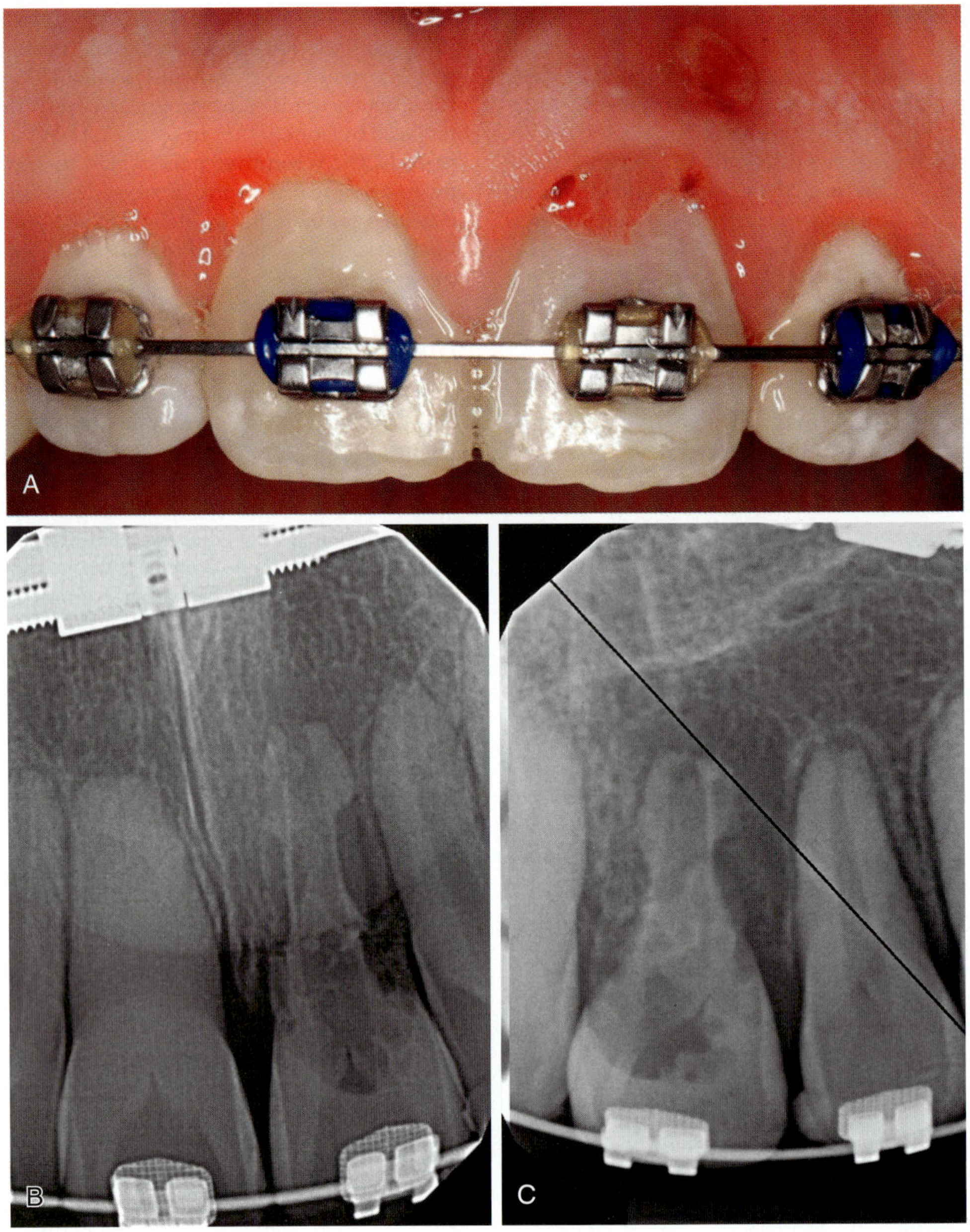

• **Fig. 11.24** A 14-year-old patient presented for consultation 5 years after avulsion of the maxillary left central incisor. A clinical photograph **(A)** and radiographic examination (**B** and **C**) revealed the presence of external inflammatory root resorption.

Enamel fracture

Smoothen sharp edges. No additional treatment is necessary.

Crown Fractures Without Pulp Exposure

If the fracture site is small, smooth the sharp edges or seal the exposed dentin with glass ionomer. If the fractured segment is larger, the tooth can be restored with a composite restoration.

Crown Fractures with Pulp Exposure

The treatment should be aimed at preserving pulp vitality. Partial pulpotomy with calcium hydroxide followed by a glass ionomer lining and a composite restoration should be the treatment of choice if possible. However, extraction may be indicated, depending on the patient's age, cooperation, and ability to cope.

Crown-Root Fractures

If the fracture involves only a small part of the root and the rest of the tooth is stable and allows for a coronal restoration, only the fractured fragment should be removed. If the crown-root fracture is large and/or exposes the pulp, extraction is indicated.

Root Fractures

If the coronal fragment is not displaced, no treatment is required unless problems develop subsequently.

If the coronal fragment is displaced, repositioning and splinting may be considered. If repositioning is not an option, then removing the coronal segment and leaving the root apex in situ is the treatment of choice. Any attempt to remove the root apex may damage the permanent tooth bud.

Alveolar Fractures

Alveolar fractures are severe injuries that may dictate treatment while the patient is under general anesthesia. The displaced segment should be repositioned and splinted for up to 4 weeks. Teeth in the fracture line should be monitored.

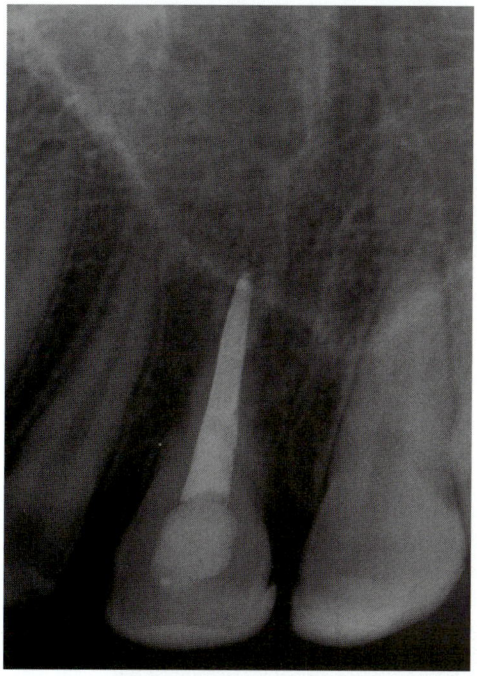

• **Fig. 11.25** Periapical radiograph of a 12-year-old patient 2 years after replantation of the maxillary right central incisor. Note the presence of replacement root resorption (dentin replaced by bone) in the absence of radiolucencies.

Luxation Injuries

Concussion and Subluxation

These injuries require no treatment other than promoting good oral hygiene to prevent healing complications. Brushing with a soft toothbrush and the use of alcohol-free 0.12% chlorhexidine topically on the affected area with a cotton swab for a week should be encouraged.

Crown discoloration could occur after some luxation injuries. This discoloration is usually the main complaint for seeking treatment. However, studies have demonstrated that the positive association between the pulp status and crown discoloration should be considered with caution and that discoloration is not considered an indication for treatment.[130-133] Discolored teeth should be followed and should be treated when signs of infection develop (e.g., sinus tract, abscess etc.). Pulp canal obliteration is the other common sequela after luxation injuries. This obliteration changes the primary crown to a darker yellow color, which is not pathologic and requires no treatment (Fig. 11.29).[127,128,134]

Extrusive Luxations

The treatment would depend on the degree of extrusion, root formation, mobility, and the ability of the child to manage the treatment procedure. For minor extrusions the tooth may be left untreated for spontaneous realignment or repositioned if there is occlusal interference. Extraction may be the treatment of choice for severely extruded teeth.

Lateral Luxations

For minor lateral luxations, the tooth may be left untreated for spontaneous realignment or repositioned if there is occlusal interference. In case of minor occlusal interferences, minor occlusal adjustment may be indicated. In cases of more severe occlusal interferences, the tooth may be repositioned after the use of local anesthesia. In cases of severe displacement (crown is displaced labially), extraction is the treatment of choice.

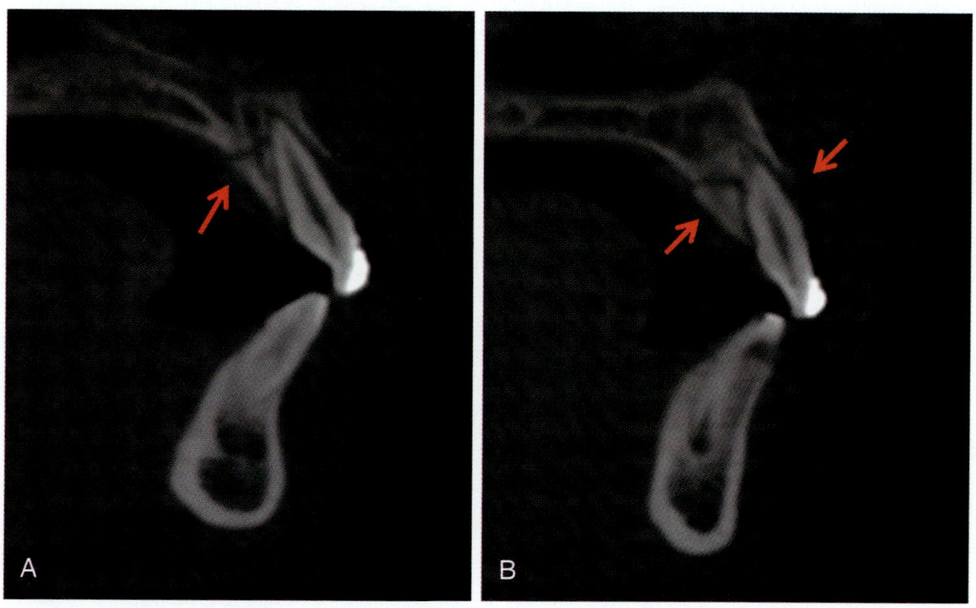

• **Fig. 11.26** Alveolar fractures of the lingual (**A** and **B**) and buccal (**B**) cortical plates.

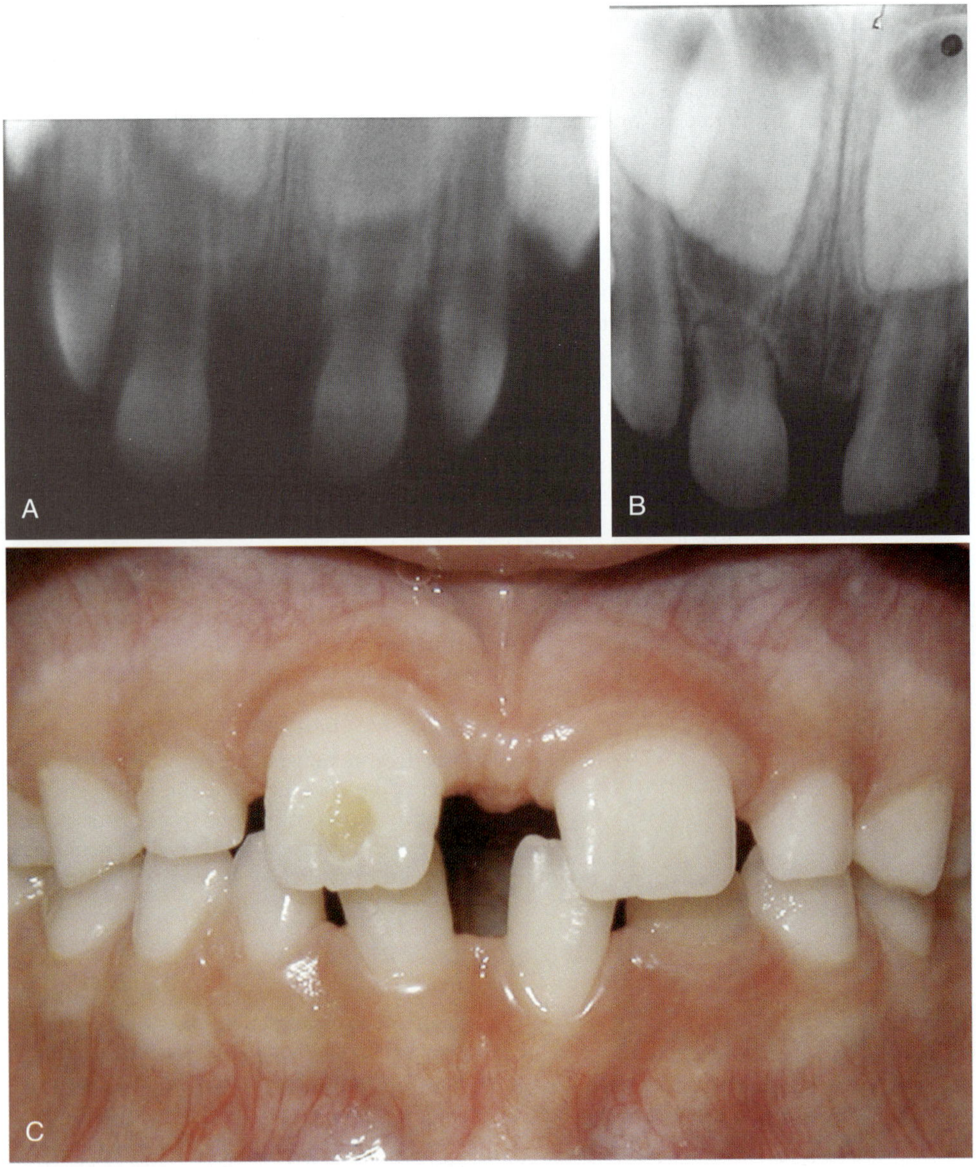

• **Fig. 11.27** Hypoplasia in a permanent incisor after avulsion and subsequent replantation of a primary central incisor. A 1-year-old boy fell and struck the central incisors against a table. The primary right central incisor was avulsed and replanted. The patient followed a 7-day course of amoxicillin. **A,** Radiograph at the time of injury shows the replanted immature central incisor. **B,** At the 3-year, 5-month follow-up control, the root has been almost completely resorbed. The contralateral tooth shows complete root formation. **C,** Crown hypoplasia of the right permanent successor at 7-year follow-up control.

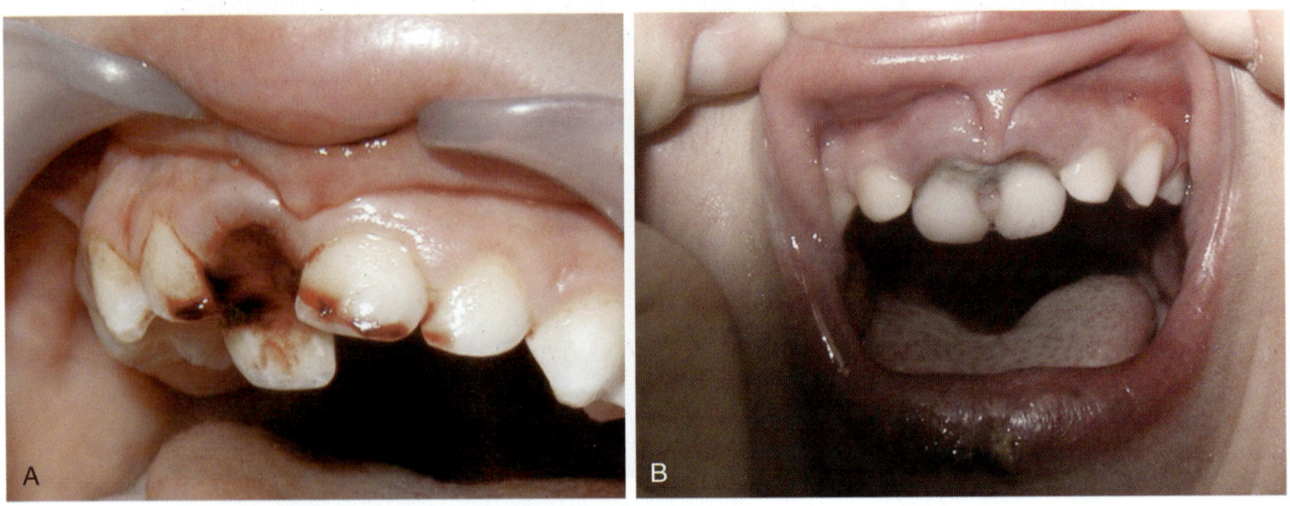

• **Fig. 11.28** Treatment priorities after traumatic injuries in the primary dentition include urgent care to alleviate pain and enable recovery of masticatory function. **A,** Severe tooth displacement. **B,** Extrusive luxation of both primary central incisors.

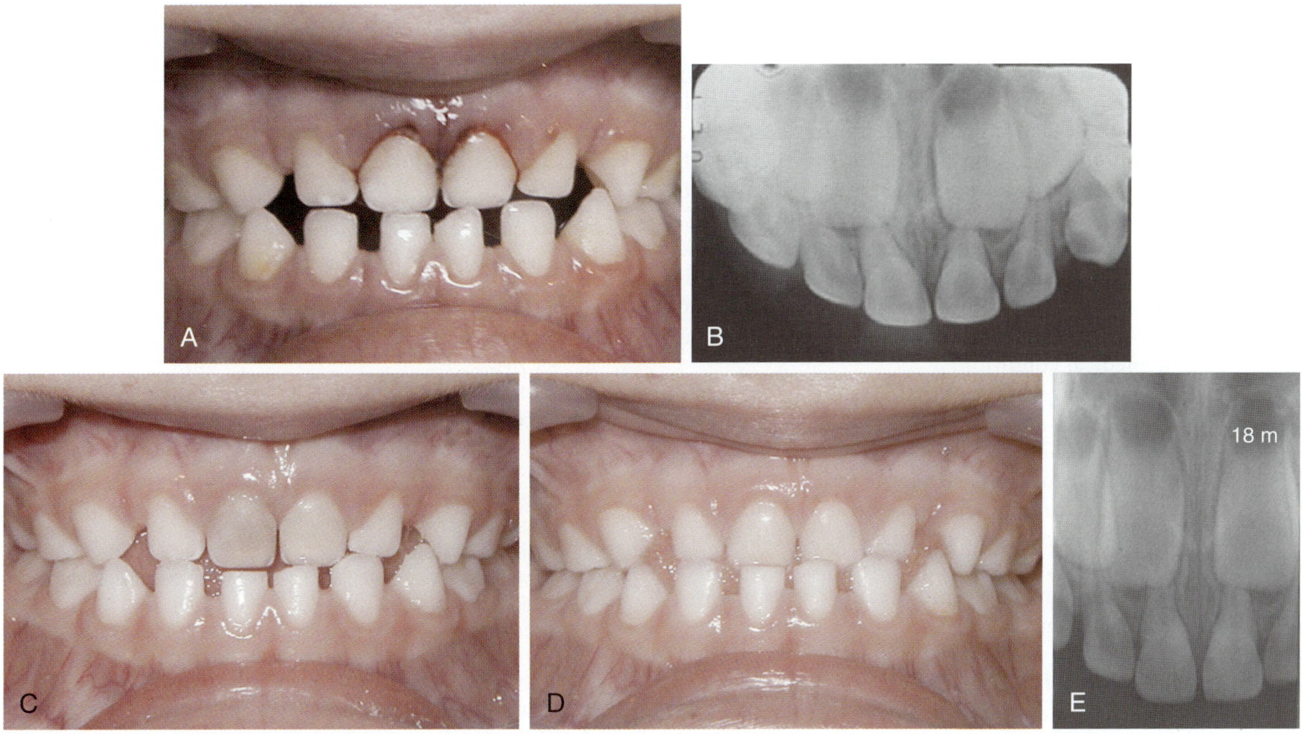

• **Fig. 11.29** Color changes in primary teeth after a subluxation injury. A 5-year-old girl fell while playing and struck her front teeth against the floor. **A,** The girl arrived in the clinic within 1 hour for clinical examination. Both central incisors were mobile but not displaced. Bleeding from the gingival crevice was observed. Because of minor occlusal interference, slight grinding of the opposite teeth was performed. Oral hygiene instructions given to the mother included topical use of chlorhexidine. **B,** Radiograph at the time of injury shows no radiographic changes. **C,** After 1 month, there was no occlusal interference, but gray discoloration is seen in both central incisors. **D,** At 18-month follow-up control, the color of the crowns had returned to normal. **E,** Periapical radiograph shows pulp canal obliteration in both traumatized teeth.

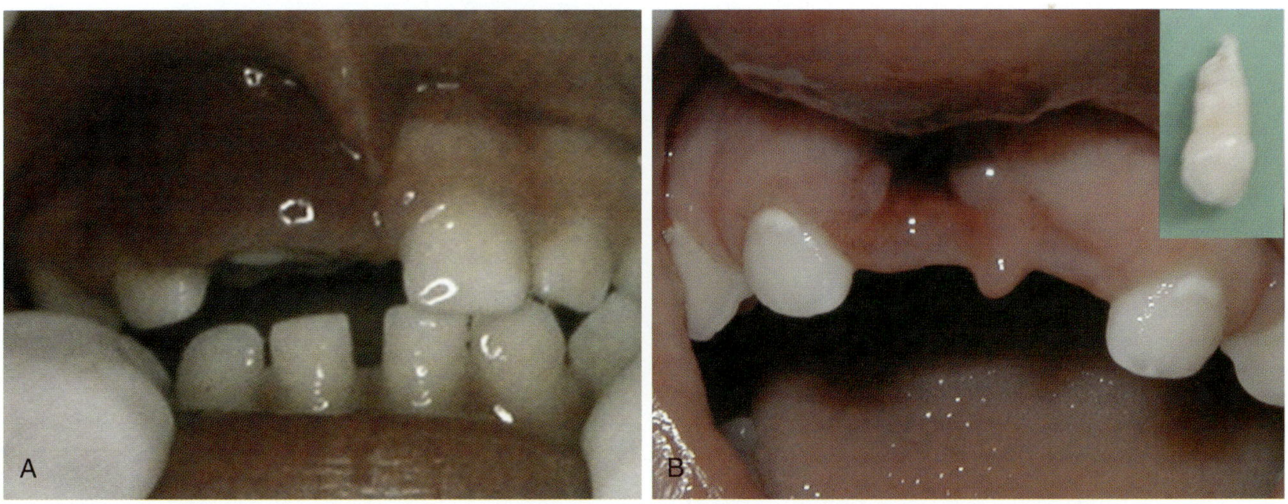

• **Fig. 11.30** Importance of accurate diagnosis after intrusions and avulsions in the primary dentition. **A,** Intrusive luxation. A maxillary right central incisor has been deeply intruded in the alveolar socket, giving the appearance of having been avulsed. **B,** Avulsion. The avulsed tooth was brought into the clinic, confirming that it was not intruded.

Intrusive Luxations

If the apex of the primary tooth is displaced toward or through the buccal bone, the tooth can be left in place for spontaneous repositioning.[126,129] The intruded tooth should be carefully extracted if it impinges on the permanent successor.

Avulsions

Replantation of avulsed primary teeth is not recommended because of the risk of damage to the permanent successor (Fig. 11.30). A radiographic examination helps with confirmation of the avulsed tooth and with the stage of development of the permanent tooth bud.

Patient Instructions

Parents should receive information about how to brush their children's teeth after an injury. Careful oral hygiene after each meal, in addition to topical use of 0.12% chlorhexidine twice per day for 1 week should be recommended. A soft diet for 10 days and restriction of the use of an intraoral pacifier are also recommended. There is no evidence to support the use of systemic antibiotics in the management of luxation injuries of the primary dentition.[127] If the child's medical status warrants antibiotic coverage, the clinician should contact the pediatrician whenever possible because pediatricians may give recommendations for a specific medical condition.

Prevention

Dental and maxillofacial trauma is common and seen in high-risk populations, which include children, athletes, individuals with disabilities, the geriatric population, and military personnel.[135-140] However, most dental traumatic injuries are preventable, and proper management can prevent adverse complications. Management involves primary management, which would involve (1) education, (2) early orthodontic treatment in predisposed children, and (3) protective devices for contact sports. Secondary prevention would entail early diagnosis and treatment of trauma before complications develop.[141]

Primary Management

Education should focus on the prevention of dental trauma, which includes addressing the known risk factors early on. Educating people regarding the implementation of therapeutic guidelines at the site of injury is also necessary. Several studies have reported the need for such an education campaign among school staff, parents, nurses, coaches, physicians, paramedics, and even dentists.[142-148] Early orthodontic treatment is necessary because dental trauma has been found to be more prevalent among children with an incisal overjet of more than 7 mm and/or with incompetent lips.[149,150] In these patients, the maxillary anterior teeth are directly exposed to any impact without interposition of soft tissues. Hence, early orthodontic treatment is also highly recommended to prevent dental trauma.

Contact sports can result in a higher likelihood of traumatic injuries to the teeth.[138,151] Dental professionals should educate patients and the public about mouthguard protection for contact sports. Studies have demonstrated that mouthguards contribute to a lower prevalence of dentoalveolar trauma among athletes who play contact sports.[152-154] Mouthguards usually fall in to one of the three categories: stock mouthguards, mouth-formed mouthguards, or custom-made mouthguards. Comfort, the ability to speak and breathe easily, esthetics, and the athlete's perception of how the mouthguard affects their image all influence which mouthguard will be selected and whether the mouthguard will actually be used.[141] Current research supports the fact that neither the mouth-formed and nor the custom-made mouthguards pose any negative effects on athletic performance and strength; however, the custom-made mouthguards were found to be more comfortable and did not cause any breathing difficulty.[155-157] Other studies have reported that the custom-made mouthguards are superior in their protective function.[141]

Secondary Management

Diagnosis and prompt treatment of trauma are necessary to avoid future complications. This chapter focused on the secondary management of trauma and discussed the diagnosis and treatment of various traumatic injuries.

Study Questions

6. What percentage of intrusive luxated teeth with closed apices undergo pulp necrosis?
   A. 5-20%
   B. 25-40%
   C. 55-70%
   D. 85-100%
7. Which of the following factors can affect the prognosis of avulsed teeth?
   A. The tooth type
   B. Time of injury
   C. Extraoral dry time
   D. Patient's lip closure
8. Which of the following statement does not describe Inflammatory Resorption?
   A. It occurs in response to the presence of infected necrotic pulp tissue.
   B. It is characterized by the loss of tooth structure.
   C. Tooth structure is resorbed and replaced by bone.
   D. It subsides after the removal of the necrotic pulp.
9. Avulsed primary teeth should always be replanted.
   A. True
   B. False
10. Which of the following factors is involved in the primary prevention of trauma?
   A. Education
   B. Early orthodontic treatment in predisposed children
   C. Protective devices for contact sports
   D. All of the above.

ANSWERS

Answer Box 11

1. Correct answer: D. All of the above.
2. Correct answer: B. Late differentiation of the Ad fibers.
3. Correct answer: A. Restoration of the missing tooth structure.
4. Correct answer: A. Removal of minimal amount of the coronal pulp.
5. Correct answer: D. All of the above.
6. Correct answer: D. 85–100%
7. Correct answer: C. Extraoral dry time
8. Correct answer: C. Tooth structure is resorbed and replaced by bone.
9. Correct answer: B. False.
10. Correct answer: D. All of the above.

References

1. Bakland L, Andreasen JO: Examination of the dentally traumatized patient, *J Calif Dent Assoc* 24(35–37):40–44, 1996.
2. Bickley L, Szilagyi PG: *Bates' guide to physical examination and history taking*, ed 12, Philadelphia, 2017, Wolters Kluwer.
3. Arnon Tetanus S: In Behrman R, Kleigman R, Arvin AM, editors: *Nelson's textbook of pediatrics*, ed 15, Philadelphia, 1995, Saunders.
4. Scorza K, Raleigh MF, O'Connor FG: Current concepts in concussion: evaluation and management, *Am Fam Physician* 85:123–132, 2012.

5. Kamboozia A, Poonia-Moorthy A: The fate of teeth in mandibular fracture lines: a clinical and radiographic follow-up study, *Int J Oral Maxillofac Surg* 22:97–101, 1993.
6. Oikarinen K, Lahti J, Raustia AM: Prognosis of permanent teeth in the line of mandibular fractures, *Endod Dent Traumatol* 6:177–182, 1990.
7. Andreasen F, Pedersen BV: Prognosis of luxated permanent teeth: the development of pulp necrosis, *Endod Dent Traumatol* 1:207–220, 1985.
8. Fulling H, Andreasen JO: Influence of maturation status and tooth type of permanent teeth upon electrometric and thermal pulp testing, *Scand J Dent Res* 84:286–290, 1976.
9. Setzer F, Challagulla P, Kataoka SH, et al.: Effect of tooth isolation on laser Doppler readings, *Int Endod J* 46(6):517–522, 2013.
10. Emshoff R, Moschen I, Strobl H: Use of laser Doppler flowmetry to predict vitality of luxated or avulsed permanent teeth, *Oral Surg Oral Med Oral Pathol Oral Radiol Endod* 98:750–755, 2004.
11. Emshoff R, Emshoff I, Moschen I, et al.: Laser Doppler flow measurements of pulpal blood flow and severity of dental injury, *Int Endod J* 37:463–467, 2004.
12. Radhakrishnan S, Munshi AK, Hegde AM: Pulse oximetry: A diagnostic instrument in pulp vitality testing, *J Clin Pediatr Dent* 26:141–145, 2002.
13. Schnettler J, Wallace JA: Pulse oximetry as a diagnostic tool of pulpal vitality, *J Endod* 17(10):488–490, 1991.
14. Noblett W, Wilcox LR, Scamman F, et al.: Detection of pulpal circulation in vitro by pulse oximetry, *J Endod* 22(1):1–5, 1996.
15. Gopikrishna V, Tinagupta K, Kandaswamy D: Evaluation of efficacy of a new custom-made pulse oximeter dental probe in comparison with the electrical and thermal tests for assessing pulp vitality, *J Endod* 33(4):411–414, 2007.
16. Gopikrishna V, Tinagupta K, Kandaswamy D: Comparison of electrical, thermal, and pulse oximetry methods for assessing pulp vitality in recently traumatized teeth, *J Endod* 33(5):531–535, 2007.
17. Pioto NR, Costa B, Gomide MR: Dental development of the permanent lateral incisor in patients with incomplete and complete unilateral cleft lip, *Cleft Palate Craniofac J* 42(5):517–520, 2005.
18. Andreasen F, Andreasen JO: Diagnosis of luxation injuries: the importance of standardized clinical, radiographic, and photographic techniques in clinical investigations, *Endod Dent Traumatol* 1(5):160–169, 1985.
19. Andreasen F, Andreasen JO, Bakland L, et al.: *Traumatic dental injuries*, ed 2, Oxford, UK, 2003, Blackwell Munksgaard.
20. Scarfe W: Imaging of maxillofacial trauma: evolutions and emerging revolutions, *Oral Surg Oral Med Oral Pathol Oral Radiol Endod* 100(2 Suppl):S75–S96, 2005.
21. Andersson L: IADT guidelines for treatment of traumatic dental injuries, *Dent Traumatol* 28(1):1, 2012.
22. Scarfe WC, Levin MD, Gane D, Farman AG: Use of cone beam computed tomography in endodontics, *Int J Dent* 634567, 2009.
23. Cohenca N, Silberman A: Contemporary imaging for the diagnosis and treatment of traumatic dental injuries: a review, *Dent Traumatol* 33(5):321–328, 2017.
24. Ludlow JB, Davies-Ludlow LE, Brooks SL, Howerton WB: Dosimetry of 3 CBCT devices for oral and maxillofacial radiology: CB Mercuray, NewTom 3G and i-CAT, *Dentomaxillofac Radiol* 35(4):219–226, 2006.
25. Ngan DC, Kharbanda OP, Geenty JP, Darendeliler MA: Comparison of radiation levels from computed tomography and conventional dental radiographs, *Aust Orthod J* 19(2):67–75, 2003.
26. Barghan S, Merrill R, Tetradis S: Cone beam computed tomography imaging in the evaluation of the temporomandibular joint, *J Calif Dent Assoc* 38(1):33–39, 2010.
27. Chanani A, Adhikari HD: Reliability of cone beam computed tomography as a biopsy-independent tool in differential diagnosis of periapical cysts and granulomas: an in vivo study, *J Conserv Dent* 20(5):326–331, 2017.
28. Rosenberg PA, Frisbie J, Lee J, et al.: Evaluation of pathologists (histopathology) and radiologists (cone beam computed tomography) differentiating radicular cysts from granulomas, *J Endod* 36(3):423–428, 2010.
29. Simon JH, Enciso R, Malfaz JM, et al.: Differential diagnosis of large periapical lesions using cone-beam computed tomography measurements and biopsy, *J Endod* 32(9):833–837, 2006.
30. Curtis DM, VanderWeele RA, Ray JJ, Wealleans JA: Clinician-centered outcomes assessment of retreatment and endodontic microsurgery using cone-beam computed tomographic volumetric analysis, *J Endod* 44(8):1251–1256, 2018.
31. Schloss T, Sonntag D, Kohli MR, Setzer FC: A Comparison of 2- and 3-dimensional healing assessment after endodontic surgery using cone-beam computed tomographic volumes or periapical radiographs, *J Endod* 43(7):1072–1079, 2017.
32. Cotti E, Vargiu P, Dettori C, Mallarini G: Computerized tomography in the management and follow-up of extensive periapical lesion, *Endod Dent Traumatol* 15(4):186–189, 1999.
33. Jacobs R, Salmon B, Codari M, et al.: Cone beam computed tomography in implant dentistry: recommendations for clinical use, *BMC Oral Health* 18(1):88, 2018.
34. Baumrind S, Carlson S, Beers A, et al.: Using three-dimensional imaging to assess treatment outcomes in orthodontics: a progress report from the University of the Pacific, *Orthod Craniofac Res* 6(Suppl 1):132–142, 2003.
35. Samandara A, Papageorgiou SN, Ioannidou-Marathiotou I, et al.: Evaluation of orthodontically induced external root resorption following orthodontic treatment using cone beam computed tomography (CBCT): a systematic review and meta-analysis, *Eur J Orthod* 41(1):67–79, 2018.
36. Cavalcanti MG: Cone beam computed tomographic imaging: perspective, challenges, and the impact of near-trend future applications, *J Craniofac Surg* 23(1):279–282, 2012.
37. Patel S, Durack C, Abella F, et al.: Cone beam computed tomography in endodontics - a review, *Int Endod J* 48(1):3–15, 2015.
38. Farik B, Munksgaard EC, Kreiborg S, et al.: Adhesive bonding of fragmented anterior teeth, *Endod Dent Traumatol* 14:119–123, 1998.
39. Diangelis A, Andreasen JO, Ebeleseder KA, et al.: International association of dental traumatology guidelines for the management of traumatic dental injuries, *Dent Traumatol* 28:2–12, 2012.
40. Cvek M: A clinical report on partial pulpotomy and capping with calcium hydroxide in permanent incisors with complicated crown fractures, *J Endod* 4:232–237, 1978.
41. Fuks A, Cosack A, Klein H, et al.: Partial pulpotomy as a treatment alternative for exposed pulps in crown-fractured permanent incisors, *Endod Dent Traumatol* 3(3):100–102, 1987.
42. Mejàre I, Cvek M: Partial pulpotomy in young permanent teeth with deep carious lesions, *Endod Dent Traumatol* 9(6):238–242, 1993.
43. Bakland L: Management of traumatically injured pulps in immature teeth using MTA, *J Calif Dent Assoc* 28:855–858, 2000.
44. Fuks A, Gavra S, Chosack A: A long-term follow-up of traumatized incisors treated by partial pulpotomy, *Pediatr Dent* 15:334–336, 1993.
45. Cohenca N, Simon JH, Roges R, et al.: Clinical Indications for digital imaging in dento-alveolar trauma, part 1: traumatic injuries, *Dent Traumatol* 23:95–104, 2007.
46. Andreasen J, Andreasen FM: Root fractures. In Andreasen J, Andreasen FM, editors: *Textbook and color atlas of traumatic injuries to the teeth*, ed 3, Copenhagen, 1994, Munksgaard.
47. Andreasen J, Andreasen FM: Classification, etiology, and epidemiology of traumatic dental injuries. In Andreasen J, Andreasen FM, editors: *Textbook and color atlas of traumatic injuries to the teeth*, ed 3, Copenhagen, 1994, Munksgaard.
48. Bender I, Freedland JB: Clinical considerations in the diagnosis and treatment of intra-alveolar root fractures, *JADA* 107:595–600, 1983.

49. May J, Cohenca N, Peters OA: Contemporary management of horizontal root fractures to the permanent dentition; diagnosis - radiologic assessment to include cone beam computed tomography, *J Endod* 39, 2013. S20–S5.
50. Andreasen F, Andreasen JO, Bayer T: Prognosis of root-fractured permanent incisors: prediction of healing modalities, *Endod Dent Traumatol* 5:11–22, 1989.
51. Andreasen J, Andreasen FM, Mejàre I, et al.: Healing of 400 intra-alveolar root fractures. Part 2: effect of treatment factors such as treatment delay, repositioning, splinting type and period and antibiotics, *Dent Traumatol* 20:203–211, 2004.
52. Andreasen J, Andreasen FM, Mejàre I, et al.: Healing of 400 intra-alveolar root fractures. Part 1: effect of pre-injury and injury factors such as sex, age, stage of root development, fracture type, location of fracture, and severity of dislocation, *Dent Traumatol* 20:192–202, 2004.
53. Welbury R, Kinirons MJ, Day P, et al.: Outcomes for root-fractured permanent incisors: a retrospective study, *Pediatr Dent* 24:98–102, 2002.
54. Andreasen J, Hjorting-Hansen E: Intra-alveolar root fractures: radiographic and histologic study of 50 cases, *J Oral Surg* 25(5):414–426, 1967.
55. Cvek M, Andreasen JO, Borum MK: Healing of 208 intra-alveolar root fractures in patients aged 7-17 years, *Dent Traumatol* 17:53–62, 2001.
56. Cvek M, Mejàre I, Andreasen JO: Conservative endodontic treatment of teeth fractured in the middle or apical part of the root, *Dent Traumatol* 20:261–269, 2004.
57. Herweijer J, Torabinejad M, Bakland LK: Healing of horizontal root fractures, *J Endod* 18:118–122, 1992.
58. Zachrisson B, Jacobsen I: Long-term prognosis of 66 permanent anterior teeth with root fracture, *Scand J Dent Res* 83:345–354, 1975.
59. Fulling HJ, Andreasen JO: Influence of maturation status and tooth type of permanent teeth upon electrometric and thermal pulp testing, *Scand J Dent Res* 84(5):286–290, 1976.
60. Bastos JV, Goulart EM, de Souza Cortes MI: Pulpal response to sensibility tests after traumatic dental injuries in permanent teeth, *Dent Traumatol* 30(3):188–192, 2014.
61. Andreasen FM: Transient apical breakdown and its relation to color and sensibility changes after luxation injuries to teeth, *Endod Dent Traumatol* 2(1):9–19, 1986.
62. Andreasen FM: Pulpal healing after luxation injuries and root fracture in the permanent dentition, *Endod Dent Traumatol* 5(3):111–131, 1989.
63. Andreasen FM, Pedersen BV: Prognosis of luxated permanent teeth—the development of pulp necrosis, *Endod Dent Traumatol* 1(6):207–220, 1985.
64. Andreasen FM, Andreasen JO: Diagnosis of luxation injuries: the importance of standardized clinical, radiographic and photographic techniques in clinical investigations, *Endod Dent Traumatol* 1(5):160–169, 1985.
65. Andreasen FM, Zhijie Y, Thomsen BL, Andersen PK: Occurrence of pulp canal obliteration after luxation injuries in the permanent dentition, *Endod Dent Traumatol* 3(3):103–115, 1987.
66. Diangelis AJ, Andreasen JO, Ebeleseder KA, et al.: Guidelines for the management of traumatic dental injuries: 1. fractures and luxations of permanent teeth, *Pediatr Dent* 39(6):401–411, 2017.
67. Nasjleti CE, Castelli WA, Caffesse RG: The effects of different splinting times on replantation of teeth in monkeys, *Oral Surg Oral Med Oral Pathol* 53(6):557–566, 1982.
68. Andreasen JO, Bakland LK, Andreasen FM: Traumatic intrusion of permanent teeth. Part 2. A clinical study of the effect of preinjury and injury factors, such as sex, age, stage of root development, tooth location, and extent of injury including number of intruded teeth on 140 intruded permanent teeth, *Dent Traumatol* 22(2):90–98, 2006.
69. Andreasen JO, Bakland LK, Matras RC, Andreasen FM: Traumatic intrusion of permanent teeth. Part 1. An epidemiological study of 216 intruded permanent teeth, *Dent Traumatol* 22(2):83–89, 2006.
70. DiAngelis AJ, Andreasen JO, Ebeleseder KA, et al.: Guidelines for the management of traumatic dental injuries: 1. fractures and luxations of permanent teeth, *Pediatr Dent* 38(6):358–368, 2016.
71. Andreasen JO, Bakland LK, Andreasen FM: Traumatic intrusion of permanent teeth. Part 3. A clinical study of the effect of treatment variables such as treatment delay, method of repositioning, type of splint, length of splinting and antibiotics on 140 teeth, *Dent Traumatol* 22(2):99–111, 2006.
72. Dumsha TC: Luxation injuries, *Dent Clin North Am* 39(1):79–91, 1995.
73. Andreasen JO, Borum MK, Jacobsen HL, Andreasen FM: Replantation of 400 avulsed permanent incisors. 4. Factors related to periodontal ligament healing, *Endod Dent Traumatol* 11(2):76–89, 1995.
74. Andreasen JO, Borum MK, Andreasen FM: Replantation of 400 avulsed permanent incisors. 3. Factors related to root growth, *Endod Dent Traumatol* 11(2):69–75, 1995.
75. Andreasen JO, Borum MK, Jacobsen HL, Andreasen FM: Replantation of 400 avulsed permanent incisors. 2. Factors related to pulpal healing, *Endod Dent Traumatol* 11(2):59–68, 1995.
76. Andreasen JO, Borum MK, Jacobsen HL, Andreasen FM: Replantation of 400 avulsed permanent incisors. 1. Diagnosis of healing complications, *Endod Dent Traumatol* 11(2):51–58, 1995.
77. Trope M: Avulsion and replantation, *Refuat Hapeh Vehashinayim* 19(2):6–15, 1993. 76, 2002.
78. Trope M: Clinical management of the avulsed tooth: present strategies and future directions, *Dent Traumatol* 18(1):1–11, 2002.
79. Is Khinda V, Kaur G, S Brar G, et al.: Clinical and practical implications of storage media used for tooth avulsion, *Int J Clin Pediatr Dent* 10(2):158–165, 2017.
80. Blomlöf L: Milk and saliva as possible storage media for traumatically exarticulated teeth prior to replantation, *Swed Dent J Suppl* 8:1–26, 1981.
81. Blomlöf L: Storage of human periodontal ligament cells in a combination of different media, *J Dent Res* 60(11):1904–1906, 1981.
82. Lindskog S, Blomlöf L: Influence of osmolality and composition of some storage media on human periodontal ligament cells, *Acta Odontol Scand* 40(6):435–441, 1982.
83. Poi WR, Sonoda CK, Martins CM, et al.: Storage media for avulsed teeth: a literature review, *Braz Dent J* 24(5):437–445, 2013.
84. Adnan S, Lone MM, Khan FR, et al.: Which is the most recommended medium for the storage and transport of avulsed teeth? A systematic review, *Dent Traumatol* 34(2):59–70, 2018.
85. Kwan SC, Johnson JD, Cohenca N: The effect of splint material and thickness on tooth mobility after extraction and replantation using a human cadaveric model, *Dent Traumatol* 28(4):277–281, 2012.
86. Cvek M, Cleaton-Jones P, Austin J, et al.: Effect of topical application of doxycycline on pulp revascularization and periodontal healing in reimplanted monkey incisors, *Endod Dent Traumatol* 6(4):170–176, 1990.
87. Cvek M, Cleaton-Jones P, Austin J, et al.: Pulp revascularization in reimplanted immature monkey incisors—predictability and the effect of antibiotic systemic prophylaxis, *Endod Dent Traumatol* 6(4):157–169, 1990.
88. Ritter AL, Ritter AV, Murrah V, et al.: Pulp revascularization of replanted immature dog teeth after treatment with minocycline and doxycycline assessed by laser Doppler flowmetry, radiography, and histology, *Dent Traumatol* 20(2):75–84, 2004.
89. Kling M, Cvek M, Mejare I: Rate and predictability of pulp revascularization in therapeutically reimplanted permanent incisors, *Endod Dent Traumatol* 2(3):83–89, 1986.
90. Shulman LB, Gedalia I, Feingold RM: Fluoride concentration in root surfaces and alveolar bone of fluoride-immersed monkey incisors three weeks after replantation, *J Dent Res* 52(6):1314–1316, 1973.

91. Hammarström L, Pierce A, Blomlöf L, et al.: Tooth avulsion and replantation—a review, *Endod Dent Traumatol* 2(1):1–8, 1986.
92. Trope M: Clinical management of the avulsed tooth, *Dent Clin North Am* 39(1):93–112, 1995.
93. National Center for Immunization and Respiratory Diseases: General recommendations on immunization—Recommendations of the Advisory Committee on Immunization Practices (ACIP), *MMWR Recomm Rep* 60(2):1–64, 2011.
94. Frank AL: Therapy for the divergent pulpless tooth by continued apical formation, *J Am Dent Assoc* 72(1):87–93, 1966.
95. Rafter M: Apexification: a review, *Dent Traumatol* 21(1):1–8, 2005.
96. Stewart GG: Calcium hydroxide-induced root healing, *Oral Health* 65(12):10–15, 1975.
97. West NM, Lieb RJ: Biologic root-end closure on a traumatized and surgically resected maxillary central incisor: an alternative method of treatment, *Endod Dent Traumatol* 1(4):146–149, 1985.
98. Valera MC, Albuquerque MT, Yamasaki MC, et al.: Fracture resistance of weakened bovine teeth after long-term use of calcium hydroxide, *Dent Traumatol* 31(5):385–389, 2015.
99. Andreasen JO, Farik B, Munksgaard EC: Long-term calcium hydroxide as a root canal dressing may increase risk of root fracture, *Dent Traumatol* 18(3):134–137, 2002.
100. Andreasen JO, Munksgaard EC, Bakland LK: Comparison of fracture resistance in root canals of immature sheep teeth after filling with calcium hydroxide or MTA, *Dent Traumatol* 22(3):154–156, 2006.
101. Witherspoon DE, Ham K: One-visit apexification: technique for inducing root-end barrier formation in apical closures, *Pract Proced Aesthet Dent* 13(6):455–460, 2001. quiz 62.
102. Bonte E, Beslot A, Boukpessi T, Lasfargues JJ: MTA versus Ca(OH)2 in apexification of non-vital immature permanent teeth: a randomized clinical trial comparison, *Clin Oral Investig* 19(6):1381–1388, 2015.
103. Cicek E, Yilmaz N, Kocak MM, et al.: Effect of mineral trioxide aggregate apical plug thickness on fracture resistance of immature teeth, *J Endod* 43(10):1697–1700, 2017.
104. Miller EK, Lee JY, Tawil PZ, et al.: Emerging therapies for the management of traumatized immature permanent incisors, *Pediatr Dent* 34(1):66–69, 2012.
105. Wigler R, Kaufman AY, Lin S, et al.: Revascularization: a treatment for permanent teeth with necrotic pulp and incomplete root development, *J Endod* 39(3):319–326, 2013.
106. Thomson A, Kahler B: Regenerative endodontics—biologically-based treatment for immature permanent teeth: a case report and review of the literature, *Aust Dent J* 55(4):446–452, 2010.
107. Cotti E, Mereu M, Lusso D: Regenerative treatment of an immature, traumatized tooth with apical periodontitis: report of a case, *J Endod* 34(5):611–616, 2008.
108. Martin MP, Pileggi R: A quantitative analysis of Propolis: a promising new storage media following avulsion, *Dent Traumatol* 20(2):85–89, 2004.
109. Trope M, Moshonov J, Nissan R, et al.: Short- vs. long-term calcium hydroxide treatment of established inflammatory root resorption in replanted dog teeth, *Endod Dent Traumatol* 11(3):124–128, 1995.
110. Rotstein I, Salehrabi R, Forrest JL: Endodontic treatment outcome: survey of oral health care professionals, *J Endod* 32(5):399–403, 2006.
111. Salehrabi R, Rotstein I: Endodontic treatment outcomes in a large patient population in the USA: an epidemiological study, *J Endod* 30(12):846–850, 2004.
112. Abd-Elmeguid A, ElSalhy M, Yu DC: Pulp canal obliteration after replantation of avulsed immature teeth: a systematic review, *Dent Traumatol* 31(6):437–441, 2015.
113. Souza BDM, Dutra KL, Kuntze MM, et al.: Incidence of root resorption after the replantation of avulsed teeth: a meta-analysis, *J Endod* 44(8):1216–1227, 2018.
114. Andreasen JO, Andreasen FM: Root resorption following traumatic dental injuries, *Proc Finn Dent Soc* 88(Suppl 1):95–114, 1992.
115. Yamashita FC, Previdelli ITS, Pavan NNO, Endo MS: Retrospective study on sequelae in traumatized permanent teeth, *Eur J Dent* 11(3):275–280, 2017.
116. Lin S, Ashkenazi M, Karawan M, et al.: Management of ankylotic root resorption following dental trauma: a short review and proposal of a treatment protocol, *Oral Health Prev Dent* 15(5):467–474, 2017.
117. Panzarini SR, Gulinelli JL, Poi WR, et al.: Treatment of root surface in delayed tooth replantation: a review of literature, *Dent Traumatol* 24(3):277–282, 2008.
118. Mahajan SK, Sidhu SS: Effect of fluoride on root resorption of autogenous dental replants. Clinical study, *Aust Dent J* 26(1):42–45, 1981.
119. Selvig KA, Bjorvatn K, Claffey N: Effect of stannous fluoride and tetracycline on repair after delayed replantation of root-planed teeth in dogs, *Acta Odontol Scand* 48(2):107–112, 1990.
120. Oikarinen K, Lahti J, Raustia AM: Prognosis of permanent teeth in the line of mandibular fractures, *Endod Dent Traumatol* 6(4):177–182, 1990.
121. Lauridsen E, Gerds T, Andreasen JO: Alveolar process fractures in the permanent dentition. Part 2. The risk of healing complications in teeth involved in an alveolar process fracture, *Dent Traumatol* 32(2):128–139, 2016.
122. Altun C, Cehreli ZC, Guven G, Acikel C: Traumatic intrusion of primary teeth and its effects on the permanent successors: a clinical follow-up study, *Oral Surg Oral Med Oral Pathol Oral Radiol Endod* 107(4):493–498, 2009.
123. Da Silva Assuncao LR, Ferelle A, Iwakura ML, Cunha RF: Effects on permanent teeth after luxation injuries to the primary predecessors: a study in children assisted at an emergency service, *Dent Traumatol* 25(2):165–170, 2009.
124. do Espirito Santo Jacomo DR, Campos V: Prevalence of sequelae in the permanent anterior teeth after trauma in their predecessors: a longitudinal study of 8 years, *Dent Traumatol* 25(3):300–304, 2009.
125. de Amorim Lde F, Estrela C, da Costa LR: Effects of traumatic dental injuries to primary teeth on permanent teeth—a clinical follow-up study, *Dent Traumatol* 27(2):117–121, 2011.
126. Colak I, Markovic D, Petrovic B, et al.: A retrospective study of intrusive injuries in primary dentition, *Dent Traumatol* 25(6):605–610, 2009.
127. Malmgren B, Andreasen JO, Flores MT, et al.: Guidelines for the management of traumatic dental injuries: 3. injuries in the primary dentition, *Pediatr Dent* 38(6):377–385, 2016.
128. Malmgren B, Andreasen JO, Flores MT, et al.: Guidelines for the management of traumatic dental injuries: 3. Injuries in the primary dentition, *Pediatr Dent* 39(6):420–428, 2017.
129. Spinas E, Melis A, Savasta A: Therapeutic approach to intrusive luxation injuries in primary dentition. A clinical follow-up study, *Eur J Paediatr Dent* 7(4):179–186, 2006.
130. Holan G, Fuks AB: The diagnostic value of coronal dark-gray discoloration in primary teeth following traumatic injuries, *Pediatr Dent* 18(3):224–227, 1996.
131. Moccelini BS, de Alencar NA, Bolan M, et al.: Pulp necrosis and crown discoloration: a systematic review and meta-analysis, *Int J Paediatr Dent*, 2018.
132. Soxman JA, Nazif MM, Bouquot J: Pulpal pathology in relation to discoloration of primary anterior teeth, *ASDC J Dent Child* 51(4):282–284, 1984.
133. Holan G: Long-term effect of different treatment modalities for traumatized primary incisors presenting dark coronal discoloration with no other signs of injury, *Dent Traumatol* 22(1):14–17, 2006.
134. Borum MK, Andreasen JO: Sequelae of trauma to primary maxillary incisors. I. Complications in the primary dentition, *Endod Dent Traumatol* 14(1):31–44, 1998.
135. Odersjo ML, Robertson A, Koch G: Incidence of dental traumatic injuries in children 0–4 years of age: a prospective study based on parental reporting, *Eur Arch Paediatr Dent* 19(2):107–111, 2018.

136. Richards D: One billion people have experienced a traumatic dental injury, *Evid Based Dent* 19(2):34–35, 2018.
137. Bagattoni S, Sadotti A, D'Alessandro G, Piana G: Dental trauma in Italian children and adolescents with special health care needs. A cross-sectional retrospective study, *Eur J Paediatr Dent* 18(1):23–26, 2017.
138. Galic T, Kuncic D, Poklepovic Pericic T, et al.: Knowledge and attitudes about sports-related dental injuries and mouthguard use in young athletes in four different contact sports–water polo, karate, taekwondo and handball, *Dent Traumatol* 34(3):175–181, 2018.
139. Shumate R, Portnof J, Amundson M, et al.: Recommendations for care of geriatric maxillofacial trauma patients following a retrospective 10-year multicenter review, *J Oral Maxillofac Surg* 76(9):1931–1936, 2018.
140. Antikainen A, Patinen P, Pakkila J, et al.: The types and management of dental trauma during military service in Finland, *Dent Traumatol* 34(2):87–92, 2018.
141. Levin L, Zadik Y: Education on and prevention of dental trauma: it's time to act!, *Dent Traumatol* 28(1):49–54, 2012.
142. Al-Sehaibany FS, Alajlan R, Almubarak D, et al.: Knowledge on management of traumatic dental injuries among Saudi mothers, *Clin Cosmet Investig Dent* 10:123–128, 2018.
143. Al-Sehaibany FS, Almubarak DZ, Alajlan RA, et al.: Elementary school staff knowledge about management of traumatic dental injuries, *Clin Cosmet Investig Dent* 10:189–194, 2018.
144. Zafar A, Aslam N, Nasir N, et al.: Knowledge, attitudes and practices of health care workers regarding needle stick injuries at a tertiary care hospital in Pakistan, *J Pak Med Assoc* 58(2):57–60, 2008.
145. Zafar K, Ghafoor R, Khan FR, Hameed MH: Awareness of dentists regarding immediate management of dental avulsion: knowledge, attitude, and practice study, *J Pak Med Assoc* 68(4):595–599, 2018.
146. Holan G, Shmueli Y: Knowledge of physicians in hospital emergency rooms in Israel on their role in cases of avulsion of permanent incisors, *Int J Paediatr Dent* 13(1):13–19, 2003.
147. Perunski S, Lang B, Pohl Y, Filippi A: Level of information concerning dental injuries and their prevention in Swiss basketball—a survey among players and coaches, *Dent Traumatol* 21(4):195–200, 2005.
148. Lin S, Levin L, Emodi O, et al.: Physician and emergency medical technicians' knowledge and experience regarding dental trauma, *Dent Traumatol* 22(3):124–126, 2006.
149. Batista KB, Thiruvenkatachari B, Harrison JE, O'Brien KD: Orthodontic treatment for prominent upper front teeth (Class II malocclusion) in children and adolescents, *Cochrane Database Syst Rev* 3:CD003452, 2018.
150. Brin I, Ben-Bassat Y, Heling I, Brezniak N: Profile of an orthodontic patient at risk of dental trauma, *Endod Dent Traumatol* 16(3):111–115, 2000.
151. Hersberger S, Krastl G, Kuhl S, Filippi A: Dental injuries in water polo, a survey of players in Switzerland, *Dent Traumatol* 28(4):287–290, 2012.
152. Fernandes LM, Neto JCL, Lima TFR, et al.: The use of mouthguards and prevalence of dento-alveolar trauma among athletes. A systematic review and meta-analysis, *Dent Traumatol* 35(1):54–72, 2019.
153. Green JI: The role of mouthguards in preventing and reducing sports-related trauma, *Prim Dent J* 6(2):27–34, 2017.
154. Knapik JJ, Marshall SW, Lee RB, et al.: Mouthguards in sport activities: history, physical properties and injury prevention effectiveness, *Sports Med* 37(2):117–144, 2007.
155. Duddy FA, Weissman J, Lee Sr RA, et al.: Influence of different types of mouthguards on strength and performance of collegiate athletes: a controlled-randomized trial, *Dent Traumatol* 28(4):263–267, 2012.
156. Gawlak D, Mierzwińska-Nastalska E, Mańka-Malara K, Kamiński T: Comparison of usability properties of custom-made and standard self-adapted mouthguards, *Dent Traumatol* 30(4):306–311, 2014.
157. Gawlak D, Mierzwińska-Nastalska E, Mańka-Malara K, Kamiński T: Assessment of custom and standard, self-adapted mouthguards in terms of comfort and users subjective impressions of their protective function, *Dent Traumatol* 31(2):113–117, 2015.

12 Root Canal Anatomy

MARCO VERSIANI, BLAINE CLEGHORN, AND WILLIAM CHRISTIE

CHAPTER OUTLINE

LEARNING OBJECTIVES

After reading this chapter, the student should be able to:

1. Recognize errors that may cause difficulties or failures in root canal treatment owing to lack of knowledge of pulp anatomy.
2. List techniques that help determine the type of root canal system.
3. Draw the eight most common canal types (Vertucci's I to VIII), the shapes of roots in cross-section, and common canal configurations in these roots.
4. Understand the two most commonly used classification systems (Vertucci and Weine) for root canal system and their limitations.
5. Describe a new classification system of root canal system morphology that uses universal tooth number along with canal number and morphology of individual roots as depicted in cleared bench specimens or clinical tomography images.
6. Know about root canal research in the past and understand how present research is helping identify the complexity and variations in ethnicity of the human root canal system.
7. Describe the most common root and root canal anatomy of each tooth.
8. For each tooth type, list the average length, number of roots, and most common root curvature directions.
9. Characterize the most frequent variations in root and root canal anatomy of each tooth group.
10. Explain why standard periapical radiographs do not present the complete picture of root and root canal anatomy.
11. Draw a representative example of the most common internal and external anatomy of each tooth in the following planes: (1) sagittal section of mesiodistal and faciolingual planes and (2) cross-section through the cervical, middle, and apical thirds.
12. Suggest methods for determining whether roots and canals are curved and the severity of the curvature.
13. Explain why many root curvatures are not apparent on standard radiographs.
14. State the tenet of the relationship of pulp-root anatomy.
15. List each tooth and the root or roots that require a search for more than one canal.
16. List and recognize the significance of iatrogenic or pathologic factors that may cause alterations in root canal anatomy.
17. Define the root canal space and list and describe its major components.
18. Describe variations in the root canal system in the apical third.
19. Describe how to determine clinically the distance from the occlusal-incisal surface to the roof of the chamber.
20. Discuss the location, morphology, frequency, and importance of accessory (lateral) canals.
21. Describe relationships between the anatomic apex, radiographic apex, and actual location of the apical foramen.
22. Describe common variations in root canal anatomy resulting from developmental abnormalities and state their significance.
23. Identify the most common root and root canal morphologic variations as they relate to ethnicity.

Introduction

The ultimate goal of endodontic therapy is to seal the root canal system after all vital or necrotic tissue, microorganisms, and their byproducts are removed from the canal space. However, this objective may be difficult to attain in reality because of the complexity of the internal anatomy of teeth. Residual bacteria and debris may remain relatively unaffected in the missed canal system or even in the unprepared canal walls, isthmuses, lateral canals, apical ramifications, and recesses from oval/flattened canals which may compromise the successful treatment outcome. Thus, a thorough understanding of the number of canals, of the inner-canal morphology, and the variations in all groups of teeth is a basic requirement for successful endodontic therapy.

In the past, several studies were performed on the range of variations in human root canal anatomy, and the findings have had a noteworthy influence on clinical practice. In recent years, significant noninvasive technological advances for imaging teeth have been introduced that allow anatomic studies to be done using large populations and evaluate specific and fine anatomic features of a tooth group. The latest morphological studies on root and root canal anatomy use high-resolution three-dimensional (3D) tomographic images to illustrate and define terminologies associated with this topic.

Gaining Knowledge and Comprehension of Root and Canal Anatomy

Textbooks and courses in dental anatomy are ideal sources for teaching a dental student about normal human tooth anatomy. These study aids can present the dental student or dental practitioner with knowledge of the ideal coronal anatomy and its relation to occlusion, the anatomy of the human tooth root, and occasionally the morphology of the pulp and root canals. But the usual dental anatomy that is shown assumes the ideal (or most frequently encountered) tooth shape. Is this enough to perform endodontic treatment for our patients, when genetic variations may have produced roots and root canal systems that vary from the normal? For example, why is the maxillary first premolar inevitably depicted as having two roots (and two canals) whereas the second premolar is illustrated as a single but oval rooted tooth with one, or maybe two canals? Studies that compare the incidence of variation in root number in different populations have shown a significant variation in morphology of the human maxillary and mandibular premolars, based on ethnicity.[1] Therefore, when it comes to performing the complex operation of root canal therapy, more detailed knowledge of root number and root canal system anatomy is required. The purpose of this chapter is to acquire that knowledge at a higher level.

The first task for a dental student, as stated, is to learn the normal anatomy of each tooth in the arch with respect to its complex root canal system. In principle, the shape of the external root will be reflected in the internal morphology of a root canal system. This is considered a tenet of the relationship of pulp-root anatomy. Each of the individual 16 types of teeth in the permanent dentition has its own individual root canal system morphology or shape. This is considered basic dental anatomy, which must then be matched clinically to what is interpreted from the two-dimensional (2D) shadow of the radiographic image.

The second task is to acquire detailed dental anatomy knowledge of possible variations from the norm. Thus one should realize that each human tooth type has a range of variation in its morphology. The shape of the root canal system is influenced by embryonic development and is controlled by each patient's genetic background. To perform successful endodontic treatment, one must anticipate variation in chamber size and depth from the occlusal surface, the canal size, shape, length, curvature, branches, lateral canals, and apical accessory canals, to mention just a few variables. These variations may or may not be clearly seen in a standard periapical radiographic image.

Methods of Study to Learn Normal and Variations in Tooth Anatomy

In the first half of the 16th century, a set of seven books written by Andreas Vesalius (1514-1564) entitled *De Humani Corporis Fabrica* was published. This was a major advance in the history of anatomy over the long-dominant works of ancient Middle Ages writers. It is noteworthy that an important anatomic aspect of teeth that had been ignored by previous authors on which, centuries later, the endodontic specialty would be born, was highlighted for the first time in the literature. In Chapter XI, there is a drawing of a sectioned two-rooted mandibular molar showing its internal anatomy (Fig. 12.1, *A*). In 1563, Bartolomeo Eustachi (c. 1520-1574), in his treatise *il Libellus de Dentibus,* made very significant contributions toward the anatomy and physiology of the dentition, including the first descriptions of the dental pulp, the periodontal ligament, the dental follicles, the trigeminal nerve, and other oral structures, based upon extensive dissections of both human and animal specimens. In Chapter XVIII, Eustachi describes the pulp cavity and its contents, and shows accurate tables in which he specified the number of roots and the external morphologic variations of all groups of human teeth (Fig. 12.1, *B*). Eustachi's book brought the macroscopic anatomy of teeth to a high degree of perfection that remained unsurpassed until the 19th century with the posthumous work of Georg Carabelli (1787-1842), who provided the most detailed description of the number and direction of the root canals at that time (Fig. 12.1, *C*). Nevertheless, it was only at the end of 19th century that some researchers finally realized the need for in-depth research on root canal morphology. In 1903, Gustav Preiswerk (1866-1908) performed a profound and comprehensive study on this subject. In his pioneering study, Wood's metal, an alloy that melts at a low temperature, was molten and injected into the canal space. After complete decalcification of the teeth, 3D metal models of the internal anatomy were obtained for the first time (Fig. 12.1, *D*). Some years later, Guido Fischer (1877-1959) presented the challenging nature of the apical root anatomy. He obtained better results than Preiswerk by filling approximately 700 teeth with a collodion solution. This solution penetrated all the branches of the root canal system and hardened in 2 or 3 weeks, providing a full 3D replica of the root canal system (Fig. 12.1, *E*). The complexity and unpredictability of the root canal morphology led Fischer to coin the term *Kanalsystem,* which has been widely used nowadays as "root canal system." It may be said that the innovative 3D anatomic studies of Preiswerk and Fischer resulted in huge advancements, adding new and significant knowledge to the dental literature and stimulating other researchers to undertake further investigations on this topic. In those later studies, large numbers of extracted teeth were collected, placed in a category and analyzed, or counted to compare their shape and size. Root numbers for the multirooted posterior teeth could even be tabulated. Data from these in vitro studies were then printed in the tables found in the earliest textbooks in dentistry. This was the first phase of research in human root anatomy.[2]

Hess wrote a landmark publication on the morphology of root canals using some 3000 permanent teeth. Canal shapes were made visible by injecting vulcanite into canal systems and dissolving the surrounding roots. This process showed graphically how complex the canal system was for each tooth (Fig. 12.1, *F*). A similar method was used for primary teeth by Zürcher, and the results were combined and reprinted in the English literature in 1925. Many variable shapes and extra canals in single rooted

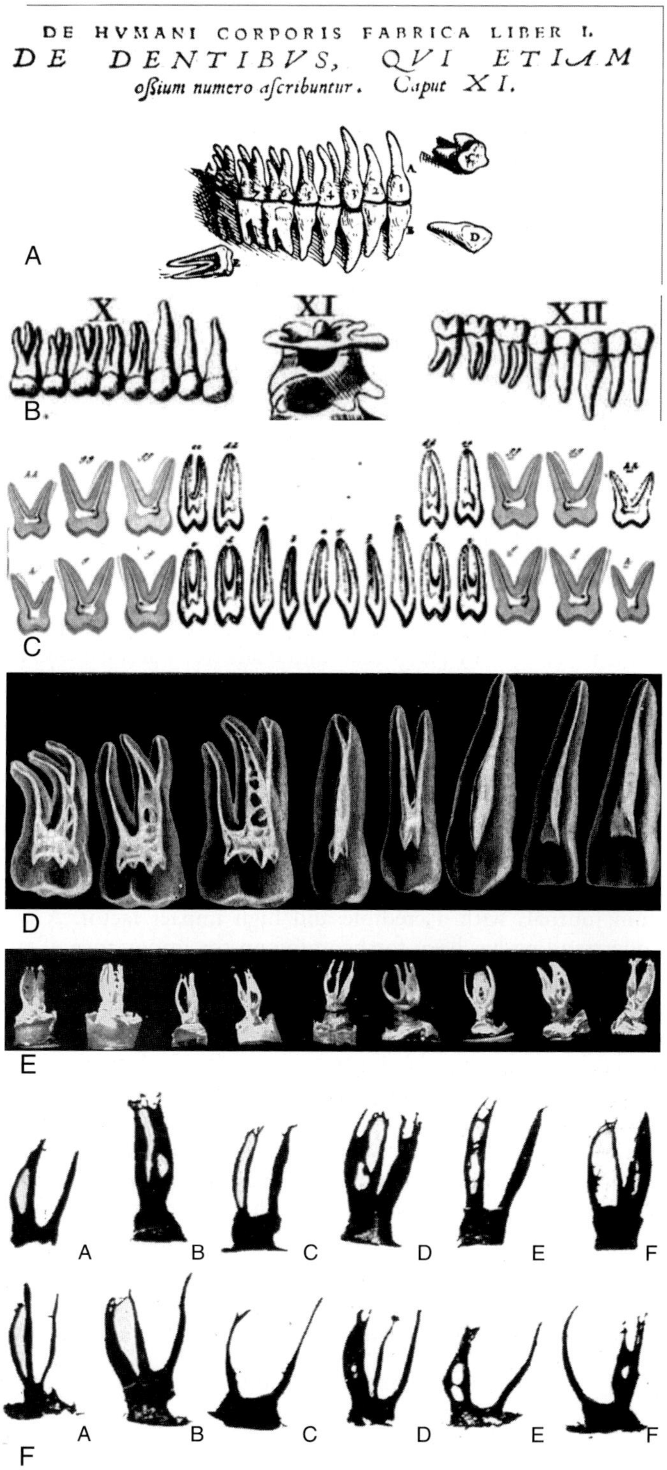

• **Fig. 12.1 Historical images of classical studies on root canal anatomy. A,** First drawing of a sectioned two-rooted mandibular molar showing its internal anatomy by Andreas Vesalius (1543); **B,** illustration depicting the number of roots and the external morphologic variations of all groups of human teeth by Eustachi (1563); **C,** illustration of the number and direction of the root canal in different groups of teeth by Carabelli (1842); **D,** 3D metal models of the internal anatomy of different teeth obtained by Preiswerk (1903); **E,** 3D models of the internal anatomy of teeth obtained by Fischer using collodion solution (1907); **F,** Canal shapes of mandibular molars obtained by injecting vulcanite into the canal systems by Hess (1925). (Courtesy Dr. Perrini.[241] Published with permission.)

teeth were shown to exist. For example, in the casts of mandibular incisor, mandibular premolar, and mandibular canine, the canals were complex and sometimes multiple in number. Illustrations in his publication are remarkable for their accuracy but were either overlooked or ignored as being abnormal variants at the time. Subsequent anatomic studies and an earlier published study have confirmed their observations.[2] More recent studies on canal numbers, both ex vivo and in vivo, have shown that former endodontic techniques in root canal therapy using less flexible instruments only available at the time had inadvertently missed many of these extra and complex canal systems.[3]

Clinical competence relies on the development of the widely recognized psychomotor aspect. Inextricably coupled with these psychomotor skills is the ability to self-evaluate the process of correction and the product itself compared with the desired outcome. Visual perception has been suggested as a prerequisite skill for determining the appropriate goals and strategy for a correction. Visual skill is required to observe normal 3D tooth morphology in detail, to differentiate normal tooth morphology from its variations. Further, motor skills are also required to execute clinically relevant dental procedures. In the development of psychomotor skills, the student must teach his or her hands to do that which his or her mind dictates as correct. Models that simulate teeth in which root canals can be visualized would serve as valuable teaching aids in offering direct visual information on the effects of instrumentation during endodontic procedures. The visual experiences afforded by these models must provide mental images, which can be transferred to the performance of endodontic procedures on actual teeth. Nowadays, most dental schools continue to present foundational knowledge of dental anatomy in lectures and to develop students' psychomotor skills through a combination of 2D drawing projects, radiographs, and exercises to carve teeth from oversized wax blocks. As a result, neither knowledge nor psychomotor skills are learned in the context of clinical practice, thus potentially hindering the student's ability to later recall and apply learning to actual patient care. On the other hand, practice on extracted teeth has been a universal method of teaching preclinical endodontics and gives students the opportunity of gaining expertise before moving to treating patients. However, infection control concerns, originated by the manipulation of extracted teeth, along with ethical factors are threatening such preclinical laboratory practice in some teaching institutions. These drawbacks have stimulated the development of alternative simulation methods for teaching root canal anatomy.[4]

Root Canal Anatomy Since the Age of Specialization in Endodontics

One must not take away from dental practitioners who revived the popularity and viability of root canal therapy after the misinformed attitudes in the age of "Focal Infection Theory." By the mid-20th century the attitudes and instruments in endodontics had changed;[5] thus standardization of instruments and techniques led to saving many more teeth, while using a recognized and effective treatment rationale. However, it was recognized that if missed canals were leading to failure to seal the entire canal system, then new studies on the variability of root and canal anatomy had to be done. New methods of study were devised that used both radiographs and bench studies of extracted teeth. This has led to the second phase of research in dental and root anatomy, which began about the time of recognition of endodontics as a specialty branch of restorative dentistry in 1964 in the United States.

These tooth anatomy studies included methods such as conventional and laboratory radiography (with or without contrast media), resin injection, macroscopic and microscopic evaluations, tooth sectioning, root clearing techniques, and scanning electron microscopy. Kuttler in 1955[6] used a dissection microscope to show that the apical foramen in teeth varied considerably in diameter. Skidmore and Bjørndal in 1971[7] illustrated casts of mandibular first molars with multiple and complex canal systems. Another example of the practical aspect of studying root morphology was the paper by Davis et al. in 1972[8] that described the use of injected silicone into standard endodontic-prepared canals, with the resulting casts showing that some areas of the canal system had not been completely shaped. All of these canal anatomy studies and more, either in physical anthropology papers or in dental journals, built on a second wave of root and canal system knowledge.[9-11]

Undoubtedly, these techniques have shown a great potential for endodontic research. However, although most of these methods required the partial or even full destruction of the studied samples rendering irreversible changes in the specimens and many artifacts, others provided only a 2D image of a 3D structure.[12] These inherent limitations have repeatedly been discussed, encouraging the search for new methods with improved possibilities.

More recently, the third phase of studies in human root and root canal anatomy is well underway. Increased computer power of digital radiographs and advanced technology are producing studies of human teeth with conventional medical computed tomography (CT), magnetic resonance microscopy, tuned-aperture CT, optical coherence tomography, volumetric or cone beam CT (CBCT; used as a clinical enhancement of practice), and micro–computed tomography (micro-CT). CT-based training replicas produced using 3D printing technology have improved the use of artificial teeth for teaching purposes (Fig. 12.2). Replicas with different root canal complexities can be printed as oversized models in a rapid prototyping printer, allowing the students to hold them in hand to observe details of the internal anatomy in different views. Additional applications of printed models in dental education also include the possibility to (1) scale the teeth for didactic purposes, (2) build a collection of 3D tooth models showing atypical or only regionally prevalent anatomies, (3) produce a large number of teeth for destructive analysis, (4) present the teeth in the form of individual substructures that need to be assembled correctly by the students, and (5) build an extensive collection of 3D models of healthy and diseased teeth using raw data made available online by researchers and dentists from all over the world.[4]

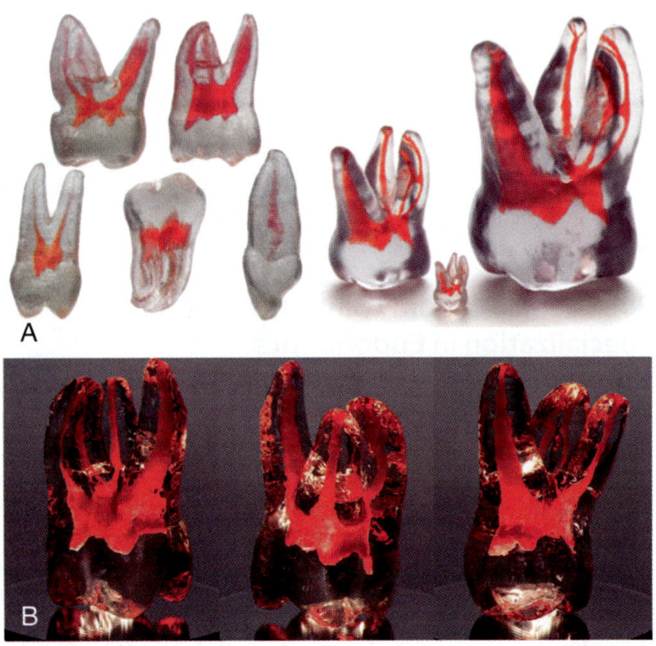

• **Fig. 12.2** Replicas of various teeth manufactured from corresponding real-tooth micro-CT scans using three-dimensional (3D) printing technology in assorted sizes for didactic or teaching purposes. **A,** True Tooth®; **B,** RepliDens®. (**A,** images available at https://dentalengineeringlab.com/truetooth/; **B,** images available at https://www.smartodont.ch/replidens/.)

As imaging has been adopted in modern dental education, it has benefited from the concurrent development of technologies that have allowed the material to be presented electronically. One of the technologies with the greatest effect has been the Internet. The Internet has increasingly been used as an educational tool as a result of its ability to provide a large volume of educational material in a single, readily accessible location and permitting flexibility in the material format.[4] Images, text, interactive quizzes, and videos can be integrated seamlessly into a comprehensive educational resource. In this way, digital images acquired from micro-CT devices could be used to generate anatomic tooth data on a large scale and made freely accessible to the public through the Internet (www.rootcanalanatomy.blogspot.com), thus circumventing the problems of individual researchers requiring access to high-cost scanning devices.[13] Therefore one of the most important aspects of the computer age of communication is the ability to find and access research from many more dental schools and dental researchers from all over the dental academic world. Although a computer search may seem quick and easy, one must rely only on reliable research publications from journals with a credible and high impact factor. A new understanding has been forthcoming on the importance of ethnicity and human dental anatomy.[14]

The misconception of thinking about "one-root equals one-canal" in endodontic treatment has been shattered by a number of classic papers that demonstrate otherwise. In fact, a number of studies have classified and described the morphology of multiple canals in a broad diameter root. This multiple canal configuration may divide, combine, and separate as it forms in root closure toward the various morphologies of the apical foramen terminus.[15] It is prudent to assume that any root that requires treatment may contain more than one canal system per root, until proved otherwise.

Multiple Canals Within a Single Root

Weine et al. in 1969[16] were the first authors to recognize and publish how commonly two canals in one root occurred, and then to classify the two canals in the mesiobuccal root of the maxillary first molar tooth as the "type specimen" (Fig. 12.3, *A*). Piñeda and Kuttler in 1972[17] used radiographs on 7275 extracted teeth to demonstrate multiple canal systems in three dimensions not usually seen in the clinical setting. Other researchers[18-20] soon added observations that confirmed this morphology was not uncommon in many other broad labiolingual or buccolingual roots, as well as, the mesiobuccal root of maxillary molars.

Vertucci et al.[21] developed a more complex classification that is better adapted to research and applied in any other tooth that is wider in the labiolingual or buccolingual dimension (Fig. 12.3, *B*). Essentially, Weine and Vertucci's configuration systems were based on the number of root canals that begin at the pulp chamber floor,

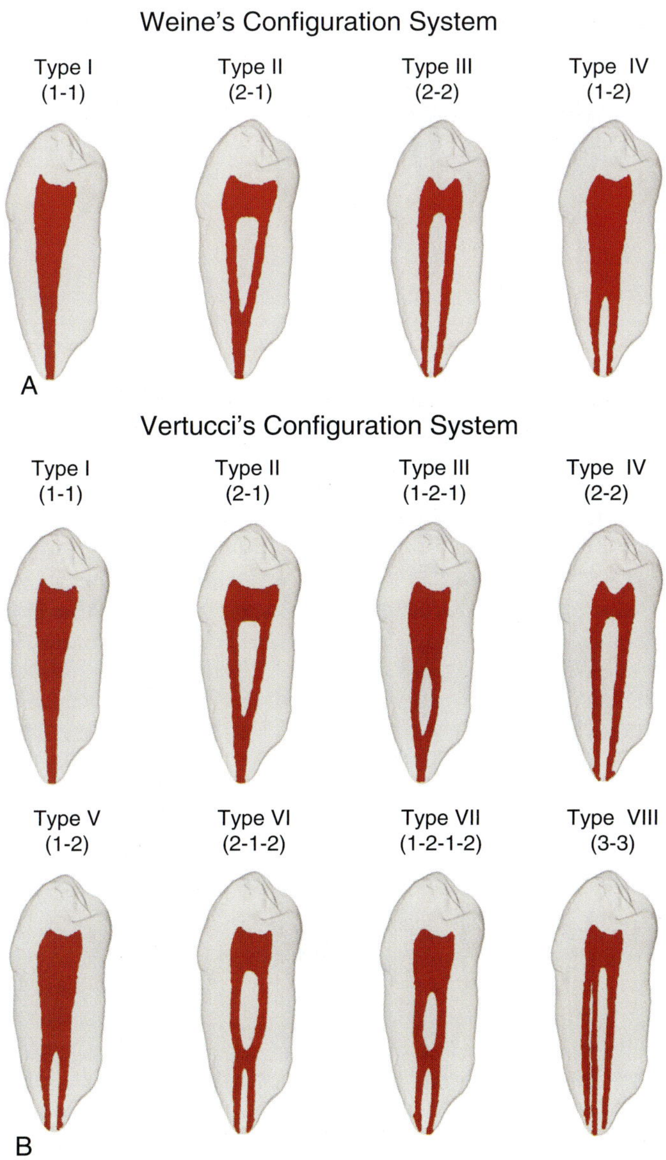

• **Fig. 12.3** **A,** Diagrammatic representations of Weine's classification for root canal morphology. Type I: A single canal from pulp chamber to the apex (1-1 configuration); Type II: Two separate canals leaving the chamber, but merging short of the apex to form a single canal (2-1 configuration); Type III: Two distinct canals from pulp chamber to the apex (2-2 configuration); Type IV: A single canal leaving the chamber and dividing into two separate canals at the apex (1-2 configuration). **B,** Diagrammatic representations of Vertucci's classification for root canal morphology. Type I: A single canal from pulp chamber to the apex (1-1 configuration); Type II: Two separate canals leaving the chamber, but merging short of the apex to form a single canal (2-1 configuration); Type III: A single canal that divides into two, and subsequently merges to exit as one (1-2-1 configuration); Type IV: Two distinct canals from pulp chamber to the apex (2-2 configuration); Type V: A single canal leaving the chamber and dividing into two separate canals at the apex (1-2 configuration); Type VI: Two separate canals leaving the pulp chamber, merging in the body of the root, and dividing again into two distinct canals short from the apex (2-1-2 configuration); Type VII: A single canal that divides, merges, and exits into two distinct canals short from the apex (1-2-1-2 configuration); Type VIII: Three distinct canals within one root from pulp chamber to the apex (3-3 configuration).

arise along the course of the canal, and open through an apical foramen. Later, Versiani and Ordinola-Zapata[22] expanded and adapted these classifications to 3D tomographic descriptions of at least 37 complex canal systems possible to be observed in a single root (Fig. 12.4). The following tables of root numbers of tooth pairings will help one understand the variation in incidence of single and multiple canal numbers based on a large sample from multiple studies. The computer-generated figures will also show graphically some of the variations in anatomy that may be found in the human dentition. Other research studies have shown that furcation canals, lateral canals, and apical ramifications have developed all too commonly.[23] Better cleansing and obturation techniques will more likely seal all portals of exit in the chamber and canal and lead to higher success rates in studies, based on evidence.

Success in root canal therapy can be achieved by first knowing the normal canal anatomy and then by being aware of the many variations that the path of the canal system can follow. One should be able to develop a 3D visualization, both in longitudinal and in cross-section while still using clinical tactile sense to guide a file toward the apical foramen or apical terminus. The following description and images will help provide that knowledge to aid one in honing that skill and expertise.

Root Canal Components and Morphology

Basically, the root canal system can be divided into two parts: the pulp chamber, commonly located within the anatomic dental crown, and the root canal space, found inside the radicular portion of the tooth.[24]

Pulp Chamber

The pulp chamber is a cavity normally situated in the center of the crown and, when there are no pathologic conditions, resembles the shape of the crown surface. In anterior teeth that have a single canal in one root, the pulp chamber and root canal are continuous whereas, in posterior teeth with multiple canals and more than one root, the pulp chamber floor separates these two components. In premolars and molars, the pulp chamber usually presents a square shape with six sides: the floor, the roof, and four axial walls identified as mesial, distal, buccal, or lingual (palatal). The pulp chamber roof usually presents projections or prominences associated with cusps, mamelons, or incisal ridges, denominated pulp horns.[22] In teeth with physiologic wear or other irritation, continuous dentin formation (either physiologic or reactionary) by primary odontoblasts may lead to a decrease in the pulpal space dimensions which, in some cases, can compromise root canal treatment.[25]

Based on the anatomic study of 500 teeth, Krasner and Rankow[26] demonstrated that specific and consistent pulp chamber anatomy exists. Then, they proposed some general rules or laws (Fig. 12.5) for aiding in the determination of the pulp chamber position and the location and number of root canal entrances in each group of teeth:

- *Law of centrality:* The floor of the pulp chamber is always located in the center of the tooth at the level of the cementoenamel junction (CEJ).
- *Law of concentricity:* The walls of the pulp chamber are always concentric to the external surface of the tooth at the level of the CEJ (i.e., the external root surface anatomy reflects the internal pulp chamber anatomy).

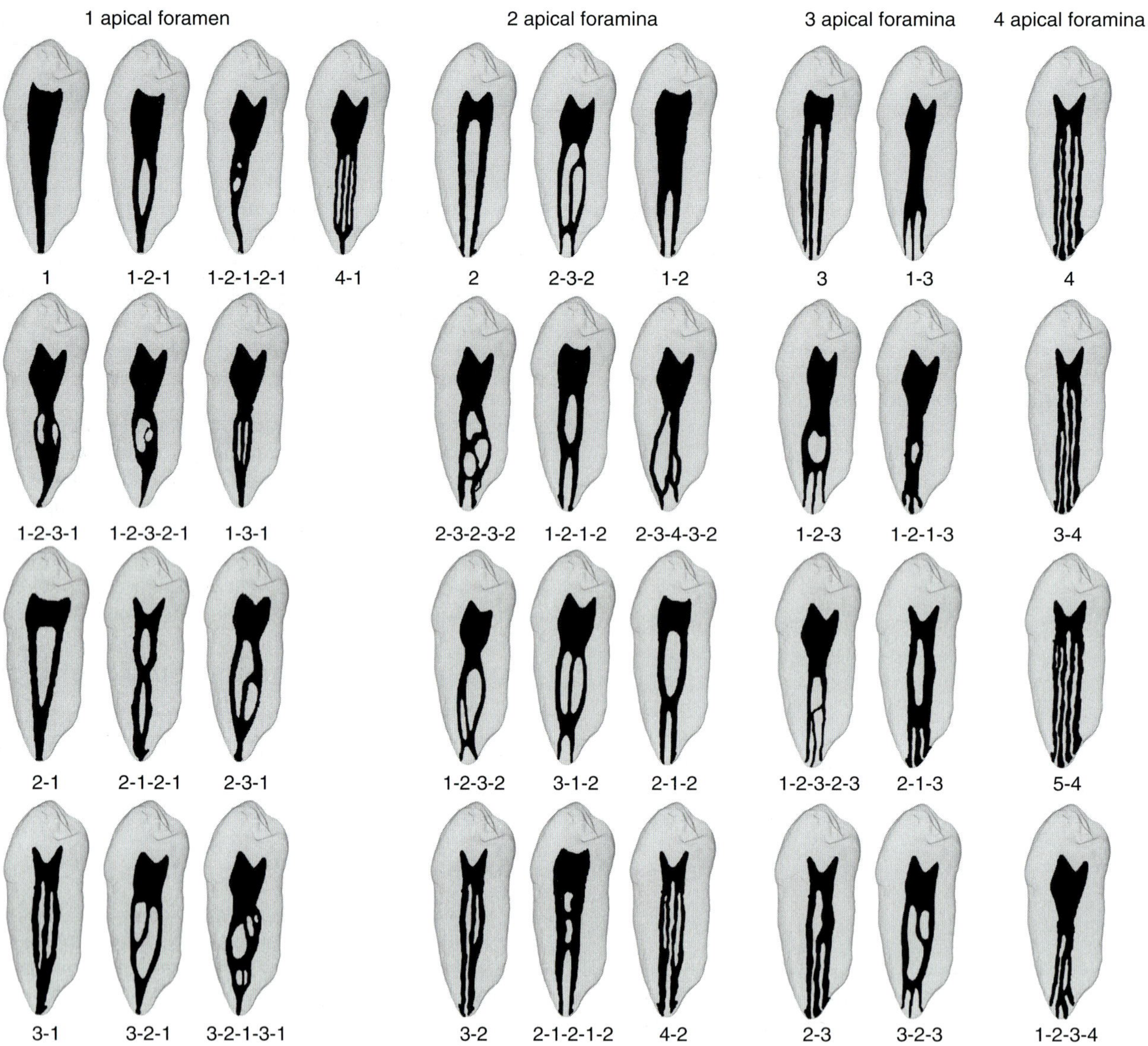

• **Fig. 12.4** Thirty-seven most common canal configurations possible to be observed in a single root, according to Versiani and Ordinola-Zapata.[22]

- *Law of the CEJ:* The distance from the external surface of the clinical crown to the wall of the pulp chamber is the same throughout the circumference of the tooth at the level of the CEJ. The CEJ is the most consistent, repeatable landmark for locating the position of the pulp chamber.
- *Law of symmetry 1:* Except for maxillary molars, the orifices of the canals are equidistant from a line drawn in a mesiodistal direction, through the pulp chamber floor.
- *Law of symmetry 2:* Except for the maxillary molars, the orifices of the canals lie on a line perpendicular to a line drawn in a mesiodistal direction across the center of the floor of the pulp chamber.
- *Law of color change:* The color of the pulp chamber floor is always darker than the walls.
- *Law of orifice location 1:* The orifices of the root canals are always located at the junction of the walls and the floor.
- *Law of orifice location 2:* The orifices of the root canals are located at the angles in the floor-wall junction.
- *Law of orifice location 3:* The orifices of the root canals are located at the terminus of the root developmental fusion lines.

In addition to knowing these laws, the use of better illumination and magnification sometimes associated with specific instruments, such as thin ultrasonic tips or special burs, would provide the best approach to explore the anatomic variations of the pulp chamber in order to locate all canal orifices and avoid missed canals.[24]

Root Canal

The root canal is the portion of the pulp canal space within the root of the tooth limited by the pulp chamber and the foramen that follows the external outline of the root (Fig. 12.6). The root canal can be subdivided into two components: the main canal, which is mostly cleaned by mechanical means, and lateral components composed by isthmuses, accessory canals (furcation, lateral and secondary canals), and some recesses of flattened- and oval-shaped canals.[24]

In longitudinal section, canals are usually broader faciolingually than in the mesiodistal plane. Traditionally, canal shape has been classified as round, oval, long oval, flattened, or irregular (Fig. 12.7).[27] Its geometric cross-sectional shape has been also quantitatively

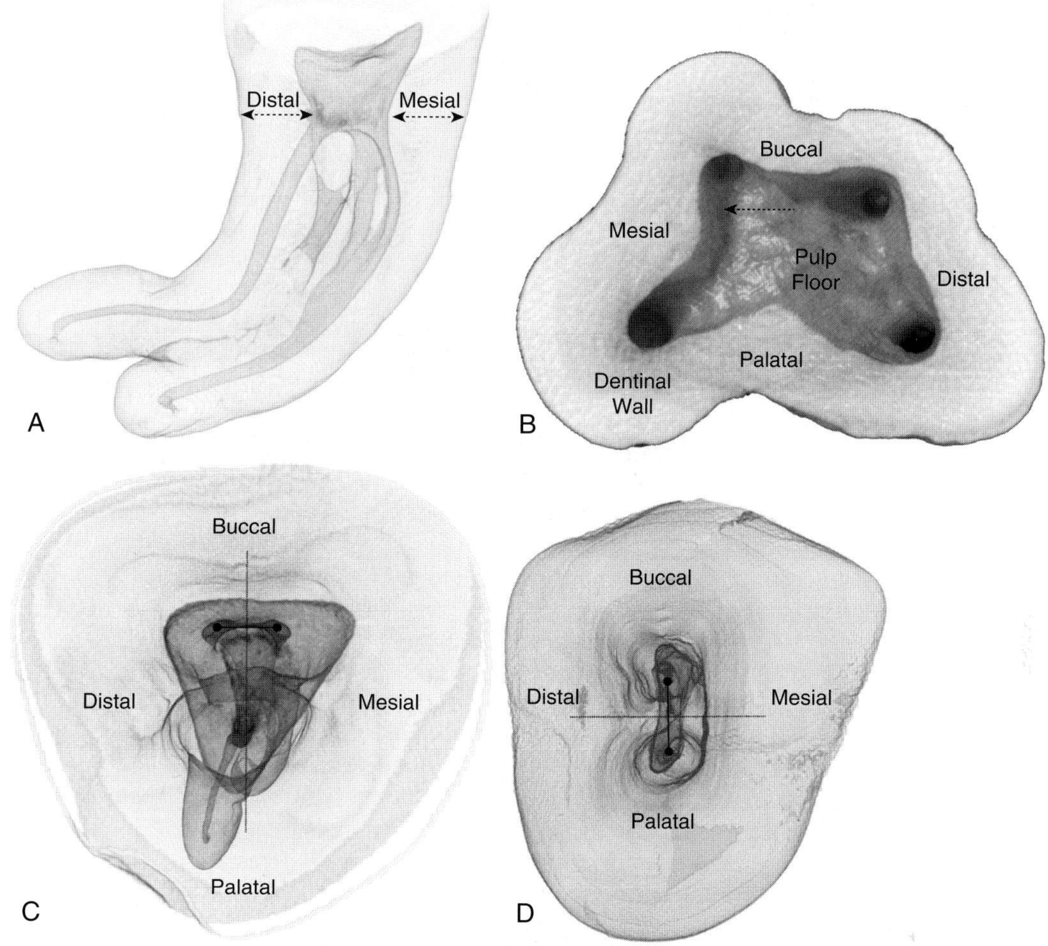

• **Fig. 12.5** Three-dimensional (3D) micro–computed tomography (micro-CT) images of posterior teeth demonstrating the **(A)** laws of centrality and concentricity, at the cementoenamel junction (CEJ) in a mandibular molar tooth; **(B)** laws of color change and orifice locations 1, 2, and 3 (*arrow*: developmental fusion lines) in a four-rooted maxillary second molar tooth; and **(C–D)** laws of symmetry 1 (three-rooted maxillary molar) and 2 (two-rooted maxillary premolar).

described by calculating the mean aspect ratio, defined as the ratio of the major to the minor canal diameters. The major diameter is the distance between the two most distant points of the canal in the buccolingual direction, whereas the minor diameter is the longest chord through the root canal that could be drawn in the direction orthogonal to that of the major diameter. Accordingly, an oval-shaped canal has an aspect ratio between 1 and 2, a long oval canal higher than 2 but lower than 4, and a flattened canal has a value higher than 4.[28] It is interesting to point out that, in a same tooth, canal cross-sections may show different shapes at different levels of the root; however, at the apical third, it is more round or slightly oval in shape in comparison with the middle and coronal thirds.[12,28] Thus, as previously mentioned, the anatomy of the root canal systems is often complex and can vary greatly in number and shape.

Isthmus

An isthmus, also called *transverse anastomosis*, is a narrow, ribbon-shaped communication between two root canals that may contain vital tissue, necrotic pulp, biofilms, or residual filling material.[29,30] Isthmuses (or isthmi) may present with different configurations (Fig. 12.8), and their prevalence is dependent on the type of teeth, the root level, and the patient's age. Hsu and Kim[31] classified the isthmuses configuration into five types:

- Type I—Two canals with no notable communication
- Type II—A hair-thin connection between the two main canals
- Type III—Differs from type II because of the presence of three canals instead of two
- Type IV—An isthmus with extended canals into the connection
- Type V—A true connection or wide corridor of tissue between two main canals.

It is noteworthy that experimental studies demonstrated the impossibility of obtaining a complete mechanical debridement or chemical disinfection of isthmuses with the current technology, mostly because of the presence of hard tissue debris packed into these areas during the mechanical preparation of the main root canal.[32-36] Clinical studies have also shown that unfilled isthmuses can be commonly observed after root-end resection in cases referred for apicoectomy treatment.[37] These limitations, however, can be surpassed in nonsurgical treatment by using chemical agents that have the ability to dissolve organic tissue at fins and isthmuses level, often associated with ultrasonic activation.[33]

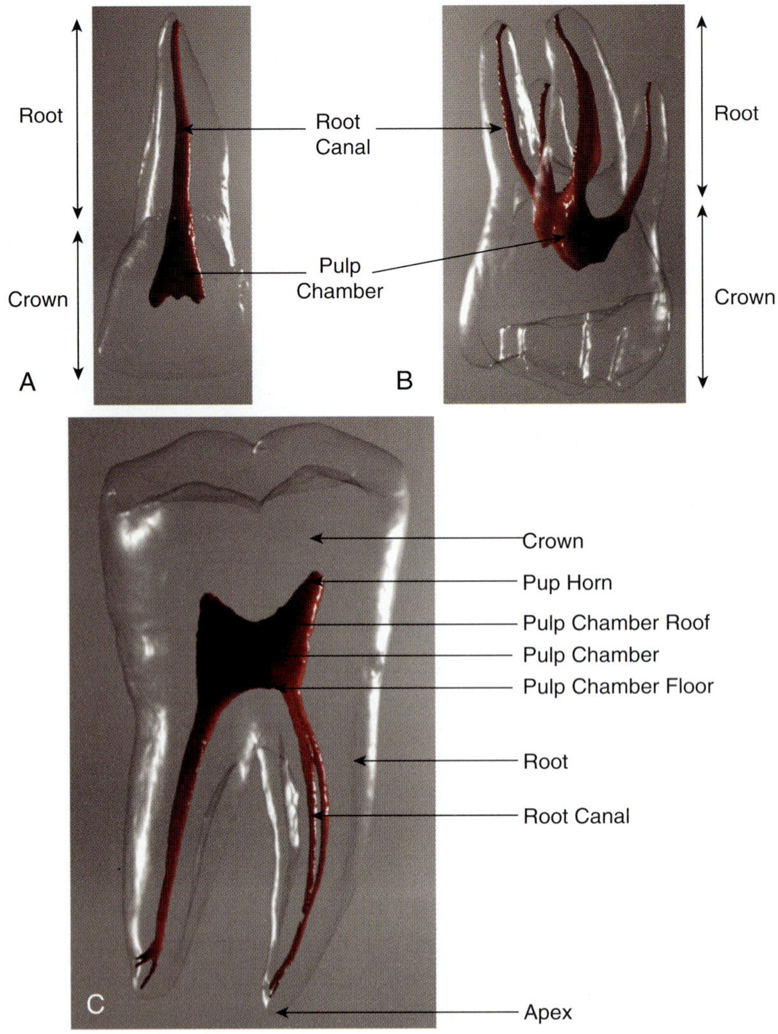

• **Fig. 12.6** Three-dimensional (3D) models of real **(A)** incisor and **(B–C)** molar teeth, obtained by micro–computed tomography (micro-CT) technology, showing the main components of the root canal system.

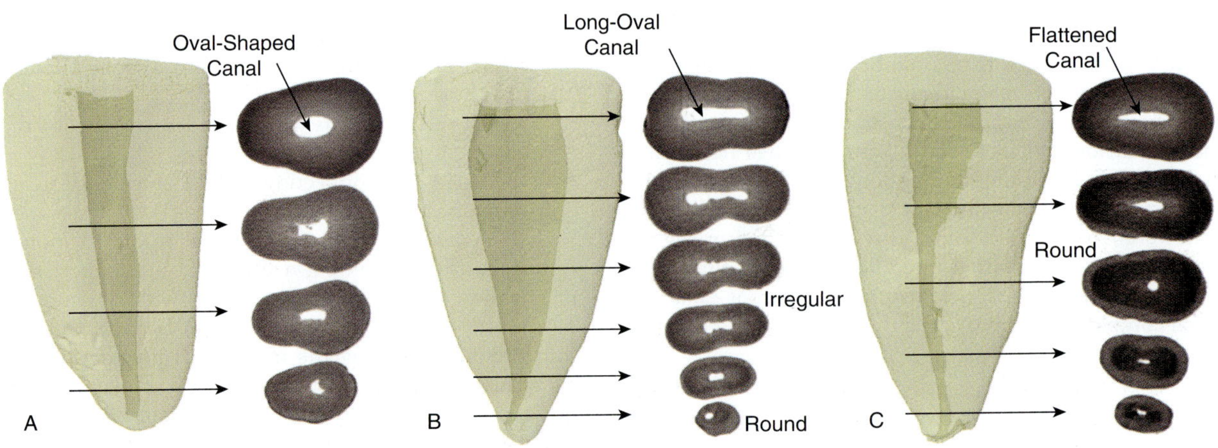

• **Fig. 12.7** Two-dimensional (2D) root canal cross-sections of three mandibular canines **(A–C)** showing that canals are usually broader buccolingually than in the mesiodistal plane, and may present different shapes at distinct levels of the root.

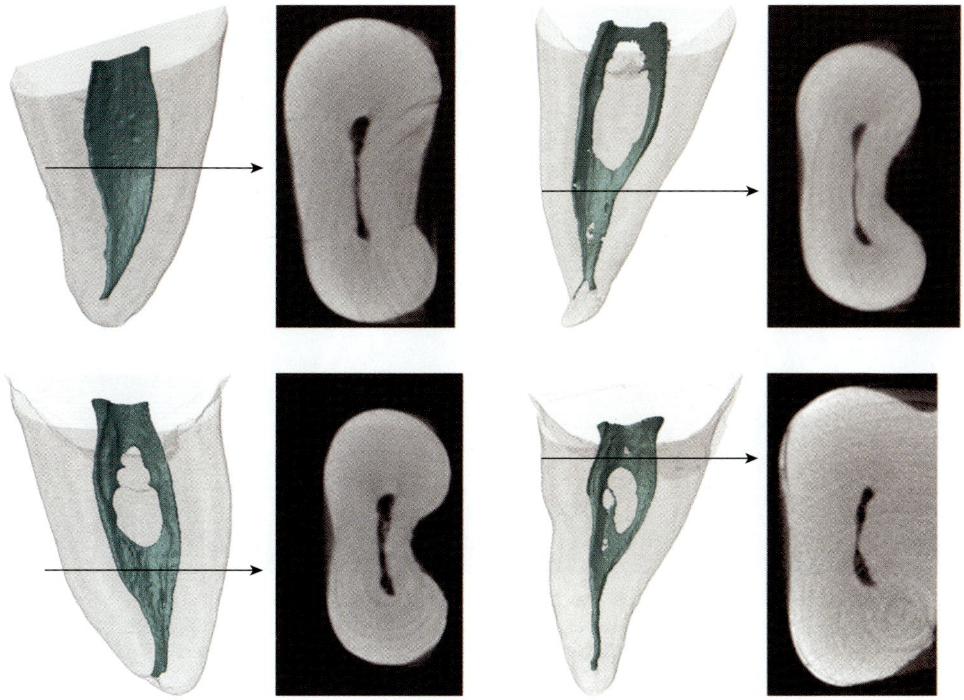

• **Fig. 12.8** Two-dimensional (2D) root canal cross-sections of four mesial roots of mandibular molars showing isthmuses with different sizes and shapes at different levels of the root.

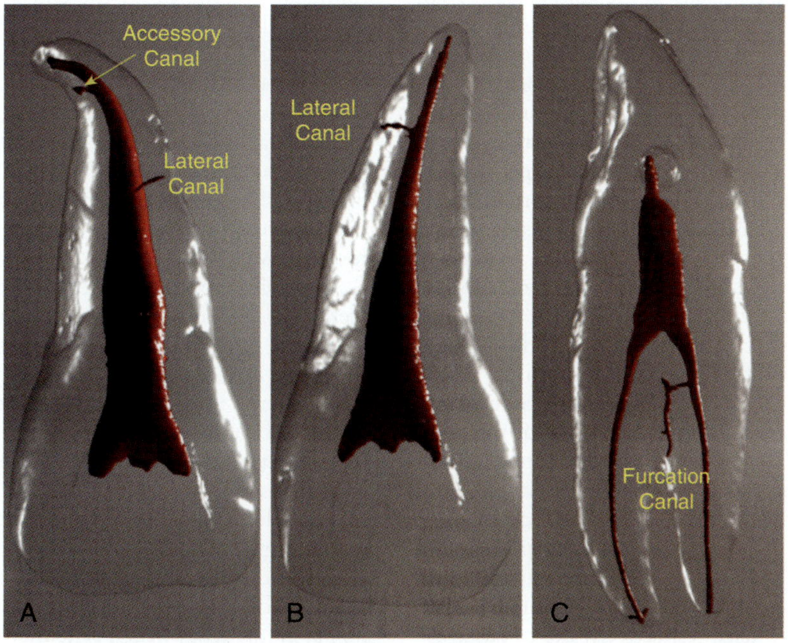

• **Fig. 12.9** Three-dimensional (3D) models of **(A–B)** two maxillary central incisors and **(C)** a two-rooted mandibular canine, obtained by micro–computed tomography (micro-CT) technology, showing the lateral components of the root canal system.

In addition, with the advent of the operatory microscope, it is possible to identify and treat most of the isthmus areas with thin ultrasonic tips, in both surgical and nonsurgical endodontic procedures, to ensure their debridement and seal.[34,35]

Accessory Canals

An accessory canal is any branch of the root canal that communicates with the periodontal ligament, whereas a lateral canal is defined as an accessory canal located at the coronal or middle third of the root (Fig. 12.9, *A* and *B*).[38] They are formed after a localized fragmentation of Hertwig's epithelial root sheath develops, leaving a small gap, or when blood vessels running from the dental sac through the dental papilla persist as collateral circulation.[39] Accessory canals represent potential pathways through which bacteria and/or their byproducts from the necrotic root canal might reach the periodontal ligament and cause disease.[39]

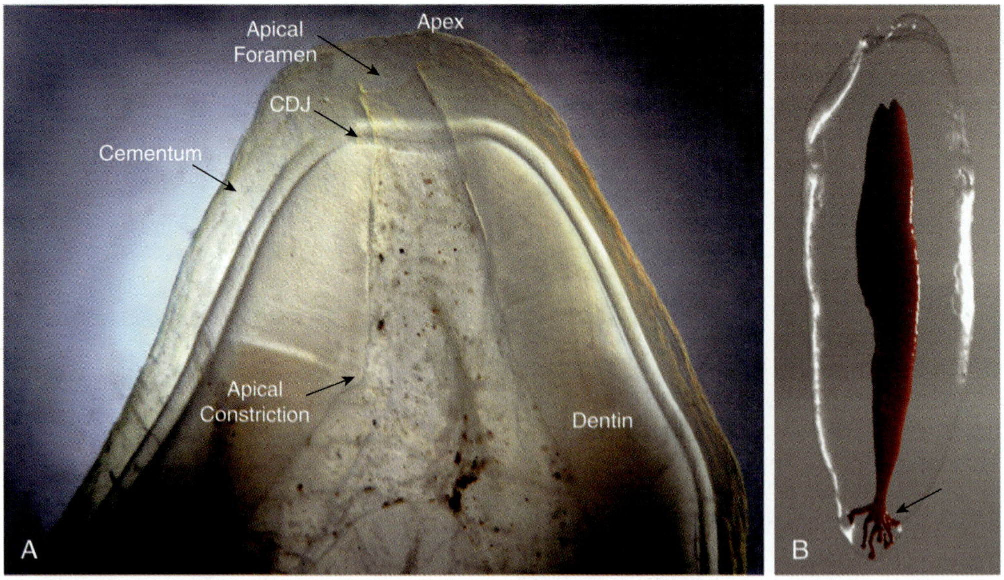

• **Fig. 12.10** **A,** Anatomic landmarks at the apex of a cleared single-rooted tooth (CDJ: cementodentinal junction). **B,** Three-dimensional (3D) micro–computed tomography (micro-CT) model of a mandibular canine presenting apical ramification (arrow). (A, Courtesy Dr. Francisco Balandrano. Published with permission.)

De Deus[23] studied the frequency, location, and direction of the accessory canals in 1140 teeth and showed that 27.4% of the sample (n = 330) had accessory canals, especially in the apical area (17%), followed by the middle (8.8%) and coronal (1.6%) thirds. Similarly, Vertucci[40] evaluated 2400 teeth and observed a lower occurrence of canal ramifications in the middle (11.4%) and coronal (6.3%) thirds compared with the apical level (73.5%). Lateral canals are not usually visible in preoperative radiographs, but their presence can be suspected when there is a localized thickening of the periodontal ligament or there is a lesion on the lateral surface of the root. Clinically, it is also relevant that lateral canals cannot be instrumented most of the time. In this way, their content can only be neutralized by means of effective irrigation with a suitable antimicrobial solution or with an additional use of intracanal medication.[24,25]

Canals connecting the pulp chamber to the periodontal ligament in the furcation region of a multirooted tooth are called furcation canals (Fig. 12.9, *C*).[38] These canals are derived from entrapment of periodontal vessels during the fusion of the parts of the diaphragm, which will become the floor of the pulp chamber. In some cases, furcation canals have been associated with primary endodontic lesions in the interradicular region of multirooted teeth. Vertucci and Williams observed the presence of furcation canals in 13% of mandibular first molars,[41] and in most of them the canal extended from the center of the pulpal floor, whereas in four and two specimens, respectively, the canals arose from the mesial and distal aspects of the floor. Later, Vertucci and Anthony[42] observed the presence of foramina on both the pulp chamber floor and the furcation surface in 36% of maxillary first molars, 12% of maxillary second molars, 32% of mandibular first molars, and 24% of mandibular second molars. Recently, micro-CT studies have also demonstrated the presence of furcation canals in two-rooted mandibular canines and three-rooted mandibular premolars.[43]

Apical Canal

The main root canal ends at the apical foramen (major foramen), which frequently opens laterally on the root surface, at a mean distance between 0.2 to 3.8 mm from the anatomic apex,[44] despite larger distances have been reported recently.[45] The anatomic apex is the tip or the end of the root as determined morphologically.[38] Depending on the type of teeth, the apical foramen can coincide with the anatomic apex in a percentage frequency ranging from 6.7% to 46% of the cases.[10,17,40,46] Its diameter has been described between 0.21 to 0.39 mm.[47] The mesial roots of mandibular molars, the maxillary premolars, and the mesiobuccal roots of maxillary molars present the highest percentage of multiple apical foramina.[47] A previous study on root apices of all groups of permanent teeth showed that the number of foramina on each root may vary from 1 to 16.[44]

The apical portion of the root canal having the narrowest diameter has been called the "apical constriction" (minor foramen).[38] From the apical constriction, the canal widens as it approaches the apical foramen. The topography of the apical constriction is not constant[12,15] and, when present, is usually located 0.5 to 1.5 mm from the center of the apical foramen.[30] The cementodentinal junction (CDJ) is the point at which the cemental surface terminates at or near the apex of a tooth and meets dentin.[38] At this histologic landmark pulp tissue ends and periodontal tissues begin (Fig. 12.10, *A*).[25]

Another relevant variation of the root canal at or near the apex is an intricate network of ramifications, also called *apical ramification of apical delta*, which is defined as a morphology in which the main canal divides into multiple accessory canals (Fig. 12.10, *B*).[38] In maxillary teeth, the percentage frequency of apical ramification ranges from 1% (central incisors) to 15.1% (second premolars), whereas in mandibular teeth its frequency varies from 5% (central incisors) to 14% (distal root of first molars).[40] In the treatment of clinical cases, the infection of this tortuous and complex anatomic configuration with several portals of exit can be related as an etiologic factor of nonsurgical failures.[39]

Canal Curvature and Size

Knowledge of the root curvature is an important factor in choosing the appropriate chemomechanical protocol for cleaning and shaping the root canal system. Before the introduction of nickel-titanium (NiTi) instruments, several iatrogenic procedures were associated with the preparation of curved canals including zips, separated instruments, ledges, and perforations.[48] Nowadays, these iatrogenic complications are no longer a problem, except for instrument separation. Therefore this is one of the factors determining the difficulty of treatment and the likelihood of iatrogenic errors and shows that preoperative recognition of canal curvature is of utmost importance.[22]

Nearly all root canals are curved in the apical third, particularly in a faciolingual direction, which is not evident on standard radiography.[30] In general, the curvature may vary from gradual curvature of the entire canal, sharp curvature of the canal near the apex, or a gradual curvature of the canal with a straight apical ending. Numerous methods have been proposed to determine root canal curvature,[49,50] but the Schneider's method has been the most widely used. Schneider[51] classified single-rooted permanent teeth according to the degree of curvature of the root, which was determined by first drawing a line parallel to the long axis of the canal, then, a second line connecting the apical foramen to the point in the first line where the canal began to leave the long axis of the tooth. The angle formed by these two lines was the angle of curvature and its degree was classified as straight (≤5 degrees), moderate (10 to 20 degrees), or severe (25 to 70 degrees).

Another method was introduced by Weine[52] that also relies on the definition of two straight lines, but it reflects the root canal curvature more accurately than Schneider's method, especially in the apical part. A third proposal, geometrically equivalent to Weine's method, was introduced by Pruett et al.,[53] but its major innovation was the concurrent measurement of the radius of curvature by the superimposition of a circular arc on the curved part of the root canal. Therefore, the Schneider angle, when used in combination with the radius and length of the curve, may provide a more precise method for describing the apical geometry of canal curvature.

Clinically, different angled views are necessary to determine the presence, direction, and severity of the root canal curvature. Schäfer et al.[54] evaluated radiographically the degree of curvature of 1163 root canals from all groups of teeth. The degree of curvature ranged from 0 to 75 degrees and from 0 to 69 degrees in clinical and proximal views, respectively. The highest degree of curvature was observed in the clinical view of the mesiobuccal canal of maxillary molars and in the mesial canals of mandibular molars. In several cases, the angles of proximal curvatures were higher than those of the clinical view. Additionally, a secondary curvature (S-shaped canal) was observed in 12.3% and 23.3% of the maxillary and mandibular teeth, respectively.

Root Canal Configuration Systems

Various classification systems have been proposed in an attempt to have a standardized root canal classification system that can be used by clinicians and researchers. The two most commonly used systems are the ones developed by Weine et al.,[16] followed by Vertucci et al. (see Fig. 12.3).[21] Weine's initial classification included three types based on a sectioning study of the mesiobuccal root of permanent maxillary first molars. The system classifies the canal configuration by two numbers. The first number is the number of canals found at the floor of the pulp chamber whereas the second number describes the canal configuration at the apex. For example, a Weine Type II canal configuration (2-1) means that two distinct canals are found at the floor of the pulp chamber and the two canals subsequently join and form a single canal at the apex. The Type IV canal configuration (1-2) was added later.[52] Vertucci's classification system was developed based on a clearing study (followed by dye injected into the canals) of 200 maxillary second premolars and eight canal types were described. Vertucci et al.[21] defined the Type VIII root canal system as three separate canals in maxillary premolars from the pulp chamber to the apex. However, the study did not specify whether the three canals were within a tooth that contained one, two, or three roots. Many studies have classified Type VIII canal configurations lumping single, double, and triple-rooted teeth together.[21,40,55,56] Some studies, though, have classified three-rooted maxillary premolars with single canals in each root as Type I canal systems in each root.[57,58] It seems logical, however, that a Type VIII canal should only be used in one broad or fused root of a tooth, and not in the separated roots and apex of the same tooth as may be shown on the radiograph.

In addition, numerous other canal types have been reported by various authors that did not fit into either classification system.[59] Recently, based on the study of hundreds of permanent teeth, Versiani and Ordinola-Zapata[60] found 37 different canal types using micro-CT technology (see Fig. 12.4). Clearly, neither the Weine nor the Vertucci classification system can adequately describe these additional complex canal configurations. A simple classification system that can be used to describe all of the possible canal configurations in all teeth has yet to be developed. However, a new canal classification system proposed by Ahmed et al.[59] shows promise because the system can accommodate any type of canal configuration by using root name and canal numbers to categorize the canal configuration in each root (Fig. 12.11).

Root Canal Anomalies and Embryologic Malformations

Anomalous root and root canal morphology can be found associated with any tooth with varying degrees and frequency in the human dentition. Dental anomalies are formative defects caused by genetic disturbances during the morphogenesis of teeth.[61] Anomalies may occur during the developmental stages of the tooth that are manifested clinically later in life once the tooth is fully formed.[62-64] Failure to diagnose teeth with anomalous anatomy may lead to misdiagnosis and a treatment plan that could cause permanent irreversible damage and loss of the tooth.[30] In this way, the clinician must be aware of the existence of some anatomic anomalies to implement an appropriate treatment plan. Major anomalies that affect endodontic practice include taurodontism, dens invaginatus, dens evaginatus, extra roots (radix), and C-shaped canals.[61]

Taurodontism

Taurodontism (or a "bull-shaped" tooth) is a dental morphologic variation in which the body of the tooth is enlarged and the roots are reduced in length.[65] A taurodont tooth presents a large pulp chamber with apical displacement of the pulpal floor and furcation of the roots (Fig. 12.12, *A* and *B*).[38] The etiology of taurodontism is unclear, but it also appears in certain genetic syndromes.[66] It is thought to be caused by the failure of Hertwig's epithelial root sheath diaphragm to invaginate at the proper horizontal level, resulting in a tooth with normal dentin, short roots, elongated body, and enlarged pulp.[63,64,67] The teeth involved are almost invariably molars or rarely premolars. It can be uni- or bilateral and may affect single or multiple teeth.[68] The condition may also present rarely in the primary dentition molar teeth.[69] Taurodontism is most famously reported to occur in high

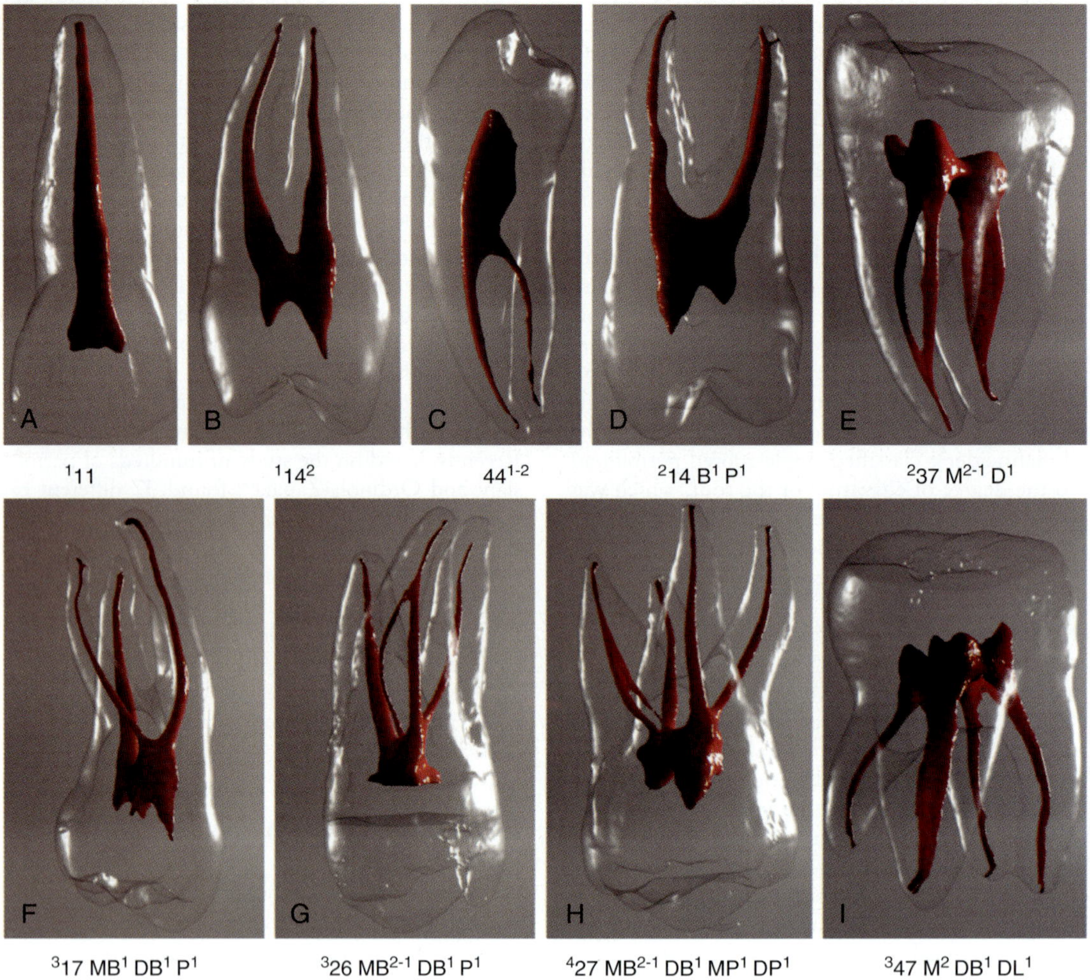

• **Fig. 12.11** Three-dimensional (3D) micro–computed tomography (micro-CT) models of **(A–C)** single-, **(D–E)** double-, and **(F–I)** multirooted teeth classified according to the new system proposal by Ahmed et al.[59] *B*, Buccal; *D*, distal; *DB*, distobuccal; *DL*, distolingual; *DP*, distopalatal; *M*, mesial; *MB*, mesiobuccal; *MP*, mesiopalatal; *P*, palatal. (Published with permission.)

incidence by Keith in 1913 as found in *Homo neanderthal* from the Krapina archaeologic find in the early 1900s.[70]

Taurodontism was classified earlier by Shaw in 1928 and has been graded according to its severity: normal (cynodont), least pronounced (hypotaurodontism), moderate (mesotaurodontism), and most severe (hypertaurodontism).[71] Clinically, the crowns of these teeth usually have normal characteristics. Therefore the diagnosis is entirely radiologic.[68] Owing to the complexity of the root canal anatomy and the proximity of the orifices to the root apex, complete filling of the root canal system in taurodontism is challenging. Because the pulp of a taurodont is usually voluminous, control of bleeding in cases of pulpitis may take some time and effort compared to teeth with normal anatomy. Additional efforts such as application of ultrasonic instrumentation combined with sodium hypochlorite (NaOCl) as an irrigant solution should be made to dissolve as much organic material as possible.[68,72,73]

Dens Invaginatus and Dens Evaginatus

Dens invaginatus (dens in dente, dilated composite odontome, dilated odontome, gestant anomaly, invaginated odontome, dilated gestant odontome, tooth inclusion, dentoid in dente) is a developmental defect resulting from invagination in the surface of the tooth crown before calcification has occurred (Fig. 12.12, *C–F*).[61] Clinically, it may appear as an accentuation of the lingual pit in anterior teeth and, in its more severe form, gives a radiographic appearance of a tooth within a tooth, hence the term *dens in dente*.[38] Its etiology is controversial and remains unclear. The affected teeth radiographically show an infolding of enamel and dentin that may extend deep into the pulp cavity and into the root and sometimes even reach the root apex.[74] The most common associated clinical finding is an early pulpal involvement, explained by the existence of a canal extending from the invagination into the pulp.[75] The invagination also allows the entry of irritants into an area that is separated from pulpal tissue by only a thin layer of enamel and dentin and presents a predisposition for the development of dental caries.[74] Therefore this condition must be recognized early and the tooth prophylactically restored.[73] The variability of its root canal system configuration is unlimited. Clinically, however, it can only be speculated upon from radiographs.[76] In this way, the most commonly referred classification was proposed by Oehlers,[77] who categorized it into three types: Type 1—the invagination is confined to the crown and does not extend beyond the CEJ; Type 2—the invagination extends past

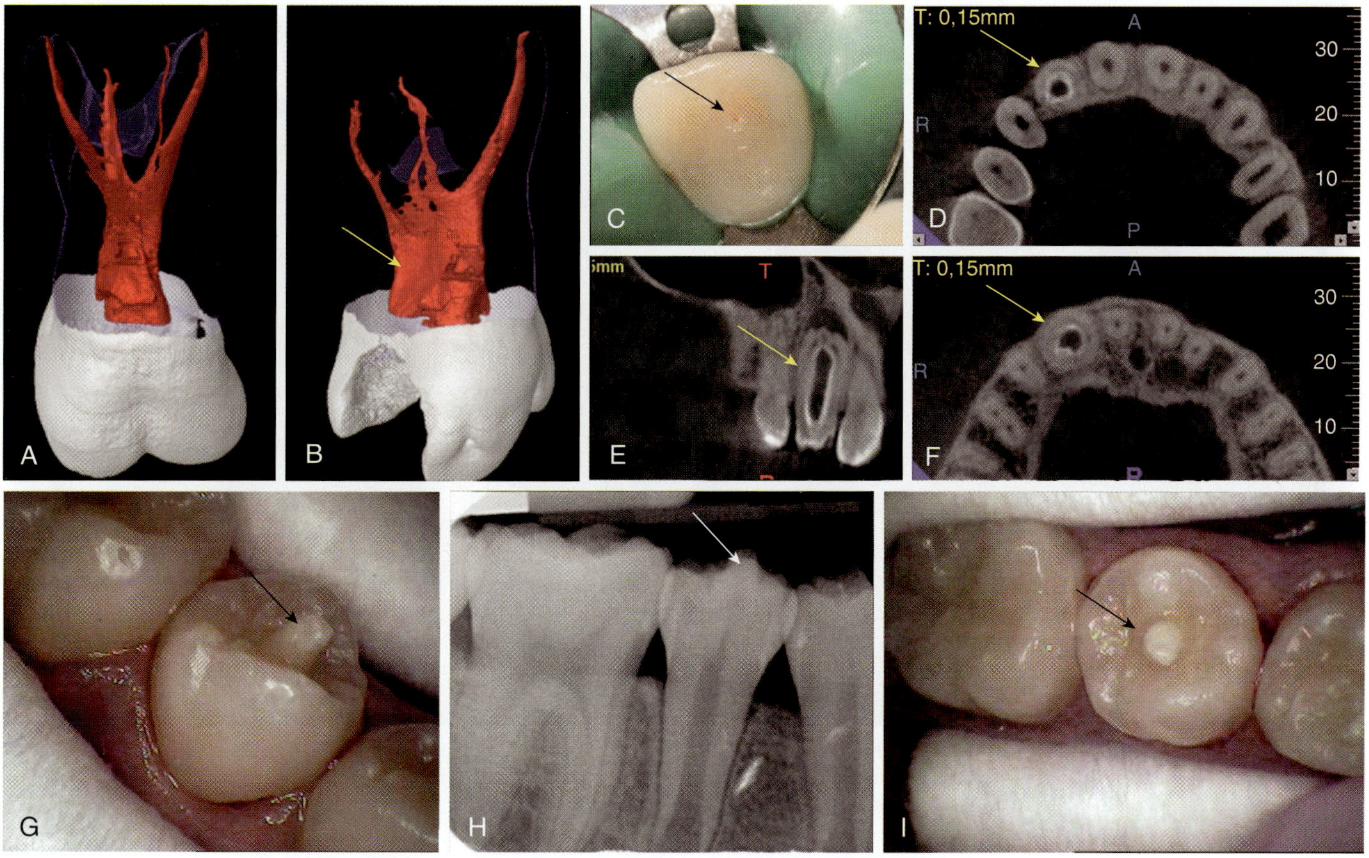

• **Fig. 12.12 Root canal anomalies and embryologic malformations. (A–B)** Taurodont maxillary second molar presenting a large pulp chamber (yellow arrow) with apical displacement of the pulpal floor and furcation of the roots; **C–F,** Clinical and tomographic views of a maxillary lateral incisor with dens invaginatus (arrows) (Courtesy of Dr. Oscar von Stetten. Published with permission); **G–I,** Clinical and radiographic views of a mandibular second premolar with dens evaginatus (arrows). (Courtesy Dr. Daniela Bololoi. Published with permission.)

the CEJ and does not involve the periradicular tissues, but may communicate with the dental pulp; and Type 3—the invagination extends beyond the CEJ and may present a second apical foramen, with no immediate communication with the pulp. In the literature, the reported prevalence of this anomaly varies from 0.25%[78] to 10%[79] and the most affected teeth are permanent maxillary lateral incisors, despite the fact that it may occur in any tooth.[74,80] This high range frequency of dens invaginatus has been associated with the study design, sample size and composition, and diagnostic criteria.[74,75]

Dens evaginatus is an anomalous outgrowth of tooth structure resulting from the folding of the inner enamel epithelium into the stellate reticulum with the projection of structure exhibiting enamel, dentin, and pulp tissue (Fig. 12.12, *G–I*).[38] It arises most frequently from the occlusal surface of involved posterior teeth, mainly maxillary and mandibular premolars, and primarily from the lingual surface of associated anterior teeth (called *talon cusps* when in this location).[81,82] Its etiology remains unclear. However, it predominantly occurs in people of Asian descent with varying estimates reported at 0.5%[83] to 15%,[84] depending on the population group studied. The presence of pulp within the cusp-like tubercle has great clinical significance. Because the tubercle may extend above the occlusal surface, malocclusion or attrition with the opposing tooth may cause abnormal wear or fracture of the tubercle, and this is how pulp exposure occurs.[82] Subsequent pulpal inflammation or infection will most likely ensue, at times when the root apex closure has not occurred in the young patient. It is important for the clinician to be able to recognize and treat the entity soon after affected teeth have erupted into the oral cavity in order to avoid the development of pathologic conditions.[82]

Radix

Radix is a Latin word for "root" and is referred to additional roots of teeth, mostly molars. In radix molars, each root usually contains a single root canal.[61]

In four-rooted maxillary molars, the palatal part of the root complex is made up of two macrostructures located mesially and distally, which are in principle cone-shaped and either separate or nonseparate in relation to each other.[85] If the mesial of the two palatal root structures has direct affinity to the mesiolingual part of the crown, which is more pronounced, the mesial root structure is identified as radix mesiolingualis, whereas the distal structure is identical with the palatal root component. If the distal of the two palatal root structures has direct affinity to the distopalatal part of the crown, the distal root structure is identified as radix distolingualis, whereas the mesial structure is identical with the palatal root component (Fig. 12.13).[86]

In mandibular molars, additional roots have been identified as radix entomolaris and radix paramolaris.[61,87] Radix entomolaris has been defined as a supernumerary root on a mandibular molar located distolingually (Fig. 12.14), whereas radix paramolaris is

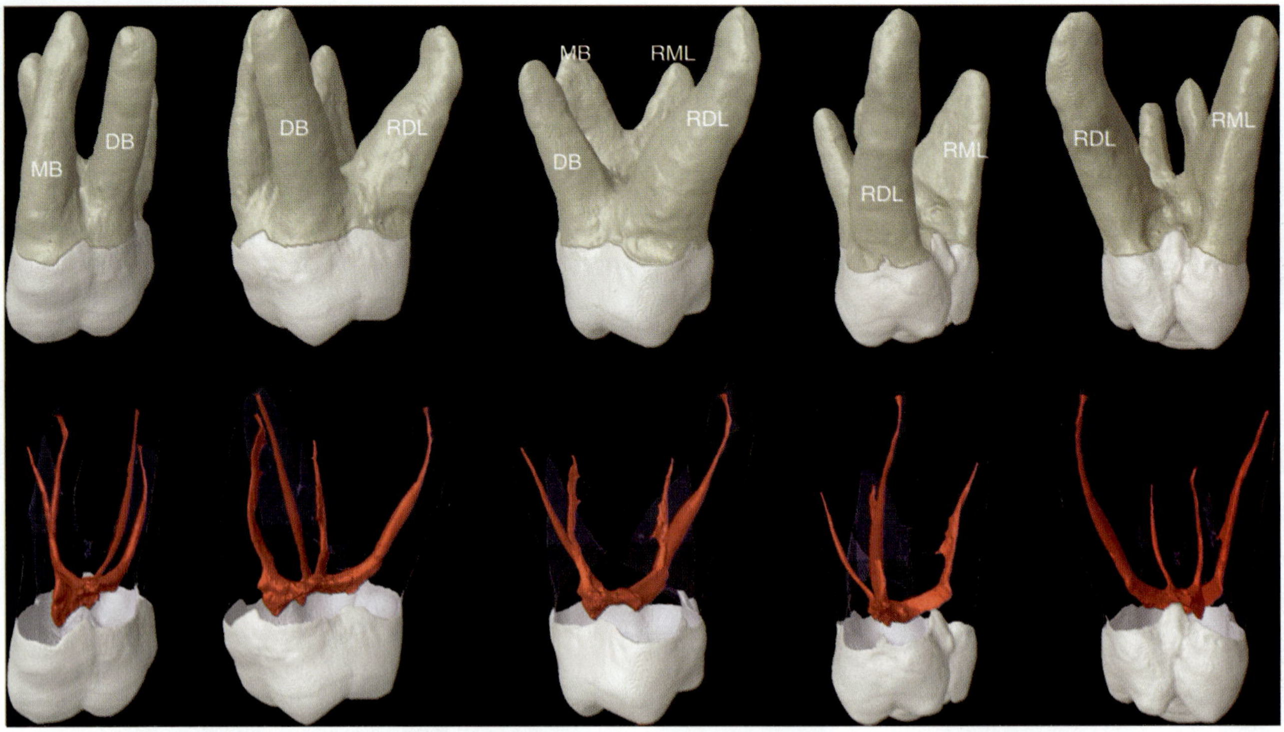

• **Fig. 12.13** Different views of a three-dimensional (3D) micro–computed tomography (micro-CT) models of the external and internal morphologies of a four-rooted maxillary molar showing radix mesiolingualis (RML) and radix distolingualis (RDL). *DB*, Distobuccal root; *MB*, mesiobuccal root.

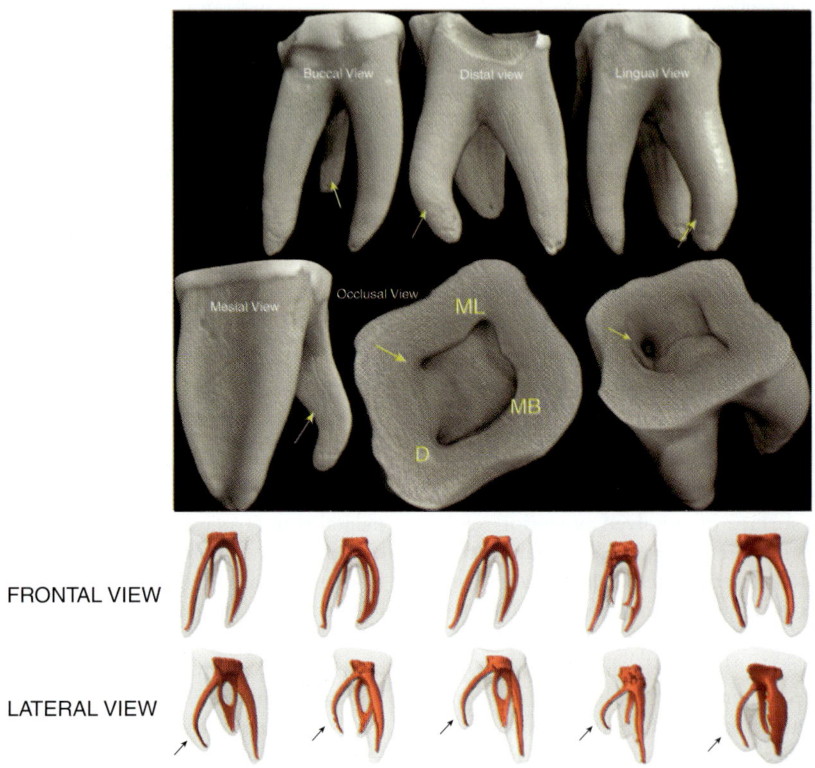

• **Fig. 12.14** Three-dimensional (3D) micro–computed tomography (CT) models of the external and internal morphologies of mandibular second molars showing radix entomolaris *(yellow arrows)*. In the lateral view, the curvature of the radix is depicted (black arrows).

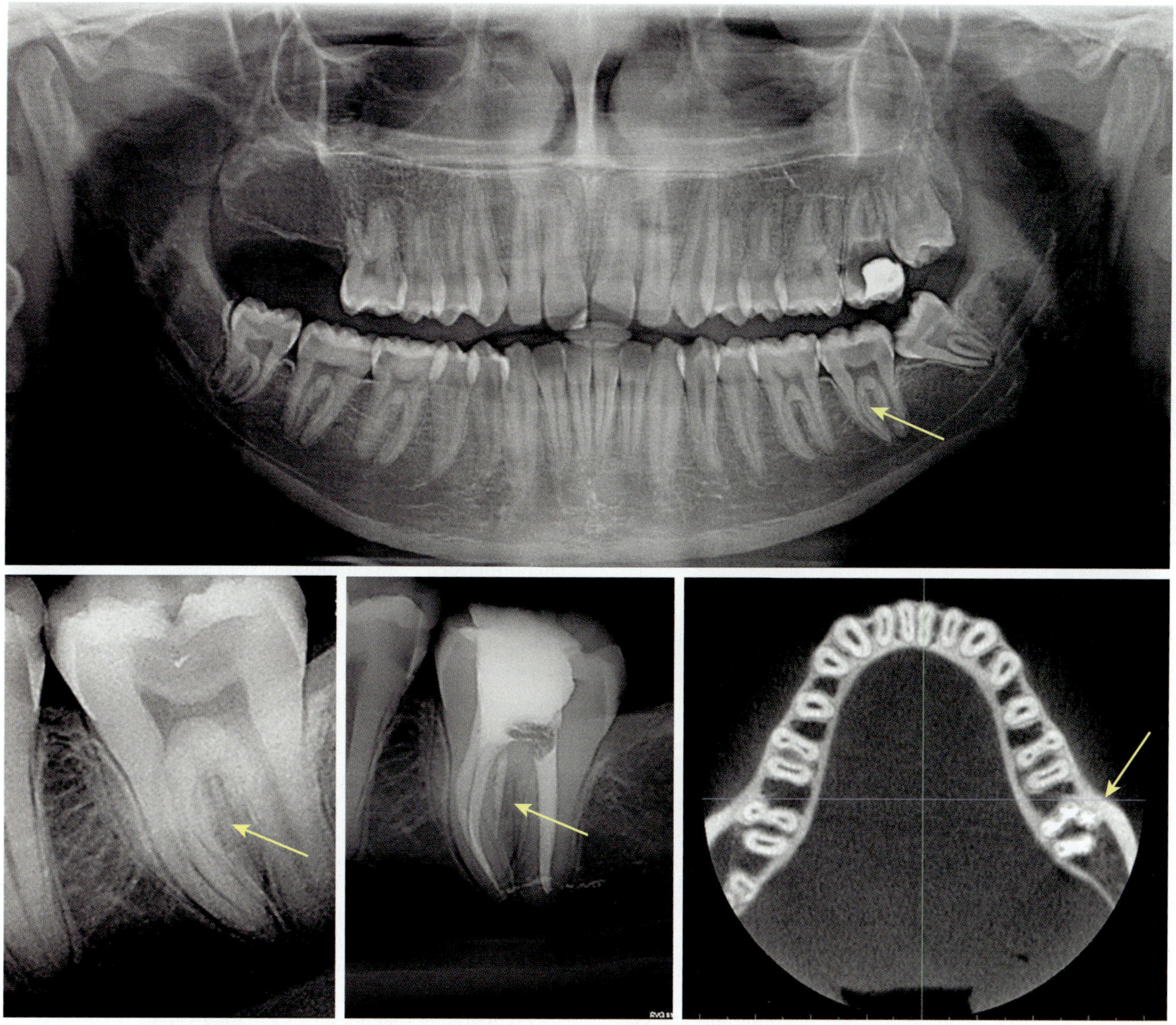

• **Fig. 12.15** Radiographic and tomographic views of a mandibular left second premolar showing a radix paramolaris *(arrows)*, before and after root canal treatment. (Courtesy Dr. Nuno Pinto. Published with permission.)

an extra root located mesiobuccally (Fig. 12.15).[38] The presence of these anatomic anomalies has been associated with certain ethnic groups such as Sino Americans, which include Chinese, Inuit, and American Indians.[88,89] Radix paramolaris is a very rare structure and its prevalence was found to be 0%, 0.5%, and 2.0% for the mandibular first, second, and third molars, respectively,[90] whereas radix entomolaris occurs with a higher frequency, ranging from 0.2%[91] to 32%[92] of the studied samples. The orifice of the radix entomolaris is located disto- to mesiolingually from the main canal or canals of the distal root, whereas the orifice of the radix paramolaris is located mesio- to distobuccally from the main mesial canals.[88] A dark line or groove from the main root canal on the pulp chamber floor leads to these orifices[89]; however, they provide a limited practical aid for its identification in clinical practice. These anatomic variations present definite challenges to therapy because of their orifice inclination and root canal curvature. In this way, preoperative periapical radiographs at different horizontal angles or a CBCT examination are required to identify this additional root, which will also result in a modified opening cavity. An accurate diagnosis of these anatomic variations is important to avoid missed canals.[87]

C-Shaped Canals

The C-shaped configuration was first reported in the endodontic literature by Cooke and Cox in 1979,[93] but this canal configuration has been well-known since the beginning of the 20th century.[94] This anatomic variation is so named for the root and root canal cross-sectional shape of the capital letter "C."[95] Its main anatomic feature is the presence of one or more isthmuses connecting individual canals, which can change the cross-sectional and 3D canal shape along the root (Fig. 12.16).[95-97] Typically, this configuration is found in teeth with fusion of the roots either on its buccal or lingual aspect, and results from the failure of Hertwig's epithelial root sheath to develop or fuse in the furcation area during the developing stage of the teeth.[63,64] Failure on the buccal side will result in a lingual groove, and the opposite cases would be possible.[63] In such teeth, the floor of the pulp chamber is frequently

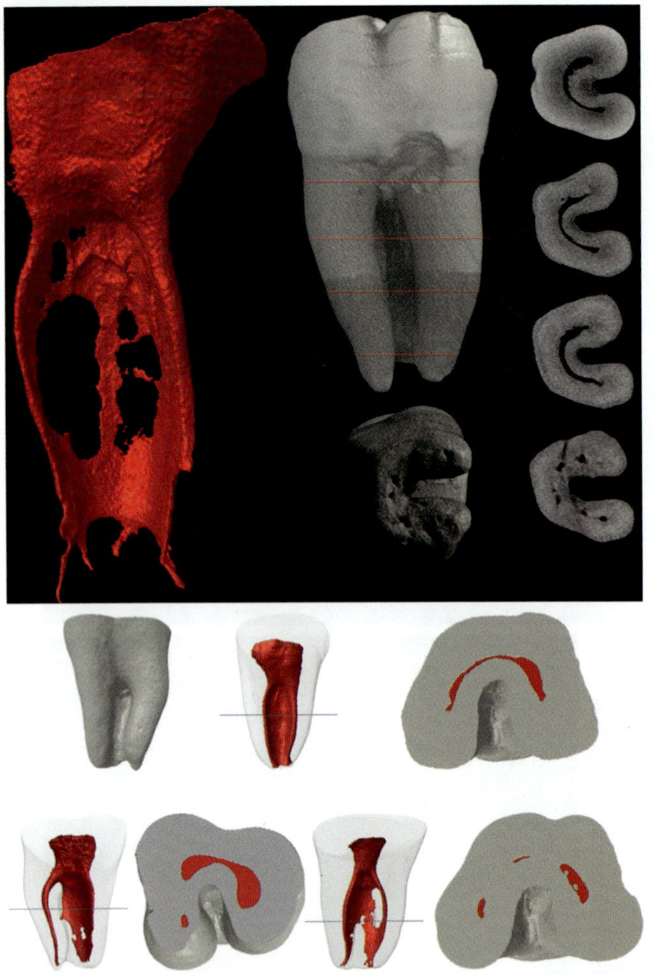

• **Fig. 12.16** Three-dimensional (3D) micro–computed tomography (CT) models of the external and internal morphologies of mandibular second molars showing different C-shaped canal configurations.

situated deeply and may assume an unusual anatomic appearance.[97] Below the orifice level, the root structure of a C-shaped tooth can harbor a wide range of anatomic variations,[95] which make it a challenge with respect to disinfection.[98] This variation may occur in different types of teeth[97,99-102]; however, it is most commonly found in mandibular second molars[103,104] with a reported prevalence ranging from 2.7%[105] to 44.5%.[106] There is significant ethnic variation in the frequency of C-shaped molar teeth, which are much more common in Asian populations than in Caucasian populations.[30] In population-based studies, the reported prevalence was 10.6% in Saudi Arabians,[107] 19.14% in Lebanese,[108] 31.5% in Chinese,[104] and 44.5% in Koreans.[106] To date, two studies have addressed the efficacy of different systems in the preparation of C-shaped mandibular molar canals showing a significant percentage of canal area unaffected by the instrumentation procedure.[98,109]

In 1991 Melton et al.[96] proposed the first classification for C-shaped canal configuration in mandibular second molars based on its cross-sectional shape. They fall into three categories: Category I—a continuous C-shaped canal running from the pulp chamber to the apex; Category II—a semicolon-shaped orifice in which dentin separates a main C-shaped canal from one mesial distinct canal; Category III—two or more discrete and separate canals which could join in the apical (subdivision I), middle (subdivision II), or coronal (subdivision III) thirds.

It is important to point out that mandibular molar teeth can present with irregularities in their canal systems throughout the root and the presence of these categories may vary from the pulp chamber to the apex.[106] In this way, Fan et al.[110] modified Melton's method and recommended to classify each portion of the same tooth using five categories:

- Category I—The shape was an uninterrupted "C" with no separation or division.
- Category II—The canal shape resembled a semicolon resulting from a discontinuation of the "C" outline.
- Category III—Two or three separate canals
- Category IV—Only one round or oval canal in the cross-section (normally found near the apex)
- Category V—No canal lumen (usually seen near the apex only)

Melton's classification[96] stated that categories II and III have separated canals, but no description was provided to differentiate them. In the modified classification,[110] one of the canals in the category II would appear as an arc and would be more likely to extend into the "fused" area of the root where the dentin wall may be quite thin.

C-shaped canal anatomy has also been reported in third molars,[111] lateral incisors,[102] mandibular first premolars,[97,99,101,112,113] mandibular first molars,[114] and maxillary first[115,116] and second[117] molars. Recently the prevalence of C-shaped canal configuration in maxillary molars with root fusion was reported to be as high as 15% (Fig. 12.17, *A*).[115] Mandibular first premolars present a variety of root canal configurations that include the presence of two or three root canals[40,113] and a C-shaped configuration system (Fig. 12.17, *B*).[118] As in mandibular molars, C-shaped canal systems in the mandibular first premolars vary among different ethnic groups, with its prevalence being reported to range from 1%[119] to 18%.[120] This configuration has been highly associated with Vertucci's type V configuration[100] (i.e., a single canal that bifurcates at the middle third and with the presence of a groove or concavity on the external root surface).[97,113] Radicular grooves on mandibular first premolars usually begin 3 mm from the CEJ and present frequently on the proximal lingual area of the middle root, not always extending to the root apex.[97,120]

Preoperative diagnosis of C-shaped canals is complex, mainly because these unique anatomic features are not easily recognized on a traditional 2D periapical radiograph.[98] With the increased use of CBCT scanning, clinicians may be able to detect C-shaped canals before endodontic treatment. Nevertheless, even when recognized, the disinfection procedure still remains a challenge, mostly because of the isthmus areas. Irregular areas in a C-shaped canal that may house soft tissue remnants or infected debris may escape thorough cleaning and may be a source of bleeding and severe pain.[121] In this way, the use of a dental microscope associated with sonic or ultrasonic instrumentation techniques may make treatment outcome more predictable.[30] Because of its challenging morphology, the C-shaped canal anatomy increases the difficulty in root canal therapy and may account for the frequent occurrence of endodontic failure on this tooth.[120]

Other Anomalies

(1) **Fusion:** It is commonly defined as the union of two distinct dental sprouts that occurs in any stage of the dental organ.[38] They are joined by the dentin, whereas pulp chambers and canals may be linked or separated depending on the developmental stage when the union occurs. This process involves epithelial and mesenchymal germ layers resulting in irregular tooth

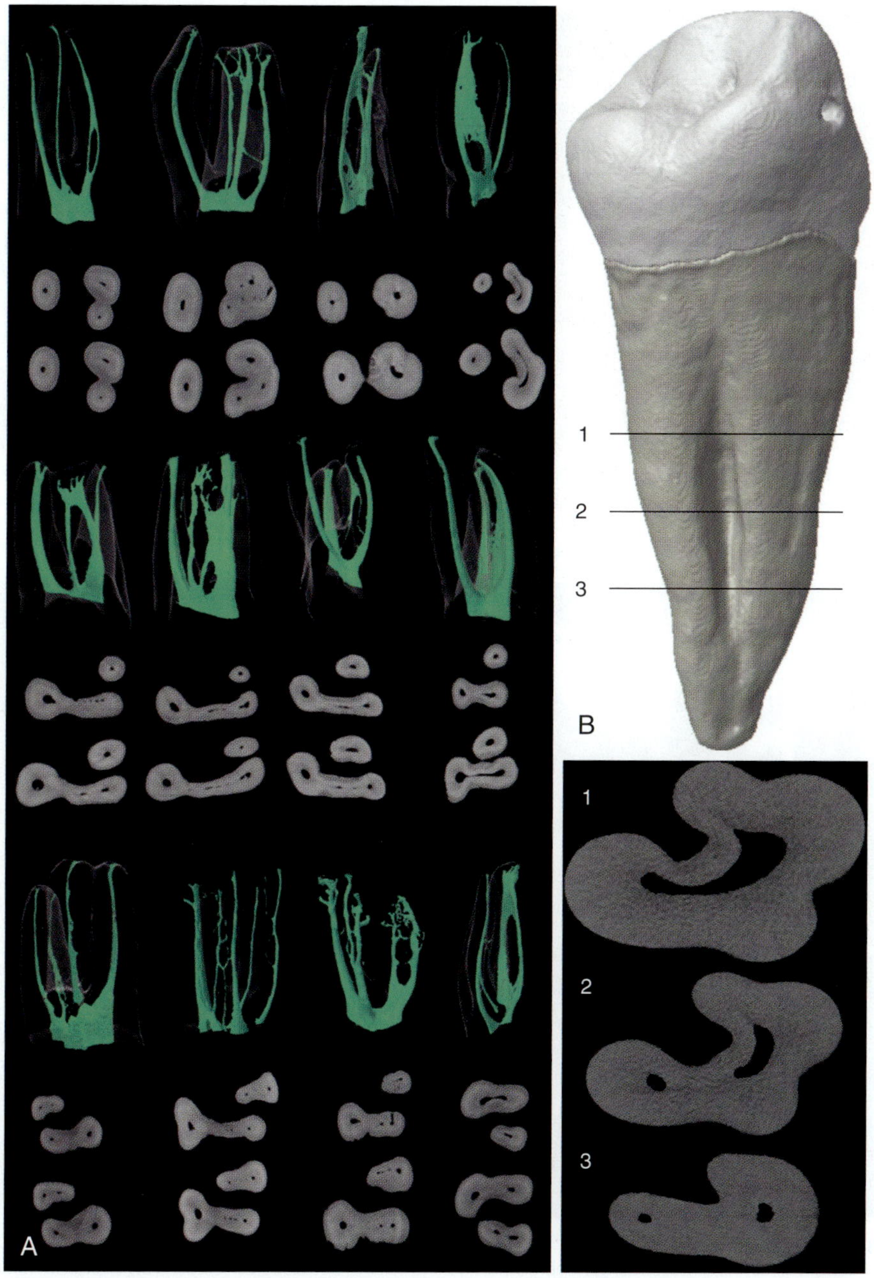

• **Fig. 12.17 A,** Three-dimensional (3D) models and two-dimensional (2D) cross-sections of maxillary second molars with fused roots. Note the complexity of the root canal system with the presence of canal interconnections, apical ramifications and C-shaped canals; **B,** 3D model and 2D cross-sections at different levels of the root of a mandibular first premolar with radicular groove and C-shaped canal configuration.

morphology and occurs more frequently in anterior teeth (Fig. 12.18).[122]

(2) **Gemination:** It is a disturbance during odontogenesis in which partial cleavage of the tooth germ occurs and results in a tooth that has a double or "twin" crown, usually not completely separated, and sharing a common root and pulp space (see Fig. 12.18).[38] The root and pulp are also irregular in morphology.

(3) **Hypercementosis:** This refers to an excessive deposition of nonneoplastic cementum over normal root cementum, which alters the root morphology macroscopic appearance.[38] Its pathogenesis is ambiguous. Most of the cases are idiopathic. Several local and systemic factors are also linked to this condition, such as Paget disease, acromegaly, or vitamin A deficiency (Fig. 12.19).[123]

(4) **Radicular Groove:** This is a developmental depression in the proximal aspect of the root surface.[124] Radicular grooves have been reported as being widespread in Africans and native Australians and are relatively rare in Western Eurasians.[125] It is relevant in clinic care because its depth may act as a reservoir for dental plaque and calculus, increasing the difficulty in the management of periodontal disease.[97,101] In mandibular premolar teeth, its presence has been associated with anatomic complexities of the root canal system, such as canal bifurcation and C-shaped configuration (Fig. 12.20).[97,99,101]

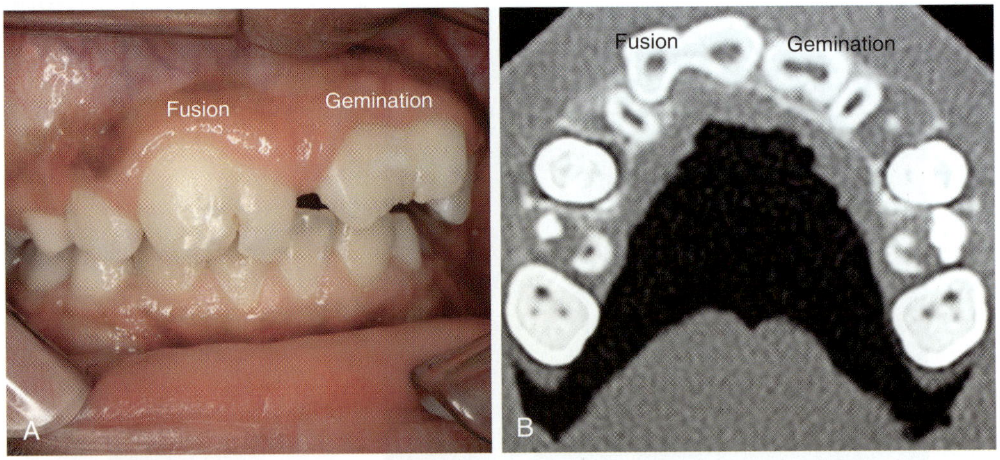

• **Fig. 12.18** **A,** Clinical and **B,** tomographic views of a patient presenting fusion and gemination at the anterior teeth. (Courtesy Dr. Antonis Chaniotis. Published with permission.)

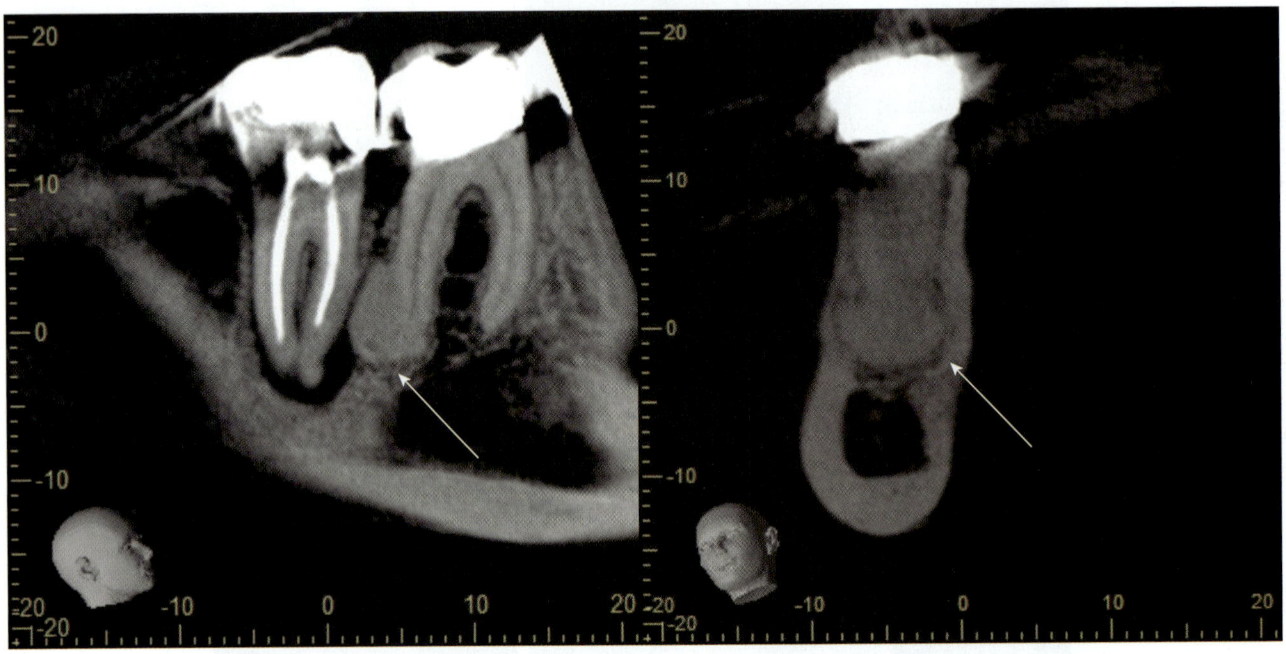

• **Fig. 12.19** Coronal and sagittal cone beam computed tomography (CBCT) images from a distal root of a mandibular first molar presenting hypercementosis *(arrow)*. (Courtesy Dr. Oscar von Stetten. Published with permission.)

Aging

The root canal anatomy is susceptible to changes over the years because of physiologic or pathologic events. Natural physiologic aging tends to modify the root canal system morphology as a result of the deposition of secondary dentin, which starts to form once the tooth erupts and is in occlusion.[126] Consequently, young patients tend to present with large single canals and pulp chambers,[127,128] whereas older patients tend to present with more sharply defined and narrow root canals.[127] Other pathologic or iatrogenic factors can also modify the deposition of dentin including occlusal trauma, periodontal disease, carious lesions, or deep restorative procedures.[129]

In the literature, CBCT imaging technology has been also used to address in vivo root canal morphologic changes caused by aging.[3] Overall, results showed no significant difference between maxillary and mandibular anterior teeth groups regarding age, despite contradictory information can be found. While in mandibular anterior teeth most studies reported a lower prevalence of multiple canals in older patients,[130,131] in maxillary and mandibular premolars and in mandibular molars[128,132] it was observed that there was a progressive decrease of Vertucci's Type I configuration with age. The prevalence of a second canal in the mesiobuccal root of maxillary first and second molars was also evaluated and most studies reported a lower prevalence of this configuration in older patients.[129,133-135]

Root Canal Anatomy of Maxillary and Mandibular Teeth

In this section, illustrations and tables of the characteristics of the anatomy of the human root and root canals are depicted. The teeth

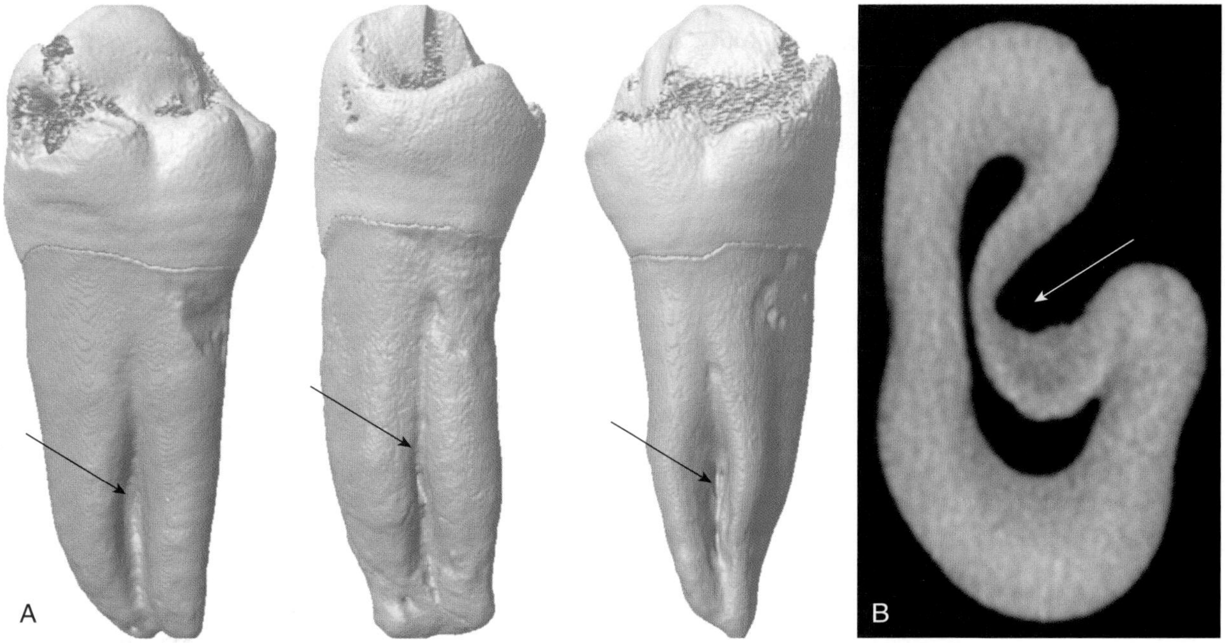

• **Fig. 12.20** **A,** Three-dimensional (3D) micro–computed tomography (micro-CT) models of mandibular premolars showing the external anatomy with the presence of radicular grooves *(arrows)*; **B,** Two-dimensional (2D) cross-section of the root of a mandibular premolar showing radicular groove *(arrow)* and a C-shaped canal configuration.

are paired to facilitate comparison among groups. Root and canal number averages are calculated from a weighted average of a large number of dental anatomy research articles published from a number of sources. Other data listed describe the canal characteristics such as average length of root and crown, canal curvature direction, canal shape, lateral canals, and apical anastomoses. Most important is the listing of the most common anomalies or variation from the normal that may be found in that tooth type. Those data are usually present in numerous case reports from a PubMed search.[3,136]

Of great interest, not only to dentists but also to the science of physical anthropology, are the ethnic variations that can be found in human populations.[11] It is true that genetics plays the main role in determining the shape of a crown and root. Bilateral symmetry is usually present in the antimere of the opposite quadrant but not necessarily so when it comes to variation in root number or anomalous tooth formation. A suite of dental variations in crown and root anatomy may be used to indicate ethnic identity in a population when a number of characteristics appear in a higher incidence of that population. The dental characteristics that are of interest to a physical anthropologist include deep lingual fossa (shoveling) of anterior teeth, dens invaginatus, dens evaginatus (talon cusp and occlusal tubercles of premolar teeth), bifurcated roots of mandibular canines, three roots of maxillary premolar teeth, fusion or single root of the maxillary premolar, multiple roots or multiple canals of mandibular premolar teeth, C-shaped molar teeth, taurodontism, fusion of roots, double canals in palatal or distal root of maxillary molars, four roots with double palatal root in maxillary second molar teeth, and radix entomolaris or the distolingual root of mandibular molar teeth.

Tratman in 1950[11] used extracted teeth to show a number of variations or traits in dental anatomy in Asian populations that varied from the generally accepted Western Eurasian dental anatomy of the time. Since then, many large population studies using full mouth radiographs or the panographic X-ray technique have identified root form variation.[1] A higher incidence of the distolingual root of both first and second mandibular molar teeth in Asian and North American aboriginal native populations is a good example. There have been only a few studies that show a variation in incidence that is gender linked.[137-139] More recently, a series of epidemiologic studies on root canal anatomy using CBCT 3D imaging technology have been published. The most important advantage of using CBCT is the possibility of performing in vivo studies analyzing the full dentition of a large number of patients collected from a specific population in a consecutive manner, addressing the influence of several variables such as ethnicity, aging, gender, and side (left or right) on teeth. Therefore, information regarding the number of roots and root canals and the most frequently observed canal configurations was depicted from a recent epidemiologic study using CBCT technology.[3]

The following tables and figures will help outline the common characteristics of each tooth type and list some variations or anomalies.

Incisors

Morphologic aspects of the root and root canal anatomy of maxillary and mandibular incisors are detailed in Table 12.1, Fig. 12.21, and Appendices 1 to 4 (Summary of Root Numbers and Root Canal Systems of the Permanent Teeth).

The maxillary central incisors are centered in the maxilla, one on either side of the midline, with the mesial surface of each in contact with the mesial surface of the other. The pulp cavity follows the general outline of the crown and root. In this way, the pulp chamber is very narrow in the incisal region and wider in the mesiodistal dimension than in the labiolingual dimension. The maxillary lateral incisor supplements the central incisor in function, and the crowns bear a close resemblance. However, the lateral incisor is smaller in all dimensions except root length.

TABLE 12.1 Morphologic Aspects of the Root and Root Canal Anatomy of Maxillary and Mandibular Incisors

	Maxillary Central Incisor	Maxillary Lateral Incisor	Mandibular Incisors
Overall length	23.6 mm (16.5-32.6 mm)	22.5 mm (17.7-28.9 mm)	C: 20.8 mm (16.9-26.7 mm) L: 22.1 mm (18.5-26.6 mm)
Root length	13.0 mm (6.3-20.3 mm)	13.4 mm (9.6-19.4 mm)	C: 12.6 mm (7.7-17.9 mm) L: 13.5 mm (9.4-18.1 mm)
Number of roots	1 (99.94%) 2 (0.06%)	1 (99.94%) 2 (0.06%)	C: 1 (100%) L: 1 (99.92%) 2 (0.08%)
Number of canals	1 (99.2%) 2 (0.8%)	1 (98.5%) 2 (1.5%)	C: 1 (86.5%) 2 (14.4%) Other (0.1%) L: 1 (79.7%) 2 (20.2%) Other (0.1%)
Canal configuration	Types I (99.2%) IV (0.5%) II (0.1%) III (0.1%) V (0.1%)	Types I (98.5%) II (0.8%) V (0.4%) III (0.2%) IV (0.1%)	C: Types I (86.5%) III (8.1%) V (2.8%) II (2%) IV (1.4%) VII (0.1%) Other (0.1%) L: Types I (79.7%) III (11.9%) V (3.8%) II (2.6%) IV (1.8%) VII (0.1%) Other (0.1%)
Accessory canals	18.9%-42.6% (coronal: 1%; middle: 6%; apical: 93%)	5.5%-26% (coronal: 1%; middle: 8%; apical: 91%)	C: 0%-20% (coronal: 3%; middle: 12%; apical: 85%) L: 0.9%-18% (coronal: 2%; middle: 15%; apical: 83%)
Apical curvature	Straight (75%) Labial (9.3%) Distal (7.8%) Mesial (4.3%) Palatal (3.6%)	Distal (49.2%) Straight (29.7%) Palatal (3.9%) Labial (3.9%) Mesial (3.1%) S-shaped (1.6%) Other (8.6%)	C: Straight (66.7%) Labial (18.8%) Distal (12.5%) S-shaped (2%) L: Straight (54%) Distal (33.3%) Labial (10.7%) S-shaped (2%)
Anomalies	2 canals[141-143] 3 canals[144] 4 canals[145] 2 roots[141-143] Radicular groove[146] Fusion/gemination[147]	2 canals[148] 3 canals[149] 4 canals[150] 2 roots[151] Radicular groove[146] Fusion/gemination[152] Dens invaginatus[153] Dens evaginatus[154] C-shaped[102]	3 canals[155] Fusion/gemination[156] Dens invaginatus[157] 2 roots[158]
Ethnic variations	Deep lingual fossa (shoveling) in Asian and North American native populations	Coronal shoveling present to a lesser degree	

C, Central; *L*, lateral.

Root canal configurations are classified according to Vertucci.[40]

Adapted from Versiani MA, Pereira MR, Pécora JD, Sousa Neto MD: Root canal anatomy of maxillary and mandibular teeth. In Versiani MA, Basrani B, Sousa Neto MD, editors: *The root canal anatomy in permanent dentition*, ed 1. Switzerland, 2018, Springer International Publishing, pp 181–240.

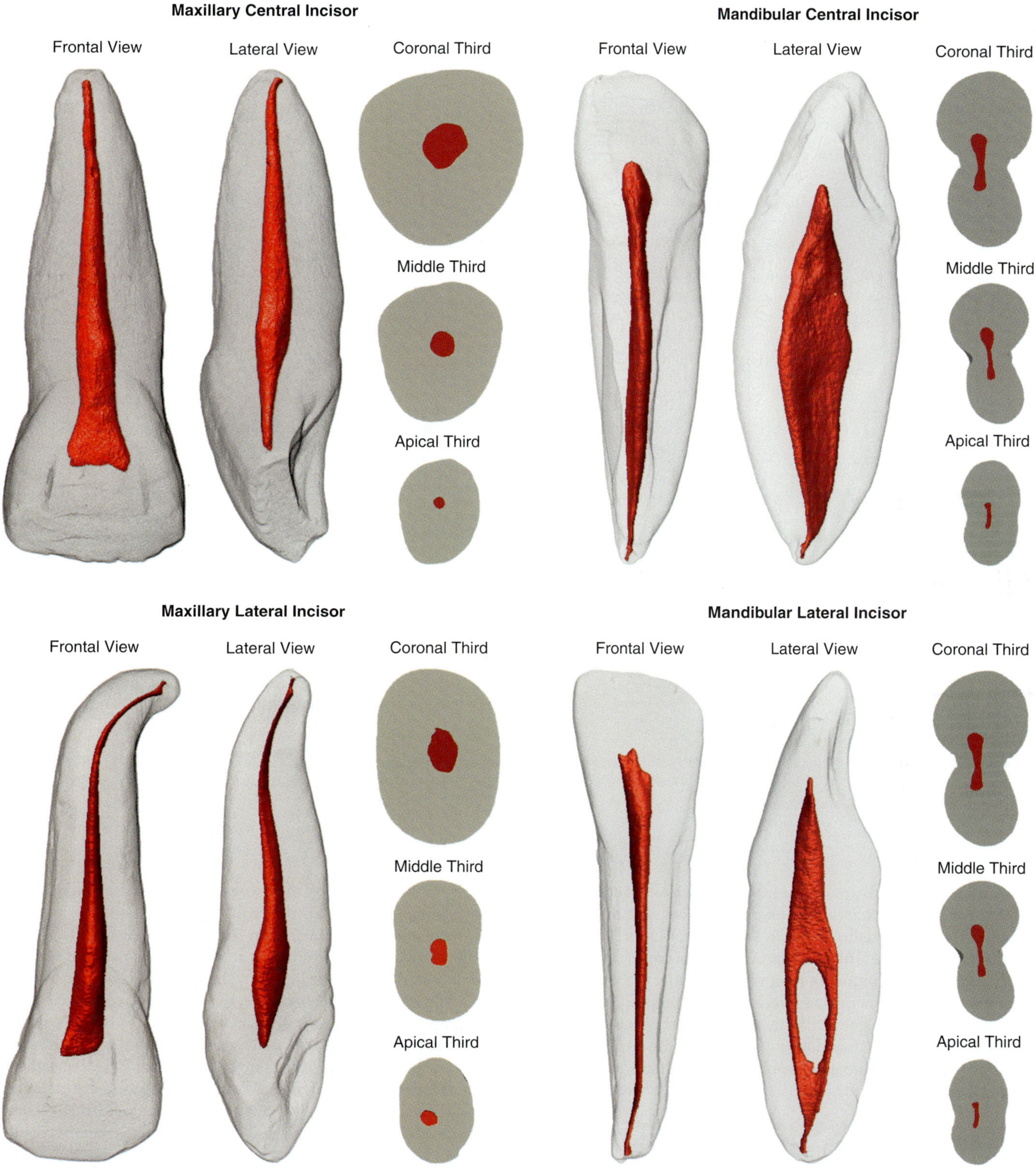

• **Fig. 12.21** Three-dimensional (3D) micro–computed tomography (micro-CT) models and two-dimensional (2D) cross-sections depicting the internal and external anatomy of maxillary and mandibular incisors.

The pulp chamber is narrow in the incisal region and may become very wide at the cervical level of the tooth, whereas pulp horns are usually prominent.[140]

The mandibular central incisors are centered in the mandible, one on either side of the midline, with the mesial surface of each one in contact with the mesial surface of the other. The right and left mandibular lateral incisors are distal to the central incisors. The mandibular central and lateral incisors have smaller mesiodistal dimensions than any of the other teeth. The central incisor is somewhat smaller than the lateral incisor, which is the reverse of the situation in

TABLE 12.2 Morphologic Aspects of the Root and Root Canal Anatomy of Maxillary and Mandibular Canines

	Maxillary Canine	Mandibular Canine
Overall length	26.4 mm (20.0-38.4 mm)	25.9 mm (16.1-34.5 mm)
Root length	16.5 mm (10.8-28.5 mm)	15.9 mm (9.5-22.2 mm)
Number of roots	1 (100%)	1 (98.57%) 2 (1.43%)
Number of canals	1 (97%) 2 (3%)	1 (92.4%) 2 (7.3%) Other (0.3%)
Canal configuration	Types I (98.5%) III (1.2%) II (0.8%) V (0.7%) IV (0.2%) Other (0.1%)	Types I (92.4%) III (2.7%) II (1.9%) IV (1.5%) V (1.2%) Other (0.3%)
Accessory canals	3.4%-30% (coronal: 0%; middle: 10%; apical: 90%)	4.5%-30% (coronal: 4%; middle: 16%; apical: 80%)
Apical curvature	Straight (38.5%) Distal (19.5%) Labial (12.8%) Mesial (12%) Palatal (6.5%) Other (10.7%)	Straight (68.2%) Distal (19.6%) Labial (6.8%) Mesial (0.8%) S-shaped (1.5%) Other (3.1%)
Anomalies	2 canals[159] Dens invaginatus[160]	2 canals[161] 3 canals[162] 2 roots[161]
Ethnic variations		Bifurcated roots in mandibular canines are most common in some Western Eurasian populations

Root canal configurations are classified according to Vertucci.[40]

Adapted from Versiani MA, Pereira MR, Pécora JD, Sousa Neto MD: Root canal anatomy of maxillary and mandibular teeth. In Versiani MA, Basrani B, Sousa Neto MD, editors.: *The root canal anatomy in permanent dentition.* ed 1. Switzerland, 2018, Springer International Publishing, pp 181–240.

the maxilla. These teeth are similar in form and have smooth crown surfaces that show few traces of developmental lines. The mandibular central incisor is the smallest tooth in the mouth, but its labiolingual root dimension is large. This tooth usually has one canal. Two ribbon-shaped canals may be found, but not very frequently (15% and 20% of central and lateral incisors, respectively). The pulp horns are well developed in this tooth group. The mandibular lateral incisor tends to be a little larger than the mandibular central incisor in all dimensions, including the pulp chamber. The pulp canal may taper gently from the apex or narrow abruptly in the last 3 to 4 mm of the root canal.[140]

Canines

Morphologic aspects of the root and root canal anatomy of maxillary and mandibular canines are detailed in Table 12.2, Fig. 12.22, and Appendices 1 to 4 (Summary of Root Numbers and Root Canal Systems of the Permanent Teeth).

Maxillary canines are the longest teeth in the mouth. The crowns are usually as long as those of the maxillary central incisors, and the single roots are longer than those of any of the other teeth. Therefore the maxillary canine has the largest labiolingual root dimension of any tooth and because the pulp cavity corresponds closely to the outline of the tooth, the size of the pulp chamber may also be the largest in the mouth.

The mandibular canine crown is narrower mesiodistally than that of the maxillary canine, although it is just as long in most instances and, in many instances, is longer by 0.5 to 1 mm. The root may be as long as that of the maxillary canine, but usually it is somewhat shorter. The pulp cavity of the mandibular canine tends to be a little shorter than that of the maxillary canine. A not rare variation in the form of the mandibular canine is bifurcated roots, and it is also not uncommon to find two roots or at least two canals. Because the presence of two canals cannot be easily detected radiographically, their presence must be ruled out clinically as well. Some mandibular canines demonstrate an abrupt narrowing of the pulp cavity when passing from the pulp chamber to the pulp canal. Other mandibular canine teeth demonstrate an abrupt narrowing of the pulp canal in the apical region.[140]

Premolars

Morphologic aspects of the root and root canal anatomy of maxillary and mandibular premolars are detailed in Tables 12.3 and 12.4, Fig. 12.23, and Appendices 1 to 4 (Summary of Root Numbers and Root Canal Systems of the Permanent Teeth).

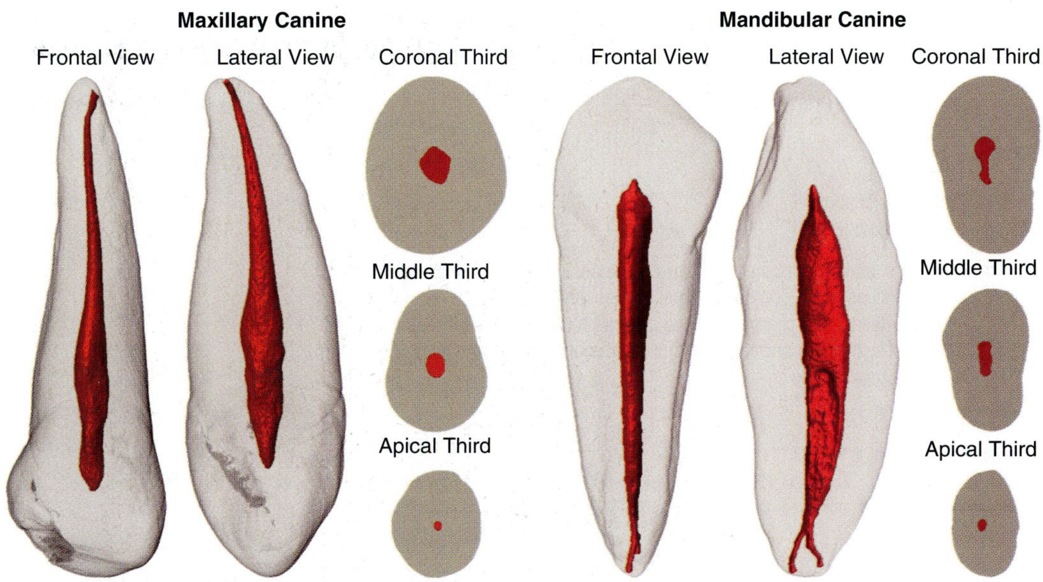

• **Fig. 12.22** Three-dimensional (3D) micro–computed tomography (micro-CT) models and two-dimensional (2D) cross-sections depicting the internal and external anatomy of maxillary and mandibular canines.

TABLE 12.3 Morphologic Aspects of the Root and Root Canal Anatomy of Maxillary Premolars

	Maxillary First Premolar	Maxillary Second Premolar
Overall length	21.5 mm (15.5-28.9 mm)	21.2 mm (15.2-28.4 mm)
Root length	13.4 mm (8.3-19.0 mm)	14.0 mm (8.0-20.6 mm)
Number of roots	2 (55.3%) 1 (43.1%) 3 (1.6%)	1 (86.2%) 2 (13.5%) 3 (0.3%)
Number of canals	2 (77.3%) 1 (20.1%) 3 (1.2%) Other (1.3%)	2 (56.7%) 1 (42.7%) 3 (0.4%) Other (0.3%)
Canal configuration	Types IV (50.1%) I (20.1%) II (17.4%) VI (4.9%) V (3%) III (1.5%) VIII (1.2%) VII (0.4%) Other (1.3%)	Types I (42.7%) II (18.7%) IV (17.6%) V (9.6%) VI (6.3%) III (4%) VII (0.5%) VIII (0.4%) Other (0.3%)
Accessory canals	17.8%-49.5% (coronal: 4.7%; middle: 10.3%; apical: 74%)	12.9%-59.5% (coronal: 4%; middle: 16.2%; apical: 78.2%)
Apical curvature	B: Palatal (36.2%) Straight (27.8%) Distal (14%) Buccal (14%) S-shaped (8%) P: Straight (44.4%) Buccal (27.8%) Distal (14%) Palatal (8.3%) S-shaped (5.5%)	Straight (37.4%) Distal (29.5%) Buccal (15.7%) S-shaped (13%) Distal (4.4%)

Continued

TABLE 12.3 Morphologic Aspects of the Root and Root Canal Anatomy of Maxillary Premolars—cont'd

	Maxillary First Premolar	Maxillary Second Premolar
Anomalies	3 canals[163] Radicular groove[164] Fusion/gemination[165] Dens evaginatus[166]	3 canals[163] Dens invaginatus[167]
Ethnic variations	Caucasian and other populations (excluding Asian and North American native populations) most commonly have 2 roots. Asian and North American native populations most commonly have a single root. Dens evaginatus on the occlusal surfaces of all premolars is more common in Asian and North American native populations	

B, Buccal root/canal; *P*, palatal root/canal.

Root canal configurations are classified according to Vertucci.[40]

Adapted from Versiani MA, Pereira MR, Pécora JD, Sousa Neto MD: Root canal anatomy of maxillary and mandibular teeth. In: Versiani MA, Basrani B, Sousa Neto MD, editors. *The root canal anatomy in permanent dentition*. ed 1. Switzerland, 2018, Springer International Publishing, pp 181–240.

TABLE 12.4 Morphologic Aspects of the Root and Root Canal Anatomy of Mandibular Premolars

	Mandibular First Premolar	Mandibular Second Premolar
Overall length	22.4 mm (17.0-28.5 mm)	22.1 mm (16.8-28.1 mm)
Root length	14.4 mm (9.7-20.2 mm)	14.7 mm (9.2-21.2 mm)
Number of roots	1 (97.5%) 2 (2.5%)	1 (98.5%) 2 (1.5%)
Number of canals	1 (71.3%) 2 (27.9%) 3 (0.1%) Other (0.7%)	1 (84.7%) 2 (15.05%) 3 (0.05%) Other (0.2%)
Canal configuration	Types I (71.3%) V (18.7%) IV (3.5%) III (2.8%) II (2.3%) VI (0.5%) VII (0.1%) VIII (0.1%) Other (0.7%)	Types I (84.7%) V (13.44%) II (0.7%) III (0.5%) IV (0.3%) VI (0.07%) VIII (0.05) VII (0.04%) Other (0.2%)
Accessory canals	8.8%-44.3% (coronal: 4.3%; middle: 16.1%; apical: 78.9%)	4%-48.3% (coronal: 3.2%; middle: 16.4%; apical: 80.1%)
Apical curvature	Straight (47.5%) Distal (34.8%) Lingual (7.1%) Buccal (2.1%) S-shaped (6.4%) Other (2.1%)	Distal (39.8%) Straight (38.5%) Buccal (10.1%) Lingual (3.4%) S-shaped (6.8%) Other (1.4%)
Anomalies	3 canals[113] 4 canals[168] Radicular groove[112] C-shaped[97] Dens evaginatus[169] Dens invaginatus[170] Fusion/gemination[171]	3 canals[172] 4 canals[173] 5 canals[174] 2 roots[175] C-shaped[99] Dens evaginatus[176] Taurodontism[174] Fusion/gemination[177]
Ethnic variations	African American population has a significantly higher incidence of two canals and two roots compared with Caucasian[1]	

Root canal configurations are classified according to Vertucci.[40]

Adapted from Versiani MA, Pereira MR, Pécora JD, Sousa Neto MD: Root canal anatomy of maxillary and mandibular teeth. In: Versiani MA, Basrani B, Sousa Neto MD, editors. The *root canal anatomy in permanent dentition*. ed 1. Switzerland, 2018, Springer International Publishing, pp 181–240.

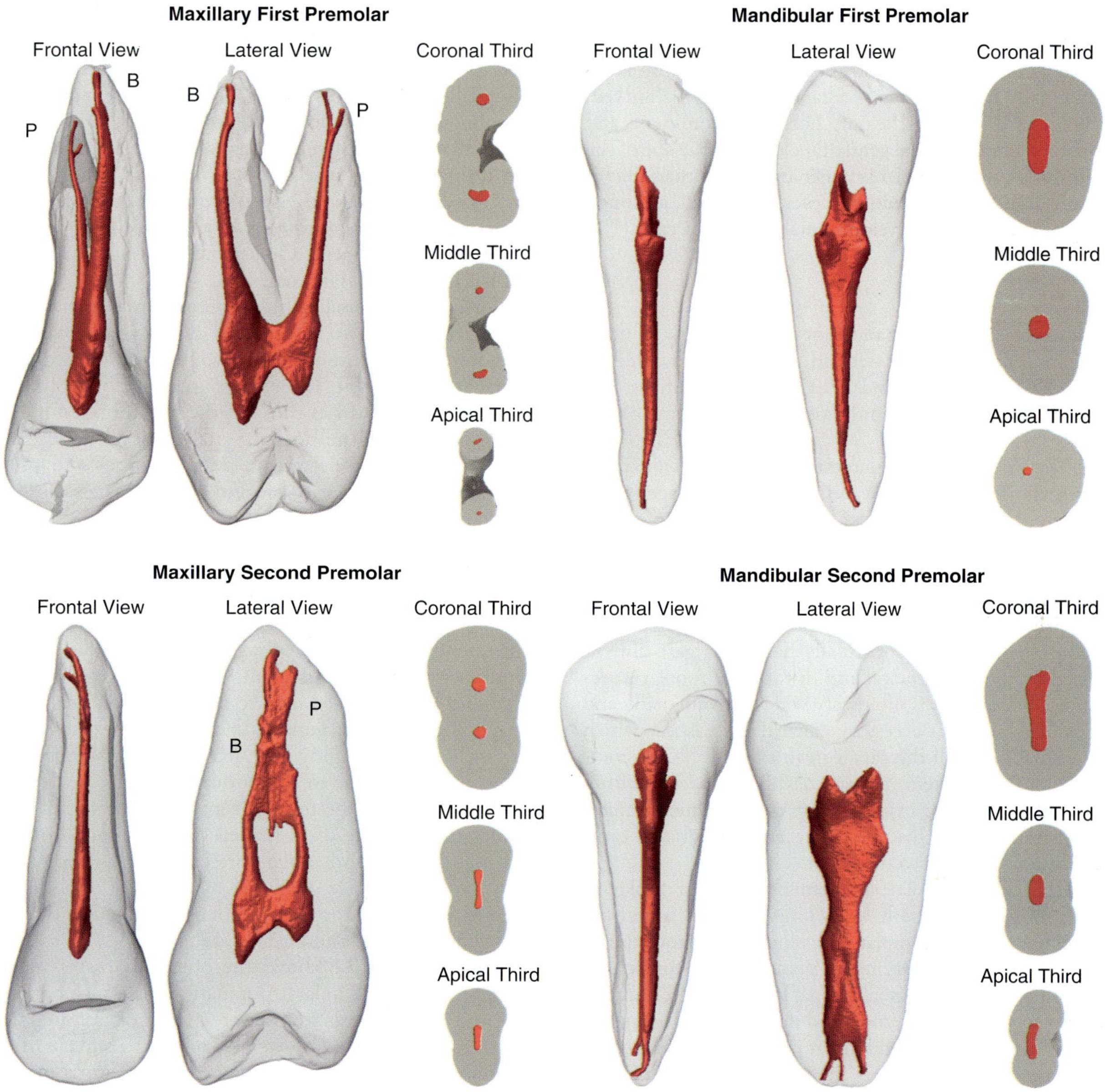

• **Fig. 12.23** Three-dimensional (3D) micro–computed tomography (micro-CT) models and two-dimensional (2D) cross-sections depicting the internal and external anatomy of maxillary and mandibular premolars.

The premolars are so named because they are anterior to the molars in the permanent dentition. The maxillary first premolar has two cusps, a buccal and a lingual, each being sharply defined. The buccal cusp is usually about 1 mm longer than the lingual cusp and, because of that, the pulp horn usually extends further occlusally under the buccal cusp than the lingual cusp. The maxillary first premolar may have two well-developed roots, two root projections that are not fully separated, or one broad root. The majority of maxillary first premolars have two root canals, but a small percentage of teeth may have three roots and three canals that may at times be difficult to see or almost undetectable radiographically. The pulp chamber floor is below the cervical level of all the variations found in this tooth group.

The maxillary second premolar supplements the maxillary first premolar in function and closely resembles it in shape. The maxillary second premolar may have a crown that is noticeably smaller cervico-occlusally and also mesiodistally. However, it may also be larger in those dimensions. Usually the root of the second premolar is as long as, if not a millimeter or so longer than, that of the first premolar. Most maxillary second premolars have only one root and canal. Two roots are possible, although two canals within a single root may also be found. The pulp cavity may demonstrate well-developed pulp horns; others may have blunted or nonexistent pulp horns. The pulp chamber and root canal are very broad in the buccolingual aspect of teeth with single canals.[140]

The mandibular first premolar is always the smallest of the two mandibular premolars, whereas the opposite is true, in many cases, of the maxillary premolars. Most of these teeth have one canal, but two or three canals are possible. The pulp chamber is usually very large, and the pulp cavity may taper gently toward the apex or abruptly as the root canal start. The root of the first premolar usually shows a deep developmental groove that has been associated with complex anatomic features including C-shaped and extra root canals.[140]

The mandibular second premolar usually has three well-formed cusps in most cases: one large buccal cusp and two smaller lingual cusps. However, two-cusped forms of this tooth are also fairly common. It usually has one root and canal that may be curved, usually in the distal direction. The pulp horns are prominent, and the pulp chamber and root canal gently taper toward the apex. The single root of the second premolar is larger and longer than that of the first premolar. The root is seldom, if ever, bifurcated, although some specimens show a deep developmental groove buccally.[140]

Molars

Morphologic aspects of the root and root canal anatomy of maxillary and mandibular first and second molars are detailed in Tables 12.5, 12.6, Figs. 12.24 and 12.25, and Appendices 1 to 4 (Summary of Root Numbers and Root Canal Systems of the Permanent Teeth).

The maxillary molars are the largest and strongest maxillary teeth, by virtue both of their bulk and of their anchorage in the jaws. The crown of this tooth is wider buccolingually than mesiodistally. The maxillary first molar is normally the largest tooth in the maxillary arch. It has four well-developed functioning cusps and one supplemental cusp (the cusp of Carabelli) that is of little practical use. The maxillary first molar normally has three roots and four canals. The palatal root usually has the largest dimensions, followed by the mesiobuccal and distobuccal roots, respectively. The mesiobuccal root is often very wide buccolingually and normally possesses an extra accessory canal named *MB2*, which usually is the smallest of all the canals in this tooth.[140] The complexity of its root canal system may surpass all other teeth within the human dentition. More extensive use of the clinical microscope has contributed to the discovery that not only a fourth canal but other additional canals also may exist.

The maxillary second molar supplements the first molar in function. The roots of this tooth are as long as, if not somewhat longer than, those of the first molar. The tendency for root fusion is greater in the second maxillary molar than in the first maxillary molar, but the palatal root is usually separate. Most often maxillary second molars possess three roots and three canals. The mesiobuccal root of the maxillary second molar is not as complex as that formed in the maxillary first molar. The tendency for a very wide mesiobuccal canal is not present in this tooth group.[140]

The mandibular first molar is usually the largest tooth in the mandibular arch. It has five well-developed cusps, two well-developed roots, one mesial and one distal, which are very broad buccolingually. These roots are widely separated at the apices. The buccolingual cross-section of the mandibular first molar demonstrates a large pulp chamber that may extend well down into the root formation. The mesial root usually has a more complicated canal system because of the presence of two canals and their interconnections. The distal root usually has one large canal, but two canals are often present. Occasionally, a fourth canal is present that has its own separate root.

Normally, the mandibular second molar has four well-developed cusps, two buccal and two lingual, of nearly equal development. The tooth has two well-developed roots, one mesial and one distal. These roots are broad buccolingually, but they are not as broad as those of the first molar, nor are they as widely separated. The buccolingual section of the mandibular second molar demonstrates a pulp chamber and pulp canals that tend to be more variable and complex than those found in the mandibular first molar.[140]

In the literature, first and second permanent molars are the most studied teeth in relation to internal and external anatomy. On the other hand, considering that third molars have variable and unpredictable morphology and also because their extraction is frequently indicated, these teeth are rarely considered for endodontic or restorative treatment. Therefore only a limited number of studies have reported data regarding the internal and external morphology of third molars. In general, these studies show an extremely varied anatomy, with maxillary third molars having one to five roots with one to six root canals, whereas the mandibular third molars have one to four roots and one to six root canals, besides the presence of C-shaped canals. In addition, maxillary and mandibular third molars present a high incidence of fused roots, with an average of 70.1% and 40.7%, respectively, which explains their variations in number, morphology, direction, and arrangement of roots and canals (Table 12.7).

Finally, Table 12.8 shows the outcomes from epidemiologic studies using CBCT in large populations, in which both data from root and root canal anatomy were evaluated, selected, and combined, aiming to offer an overview of the percentage frequency of different number of roots and root canal configuration types in all groups of teeth.

TABLE 12.5 Morphologic Aspects of the Root and Root Canal Anatomy of Maxillary First and Second Molars

	Maxillary First Molar	Maxillary Second Molar
Overall length	20.1 mm (17.0-27.4 mm)	20.0 mm (16.0-26.2 mm)
Root length	MB:12.9 mm (8.5-18.8 mm) DB: 12.2 mm (8.9-15.5mm) P: 13.7 mm (10.6-17.5 mm)	MB: 12.9 mm (9.0-18.2 mm) DB: 12.1 mm (9.0-16.3mm) P: 13.5 mm (9.8-18.8 mm)
Number of roots	3 (97.7%) 2 (1.8%) 4 (0.3%) 1 (0.2%)	3 (73.7%) 2 (14.9%) 1 (10.7%) 4 (0.7%)

TABLE 12.5 Morphologic Aspects of the Root and Root Canal Anatomy of Maxillary First and Second Molars—cont'd

	Maxillary First Molar	Maxillary Second Molar
Number of canals	MB: 2 (60.4%) 1 (29.3%) 3 (0.1%) Other (0.4%) DB: 1 (98.6%) 2 (1.4%) P: 1 (99.26%) 2 (0.7%) Other (0.04%)	MB: 1 (66.1%) 2 (33.7%) 3 (0.05%) Other (0.2%) DB: 1 (99.6%) 2 (0.4%) P: 1 (99.67%) 2 (0.35%) 3 (0.01%) Other (0.01%)
Canal configuration	MB: Types I (39.1%) II (29.3%) IV (26%) V (2%) III (1.6%) VI (1.4%) VII (0.1%) VIII (0.1%) Other (0.4%) DB: Types I (98.6%) II (0.4%) V (0.4%) III (0.3%) IV (0.2%) VI (0.1%) P: Types I (99.26%) II (0.3%) III (0.2%) IV (0.1%) V (0.1%) Other (0.04%)	MB: Types I (39.1%) II (29.3%) IV (26%) V (2%) III (1.6%) VI (1.4%) VII (0.1%) VIII (0.1%) Other (0.4%) DB: Types I (98.6%) II (0.4%) V (0.4%) III (0.3%) IV (0.2%) VI (0.1%) P: Types I (99.26%) II (0.3%) III (0.2%) IV (0.1%) V (0.1%) Other (0.04%)
Accessory canals	MB: 51% (coronal: 10.7%; middle: 13.1%; apical: 58.2%) DB: 36% (coronal: 10.1%; middle: 12.3%; apical: 59.6%) P: 48% (coronal: 9.4%; middle: 11.3%; apical: 61.3%)	MB: 50% (coronal: 10.1%; middle: 14.1%; apical: 65.8%) DB: 29% (coronal: 9.1%; middle: 13.3%; apical: 67.6%) P: 42% (coronal: 8.7%; middle: 11.2%; apical: 70.1%)
Apical Curvature	MB: Distal (78%) Straight (21%) S-shaped (1%) DB: Straight (54%) Mesial (19%) Distal (17%) S-shaped (10%) P: Buccal (55%) Straight (40.7%) Mesial (3.2%) Distal (1.1%)	MB: Distal (54%) Straight (22%) Others (24%) DB: Straight (54%) Mesial (17%) Others (29%) P: Straight (63%) Buccal (37%)
Anomalies	1 canal[178] 5 canals[179] 6 canals[180] 7 canals[181] 8 canals[182] C-shaped[116] 4 roots[85] Taurodontism[68]	1 or 2 canals[183] 5 canals[184] Fusion/gemination[185] Taurodontism[186]
Ethnic variations		

MB, Mesiobuccal root/canal; *DB*, distobuccal root/canal; *P*, palatal root/canal.

Root canal configurations are classified according to Vertucci.[40]

Adapted from Versiani MA, Pereira MR, Pécora JD, Sousa Neto MD: Root canal anatomy of maxillary and mandibular teeth. In Versiani MA, Basrani B, Sousa Neto MD, editors. *The root canal anatomy in permanent dentition.* ed 1. Switzerland, 2018, Springer International Publishing, pp 181–240.

TABLE 12.6 Morphologic Aspects of the Root and Root Canal Anatomy of Mandibular First and Second Molars

	Mandibular First Molar	Mandibular Second Molar
Overall length	20.9 mm (17.0-27.7 mm)	20.6 mm (15.5-25.5 mm)
Root length	M: 14.0 mm (10.6-20.0 mm) D: 13.0 mm (8.1-17.7 mm)	M: 13.9 mm (9.3-18.3 mm) D: 13.0 mm (8.5-18.3 mm)
Number of roots	2 (86.9%) 3 (12.5%) 1 (0.55%) 4 (0.05%)	2 (78.6%) 1 (19%) 3 (2.2%) 4 (0.2%)
Number of canals	M: 1 (2.37%) 2 (96.59%) 3 (0.03%) Other (1.01%) D: 1 (70.3%) 2 (29.56%) Other (0.14%)	M: 2 (87.1%) 1 (12.5%) D: 1 (92.56%) 2 (7.44%)
Canal configuration	M: Types IV (71.3%) II (19.9%) III (2.9%) I (2.37%) V (2.1%) VI (0.3%) VII (0.09%) VIII (0.03%) Other (1.01%) D: Types I (70.3%) II (13%) IV (10.1%) III (3.6%) V (2.7%) VI (0.08%) VII (0.08%) Other (0.14%)	M: Types IV (47.8%) II (32.8%) I (12.5%) III (3.27%) V (3%) VI (0.2%) VII (0.1%) Other (0.33%) D: Types I (92.56%) II (4.4%) IV (2%) III (0.5%) V (0.5%) VI (0.04%)
Accessory canals	M: 45% (coronal: 10.4%; middle: 12.2%; apical: 54.4%) D: 30% (coronal: 8.7%; middle: 10.4%; apical: 57.9%)	M: 49% (coronal: 10.1%; middle: 13.1%; apical: 65.8%) D: 34% (coronal: 9.1%; middle: 11.6%; apical: 68.3%)
Apical curvature	M: Distal (84%) Straight (16%) D: Straight (73.5%) Distal (18%) Mesial (8.5%)	M: Distal (60.8%) Straight (27.2%) Buccal (4%) S-shaped (8%) D: Straight (57.6%) Distal (18.4%) Mesial (13.6%) Buccal (4%) S-shaped (6.4%)
Anomalies	5 canals[187] 6 canals[188] 7 canals[189] Radix[89] Taurodontism[190] Fusion/gemination[191] Isthmus[192] 3 roots[193] C-shaped[194] 3 canals in the distal root[195]	1 canal[196] 2 canals[197] 5 canals[198] Fusion/gemination[199] Isthmus[192] C-shaped[110]
Ethnic variations	Radix entomolaris is most common in Asian and North American native populations	

M, Mesial root/canal; D, distal root/canal.

Root canal configurations are classified according to Vertucci.[40]

Adapted from Versiani MA, Pereira MR, Pécora JD, Sousa Neto MD: Root canal anatomy of maxillary and mandibular teeth. In Versiani MA, Basrani B, Sousa Neto MD, editors: *The root canal anatomy in permanent dentition*, ed 1, Switzerland, 2018, Springer International Publishing, pp 181–240.

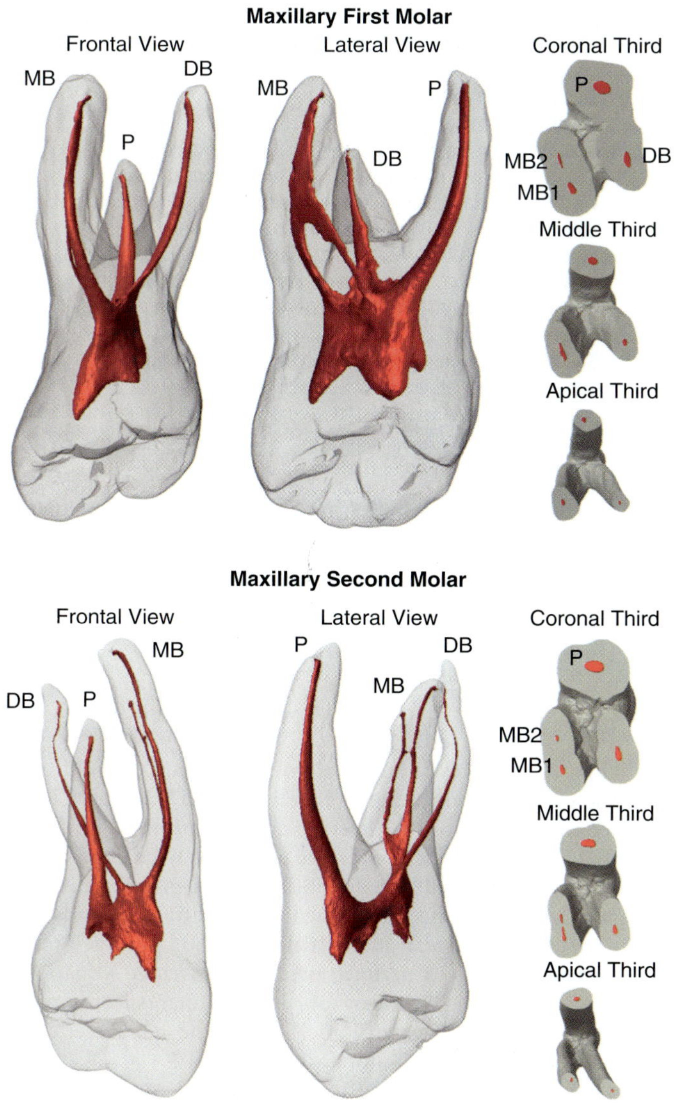

• **Fig. 12.24** Three-dimensional (3D) micro–computed tomography (micro-CT) models and two-dimensional (2D) cross-sections depicting the internal and external anatomy of maxillary molars.

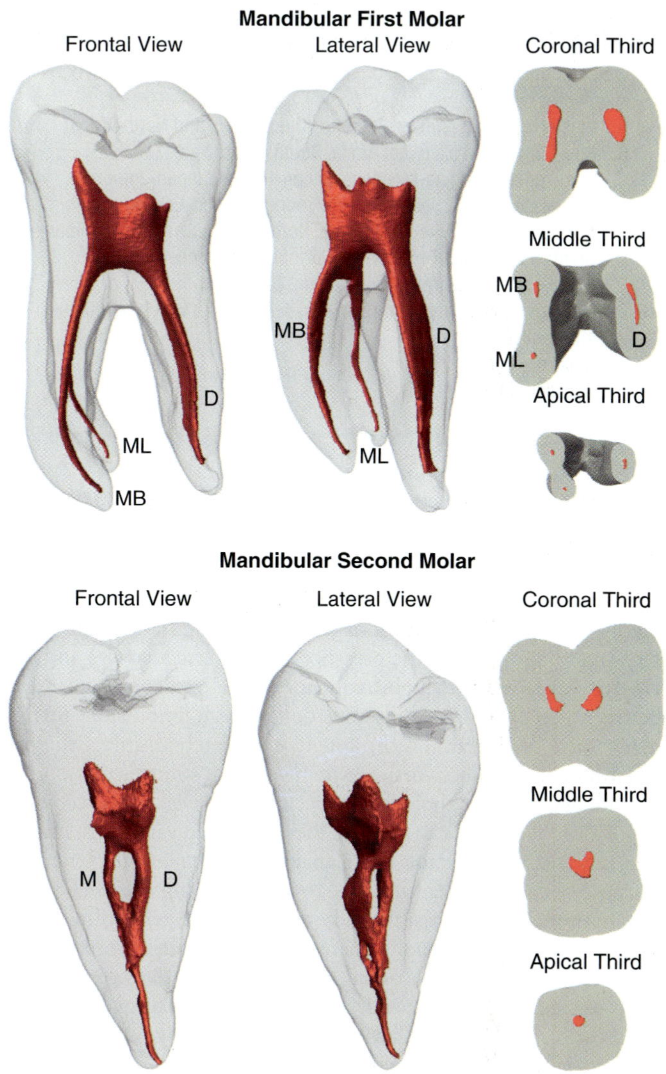

• **Fig. 12.25** Three-dimensional (3D) micro–computed tomography (micro-CT) models and two-dimensional (2D) cross-sections depicting the internal and external anatomy of mandibular molars.

Study Questions

1. Why is there a need for a new root canal morphology classification system?
   A. The Weine's classification system is limited and cannot classify all types of canal configurations.
   B. The Type VIII canal system in the Vertucci classification is unclear.
   C. The Vertucci system does not include all types of canal configurations.
   D. All of the above are correct.
2. Which anterior tooth in the permanent dentition has the highest incidence of two roots with two bifid root apices?
   A. Maxillary central incisor
   B. Maxillary lateral incisor
   C. Maxillary canine
   D. Mandibular central incisor
   E. Mandibular lateral incisor
   F. Mandibular canine
3. Which of the following ethnic groups has the highest incidence of radix entomolaris?
   A. Western Eurasia (Western Europe, Middle East, and North Africa)
   B. Sub-Saharan Africa (West Africa, South Africa, San)
   C. Sino-America (China-Mongolia, Japan-Recent, Japan-Jomon, Northeast Siberia, South Siberia, American Arctic-Eskimo-Aleuts, Northwest North America-Indians, North and South America-Indians)
   D. Sunda-Pacific (South East Asia, Polynesia, Micronesia)
   E. Sahul-Pacific (Australia, New Guinea, Melanesia)
4. Which permanent teeth or roots of permanent teeth is there a high likelihood of finding two or more canals?
   A. Maxillary central incisor
   B. Maxillary first premolar
   C. Maxillary second premolar
   D. Mandibular first premolar
   E. Mandibular second premolar
   F. Mesiobuccal root of the maxillary first molar
   G. Palatal root of the maxillary first molar
   H. Mesial root of the mandibular first molar
   I. Distal root of the of the mandibular first molar
   J. Mesial root of the mandibular second molar
   K. Distal root of the mandibular second molar

Continued

Study Questions—cont'd

5. Which of the following ethnic groups has the highest incidence of dens evaginatus?
   A. Western Eurasia (Western Europe, Middle East, and North Africa)
   B. Sub-Saharan Africa (West Africa, South Africa, San)
   C. Sino-America (China-Mongolia, Japan-Recent, Japan-Jomon, Northeast Siberia, South Siberia, American Arctic-Eskimo-Aleuts, Northwest North America-Indians, North and South America-Indians)
   D. Sunda-Pacific (South East Asia, Polynesia, Micronesia)
   E. Sahul-Pacific (Australia, New Guinea, Melanesia)
6. Dens invaginatus is most commonly associated with which permanent anterior tooth?
   A. Maxillary central incisor
   B. Maxillary lateral incisor
   C. Maxillary canine
   D. Mandibular central or lateral incisor
   E. Mandibular canine
7. Which of the following ethnic groups has the highest incidence of bifurcated permanent mandibular canine root morphology?
   A. Western Eurasia (Western Europe, Middle East, and North Africa)
   B. Sub-Saharan Africa (West Africa, South Africa, San)
   C. Sino-America (China-Mongolia, Japan-Recent, Japan-Jomon, Northeast Siberia, South Siberia, American Arctic-Eskimo-Aleuts, Northwest North America-Indians, North and South America-Indians)
   D. Sunda-Pacific (South East Asia, Polynesia, Micronesia)
   E. Sahul-Pacific (Australia, New Guinea, Melanesia)

Influence of Root Canal Anatomy in Endodontic Procedures

Outcomes of nonsurgical and surgical endodontic procedures are highly influenced by variations in canal configuration and cross-sectional shapes and by the presence of canal irregularities and curvatures. Moreover, the high frequency of fins and communications between canals within the same root make it impossible for any mechanical or chemical technique to completely disinfect the root canal system. It is noteworthy to point out that some factors, such as physiologic aging, pathology, and occlusion, as well as the secondary deposition of dentin, can increase the mentioned variations, making shaping and cleaning the root canals a real challenge. Hence, the purpose of the treatment must be toward reducing the level of contamination as far as possible and entombing the remaining microorganisms. Clinicians ought, therefore, to be aware of complex root canal structures, cross-sectional dimensions, and iatrogenic alterations of canal anatomy. In this way, it is advisable to make a careful diagnostic interpretation based on angled radiographs or tomographic examinations, proper access preparation, and a detailed inspection of the pulp chamber floor. Ideally the search for root canal orifices should be under magnification with high intensity lighting, aiming to improve the treatment outcome.[22]

Essentially, there are three conditions that the clinician faces routinely when undertaking root canal treatment: teeth with vital and irreversibly inflamed pulps, teeth with necrotic pulps with or without primary apical periodontitis, and retreatment cases because of posttreatment apical periodontitis. In teeth with irreversible pulpitis, infection is usually restricted to the coronal parts of the canal and is easily controlled by abundant irrigation of the pulp chamber with sodium hypochlorite (NaOCl) after completion of the access cavity preparation. Then, under strict aseptic conditions, the clinician needs to clean the canal by removing the inflamed vital pulp tissue as much as possible.[216] In necrotic untreated teeth and treated teeth referred for retreatment because of posttreatment apical periodontitis an infection is established in the root canal system. In these cases, in addition to cleaning the canal from the necrotic pulp tissue or the previous filling material, the clinician also needs to combat infection. The successful treatment outcome will depend on how effective the clinician is in achieving these goals.[217]

One of the main steps of root canal treatment involved with disinfection of the root canal system is chemomechanical preparation. This procedure is of utmost importance for cleaning and disinfection, because instruments and irrigants act primarily in the main canal. Numerous studies have shown that instrumentation and irrigation are highly effective in reducing the intracanal bacterial populations.[218-220] Clinical[219,221] and in vitro studies[222,223] have clearly demonstrated that preparation using an antibacterial irrigating solution such as NaOCl significantly enhances disinfection compared with irrigation with saline or water. Most canals instrumented and irrigated with 2.5% NaOCl have the number of bacteria reduced 10^2 to 10^5 fold, which has resulted in an overall reduction of bacterial counts of 95% to 99%.[222,224] Regular exchange and the use of large volumes of irrigants should maintain the optimum antibacterial effectiveness of the NaOCl solution, compensating for the effects of concentration.[222] It has been reported that the beneficial effects of using NaOCl compared with saline are only observed after significant apical enlargement.[219,221] Several studies agree that supplementary irrigation methods using laser- or ultrasonic-activated irrigation and positive-pressure pulsed-delivery systems perform better than syringe irrigation in the removal of dentin debris or soft tissue remnants from fins and noninstrumented oval extensions,[33-35] but the relative effectiveness of each method is still unclear.[216]

Accessory canals and dentinal tubules present similar challenges for root canal irrigation but at a different length scale. Accessory canals (10 µm to 200 µm) are perceived to be smaller than the main canal but larger than dentinal tubules (0.5 µm to 3.2 µm).[25] Irrigant flow in accessory canals and dentinal tubules is driven by the flow in the main canal and appears to be limited to a depth approximately twice their diameter, whereas diffusion dominates irrigant transport beyond that point. Therefore optimum irrigant refreshment in the main canal to maintain a favorable concentration gradient, any increase in the temperature of the irrigants, and a longer application period could enhance particle transport. Nevertheless, the importance of accessory canal and dentinal tubule cleaning for the success of root canal treatment has been debated.[225]

Despite the optimal antibacterial effect obtained by chemomechanical preparation, clinical bacteriologic studies have demonstrated that 30% to 60% of the previously infected root canals still have detectable levels of bacteria after instrumentation.[218-220,226-228] The main reasons for bacteria to persist after chemomechanical procedures is that they are resistant to treatment or they are unaffected by instruments/irrigants. Although some microorganisms have been shown to be resistant to some endodontic antimicrobial agents,[229] resistance both to debridement and to NaOCl is highly unlikely to occur. Bacteria usually survive after treatment procedures not because they are more

TABLE 12.7 **Summary of the Studies on Root and Root Canal Anatomy of Third Molars**

				NUMBER OF ROOTS (%)				NUMBER OF ROOT CANALS (%)				
References	Population	Study Type	Sample	1	2	3	≥4	1	2	3	4	≥5
Maxillary Third Molars												
Barret[200]	USA	Sectioning	32	28.1	34.4	37.5	-	-	-	-	-	-
Piñeda & Kuttler[17]	Mexico	Radiograph	292	-	-	-	-	21.4	51.7	21.0	5.9	-
Green[18]	USA	Sectioning	100 MB	-	-	-	-	63.0	37.0	-	-	-
Hession[201]	Australia	Radiograph	12	-	-	-	-	16.7	25.0	58.3	-	-
Pécora et al.[202]	Brazil	Clearing	50	-	-	-	-	-	-	68.0	32.0	-
Guerisoli et al.[203]	Brazil	Clearing	155	12.3	1.9	81.9	3.8[a]	4.5	11.6	67.8	14.2	1.9
Stropko[204]	USA	Retrospective	25	-	-	-	-	-	20.0	60.0	20.0	-
Sidow et al.[111]	USA	Clearing	150	15.3	32	45.3	7.4	7.4[c]	3.3	57.3	27.3	4.7[d]
Ng et al.[205]	Burma	Clearing	72	19.4	19.4	55.6	5.6	5.6	25.0	47.2	22.2	-
Alavi et al.[206]	Thailand	Clearing	151	1.3	6.6	88.1	4.0	9.9	11.3	48.3	29.1	1.3
Weng et al.[207]	China	Clearing	43	-	-	-	-	27.9	11.6	44.2	16.3	-
Sert et al.[208]	Turkey	Clearing	290	35.5	28.6	34.1	1.7	12.4	29.7	46.9	11.0	-
Cosic et al.[209]	Croatia	Sectioning	56	8.9	5.4	83.9	1.8	7.1	7.1	75.0	10.8	-
Tomaszewska et al.[210]	Poland	Micro-CT	78	38.5	-	61.5	-	23.1	15.4	46.1	15.4	-
Mandibular Third Molars												
Barret[200]	USA	Sectioning	32	15.6	71.9	12.5	-	-	-	-	-	-
Piñeda & Kuttler[17]	Mexico	Radiograph	259	-	-	-	-	-	65.8	26.4	7.8	-
Green[18]	USA	Sectioning	100 MR	-	-	-	-	74.0	26.0	-	-	-
Hession[201]	Australia	Radiograph	3	-	-	-	-	-	33.3	66.7	-	-
Zakhary et al.[211]	Egypt	Radiograph	374	11.8	82.3	5.9	-	11.8	17.6	64.7	5.9	-
Guerisoli et al.[203]	Brazil	Clearing	114	51.8	46.4	1.8	-	12.3	69.3	18.4	-	-
Sidow et al.[111]	USA	Clearing	150	16.7	76.7	5.3	1.3	7.3[e]	16.7	55.3	16.7	4.0[d]
Gulabivala et al.	Burma	Clearing	58	-	100	-	-	1.7	51.7	44.8	1.7	-
Gulabivala et al.[212]	Thailand	Clearing	173	11.6	86.7	21.2	0.6	6.4	64.1	28.3	5.2	-
Sert et al.[208]	Turkey	Clearing	370	24.9	69.5	5.4	0.3	10.8	52.7	17.3	18.6	0.5
Kuzekanani et al.[213]	Iran	Clearing	150	21.4	72.6	5.3	0.7	10.0[f]	52.0	32.7	5.3	-
Cosic et al.[209]	Croatia	Sectioning	50	56.0	44.0	-	-	4.0	6.0	90.0	-	-
Park et al.[214]	South Korea	Tomography	214	41.6[b]	56.5	1.9	-	-	-	-	-	-

MB, Mesiobuccal root; *micro-CT*, micro–computed tomography; *MR*, mesial root.
[a]0.6% of the sample had five roots; [b]3.7% of the sample had C-shaped canals;
[c]4.7% of the sample had C-shaped canals; [d]0.7% of the sample had six canals;
[e]4.0% of the sample had C-shaped canals; [f]3.3% of the sample had C-shaped canals.
Adapted from Ahmad IA, Azzeh MM, Zwiri AMA, Haija MASA, Diab MM: Root and root canal morphology of third molars in a Jordanian subpopulation, *Saudi Endod J* 6:113, 2016.[215]

TABLE 12.8 Combined Data From CBCT Studies on Root and Root Canal Morphology of Maxillary and Mandibular Permanent Teeth

	Number of	NUMBER OF ROOTS (%)				ROOT CANAL CONFIGURATION (%)								
Maxillary	**Teeth**	**1**	**2**	**3**	**4**	**I**	**II**	**III**	**IV**	**V**	**VI**	**VII**	**VIII**	**Other**
Central incisor	3125	99.94	0.06	0	0	99.20	0.1	0.1	0.5	0.1	0	0	0	0
Lateral incisor	3068	99.94	0.06	0	0	98.50	0.8	0.2	0.1	0.4	0	0	0	0
Canine	3148	100	0	0	0	97.0	0.8	1.2	0.2	0.7	0	0	0	0.1
1st premolar	2575	43.1	55.3	1.6	0	20.10	17.4	1.5	50.1	3.0	4.9	0.4	1.2	1.3
2nd premolar	2345	86.2	13.5	0.3	0	42.70	18.7	4.0	17.6	9.6	6.3	0.5	0.4	0.3
1st molar	8934	0.2	1.8	97.7	0.3									
MB root	8934					39.10	29.3	1.6	26.0	2.0	1.4	0.1	0.1	0.4
DB root	7473					98.60	0.4	0.3	0.2	0.4	0.01	0	0	0
P root	8445					99.26	0.3	0.2	0.1	0.1	0	0	0	0.04
2nd molar	9570	10.7	14.9	73.7	0.7									
MB root	9353					66.10	15.3	2.8	13.0	1.9	0.6	0.1	0.05	0.2
DB root	9570					99.60	0.2	0.07	0.1	0.03	0	0	0	0
P root	9570					99.67	0.1	0.1	0.1	0.05	0	0	0.01	0.01
Mandibular		**1**	**2**	**3**	**4**	**I**	**II**	**III**	**IV**	**V**	**VI**	**VII**	**VIII**	**Other**
Central incisor	11860	100	0	0	0	86.5	2.0	8.1	1.4	2.8	0	0.1	0	0.1
Lateral incisor	11805	99.92	0.08	0	0	79.7	2.6	11.9	1.8	3.8	0	0.1	0	0.1
Canine	10009	98.57	1.43	0	0	92.4	1.9	2.7	1.5	1.2	0	0	0	0.3
1st premolar	6043	97.5	2.5	0	0	71.3	2.3	2.8	3.5	18.7	0.5	0.1	0.1	0.7
2nd premolar	6350	98.5	1.5	0	0	84.7	0.7	0.5	0.3	13.4	0.07	0.04	0.05	0.2
1st molar	7388	0.55	86.9	12.5	0.05									
Mesial root	7388					2.37	19.9	2.9	71.3	2.1	0.3	0.09	0.03	1.01
Distal root	6712					70.3	13.0	3.6	10.1	2.7	0.08	0.08	0	0.14
2nd molar	7439	19.0	78.6	2.2	0.2									
Mesial root	6734					12.5	32.8	3.27	47.8	3.0	0.2	0.1	0	0.33
Distal root	7439					92.56	4.4	0.5	2.0	0.5	0.04	0	0	0

Root canal configurations are classified according to Vertucci.[40]

CBCT, Cone beam computed tomography; *DB,* distobuccal; *MB,* mesiobuccal; *P,* palatal.

Adapted from Versiani MA, Pereira MR, Pécora JD, Sousa Neto MD: Root canal anatomy of maxillary and mandibular teeth. In Versiani MA, Basrani B, Sousa Neto MD, editors. *The root canal anatomy in permanent dentition.* ed 1. Switzerland, 2018, Springer International Publishing, pp 181–240.

resistant but because they were not affected by instruments and irrigants. Bacteria remain unaffected because treatment was inadequately carried out (small instrumentation, too short of the apex, poor irrigation, etc.) or because bacteria were located in difficult-to-reach anatomic areas. In fact, the latter is the main reason for bacterial persistence even after diligent endodontic treatment. Canals that are flattened or oval-shaped are often not properly cleaned and disinfected by current hand or rotary NiTi instrumentation using reaming motions.[230,231] Recesses are commonly left untouched at the extremities of the canal's largest diameter (Fig. 12.26).[232,233] In addition to harboring remnants of pulp tissue or bacterial biofilms, such recesses may also be packed with dentin chips generated and pushed therein by rotating instruments.[32,33] Packed debris can interfere with the quality of obturation and, in infected root canals, can harbor bacteria to serve as a potential source of persistent infection.[234]

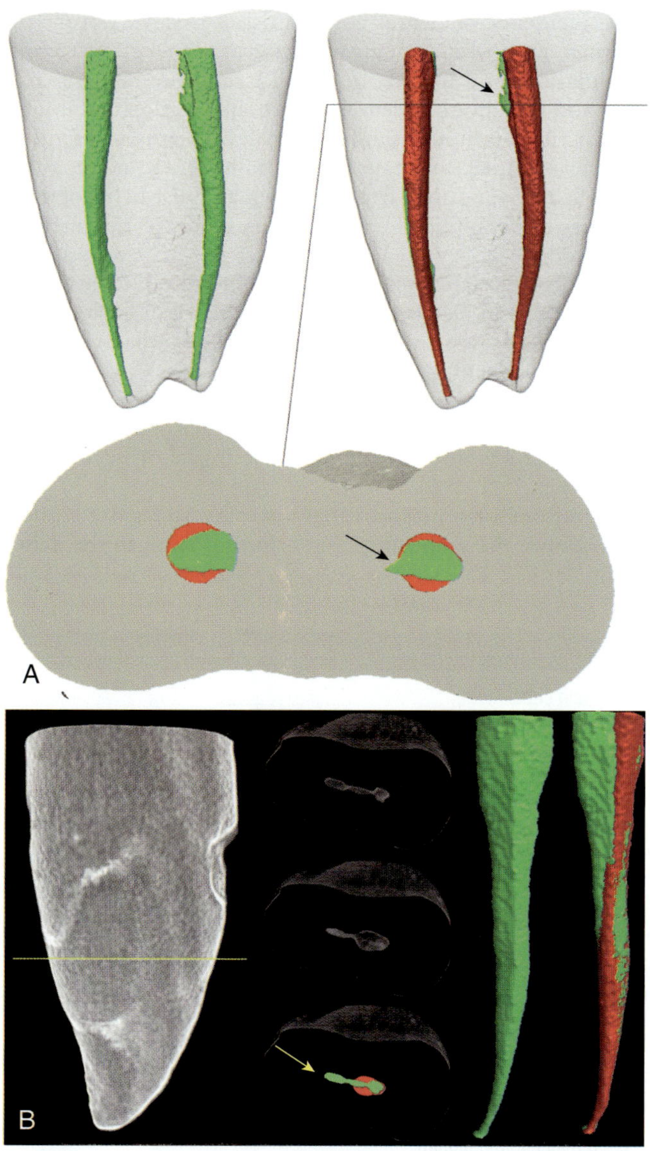

• **Fig. 12.26** Three-dimensional (3D) micro–computed tomography (micro-CT) models and two-dimensional (2D) cross-sections of a **(A)** mesial root of mandibular molar and **(B)** a mandibular canine showing the superimposed root canal system before *(in green)* and after *(in red)* preparation with rotary nickel-titanium (NiTi) instruments, depicting the irregularities of the root canal shape left untouched *(arrows)*.

In summary, anatomic complexities represent physical constraints that pose a serious challenge to adequate disinfection. The main root canal lumen and minor anatomic irregularities are usually incorporated into preparation and affected by NaOCl, but bacteria and organic tissue may remain in areas not reached by instruments and irrigants.[234-236] Unaffected areas include root canal walls untouched by instruments, recesses, dentinal tubules, isthmuses, lateral canals, and apical ramifications.[230,235-237] These areas are usually not affected because of the inherent physical limitations of instruments and the short retention time of irrigants within the root canal system. If bacterial biofilms remain in untouched and unaffected canal areas, the treatment outcome is put at risk.[217]

Clinical Outcome Remarks

Diagnosis and treatment planning for endodontic therapy involves the reading of clinical radiographs to determine the morphology of the root and root canals. Perhaps the most important aspect of assessing the degree of difficulty of an endodontic treatment is to know the dental anatomy of the tooth requiring treatment. A thorough cleaning and shaping of a canal system is accomplished by observing and anticipating the complexity of the internal pulpal anatomy. The Washington Study[238] and others since[239,240] have shown that not all teeth that received endodontic treatment enjoyed the same degree of success. By inference, it was the realization that all teeth in the dental arch did not have a simple, single "hollow-tube" to the apical foramen and differed in root morphology in many ways.

The dental literature is replete with examples of complex dental root anatomy, and many of the cases are a result of endodontic failure to heal because of missed, poorly filled, or unfilled canal systems. The importance of learning both the normal and variations from the normal morphology of roots and root canals in the human dentition cannot be overemphasized. The dental anatomy research of root number and root shape will help the clinician in a search for canal systems within the pulp chamber or along the canal length.

Teeth that have a broad diameter, usually in the labiolingual or buccolingual direction, have been shown to have a high incidence of double or even multiple canal numbers and apical foramen outlets. Multiple root canal classification systems have been proposed over the years, each with their own advantages and shortcomings. Standard radiographs may only give clues to the complexity of canal systems. Even 3D radiographs like the CBCT need a high resolution and a degree of skill in interpreting the image of a root canal system. The clinicians who know their ability and can anticipate a complex root canal system during instrumentation can be more thorough in cleansing and shaping the entire root canal space. The highest success rate and the lowest number of failed treatments will result as a treatment outcome when dental anatomy is taken into account.

Conclusions

Knowledge of both normal root and root canal anatomy is most critically important to perform successful endodontic treatment. The science of dental anatomy of the human dentition helps a dentist not only in restorative dentistry for coronal anatomy, but also in endodontic therapy with root and root canal anatomy research. A number of conclusions may be drawn from reading the information in this chapter about human root canal anatomy as it relates to a proposed endodontic treatment:

- The study of human anatomy of teeth started in the 16th century. Root anatomy and canal anatomy research specifically was the interest of dental anatomists for over a century, as shown by a perusal of the important early dental literature. However, its importance in performing root canal treatment has made this the province of modern endodontology.
- One can see the progression of knowledge and introduction of new techniques when the historical perspective is taken into account, with three loosely defined phases of root canal morphology research.
- The two most popular canal classification systems by Weine or Vertucci and more lately by Ahmed et al. using the Universal Tooth Number system all have their advantages and difficulties when applied to clinical or laboratory root anatomy research. Nonetheless, our understanding of the complexity of the morphology of pulp space has expanded from the earlier studies.

- The root canal components consist of the coronal pulp chamber, which is continuous with the radicular root canal space in anterior teeth. Posterior teeth may have a chamber floor when the radicular roots form in their embryonic development.
- The morphology of the pulp space is distinctive for each tooth in the arch, but each tooth also has its own unique morphology of root shape and canal number as controlled by many genetic factors.
- By analyzing the detailed description and tables of root number and canal number for each tooth in the dental arch, one can see the relative likelihood of finding more than one canal per root in a clinical situation.
- Radix entomolaris, or the extra distal root on the lingual aspect of mandibular molar teeth, is most common in Asian and North American native indigenous populations, and the incidence may be as high as 20% in some populations.
- A comparison of root number, canal number, root size, and many other variable features of the human dentition in the printed tables shows that the more posterior tooth is slightly smaller and less distinctive in its dental characteristics.
- The incidence of dental characteristics that vary from the normal may occur in greater numbers in certain ethnic populations and include things like root number in maxillary and mandibular premolar teeth, bifurcation and double canals in mandibular canines, dens evaginatus in premolar teeth, C-shaped, and taurodont anomalies, to name a few. All of these variations from the average must be recognized as possible complications before endodontic treatment is initiated.
- Root canal anatomy influences treatment procedures in a number of ways and may result in a high degree of difficulty, which would be a reason to refer treatment to a specialist for endodontic treatment.
- One of the most common reasons for a failed root canal treatment is to not anticipate or locate the double or multiple canal system in roots that have a wide labiolingual or buccolingual diameter.
- Illustrations of root and canal anatomy will aid a student to visualize the shape and dimensions of teeth in the dental arch.

Study Questions

8. When a tooth requires endodontic therapy, which of the following statements is correct with respect to root canal morphology?
   A. There is usually one straight canal within any given root.
   B. The canal is usually positioned more to the facial.
   C. Assume that each root may contain more than one canal system.
   D. Canals tend to become larger with age.
9. The resurgence of studies of human root and canal anatomy may be attributed to:
   A. Newer laboratory and clinical radiographic techniques such as CBCT
   B. Additional populations to be studied in dental schools outside of North America and Europe
   C. A growing interest in endodontics and realization that knowledge of variations in dental root anatomy is the key to successful treatment
   D. The resurrection of practitioners wanting to prove the "theory of focal infection" and the inability to seal root canals 100%
10. Krasner and Rankow proposed a series of laws to aid in determining the position of the pulp chamber and the location and number of canal entrances. The "law of centrality" means that the pulp chamber is centered in the tooth:
    A. At the midpoint of the crown
    B. At the level of the cementoenamel junction
    C. 1 mm occlusal to the furcation
    D. But it is highly variable in its vertical position
11. Krasner and Rankow proposed a series of laws to aid in determining the position of the pulp chamber and the location and number of canal entrances. The "law of color change" means that:
    A. The walls are darker than the floor of the pulp chamber.
    B. The walls are lighter than the floor of the pulp chamber.
    C. Both the walls and floor become lighter in color with secondary dentin with age.
12. Which of the following are routinely used for the identification of all canal orifices during molar root canal therapy during routine access opening procedure?
    A. Good illumination
    B. Magnification
    C. CBCT imaging
    D. Specialized instruments
13. Which of the following components of the root canal system are primarily cleansed by chemomechanical means?
    A. Accessory canals.
    B. Lateral canals.
    C. Main canal.
    D. Furcation canals.
14. In cross-section, root canal shapes are classified as:
    A. Oval
    B. Round
    C. Long oval
    D. Flattened
    E. Irregular
    F. Regular
15. Which of the following are consistent with a transverse anastomosis as found in some ovoid-shaped roots, which contain two or more canal systems?
    A. It is also called an isthmus.
    B. It is a narrow, ribbon-shaped communication between two root canals.
    C. It always contains vital tissue.
    D. It can contain necrotic debris.
    E. It may contain biofilm.
16. In the study by Schäfer and colleagues that measured the degree of curvature of more than 1000 root canals from all groups of teeth by using radiographs, the highest degree of curvature was found in the:
    A. Mesiobuccal canal of maxillary molars
    B. Distobuccal canal of maxillary molars
    C. Mesial canals of mandibular molars
    D. Distal canals of mandibular molars
17. Which of the following developmental anomaly condition is characterized by an enlarged pulp chamber and root trunk and a shortening of the roots?
    A. Dens invaginatus
    B. Dens evaginatus
    C. Taurodontism
    D. Radix entomolaris
    E. C-shaped canal system
18. Which of the following root canal anatomy factors are known to affect the outcome of surgical and nonsurgical endodontics?
    A. Canal irregularities
    B. Canal curvature
    C. The presence of fins
    D. The deposition of secondary and tertiary dentin with age

ANSWERS

Answer Box 12

1. Correct Answer: D. Both the Weine and Vertucci classification systems have limitations because neither can classify all canal system configurations. The Vertucci classification system has sometimes been used inconsistently. One example is how a three-rooted maxillary first premolar with a single canal in each root is classified. Some authors classify this as Type VIII, whereas others classify the canal system in each root (mesiobuccal, distobuccal, and palatal) as Type I canal systems.
2. Correct answer: F. The mandibular canine is the most common anterior tooth to have a bifurcated root. The root bifurcates into a labial and lingual root and can have an incidence of 3% to 5%, especially in some Western Eurasian populations.
3. Correct answer: C. Radix entomolaris is an extra root found in a lingual position of the permanent mandibular molar. Therefore a mandibular molar would have three roots (mesial, distolingual, and distobuccal) instead of the typical two roots (mesial and distal). This is most common in Asian and North American aboriginal populations in the permanent mandibular first molar. The incidence can be 20% or more in these populations.
4. Correct answers: B, F, H and J. Each of these teeth or roots of teeth generally have a significantly high incidence of two canals.
5. Correct answer: C. Dens evaginatus presents as a tubercle on the occlusal surface of any of the premolars and has the highest incidence in Asian and North American aboriginal populations.
6. Correct answer: B. This infolding of enamel can be mild to severe. Oehlers classified dens invaginatus as Types 1, 2, and 3 with the most severe form being Type 3. The permanent maxillary lateral incisor is the tooth that is most commonly affected with this developmental anomaly.
7. Correct answer: A. Although the incidence of bifurcated permanent mandibular canines is relatively low, it is highest in the Western Eurasian ethnic group (approximately 5% to 6%) in both ancient and modern populations.
8. Correct answer: C. It is critically important to always assume that a root has more than one canal until proven otherwise. Failure to find, cleanse, instrument, and obturate the entire root canal system in any given tooth will likely result in treatment failure. Although some roots and some teeth may be more likely to be elongated in cross-section and not round, there are a few rare anomalies of double canal formation that may not appear on a standard radiograph.
9. Correct answer: D. Only statement "D" is incorrect. The practitioners who are trying to discredit the safety and successfulness of current endodontic treatment use the century-old and faulty research methods and papers. The third phase of human root anatomy research uses modern imaging systems and have expanded to include worldwide dental schools and touch on all ethnicities.
10. Correct answer: B. Understanding the series of laws outlined by Krasner and Rankow is critical to endodontic treatment success and conversely, avoiding iatrogenic errors that could lead to adverse treatment outcome.
11. Correct answer: B. Understanding the series of laws outlined by Krasner and Rankow is critical to endodontic treatment success and conversely, avoiding iatrogenic errors that could lead to adverse treatment outcome.
12. Correct answers: A, B and D. Although CBCT can be a valuable adjunct in endodontics, it should be used selectively where indicated. The standard of practice and ALARA concept (As Low As Reasonably Achievable) do not dictate special imaging techniques in routine operations.
13. Correct answer: C. Accessibility, location, and orientation of the main canal in a tooth receiving endodontic therapy are the primary reasons for the importance of mechanical means in canal cleansing.
14. Correct answer: A, B, C, D and E. The internal shape of the root canal system mirrors the external shape of the root, which is variable in its morphology throughout the dentition.
15. Correct answers: A, B, D and E. The four answers describe a root canal system transverse anastomosis. This difficult to reach region of a root canal system is contaminated both in necrotic therapy and in retreatment endodontics and thus difficult to seal effectively.
16. Correct answers: A and C. The greater the canal curvature, the more complex the endodontic treatment of that canal becomes. Also, age leads to narrower canal systems, which compounds the complexity.
17. Correct answer: C. This accurately describes taurodontism. Teeth most commonly involved are the molars and possibly premolars. As a result of the large volume of pulp contained in the large pulp chamber, excess bleeding may be challenging to manage on performing an access opening when the pulp is highly inflamed.
18. Correct answer: A, B, C and D. All of the factors listed previously contribute to increasing the complexity of root canal treatment and the clinical outcome.

References

1. Trope M, Elfenbein L, Tronstad L: Mandibular premolars with more than one root canal in different race groups, *J Endod* 12(8):343–345, 1986.
2. Perrini N, Versiani MA: Historical overview of the studies on root canal anatomy. In Versiani MA, Basrani B, Sousa Neto MD, editors: *The root canal anatomy in permanent dentition*, ed 1, Switzerland, 2018, Springer International Publishing, pp 3–16.
3. Martins JN, Versiani MA: CBCT and micro-CT on the study of root canal anatomy. In Versiani MA, Basrani B, Sousa Neto MD, editors: *The root canal anatomy in permanent dentition*, ed 1, Switzerland, 2018, Springer International Publishing, pp 89–180.
4. Basrani B, Versiani MA: Contemporary strategies for teaching internal anatomy of teeth. In Versiani MA, Basrani B, Sousa Neto MD, editors: *The root canal anatomy in permanent dentition*, ed 1, Switzerland, 2018, Springer International Publishing, pp 373–390.
5. Ingle JI: The need for endodontic instrument standardization, *Oral Surg Oral Med Oral Pathol* 8(11):1211–1213, 1955.
6. Kuttler Y: Microscopic investigation of root apexes, *J Am Dent Assoc* 50(5):544–552, 1955.
7. Skidmore AE, Bjorndal AM: Root canal morphology of the human mandibular first molar, *Oral Surg Oral Med Oral Pathol* 32(5):778–784, 1971.
8. Davis SR, Brayton SM, Goldman M: The morphology of the prepared root canal: a study utilizing injectable silicone, *Oral Surg Oral Med Oral Pathol* 34(4):642–648, 1972.
9. Green D: Morphology of the pulp cavity of the permanent teeth, *Oral Surg Oral Med Oral Pathol* 8(7):743–759, 1955.
10. Green D: A stereomicroscopic study of the root apices of 400 maxillary and mandibular anterior teeth, *Oral Surg Oral Med Oral Pathol* 9(11):1224–1232, 1956.
11. Tratman EK: A comparison of the teeth of people; Indo-European racial stock with the Mongoloid race stock, *Dent Rec (London)* 70(3):63–68, 1950.
12. Versiani MA, Pécora JD, Sousa-Neto MD: Microcomputed tomography analysis of the root canal morphology of single-rooted mandibular canines, *Int Endod J* 46(9):800–807, 2013.

13. Kato A, Ohno N: Construction of three-dimensional tooth model by micro-computed tomography and application for data sharing, *Clin Oral Investig* 13(1):43–46, 2009.
14. Scott R, Turner II C: *The anthropology of modern human teeth*, Cambridge, 2000, Cambridge University Press.
15. Dummer PM, McGinn JH, Rees DG: The position and topography of the apical canal constriction and apical foramen, *Int Endod J* 17(4):192–198, 1984.
16. Weine FS, Healey HJ, Gerstein H, Evanson L: Canal configuration in the mesiobuccal root of the maxillary first molar and its endodontic significance, *Oral Surg Oral Med Oral Pathol* 28(3):419–425, 1969.
17. Piñeda F, Kuttler Y: Mesiodistal and buccolingual roentgenographic investigation of 7,275 root canals, *Oral Surg Oral Med Oral Pathol* 33(1):101–110, 1972.
18. Green D: Double canals in single roots, *Oral Surg Oral Med Oral Pathol* 35(5):689–696, 1973.
19. Piñeda F: Roentgenographic investigation of the mesiobuccal root of the maxillary first molar, *Oral Surg Oral Med Oral Pathol* 36(2):253–260, 1973.
20. Seidberg BH, Altman M, Guttuso J, Suson M: Frequency of two mesiobuccal root canals in maxillary permanent first molars, *J Am Dent Assoc* 87(4):852–856, 1973.
21. Vertucci F, Seelig A, Gillis R: Root canal morphology of the human maxillary second premolar, *Oral Surg Oral Med Oral Pathol* 38(3):456–464, 1974.
22. Versiani MA, Ordinola-Zapata R: Root canal anatomy: implications in biofilm disinfection. In Chavez de Paz L, Sedgley C, Kishen A, editors: *Root canal biofilms*, ed 1, Toronto, 2015, Springer International Publishing AG, pp 23–52.
23. De Deus QD: Frequency, location, and direction of the lateral, secondary, and accessory canals, *J Endod* 1(11):361–366, 1975.
24. Ordinola-Zapata R, Versiani MA, Bramante CM: Root canal components. In Versiani MA, Basrani B, Sousa Neto MD, editors: *The root canal anatomy in permanent dentition*, ed 1, Switzerland, 2018, Springer International Publishing, pp 31–46.
25. Tjäderhane L: Dentin basic structure, composition, and function. In Versiani MA, Basrani B, Sousa Neto MD, editors: *The root canal anatomy in permanent dentition*, ed 1, Switzerland, 2018, Springer International Publishing, pp 17–30.
26. Krasner P, Rankow HJ: Anatomy of the pulp-chamber floor, *J Endod* 30(1):5–16, 2004.
27. Jou YT, Karabucak B, Levin J, Liu D: Endodontic working width: current concepts and techniques, *Dent Clin North Am* 48(1):323–335, 2004.
28. Wu MK, R'oris A, Barkis D, Wesselink PR: Prevalence and extent of long oval canals in the apical third, *Oral Surg Oral Med Oral Pathol Oral Radiol Endod* 89(6):739–743, 2000.
29. Weller RN, Niemczyk SP, Kim S: Incidence and position of the canal isthmus. Part 1. Mesiobuccal root of the maxillary first molar, *J Endod* 21(7):380–383, 1995.
30. Vertucci FJ: Root canal morphology and its relationship to endodontic procedures, *Endod Topics* 10(1):3, 2005.
31. Hsu YY, Kim S: The resected root surface. The issue of canal isthmuses, *Dent Clin North Am* 41(3):529–540, 1997.
32. De-Deus G, Marins J, Silva EJ, et al.: Accumulated hard tissue debris produced during reciprocating and rotary nickel-titanium canal preparation, *J Endod* 41(5):676–681, 2015.
33. Versiani MA, Alves FR, Andrade-Junior CV, et al.: Micro-CT evaluation of the efficacy of hard-tissue removal from the root canal and isthmus area by positive and negative pressure irrigation systems, *Int Endod J* 49(11):1079–1087, 2016.
34. Keleş A, Alcin H, Sousa-Neto MD, Versiani MA: Supplementary steps for removing hard tissue debris from isthmus-containing canal systems, *J Endod* 42(11):1677–1682, 2016.
35. Leoni GB, Versiani MA, Silva-Sousa YT, et al.: Ex vivo evaluation of four final irrigation protocols on the removal of hard-tissue debris from the mesial root canal system of mandibular first molars, *Int Endod J* 50(4):398–406, 2017.
36. Perez R, Neves AA, Belladonna FG, et al.: Impact of the needle insertion depth on the removal of hard-tissue debris, *Int Endod J* 50(6):560–568, 2016.
37. von Arx T: Frequency and type of canal isthmuses in first molars detected by endoscopic inspection during periradicular surgery, *Int Endod J* 38(3):160–168, 2005.
38. American Association of Endodontists: *Glossary of endodontics terms*, ed 9, Chicago, 2016, American Association of Endodontists.
39. Ricucci D, Siqueira Jr JF: Fate of the tissue in lateral canals and apical ramifications in response to pathologic conditions and treatment procedures, *J Endod* 36(1):1–15, 2010.
40. Vertucci FJ: Root canal anatomy of the human permanent teeth, *Oral Surg Oral Med Oral Pathol* 58(5):589–599, 1984.
41. Vertucci FJ, Williams RG: Root canal anatomy of the mandibular first molar, *J N J Dent Assoc* 45(3):27–28, 1974.
42. Vertucci FJ, Anthony RL: A scanning electron microscopic investigation of accessory foramina in the furcation and pulp chamber floor of molar teeth, *Oral Surg Oral Med Oral Pathol* 62(3):319–326, 1986.
43. Versiani MA, Pécora JD, Sousa-Neto MD: Update in root canal anatomy of permanent teeth using microcomputed tomography. In Basrani B, editor: *Endodontic irrigation: chemical disinfection of the root canal system*, ed 1, Switzerland, 2015, Springer International Publishing AG, pp 15–44.
44. Gutierrez JH, Aguayo P: Apical foraminal openings in human teeth. Number and location, *Oral Surg Oral Med Oral Pathol Oral Radiol Endod* 79(6):769–777, 1995.
45. Versiani MA, Ahmed HM, Sousa-Neto MD, et al.: Unusual deviation of the main foramen from the root apex, *Braz Dent J* 27(5):589–591, 2016.
46. Mizutani T, Ohno N, Nakamura H: Anatomical study of the root apex in the maxillary anterior teeth, *J Endod* 18(7):344–347, 1992.
47. Morfis A, Sylaras SN, Georgopoulou M, et al.: Study of the apices of human permanent teeth with the use of a scanning electron microscope, *Oral Surg Oral Med Oral Pathol* 77(2):172–176, 1994.
48. Marceliano-Alves MF, Sousa-Neto MD, Fidel SR, et al.: Shaping ability of single-file reciprocating and heat-treated multifile rotary systems: a micro-CT study, *Int Endod J* 48(12):1129–1136, 2015.
49. Nagy CD, Szabó J, Szabó J: A mathematically based classification of root canal curvatures on natural human teeth, *J Endod* 21(11):557–560, 1995.
50. Weine FS: *Endodontic therapy*, ed 5, St. Louis, 1996, Mosby-Yearbook, Inc.
51. Schneider SW: A comparison of canal preparations in straight and curved root canals, *Oral Surg Oral Med Oral Pathol* 32(2):271–275, 1971.
52. Weine FS: *Endodontic therapy*, ed 3, St. Louis, 1982, Mosby.
53. Pruett JP, Clement DJ, Carnes Jr DL: Cyclic fatigue testing of nickel-titanium endodontic instruments, *J Endod* 23(2):77–85, 1997.
54. Schäfer E, Diez C, Hoppe W, Tepel J: Roentgenographic investigation of frequency and degree of canal curvatures in human permanent teeth, *J Endod* 28(3):211–216, 2002.
55. Peiris R: Root and canal morphology of human permanent teeth in a Sri Lankan and Japanese population, *Anthropol Sci* 116(2):123–133, 2008.
56. Gupta S, Sinha DJ, Gowhar O, et al.: Root and canal morphology of maxillary first premolar teeth in North Indian population using clearing technique: an in vitro study, *J Conserv Dent* 18(3):232–236, 2015.
57. Bulut DG, Kose E, Ozcan G, et al.: Evaluation of root morphology and root canal configuration of premolars in the Turkish individuals using cone beam computed tomography, *Eur J Dent* 9(4):551–557, 2015.
58. Elnour M, Khabeer A, AlShwaimi E: Evaluation of root canal morphology of maxillary second premolars in a Saudi Arabian subpopulation: an in vitro microcomputed tomography study, *Saudi Dent J* 28(4):162–168, 2016.
59. Ahmed HMA, Versiani MA, De-Deus G, Dummer PMH: A new system for classifying root and root canal morphology, *Int Endod J* 50(8):761–770, 2017.

60. Versiani MA, Ordinola-Zapata R, Keleş A, et al.: Middle mesial canals in mandibular first molars: a micro-CT study in different populations, *Arch Oral Biol* 61(1):130–137, 2016.
61. Versiani MA, Martins JN, Basrani B: 3D visual glossary of terminology in root and root canal anatomy. In Versiani MA, Basrani B, Sousa Neto MD, editors: *The root canal anatomy in permanent dentition*, ed 1, Switzerland, 2018, Springer International Publishing, pp 391–422.
62. Hargreaves KM, Cohen S: *Cohen's pathways of the pulp*, ed 10, St. Louis, 2011, Mosby.
63. Nanci A, Ten Cate AR: *Ten Cate's oral histology: development, structure, and function*, ed 8, St. Louis, 2013, Elsevier.
64. Woelfel JB, Scheid RC: *Dental anatomy: its relevance to dentistry*, ed 6, Philadelphia, 2002, Lippincott Williams & Wilkins.
65. Jafarzadeh H, Azarpazhooh A, Mayhall JT: Taurodontism: a review of the condition and endodontic treatment challenges, *Int Endod J* 41(5):375–388, 2008.
66. Gardner DG, Girgis SS: Taurodontism, shovel-shaped incisors and the Klinefelter syndrome, *Dent J* 44(8):372–373, 1978.
67. Regezi JA, Sciubba JJ, Jordan RCK: *Oral pathology: clinical pathologic correlations*, ed 5, St. Louis, 2008, Saunders/Elsevier.
68. Sert S, Bayrl G: Taurodontism in six molars: a case report, *J Endod* 30(8):601–602, 2004.
69. Mjör IA: The structure of taurodont teeth, *ASDC J Dent Child* 39(6):459–463, 1972.
70. Keith A: Problems relating to the teeth of the earlier forms of prehistoric man, *Proc R Soc Med* 6(Odontol Sect):103–124, 1913.
71. Shaw JC: Taurodont teeth in South African races, *J Anat* 62(Pt 4):476–498, 1928.
72. Tsesis I, Shifman A, Kaufman AY: Taurodontism: an endodontic challenge. Report of a case, *J Endod* 29(5):353–355, 2003.
73. Metgud S, Metgud R, Rani K: Management of a patient with a taurodont, single-rooted molars associated with multiple dental anomalies: a spiral computerized tomography evaluation, *Oral Surg Oral Med Oral Pathol Oral Radiol Endod* 108(2):e81–e86, 2009.
74. Hülsmann M: Dens invaginatus: aetiology, classification, prevalence, diagnosis, and treatment considerations, *Int Endod J* 30(2):79–90, 1997.
75. Ridell K, Mejáre I, Matsson L: Dens invaginatus: a retrospective study of prophylactic invagination treatment, *Int J Paediatr Dent* 11(2):92–97, 2001.
76. Rotstein I, Stabholz A, Heling I, Friedman S: Clinical considerations in the treatment of dens invaginatus, *Endod Dent Traumatol* 3(5):249–254, 1987.
77. Oehlers FA: Dens invaginatus (dilated composite odontome). I. Variations of the invagination process and associated anterior crown forms, *Oral Surg Oral Med Oral Pathol* 10(11):1204–1218, 1957.
78. Poyton HG, Morgan GA: Dens in dente, *Dent Radiogr Photogr* 39(2):27–33, 1966.
79. Ruprecht A, Sastry KA, Batniji S, Lambourne A: The clinical significance of dental invagination, *J Pedod* 11(2):176–181, 1987.
80. Oehlers FA: Dens invaginatus (dilated composite odontome). II. Associated posterior crown forms and pathogenesis, *Oral Surg Oral Med Oral Pathol* 10(12):1302–1316, 1957.
81. Oehlers FA, Lee KW, Lee EC: Dens evaginatus (evaginated odontome). Its structure and responses to external stimuli, *Dent Pract Dent Rec* 17(7):239–244, 1967.
82. Levitan ME, Himel VT: Dens evaginatus: literature review, pathophysiology, and comprehensive treatment regimen, *J Endod* 32(1):1–9, 2006.
83. Kocsis G, Marcsik A, Kókai E, Kocsis K: Supernumerary occlusal cusps on permanent human teeth, *Acta Biol Szeged* 46(1-2):71–82, 2002.
84. Merrill RG: Occlusal anomalous tubercles on premolars of Alaskan Eskimos and Indians, *Oral Surg Oral Med Oral Pathol* 17(4):484–496, 1964.
85. Versiani MA, Pécora JD, Sousa-Neto MD: Root and root canal morphology of four-rooted maxillary second molars: a micro-computed tomography study, *J Endod* 38(7):977–982, 2012.
86. Carlsen O, Alexandersen V: Radix mesiolingualis and radix distolingualis in a collection of permanent maxillary molars, *Acta Odontol Scand* 58(5):229–236, 2000.
87. Souza-Flamini LE, Leoni GB, Chaves JF, et al.: The radix entomolaris and paramolaris: a micro-computed tomographic study of 3-rooted mandibular first molars, *J Endod* 40(10):1616–1621, 2014.
88. Calberson FL, De Moor RJ, Deroose CA: The radix entomolaris and paramolaris: clinical approach in endodontics, *J Endod* 33(1):58–63, 2007.
89. De Moor RJ, Deroose CA, Calberson FL: The radix entomolaris in mandibular first molars: an endodontic challenge, *Int Endod J* 37(11):789–799, 2004.
90. Carlsen O, Alexandersen V: Radix paramolaris in permanent mandibular molars: identification and morphology, *Scan J Dent Res* 99(3):189–195, 1991.
91. Tratman EK: Three-rooted lower molars in man and their racial distribution, *Br Dent J* 64:264–274, 1938.
92. Turner 2nd CG: Three-rooted mandibular first permanent molars and the question of American Indian origins, *Am J Phys Anthropol* 34(2):229–241, 1971.
93. Cooke 3rd HG, Cox FL: C-shaped canal configurations in mandibular molars, *J Am Dent Assoc* 99(5):836–839, 1979.
94. Keith A, Knowles FH: The description of teeth of palaeolithic man from Jersey, *J Anat Physiol* 46(pt 1):12–27, 1911.
95. Jafarzadeh H, Wu YN: The C-shaped root canal configuration: a review, *J Endod* 33(5):517–523, 2007.
96. Melton DC, Krell KV, Fuller MW: Anatomical and histological features of C-shaped canals in mandibular second molars, *J Endod* 17(8):384–388, 1991.
97. Fan B, Yang J, Gutmann JL, Fan M: Root canal systems in mandibular first premolars with C-shaped root configurations. Part I: microcomputed tomography mapping of the radicular groove and associated root canal cross-sections, *J Endod* 34(11):1337–1341, 2008.
98. Solomonov M, Paqué F, Fan B, et al.: The challenge of C-shaped canal systems: a comparative study of the self-adjusting file and ProTaper, *J Endod* 38(2):209–214, 2012.
99. Cleghorn BM, Christie WH, Dong CC: Anomalous mandibular premolars: a mandibular first premolar with three roots and a mandibular second premolar with a C-shaped canal system, *Int Endod J* 41(11):1005–1014, 2008.
100. Fan B, Ye W, Xie E, et al.: Three-dimensional morphological analysis of C-shaped canals in mandibular first premolars in a Chinese population, *Int Endod J* 45(11):1035–1041, 2012.
101. Gu YC, Zhang YP, Liao ZG, Fei XD: A micro-computed tomographic analysis of wall thickness of C-shaped canals in mandibular first premolars, *J Endod* 39(8):973–976, 2013.
102. Bóveda C, Fajardo M, Millán B: Root canal treatment of an invaginated maxillary lateral incisor with a C-shaped canal, *Quintessence Int* 30(10):707–711, 1999.
103. Manning SA: Root canal anatomy of mandibular second molars. Part II. C-shaped canals, *Int Endod J* 23(1):40–45, 1990.
104. Yang ZP, Yang SF, Lin YC, et al.: C-shaped root canals in mandibular second molars in a Chinese population, *Endod Dent Traumatol* 4(4):160–163, 1988.
105. Weine FS, Pasiewicz RA, Rice RT: Canal configuration of the mandibular second molar using a clinically oriented in vitro method, *J Endod* 14(5):207–213, 1988.
106. Jin GC, Lee SJ, Roh BD: Anatomical study of C-shaped canals in mandibular second molars by analysis of computed tomography, *J Endod* 32(1):10–13, 2006.
107. Al-Fouzan KS: C-shaped root canals in mandibular second molars in a Saudi Arabian population, *Int Endod J* 35(6):499–504, 2002.
108. Haddad GY, Nehme WB, Ounsi HF: Diagnosis, classification, and frequency of C-shaped canals in mandibular second molars in the Lebanese population, *J Endod* 25(4):268–271, 1999.
109. Cheung LH, Cheung GS: Evaluation of a rotary instrumentation method for C-shaped canals with micro-computed tomography, *J Endod* 34(10):1233–1238, 2008.

110. Fan B, Cheung GS, Fan M, et al.: C-shaped canal system in mandibular second molars: Part I—Anatomical features, *J Endod* 30(12):899–903, 2004.
111. Sidow SJ, West LA, Liewehr FR, Loushine RJ: Root canal morphology of human maxillary and mandibular third molars, *J Endod* 26(11):675–678, 2000.
112. Gu Y, Zhang Y, Liao Z: Root and canal morphology of mandibular first premolars with radicular grooves, *Arch Oral Biol* 58(11):1609–1617, 2013.
113. Ordinola-Zapata R, Bramante CM, Villas-Boas MH, et al.: Morphologic micro–computed tomography analysis of mandibular premolars with three root canals, *J Endod* 39(9):1130–1135, 2013.
114. Rice RT, Gilbert Jr BO: An unusual canal configuration in a mandibular first molar, *J Endod* 13(10):513–515, 1987.
115. Martins JN, Quaresma S, Quaresma MC, Frisbie-Teel J: C-shaped maxillary permanent first molar: a case report and literature review, *J Endod* 39(12):1649–1653, 2013.
116. De Moor RJ: C-shaped root canal configuration in maxillary first molars, *Int Endod J* 35(2):200–208, 2002.
117. Yang ZP, Yang SF, Lee G: The root and root canal anatomy of maxillary molars in a Chinese population, *Endod Dent Traumatol* 4(5):215–218, 1988.
118. Ordinola-Zapata R, Monteiro Bramante C, Gagliardi Minotti P, et al.: Micro-CT evaluation of C-shaped mandibular first premolars in a Brazilian subpopulation, *Int Endod J* 48(8):807–813, 2015.
119. Yu X, Guo B, Li KZ, et al.: Cone-beam computed tomography study of root and canal morphology of mandibular premolars in a western Chinese population, *BMC Med Imaging* 12(18), 2012.
120. Lu TY, Yang SF, Pai SF: Complicated root canal morphology of mandibular first premolar in a Chinese population using the cross section method, *J Endod* 32(10):932–936, 2006.
121. Fan B, Min Y, Lu G, Yang J, et al.: Negotiation of C-shaped canal systems in mandibular second molars, *J Endod* 35(7):1003–1008, 2009.
122. Camargo AJ, Arita ES, Watanabe PC: Fusion or gemination? An unusual mandibular second molar, *Int J Surg Case Rep* 21:73–77, 2016.
123. Shoor H, Sujir N, Mutalik S, Pai KM: Hypercementosis: a rare finding in a patient with systemic lupus erythematosus, *BMJ Case Rep* pii:bcr2013202370, 2014. https://doi.org/10.1136/bcr-2013-202370.
124. Tomes CS: *A manual of dental anatomy, human and comparative*, ed 8, New York, 1923, MacMillan Co.
125. Cleghorn B, Christie W, Dong C: The root and root canal morphology of the human mandibular first premolar: a literature review, *J Endod* 33(5):509–516, 2007.
126. Johnstone M, Parashos P: Endodontics and the ageing patient, *Aust Dent J* 60(Suppl 1):20–27, 2015.
127. Gani OA, Boiero CF, Correa C, et al.: Morphological changes related to age in mesial root canals of permanent mandibular first molars, *Acta Odontol Latinoam* 27(3):105–109, 2014.
128. Thomas RP, Moule AJ, Bryant R: Root canal morphology of maxillary permanent first molar teeth at various ages, *Int Endod J* 26(5):257–267, 1993.
129. Lee JH, Kim KD, Lee JK, et al.: Mesiobuccal root canal anatomy of Korean maxillary first and second molars by cone-beam computed tomography, *Oral Surg Oral Med Oral Pathol Oral Radiol Endod* 111(6):785–791, 2011.
130. Kayaoglu G, Peker I, Gumusok M, et al.: Root and canal symmetry in the mandibular anterior teeth of patients attending a dental clinic: CBCT study, *Braz Oral Res* 29(1):1–7, 2015.
131. Zhengyan Y, Keke L, Fei W, et al.: Cone-beam computed tomography study of the root and canal morphology of mandibular permanent anterior teeth in a Chongqing population, *Ther Clin Risk Manag* 12:19–25, 2016.
132. Martins J, Ordinola-Zapata R, Marques D, et al.: Differences in root canal system configuration in human permanent teeth within different age groups, *Int Endod J* 51(8):931–941, 2018.
133. Falcão CA, Albuquerque VC, Amorim NL, et al.: Frequency of the mesiopalatal canal in upper first permanent molars viewed through computed tomography, *Acta Odontol Latinoam* 29(1):54–59, 2016.
134. Naseri M, Safi Y, Akbarzadeh Baghban A, et al.: Survey of anatomy and root canal morphology of maxillary first molars regarding age and gender in an Iranian population using cone-beam computed tomography, *Iran Endod J* 11(4):289–303, 2016.
135. Ratanajirasut R, Panichuttra A, Panmekiate S: A cone-beam computed tomographic study of root and canal morphology of maxillary first and second permanent molars in a Thai population, *J Endod* 44(1):56–61, 2018.
136. Versiani MA, Pereira MR, Pécora JD, Sousa Neto MD: Root canal anatomy of maxillary and mandibular teeth. In Versiani MA, Basrani B, Sousa Neto MD, editors: *The root canal anatomy in permanent dentition*, ed 1, Switzerland, 2018, Springer International Publishing, pp 181–240.
137. Fogel HM, Peikoff MD, Christie WH: Canal configuration in the mesiobuccal root of the maxillary first molar: a clinical study, *J Endod* 20(3):135–137, 1994.
138. Ross IF, Evanchik PA: Root fusion in molars: incidence and sex linkage, *J Periodontol* 52(11):663–667, 1981.
139. Sert S, Bayirli GS: Evaluation of the root canal configurations of the mandibular and maxillary permanent teeth by gender in the Turkish population, *J Endod* 30(6):391–398, 2004.
140. Nelson SJ, Ash Jr MM: *Wheeler's dental anatomy, physiology, and occlusion*, ed 9, St. Louis, 2010, Saunders Elsevier.
141. González-Plata RR, González-Plata EW: Conventional and surgical treatment of a two-rooted maxillary central incisor, *J Endod* 29(6):422–424, 2003.
142. Lambruschini GM, Camps J: A two-rooted maxillary central incisor with a normal clinical crown, *J Endod* 19(2):95–96, 1993.
143. Lin WC, Yang SF, Pai SF: Nonsurgical endodontic treatment of a two-rooted maxillary central incisor, *J Endod* 32(5):478–481, 2006.
144. Gondim Jr E, Setzer F, Zingg P, Karabucak B: A maxillary central incisor with three root canals: a case report, *J Endod* 35(10):1445–1447, 2009.
145. Mangani F, Ruddle CJ: Endodontic treatment of a "very particular" maxillary central incisor, *J Endod* 20(11):560–561, 1994.
146. Pécora JD, da Cruz Filho AM: Study of the incidence of radicular grooves in maxillary incisors, *Braz Dent J* 3(1):11–16, 1992.
147. Libfeld H, Stabholz A, Friedman S: Endodontic therapy of bilaterally geminated permanent maxillary central incisors, *J Endod* 12(5):214–216, 1986.
148. Pécora JD, Santana SV: Maxillary lateral incisor with two roots—case report, *Braz Dent J* 2(2):151–153, 1992.
149. Peix-Sánchez M, Miñana-Laliga R: A case of unusual anatomy: a maxillary lateral incisor with three canals, *Int Endod J* 32(3):236–240, 1999.
150. Kottoor J, Murugesan R, Albuquerque DV: A maxillary lateral incisor with four root canals, *Int Endod J* 45(4):393–397, 2012.
151. Fried IL, Winter AA: Diagnosis and treatment of a two-rooted maxillary lateral incisor, *Periodontal Case Rep* 6(2):40–44, 1984.
152. Wong M: Treatment considerations in a geminated maxillary lateral incisor, *J Endod* 17(4):179–181, 1991.
153. Pécora JD, Saquy PC, de Souza JE, Sousa-Neto MD: Endodontic treatment of a maxillary lateral incisor presenting dens invaginatus and transposition to the region of the canine - case report, *Braz Dent J* 2(1):5–8, 1991.
154. Mupparapu M, Singer SR, Goodchild JH: Dens evaginatus and dens invaginatus in a maxillary lateral incisor: report of a rare occurrence and review of literature, *Aust Dent J* 49(4):201–203, 2004.
155. Leoni GB, Versiani MA, Pécora JD, Damião de Sousa-Neto MD: Micro–computed tomographic analysis of the root canal morphology of mandibular incisors, *J Endod* 40(5):710–716, 2013.
156. Sachdeva GS, Malhotra D, Sachdeva LT, et al.: Endodontic management of mandibular central incisor fused to a supernumerary tooth associated with a talon cusp: a case report, *Int Endod J* 45(6):590–596, 2012.
157. Khabbaz MG, Konstantaki MN, Sykaras SN: Dens invaginatus in a mandibular lateral incisor, *Int Endod J* 28(6):303–305, 1995.

158. Loushine RJ, Jurcak JJ, Jeffalone DM: A two-rooted mandibular incisor, *J Endod* 19(5):250–251, 1993.
159. Barkhordar RA, Nguyen NT: Maxillary canine with two roots, *J Endod* 11(5):224–227, 1985.
160. Sousa Neto MD, Zuccolotto WG, Saquy PC, et al.: Treatment of dens invaginatus in a maxillary canine case report, *Braz Dent J* 2(2):147–150, 1992.
161. Versiani MA, Pécora JD, Sousa-Neto MD: The anatomy of two-rooted mandibular canines determined using micro-computed tomography, *Int Endod J* 44(7):682–687, 2011.
162. Orguneser A, Kartal N: Three canals and two foramina in a mandibular canine, *J Endod* 24(6):444–445, 1998.
163. Soares JA, Leonardo RT: Root canal treatment of three-rooted maxillary first and second premolars – a case report, *Int Endod J* 36(10):705, 2003.
164. Lammertyn PA, Rodrigo SB, Brunotto M, Crosa M: Furcation groove of maxillary first premolar, thickness, and dentin structures, *J Endod* 35(6):814–817, 2009.
165. Nahmias Y, Rampado ME: Root-canal treatment of a trifid crown premolar, *Int Endod J* 35(4):390–394, 2002.
166. Çolak H, Aylikçi BU, Keklik H: Dens evaginatus on maxillary first premolar: report of a rare clinical case, *J Nat Sci Biol Med* 3(2):192–194, 2012.
167. Rotstein I, Stabholz A, Friedman S: Endodontic therapy for dens invaginatus in a maxillary second premolar, *Oral Surg Oral Med Oral Pathol* 63(2):237–240, 1987.
168. Vaghela DJ, Sinha AA: Endodontic management of four rooted mandibular first premolar, *J Conserv Dent* 16(1):87–89, 2013.
169. Stecker S, DiAngelis AJ: Dens evaginatus: a diagnostic and treatment challenge, *J Am Dent Assoc* 133(2):190–193, 2002.
170. Tavano SM, de Sousa SM, Bramante CM: Dens invaginatus in first mandibular premolar, *Endod Dent Traumatol* 10(1):27–29, 1994.
171. Aryanpour S, Bercy P, Van Nieuwenhuysen JP: Endodontic and periodontal treatments of a geminated mandibular first premolar, *Int Endod J* 35(2):209–214, 2002.
172. De Moor RJ, Calberson FL: Root canal treatment in a mandibular second premolar with three root canals, *J Endod* 31(4):310–313, 2005.
173. Farmakis ET: Four-rooted mandibular second premolar, *Aust Endod J* 34(3):126–128, 2008.
174. Demiryürek EÖ, Gönülol N, Bulucu B: Endodontic treatment of a taurodontic premolar with five canals, *Aust Endod J* 39(2):81–84, 2013.
175. Goswami M, Chandra S, Chandra S, Singh S: Mandibular premolar with two roots, *J Endod* 23(3):187, 1997.
176. Koh ET, Ford TR, Kariyawasam SP, et al.: Prophylactic treatment of dens evaginatus using mineral trioxide aggregate, *J Endod* 27(8):540–542, 2001.
177. Muthukumar RS, Arunkumar S, Sadasiva K: Bilateral fusion of mandibular second premolar and supernumerary tooth: a rare case report, *J Oral Maxillofac Pathol* 16(1):128–130, 2012.
178. Gopikrishna V, Bhargavi N, Kandaswamy D: Endodontic management of a maxillary first molar with a single root and a single canal diagnosed with the aid of spiral CT: a case report, *J Endod* 32(7):687–691, 2006.
179. Beatty RG: A five-canal maxillary first molar, *J Endod* 10(4):156–157, 1984.
180. Albuquerque DV, Kottoor J, Dham S, et al.: Endodontic management of maxillary permanent first molar with 6 root canals: 3 case reports, *Oral Surg Oral Med Oral Pathol Oral Radiol Endod* 110(4):e79–e83, 2010.
181. Kottoor J, Velmurugan N, Sudha R, Hemamalathi S: Maxillary first molar with seven root canals diagnosed with cone-beam computed tomography scanning: a case report, *J Endod* 36(5):915–921, 2010.
182. Kottoor J, Velmurugan N, Surendran S: Endodontic management of a maxillary first molar with eight root canal systems evaluated using cone-beam computed tomography scanning: a case report, *J Endod* 37(5):715–719, 2011.
183. Peikoff MD, Christie WH, Fogel HM: The maxillary second molar: variations in the number of roots and canals, *Int Endod J* 29(6):365–369, 1996.
184. Kottoor J, Hemamalathi S, Sudha R, Velmurugan N: Maxillary second molar with 5 roots and 5 canals evaluated using cone beam computerized tomography: a case report, *Oral Surg Oral Med Oral Pathol Oral Radiol Endod* 109(2):e162–e165, 2010.
185. Koenen DJ, Pahncke D: Gemination or fusion: use of a CT scan to assist in diagnosis and endodontic treatment of a maxillary second molar - a case report, *ENDO* 2(2):145–151, 2008.
186. Radwan A, Kim SG: Treatment of a hypertaurodontic maxillary second molar in a patient with 10 taurodonts: a case report, *J Endod* 40(1):140–144, 2013.
187. Friedman S, Moshonov J, Stabholz A: Five root canals in a mandibular first molar, *Endod Dent Traumatol* 2(5):226–228, 1986.
188. Ryan JL, Bowles WR, Baisden MK, McClanahan SB: Mandibular first molar with six separate canals, *J Endod* 37(6):878–880, 2011.
189. Reeh ES: Seven canals in a lower first molar, *J Endod* 24(7):497–499, 1998.
190. Ashwin R, Arathi R: Taurodontism of deciduous and permanent molars: report of two cases, *J Indian Soc Pedod Prev Dent* 24(1):42–44, 2006.
191. Tsesis I, Steinbock N, Rosenberg E, Kaufman AY: Endodontic treatment of developmental anomalies in posterior teeth: treatment of geminated/fused teeth – report of two cases, *Int Endod J* 36(5):372, 2003.
192. Fan B, Pan Y, Gao Y, et al.: Three-dimensional morphologic analysis of isthmuses in the mesial roots of mandibular molars, *J Endod* 36(11):1866–1869, 2010.
193. Schäfer E, Breuer D, Janzen S: The prevalence of three-rooted mandibular permanent first molars in a German population, *J Endod* 35(2):202–205, 2009.
194. Bolger WL, Schindler WG: A mandibular first molar with a C-shaped root configuration, *J Endod* 14(10):515–519, 1988.
195. Filpo-Perez C, Bramante CM, Villas-Boas MH, et al.: Micro-computed tomographic analysis of the root canal morphology of the distal root of mandibular first molar, *J Endod* 41(2):231–236, 2015.
196. Fava LR, Weinfeld I, Fabri FP, Pais CR: Four second molars with single roots and single canals in the same patient, *Int Endod J* 33(3):138–142, 2000.
197. Chokshi S, Mehta J, Chokshi P, Vaidya R: Morphological variations in the root canal system of mandibular second molar: a case series, *Endodontology* 25:135, 2013.
198. Beatty RG, Krell K: Mandibular molars with five canals: report of two cases, *J Am Dent Assoc* 114(6):802–804, 1987.
199. Ballal S, Sachdeva G, Kandaswamy D: Endodontic management of a fused mandibular second molar and paramolar with the aid of spiral computed tomography: a case report, *J Endod* 33(10):1247–1251, 2007.
200. Barrett MT: The internal anatomy of the teeth with special reference to the pulp with its branches, *Dent Cosmos* 67:581, 1925.
201. Hession RW: Endodontic morphology. II. A radiographic analysis, *Oral Surg Oral Med Oral Pathol* 44(4):610–620, 1977.
202. Pécora JD, Woelfel JB, Sousa Neto MD, Issa EP: Morphologic study of the maxillary molars. Part II: Internal anatomy, *Braz Dent J* 3(1):53–57, 1992.
203. Guerisoli DM, de Souza RA, de Sousa Neto MD, Silva RG, Pécora JD: External and internal anatomy of third molars, *Braz Dent J* 9(2):91–94, 1998.
204. Stropko JJ: Canal morphology of maxillary molars: clinical observations of canal configurations, *J Endod* 25(6):446–450, 1999.
205. Ng YL, Aung TH, Alavi A, Gulabivala K: Root and canal morphology of Burmese maxillary molars, *Int Endod J* 34(6):620–630, 2001.
206. Alavi AM, Opasanon A, Ng YL, Gulabivala K: Root and canal morphology of Thai maxillary molars, *Int Endod J* 35(5):478–485, 2002.

207. Weng XL, Yu SB, Zhao SL, et al.: Root canal morphology of permanent maxillary teeth in the Han nationality in Chinese Guanzhong area: a new modified root canal staining technique, *J Endod* 35(5):651–656, 2009.
208. Sert S, Sahinkesen G, Topçu FT, et al.: Root canal configurations of third molar teeth. A comparison with first and second molars in the Turkish population, *Aust Endod J* 37(3):109–117, 2011.
209. Cosić J, Galić N, Vodanović M, et al.: An in vitro morphological investigation of the endodontic spaces of third molars, *Coll Antropol* 37(2):437–442, 2013.
210. Tomaszewska IM, Leszczyński B, Wróbel A, et al.: A micro-computed tomographic (micro-CT) analysis of the root canal morphology of maxillary third molar teeth, *Ann Anat* 215:83–92, 2018.
211. Zakhary SY, Fahim OM, Gorgy AA: Morphologic characteristics of lower third molar as related to successful endodontic therapy, *Egypt Dent J* 34(4):323–337, 1988.
212. Gulabivala K, Opasanon A, Ng YL, Alavi A: Root and canal morphology of Thai mandibular molars, *Int Endod J* 35(1):56–62, 2002.
213. Kuzekanani M, Haghani J, Nosrati H: Root and canal morphology of mandibular third molars in an Iranian population, *J Dent Res Dent Clin Dent Prospects* 6(3):85–88, 2012.
214. Park JB, Kim N, Park S, et al.: Evaluation of root anatomy of permanent mandibular premolars and molars in a Korean population with cone-beam computed tomography, *Eur J Dent* 7(1):94–101, 2013.
215. Ahmad IA, Azzeh MM, Zwiri AMA, et al.: Root and root canal morphology of third molars in a Jordanian subpopulation, *Saudi Endod J* 6(3):113–121, 2016.
216. Siqueira Jr JF: Roças IN, Ricucci D: Internal tooth anatomy and root canal instrumentation. In Versiani MA, Basrani B, Sousa Neto MD, editors: *The root canal anatomy in permanent dentition*, ed 1, Switzerland, 2018, Springer International Publishing, pp 277–302.
217. Siqueira Jr JF, Roças IN: Clinical implications and microbiology of bacterial persistence after treatment procedures, *J Endod* 34(11):1291–1301, 2008.
218. McGurkin-Smith R, Trope M, Caplan D, Sigurdsson A: Reduction of intracanal bacteria using GT rotary instrumentation, 5.25% NaOCl, EDTA, and Ca(OH)2, *J Endod* 31(5):359–363, 2005.
219. Shuping GB, Ørstavik D, Sigurdsson A, Trope M: Reduction of intracanal bacteria using nickel-titanium rotary instrumentation and various medications, *J Endod* 26(12):751–755, 2000.
220. Siqueira Jr JF, Paiva SS, Rôças IN: Reduction in the cultivable bacterial populations in infected root canals by a chlorhexidine-based antimicrobial protocol, *J Endod* 33(5):541–547, 2007.
221. Rodrigues RCV, Zandi H, Kristoffersen AK, et al.: Influence of the apical preparation size and the irrigant type on bacterial reduction in root canal–treated teeth with apical periodontitis, *J Endod* 43(7):1058–1063, 2017.
222. Siqueira Jr JF, Rôças IN, Favieri A, Lima KC: Chemomechanical reduction of the bacterial population in the root canal after instrumentation and irrigation with 1%, 2.5%, and 5.25% sodium hypochlorite, *J Endod* 26(6):330–334, 2000.
223. Siqueira Jr JF, Rôças IN, Santos SR, et al.: Efficacy of instrumentation techniques and irrigation regimens in reducing the bacterial population within root canals, *J Endod* 28(3):181–184, 2002.
224. Rôças IN, Provenzano JC, Neves MA, Siqueira Jr JF: Disinfecting effects of rotary instrumentation with either 2.5% sodium hypochlorite or 2% chlorhexidine as the main irrigant: a randomized clinical study, *J Endod* 42(6):943–947, 2016.
225. Boutsioukis C: Internal tooth anatomy and root canal irrigation. In Versiani MA, Basrani B, Sousa Neto MD, editors: *The root canal anatomy in permanent dentition*, ed 1, Switzerland, 2018, Springer International Publishing, pp 303–322.
226. Paquette L, Legner M, Fillery ED, Friedman S: Antibacterial efficacy of chlorhexidine gluconate intracanal medication in vivo, *J Endod* 33(7):788–795, 2007.
227. Siqueira Jr JF, Guimarães-Pinto T, Rôças IN: Effects of chemomechanical preparation with 2.5% sodium hypochlorite and intracanal medication with calcium hydroxide on cultivable bacteria in infected root canals, *J Endod* 33(7):800–805, 2007.
228. Siqueira Jr JF, Rôças IN, Paiva SS, et al.: Bacteriologic investigation of the effects of sodium hypochlorite and chlorhexidine during the endodontic treatment of teeth with apical periodontitis, *Oral Surg Oral Med Oral Pathol Oral Radiol Endod* 104(1):122–130, 2007.
229. Sirén EK, Haapasalo MP, Waltimo TM, Ørstavik D: *In vitro* antibacterial effect of calcium hydroxide combined with chlorhexidine or iodine potassium iodide on *Enterococcus faecalis*, *Eur J Oral Sci* 112(4):326–331, 2004.
230. Paqué F, Balmer M, Attin T, Peters OA: Preparation of oval-shaped root canals in mandibular molars using nickel-titanium rotary instruments: a micro-computed tomography study, *J Endod* 36(4): 703–707, 2010.
231. De-Deus G, Barino B, Zamolyi RQ, et al.: Suboptimal debridement quality produced by the single-file F2 ProTaper technique in oval-shaped canals, *J Endod* 36(11):1897–1900, 2010.
232. Versiani MA, Leoni GB, Steier L, et al.: Micro-computed tomography study of oval-shaped canals prepared with the Self-adjusting File, Reciproc, WaveOne, and ProTaper universal systems, *J Endod* 39(8):1060–1066, 2013.
233. Versiani MA, Pécora JD, de Sousa-Neto MD: Flat-oval root canal preparation with self-adjusting file instrument: a micro-computed tomography study, *J Endod* 37(7):1002–1007, 2011.
234. Ricucci D, Siqueira Jr JF, Bate AL, Pitt Ford TR: Histologic investigation of root canal-treated teeth with apical periodontitis: a retrospective study from twenty-four patients, *J Endod* 35(4):493–502, 2009.
235. Nair PN, Henry S, Cano V, Vera J: Microbial status of apical root canal system of human mandibular first molars with primary apical periodontitis after "one-visit" endodontic treatment, *Oral Surg Oral Med Oral Pathol Oral Radiol Endod* 99(2):231–252, 2005.
236. Vera J, Siqueira Jr JF, Ricucci D, et al.: One- versus two-visit endodontic treatment of teeth with apical periodontitis: a histobacteriologic study, *J Endod* 38(8):1040–1052, 2012.
237. Siqueira Jr JF, Alves FR, Versiani MA, et al.: Correlative bacteriologic and micro-computed tomographic analysis of mandibular molar mesial canals prepared by self-adjusting file, Reciproc, and twisted file systems, *J Endod* 39(8):1044–1050, 2013.
238. Ingle JI, Taintor JF: The Washington study. In Ingle JI, Taintor JF, editors: *Endodontics*, ed 3, Philadelphia, 1985, Lea & Febiger, pp 27–53.
239. Seltzer S, Bender IB, Turkenkopf S: Factors affecting successful repair after root canal therapy, *J Am Dent Assoc* 67:651–652, 1963.
240. Crump MC: Differential diagnosis in endodontic failure, *Dent Clin North Am* 23(4):617–635, 1979.
241. Perrini N: *Storia anatomica del sistema dei canali radicolari*, Milan, 2010, Società Italiana di Endodonzia.

13

Isolation, Endodontic Access, and Length Determination

FABRICIO B. TEIXEIRA, ANNE E. WILLIAMSON, AND SHAHROKH SHABAHANG

CHAPTER OUTLINE

LEARNING OBJECTIVES

After reading this chapter the student should be able to:

1. Describe the rationale for rubber dam isolation during endodontic procedures.
2. Describe techniques for application of the clamp and rubber dam.
3. Recognize situations in which special isolation approaches are necessary and identify isolation techniques for unusual situations.
4. Identify patients who should be considered for referral.
5. Identify major objectives of endodontic access preparation, including importance of dentin preservation.
6. Relate reasons and indications for removing caries or restorations before access.
7. Describe the technical procedure, materials used, and sequence to properly access all teeth.
8. Demonstrate the step-by-step technique for obtaining estimated and correct working lengths.
9. Describe the practice and accuracy of electronic apex locators.
10. Illustrate the portions of the tooth that must be removed to attain access to the canals.

Chapters 14 and 15 address the technical aspects of nonsurgical root canal treatment. Areas presented include isolation, access, length determination, cleaning and shaping, and obturation. A number of instruments and techniques are advocated for treatment procedures. These chapters introduce concepts and principles that are important for successful treatment. These building blocks are based on the best available evidence and provide a basis for incorporating more complex and alternative techniques.

Rubber Dam Isolation

Application

Application of the rubber dam for isolation during endodontic treatment has many distinct advantages and is mandatory for legal considerations.[1] Expert testimony is not required in cases involving patients who swallowed or aspirated instruments or materials, because juries are considered competent to determine negligence. Failure to use a rubber dam indicates that the clinician does not understand the need to protect the patient from aspiration or swallowing instruments, the protection afforded the dental staff from contaminated aerosols, the microbial nature of the disease process, and the decreased success rate for treatment when strict asepsis is not used.

Evidence exists that many general dentists unnecessarily place themselves at risk by not using the rubber dam when performing endodontic procedures.[2] Although the use of the rubber dam in the United States is considered the standard of care, recent studies have shown that is not universal among general dentists. A survey conducted in 2013 reported that only 44% of general dentists who perform root canal therapy (RCT) use rubber dam isolation. Moreover, 15% reported that they do not use a rubber dam for any of the RCTs that they provide.[2] Considering that the use of rubber dam significantly increases the tooth survival rates after initial

RCT, its constant usage will improve the infection control—and in consequence the outcome—of endodontic treatment.[3]

The rubber dam provides protection for the patient and creates an aseptic environment; it enhances visibility, retracts tissues, and makes treatment more efficient. Soft tissues are protected from laceration by rotary instruments, chemical agents, and medicaments. Irrigating solutions are confined to the operating field. Most important, rubber dam isolation protects the patient from swallowing or aspirating instruments and materials (Fig. 13.1).[4] An additional advantage is that the dentist and auxiliary employees are also protected.[5-7] The risk from aerosols is minimized,[8,9] and the dam provides a barrier against the patient's saliva and oral bacteria. Application of the rubber dam may also reduce the potential for transmission of systemic diseases, such as acquired immunodeficiency syndrome (AIDS), hepatitis, and tuberculosis.[5,9]

The rubber dam is manufactured from latex; however, nonlatex rubber dam material is available for patients with latex allergy and is used exclusively in many institutions (Fig. 13.2).[10] The rubber dam can be obtained in a variety of colors that provide contrast to the tooth. The thickness also varies (light, medium, heavy, and extra heavy). A medium-weight dam is recommended because a lightweight dam is easily torn during the application process. Also, the medium material fits better at the gingival margin and provides good retraction.

The design of the rubber dam frames also varies. For endodontics, plastic frames are recommended; they are radiolucent and do not require complete removal during exposure of interim images, such as the working length and master cone radiographs.

Rubber Dam Retainers

Rubber dam clamps fit the various tooth groups. During routine treatment, metal clamps are adequate; however, they may damage tooth structure[11] or existing restorations. Some have serrated edges to enhance retention when minimal coronal tooth structure remains. Plastic clamps are manufactured and have the advantage of being radiolucent. This radiolucency is an advantage in difficult cases in which the pulp chamber and canal cannot be located. When using a plastic clamp, the rubber dam can remain in place. The plastic clamps are less likely than metal ones to damage tooth structure or existing restorations.[12]

Types

Different styles and shapes of rubber dam clamps are available for specific situations. The following selection is recommended: (1) for anterior teeth: Ivory No. 9 or 212; for premolars: No. 0 and 2; and for *molars:* No. 14, 14A, 56, and 205. Clamps that will manage most isolation situations during root canal treatment are shown in Fig. 13.3. Winged clamps permit the application of the rubber dam as a single unit during single-tooth isolation (Fig. 13.4).[13]

Universal Clamp Designs

Two designs (see Fig. 13.3), the "butterfly" Ivory No. 9 and the Ivory No. 56, are suitable for most isolations. The butterfly design (No. 9) has small beaks, is deep reaching, and can be applied to most anterior and premolar teeth. The No. 56 clamp can isolate most molars.

With teeth that are smaller, reduced by crown preparation, or abnormally shaped, a clamp with smaller radius beaks (No. 0, 9, or 14) is necessary. Small-radius beaks can be positioned farther apically on the root, which stretches the dam cervically in the interproximal space.

Additional Designs

Clamps that may be most useful when little coronal tooth structure remains have beaks that are inclined apically. These are termed *deep-reaching clamps.* Clamps with serrated edges are also available for cases involving minimal coronal structure. These clamps should not be placed on porcelain surfaces because damage may occur.[11]

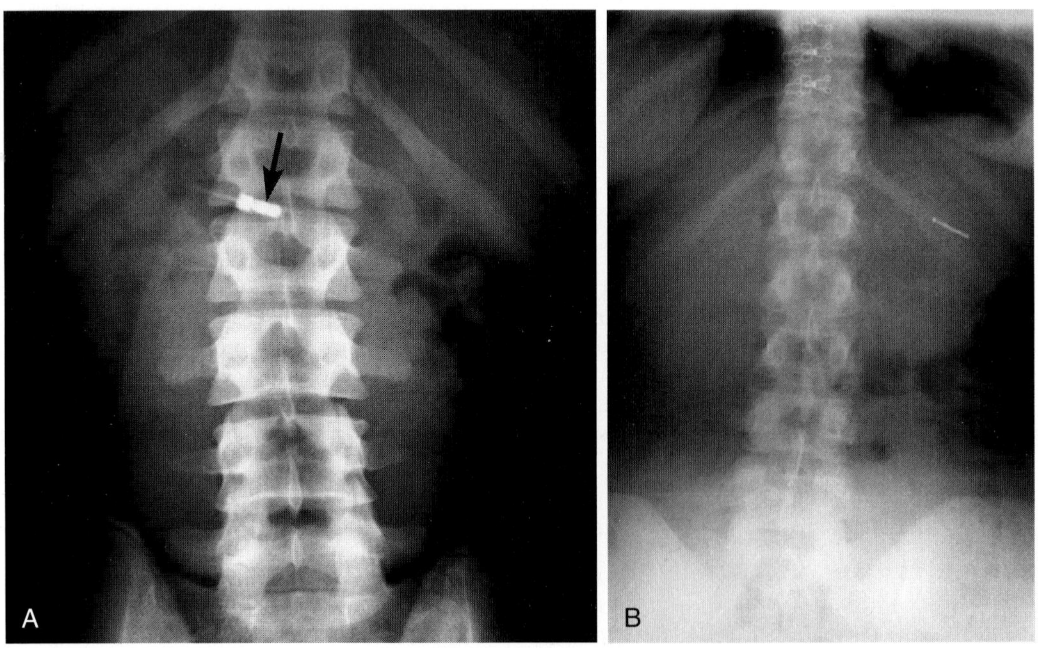

• **Fig. 13.1 A,** A file *(arrow)* that a patient swallowed during endodontic treatment. **B,** A bur that a patient also swallowed due to the lack of proper protection with rubber dam.

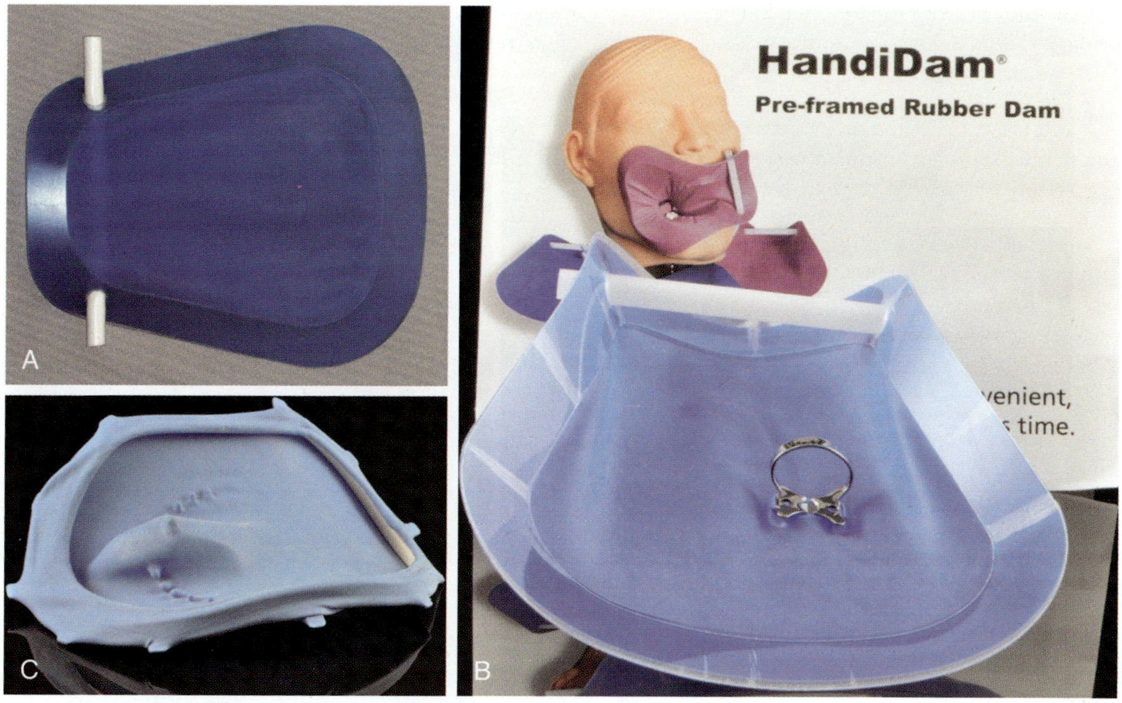

• **Fig. 13.2** **A** and **B,** Disposable rubber dam systems; **C**, OptiDam, a three-dimensional rubber dam.

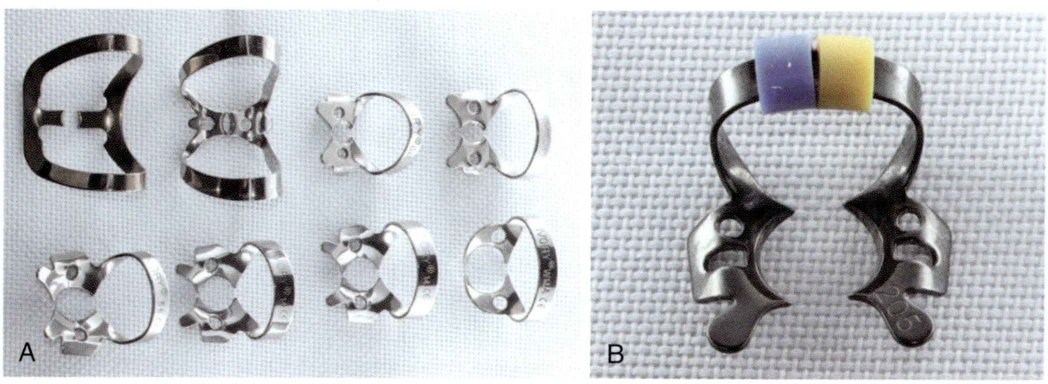

• **Fig. 13.3** **A**, The retainers in the bottom left (No. 212 and 9) are designed for anterior teeth but are useful for premolars. The two clamps in the bottom right (No. 56 and 14) are for molars and anterior teeth. The upper left clamps (No. 0 and 2) are for premolars. No. W14A and 14 are deeper reaching than the No. 56. **B**, Clamp No. 205 can be used for most of the molars.

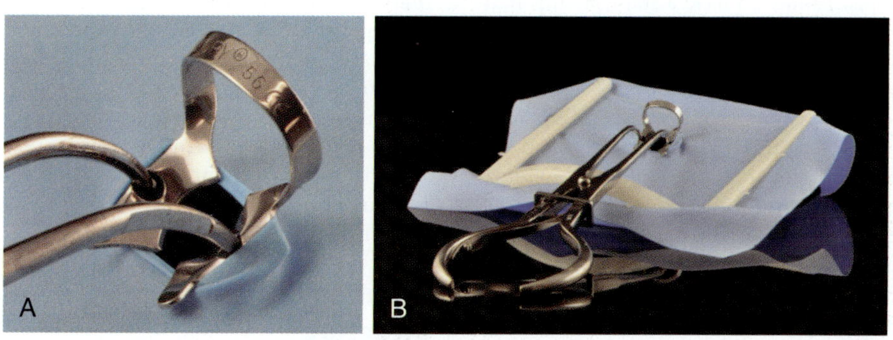

• **Fig. 13.4** **A,** Placement of the rubber dam as a single unit requires the use of a winged clamp. A hole is punched in the rubber dam and then stretched over the wings of the appropriate clamp. **B,** The rubber dam is attached to a plastic radiolucent frame, and the rubber dam forceps is then used to carry the unit to the tooth.

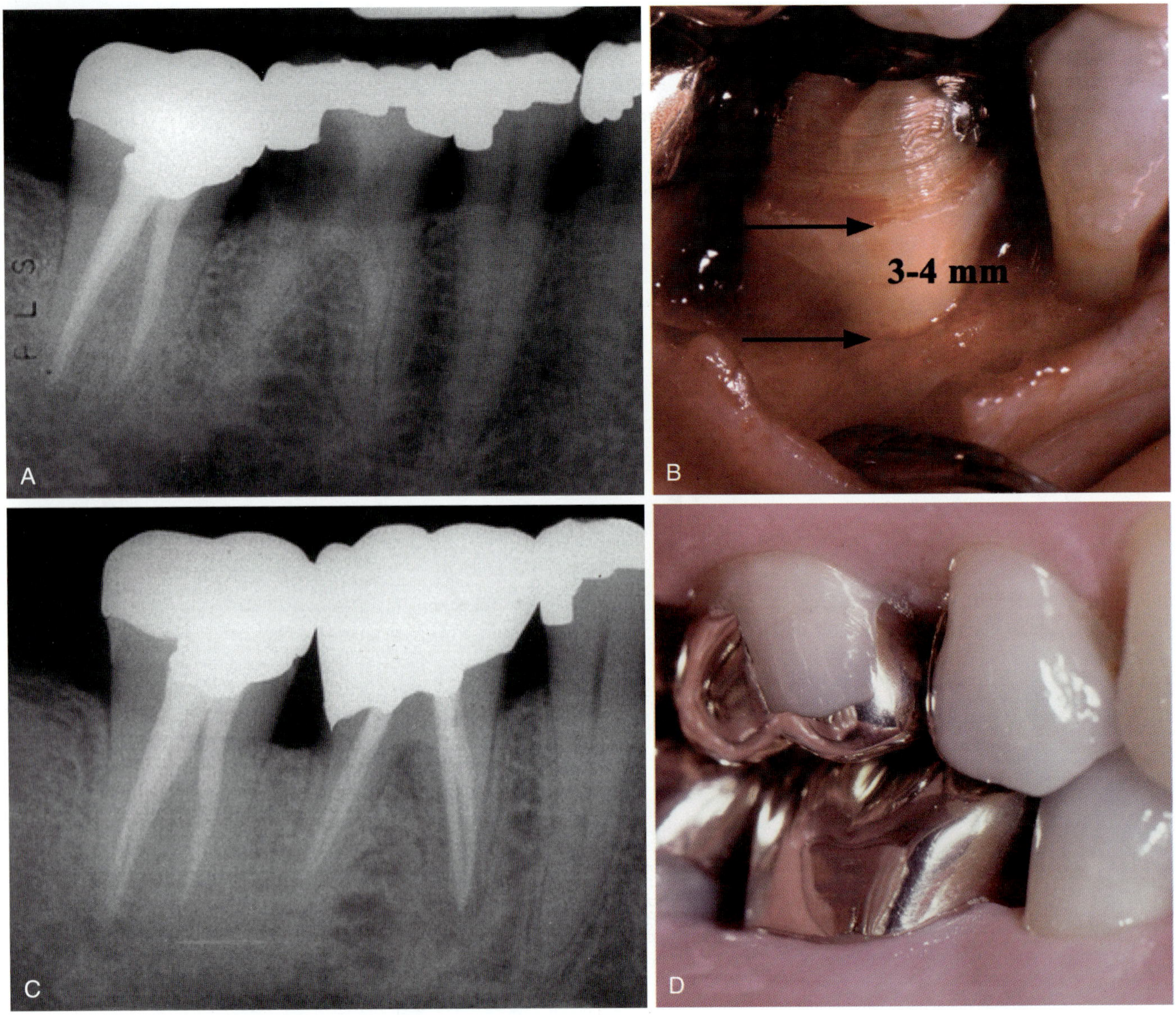

• **Fig. 13.5** **A,** The first molar shows extensive caries on the distal extending to the crestal bone. **B,** A full-thickness, mucoperiosteal flap and osseous reduction are performed after caries excavation and preparation for a provisional crown; then, 3 to 4 mm of tooth structure coronal to the osseous crest restores the biologic width. **C,** Root canal treatment and placement of the crown. **D,** The definitive restoration.

For stability, the clamp selected must have four-point contact between the tooth and beaks. Failure to have a stable clamp may result in damage to the gingival attachment and coronal structure,[11,14] or the clamp may be dislodged. Clamps may also be modified by grinding to adapt to unusual situations.[15]

Placement of the rubber dam as a single unit is fast and efficient. Once in place, the dam is flossed through the contacts, and the facial and lingual portions of the dam are flipped under the wings.

Identification of the tooth requiring treatment is usually routine. However, if no caries or restorations are present, the operator may clamp the wrong tooth. This error can be avoided by marking the tooth before rubber dam application or by beginning the access after placement of a throat pack without the rubber dam in place.

Preparation for Rubber Dam Placement

Before treatment is initiated, the degree of difficulty in obtaining adequate isolation must be assessed. Often, teeth requiring root canal treatment have large restorations, caries, or minimal remaining tooth structure that may present complications during isolation and access. Adequate isolation requires that caries, defective restorations, and restorations with leaking margins be removed before treatment. Removal of all existing restorations has been advocated to improve the ability to assess restorability, pathogenesis of disease, and prognosis.[24]

Once the treatment plan has been finalized, it may be necessary to perform ancillary procedures to allow for placement of the rubber dam.[16,17]

Isolation of Teeth with Inadequate Coronal Structure

Ligation, the use of deep-reaching clamps, bonding, or building up before access are the major methods of isolating teeth without adequate coronal tooth structure. Surgical management may also be required (Fig. 13.5).

In the case of inability to obtain appropriate isolation, the patient should be referred to an endodontic specialist.

Ligation

Inadequate coronal structure is not always the cause of lack of retention. In young patients the tooth may not have erupted sufficiently to make the cervical area available for clamp retention. In these cases, ligation with floss or the use of interproximal rubber Wedjets is indicated (see Fig. 13.15, *D*). Another approach is multiple tooth isolation (see Fig. 13.2, *C*, OptiDam 3D rubber dam).

Deep-Reaching Clamps

When the loss of tooth structure extends below the gingival tissues but there is adequate structure above the crestal bone, a deep-reaching clamp is indicated. It may be necessary to use a caulking material or resin around the clamp to provide an adequate seal (Fig. 13.6). Another option is the use of an anterior retainer regardless of the tooth type.

Bonding

When there is missing tooth structure, including the natural height of contour, retention can be increased by bonding resin on the facial and lingual surfaces of the remaining tooth structure.[18] The clamp is placed apical to the resin undercut. After treatment the resin is easily removed. This technique is preferred over the more invasive technique of cutting horizontal grooves in the facial and lingual surfaces for the prongs of the clamp.

Replacement of Coronal Structure

Temporary Restorations

When there is missing tooth structure but adequate retention, missing structure can be restored with reinforced intermediate restorative material (IRM) containing zinc oxide–eugenol, glass ionomers, or resins. These materials provide an adequate coronal seal and are stable until the definitive restoration is placed. Bonded materials provide a better seal with improved strength and esthetics.

Band Placement

Placement of orthodontic bands may be indicated in cases of cracked or fractured teeth to provide protection and support until a definitive restoration can be placed. The bands are available in various sizes and are appropriately contoured. A band can be cemented, and the missing tooth structure replaced with IRM (see Fig. 13.39). During the placement procedure, it is important to protect the canals and pulp chamber.

Provisional Crowns

Placement of temporary crowns is an option; however, they reduce visibility, result in the loss of anatomic landmarks, and may change the orientation for access and canal location. Often temporary crowns are displaced during treatment by the rubber dam clamp. In general, when provisional crowns are placed, they should be removed before endodontic treatment to provide the correct orientation and maintain the remaining tooth structure.

Rubber Dam Placement

Placement as a Unit

Placement of the rubber dam, clamp, and frame as a unit is preferred (see Fig. 13.4). This method is most efficient and is applicable in most cases. A traditional dam and frame can be used, or proprietary disposable systems are available (see Fig. 13.2). The steps in this process are as follows:

1. The dam is placed on the frame so that it is stretched tightly across the top and bottom but has slack horizontally in the middle.
2. A hole is punched in the dam, and then the clamp wings are attached to the dam.
3. The dam, frame, and clamp are placed as a unit to engage the tooth near the gingival margin.
4. The dam is released apically off the clamp wings to allow it to constrict around the tooth neck. The dam is then flossed through the contacts.

Placement of a Clamp, Followed by the Dam and Then the Frame

Placement of a clamp followed by the dam and frame is seldom used but may be necessary when an unobstructed view is required while the clamp is positioned. The clamp is first placed on the tooth and secured. The rubber dam is then stretched over the clamp and the frame affixed.[5]

Placement of the Rubber Dam and Frame and Then the Clamp

The preferred method for applying a butterfly clamp that does not have wings (No. 212) is to place the dam and frame and then the clamp. improved visibility is possible when the hole is stretched over the tooth and gingiva first by the operator or dental assistant, and the clamp is then placed. The No. 212 clamp has narrow beaks and is often used in situations in which wing clamps are unstable or cannot be retained.

Rubber Dam Leakage

Several proprietary products are available for placement around the rubber dam at the tooth–dam interface should leakage occur (see Fig. 13.6). These are caulklike materials, putty, or light-cured resins; they are easily applied and removed after treatment and are especially useful for isolation of an abutment for a fixed partial denture or for a tooth that is undergoing active orthodontic treatment.

The material can be placed on the gingival tissues at the dam–tooth interface after isolation. The caulking and putty materials adhere to wet surfaces, although the putty has a stiffer consistency.

Disinfection of the Operating Field

Various methods and techniques are used to disinfect the tooth, clamp, and surrounding rubber dam after placement. These disinfectants include alcohol, quaternary ammonium compounds, sodium hypochlorite, organic iodine, mercuric salts, chlorhexidine, and hydrogen peroxide. An effective technique is as follows: (1) plaque is removed by rubber cup and pumice; (2) the rubber dam is placed; (3) the tooth surface, clamp, and surrounding rubber dam are scrubbed with 30% hydrogen peroxide; and (4) the surfaces are swabbed with 5% tincture of iodine or with sodium hypochlorite.[19]

Access Openings

Endodontic access openings are based on the anatomy and morphology of each individual tooth group. In general, the pulp

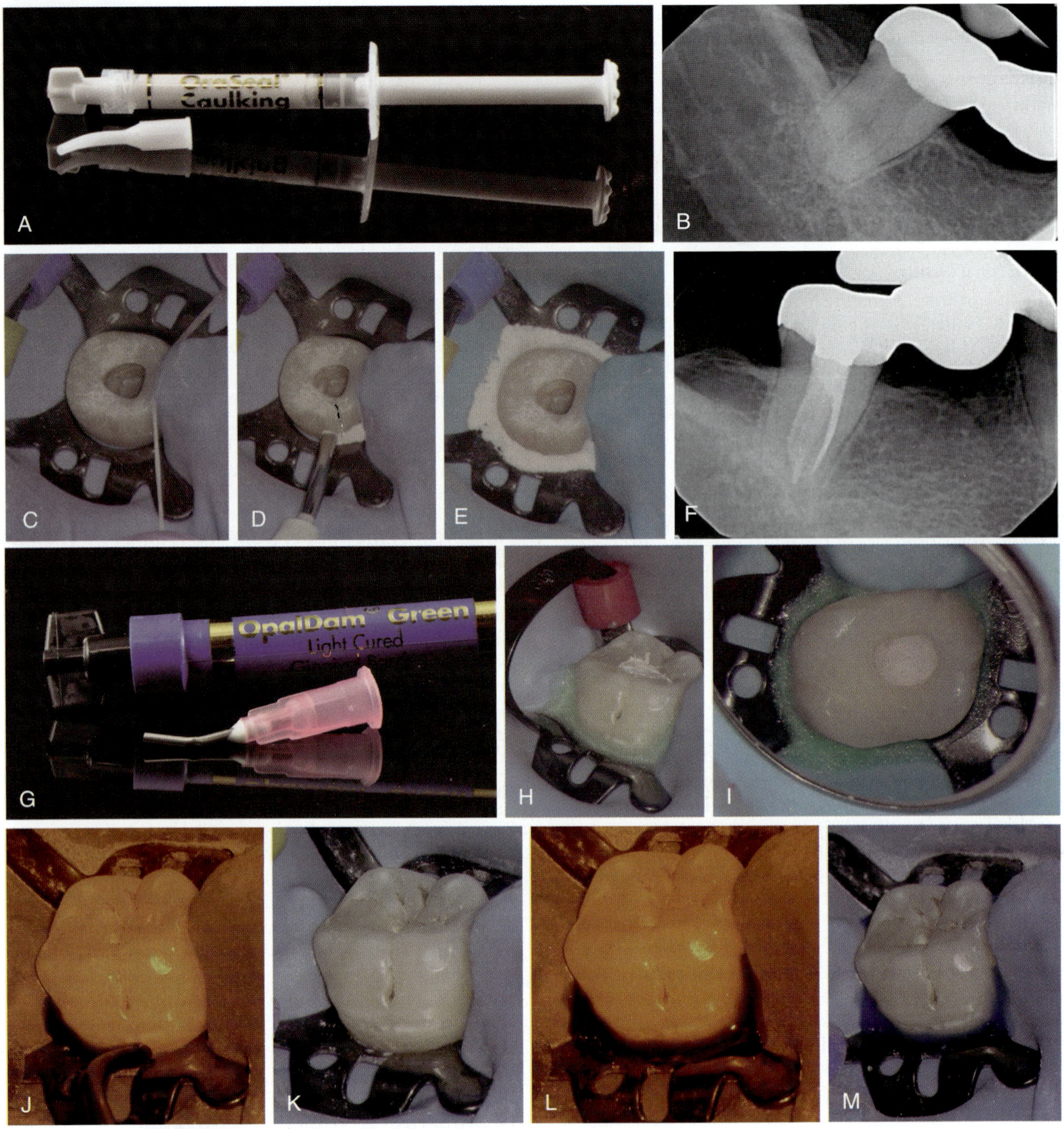

• **Fig. 13.6** **A,** Caulking and putty materials are available to prevent leakage after rubber dam application. **B,** Preoperative radiograph and **C,** demonstration of lack of isolation with dental floss. **D,** Application of the caulk. **E,** The sealed dam. **F,** Postoperative radiograph. **G,** OpalDam. **H, I,** Two teeth sealed with OpalDam after light curing. **J,** LC Block-Out. **K,** Before the sealing. **L,** Placing the Block-Out under the microscope (yellow filter to avoid the material setting). **M,** Final seal after light curing.

number of root canals dictates the final design of the access preparation. The internal anatomy is projected onto the external surface. Internal pulp chamber morphology varies with the patient's age and secondary or tertiary dentin deposition. In anterior teeth and premolars with a single root, calcification occurs in a coronal to apical direction with the chamber receding. In posterior teeth with bifurcations and trifurcations, secondary dentin is deposited preferentially on the floor of the chamber, decreasing the cervical to apical dimension of the chamber.[20,21] The mesiodistal and buccolingual dimensions remain relatively the same, as does the cusp-to-roof distance. Dystrophic calcifications related to caries, restorations, attrition abrasion, and erosion also can occur. In general, the pulp chamber is located at the cementoenamel junction (CEJ).[22,23] In young teeth, the pulp horns are at approximately the level of the height of contour.

The major objectives of the access openings include (1) removal of the chamber roof and all coronal pulp tissue, (2) locating all canals, (3) unimpeded straight-line access of the instruments in the canals to the apical one third or the first curve (if present), and (4) conservation of tooth structure.

Before initiating treatment, the clinician should assess the existing coronal structure; restorations present; tooth angulation in the arch; and the position, size, depth, and shape of the pulp chamber. A parallel preoperative radiograph or digital image is essential. Additional angled radiographs or digital images may aid the identification of additional canals and roots. Bitewing radiographs and digital images offer the most accurate and distortion-free information on chamber anatomy in posterior teeth. Recent advances in cone beam computed tomography (CBCT) imaging allow three-dimensional (3D) viewing of the pulp chamber and radicular space.[25,26] Conservation of tooth structure is important for subsequent restorative treatment and the long-term prognosis.[27] Maintaining adequate structure in the cervical region is assured by not extending the access preparation beyond the natural external chamber walls. The distance from the surface of the clinical crown to the peripheral vertical wall of the pulp chamber is the same throughout the circumference of the tooth at the level of the CEJ, and the orifices of the root canals are located at the angles in the floor–wall junction.[28,29]

General Principles

A broad discussion about the preservation of dentin during the endodontic procedures, including the conventional access, has been subjected to debate in the literature.[27] The traditional endodontic access underscores the concept of straight-line preparation to improve the mechanical débridement of root canals and to minimize procedural errors. However, the excessive removal of tooth structure has been associated with the increased risk of fracture and loss of the tooth as consequences. Lately, investigators have associated the survivability of the endodontically treated tooth with conservative approaches such as contracted endodontic cavities.[30] Even though this concept has been questioned and not completely proved to be the predictable treatment method,[31-33] we deem that dentin preservation must be taken in consideration in all procedures to increase the long-term survival rate of endodontically treated teeth.

Contemplating the debate on preservation of tooth structure and the lack of a comprehensive opinion of the straight-line access significance, the general principles for endodontic access remain (1) outline form, (2) convenience form, (3) caries removal, and (4) cleaning the periphery of the preparation to ensure it is free of any debris or objects that could fall into the canals upon access.

Outline form is the recommended shape for access preparation of a normal tooth with radiographic evidence of a pulp chamber and canal space. The outline form ensures the correct shape and location and provides straight-line access to the apical portion of the canal or to the first curvature. The access preparation must remove tooth structure that would impede the cleaning and shaping of the canal or canals. The outline form is a projection of the internal tooth anatomy onto the external root structure. The form can change with time. As an example, in anterior teeth with mesial and distal pulp horns, the access is triangular. In older individuals with chamber calcification, the pulp horns are absent, so the access is ovoid.

Convenience form allows modification of the ideal outline form to facilitate unstrained instrument placement and manipulation. As an example, the use of nickel–titanium rotary instruments requires straight-line access. An access might be modified to permit placement and manipulation of the nickel–titanium instruments. Another example is a premolar exhibiting three roots. The outline form might be made more triangular to facilitate canal location.

Caries removal is essential for several reasons. First, removing caries permits the development of an aseptic environment before entering the pulp chamber and radicular space. Second, it allows assessment of restorability before treatment. Third, caries removal provides sound tooth structure so that an adequate provisional restoration can be placed. Unsupported tooth structure is removed to ensure a coronal seal during and after treatment so that the reference point for length determination is not lost should fracture occur.

Cleaning the periphery involves preventing materials and objects from entering the chamber and canal space. A common error is entering the pulp chamber before the coronal structure or restorative materials have been adequately prepared. As a result, these materials enter the canal space and may block the apical portion of the canal.

Canal Morphologies

Five major canal morphologies have been identified (Fig. 13.7).[34] They include round, ribbon or figure eight, ovoid, bowling pin, kidney bean, and C-shape. With the exception of the round morphologic shape, each presents unique problems for adequate cleaning and shaping.

General Considerations

In difficult cases the access can be prepared without the rubber dam in place. This preparation allows visualization of the tooth shape, orientation, and position in the dental arch. When the canal or chamber is located, the rubber dam is applied. *Caution:* Until the rubber dam is in place, broaches and files cannot be used (see Fig. 13.1).

Care must be taken to prevent tooth structure or restorative materials from entering the radicular portion of the root if additional expansion of the access is necessary after the chamber is exposed. When an access is to be enlarged or restorative materials removed after chamber exposure, the radicular space must be protected. The canal orifice and chamber floor can be blocked by placing gutta-percha temporary stopping. The material is heated and then compacted with a plugger. The temporary stopping is removed with heat (preferred) or solvents after completion of the access preparation.

Before beginning the access, the clinician should assess the preoperative images to determine the degree of case difficulty. At this stage the estimated depth of access is calculated. This calculation is a measurement from the incisal edge of anterior teeth and the occlusal surface of posterior teeth to the coronal portion of the pulp chamber. Calculated in millimeters, this information is then transferred to the access bur and provides information on the depth necessary to expose the pulp. If the estimated depth of access is reached and the pulp has not been encountered, the access depth and orientation must be reevaluated. A parallel image exposed with the rubber dam removed helps determine the depth and orientation so that perforations and unnecessary removal of tooth structure can be avoided (see Fig. 13.33).

The estimated depth of access for anterior teeth is similar in different tooth groups.[35] The maxillary central and lateral incisors average 5.5 mm for the central incisor and 5 mm for the lateral incisor. The mandibular central and lateral incisors average 4.5 mm for the central incisor and 5 mm for the lateral incisor. The maxillary canine averages 5.5 mm, and the mandibular canine, with its longer clinical crown, averages 6 mm. In maxillary furcated premolars, the

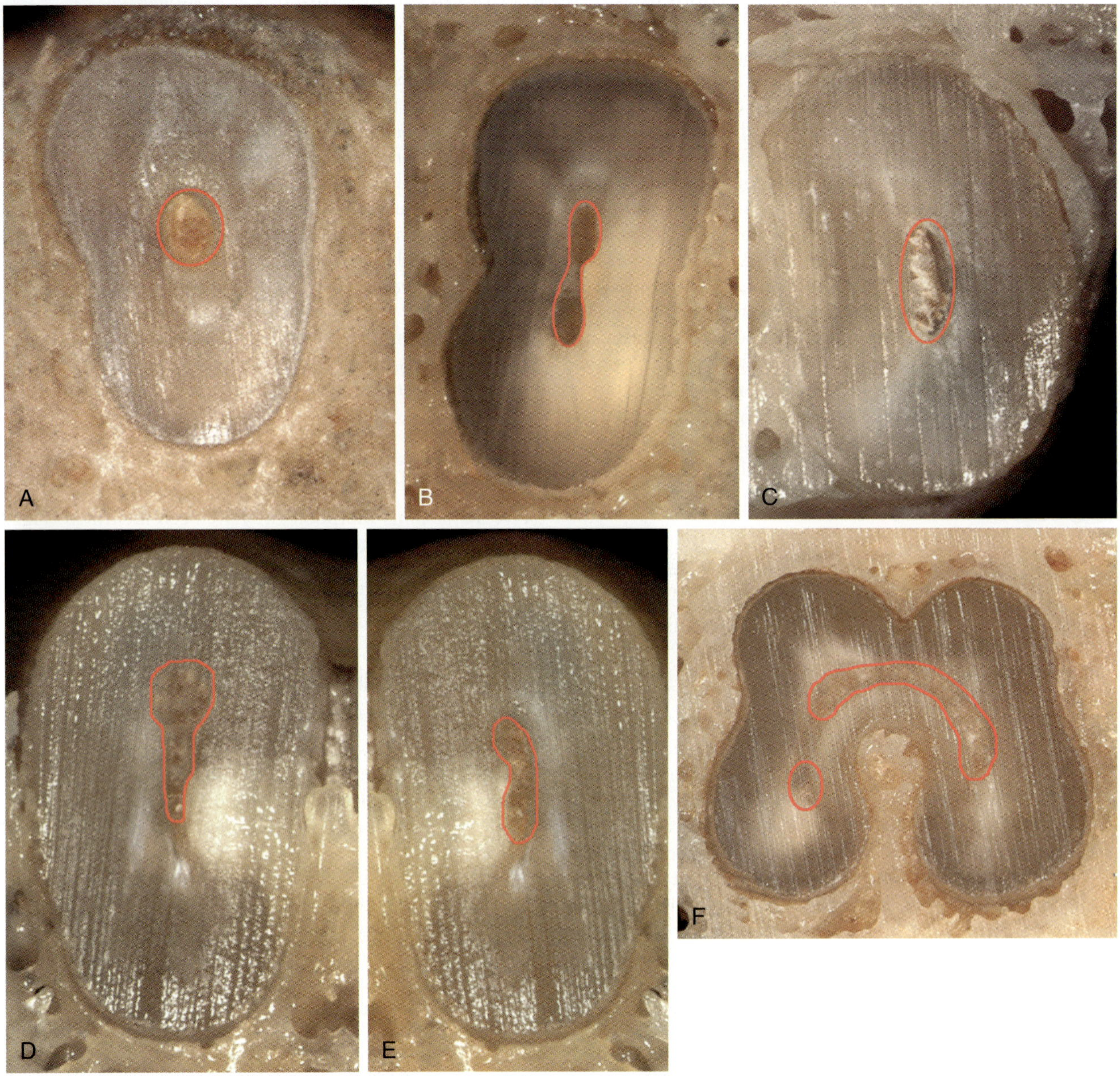

• **Fig. 13.7** Common canal morphologies. **A,** Round. **B,** Ribbon shaped (hourglass). **C,** Ovoid. **D,** Bowling pin. **E,** Kidney bean shaped. **F,** C-shaped.

average distance from the buccal cusp tip to the roof of the chamber is 7 mm.[35] For maxillary molars, the distance is 6 mm, and for the mandibular molars, it is 6.5 mm. With an average pulp chamber height of 2 mm, the access depth for most molars should not extend beyond 8 mm (the floor of the chamber).[23]

Access openings are best accomplished using fissure burs in the high-speed handpiece. A number of special burs are also available for access. No single bur type is superior. For the clinician with knowledge of anatomy and morphology and the appropriate clinical skills and judgment, bur selection is a personal choice (Figs. 13.8 and 13.9). Regardless of the high-speed bur chosen, the bur is placed in the chamber and removed while rotating. High-speed burs are not used in the canals. Failure to follow these principles can result in breakage (Fig. 13.10).

Visualization of the internal anatomy is enhanced during access by using a fiberoptic handpiece and microscopy.[36] Illumination is the key. A sharp endodontic explorer is used to detect the canal orifice or to aggressively dislodge calcifications. When a canal is located, a small file or pathfinding instrument (0.06, 0.08, or 0.10 stainless steel file) is used to explore the canal and determine canal patency close to the apical foramen. Care should be exercised during this process to avoid forcing tissue apically, which might result in canal blockage (Fig. 13.11). This procedure is performed in the presence of irrigant or lubricant.

Removal of restorative materials during access is often indicated, with the knowledge that after treatment a new restoration will be placed. Removal enhances visibility and may reveal undetected canals, caries, or coronal fractures. When difficulties occur with calcifications or extensive restorations, the operator may become disoriented. The discovery of one canal can serve as a reference in locating the remaining canals. A file can be inserted and an angled image exposed to reveal which canal has been located.

It is important not to violate marginal ridges during access preparation in any of the tooth groups.

Complex restorations, such as crowns and fixed partial dentures, may have changed the coronal landmarks used in canal location. A tipped tooth might be "uprighted" or a rotated tooth "realigned." Loss

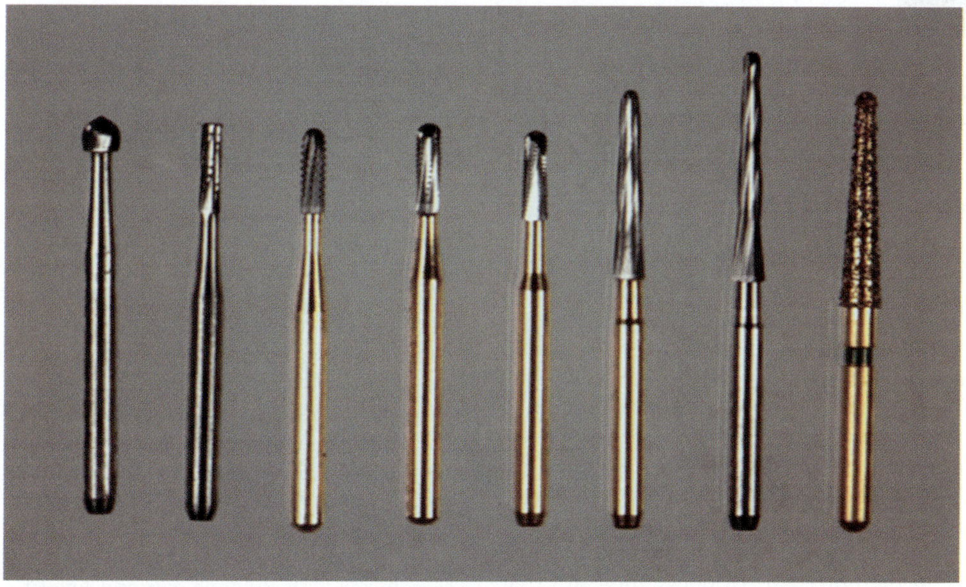

• **Fig. 13.8** Examples of access burs. *Left to right,* No. 4 round carbide, No. 557 carbide, Great White, Beaver bur, Transmetal, Multipurpose bur, Endo Z bur, and Endo Access bur.

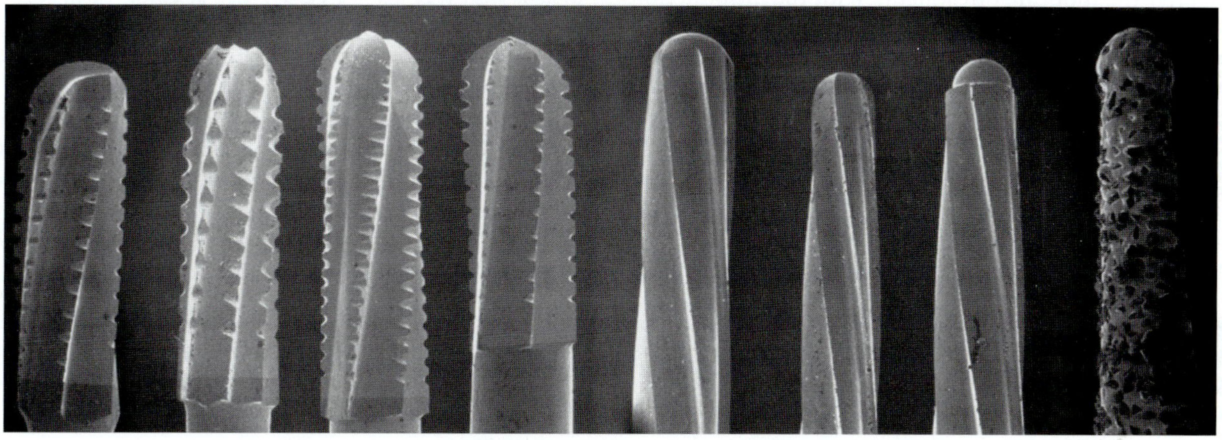

• **Fig. 13.9** Muller discovery Access burs.

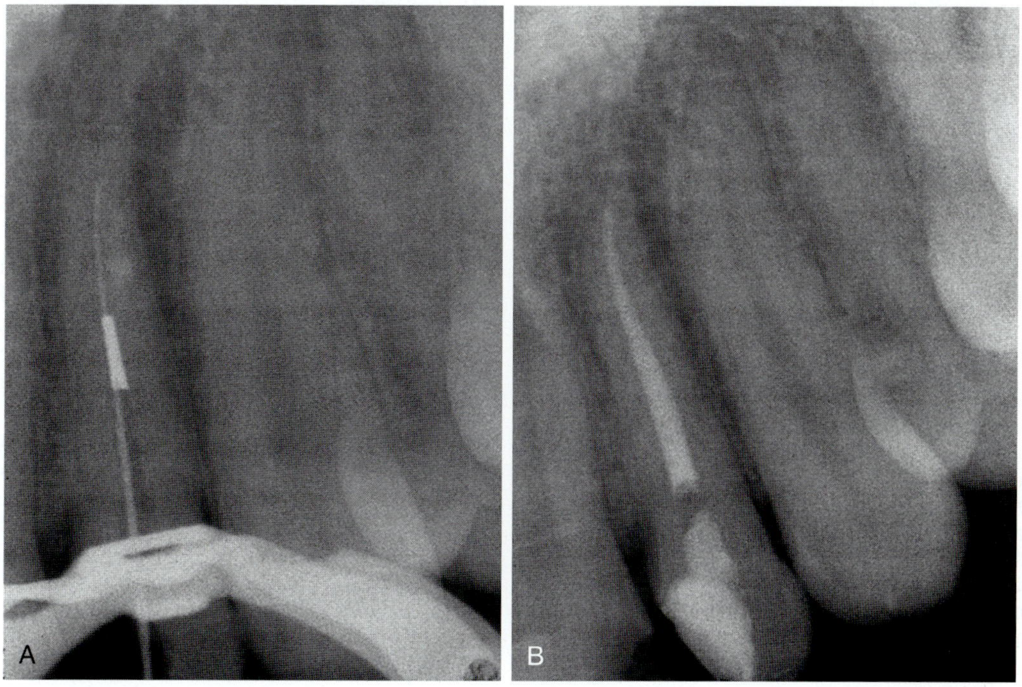

• **Fig. 13.10** **A,** Fractured fissure bur and working length file bypassing the obstruction. **B,** After the bur was removed with files and ultrasonics.

of orientation can result in incorrect identification of a canal, and searching for the other canals in the wrong direction results in excessive removal of tooth structure, perforation, or failure to locate and débride all canals.

Access through crowns with extensive foundations may make visibility difficult. Class V restorations may have induced coronal calcification or could have been placed directly into the pulp space or the canals. In some instances, it may be best to remove restorative materials that interfere with visibility before initiating root canal treatment.

A modification of the armamentarium for teeth restored with crowns has been advocated for all-ceramic crowns. The initial outline and penetration through ceramic (porcelain) restorative material are made with a round diamond bur in the high-speed handpiece with water coolant. After penetration into dentin, a fissure bur is used. In teeth with porcelain-fused-to-metal restorations, a metal cutting bur is recommended. When possible, the access should remain in metal to reduce the potential for fracture in the porcelain. Evidence indicates that with a water coolant and careful instrumentation, diamond and carbide burs are equally effective.[37] The access is restored with amalgam after the root canal treatment. With the introduction of all-ceramic and zirconia crowns, specialized burs have been fabricated to facilitate access through these very hard materials.

In summary, aids in canal location include a knowledge of pulp anatomy and morphology; parallel straight-on and angled radiographs or digital images; a sharp endodontic explorer; interim radiographs or digital images; long-shanked, slow-speed burs (Fig. 13.12); ultrasonic instruments for troughing; dye staining; irrigation; transillumination; and enhanced vision with loupes or microscopy.[38] Additional aids include CBCT imaging.[25,26]

Study Questions

1. Avoidance of rubber dam isolation can place patients and clinicians at unnecessary risk.
   a. True
   b. False
2. Rubber dam isolation serves the following purpose:
   a. Protects patient from instruments
   b. Provides a more aseptic field of work
   c. Enhances visibility
   d. Retracts tissues
   e. All of the above
3. If adequate tooth structure is not remaining for clamp placement, which of the following is not acceptable?
   a. Rubber dam placement may be avoided.
   b. The tooth may require placement of a buildup to enhance remaining structure.
   c. The tooth may require crown lengthening procedure.
   d. Patient may need to be referred to a specialist.
   e. A deep-reaching clamp may be required.
4. What is the best time to assess difficulties and challenges in tooth isolation and placement of a rubber dam?
   a. Before initiation of treatment
   b. At the time of placement of the clamp
   c. After access preparation
   d. After caries removal
5. Which of the following is correct with respect to access preparation?
   a. Endodontic access openings are based on the anatomy and morphology of each tooth.
   b. The pulp number of root canals dictates the final design.
   c. Typically, the internal anatomy is projected onto the external surface.
   d. Age may affect the internal anatomy of the pulp chamber.
   e. All of the above.

Access Openings and Canal Location*

Maxillary Central and Lateral Incisors

The maxillary central incisor has one root and one canal.[41] In young individuals, the prominent pulp horns require a triangular outline form to ensure that tissue and obturation materials, which otherwise might cause coronal discoloration, are removed (Fig. 13.13). Although the canal is centered in the root at the CEJ and when the tooth is viewed from a mesial to distal orientation, it is evident that the crown is not directly in line with the long axis of the root (Fig. 13.14). For this reason, the establishment of the outline form and initial penetration into enamel are made with the bur perpendicular to the lingual surface of the tooth. This outline form is made in the middle third of the lingual surface (Figs. 13.15 and Figs. 13.16). After penetration to the depth of 2 to 3 mm, the bur is reoriented to coincide with the long axis and lingual orientation of the root.

After penetration to a depth of 2 to 3 mm, the bur is reoriented to coincide with the long axis and lingual orientation of the root. This reorientation reduces the risk of a lateral perforation through the facial surface. An additional common error is failure to remove the lingual shelf (see Fig. 13.15, *C*), which results in inadequate access to the entire canal. The canal is located by using a sharp endodontic explorer. When calcification has occurred, long-shanked burs in a slow-speed handpiece can be used (see Figs. 13.12 and 13.24, *D*). These burs move the head of the handpiece away from the tooth and enhance the ability to see exactly where the bur is placed in the tooth.

Access for the maxillary lateral incisor is similar to that for the central incisor. A triangular access is indicated in young patients with pulp horns (Fig. 13.17); as the pulp horns recede, the outline form becomes ovoid (Fig. 13.18).

Dens invaginatus (or dens en dente) is a common developmental defect in the maxillary lateral incisor that results in pulp necrosis.[40-42] Additionally, a lingual groove may be found in maxillary lateral incisors, as evidenced by a narrow probing defect. These developmental defects complicate treatment and affect the prognosis.

Maxillary Canines

The maxillary canines have one canal in a single root. In general, pulp horns are absent, so the outline form is ovoid in the middle third of the lingual surface (Figs. 13.19 and 13.20). As attrition occurs, the chamber appears to move more incisally because of the loss of structure. In cross-section, the pulp is wide in a faciolingual direction compared with the mesiodistal dimension.

Maxillary Premolars

The maxillary first and second premolars have a similar coronal structure; therefore the outline form is similar for these two teeth. It is centered in the crown and has an ovoid shape in the faciolingual direction (Figs. 13.21 and 13.22). An important anatomic consideration with these teeth is the mesial concavity at the CEJ. In this area, a lateral perforation is likely to occur. When two canals are present, the canal orifices are located under the buccal and lingual cusp tips, equidistant from a line drawn through the center of the chamber in a mesial to distal direction. The cross-sectional morphology shows a kidney bean– or ribbon-shaped configuration. In rare instances when three canals are present, the outline form is triangular, with the base to the facial and the apex toward the lingual.

*See Appendix, Pulpal Anatomy and Access Preparations, for color illustrations showing the size, shape, and location of the pulp space in each tooth.

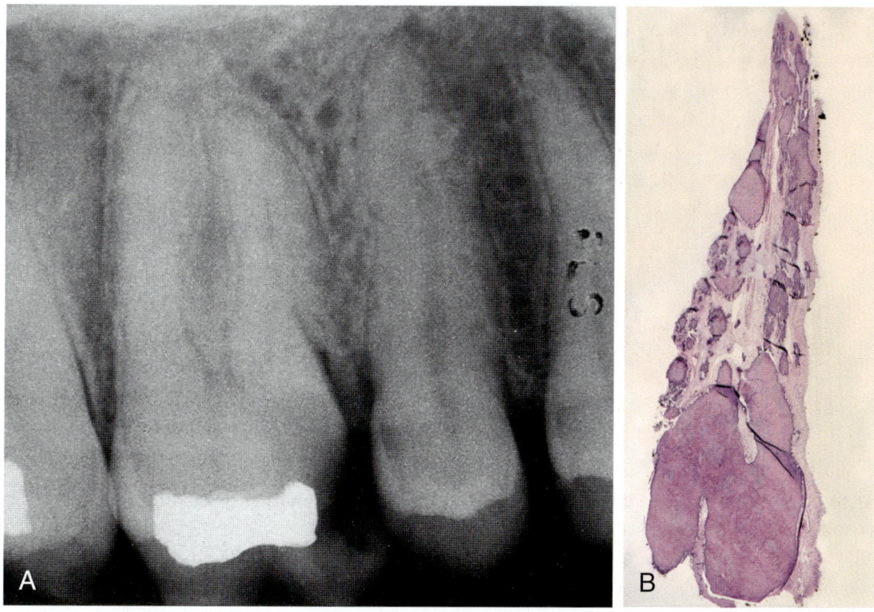

• **Fig. 13.11 A,** Maxillary first molar shows extensive mesial caries. **B,** Histologic section of pulp tissue from the palatal canal reveals extensive calcification. Early canal exploration should be done with small files to avoid forcing the tissue and calcification apically and blocking the canal.

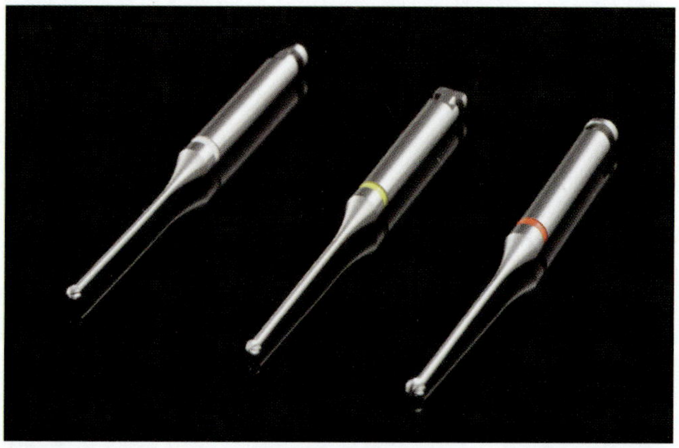

• **Fig. 13.12** Mueller burs have a round cutting head attached to a long shank. The long shank is not designed to drill deep into the root, but rather to extend the head of the slow-speed handpiece away from the tooth and permit better visibility.

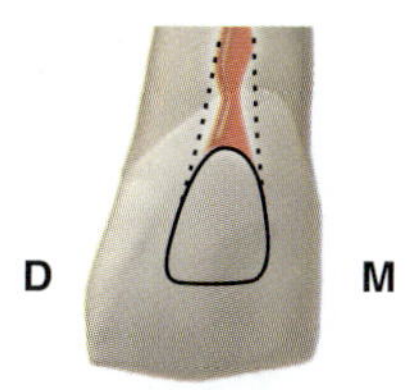

• **Fig. 13.13** A triangular outline form for access of the maxillary central incisor.

Maxillary Molars

The maxillary first and second molars have similar access outline forms. The outline form is triangular and located in the mesial half of the tooth, with the base to the facial and the apex toward the lingual (Figs. 13.23 and 13.24). The transverse or oblique ridge is left mostly intact. The external references for canal location serve as a guide in developing the outline form. The mesiobuccal canal orifice lies slightly distal to the mesiobuccal cusp tip. The distobuccal canal orifice lies distal and slightly lingual to the main mesiobuccal canal and is in line with the buccal groove. The lingual or palatal canal orifice generally exhibits the largest orifice and lies slightly distal to the mesiolingual cusp tip. The mesiobuccal root is very broad in a buccolingual direction; thus a small second canal is common.[43-47] The mesiolingual canal orifice (commonly referred to as the *MB2 canal*) is located 1 to 3 mm lingual to the main mesiobuccal canal *(MB1 canal)* and is slightly mesial to a line drawn from the mesiobuccal to the lingual or palatal canal. The initial movement of the canal from the chamber is often not toward the apex but laterally toward the mesial (Fig. 13.25).

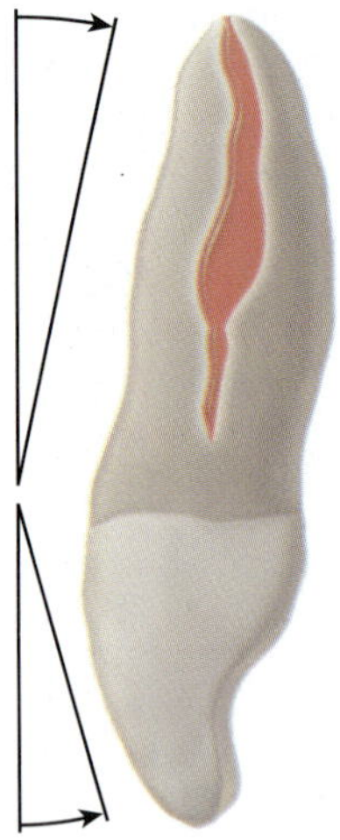

• **Fig. 13.14** Note the lingual inclination of the root in relation to the crown. In addition, the pattern of calcification occurs from the coronal portion of the pulp apically.

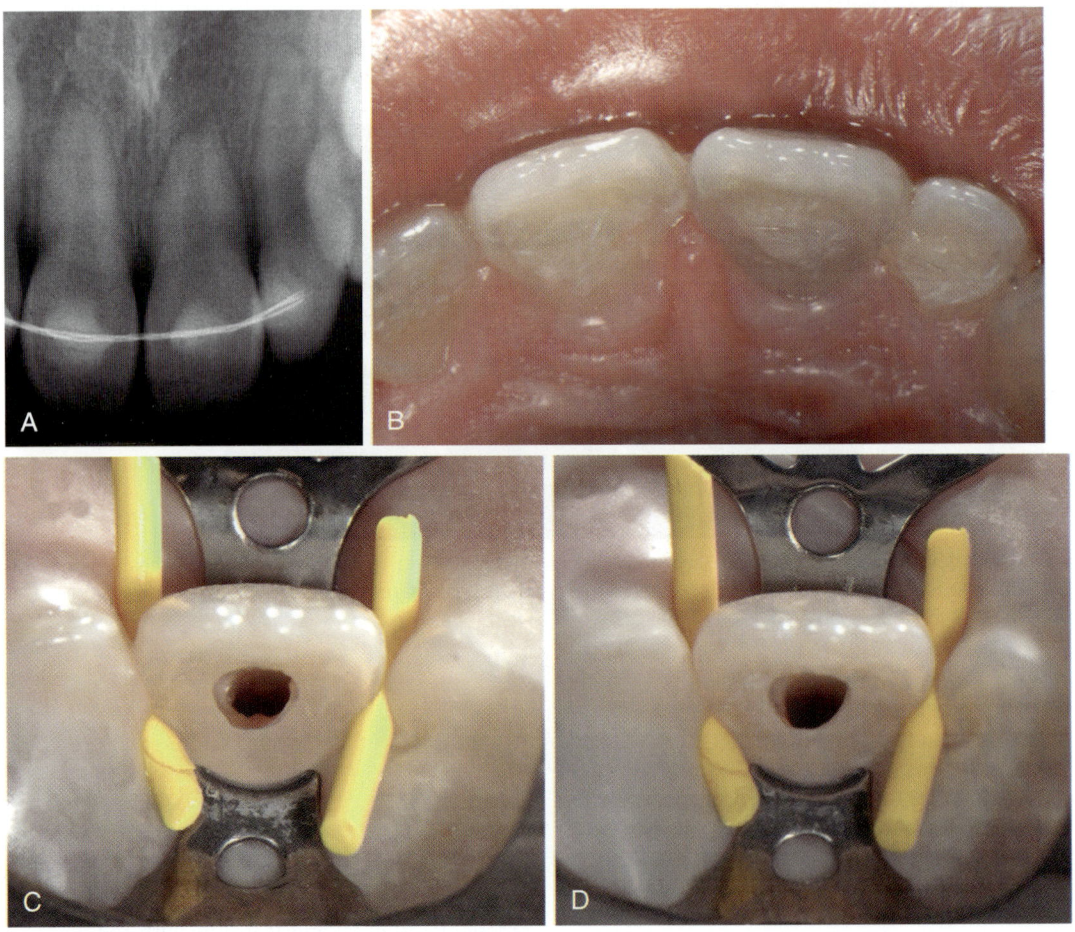

• **Fig. 13.15** A maxillary left central incisor showing pulp necrosis. **A,** A large pulp space with pulp horns that requires a triangular access outline. **B,** The lingual surface after removal of the orthodontic retaining wire. Note that tooth #9 is slightly discolored. **C,** The initial triangular access form exposing the chamber. Note that the lingual shelf has not been removed to expose the lingual wall. **D,** Removal of the lingual shelf and completed access.

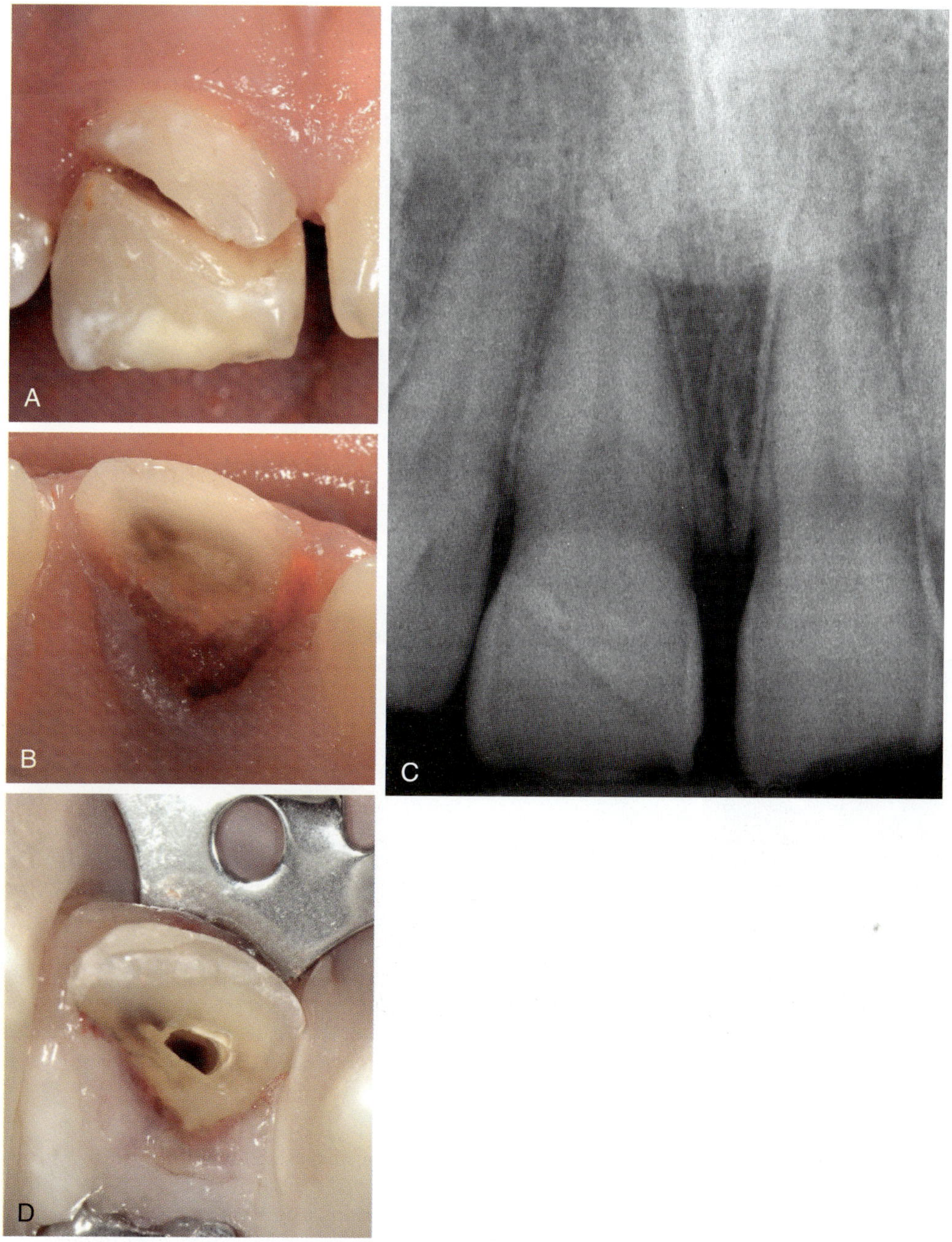

• **Fig. 13.16** Crown-root fracture. **A,** Initial presentation demonstrating fragment separation. **B,** The lingual surface with the segment removed. **C,** Preoperative radiograph. **D,** The extent of the fracture subgingivally requires a unique approach to isolation. Note that a premolar clamp is placed on the gingival tissues for isolation.

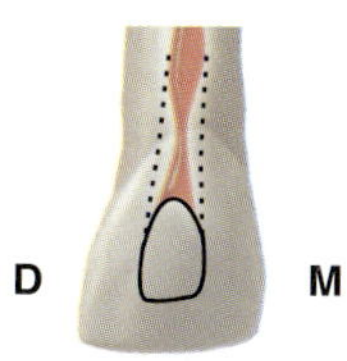

• **Fig. 13.17** Triangular outline form of the maxillary lateral incisor.

Removal of the coronal dentin (cornice) in this area permits exposure of the canal as it begins to move apically and facilitates negotiation (Figs. 13.26 and 13.27; also see Figs. 13.24 and 13.25).[47] The operating microscope is a valuable aid.[36,38,39]

Mandibular Central and Lateral Incisors

The mandibular incisors are narrow in the mesiodistal dimension and broad faciolingually. There may be one canal with an ovoid or a ribbon-shaped configuration; often two canals are present. When there are two canals, the facial canal is easier to locate and is generally straighter than the lingual canal, which is often shielded

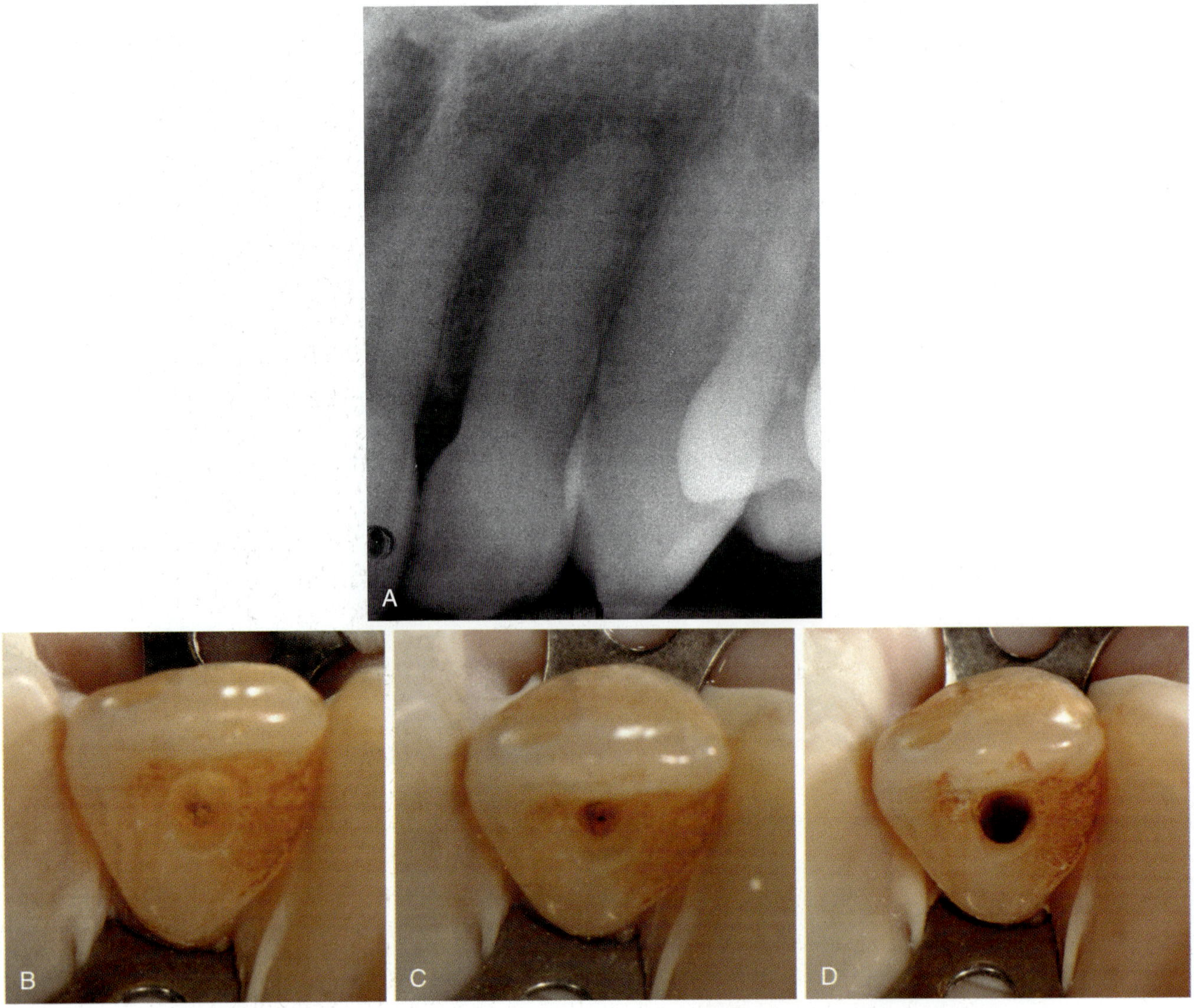

• **Fig. 13.18** **A,** Lateral incisor with a receded pulp chamber. **B,** Initial ovoid outline form is initiated. **C,** Coronal calcification is indicated by the color change. **D,** Completed access.

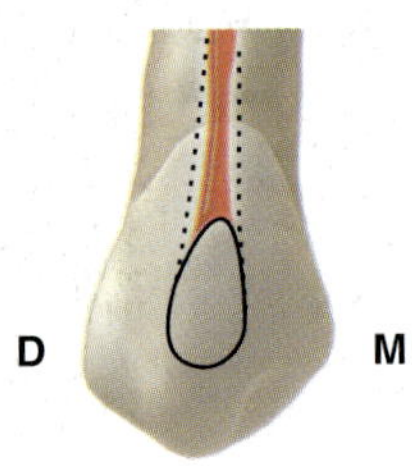

• **Fig. 13.19** Outline form for the maxillary canine.

by a lingual bulge. Because the tooth is often tipped facially, the lingual canal is difficult to locate; perforations primarily occur on the facial surface.

The narrow mesiodistal dimension of these teeth makes access and canal location difficult. In young patients with mesiodistal pulp horns, the outline form is triangular with the base incisally and the apex gingivally. As the pulp recedes over time and the pulp horns disappear, the shape becomes more ovoid. The access is positioned in the middle third of the lingual surface (Figs. 13.28 and 13.29). Because of the small size of these teeth and the presence of mesiodistal concavities, access must be precisely positioned. The initial outline form is established into dentin with the bur perpendicular to the lingual surface. At a depth of 2 to 3 mm, the bur is reoriented along the long axis of the root. Because the percentage of teeth with two canals is reported to be 25% to 40%,[48,49] the lingual surface of the chamber and canal must be diligently explored with a small, precurved stainless steel file. A Gates Glidden drill or orifice shaper is used on the lingual to remove the dentin bulge.

In cases of attrition, the access moves toward the incisal surface. With the use of nickel–titanium rotary and reciprocating instruments, straight-line access is imperative. A more incisal approach on the lingual or facial surface is justified.[50] A modification of the access for the incisors is a facial approach.[51] This approach provides better visibility and can be used when there is crowding or when the canal is receded below the CEJ.

Mandibular Canines

The mandibular canines usually have a long, slender crown in comparison with the maxillary canine, which is shorter and wider in a mesiodistal direction. The tooth may have one or two roots. The root is broad in a faciolingual dimension and therefore may

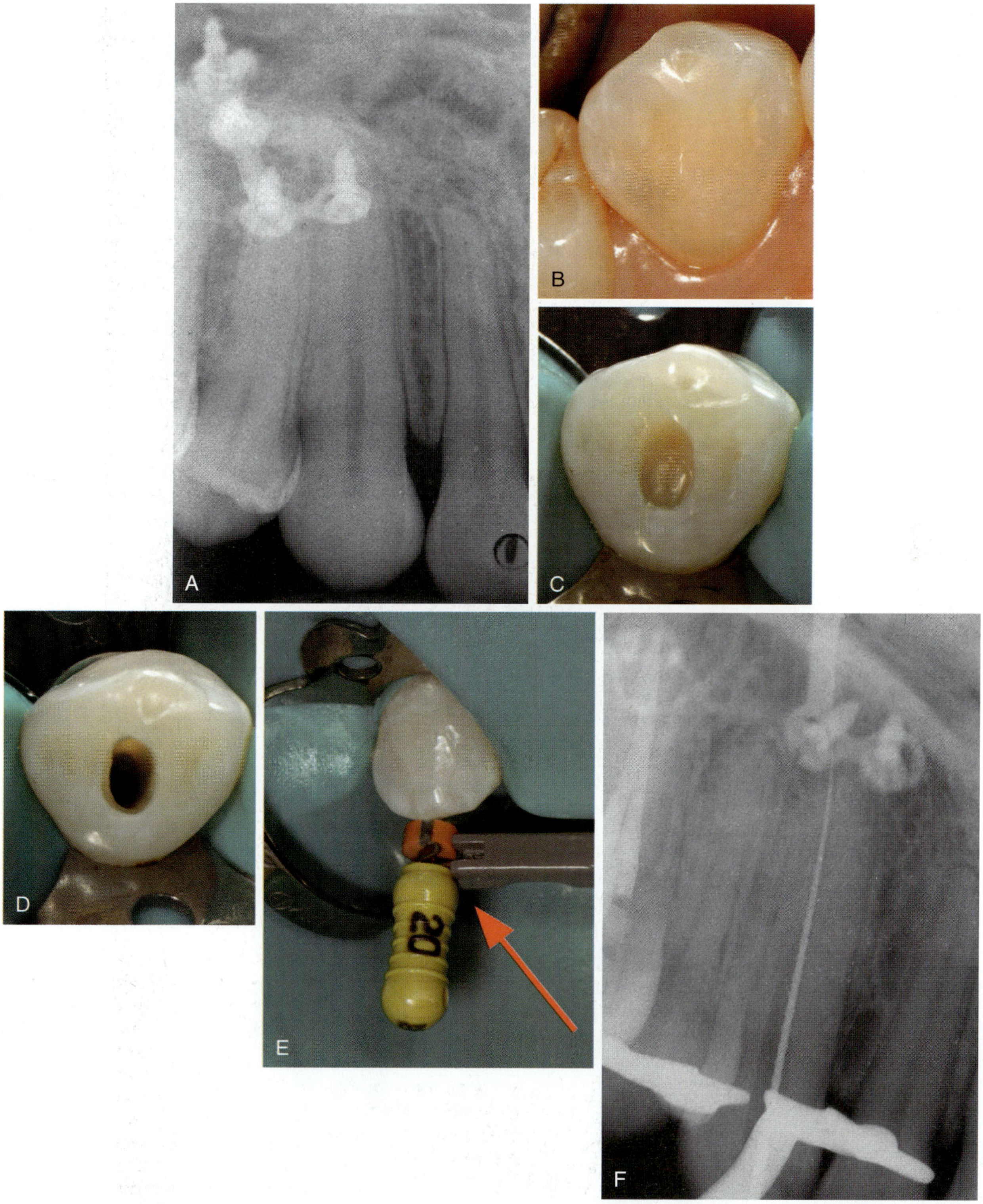

• **Fig. 13.20** **A,** The apex is obscured by the screws placed during a maxillary surgical advancement. **B,** Lingual surface. **C,** Initial access outline into dentin. **D,** Access is finalized. **E,** Apex locator *(arrow)*. **F,** Working length.

contain two canals.[49] The outline form is ovoid and positioned in the middle third of the crown on the lingual surface (Figs. 13.30 and 13.31). On access opening into the chamber, the lingual surface should be explored for the presence of a lingual canal. As attrition occurs, the access must be more incisal, and in severe cases it may include the incisal edge of the tooth.

Mandibular Premolars

The mandibular premolars appear to be easy to treat, but the anatomy may be complex. One, two, or three roots are possible, and canals often divide deep within the root in these complex morphologic configurations.[49,52] The crown of the first premolar has

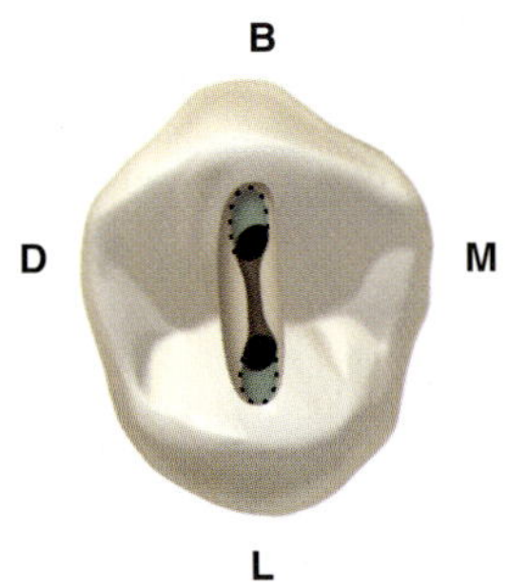

• **Fig. 13.21** Ovoid outline form for the maxillary premolars.

a prominent buccal cusp and a vestigial lingual cusp. In addition, there is a lingual constriction. Mesiodistal projections reveal that the chamber and canal orifice are positioned buccally. The access is therefore ovoid in a buccolingual dimension and positioned buccal to the central groove (Figs. 13.32 and 13.33). It extends just short of the buccal cusp tip. The mandibular second premolar has a prominent buccal cusp, but the lingual cusp can be more prominent than with the first premolar. There is also a lingual constriction, so the outline form is ovoid from buccal to lingual and positioned centrally (Fig. 13.34).

Mandibular Molars

The mandibular molars are similar in anatomic configuration; however, there are subtle differences. The most common mandibular first molar configuration is two canals in the mesial root, although three have been reported,[53] and one canal in the distal root. A second canal is present in the distal root in 30% to 35% of

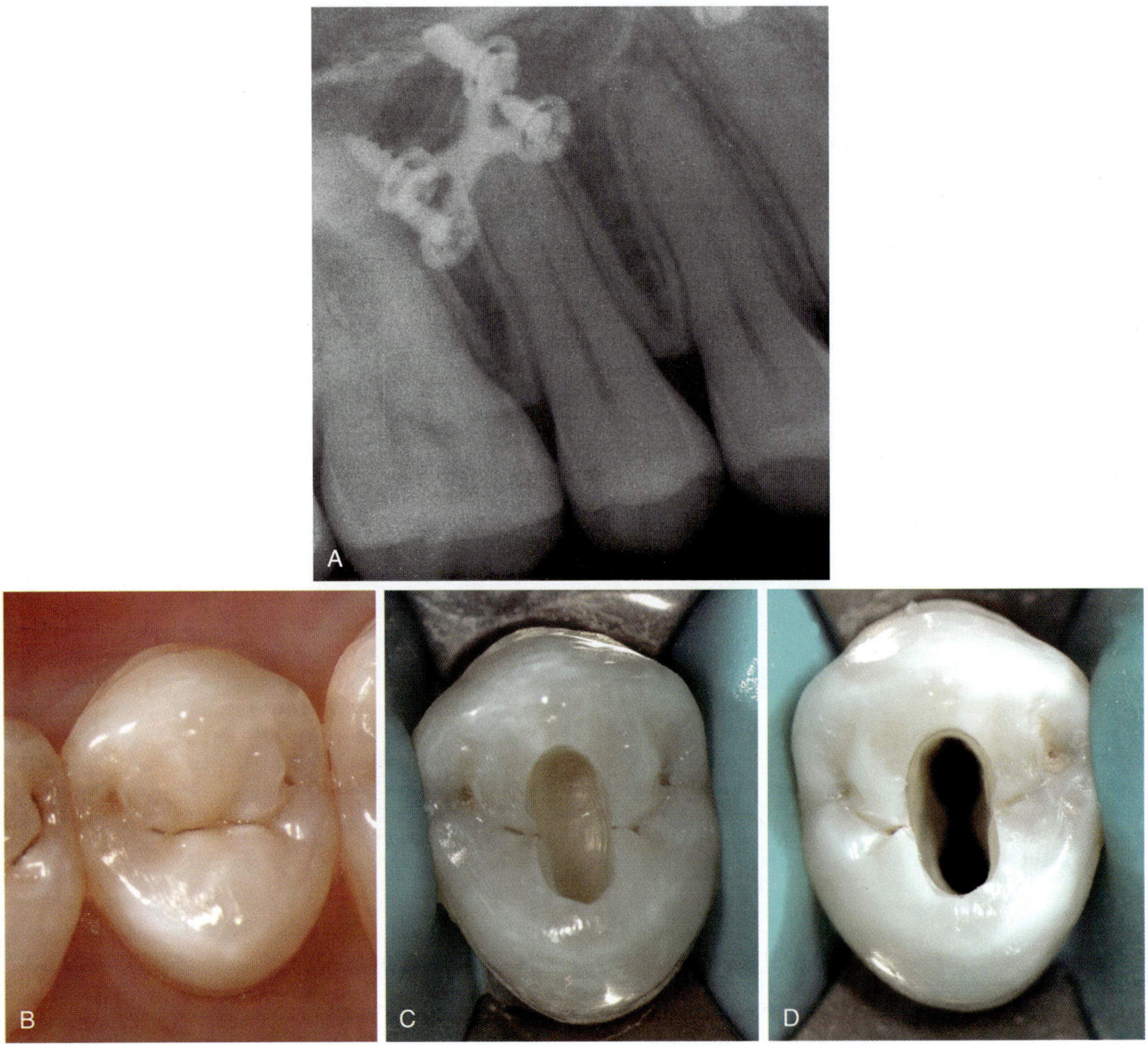

• **Fig. 13.22 A,** Note the obstructed view of the apical region. **B,** Maxillary right second premolar. **C,** The initial outline form prepared into dentin. **D,** The chamber and canals are accessed.

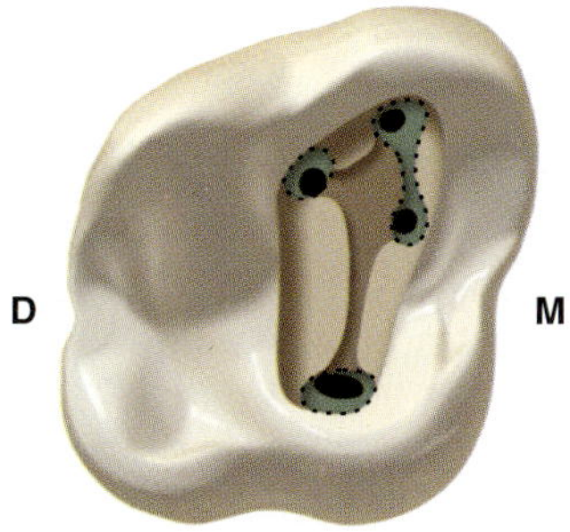

• Fig. 13.23 Triangular outline form for access of the maxillary molar.

cases (Fig. 13.35).[53,55] The roots often have a kidney bean shape in cross section with the concavity in the furcal region. The most common configuration for the mandibular second molar is two canals in the mesial root and one canal in the distal root. The incidence of four canals is low.[54]

The coronal reference points for canal location in the mandibular molar roots are influenced by the position of the crown on the root and by the lingual tipping of these teeth in the arch (Fig. 13.36). The mesiobuccal canal orifice is located slightly distal to the mesiobuccal cusp tip. The mesiolingual canal orifice is located in the area of the central groove area and slightly distal compared with the mesiobuccal canal. The distal canal is located near the intersection of the buccal, lingual, and central grooves. When a distobuccal canal is present, the orifice can be found buccal to the main distal canal and often is slightly more mesial. The mandibular first molar may even have a distinct separate extra distal root. Because of these anatomic relationships, the access outline form is rectangular or trapezoidal and positioned in the mesiobuccal portion of the crown (Fig. 13.37). An additional variation in mandibular molars is the presence of a middle mesial canal (Fig. 13.38).

During access preparation, the cervical bulge that overlies the canal orifices of the mesiobuccal and mesiolingual canals is removed (Fig. 13.39), permitting straight-line access to the first curve or apical portion of the root by reducing the emergence profile. This technique also enhances entry into the canals.

Errors in Access

Inadequate Preparation

Errors in access preparations are varied (Fig. 13.40). A common error is inadequate preparation, which has several significant consequences. Direct effects are decreased access and visibility, which prevent the clinician from locating the canals. The ability to remove the coronal pulp tissue and subsequent obturation materials is limited, and straight-line access cannot be achieved. Inadequate straight-line access can indirectly lead to errors during the cleaning and shaping. When files are deflected by coronal interferences, procedural errors, such as loss of working length, apical transportation, ledging, and apical perforation, are likely in curved canals. A No. 25 file or above has a straightening force that overcomes the confining resistance of the dentin wall. The file cuts on the outer surface apical to the curvature and the inner wall coronal to the curve. Adequate straight-line access decreases the canal curvature and reduces the coronal interferences, allowing the instrument to work more freely in the canal.[55]

Excessive Removal of Tooth Structure

The excessive removal of tooth structure has direct consequences and unlike inadequate preparation is irreversible and cannot be corrected. A minimum consequence is weakening of the tooth and subsequent coronal fracture. Evidence indicates that appropriate access and strategic removal of tooth structure that does not involve the marginal ridges do not significantly weaken the remaining coronal structure.[56] The marginal ridges provide the faciolingual strength to the crown[57]; access openings do not require removal of tooth structure in this area.[58]

The ultimate result of removing excessive tooth structure is perforation. Perforations in single-rooted teeth are located on the lateral surface. In multirooted teeth, perforations may be lateral or furcal (see Chapter 18).

Length Determination

Radiographic Evaluation

The *working length* is defined as the distance from a predetermined coronal reference point (usually the incisal edge in anterior teeth and a cusp tip in posterior teeth) to the point where the cleaning and shaping and obturation should terminate. The reference point must be stable so that fracture does not occur between visits. Unsupported cusps that are weakened by caries or restorations should be reduced. The point of termination is empirical and based on anatomic studies; it should be 1 mm from the radiographic apex.[59,60] This distance accounts for the deviation of the foramen from the apex, and the distance from the major diameter of the foramen to the area where a dentinal matrix can be established apically.

Before access, an estimated working length is calculated either by measuring the total length of the tooth on the diagnostic parallel radiograph or digital image or with the use of an electronic apex locater. Violation of the apex may result in inoculation of the periapical tissues with necrotic tissue, debris, and bacteria[61] and can lead to extrusion of materials during obturation[62,63] and a less favorable prognosis.[64]

After access preparation, a small file is used to explore the canal and establish patency to the estimated working length. The largest file to bind is then inserted to this estimated length; a file that is loose in the canal may be displaced during film exposure or forced beyond the apex if the patient bites down inadvertently. Millimeter markings on the file shaft or rubber stops on the instrument shaft are used for length control. A sterile millimeter ruler or measuring device can be used to adjust the stops on the file. To ensure accurate measurement and length control during canal preparation, the stop must physically contact the coronal reference point. To obtain an accurate measurement, the minimum size of the working length should be a No. 20 file. With files smaller than No. 20, it is difficult to interpret the location of the file tip on the working length film or digital image. In multirooted teeth, files are placed in all canals before the image is made.

Angled films or digital images are necessary to separate superimposed files and structures (Fig. 13.41),[65] to provide an efficient method of determining the working length, and to reduce radiation to the patient. It is imperative that the rubber dam be left in place during working length determination to ensure an aseptic environment and to protect the patient from swallowing or aspirating instruments. The film/digital sensor can be held with a hemostat or a positioning device (Fig. 13.42).

A modified paralleling technique is used to position the film/digital sensor and the cone; this has been shown to be superior to the bisecting-angle technique.[66,67] With the modified paralleling

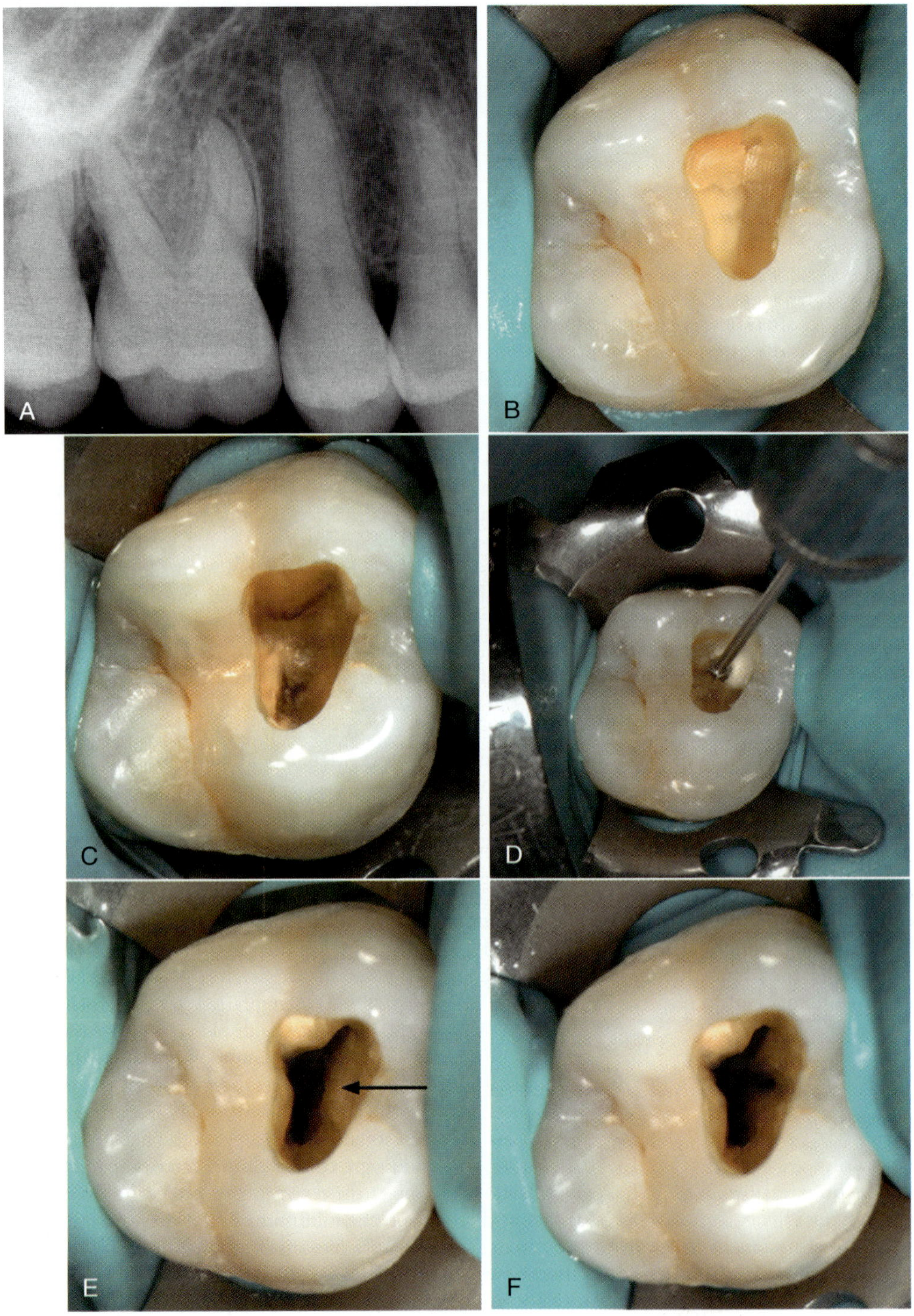

• **Fig. 13.24** **A,** Maxillary left first molar. Note the calcification in the chamber. **B,** The outline form established and dentin removed apically in layers. **C,** Exposure of the pulp horns. **D,** Use of a Mueller bur to completely unroof the chamber. Note the visibility and ability for precise removal of dentin. **E,** The completed access. The mesiobuccal canal is evident under the mesiobuccal cusp tip, the distobuccal canal is found opposite the buccal groove and slightly lingual to the main mesiobuccal canal, and the palatal canal is located under the mesiolingual cusp tip. Note the identification of the mesiolingual canal *(arrow)*. **F,** Removal of the dentinal cornice that covers the mesiolingual canal to reveal the canal orifice. (See Appendix, Pulpal Anatomy and Access Preparations, for color illustrations showing the size, shape, and location of the pulp space within each tooth.)

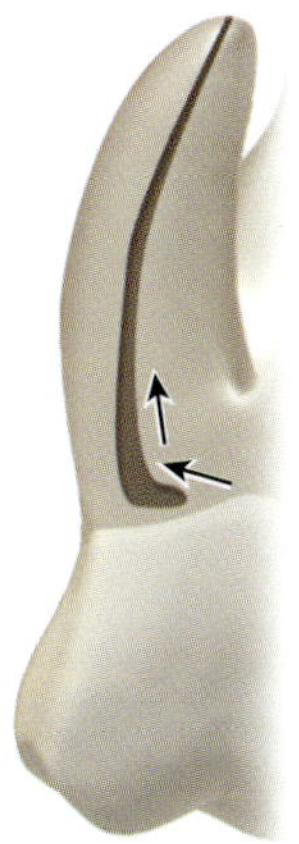

• **Fig. 13.25** The mesiolingual canal as it leaves the pulp chamber. Canals that are not negotiable but detected by an explorer may move laterally before proceeding apically.

technique, the film/digital sensor is positioned by using a hemostat approximately parallel to the long axis of the tooth. The cone is then positioned so that the central beam strikes the film at a 90-degree angle (Fig. 13.43). Although this technique is reliable, it is not foolproof.[68]

Other clinical factors should be considered in establishing the corrected working length. These include tactile sensation,[69] the patient's response, and hemorrhage. The use of tactile sensation may be valuable in large tapering canals; however, in small cylindrical canals, the rate of taper of the files may exceed the rate of taper of the canal, and binding occurs coronally, giving the false sense of constriction. Preflaring the canal before length determination increases the tactile sensation significantly compared with unflared canals.[70]

After the film or sensor exposure, the corrected working length is calculated. The distance from the file tip to the radiographic apex is determined. If the distance is greater than 1 mm, a calculation is made (adding or subtracting length) so that the file tip is positioned 1 mm from the radiographic apex. If the correction is greater than 3 mm, a second working length radiograph or digital image should be made with the file placed at the adjusted length.

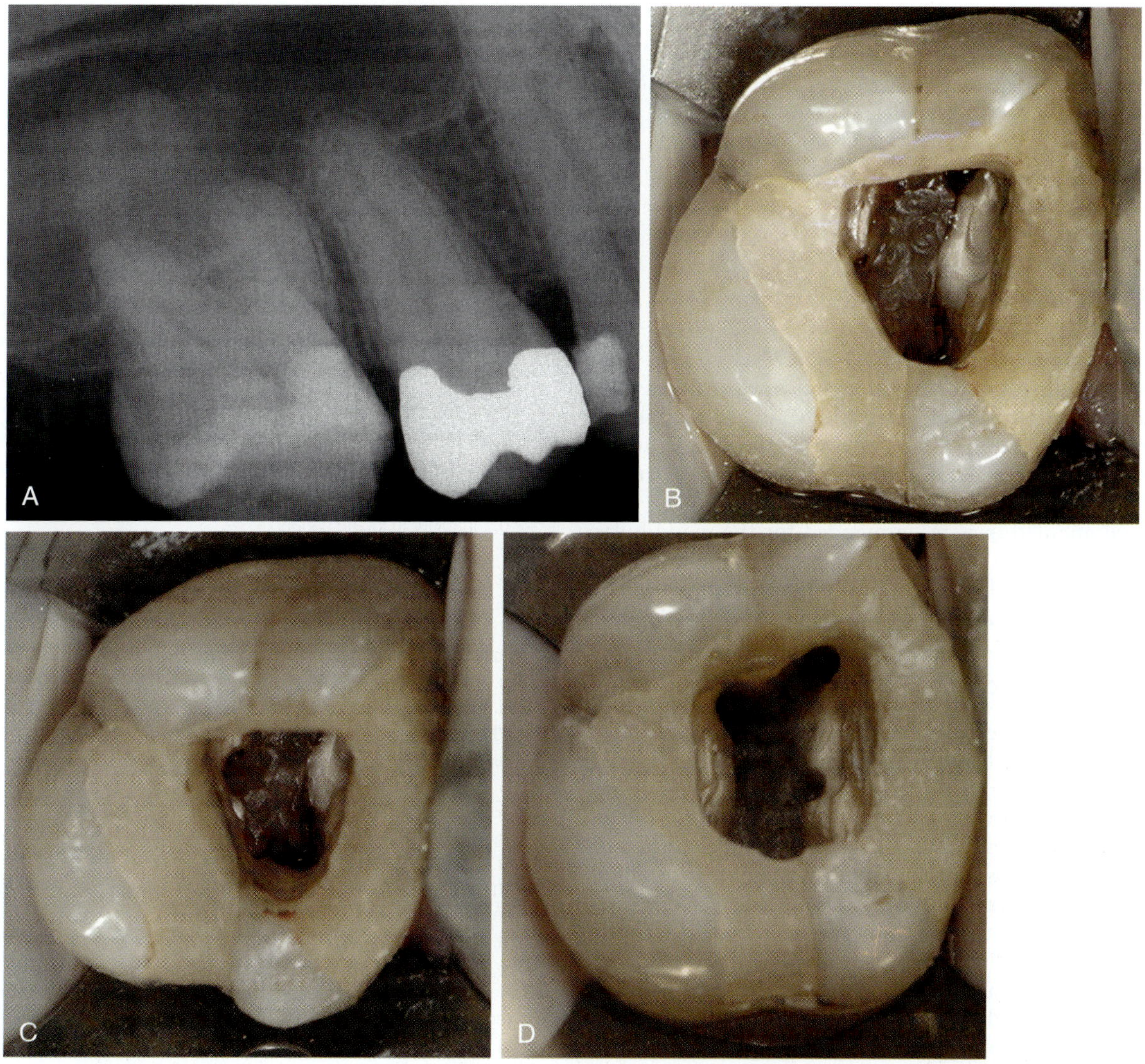

• **Fig. 13.26** **A,** Maxillary left first molar showing calcification. **B** and **C,** Initial access and identification of a pulp stone. Color and a thin line surrounding the periphery identify the hemorrhage. **D,** The pulp chamber with the stone removed. (See Appendix, Pulpal Anatomy and Access Preparations, for color illustrations showing the size, shape, and location of the pulp space within each tooth.)

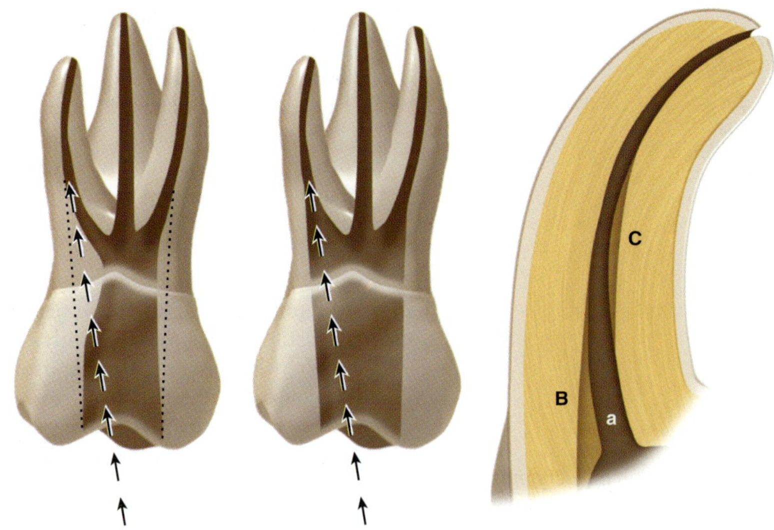

• **Fig. 13.27** **A,** The dashed lines show where dentin must be removed to achieve straight-line access. **B,** The access completed. **C,** The original canal *(a)* is modified using Gates Glidden burs to remove tooth structure at *(B)* and *(C)*.

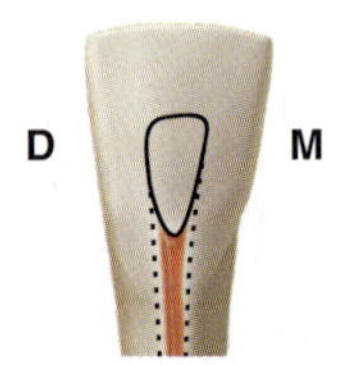

• **Fig. 13.28** Lingual outline form for the mandibular incisor.

With angled radiographs or digital images, the canal determination is based on the buccal object or SLOB rule (same lingual, opposite buccal; see Chapter 3).[71,72] Because maxillary anterior teeth have only one canal, no angle is necessary. Mesial angles are recommended for premolars and maxillary molars (Fig. 13.44). Distal angulation is recommended for the mandibular incisors and molars (Fig. 13.45). For maxillary posterior teeth, the film should be placed on the opposite side of the midline to facilitate capture of the palatal roots on the film (see Fig. 13.43).

Electronic Apex Locators

Apex locators are also used in determining length.[73,74] Contemporary apex locators are based on the principle that the flow of higher frequencies of alternating current is facilitated in a biologic environment compared with lower frequencies. Passing two differing frequencies through the canal results in the higher frequency impeding the lower frequency (Fig. 13.46). The impedance values that change relative to each other are measured and converted to length information. At the apex, the impedance values are at their maximum differences. Unlike previous models, the impedance apex locator operates accurately in the presence of electrolytes.[75] Apex locators are helpful in length determination but must be confirmed with radiographs. Films or digital images help confirm the appropriate length and can identify missed canals. If the file is not centered in the root, a second canal is likely to be present.

An apex locator is very helpful in patients with structures or objects that obstruct visualization of the apex, patients who have a gag reflex and cannot tolerate films, and patients with medical problems that prohibit the holding of a film or sensor.

The use of apex locators and electric pulp testers in patients with cardiac pacemakers has been questioned.[76-81] In a recent study involving 27 patients with either implanted cardiac pacemakers or cardioverter/defibrillators, two impedance apex locators and one electric pulp tester did not interfere with the functioning of any of the cardiac devices.[82] However, it may be advisable not to use these devices in these patients; other means of length determination and pulp testing are available.

Study Questions

6. Name the potential issues related to inadequate access preparation.
   a. Less visibility
   b. Inability to locate canals
   c. Inability to completely remove pulp tissues from the pulp chamber
   d. Instrumentation errors caused by lack of straight-line access
   e. All of the above
7. The ridges should be preserved during access preparation whenever possible.
   a. True
   b. False
8. Which of the following is correct regarding working length determination?
   a. Placement of the smallest file to the apex
   b. Placement of the largest file that binds at the apex
   c. Removal of the file stopper before placement of the file in the canal
   d. Use of files no larger than #
9. The rubber dam may be removed during radiographic working length determination.
   a. True
   b. False
10. During radiographic working length determination, a new radiograph is required if:
   a. The file is within 1 mm of the apex.
   b. The file is at the apex.
   c. The file is more than 2 mm from the apex.
   d. The file is at the apex.

ANSWERS

Answer Box 13

1 a. True
2 e. All of the above.
3 a. Rubber dam placement may be avoided.
4 a. Before initiation of treatment
5 e. All of the above
6 e. All of the above
7 a. Truex
8 b. Placement of the largest file that binds at the apex
9 b. False
10 c. The file is more than 2 mm from the apex.

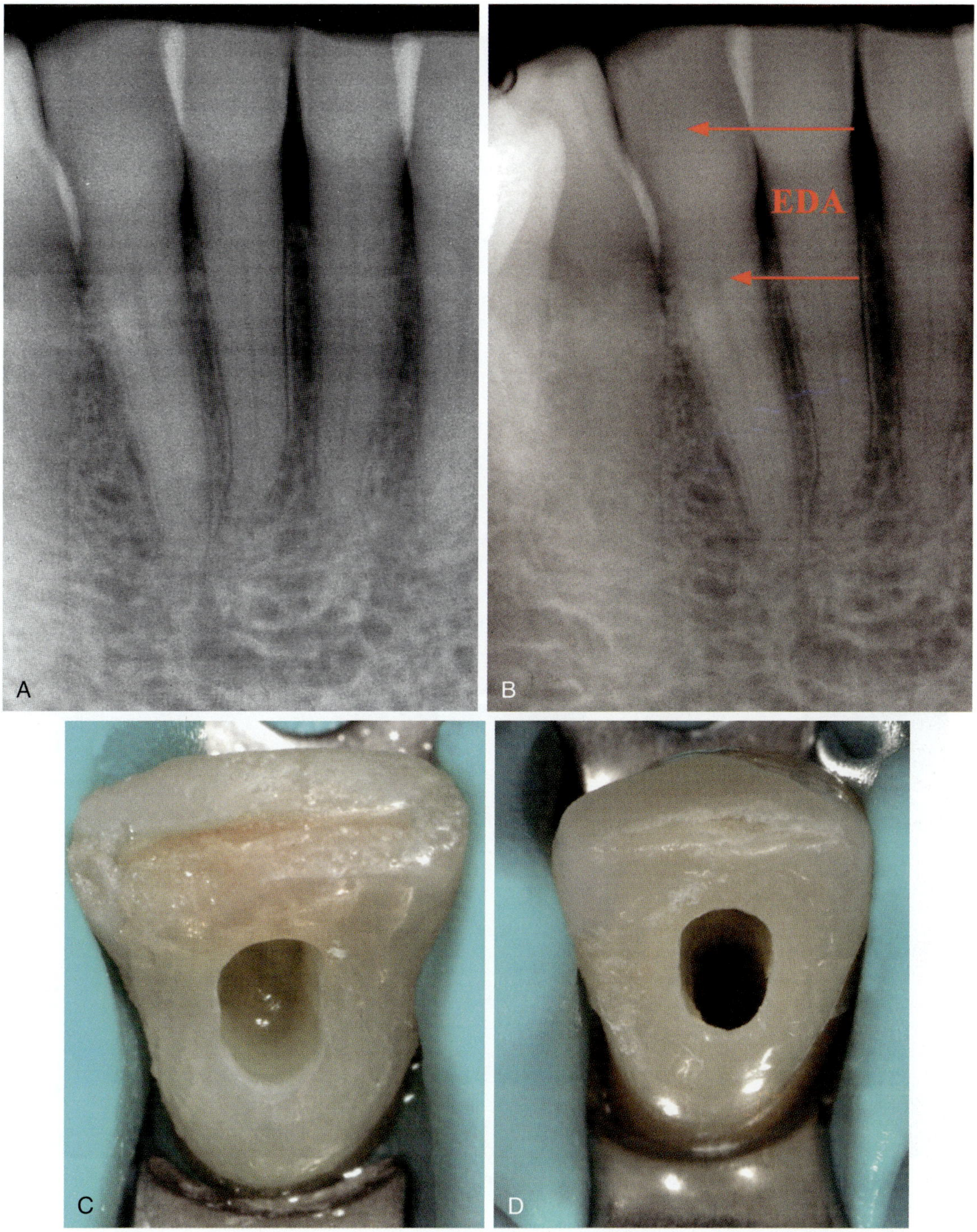

• **Fig. 13.29** **A,** Mandibular lateral incisor. **B,** Calculation of the estimated depth of access from the middle of the lingual surface to the coronal extent of the pulp. **C,** The initial outline form is more oval due to the receded chamber. **D,** Completed access.

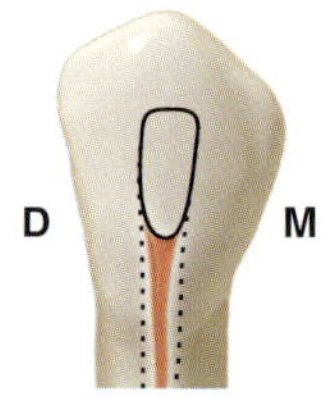

• **Fig. 13.30** Lingual ovoid outline form for the mandibular canine.

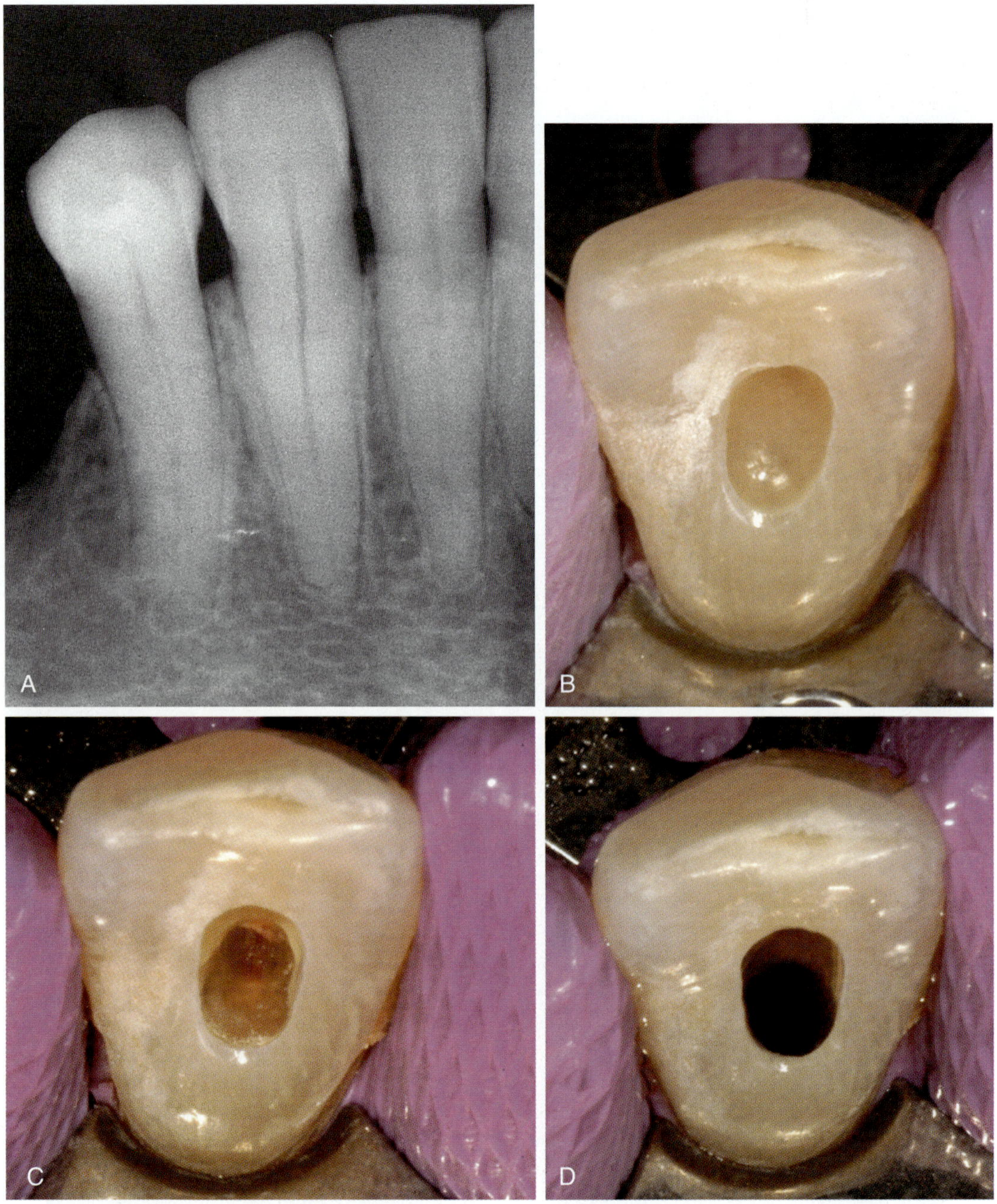

• **Fig. 13.31** **A,** Mandibular canine. **B,** The initial outline form is established into dentin. **C,** Exposure of the coronal pulp. **D,** The completed access opening.

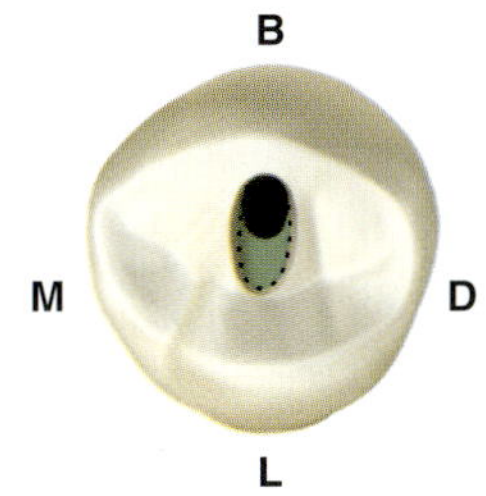

• **Fig. 13.32** Ovoid outline form for the mandibular first premolar. Note that the access is buccal to the central groove.

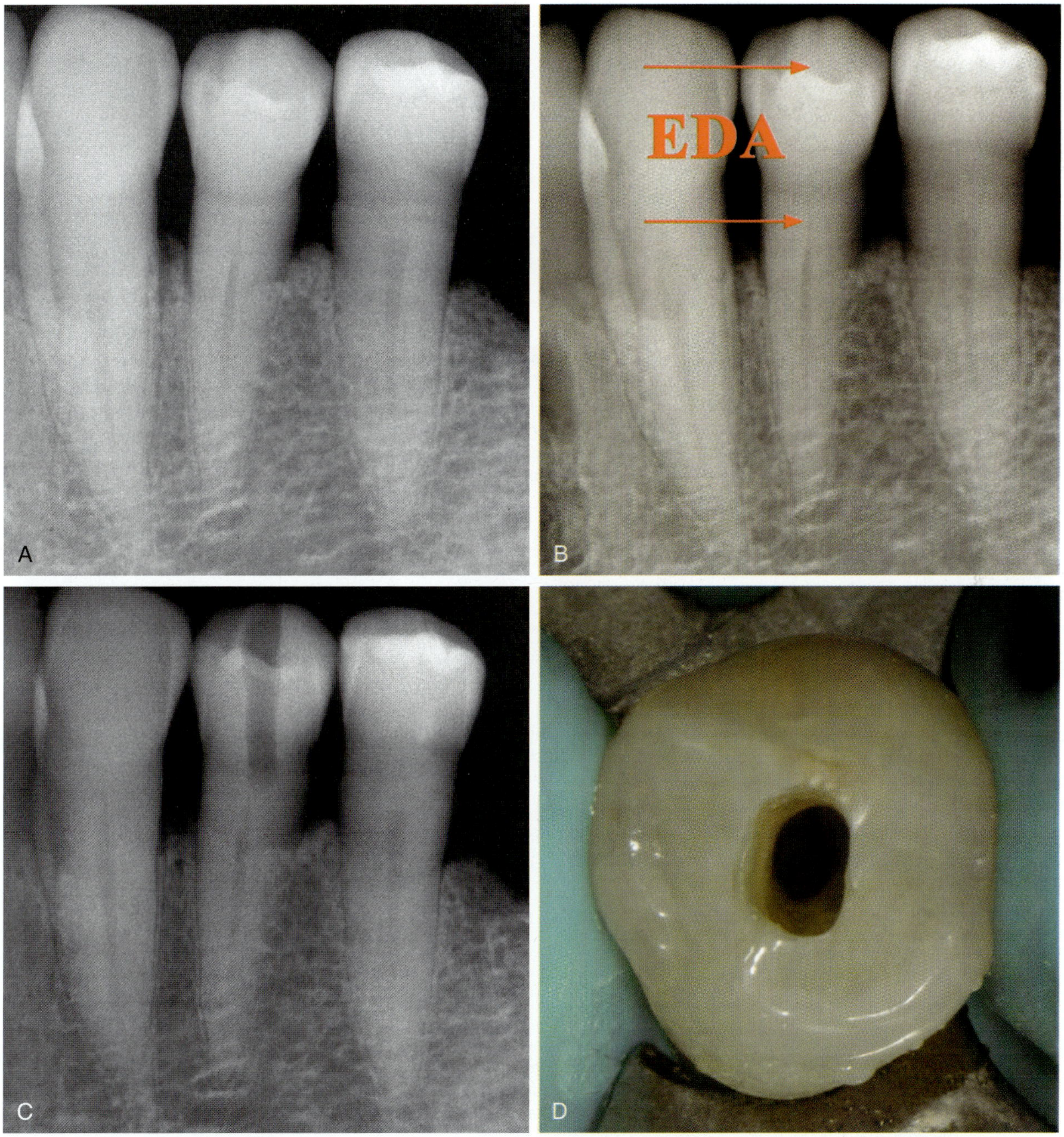

• **Fig. 13.33** **A,** Mandibular right first premolar. Note the receded pulp space. **B,** Calculation of the estimated depth of access. **C,** The estimated depth of access is reached, and the canal is not located. The rubber dam is removed and a straight-on parallel radiograph exposed. The film/digital image indicates that the canal is located mesial to the opening. **D,** The completed access.

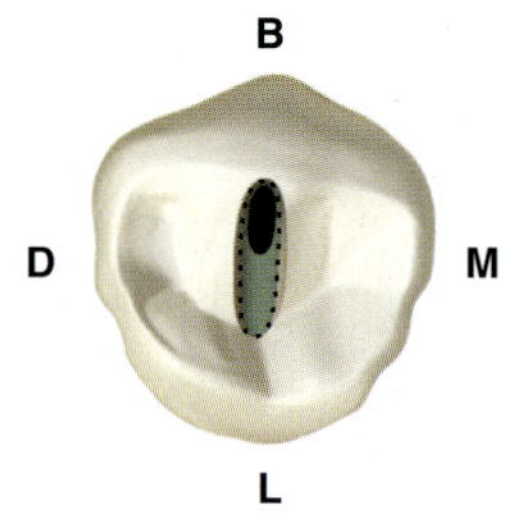

• **Fig. 13.34** Ovoid outline form for the mandibular second premolar.

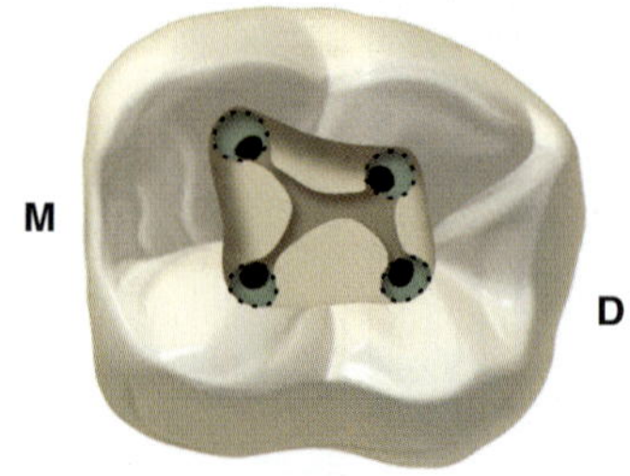

• **Fig. 13.35** Rectangular outline form for the mandibular first molar. Note that the mesiobuccal canal is located under the mesiobuccal cusp, and the mesiolingual canal lies centrally in relation to the crown and slightly to the distal of the mesiobuccal canal. The distolingual canal is located centrally, and the distobuccal canal lies more buccal and mesial to the main canal.

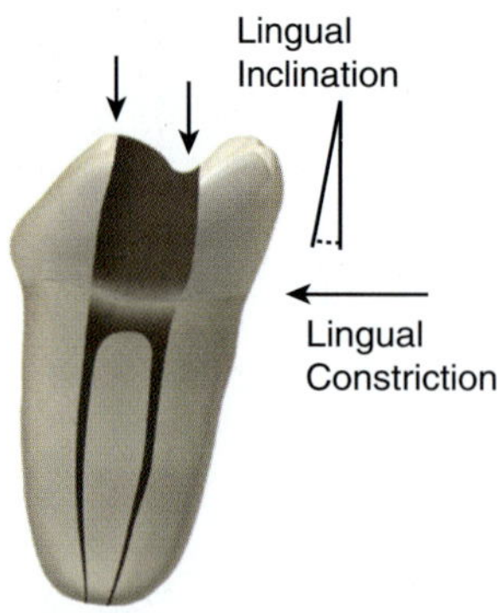

• **Fig. 13.36** Proximal view of a mandibular molar demonstrating the lingual inclination in the dental arch and a lingual constriction of the crown at the cementoenamel junction. Note that the mesiobuccal and mesiolingual canals are uniformly spaced within the root. However, with coronal access, the external reference points for the canal's location are the mesiobuccal cusp tip and the central groove as it crosses the mesial marginal ridge.

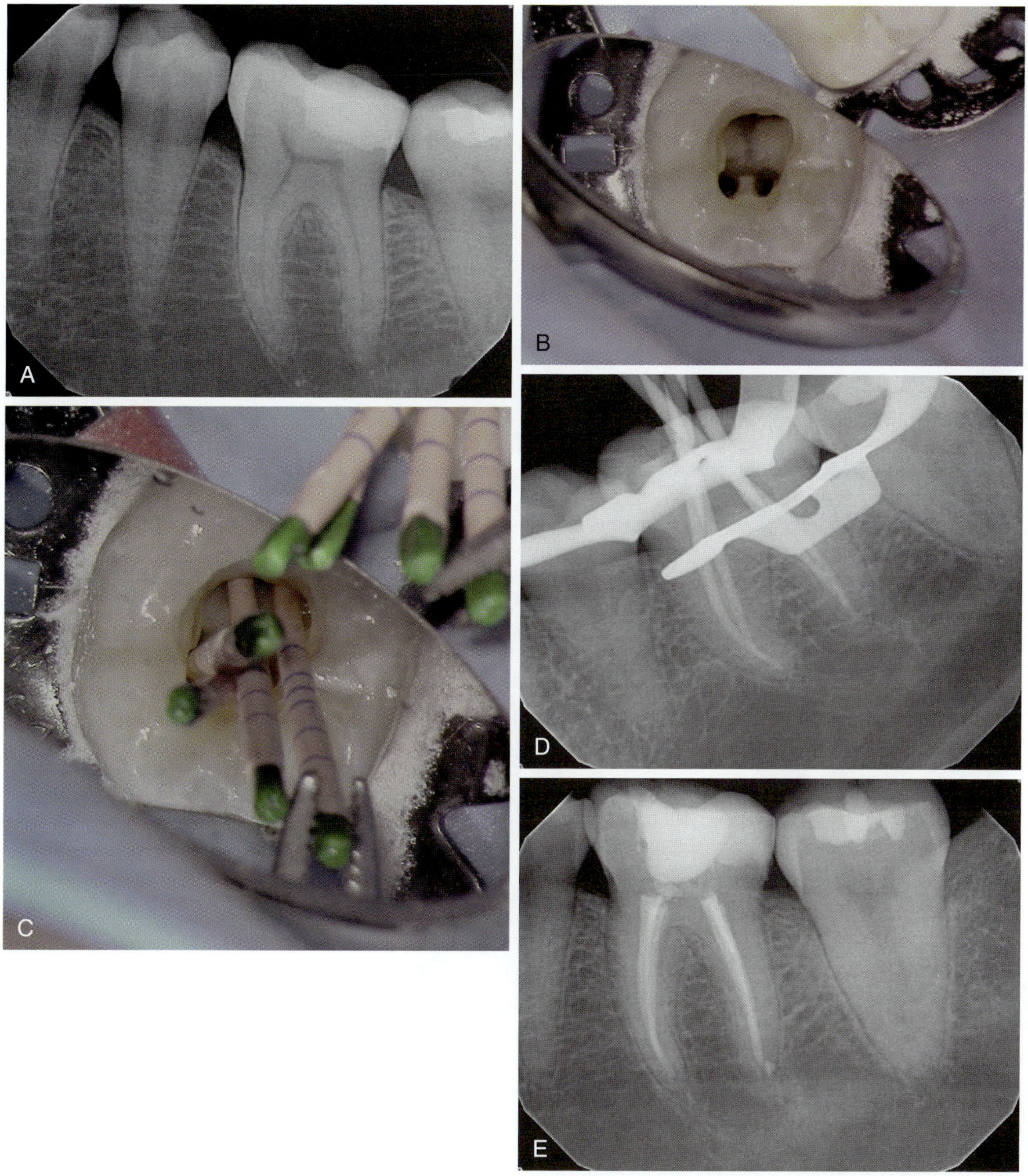

• **Fig. 13.37** **A,** The preoperative radiograph of a mandibular first molar. **B,** The completed access cavity demonstrating the two mesial canals and the single distal canal. **C,** Cone fit. **D,** Cone fit radiograph. **E,** postoperative radiograph. (See Appendix, Pulpal Anatomy and Access Preparations, for color illustrations showing the size, shape, and location of the pulp space within each tooth.)

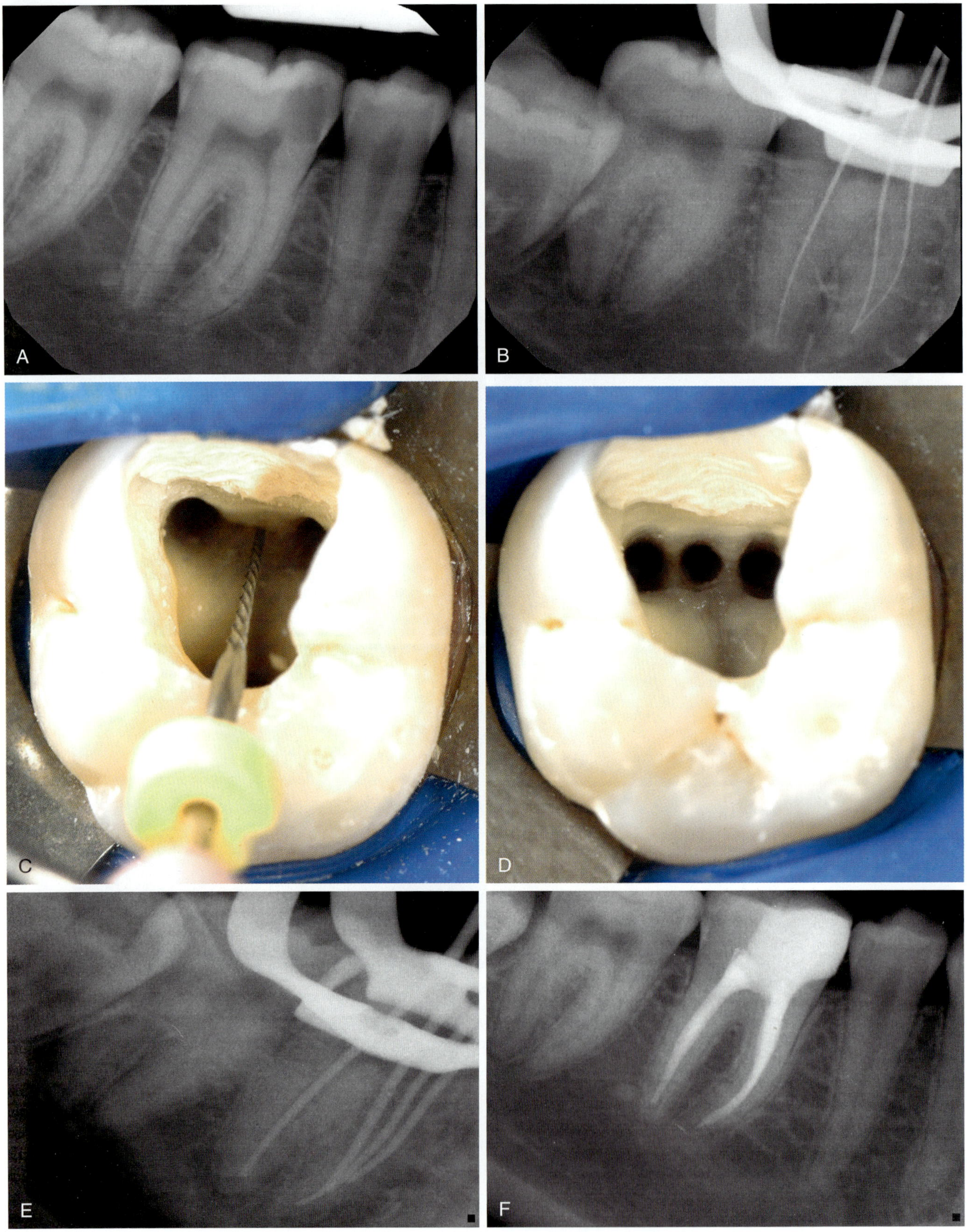

• **Fig. 13.38** A, Preoperative radiograph of a mandibular first molar with a middle mesial canal. **B,** Original working length radiographic image. **C,** Middle mesial canal located. **D,** Prepared canal. **E,** Master cone radiographic image. **F,** Postoperative radiographic image of tooth #30.

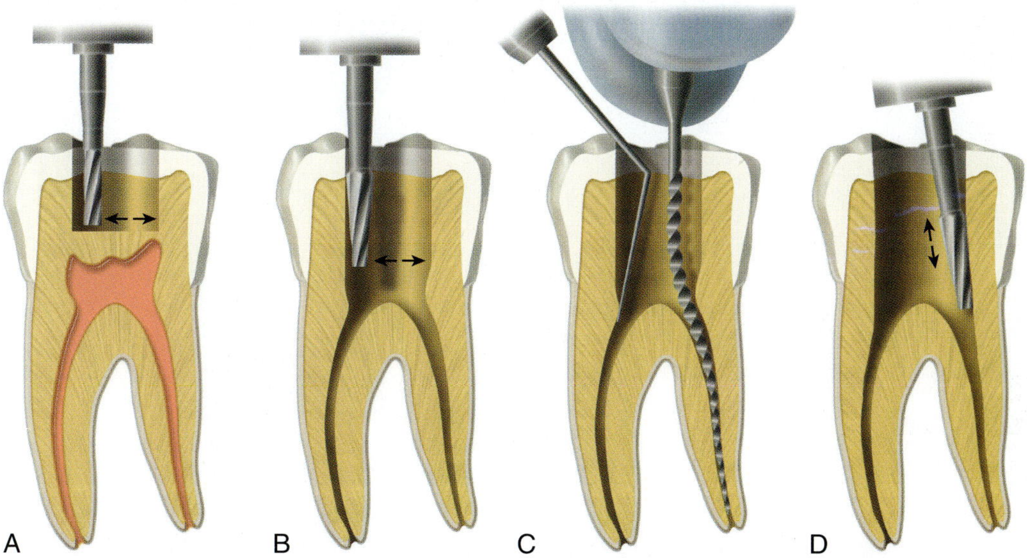

A B C D

• **Fig. 13.39** Basic steps in access preparation. **A,** The access cavity is outlined deep into dentin and close to the estimated depth of access with the high-speed handpiece. **B,** Penetration and unroofing are achieved by fissure high-speed bur or slow-speed latch-type burs. Other bur configurations are acceptable. **C** and **D,** Canal orifices are located and identified with an endodontic explorer. Small files are used to negotiate to the estimated working length. The dentin shelf that overlies and obscures the orifices is removed.

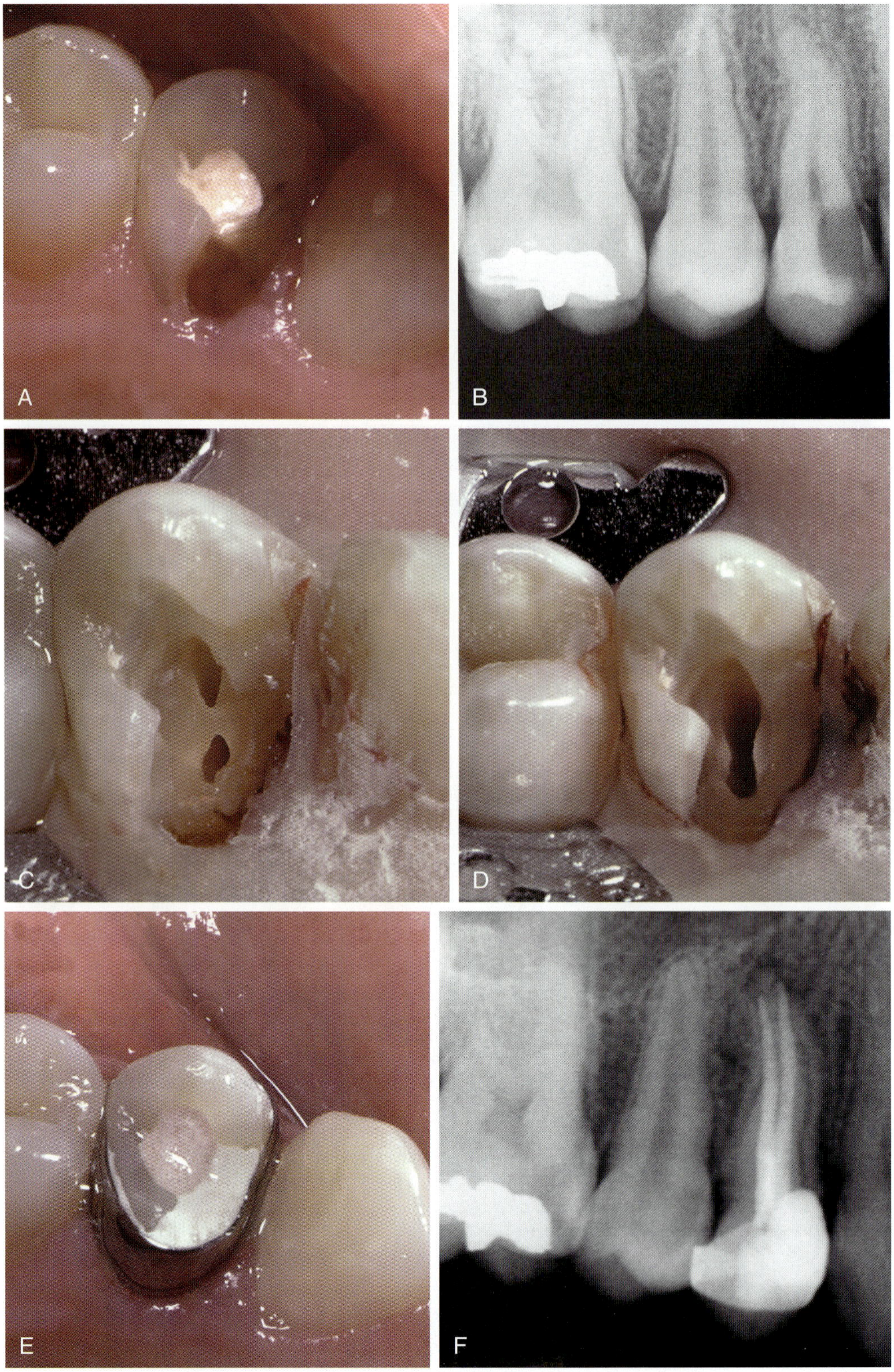

• **Fig. 13.40** **A,** Access made through gross mesial caries. **B,** Caries at the level of the crestal bone. **C,** Caries removal provides an aseptic operating field and allows assessment of restorability. Note that the previous access failed to deroof the chamber. **D,** Appropriate access reveals a ribbon-shaped pulp chamber. **E,** An orthodontic band placed to provide isolation. **F,** Post obturation.

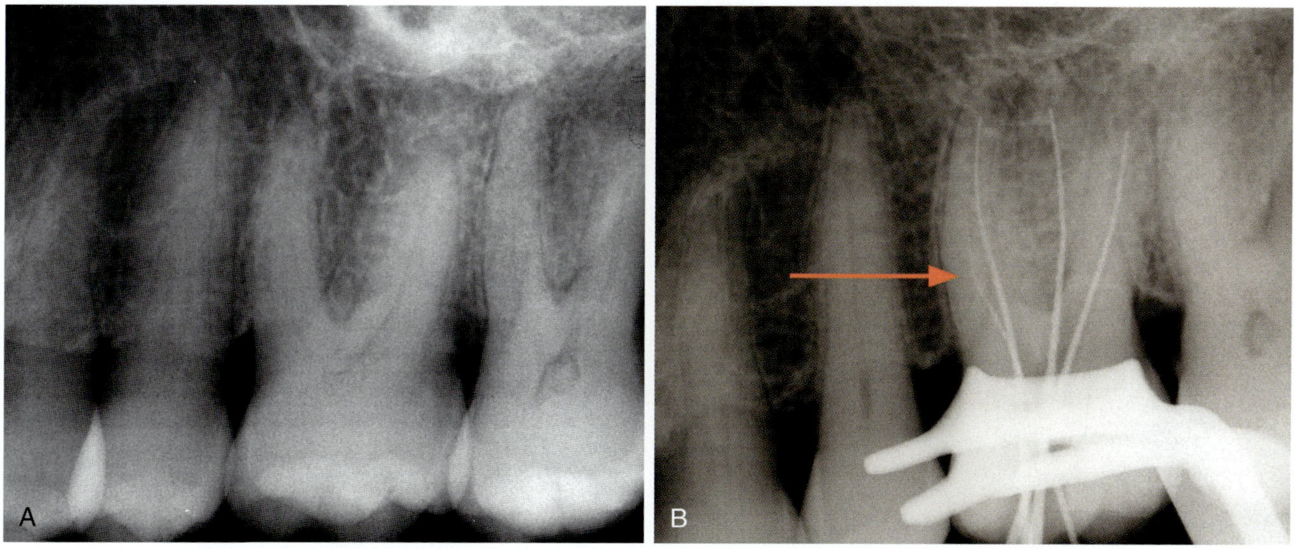

• **Fig. 13.41** **A,** Parallel preoperative radiograph. **B,** The mesial working length film is made correctly. The apices and file tips are clearly visible. Note the mesiolingual canal *(arrow).*

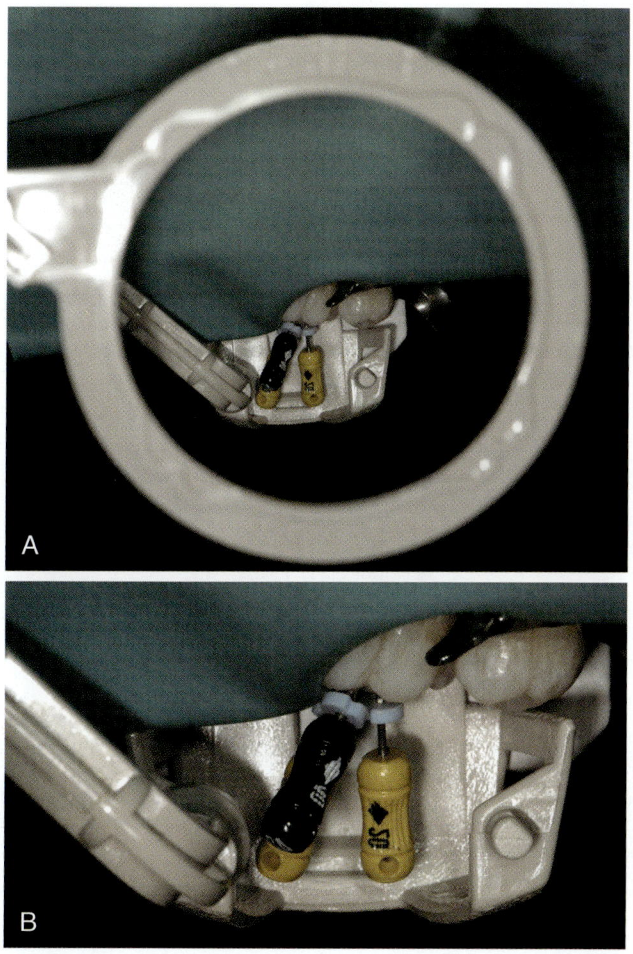

• **Fig. 13.42** **A,** Positioning device for holding working films. The ring assists in cone alignment. **B,** Close-up view of the device in position.

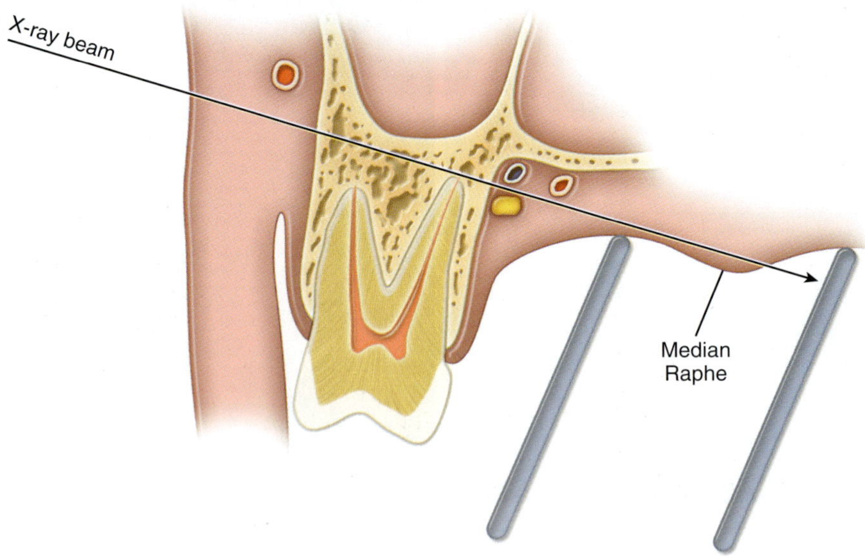

• **Fig. 13.43** Proper positioning of the radiograph when making a working length radiograph. To capture the palatal root, the film should be placed on the opposite side of the midline.

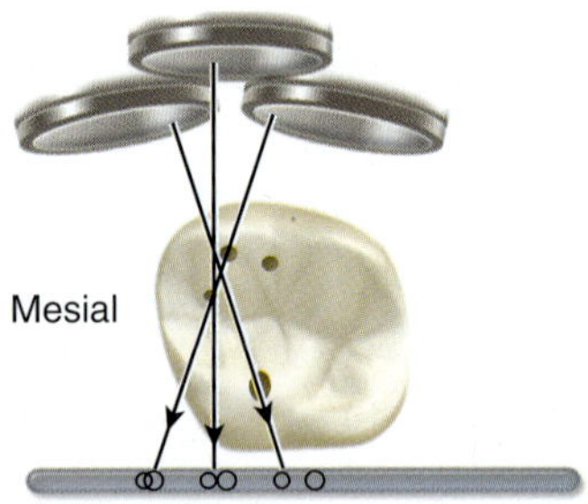

• **Fig. 13.44** Separation of the mesiobuccal and mesiolingual canals achieved by varying the horizontal angle. With maxillary molars, maximum separation occurs with a mesial cone angulation because of the mesial location of the mesiolingual canal in relation to the mesiobuccal canal.

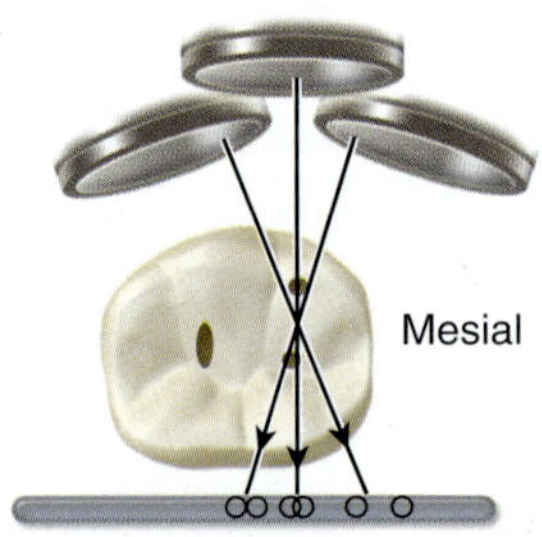

• **Fig. 13.45** Separation of the mesiobuccal and mesiolingual canals achieved by varying the horizontal angle. With mandibular molars, maximum separation occurs with a distal orientation because of the mesial location of the mesiobuccal canal in relation to the mesiolingual canal.

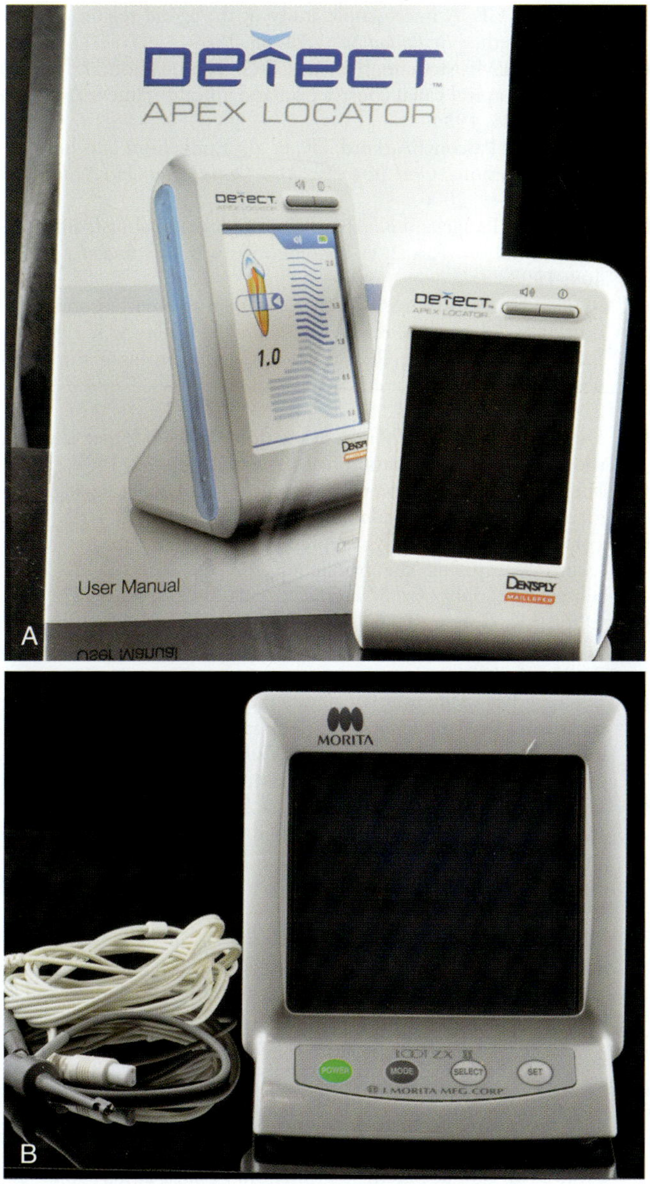

• **Fig. 13.46** **A** and **B**, Two impedance apex locators.

References

1. Cohen S, Schwartz S: Endodontic complications and the law, *J Endod* 13:191–197, 1987.
2. Anabtawi MF, Gilbert GH, Bauer MR, et al.: Rubber dam use during root canal treatment: findings from the dental practice-based research network, *J Am Dent Assoc* 144:179–186, 2013.
3. Lin P, Huang S, Chang H, et al.: The effect of rubber dam usage on the survival rate of teeth receiving root canal treatment: A nationwide population-based study, *J Endod* 40:1733–1737, 2014.
4. Taintor JF, Biesterfeld RC: A swallowed endodontic file: case report, *J Endod* 4:254–255, 1978.
5. Forrest WR, Perez RS: AIDS and hepatitis prevention: the role of the rubber dam, *Oper Dent* 11:159, 1986.
6. Cochran MA, Miller CH, Sheldrake MA: The efficacy of the rubber dam as a barrier to the spread of microorganisms during dental treatment, *J Am Dent Assoc* 119:141–144, 1989.
7. Samaranayake LP, Reid J, Evans D: The efficacy of rubber dam isolation in reducing atmospheric bacterial contamination, *ASDC J Dent Child* 56:442–444, 1989.
8. Miller RL, Micik RE: Air pollution and its control in the dental office, *Dent Clin North Am* 22:453–476, 1978.
9. Wong RC: The rubber dam as a means of infection control in an era of AIDS and hepatitis, *J Indiana Dent Assoc* 67:41–43, 1988.
10. de Andrade ED, Ranali J, Volpato MC, et al.: Allergic reaction after rubber dam placement, *J Endod* 26:182–183, 2000.
11. Madison S, Jordan RD, Krell KV: The effects of rubber dam retainers on porcelain fused-to-metal restorations, *J Endod* 12:183–186, 1986.
12. Zerr M, Johnson WT, Walton RE: Effect of rubber-dam retainers on porcelain fused to metal, *Gen Dent* 44:132–134, 1996; quiz, 41–42.
13. Schwartz SF, Foster Jr JK: Roentgenographic interpretation of experimentally produced bony lesions. I, *Oral Surg Oral Med Oral Pathol* 32:606–612, 1971.
14. Jeffrey IW, Woolford MJ: An investigation of possible iatrogenic damage caused by metal rubber dam clamps, *Int Endod J* 22:85–91, 1989.
15. Weisman MI: A modification of the No. 3 rubber dam clamp, *J Endod* 9:30–31, 1983.
16. Liebenberg WH: Access and isolation problem solving in endodontics: anterior teeth, *J Can Dent Assoc* 59:663–667, 1993. 70–71.
17. Liebenberg WH: Access and isolation problem solving in endodontics: posterior teeth, *J Can Dent Assoc* 59:817–822, 1993.
18. Wakabayashi H, Ochi K, Tachibana H, et al.: A clinical technique for the retention of a rubber dam clamp, *J Endod* 12:422–424, 1986.
19. Hermsen KP, Ludlow MO: Disinfection of rubber dam and tooth surfaces before endodontic therapy, *Gen Dent* 35:355–356, 1987.
20. Tidmarsh BG: Micromorphology of pulp chambers in human molar teeth, *Int Endod J* 13:69–75, 1980.
21. Shaw L, Jones AD: Morphological considerations of the dental pulp chamber from radiographs of molar and premolar teeth, *J Dent* 12:139–145, 1984.
22. Patel S, Rhodes J: A practical guide to endodontic access cavity preparation in molar teeth, *Br Dent J* 203:133–140, 2007.
23. Deutsch AS, Musikant BL: Morphological measurements of anatomic landmarks in human maxillary and mandibular molar pulp chambers, *J Endod* 30:388–390, 2004.
24. Abbott PV: Assessing restored teeth with pulp and periapical diseases for the presence of cracks, caries and marginal breakdown, *Aust Dent J* 49(1):33–39, 2004.
25. Patel S, Dawood A, Ford TP, et al.: The potential applications of cone beam computed tomography in the management of endodontic problems, *Int Endod J* 40:818–830, 2007.
26. Scarfe WC, Levin MD, Gane D, et al.: Use of cone beam computed tomography in endodontics, *Int J Dent* 10:20–25, 2009.
27. Clark D, Khademi J: Modern molar endodontic access and directed dentin conservation, *Dent Clin North Am* 54:249–273, 2010.
28. Krasner P, Rankow HJ: Anatomy of the pulp-chamber floor, *J Endod* 30:5–16, 2004.
29. Weine FS: *Endodontic therapy*, ed 6, St. Louis, 2004, Mosby.
30. Moore B, Verdelis K, Kishen A, et al.: Impacts of contracted endodontic cavities on instrumentation efficacy and biomechanical responses in maxillary molars, *J Endod* 42(2):1779–1783, 2016.
31. Rover G, Belladonna FG, Bortoluzzi EA, et al.: Influence of access cavity design on root canal detection, instrumentation efficacy, and fracture resistance assessed in maxillary molars, *J Endod* 43(10):11657–11662, 2017.
32. Sabeti M, Kazem M, Dianat, et al.: Impact of access cavity design and root canal taper on fracture resistance of endodontically treated teeth: an ex vivo investigation, *J Endod* 44(9):1402–1406, 2018.
33. Silva EJNL, Rover G, Belladonna FG, et al.: Impact of contracted endodontic cavities on fracture resistance of endodontically treated teeth: a systematic review of in vitro studies, *Clin Oral Investig* 22(1):109–118, 2018.
34. Lee MM, Rasimick BJ, Turner AM, et al.: Morphological measurements of anatomic landmarks in pulp chambers of human anterior teeth, *J Endod* 33:129–131, 2007.

35. Deutsch AS, Musikant BL, Gu S, et al.: Morphological measurements of anatomic landmarks in pulp chambers of human maxillary furcated bicuspids, *J Endod* 31:570–573, 2005.
36. Baldassari-Cruz LA, Lilly JP, Rivera EM: The influence of dental operating microscope in locating the mesiolingual canal orifice, *Oral Surg Oral Med Oral Pathol Oral Radiol Endod* 93:190–194, 2002.
37. Haselton DR, Lloyd PM, Johnson WT: A comparison of the effects of two burs on endodontic access in all-ceramic high lucite crowns, *Oral Surg Oral Med Oral Pathol Oral Radiol Endod* 89:486–492, 2000.
38. de Carvalho MC, Zuolo ML: Orifice locating with a microscope, *J Endod* 26:532–534, 2000.
39. Kasahara E, Yasuda E, Yamamoto A, et al.: Root canal system of the maxillary central incisor, *J Endod* 16:158–161, 1990.
40. Dankner E, Harari D, Rotstein I: Dens evaginatus of anterior teeth: literature review and radiographic survey of 15,000 teeth, *Oral Surg Oral Med Oral Pathol Oral Radiol Endod* 81:472–475, 1996.
41. Gound TG: Dens invaginatus: a pathway to pulpal pathology—a literature review, *Pract Periodontics Aesthet Dent* 9:585–594, 1997; quiz, 96.
42. Green D: Double canals in single roots, *Oral Surg Oral Med Oral Pathol* 35:689–696, 1973.
43. Kulild JC, Peters DD: Incidence and configuration of canal systems in the mesiobuccal root of maxillary first and second molars, *J Endod* 16:311–317, 1990.
44. Pineda F: Roentgenographic investigation of the mesiobuccal root of the maxillary first molar, *Oral Surg Oral Med Oral Pathol* 36:253–260, 1973.
45. Stropko JJ: Canal morphology of maxillary molars: clinical observations of canal configurations, *J Endod* 25:446–450, 1999.
46. Weine FS, Healey HJ, Gerstein H, et al.: Canal configuration in the mesiobuccal root of the maxillary first molar and its endodontic significance, *Oral Surg Oral Med Oral Pathol* 28:419–425, 1969.
47. Acosta Vigouroux SA, Trugeda Bosaans SA: Anatomy of the pulp chamber floor of the permanent maxillary first molar, *J Endod* 4:214–219, 1978.
48. Benjamin KA, Dowson J: Incidence of two root canals in human mandibular incisor teeth, *Oral Surg Oral Med Oral Pathol* 38:122–126, 1974.
49. Rankine-Wilson RW, Henry P: The bifurcated root canal in lower anterior teeth, *J Am Dent Assoc* 70:1162–1165, 1965.
50. Mauger MJ, Waite RM, Alexander JB, et al.: Ideal endodontic access in mandibular incisors, *J Endod* 25:206–207, 1999.
51. Clements RE, Gilboe DB: Labial endodontic access opening for mandibular incisors: endodontic and restorative considerations, *J Can Dent Assoc* 57:587–589, 1991.
52. Vertucci FJ: Root canal morphology of mandibular premolars, *J Am Dent Assoc* 97:47–50, 1978.
53. Vertucci FJ: Root canal anatomy of the human permanent teeth, *Oral Surg Oral Med Oral Pathol* 58:589–599, 1984.
54. Hartwell G, Bellizzi R: Clinical investigation of in vivo endodontically treated mandibular and maxillary molars, *J Endod* 8:555–557, 1982.
55. Skidmore AE, Bjorndal AM: Root canal morphology of the human mandibular first molar, *Oral Surg Oral Med Oral Pathol* 32:778–784, 1971.
56. Reeh ES, Messer HH, Douglas WH: Reduction in tooth stiffness as a result of endodontic and restorative procedures, *J Endod* 15:512–516, 1989.
57. Sedgley CM, Messer HH: Are endodontically treated teeth more brittle? *J Endod* 18:332–335, 1992.
58. Wilcox LR, Walton RE: The shape and location of mandibular premolar access openings, *Int Endod J* 20:223–227, 1987.
59. Chapman CE: A microscopic study of the apical region of human anterior teeth, *J Br Endod Soc* 3:52–58, 1969.
60. Dummer PM, McGinn JH, Rees DG: The position and topography of the apical canal constriction and apical foramen, *Int Endod J* 17:192–198, 1984.
61. Ricucci D, Pascon EA, Ford TR, et al.: Epithelium and bacteria in periapical lesions, *Oral Surg Oral Med Oral Pathol Oral Radiol Endod* 101:239–249, 2006.
62. Ricucci D, Langeland K: Apical limit of root canal instrumentation and obturation. Part 2. A histological study, *Int Endod J* 31:394–409, 1998.
63. Ricucci D: Apical limit of root canal instrumentation and obturation. Part 1. Literature review, *Int Endod J* 31:384–393, 1998.
64. Schaeffer MA, White RR, Walton RE: Determining the optimal obturation length: a meta-analysis of literature, *J Endod* 31:271–274, 2005.
65. Dummer PM, Lewis JM: An evaluation of the endometric probe in root canal length estimation, *Int Endod J* 20:25–29, 1987.
66. Forsberg J: A comparison of the paralleling and bisecting-angle radiographic techniques in endodontics, *Int Endod J* 20:177–182, 1987.
67. Forsberg J: Radiographic reproduction of endodontic "working length" comparing the paralleling and the bisecting-angle techniques, *Oral Surg Oral Med Oral Pathol* 64:353–360, 1987.
68. Olson AK, Goerig AC, Cavataio RE, et al.: The ability of the radiograph to determine the location of the apical foramen, *Int Endod J* 24:28–35, 1991.
69. Seidberg BH, Alibrandi BV, Fine H, et al.: Clinical investigation of measuring working lengths of root canals with an electronic device and with digital-tactile sense, *J Am Dent Assoc* 90:379–387, 1975.
70. Stabholz A, Rotstein I, Torabinejad M: Effect of preflaring on tactile detection of the apical constriction, *J Endod* 21:92–94, 1995.
71. Goerig AC, Neaverth EJ: A simplified look at the buccal object rule in endodontics, *J Endod* 13:570–572, 1987.
72. Richards AG: The buccal object rule, *Dent Radiogr Photogr* 53:37, 1980.
73. McDonald NJ: The electronic determination of working length, *Dent Clin North Am* 36:293–307, 1992.
74. Pratten DH, McDonald NJ: Comparison of radiographic and electronic working lengths, *J Endod* 22:173–176, 1996.
75. Fouad AF, Rivera EM, Krell KV: Accuracy of the Endex with variations in canal irrigants and foramen size, *J Endod* 19:63–67, 1993.
76. Beach CW, Bramwell JD, Hutter JW: Use of an electronic apex locator on a cardiac pacemaker patient, *J Endod* 22:182–184, 1996.
77. Garofalo RR, Ede EN, Dorn SO, et al.: Effect of electronic apex locators on cardiac pacemaker function, *J Endod* 28:831–833, 2002.
78. Moshonov J, Slutzky-Goldberg I: Apex locators: update and prospects for the future, *Int J Comput Dent* 7:359–370, 2004.
79. Simon AB, Linde B, Bonnette GH, et al.: The individual with a pacemaker in the dental environment, *J Am Dent Assoc* 91:1224–1229, 1975.
80. Woolley LH, Woodworth J, Dobbs JL: A preliminary evaluation of the effects of electrical pulp testers on dogs with artificial pacemakers, *J Am Dent Assoc* 89:1099–1101, 1974.
81. Gomez G, Duran-Sindreu F, Jara Clemente F, et al.: The effects of six electronic apex locators on pacemaker function: an in vitro study, *Int Endod J* 46:399–405, 2013.
82. Wilson BL, Broberg C, Baumgartner JC, et al.: Safety of electronic apex locators and pulp testers in patients with implanted cardiac pacemakers or cardioverter/defibrillators, *J Endod* 32:847–852, 2006.

14

Cleaning and Shaping

OVE A. PETERS, ANA ARIAS, AND SHAHROKH SHABAHANG

CHAPTER OUTLINE

LEARNING OBJECTIVES

After reading this chapter, the student will be able to:

1. State reasons and describe strategies for enlarging the cervical portion of the canal to promote straight-line access.
2. Define how to determine the appropriate size of the master apical file.
3. Describe objectives for biomechanical cleaning and shaping and explain how to determine when these have been achieved.
4. Illustrate shapes of differently created preparations and draw these both in longitudinal and cross-sectional diagrams.
5. Describe techniques for shaping canals that have irregular shapes, such as round, oval, hourglass, bowling pin, kidney bean, or ribbon.
6. Distinguish between apical stop, apical seat, and open apex, and discuss how to manage obturation in each.
7. Describe appropriate techniques for removing the pulp.
8. Characterize the difficulties of preparation in the presence of anatomic aberrations that make complete débridement difficult.
9. Describe techniques for negotiating severely curved, "blocked," "ledged," or constricted canals.
10. Discuss the properties and role of intracanal, interappointment medicaments.

Successful long-term outcomes of root canal treatment are based on establishing an accurate diagnosis and developing an appropriate treatment plan; applying knowledge of tooth anatomy and morphology (shape); and performing débridement, disinfection, and obturation of the entire root canal system while maintaining the strength of the tooth. Historically, emphasis was on obturation and sealing the radicular space. However, no technique or material provides a seal that is completely impervious to moisture from either the apical or coronal aspects. Early studies on prognosis indicated failures were attributable to incomplete obturation.[1] This proved fallacious as obturation merely reflects the adequacy of the cleaning and shaping. Canals that are poorly obturated may be incompletely cleaned and shaped. Adequate cleaning and shaping and establishing a coronal seal are essential elements for successful treatment, with obturation being less important for short-term success.[2] Elimination (or significant reduction) of inflamed or necrotic pulp tissue and microorganisms are the most critical factors. The role of obturation in long-term success has not been established but may be significant in preventing recontamination either from the coronal or apical direction. Sealing the canal space after cleaning and shaping will help to entomb any remaining organisms[3] and, with the coronal seal, prevent or at least delay recontamination of the canal and periradicular tissues. However, some bacterial species have been shown to survive entombment.[4]

These classic concepts define success in endodontics by healing of apical periodontitis if present preoperatively or the prevention of its occurrence in case that began with normal periapical tissues. However, in recent years, it has been demonstrated that vertical fracture or other nonendodontic causes are the major reasons for the eventual loss of root canal–treated teeth.[5] As a result, a more patient-centered outcome as increased susceptibility to fracture should be considered. Functional retention of the endodontically treated tooth may serve as a relevant endpoint in endodontic treatment,[6] which may compliment but should not replace the traditional focus on healing or prevention of apical periodontitis.

Principles of Cleaning and Shaping

Nonsurgical root canal treatment is a predictable method of retaining a tooth that otherwise would require extraction. Success

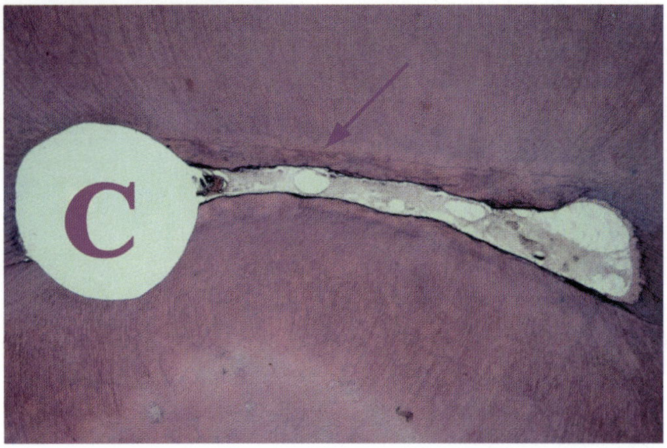

• **Fig. 14.1** Cross-section through a root showing the main canal (C) and a fin *(arrow)* and associated cul-de-sac after cleaning and shaping using files and sodium hypochlorite. Note the tissue remnants in the fin.

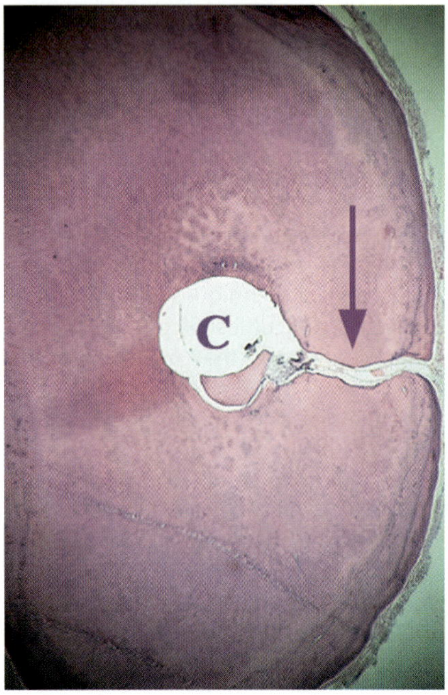

• **Fig. 14.2** The main canal (C) has a lateral canal *(arrow)* extending to the root surface. After cleaning and shaping with sodium hypochlorite irrigation, tissue remains in the lateral canal.

of root canal treatment in a tooth with a vital pulp is higher than that of a tooth diagnosed with necrotic pulp and periradicular pathosis.[7]

The reason for this difference in outcome is the persistent presence of microorganisms and their metabolic byproducts. The most significant factors affecting the clinician's inability to completely remove intracanal microorganisms are tooth anatomy and morphology. Instruments are believed to contact and plane the canal walls to débride the canal (Figs. 14.1 to 14.4), aided by irrigating solutions. Morphologic factors include lateral (see Fig. 14.2) and accessory canals, canal curvatures, canal wall irregularities, fins, cul-de-sacs (see Fig. 14.1), and isthmuses. These aberrations render full wall contact and therefore complete débridement virtually impossible. Consequently, a practical objective of cleaning is to significantly reduce the irritants, not totally eliminate them. Frequent and effective irrigation is necessary to achieve this goal. At the same time, root canals need to be enlarged to allow irrigants to properly clean the canal and to remove contaminated dentin. Irrigants readily remove microorganisms from the coronal third of a root canal, but further shaping is necessary to eliminate bacteria in less accessible canal areas. Meanwhile, the mechanical action of instruments generates debris that is typically pushed into accessory anatomy and may block the access to subsequent irrigation. This debris also needs to be flushed and removed. Therefore it is imperative to use mechanical shaping and irrigation in synergy to maximize antibacterial efficacy of endodontic procedures.

Apart from enhancing cleaning procedures, another purpose of shaping is to provide space for an effective filling of the root canal space. The main mechanistic objective of shaping is to maintain or develop a continuously tapering funnel from the canal orifice to the apex. Conceptually, the degree of enlargement is partly dictated by the method of obturation. For lateral compaction of gutta-percha, the canal should be enlarged sufficiently to permit placement of the spreader to within 1 to 2 mm of the working length (WL).[8] For warm vertical compaction techniques, the coronal enlargement must permit the placement of pluggers to within 3 to 5 mm of the WL.[9]

However, the more dentin is removed from the canal walls, the less resistant to fracture the root becomes.[10] Micronized gutta-percha points for vertical compaction that allows melting at larger distances from the heat source are now available in order to allow proper obturation of more conservative preparations. New materials based on the concept of so-called hydraulic obturation techniques are also marketed for the same purpose. However, as always, clinicians should select an obturation technique judiciously, based on available evidence.

Ideally, the degree of shaping should be tooth dependent and not depend on the obturation technique. As an example, narrow thin roots, such as mandibular incisors, may not permit the same degree of enlargement as more bulky roots, such as the maxillary central incisors.

Apical Canal Preparation

Termination of Cleaning and Shaping

Although the concept of cleaning and shaping the root canal space appears to be straightforward, there are areas where consensus does not exist. The first is the extent of the apical preparation. Early studies identified the dentinocemental junction as the area where the pulp ends and the periodontal ligament begins. Unfortunately, this is a histologic landmark and the position (which is irregular within the canal) cannot be determined clinically.

Traditionally, the apical point of termination, also known as *WL*, has been 1 mm from the radiographic apex. A classic study described the apical portion of the canal with the major diameter of the foramen and the minor diameter of the constriction (Fig. 14.4).[11] The apical constriction is defined as the narrowest portion of the canal, and the average distance from the foramen to the constriction was found to be 0.5 mm. Another study found the classic apical constriction to be present in only 46% of the teeth and, when present, varied in shape and in relation to the apical foramen.[12] Variations from the classic appearance consist of the tapering constriction, multiple constrictions, and a parallel apical canal part.[12] To complicate the issue, the foramen is rarely located at the anatomic apex. Convincing micro–computed tomography data provide a more realistic portrait of apical canal morphology (Fig. 14.5).

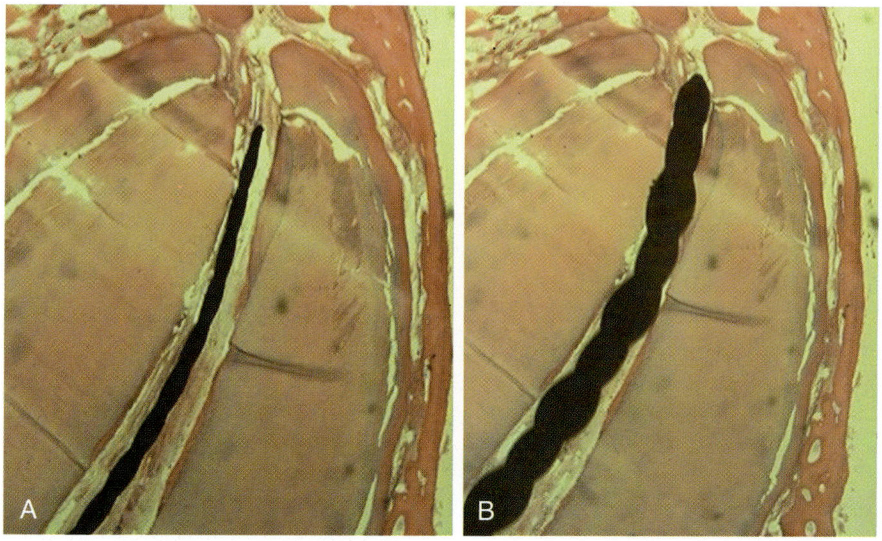

• **Fig. 14.3** **(A)** No. 15 file in the apical canal space. Note the size is inadequate for planing the walls. **(B)** No. 40 file more closely approximates the canal morphology. (Courtesy Dr. Randy Madsen.)

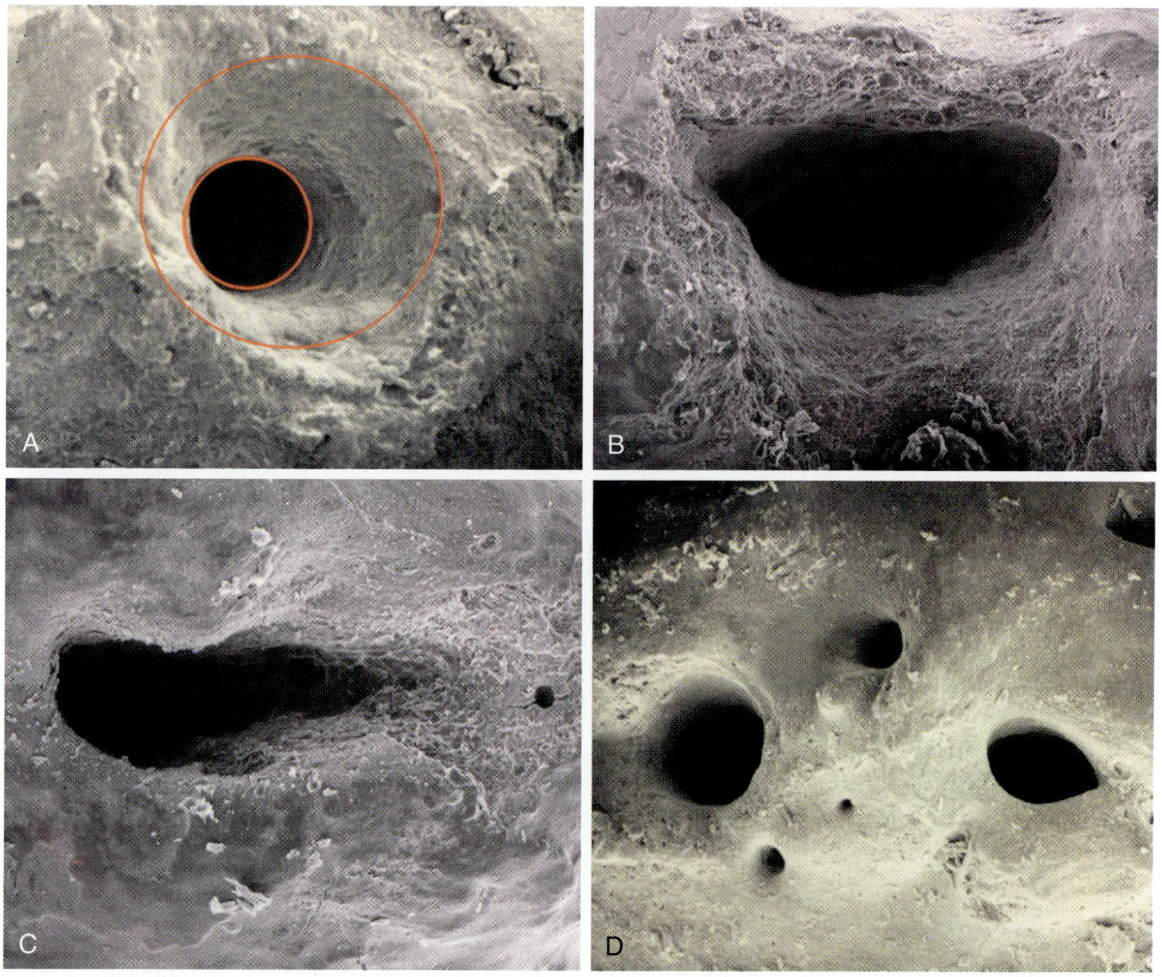

• **Fig. 14.4** **(A)** The classic apical anatomy consisting of the major diameter of the foramen and the minor diameter of the constriction. **(B)** An irregular ovoid apical canal shape and external resorption. **(C)** A bowling pin apical morphology and an accessory canal. **(D)** Multiple apical foramina.

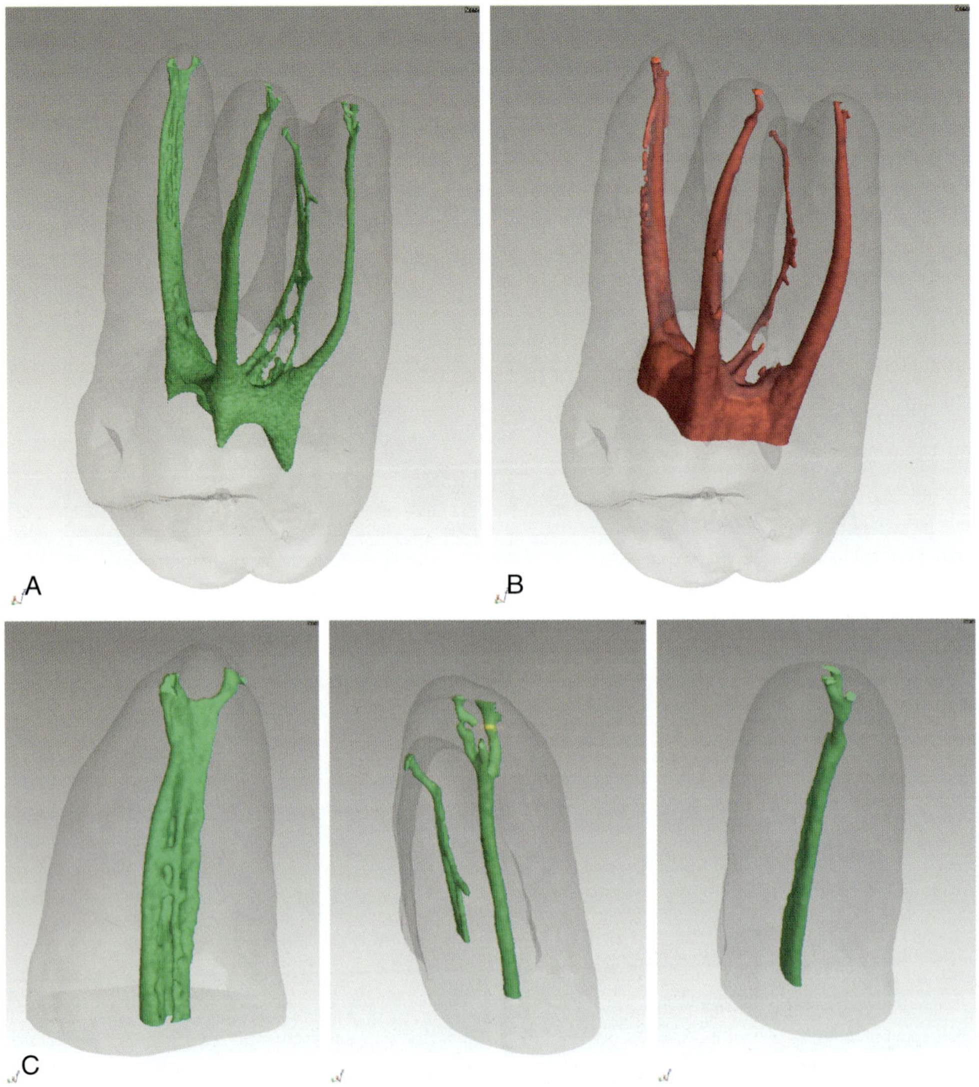

• **Fig. 14.5** **(A)** Micro–computed tomography (micro-CT) reconstruction of an unprepared root canal system of a maxillary molar. **(B)** Prepared canal system, enlarged to an apical size 30 in the palatal and 25 in the mesiobuccal and distobuccal canal. **(C)** Magnified view of the initial canal configuration for all three apices.

Apical anatomy has also been shown to be quite variable (see Figs. 14.4, *B*, and 14.5). A study found no typical pattern for foraminal openings and that no foramen coincided with the apex of the root.[13] The same group reported the foramen to apex distance to range from 0.20 to 3.8 mm.

It has also been noted that the foramen to constriction distance increases with age,[11] and root resorption may destroy the classic anatomic constriction.[14] Resorptive processes are common with pulp necrosis and apical bone resorption. Therefore root resorption is an additional factor to consider in length determination.

In a prospective study, significant adverse factors influencing success and failure were the presence of a perforation, preoperative periradicular disease, and incorrect length of the root canal filling.[15,16] The authors speculated that canals filled more than 2.0 mm short harbored necrotic tissue, bacteria, and irritants that when retreated could be cleaned and sealed.[15] A meta-analysis evaluation of success and failure indicated a better success rate when the obturation was confined to the canal space.[17] A review of several studies on endodontic outcomes confirms that extrusion of materials decreases success.[7,18,19] In one study examining cases with pulp necrosis, better success was achieved when the procedures terminated at or within 2 mm of the radiographic apex. Obturation shorter than 2 mm from the apex or past the apex resulted in a decreased success rate. In teeth with vital inflamed pulp tissue, termination between 1 and 3 mm was acceptable.[18] Two larger studies confirmed that overfill was associated with inferior outcomes.[7,19]

At the same time, working short presents higher risks of accumulation and retention of debris, which in turn may result in apical blockage and may contribute to procedural errors in the first place; furthermore, infected debris, bacteria, and their byproducts can remain in the most apical portion of the canal in cases with pulpal necrosis jeopardizing apical healing and contributing to a persistent or recurrent apical periodontitis[20,21] or posttreatment disease.[22,23]

Most publications on outcomes that extrapolate the effect of apical termination are retrospective. On the other hand, a recent prospective study demonstrated that not only the maintenance of apical patency, but also the apical extent of canal cleaning, is a significant prognostic factor for root canal treatment, recommending extending canal cleaning as close as possible to its apical terminus. In that study, the odds of success were reduced by 12% for every 1 mm of the canal short of the terminus remaining "uninstrumented."[7]

Therefore the exact clinical point of apical termination of the preparation and obturation remains a matter of debate. The need to compact the gutta-percha and sealer against the apical dentin matrix (constriction of the canal) is important in creating a seal. The decision of where to terminate the preparation is based on knowledge of apical anatomy, tactile sensation, radiographic interpretation, apex locators, apical bleeding, and the patient's response. To prevent extrusion, the cleaning and shaping procedures should be confined to the radicular space. Canals filled to the radiographic apex are actually slightly overextended.[13]

Degree of Apical Enlargement

Generalizations can be made regarding tooth anatomy and morphology, although each tooth is unique. Length of canal preparation is often emphasized with little consideration given to important factors such as canal diameter and shape. Because morphology is variable, there is no standardized apical canal size. Traditionally, preparation techniques were determined by the desire to limit procedural errors and by the method of obturation. Small apical preparation reduces the incidence of preparation errors (as is discussed in the following section) but may decrease antimicrobial efficacy of cleaning procedures. It appears that with traditional hand instruments, apical transportation occurs in many curved canals enlarged beyond a No. 20 stainless steel file.[24]

The criteria for cleaning and shaping should be based on the ability to adequately deliver sufficient amounts of irrigant and not on a specific obturation technique. The ability of irrigants to reach the apical portion of the root canal depends on canal's size, taper, and the irrigation device used.[25-27]

Larger preparation sizes have been shown to provide adequate irrigation and debris removal and significantly decrease the number of microorganisms.[28-31] However, any removal of dentin has the potential to weaken radicular structure and therefore the use of an irrigation adjunct designed to promote irrigation efficacy in smaller canals may be advantageous.[32,33]

In principle there may to be a relationship between increasing the size of the apical preparation and canal cleanliness[34] and bacterial reduction.[35,36] Instrumentation techniques that advocate minimal apical preparation may be ineffective at achieving the goal of cleaning and disinfecting the root canal space.[34,36] However, this concept reaches its limits when too large a preparation leads to procedural errors[37,38] and when modifications created in the hard tissue block the very anatomy that was to be cleaned (Fig. 14.6).[39]

A variety of microbial species can penetrate deep into dentinal tubules.[40] These intratubular organisms are sheltered from endodontic instruments, the action of irrigants, and intracanal medicaments. Dentin removal appears to be the primary method for decreasing

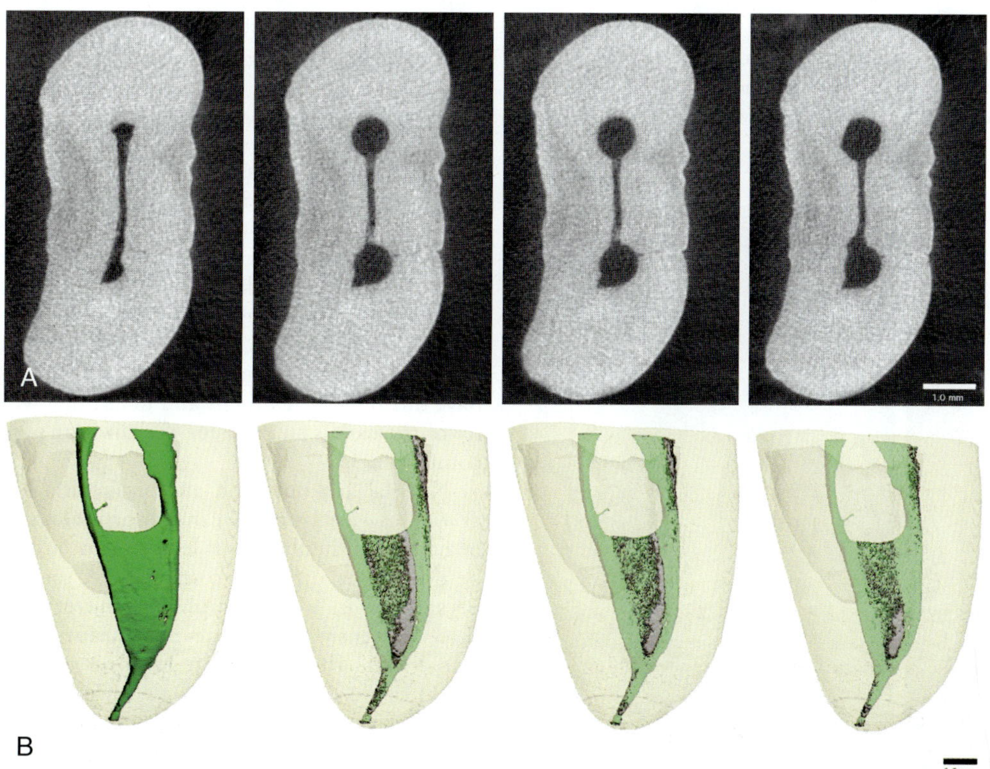

• **Fig. 14.6 (A)** Individual micro–computed tomography scans from the apical root third of a typical specimen before and after root canal preparation and irrigation with sodium hypochlorite (NaOCl), subsequent irrigation with ethylenediaminetetraacetic acid and final passive ultrasonic irrigation using again NaOCl (from left to right). **(B)** The corresponding three-dimensional reconstructions of the whole canal system are depicted below. (Reprinted from Paqué F, Boessler C, Zehnder M: Accumulated hard tissue débris levels in mesial roots of mandibular molars after sequential irrigation steps, *Int Endod J* 44(2):148, 2011 with permission.[39])

their numbers. However, it may not be possible to remove bacteria that are deep in the tubules, regardless of the technique. There is a correlation between the number of organisms present and the depth of tubular penetration[41]; in teeth with apical periodontitis, bacteria may penetrate the tubules to the periphery of the root.[42,43]

Elimination of Etiology

The development of nickel-titanium (NiTi) instruments has dramatically changed the techniques of cleaning and shaping; these instruments have been rapidly adopted by clinicians in many countries.[44-46] The primary advantage to using these flexible instruments is related to shaping, specifically a significant reduction in the incidence of preparation errors.[37]

Neither hand instruments nor rotary files have been shown to completely débride the canal.[29,47,48] Mechanical enlargement of the canal space dramatically decreases the presence of microorganisms present in the canal[49] but cannot render the canal sterile.[29] Therefore antimicrobial irrigants have been recommended in addition to mechanical preparation techniques.[50] There is currently no consensus on the most appropriate irrigant or concentration of solution, although sodium hypochlorite (NaOCl) is the most widely used irrigant.[51]

Unfortunately, solutions such as NaOCl that are designed to kill bacteria[50,52,53] are often toxic for the host cells,[54-57] and therefore extrusion beyond the canal space is to be avoided.[58,59] A major factor related to effectiveness is the volume of irrigant used during the procedure. Increasing the volume produces cleaner preparations.[60]

Apical Patency

Apical patency is a technique that advocated the repeated placement of small hand files to or slightly beyond the apical foramen during canal preparation (Fig. 14.7). A benefit of this technique during cleaning and shaping procedures is to ensure that WL is not lost and that the apical portion of the root is not packed with tissue, dentin debris, and bacteria (see Fig. 14.6, *A*). The patency concept has historically been controversial; indeed, concerns regarding possible extrusion of dentinal debris, bacteria, and irrigants have been raised,[61] a condition often considered to result in postoperative pain and possibly delayed healing.[62]

However, a large retrospective study identified the presence of apical patency as a factor possibly associated with higher success rates.[7] Moreover, at least in vitro, microorganisms do not appear to be transported beyond the confines of the canal by patency filing.[63] Small files are not directly effective in débridement (see Fig. 14.3) but achieving patency may be helpful in enhancing irrigation efficacy,[64] determining electronic WL, minimizing the risk of loss of length, reducing shaping mishaps such as canal transportation and ledges,[65] better maintaining the anatomy of the apical constriction,[66] and improving clinicians' tactile sense during apical shaping.[67]

Studies evaluating treatment failure have noted, besides several other factors, presence of bacteria outside the radicular space,[20] and bacteria have in some cases been shown to exist as plaques or biofilms on the external root structure.[68] It has been shown in vitro that maintaining patency may be connected to small amounts of irrigant to reach the periodontium, but this did not appear to increase the chance of irrigation accidents in the clinic.[69]

Moreover, a recently published systematic review concluded that maintaining apical patency was not associated with postoperative pain in teeth with either vital or nonvital pulp.[70] For all these reasons the benefits of maintaining apical patency seem to outweigh possible risks.

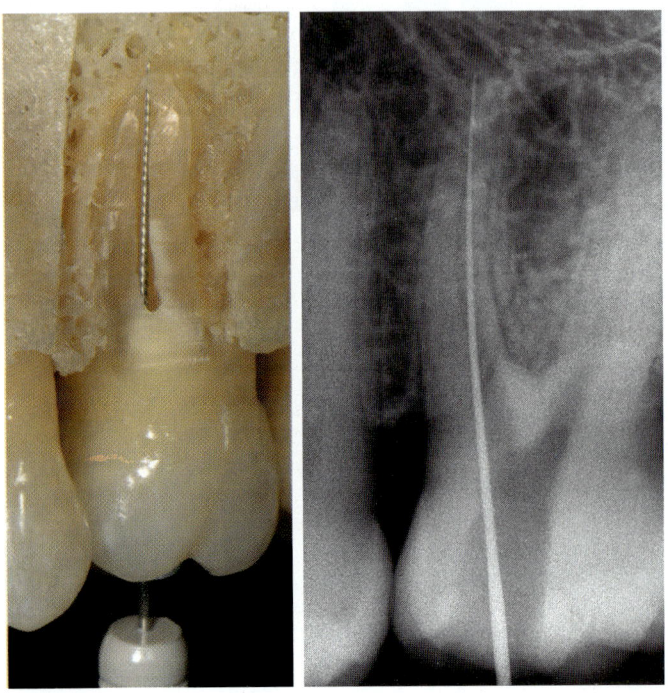

• **Fig. 14.7** A small file (No. 10 or 15) is placed beyond the radiographic apex to maintain patency of the foramen. Note the tip extends beyond the apical foramen.

Pretreatment Evaluation

Before treatment, each case should be evaluated for its degree of difficulty. The American Association of Endodontists has developed *The Endodontic Case Difficulty Assessment Form*, a practical tool that helps practitioners to identify the complexities that should not be overlooked before starting a root canal treatment. All three, patient, diagnostic, and treatment aspects, are considered to identify the level of difficulty of a specific case and help in 3 minutes to both anticipate problems the clinician may have during the treatment and determine whether the complexity of the case is suitable for the clinician's level of expertise and comfort.

Normal anatomy and anatomic variations are determined, as well as variations in canal morphology.[71] The mishandling of natural difficulties will lead to procedural mishaps that will be even more difficult to manage. A root canal that seems to be straight in a radiograph may have multiple curvatures in three dimensions that are not captured using a two-dimensional film. Therefore more than one preoperative radiograph might be needed for a proper assessment; a cone beam scan or cone beam computed tomography (CBCT) may also help to determine the best strategy to shape the most difficult canal anatomies.

Specifically, the longer a root, the more difficult it is to treat; apically, a narrow, curved root is susceptible to perforation; in multirooted teeth, a narrow area midroot could result in a stripping perforation toward the root concavity. The degree and location of curvature are determined. Canals are seldom straight, and curvatures in a buccolingual direction are normally not visible on the radiograph. Sharp curvatures or dilacerations are more difficult to manage than a continuous gentle curve. Roots with an S-shape or bayonet configuration are very difficult to treat. Intracanal mineralization will also complicate treatment. Such mineralization generally occurs in a coronal to apical direction, thus a large tapering canal may become more cylindrical with irritation or age.

The presence of resorption also will complicate treatment. With internal resorption, it is difficult to pass instruments through the coronal portion of the canal and the resorptive defect and into the apical portion. Also, files will not remove tissue, necrotic debris, and bacteria from such a resorptive defect. External resorption may perforate the canal space and present problems with hemostasis and isolation. Restorations may obstruct access and visibility, as well as change the orientation of the crown in relation to the root.

Principles of Cleaning and Shaping Techniques

Cleaning and shaping are separate and distinct concepts but are performed concurrently. The criteria of canal preparation include developing a continuously tapered funnel, maintaining the original shape of the canal, maintaining the apical foramen in its original position, keeping the apical opening as small as possible, and developing glassy smooth walls.[9] The cleaning and shaping procedures are designed to maintain an apical matrix for compacting the obturating material regardless of the obturation technique.[9]

Knowledge of a variety of techniques and instruments for treatment of the myriad variations in canal anatomy is required. There is no consensus or clinical evidence on which technique or instrument design or type is clinically superior.[38,72]

NiTi files have been incorporated into endodontics because of their flexibility and resistance to cyclic fatigue.[73] The resistance to cyclic fatigue permits these instruments to be used in a rotary handpiece, which gives them an advantage over stainless steel files. NiTi files are manufactured in both hand and rotary versions and have been demonstrated to produce superior shaping compared with stainless steel hand instruments.[37,72,74]

NiTi instruments are available in a variety of designs, many with increased taper compared with .02 mm standardized stainless steel files. The superelasticity of NiTi alloy enabled the manufacturing of more tapered instruments still flexible enough to properly shape canals with different angles and radius of curvature. The increase in the taper provides better and more continuous shapes with the use of fewer instruments and in a shorter period of time. Common tapers are .04 and .06, and the tip diameters may or may not conform to the traditional manufacturing specifications. The file systems can vary the taper while maintaining the same tip diameter or they can employ varied tapers with International Organization for Standardization (ISO) standardized tip diameters; some NiTi instruments have multiple tapers along their cutting portions, with more recent instruments featuring smaller maximum fluted diameters of less than 1 mm at the end of the fluted instrument portion.

A rational concept of root canal preparation using current instruments unfolds in stages. Classically, Stage 1 is a defined preflaring, before bringing any hand file to the apical third of the canal. Depending on the expected canal difficulty, instruments may reach WL during Stage 2; for example, if there is only one curvature. If preoperative assessments have indicated that an S-shape or multiple curvatures are present, it may be useful to introduce a Stage 3 that finally reaches the estimated WL, whereas Stage 2 provides additional enlargement into the secondary curvature.[75]

However, the appearance of proprietary thermal treatments of NiTi alloys with different series of heating and cooling treatments has led to the enhancement of the mechanical properties of contemporary rotary instruments by optimizing the microstructural characteristics of the alloy. The higher flexibility and cyclic fatigue resistance of these new instruments provides better clinical behavior and allows dentin preservation in the coronal third of many cases with a minimal orifice modification in Stage 1. Scientific evidence suggests that preserving pericervical dentin (4 mm above and below the crestal bone) is crucial for the distribution of functional stresses and the maintenance of the strength of the tooth and long-term survival.[76] Computational simulations with finite element analysis showed that masticatory stresses are reduced even when small amounts of this pericervical dentin are preserved.[77]

The authors strongly believe in this minimally invasive component of the technique because overflaring is liable to reduce dentinal wall thickness and structural strength and perhaps overall restorability (see Fig. 14.8). On the other hand, when it is performed with an instrument that allows a selective removal of dentin because of a limited maximum fluted diameter (MFD) that provides a conservative coronal preparation, early coronal flaring is also beneficial for the earlier access of disinfecting irrigation solutions, better tactile control of hand instruments during negotiation, and the easier placement of files in the delicate apical third.[78]

In general, the use of NiTi rotary instruments to WL should be preceded by a manual exploration of the canal to the desired preparation length, also known as glide path verification. This step is performed with one or more small K-files that are not precurved. In recent years, NiTi rotary instruments have been specifically designed to simplify the process of glide path preparation after a negotiating file has previously reached WL. If it is possible to predictably reach WL without precurving, rotary instruments may be used to the desired length. However, caution should be exercised in S-shaped canals, canals that join within a single root, and canals with severe dilacerations. Canals in which ledge formation is present, and very large canals where instruments fail to contact the canal walls, do not lend themselves to rotary preparation.

Instrument fracture can occur as a result of torsional loading or cyclic fatigue.[38] Torsional forces develop because of frictional resistance; therefore as the surface area increases along the flutes, the greater the friction and the more potential for fracture. Torsional stress can be reduced by limiting file contact, using a crown-down preparation technique, by verifying a glide path to WL, and with the presence of liquid irrigants such as NaOCl during shaping procedures.

Cyclic fatigue occurs as a file rotates in a curved canal.[79] At the point of curvature the outer surface of the file is under tension while the inner surface of the instrument is compressed. As the instrument rotates, the areas of tension and compression alternate, crack initiation begins, ultimately leading to fracture. There is often no visible evidence that fracture is imminent.

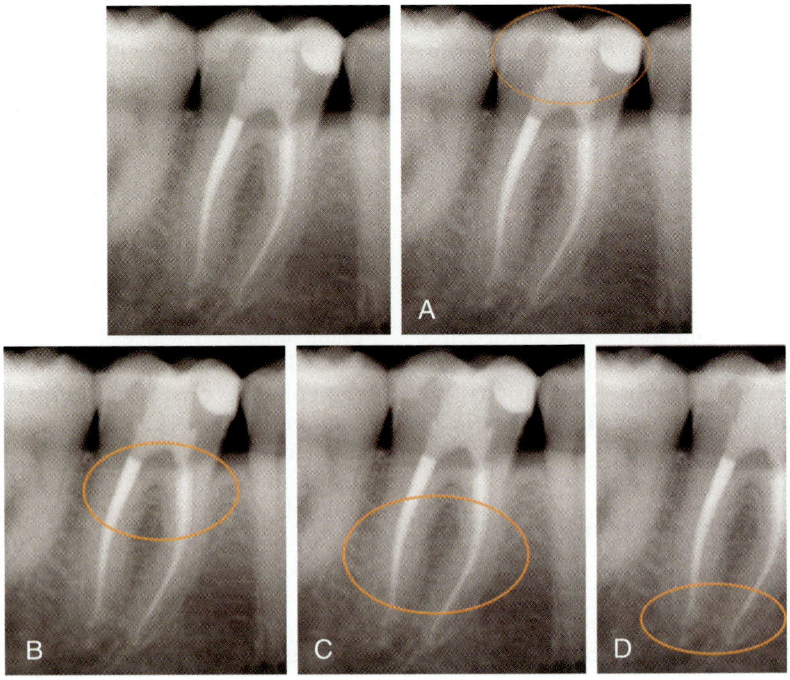

• **Fig. 14.8** An endodontically treated mandibular molar through constricted access and limited shaping, highlighting its guidelines by area: **(A)** coronal, **(B)** pericervical, **(C)** radicular body, and **(D)** apical. (Reprinted from Boveda C, Kishen A: Contracted endodontic cavities: the foundation for less invasive alternatives in the management of apical periodontitis. *Endod Topics* 33:169, 2015 with permission.)

Study Questions

1. Endodontic treatment failures result from all except which of the following?
   a. Inadequate root canal débridement
   b. Use of hand instrumentations
   c. Coronal leakage
   d. Bacteria that are more resistant to treatment protocols
2. Use of antimicrobial irrigants is an optional component of root canal débridement because new technologic advancements in file design allow better adaptation to canal irregularities.
   a. True
   b. False
3. Precise location of the apical constriction may be difficult to identify because of which of the following?
   a. The location of the apical foramen may vary
   b. The apical constriction can be altered by inflammatory changes
   c. The canal terminus is not always located at the root apex
   d. All of the above
3. Iatrogenic root perforation can adversely affect endodontic treatment outcome.
   a. True
   b. False
4. Maintenance of pericervical dentin contributes to the resistance to fractures that may be caused by masticatory forces.
   a. True
   b. False

Although new thermomechanical processed alloys have improved lifespan of instruments, it is still advised that the use of NiTi instruments be monitored[80] and limited to a reduced number of cases. For difficult or calcified or severely curved canals, it is recommended the instruments be used only once.[72]

Smear Layer Management

During cleaning and shaping, organic components of pulp tissue and inorganic dentinal debris accumulate that are not only pressed into accessory canals, fins, and isthmuses (Fig. 14.6) but also deposited on the radicular canal wall, producing an amorphous, irregular smear layer (Fig. 14.9).[81] With pulp necrosis, the smear layer may be contaminated with bacteria and their metabolic byproducts. The smear layer is superficial, with a thickness of 1 to 5 μm, and debris can be packed into the dentinal tubules to varying distances.[82]

There is not a consensus on removing the smear layer before obturation.[81,83,84] The advantages and disadvantages of the smear layer removal remain controversial; however, evidence generally supports removing the smear layer before obturation.[81,85] The organic debris present in the smear layer might constitute substrate for bacterial growth, and it has been suggested that the smear layer prohibits sealer contact with the canal wall, which permits leakage. In addition, viable microorganisms in the dentinal tubules may use the smear layer as a substrate for sustained growth. When the smear layer is not removed, it may slowly disintegrate with leaking obturation materials, or it may be removed by acids and enzymes that are produced by viable bacteria left in the tubules or that enter via coronal leakage.[3] The presence of a smear layer may also interfere with the action and effectiveness of root canal irrigants and interappointment disinfectants.[53]

With smear layer removal, filling materials adapt better to the canal wall.[86,87] Removal of the smear layer also enhances the adhesion of sealers to dentin and tubular penetration[83,86-88] and permits the penetration of all sealers to varying depths.[89] Removal of the smear layer reduces both coronal and apical leakage.[85,90]

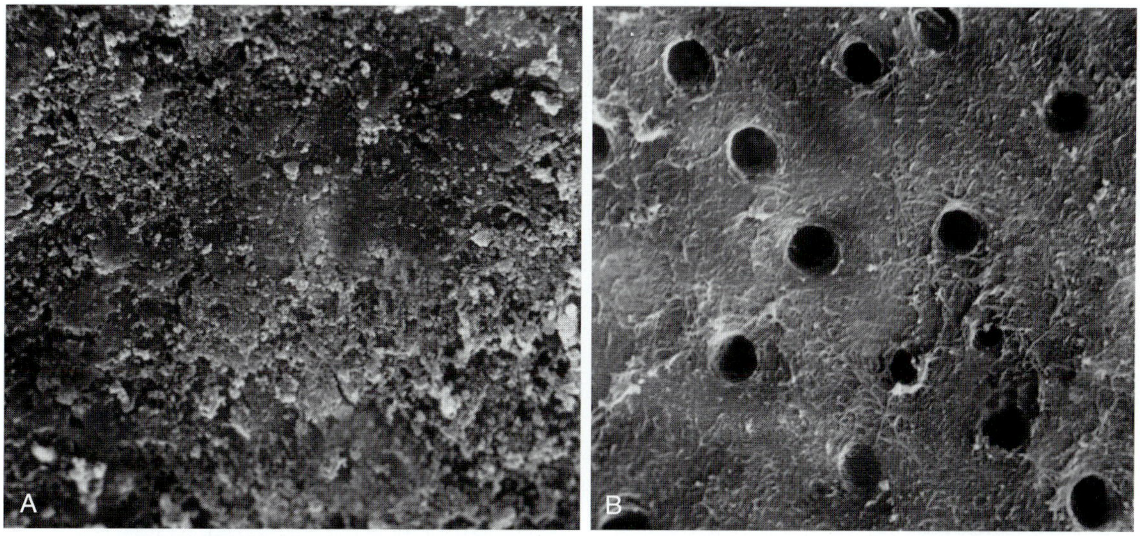

• **Fig. 14.9** **(A)** A canal wall with the smear layer present. **(B)** The smear layer removed with 17% ethylene-diaminetetraacetic acid.

• BOX 14.1 Properties of an Ideal Irrigant

Organic tissue solvent
Inorganic tissue solvent
Antimicrobial action
Nontoxic
Low surface tension
Lubricant

Irrigants

The ideal properties for an endodontic irrigant are listed in Box 14.1.[81] Currently, no solution meets all the requirements outlined. In fact, no techniques appear able to completely clean the root canal space.[39,91-93] Frequent irrigation is necessary to flush and remove the debris generated by the mechanical action of the instruments. At the same time, preparation of radicular wall creates hard tissue debris that is typically pushed into accessory anatomy, blocking access for subsequent irrigation.[39] Therefore it is imperative to use mechanical shaping and irrigation in synergy to maximize antibacterial efficacy of endodontic procedures.

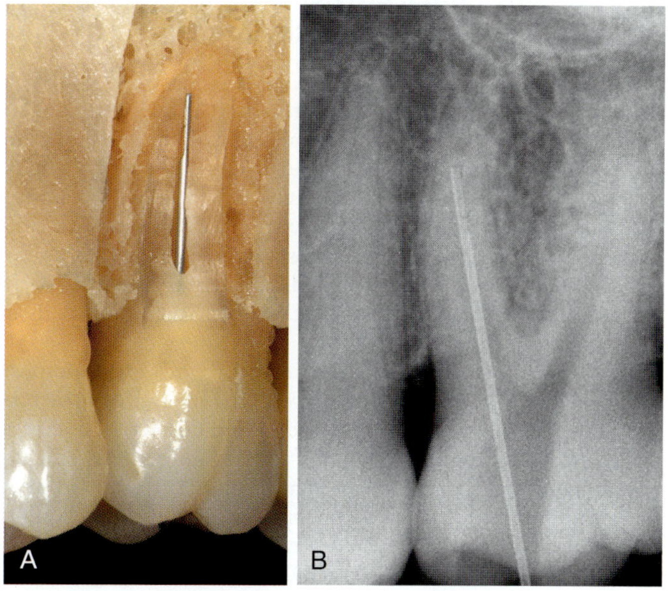

• **Fig. 14.10** **(A and B)** For effective irrigation the needle must be placed in the apical one-third of the root and must not bind.

Sodium Hypochlorite

The most common irrigant is NaOCl, which is also known as household bleach. Advantages to NaOCl include the mechanical flushing of debris from the canal, the ability of the solution to dissolve vital[94] and necrotic tissue,[95] the antimicrobial action of the solution,[47] and the lubricating action.[96] In addition, it is inexpensive and readily available.[97]

Free chlorine in NaOCl dissolves necrotic tissue by breaking down proteins into amino acids. There is no proven appropriate concentration of NaOCl, but concentrations ranging from 0.5% to 5.25% have been recommended. A common concentration is 2.5%, which decreases the potential for toxicity yet still maintains some tissue dissolving and antimicrobial activity.[98,99] Because the action of the irrigant is related to the amount of free chlorine, decreasing the concentration can be compensated by increasing the volume. Warming the solution can also increase the effectiveness of the solution.[100,101] However, NaOCl has limitations to tissue dissolution in the canal, because of limited contact with tissues in all areas of the canal.

Because of toxicity, extrusion is to be avoided.[55,59,102] The irrigating needle must be placed loosely in the canal (Fig. 14.10), and the use of side-vented needles specifically designed for endodontic irrigation is recommended in order to avoid accidents. Insertion to binding and slight withdrawal minimizes the potential for possible extrusion and an NaOCl accident (Fig. 14.11). Special care should be exercised when irrigating a canal with an open apex. To control the depth of insertion the needle is bent slightly at the appropriate length or a rubber stopper is placed on the needle.

Most likely, any irrigant does not travel apically more than 1 mm beyond the irrigation tip, so deep placement with small-gauge needles enhances irrigation (see Fig. 14.10).[103] During rinsing, the needle is moved up and down constantly to produce agitation and prevent binding or wedging of the needle.

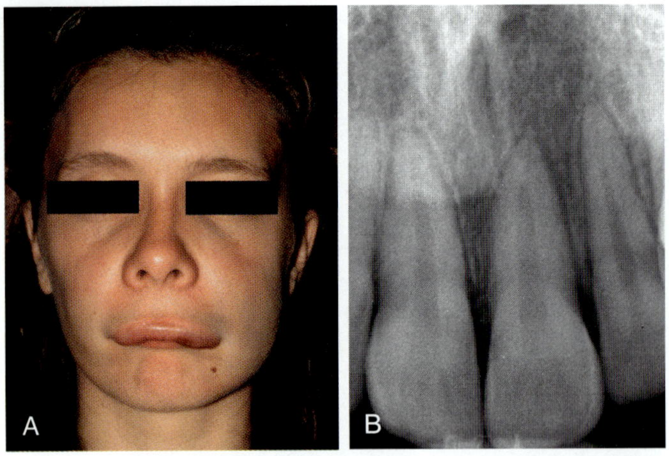

• **Fig. 14.11 (A and B)** A sodium hypochlorite accident during treatment of the maxillary left central incisor. Extensive edema occurred in the upper lip and was accompanied by severe pain.

Chelating Irrigants: Ethylenediaminetetraacetic Acid, Citric Acid, Hydroxyethylidene Bisphosphonate

As described previously, NaOCl is the most effective irrigant for organic tissue dissolution and elimination of bacteria biofilm; however, it does not remove inorganic tissue. For this reason, it needs to be combined with a chelating agent, such as ethylenediaminetetraacetic acid (EDTA), citric acid, or the more recently suggested hydroxyethylidene bisphosphonate (HEPB), also called etidronate. The chelating activity is directed toward removal of the smear layer because, in fact, these chelators have minimal tissue dissolution capacity.[104]

EDTA [105] is the most frequently used irrigant for this purpose. However, chemical interactions between EDTA and NaOCl have been described, and when combined, tissue dissolution ability of NaOCl may be affected as a result of a reduction in the active chlorine content.[106,107] For this reason, when using EDTA, the irrigation protocol recommended includes an irrigation with 17% EDTA for 1 minute at the end of the shaping procedure followed by a final rinse with NaOCl.[108] Chelators such as EDTA remove the inorganic components and leave the organic tissue elements intact. NaOCl is then necessary for removal of the remaining organic components; however, the additional use of NaOCl after chelating agents may lead to excessive demineralization of radicular wall dentin.[109]

Demineralization results in removal of the smear layer and plugs and enlargement of the tubules.[110,111] The action is most effective in the coronal and middle thirds of the canal whereas the effect is diminished in the apical third.[105,112]

Reduced efficacy may be a reflection of canal size[113] or anatomic variations such as irregular or sclerotic tubules.[114,115] The variable structure of the apical dentin presents a challenge during endodontic obturation with adhesive materials.

The recommended time for removal of the smear layer with EDTA is 1 minute.[105,116,117] The small particles of the smear layer are primarily inorganic with a high surface to mass ratio, which facilitates removal by acids and chelators. EDTA exposure over 10 minutes causes excessive removal of both peritubular and intratubular dentin.[117] A 10% solution of citric acid has also been shown to be an effective method for removing the smear layer, although it also reduces available chlorine in NaOCl solutions.[118,119]

A possible alternative to citric acid or EDTA recently suggested is HEBP. HEBP is a weak and biocompatible chelator that prevents bone resorption and is used systemically in patients suffering from osteoporosis or Paget's disease.[98] In contrast with EDTA or citric acid, HEBP appeared to reduce NaOCl active chlorine content after 1 hour and reduction continued over time, but the mixture seemed not to interfere with the dissolving properties of NaOCl. Therefore it may be mixed and used in combination with NaOCl, reducing the formation of smear layer during the mechanical preparation of the root canal. It seems that 7% to 10% HEBP could be mixed chair-side with NaOCl, without fearing any loss of NaOCl activity and administered during the whole course of root canal preparation.[107]

Chlorhexidine

Chlorhexidine possesses a broad spectrum of antimicrobial activity, provides a sustained action,[102,120] and has little toxicity.[121-124] Two percent chlorhexidine has similar antimicrobial action as 5.25% NaOCl[121] and is more effective against *Enterococcus faecalis.*[102] NaOCl and chlorhexidine are synergistic in their ability to eliminate microorganisms.[122] A disadvantage of chlorhexidine is its inability to dissolve necrotic tissue and remove the smear layer. Moreover, clinical studies do not confirm that the use of chlorhexidine is associated with better outcomes.[7]

Moreover, the interaction between chlorhexidine and NaOCl produced a precipitate that may have detrimental consequences for endodontic therapy; among them it may produce discoloration and potential toxic substances for periradicular tissues. At the same time, when chlorhexidine interacted with EDTA a precipitate was also produced.[106,125]

MTAD

An alternative method for disinfecting while at the same time removing the smear layer employs a mixture of a tetracycline isomer, an acid, and a detergent (MTAD) as a final rinse to remove the smear layer.[126] The effectiveness of MTAD to completely remove the smear layer is enhanced when low concentrations of NaOCl are used as an intracanal irrigant before the use of MTAD.[127] A 1.3% concentration is recommended. MTAD may be superior to NaOCl in antimicrobial action.[128,129] MTAD has been shown to be effective in killing *E. faecalis*, an organism commonly found in failing treatments, and may prove beneficial during retreatment. It is biocompatible,[130] does not alter the physical properties of the dentin,[130] and enhances bond strength.[131] Although there are encouraging in vitro data, MTAD has not been shown to be clinically beneficial at this point.[132]

QMix

A chlorhexidine-based mixture, marketed as QMix,[133] employs a similar underlying strategy with the potential to not only remove smear layer but also to provide antibiofilm activity. QMix consists of a proprietary mix of chlorhexidine, EDTA, and a surface-active agent. Nothing is known about its contribution to clinical outcomes, but it appears that smear layer removal is similar to 17% EDTA,[134] and antimicrobial effects are adequate.[135,136] However, tissue dissolution with prior canal shaping and use of NaOCl are still required.[137]

Irrigants for Cryotherapy

A new use of irrigant solution has been recently described in root canal treatment. Posttreatment pain is a very common situation, especially in teeth presenting with preoperative pain, pulp necrosis, and symptomatic apical periodontitis. Postoperative pain has traditionally been controlled with paracetamol, nonsteroidal antiinflammatory medication, opioids, and/or corticosteroids. In other fields of medicine, other alternatives have been suggested in search of a greater efficacy for pain control while avoiding secondary effects, cryotherapy among them. A controlled irrigation with cold saline after cleaning and shaping procedures has been recently suggested to reduce incidence and intensity of postoperative pain in those patients presenting symptomatic apical periodontitis.[138] The authors suggested a final irrigation after cleaning and shaping with cold (2.5°C) sterile saline solution, also using a cold (2.5°C) sterile microcannula attached to the Endovac negative pressure irrigation system for 5 minutes. Recently different cryotherapy applications have also resulted in lower postoperative pain levels (intracanal, intraoral, and extraoral).[139]

Ultrasonics

There are many uses of ultrasonics in root canal treatment; for example, refinement of access cavity preparations for a more conservative approach, orifice location, pulp stone removal, removal of materials from the inside of the root canal (including posts, separated instruments, silver cones), enhancing irrigation, thermoplastic obturation, and root-end preparation during surgery;[140] however, shaping curved root canals with ultrasonic instruments has been shown to create preparation errors and is no longer recommended.[141-143]

In terms of enhancing irrigation, agitation techniques allow an irrigation solution to reach the apical third and irregularities in the root canal system, and hence improve cleaning efficiency. The use of ultrasonics,[144] sonic devices,[145] or apical negative pressure[146] irrigation has been recommended. Many other devices or instruments are continuously being marketed for further disinfection of root canal system; however, cost-effectiveness still needs to be scientifically demonstrated.

The main mechanism of adjunctive cleaning with ultrasonics is acoustic microstreaming,[147] which is described as complex steady-state streaming patterns in vortex-like motions or eddy flows that are formed close to the instrument. Agitation of the irrigant with an ultrasonically activated instrument after completion of cleaning and shaping has the benefit of increasing the effectiveness of the solution.[113,148-150]

Lubricants

Lubricants facilitate manipulation of hand files during cleaning and shaping. They are an aid in initial canal negotiation, especially in small and constricted canals without taper. The use of lubricants during negotiation helps to avoid pulp tissue blockage. Especially in vital teeth, pulp tissue may block the root canal during negotiation. This type of blockage is difficult to bypass but very easy to prevent by filling the pulp chamber with viscous lubricants that will enhance the advancement of the small file without apically pushing the pulp tissue remnants.[151]

Glycerin is a mild alcohol that is inexpensive, nontoxic, aseptic, and somewhat soluble. A small amount can be placed along the shaft of the file or deposited in the canal orifice. Counterclockwise rotation of the file carries the material apically. The file can then be worked to length using a watch winding motion.

Paste lubricants can incorporate chelators. One advantage to paste lubricants is that they can suspend dentinal debris and prevent apical compaction. One proprietary product consists of glycol, urea peroxide, and EDTA in a special water-soluble base. It has been demonstrated to exhibit an antimicrobial action.[152] Another type is composed of 19% EDTA in a water-soluble viscous solution.

A disadvantage to these EDTA compounds appears to be the deactivation of NaOCl by reducing the available chlorine[153] and potential toxicity.[154] The addition of EDTA to the lubricants has not proved to be effective.[155] In general, files remove dentin faster than the chelators can soften the canal walls. Aqueous solutions, such as NaOCl, should always be used instead of paste lubricants when using NiTi rotary techniques to reduce torque.[96]

Preparation Errors

Regardless of the technique used in root canal preparation, procedural errors can occur (see Chapter 18). These include loss of WL, apical transportation, apical perforation, instrument fracture, and stripping perforations.

Loss of WL has several causes, including failure to have an adequate reference point from which the WL is determined, packing tissue and debris in the apical portion of the canal, ledge formation, and inaccurate measurements of files.

The selection of an adequate coronal reference point is very important. Some clinicians advocate for using the same coronal reference for all root canals in the same tooth to ease the procedure; however, the proper determination of a straight and stable reference localized in the original path of the instrument when shaping each canal will avoid procedural mishaps during canal preparation. Moreover, the more visible the reference point, the less stress for the rotary instrument when the clinician checks the proper shaping length.

On the other hand, the most predictable method to prevent any kind of blockage in the apical portion of the canal is to regularly use the so-called patency file during cleaning and shaping procedures. Not only does it minimize the risk of loss of length, but it also reduces further mishaps occurring when trying to force an instrument to go back to the initial length.

And lastly, the reconfirmation of the WL electronically with an apex locator after preparation of the coronal third will also help to maintain the correct length during the whole shaping procedure.

Apical transportation and zipping occur when relatively inflexible files are used to prepare curved canals. The restoring force of the file (the tendency to return to the original straight shape of the file) exceeds the threshold for cutting dentin in a curved canal (Figs. 14.12 and 14.13).[156] When this apical transportation continues with larger and larger files, a "teardrop" shape develops, and apical perforation can occur on the lateral root surface (see Fig. 14.12). Transportation in curved canals already begins with a No. 25 file.[24] Enlargement of curved canals at the WL beyond a No. 25 file can be done only when an adequate coronal flare is developed. Moreover, when shaping a difficult root canal, the most challenge anatomy is often located in the apical third. The potential of avoiding accidents in this delicate portion starts with a proper negotiation after removing the restrictive dentin in the coronal and middle third if the root canal presents great curvatures or S-shaped root canals. Choosing flexible and resistant rotary instruments is very important not to deform the apical third of root canals with complicated anatomy.

As stated before, instrument fracture occurs with torsional and cyclic fatigue. Locking the flutes of a file in the canal wall while continuing to rotate the coronal portion of the instrument is an example of torsional failure (Fig. 14.14). Conversely, cyclic fatigue results when repetitive low-level strain develops in the metal. File fracture occurs more frequently with rotaries but may also involve hand instruments such as K-type and Hedström files.[157]

Working under the operating microscope, using specific ultrasonic tips and specifically designed armamentarium will help to retrieve broken instruments from the root canal, but it is a difficult task and in most situations leads to a weakening of the tooth caused by excessive removal of dentin, allowing the instrument to disengage from the dentin and finding a path for the exit. Therefore the best way to deal with instrument fracture is prevention. To avoid NiTi rotary instruments separation some strategies are recommended: optimal case selection; understanding the

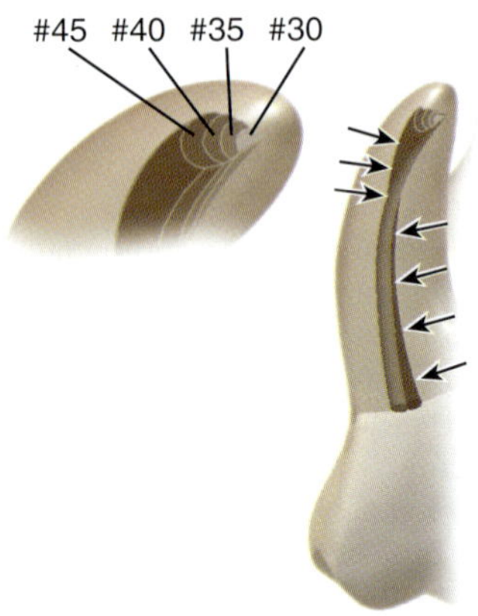

• **Fig. 14.12** Procedural errors of canal transportation, zipping, and strip perforation occur during standardized preparation when files remove dentin from the outer canal wall apical to the curve and from the inner wall coronal to the curve. This is related to the restoring force (stiffness) of the files. Note in the apical portion the transportation takes the shape of a tear drop as the larger files are used.

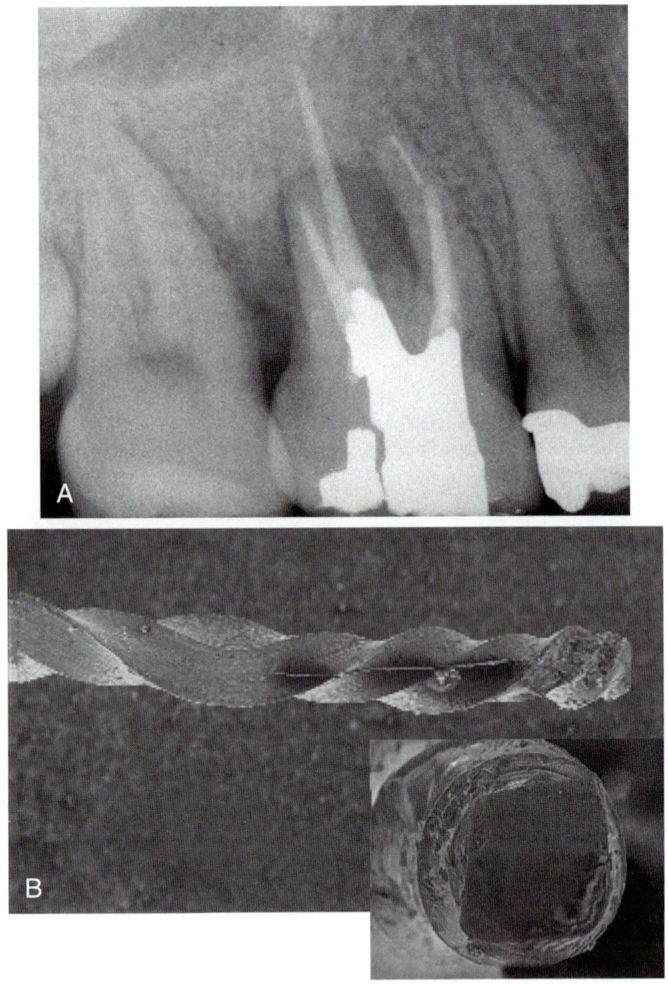

• **Fig. 14.14** **(A)** No. 35 file fractured in the mesiobuccal canal. **(B)** Scanning electron microscope examination reveals torsional failure at the point of fracture. Note the tightening of the flutes near the fracture and the unwinding of the flutes along the shaft.

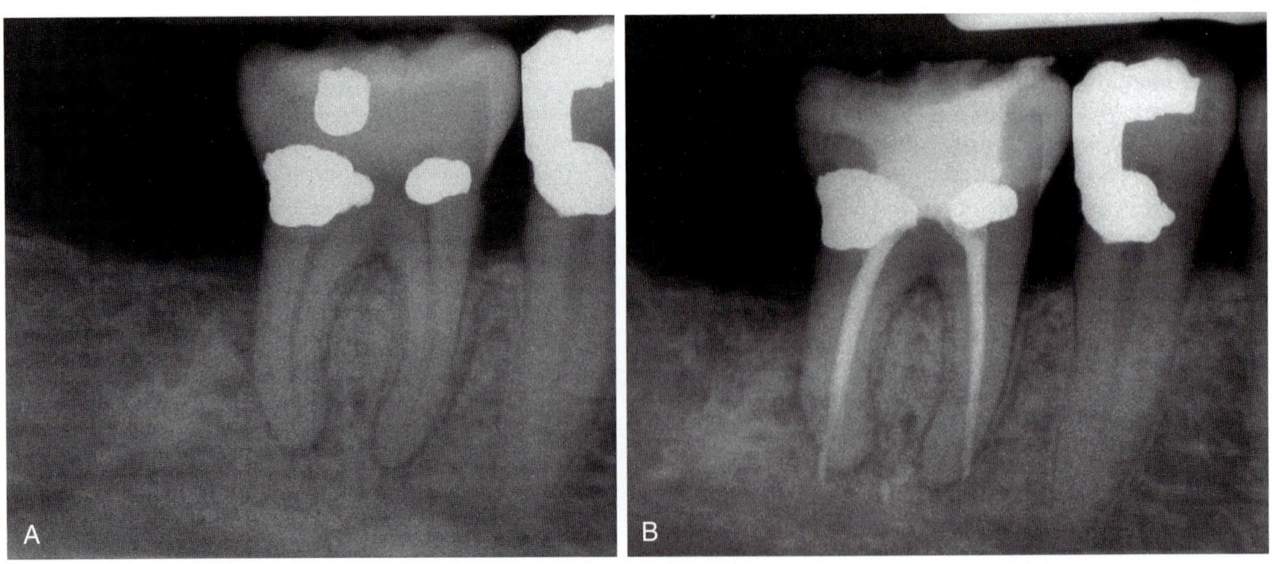

• **Fig. 14.13** A typical procedural error in shaping of curved root canals is straightening or transportation. A comparison of **(A)** preoperative and **(B)** postoperative radiographs in this case reveals that mesial and distal canals have been transported, and there are apical perforations.

characteristics and limitations of the selected instrument; limiting the use of instruments; prematurely eliminating coronal interference before taking rotary instruments to the full root canal length; ensuring a correct glide path; using the instruments following the recommended directions for use in terms of rotational speed, torque, and motion; not forcing instruments in an apical direction to avoid taper-lock; recapitulating if the instrument is not able to advance in the root canal; and not inserting the instrument in the root canal if the active cutting surface of the instrument is blocked with debris (use gauzes to clean the flutes).[78]

Stripping perforations occur toward the furcal region of curved roots and frequently in the mesial roots of maxillary and mandibular molars (Figs. 14.15 and 14.16). The canal in this area of the root is not always centered in cross-sections; before preparation, the average distance to the furcal wall (danger zone) is less than the distance to the bulky outer wall (safety zone). An additional complicating factor is the furcal concavity of the root.[158]

Preparation Techniques

Working Length Determination

A major step in clinical endodontics, regardless of the instruments used, is the determination of the apical termination of cleaning and shaping, as well as obturation procedures. Using diagnostic radiographs, an estimate of the WL can be obtained. With a staged

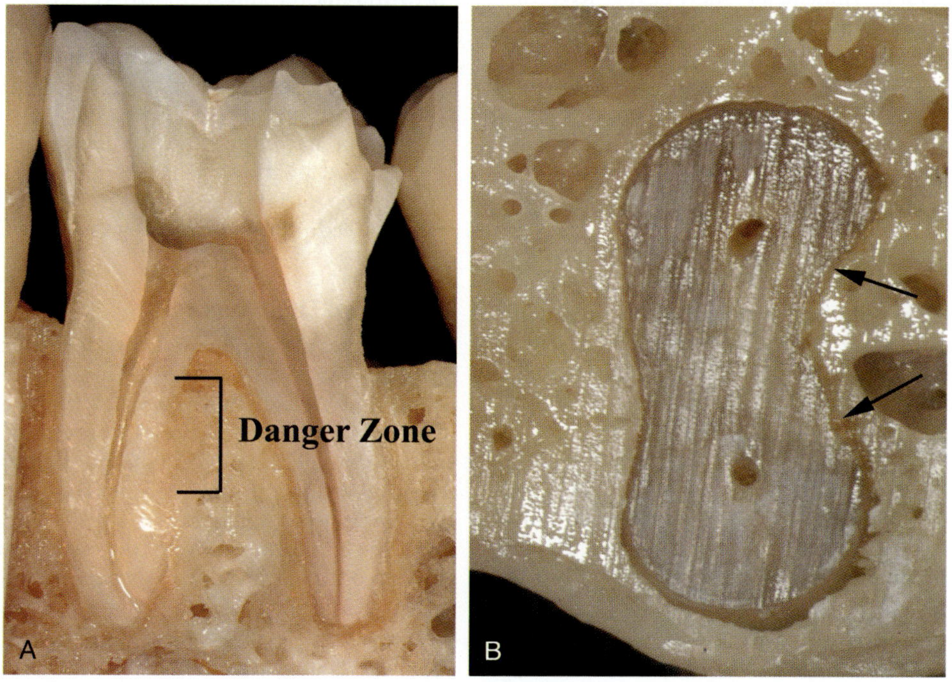

• **Fig. 14.15** **(A)** The furcal region of molars at the level of the curvature (danger zone) is a common site for stripping perforation. **(B)** Note the concavity *(arrows)* in the furcation area of this mandibular molar.

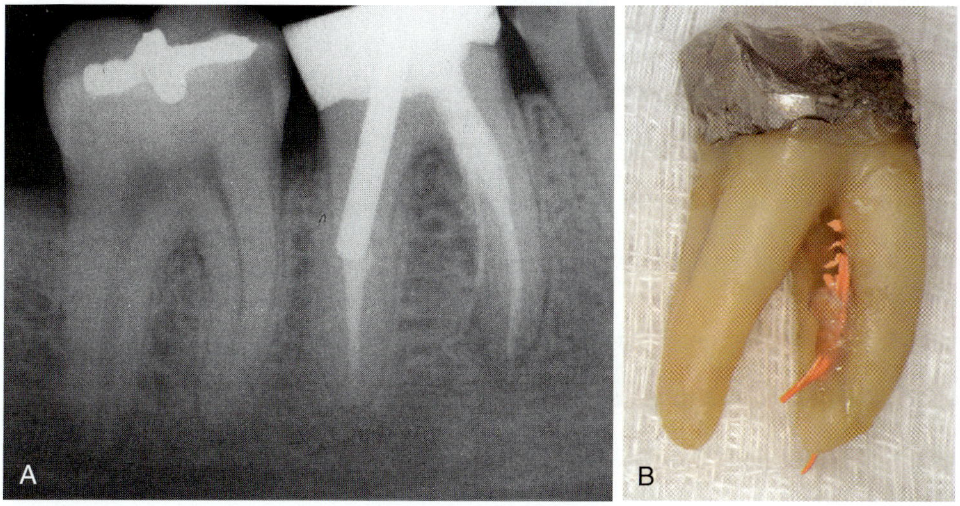

• **Fig. 14.16** Straight-line access can result in stripping perforations in the furcal areas of molars. **(A)** The use of large Gates-Glidden drills and overpreparation has resulted in the stripping perforation. **(B)** Note that the perforation is in the concavity of the furcation.

preparation sequence as detailed before, initial files will not be placed into the root canal as to reach WL, as their use is restricted to the coronal and middle thirds of the canal. However, during all shaping stages care should be taken not to inadvertently overextend the instruments. As soon as a small file appears to reach the estimated termination point, the use of an electronic apex locator is recommended. These units typically provide an accurate assessment of the location of the narrowest canal diameter and can detect the position of the test file relative to the periodontal ligament. Exposing a radiograph with the test file in place then verifies the measurement.

Based on this information clinicians may note the WL for this canal as the distance between a coronal reference point and the apical termination point. Based on clinical evidence[7,19] as well as classic studies[159] WL should terminate just short of the electronically measured canal length. During canal preparation, WLs tend to shorten as a result of the fact that the enlarged canal provides a straighter path to the apical termination point; however, this effect is minimized with coronal flaring. Nevertheless, it is recommended to periodically check the WL and correct it if needed.

Hand Instrumentation

Watch Winding

Watch winding is reciprocating back and forth (clockwise/counterclockwise) rotation of the instrument in an arch and is used to negotiate canals and to work files to place. The first file that reaches tentative WL and slightly binds is called initial apical file (IAF). Light apical pressure is applied to move the file deeper into the canal.

Reaming

Reaming is defined as the clockwise cutting rotation of the file. Generally, the instruments are placed into the canal until binding is encountered. The instrument is then rotated clockwise 180 to 360 degrees to plane the walls and enlarge the canal space.

Filing

Filing is defined as placing the file into the canal and pressing it laterally while withdrawing it along the path of insertion to scrape (plane) the wall. A modification is the quarter-turn-pull technique. This involves placing the file to the point of binding, rotating the instrument 90 degrees, and pulling the instrument along the canal wall. Any filing technique has a tendency to straighten curved canals.

Circumferential Filing

Circumferential filing is used for canals that are larger and/or not round. The file is placed into the canal and withdrawn in a directional manner sequentially against the mesial, distal, buccal, and lingual walls. Circumferential filing is not very effective beyond the coronal third of a root canal.[160,161]

• BOX 14.2 Descriptors for Files During Root Canal Preparation

Working length (WL)
Initial apical file (IAF)
Master apical file (MAF)
Final file (FF)
Final apical file (FAF)

Standardized Preparation

After 1961 instruments were manufactured with a standard formula. Clinicians utilized a preparation technique of sequentially enlarging the canal space with smaller to larger instruments at the WL.[162] In theory, this created a standardized preparation of uniform taper. Unfortunately, in cylindrical and small curved canals, procedural errors were identified with the technique (Box 14.2).[163]

Step-Back Technique

The step-back technique reduces procedural errors and improves débridement.[163,164] It involves that, after coronal flaring, the apical canal diameter is determined with the IAF (the first file that binds at WL). Subsequent preparation to WL up to the master apical file (MAF) creates the apical preparation size, for example, size No. 35; the succeeding larger files are shortened by 0.5- or 1-mm increments from the previous file length (Figs. 14.17 and 14.18) up to the final file (FF), for example, size No. 60. This step-back process creates a flared, tapering preparation while reducing procedural errors. The last file used in the step-back sequence becomes the FF. This type of preparation is superior to standardized serial filing and reaming techniques in débridement and maintaining the canal shape.[164]

Step-Down Technique

The step-down technique is advocated for cleaning and shaping procedures as it removes coronal interferences and provides coronal taper. Originally advocated for hand-file preparation,[165] the step-down technique has been incorporated into those techniques employing NiTi files. With the pulp chamber filled with irrigant or lubricant, the canal is explored with a small instrument to assess morphology (curvature). The WL can be established at this time. The coronal one third of the canal is then flared with Gates-Glidden drills or NiTi orifice shapers. A large file (such as No. 60) is then placed in the canal, and a watch-winding motion is used until resistance is encountered.[165] The process is repeated with sequentially smaller files until the apical portion of the canal is

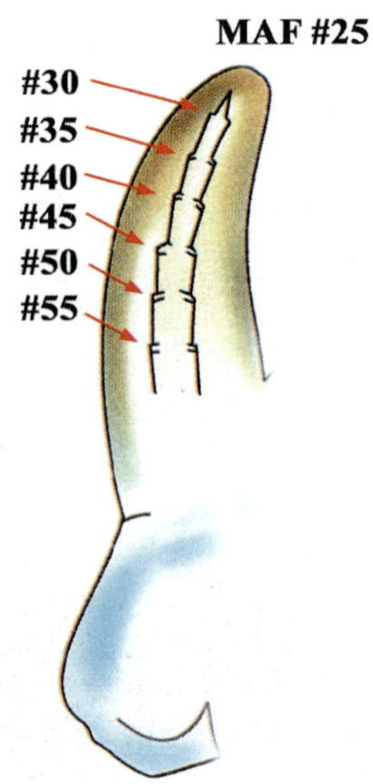

• **Fig. 14.17** The step-back preparation is designed to provide a tapering preparation. The process begins with one file size larger than the master apical file with incremental shortening of either 0.5 or 1 mm.

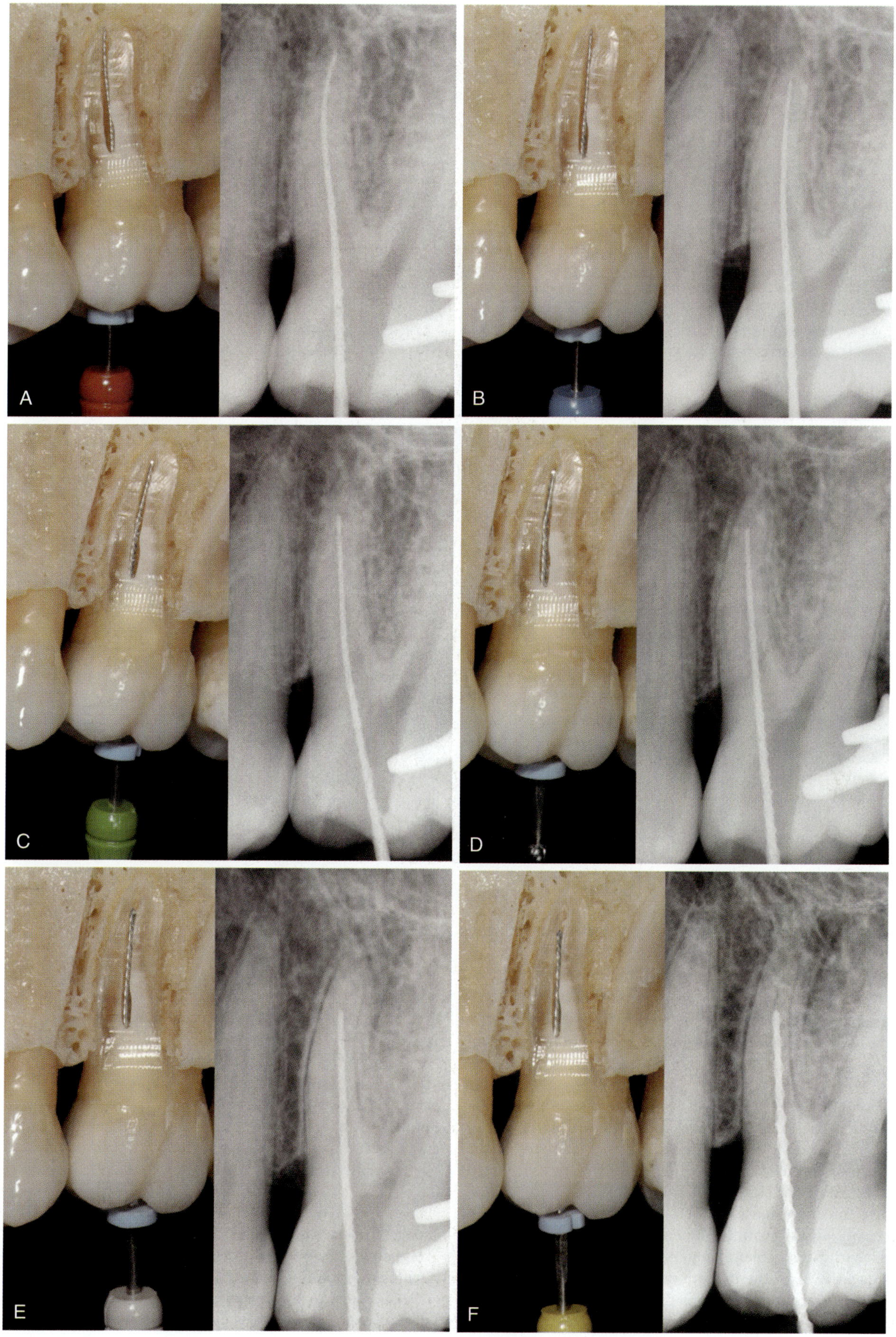

• **Fig. 14.18** An example of step-back preparation in a moderately curved canal. **(A)** The No. 25 master apical file at the corrected working length of 21 mm. **(B)** The step-back process begins with the No. 30 file at 20.5 mm. **(C)** No. 35 file at 20 mm. **(D)** No. 40 file at 19.5 mm. **(E)** No. 45 file at 19 mm. **(F)** No. 50 file at 18.5 mm.

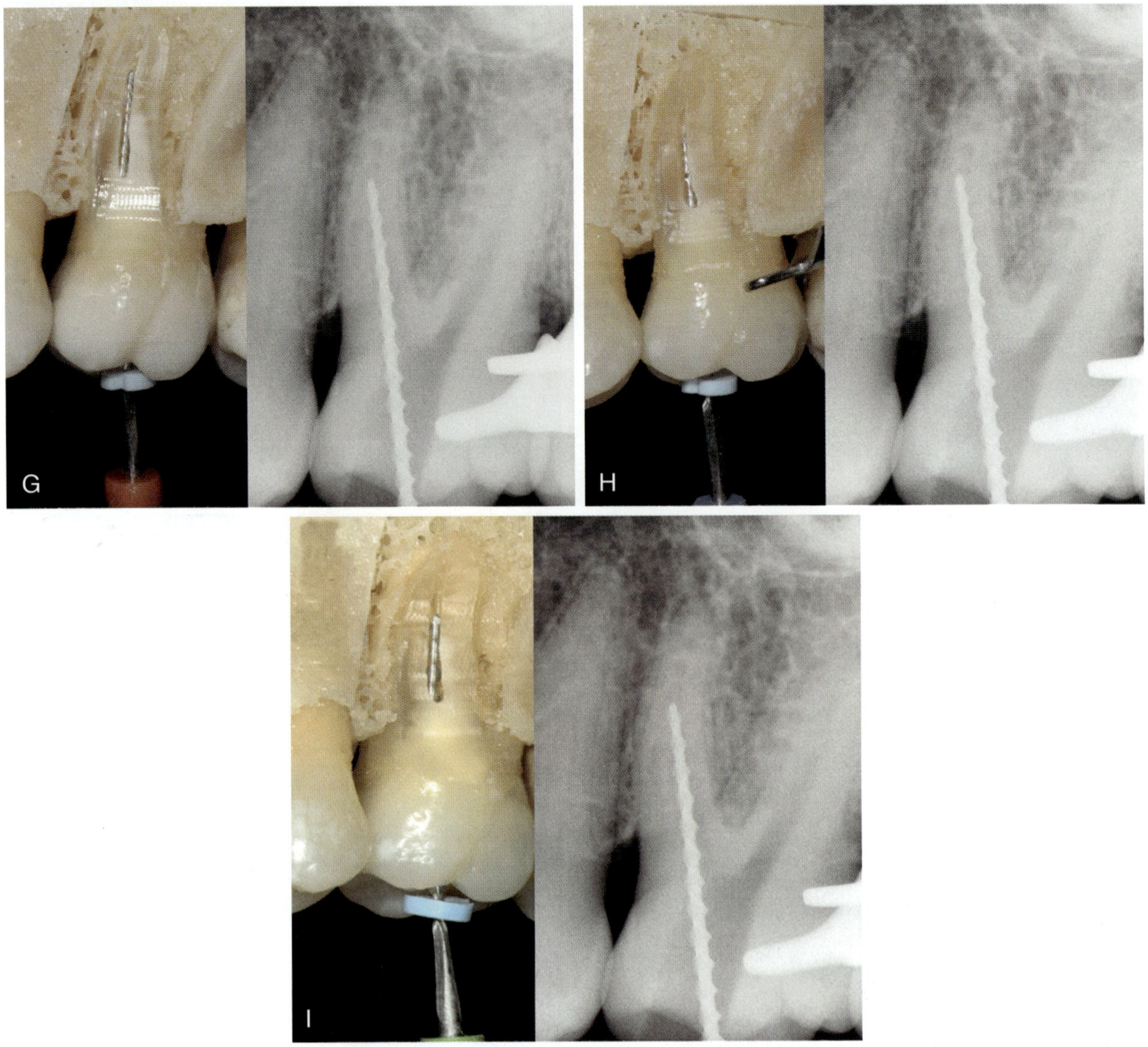

• **Fig. 14.18, cont'd** **(G)** No. 55 file at 18 mm. **(H)** No. 60 file at 17.5 mm. **(I)** No. 70 file at 17 mm.

reached. The WL and the IAF (the first file that binds at WL) can be determined whether this was not accomplished initially. The apical portion of the canal can now be prepared by enlarging the canal to the MAF at the WL. Apical taper is accomplished using a step-back technique.

Passive Step-Back Technique

The passive step-back technique is a modification of the incremental step-back technique.[9,166] After the apical diameter of the canal has been determined, the next higher instrument is inserted until it first makes contact (binding point). It is then rotated one-half turn and removed (Fig. 14.19). The process is repeated with larger and larger instruments being placed to their binding point. This entire instrument sequence is then repeated. With each sequence, the instruments drop deeper into the canal, creating a tapered preparation. Advantages to the technique include knowledge of canal morphology, removal of debris and minor canal obstructions, and a gradual passive, slight enlargement of the canal in an apical to coronal direction.

Anticurvature Filing

Anticurvature filing is advocated during coronal flaring procedures to preserve the furcal wall in the treatment of molars (Fig. 14.20). As stated before, canals are often not centered in mesial roots of maxillary and mandibular molars; instead, they are located closer to the furcation. Stripping perforations occur primarily during use of the Gates-Glidden drills but also with overzealous use of hand instruments. To prevent this procedural error, the Gates-Glidden drills should be confined to the canal space coronal to the root curvature and used in a step-back or step-down manner (Figs. 14.21 and 14.22). Gates-Glidden drills and laterally cutting NiTi orifice shapers can also be used directionally in an anticurvature fashion to selectively remove dentin from the bulky wall (safety zone) toward the line angle,

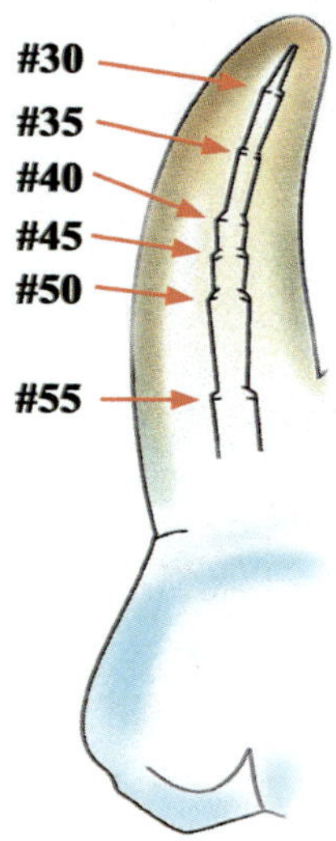

• **Fig. 14.19** Passive step-back. Smaller to larger files are inserted to their initial point of binding and then rotated 180 to 360 degrees and withdrawn. This process creates slight taper and coronal space and permits larger instruments to reach the apical one third.

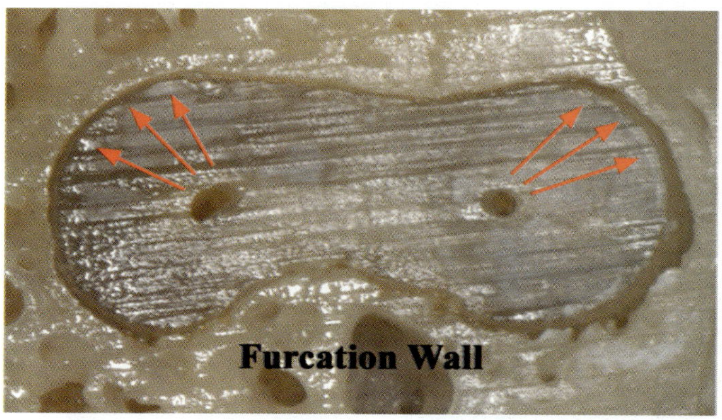

• **Fig. 14.20** The anticurvature filing technique. Instruments are directed away from the furcal danger zone toward the line angles (safety zone) where the bulk of dentin is greater.

protecting the inner or furcal wall (danger zone) coronal to the curve (see Fig. 14.20).

Balanced Force Technique

The balanced force technique recognizes the fact that instruments are guided by the canal walls when rotated.[167] Because files with a symmetric cross-section will cut in both a clockwise and counterclockwise rotation, the balanced force concept of instrumentation consists of placing the file to length and then a clockwise rotation (less than 180 degrees) engages dentin. This is followed by a counterclockwise rotation (at least 120 degrees) with apical pressure to cut and enlarge the canal. The degree of apical pressure varies from light pressure with small instruments to heavy pressure with large instruments. The clockwise rotation pulls the instrument into the canal in an apical direction. The counterclockwise cutting rotation forces the file in a coronal direction while cutting circumferentially. After the cutting rotation, the file is repositioned, and the process is repeated until the WL is reached. At this point, a final clockwise rotation is employed to evacuate the debris. The balanced force concept is considered the most effective hand instrumentation technique.[74,91]

Recapitulation

Recapitulation is important regardless of the technique selected (Fig. 14.23) and is accomplished by taking a small file to the WL to loosen accumulated debris and then flushing it with 1 to 2 mL of irrigant. Recapitulation is performed between each successive enlarging instrument regardless of the cleaning and shaping technique.

Shaping Modifications

The apical configuration in a given case may be recognized as an apical stop, apical seat, or open apex. In addition to the assessment of a diagnostic radiograph these configurations are detected by placing the MAF to the corrected WL after shaping is completed. If the MAF easily extends past WL, the apical configuration is open. If the MAF stops at WL, a file one or two sizes smaller is placed to the same depth. If this file stops as well, the apical configuration is called an apical stop. When the smaller file goes past the corrected WL, the apical configuration is a seat.

In a small curved canal, enlargement should be restricted to three sizes larger than the IAF to decrease the potential for transportation. In a straight canal, it may be larger without producing a procedural error. Because a properly prepared canal exhibits taper, the small files at the corrected WL can be used to enlarge the canal without transportation. Additional apical enlargement is performed with an irrigant in the canal and employs a reaming action at the corrected WL. The last file used becomes the so-called final apical file (FAF). Because this file is only contacting the apical portion of the canal, the technique may result in a less irregular apical preparation. The canal is then irrigated, the smear layer is removed with a decalcifying agent, and the canal dried with paper points.

Engine-Driven Instruments

Gates-Glidden Drills

Gates-Glidden drills have been historically used to enlarge canal orifices, preferably in pairs such as size Nos. 3 and 2 (diameters 0.7 and 0.9 mm, respectively) (see Figs. 14.21 and 14.22). If the canal orifice cannot accommodate a No. 50 file, careful hand instrumentation should be performed to provide adequate initial coronal space. To prevent stripping perforations, Gates-Glidden drills should not be placed apical to canal curvatures. Moreover, with the advancement of NiTi rotary instruments and the concept of minimally invasive endodontics, the use of Gates-Glidden drills should be reconsidered. The amount of dentin removed in the coronal third makes Gates-Glidden drills an unsuitable instrument for modern endodontics.

NiTi Rotary Instruments

As stated previously, NiTi rotary preparation is typically performed in a staged approach using coronal flaring; however, the specific technique is based on the instrument system selected. One instrument sequence uses NiTi files in a crown down approach, with a constant taper and variable ISO tip sizes (Fig. 14.24). With this technique, a 0.06 taper is selected. Initially a size .06/45 file is used until resistance, followed by the .06/40, .06/35, .06/30, .06/25, and .06/20. In a second technique, NiTi files with a constant tip diameter are used also in a crown down sequence. The initial file is a .10/20 instrument, the second a .08/20, the third

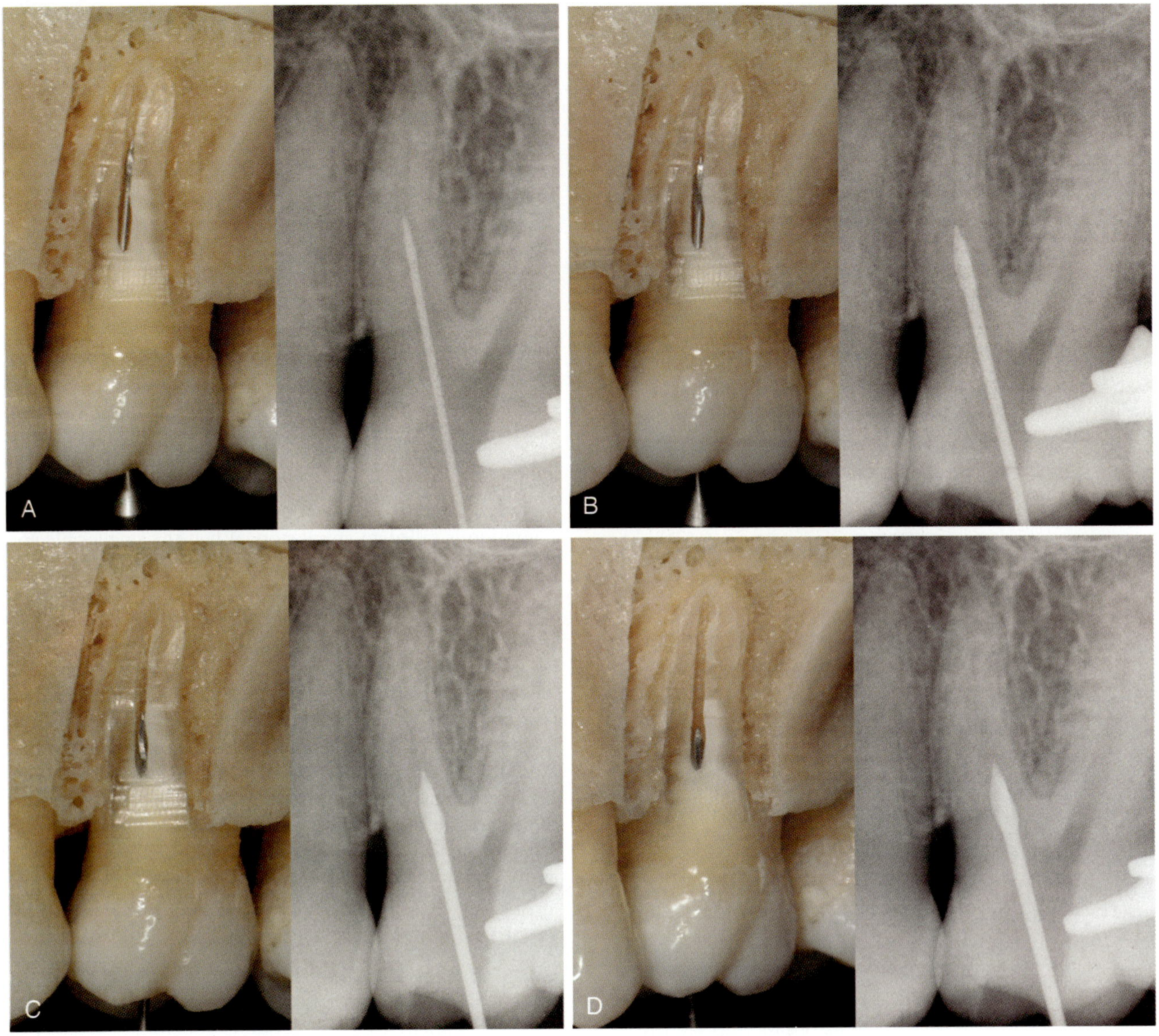

• **Fig. 14.21** Straight-line access in a maxillary left first molar with Gates-Glidden drills used in a slow-speed handpiece using a step-back technique. **(A)** The No. 1 Gates is used until resistance. **(B)** This is followed by the No. 2, which should not go past the first curvature. **(C)** The No. 3 Gates is used 3 to 4 mm into the canal **(D)** Followed by the No. 4 instrument.

a .06/20, and the fourth a .04/20 (see Fig. 14.24). Many variations of these basic approaches have been recommended for different file designs. More recently introduced systems try to limit the number of file sizes, up to the point of using only one size for the majority of canals. Obviously, one size will not fit all canal shapes, and modifications will frequently need to be made when such a system is used.

Critical for all rotaries is the handling of these files. Besides manufacturer guidelines for individual files there are several general principles that should be followed.[72,168] For example, instrument insertions should follow an in-and-out pattern; each instrumentation step should consist of three to five movements and should not exceed 10 to 15 seconds. Apically directed force should typically not exceed the force required to bend the rotary when placed on a tabletop. Most NiTi files are made of austenitic alloy and work best with lower rather than higher rotational speed (e.g., 250 rpm). However, martensitic rotaries work better with higher speeds, for example, 500 rpm.[169]

Currently marketed electric motors have the torque setting already programmed. These settings are a reasonable protection against instrument breakage caused by torsional loading but are less effective with greater tapers, such as .06 and .08.[38] All rotaries work best in canals flooded with irrigation solution and not in the presence of a gel-type lubricant such as RC Prep.[96]

NiTi rotaries should not be placed into an unexplored canal but rather follow hand instruments. These hand instruments establish a glide path that then can be followed by rotaries.[170] It is important to note that hand files for glide path preparation should not be precurved; only then can rotaries predictably follow.

Frequently NiTi rotaries are combined with hand files or other rotary instruments. One such combination technique

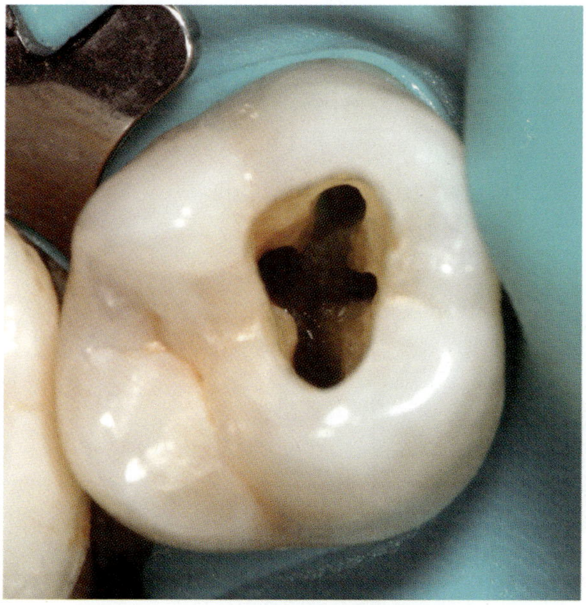

• **Fig. 14.22** A maxillary first molar following straight-line access with the Gates-Glidden drills.

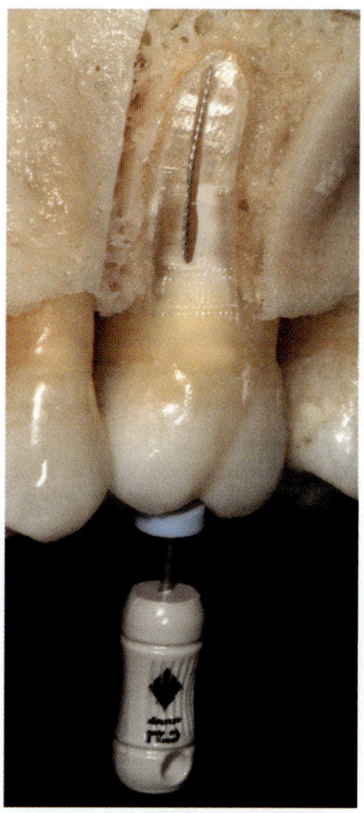

• **Fig. 14.23** Recapitulation is accomplished between each instrument by reaming with the master apical file or a smaller instrument, minimizing packing of debris and loss of length.

utilizes the following steps: coronal flaring, NiTi rotary preparation to WL, and additional apical enlargement (Box 14.3). After access, the irrigated canal is explored with a No. 10 or 15 K-file into the midroot area. Sometimes a canal is already naturally flared and wide, for example a maxillary central incisor or canine in a younger patient. Then a size No. 10 file may immediately be placed to the estimated WL and a WL radiograph can be obtained (see Fig. 14.25). For more constricted canals, NiTi orifice modifiers can be used to accomplish early coronal enlargement. This step facilitates irrigation and removes coronal interferences, which in turn permits easier access to the apical portion of the root canal and more accurate determination of apical constriction location[171] as well as size.[172]

In the presence of irrigant or gel-based lubricant, the canal is negotiated to full length with a hand file used in watch-winding motion. If an impediment is felt, the negotiation files need to be precurved. However, in order to secure a glide path for subsequent rotary use, it must be confirmed that a straight small K-file (e.g., size No. 10 or 15) reaches the corrected WL. The tightness of fit of the negotiation file at WL gives an estimate of the canal size; however, coronal interferences do not permit a more accurate assessment at this point.

Then, the middle and apical portions of the canal are prepared using NiTi rotary instruments (see Figs. 14.24 and 14.25). Rotary files are used with a crown-down approach to reach the corrected WL. Using this approach with continuously tapered rotaries creates coronal taper and reduces the contact area of the file so torsional forces are reduced.[173] Differently designed NiTi rotaries may follow a single-length principle, according to the manufacturers' recommendations.

Emphasis has traditionally been placed on determining the canal length with comparatively little consideration of the canal diameter in the apical portion of the root. Because every canal is unique in its morphology, apical canal diameters must be assessed. After initial preparation to length the size of the apical portion of the canal is determined by placing successively larger instruments to the corrected WL until slight binding is encountered (Fig. 14.26). Often, the next larger instrument will not go to the corrected WL. If it does go to length, a subjective estimation of the apical diameter must be made depending on the degree of binding. This file will be the IAF (initial file to bind). It is defined as the largest file to bind slightly at the corrected WL after straight-line access. This file size provides an estimate of the canal diameter before cleaning and shaping. A shaping target is set, the MAF, which is the point where the step-back preparation begins. It should be considered that this approach may underestimate actual constriction diameters,[174] and therefore additional apical enlargement may be reconsidered.

When the body of the canal has been shaped, the apical portion may be additionally prepared using hand or rotary files (Fig. 14.27). The first instrument selected for this portion of the shaping process is one size larger than the MAF (estimated canal diameter at WL). Recently, clinical evidence suggests that such an enlargement may be beneficial for outcome.[175]

Regardless, NiTi instruments continue to evolve and shaping with modern instruments that are more flexible allows better preparations and respect to natural anatomies. First, manufacturers focused on enhancing design characteristics such as different cross-sections, tip designs, and progressive tapers over the length of the cutting blades to improve the properties of rotary instruments. Second, they suggested reciprocation motions that seemed to enhance cyclic fatigue resistance. Third, proprietary thermal treatments optimized the mechanical properties of NiTi by improving its microstructure through different series of heating and cooling treatments (M-wire, CM-Wire, Blue and Gold alloys are some examples of improved alloys). At the same time, manufacturers have also developed different manufacturing methods to the traditional

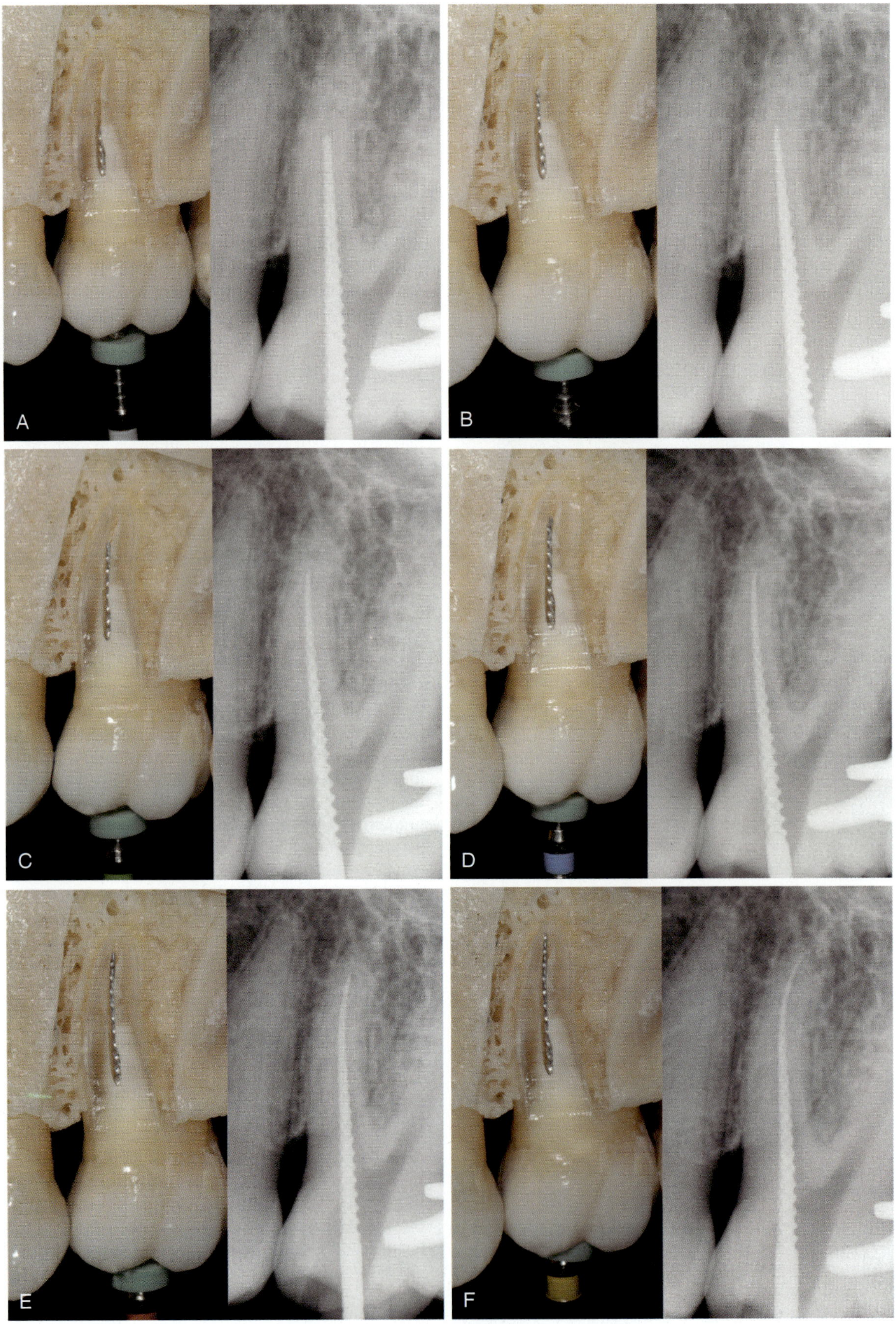

• **Fig. 14.24** The mesiobuccal canal is prepared using nickel-titanium rotary files using a crown-down technique. In this sequence, each instrument exhibits the same .06 taper with varied International Organization for Standardization standardized tip diameters. Instruments were used to resistance. **(A)** The process begins with a .06/45 file to resistance at 16.0 mm. **(B)** Followed by a .06/40 instrument at 17.0 mm. **(C)** The .06/35 file is used to 18.0 mm. **(D)** The .06/30 at 19.0 mm. **(E)** The .06/25 at 20.0 mm. **(F)** The .06/20 file is to the corrected working length of 21.0 mm.

grinding method (twisting, shape-setting, and electric discharge machining are some examples). Taking advantage of all these developments together, the last generation of rotary instruments, the so-called 3D conforming instruments (as a result of a characteristic nonflat morphology), better address nonround cross sections[176] and also better respect coronal dentin compared with traditional rotaries.[177]

• BOX 14.3 Combination Technique Steps

Canal exploration
Coronal flaring
Canal negotiation
Working length determination
Initial rotary preparation to WL
Master apical file determination
Additional apical enlargement

Criteria for Evaluating Cleaning and Shaping

After cleaning and shaping procedures, the canal should exhibit "glassy smooth" walls, and there should be no evidence of dentin filings, debris, or irrigant in the canal. This can be directly determined in the coronal root canal portion when an operating microscope is used to visualize endodontic procedures; it can only be indirectly determined in the more apical portion of the root canal by tactile feedback during instrumentation.

Shaping is evaluated by assessing the canal taper and identifying the apical configuration in size and shape. For obturation with lateral compaction, a small finger spreader should go ideally to

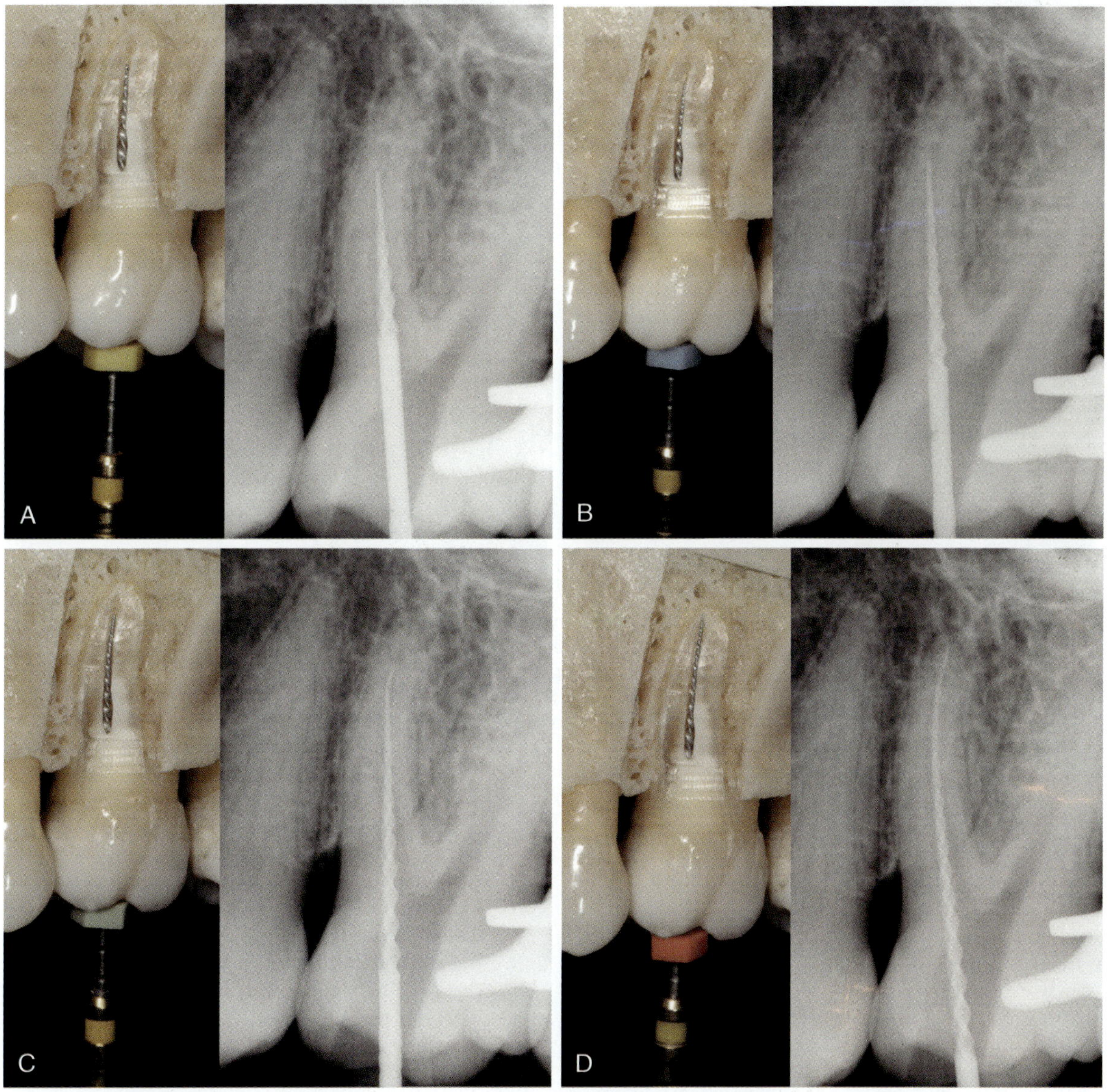

• **Fig. 14.25** Nickel-titanium rotary files with a standardized International Organization for Standardization tip diameter and variable tapered files can be used in canal preparation. In this sequence, the instruments have a standardized tip diameter of .20 mm. **(A)** Initially a 1.0/.20 file is used. **(B)** This is followed by .08/.20. **(C)** The third instrument is a .06/.20. **(D)** The final instrument is a .04/.20 file to the corrected working length of 21 mm.

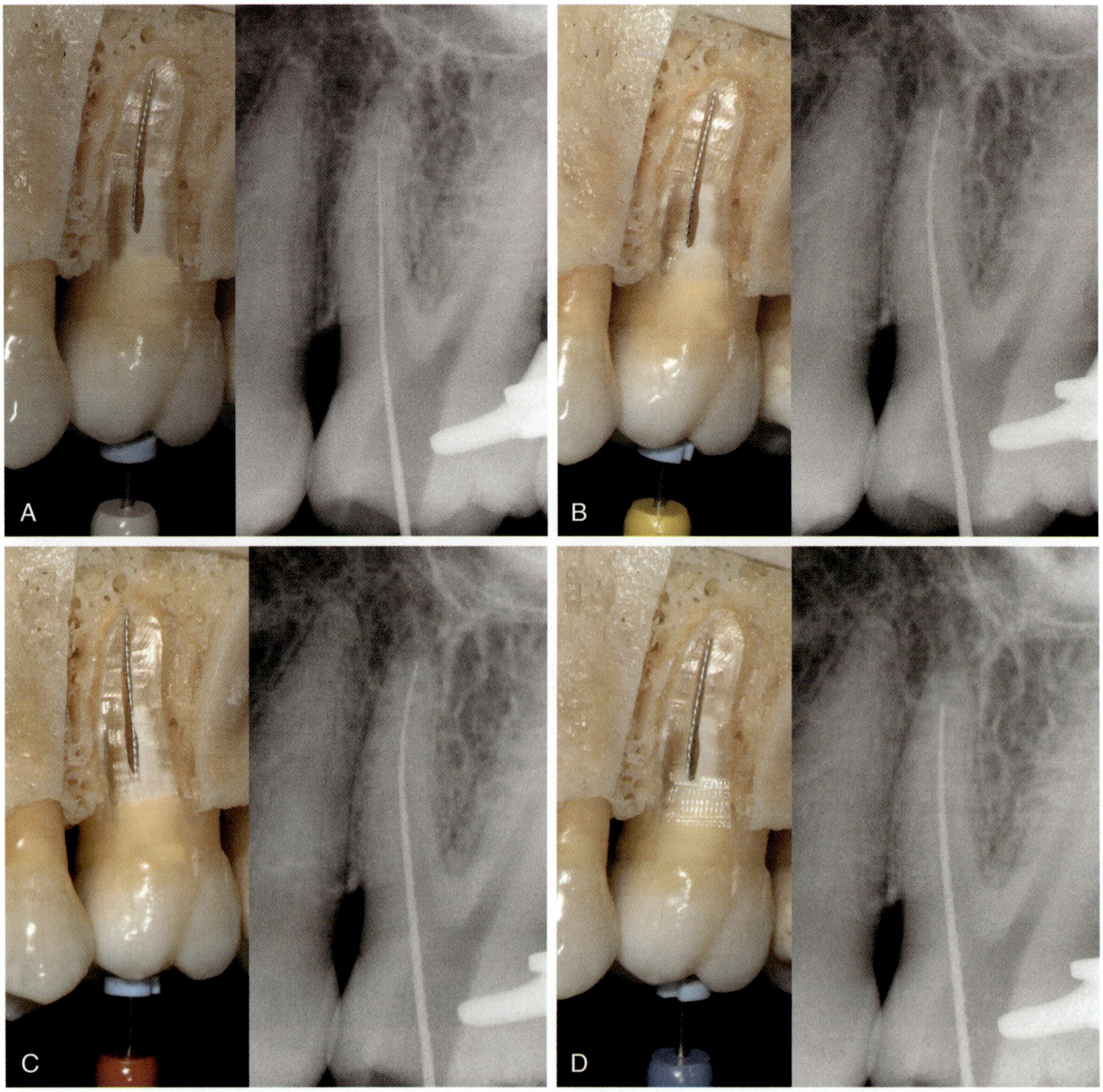

• **Fig. 14.26** After straight-line access in this maxillary molar, the actual constriction size is determined by successively placing small to larger files to the corrected working length. **(A)** No. 15 stainless steel file is placed to 21.0 mm without resistance. **(B)** No. 20 is placed to 21.0 mm without resistance. **(C)** The No. 25 file reaches 21 mm with slight binding. **(D)** No. 30 file is then placed and does not go the corrected working length, indicating the initial canal size in the apical portion of the canal is No. 25.

within 1 mm of the corrected WL without binding. For warm vertical compaction, the plugger should reach to within 5 mm of the corrected WL (Fig. 14.28).

The following principles and concepts should be applied regardless of the instruments or technique selected:

1. Initial canal exploration is always performed with smaller hand files to gauge canal size, shape, and configuration.
2. Copious irrigation must be provided between instruments in the canal.
3. Coronal preflaring will facilitate placing larger files to WL (either hand or rotary) and will reduce procedural errors such as loss of WL and canal transportation.
4. Apical canal enlargement is gradual, using sequentially larger files, regardless of flaring technique.
5. Debris is loosened and dentin is removed from all walls on the outstroke or with a rotating action at or close to WL.
6. Instrument binding or dentin removal on insertion should be avoided. Files are teased to length using a watch-winding action. This is a back-and-forth rotating motion of the files between the thumb and forefinger, continually working the file apically. Careful file manipulation in an irrigant-filled canal will help to avoid apical packing of debris and minimize extrusion of debris into the periradicular tissues.
7. Circumferential filing is used for canals that exhibit cross-sectional shapes that are not round. The file is placed into the canal and withdrawn in a directional manner against the mesial, distal, buccal, and lingual walls.

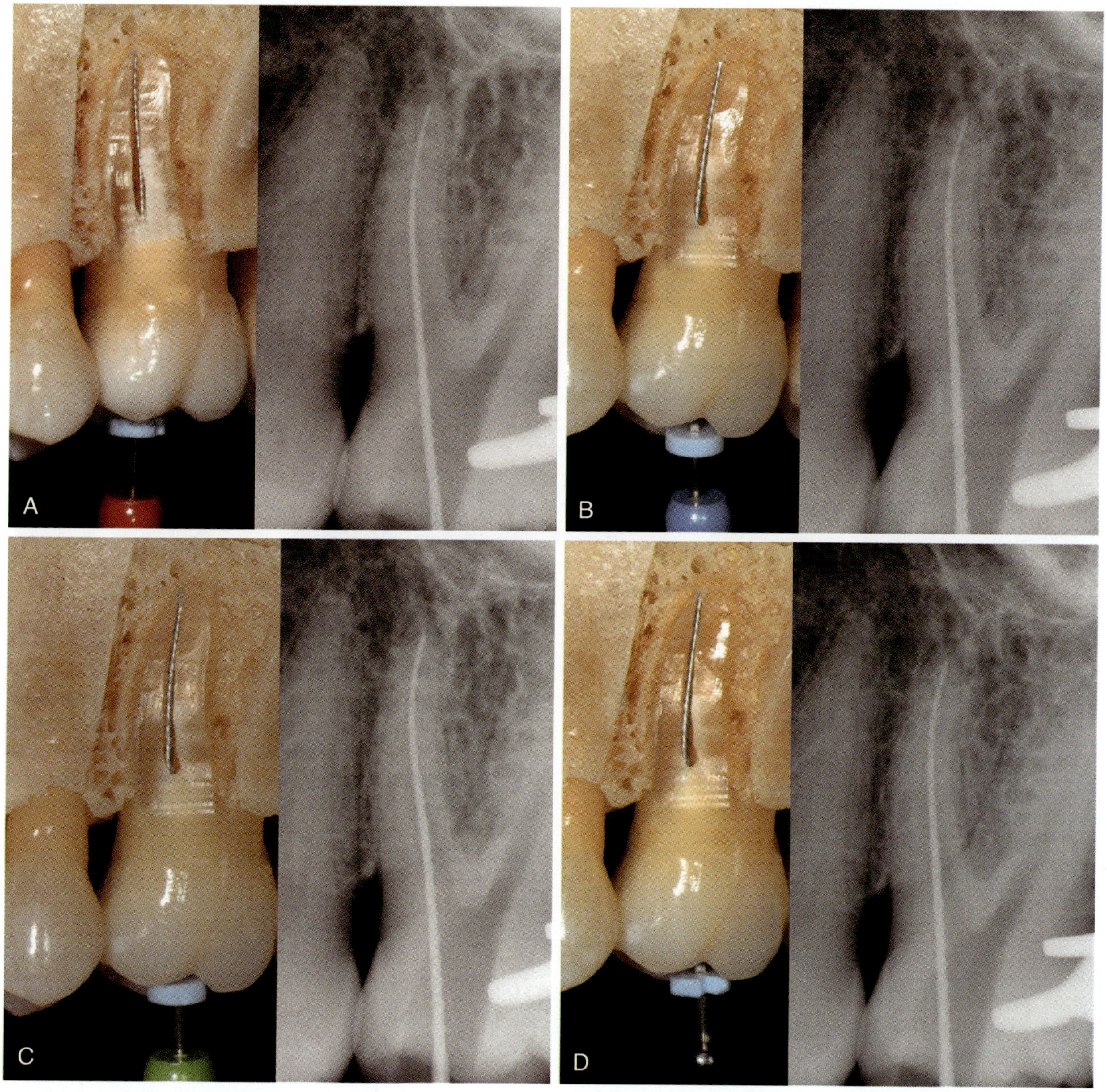

• **Fig. 14.27** Final apical enlargement. **(A)** The master apical file No. 25 at the corrected working length of 21.0 mm. **(B)** Enlargement with a No. 30 file to the corrected working length of 21.0 mm. **(C)** Further enlargement with a No. 35 file. **(D)** Final enlargement to a No. 40 file. The final instrument used becomes the final apical file (FAF).

8. After each insertion the file is removed and the flutes are cleaned of debris; the file can then be reinserted into the canal to plane the next wall. Debris is removed from the file by wiping it with an alcohol-soaked gauze or a cotton roll.[178]
9. Recapitulation is done to loosen debris by placing a small-size file to the corrected WL followed by irrigation to mechanically remove the material. During recapitulation, the canal walls are not planed, and the canal is not enlarged.
10. Small, long, and curved canals are the most difficult and tedious to enlarge. They require extra caution during preparation because they are the most prone to loss of length and transportation.
11. Overenlargement of curved canals by files attempting to straighten themselves will to lead to procedural errors (see Fig. 14.12).
12. Overpreparation of canal walls toward the furcation may result in a stripping perforation in the danger zone where root dentin is thinner (see Fig. 14.13).
13. Instruments, irrigants, debris, and obturating materials should be contained within the canal. These are all known physical or chemical irritants that will induce periradicular inflammation and may delay or compromise healing.
14. Creation of an apical stop may be impossible if the apical foramen is already very large. An apical taper (seat) is attempted but with care. Overusing large files aggravates the

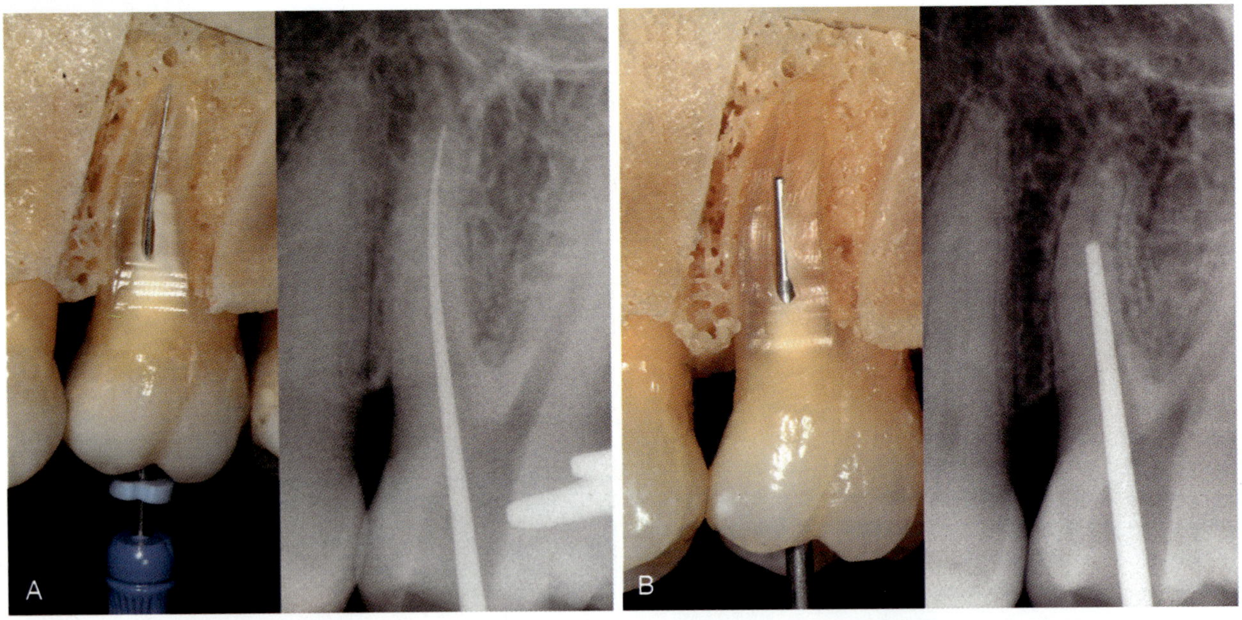

• **Fig. 14.28** The coronal taper is assessed using the spreader or plugger depth of penetration. **(A)** With lateral compaction, a finger spreader should fit loosely 1.0 mm from the corrected working length with space adjacent to the spreader. **(B)** For warm vertical compaction, the plugger should go to within 5.0 mm of the corrected working length.

problem by creating an even larger apical opening. A resistance form along the root canal should allow proper warm vertical obturation with no need of an apical stop.

15. Forcing or locking (binding) files into dentin produces unwanted torsional force. This tends to untwist or "wrap up" and will weaken and break the instrument.

Intracanal Medicaments

Intracanal medicaments have a long history of use as interim appointment dressings. They have been employed for the following three purposes: (1) to reduce interappointment pain, (2) to decrease the bacterial count and prevent regrowth, and (3) to render the canal contents inert. Some common agents are listed in Box 14.4.

Clinical evidence of the effectiveness of these agents is mixed; this has led to increased interest in the efficacy of so-called single visit endodontic therapy. There are only few prospective studies directly comparing these two treatment modalities, with a meta-analysis favoring single-visit treatment.[179] Two well-done clinical studies[180,181] showed remaining microorganisms in accessory anatomy and isthmi, but also in the main canal, remaining after single visit treatment as well as in the majority of the cases with calcium hydroxide placement.

• BOX 14.4 Groupings of Commonly Used Intracanal Medicaments

Calcium hydroxide
Phenolics
Aldehydes
Halides
Steroids
Antibiotics
Combinations

Calcium Hydroxide

One intracanal agent that is effective in inhibiting microbial growth in canals is calcium hydroxide.[182] Calcium hydroxide has antimicrobial activity that is a result of the alkaline pH, and it may aid in dissolving necrotic tissue remnants and bacteria and their byproducts.[183-185] Interappointment calcium hydroxide in the canal demonstrates no pain-reduction effects.[186] Calcium hydroxide has been recommended for use in teeth with necrotic pulp tissue and bacterial contamination. It probably has little benefit in teeth with vital pulps. Calcium hydroxide should be placed as a powder mixed with a liquid such as local anesthetic solution, saline, or sterile water, to form a slurry; or as a proprietary paste supplied in a syringe (see Fig. 14.29). A lentulo spiral is effective and efficient for placement.[187-189] Spinning the paste into the canal by rotating a file counterclockwise and using an injection technique is not as effective. It is important to place the material deeply and densely for maximum effectiveness. To accomplish this, straight-line access should be performed, and the apical portion of the canal prepared to a No. 25 file or greater. Removal after placement is difficult,[190] and this is especially true in the apical portion of the root.

Phenols and Aldehydes

The majority of these medicaments exhibit nonspecific action and can destroy host tissues, as well as microbes.[191-193] Historically, it was thought that these agents were effective, although their use was based on opinion and empiricism. The phenols and aldehydes are toxic, and the aldehydes are fixative agents.[194,195] When placed in the radicular space, they have access to the periradicular tissues and the systemic circulation.[196,197] Research has demonstrated that their clinical use is not justified.[198-202] Clinical studies assessing the ability of these agents to prevent or control interappointment pain indicate that they are not effective.[203-206]

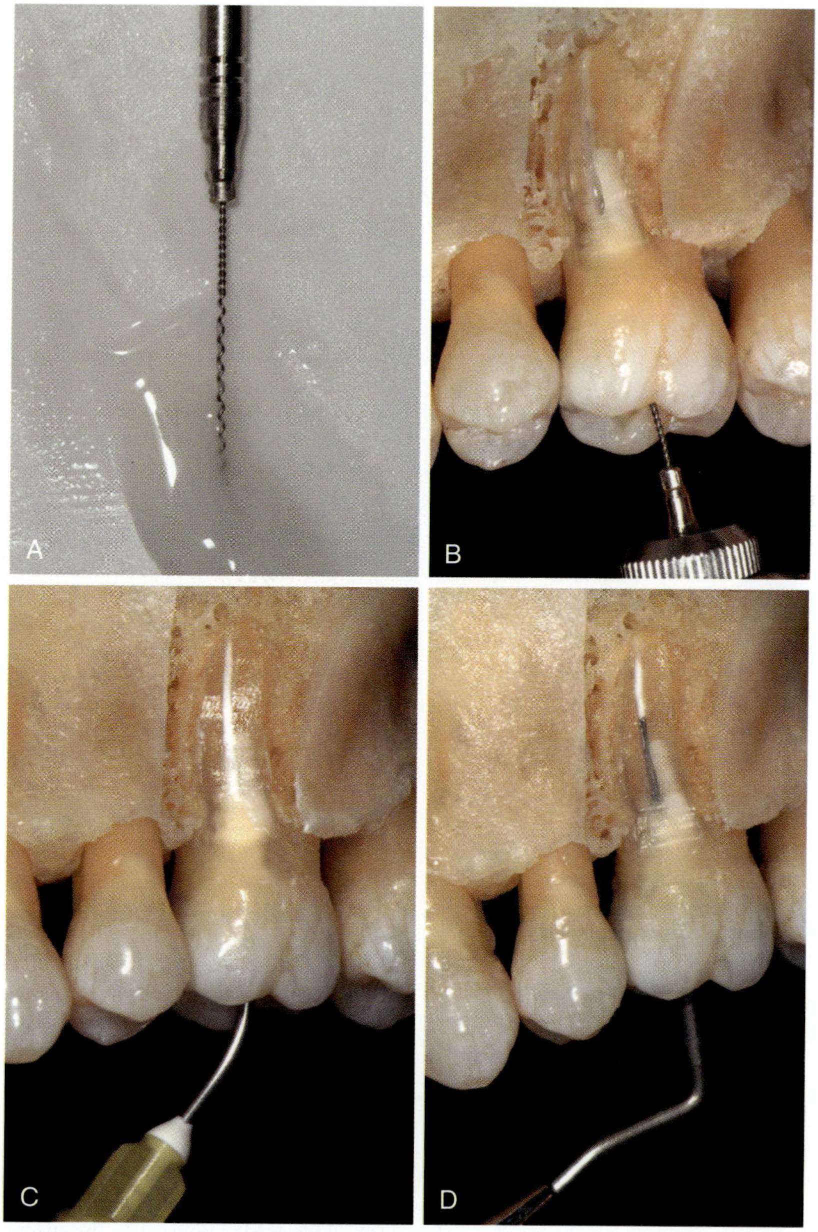

• **Fig. 14.29** Calcium hydroxide placement. **(A)** Calcium hydroxide mixed with glycerin to form a thick paste. **(B)** Placement with a lentulo spiral. **(C)** Injection of a proprietary paste. **(D)** Compaction of calcium hydroxide powder with a plugger.

Corticosteroids

Corticosteroids are antiinflammatory agents that have been advocated for decreasing postoperative pain by suppressing inflammation. The use of corticosteroids as intracanal medicaments may decrease lower-level postoperative pain in certain situations;[207] however, evidence also suggests that they may be ineffective, particularly with greater pain levels.[206] Cases of irreversible pulpitis and cases in which the patient is experiencing acute apical periodontitis are examples where steroid use might be beneficial.[207-209]

Chlorhexidine

Chlorhexidine has recently been advocated as an intracanal medicament.[210,211] A 2% gel is recommended, which can be used alone in gel form or mixed with calcium hydroxide. When used with calcium hydroxide, the antimicrobial activity is greater than when calcium hydroxide is mixed with saline,[212] and periradicular healing in animal models appears to be enhanced.[213] However, a recent randomized clinical trial did not show that the combination of calcium hydroxide and 2% chlorhexidine was advantageous compared with single appointment treatment in cases with periapical lesions, after 1 year of observation.[187]

Study Questions

6. Although removal of the smear layer is not universally advocated before root canal obturation, those advocating its removal cite the following rationale.
   a. Smear layer provides an improved seal of the canal during obturation
   b. The organic component of smear layer is antimicrobial
   c. Maintenance of the smear layer strengthens root structure
   d. Smear layer may contain bacterial contaminants
7. NaOCl is effective in removing the smear layer.
   a. True
   b. False
8. Which of the following irrigants may reduce postoperative pain?
   a. NaOCl
   b. EDTA
   c. Cold saline
   d. Chlorhexidine
9. Select the method that is most effective in maintaining canal patency.
   a. Radiographic root length determination
   b. Electronic root length determination
   c. Use of patency file
   d. Selection of correct reference point
10. Select the most commonly used intracanal medication placed when endodontic treatment is not completed.
    a. NaOCl
    b. Calcium hydroxide
    c. Phenolic products
    d. Chlorhexidine

ANSWERS

Answer Box 14

1 b. Use of hand instrumentations
2 b. False
3 d. All of the above
4 a. True
5 a. True
6 d. Smear layer may contain bacterial contaminants
7 b. False
8 c. Cold saline
9 c. Use of patency file
10 b. Calcium hydroxide

References

1. Ingle JI: *Endodontics*, ed 5, London ON, 2002, BC Decker.
2. Sabeti MA, Nekofar M, Motahhary P, et al.: Healing of apical periodontitis after endodontic treatment with and without obturation in dogs, *J Endod* 32(7):628, 2006.
3. Delivanis PD, Mattison GD, Mendel RW: The survivability of F43 strain of *Streptococcus sanguis* in root canals filled with gutta-percha and Procosol cement, *J Endod* 9(10):407, 1983.
4. Sedgley CM, Lennan SL, Applebe OK: Survival of *Enterococcus faecalis* in root canals ex vivo, *Int Endod J* 38(10):735, 2005.
5. Landys Boren D, Jonasson P, Kvist T: Long-term survival of endodontically treated teeth at a public dental specialist clinic, *J Endod* 41(2), 2015.
6. Salehrabi R, Rotstein I: Endodontic treatment outcomes in a large patient population in the USA: an epidemiological study, *J Endod* 30(12), 2004.
7. Ng YL, Mann V, Gulabivala K: A prospective study of the factors affecting outcomes of nonsurgical root canal treatment: part 1: periapical health, *Int Endod J* 44(7):583, 2011.
8. Allison DA, Weber CR, Walton RE: The influence of the method of canal preparation on the quality of apical and coronal obturation, *J Endod* 5(10):298, 1979.
9. Schilder H: Cleaning and shaping the root canal, *Dent Clin North Am* 18(2):269, 1974.
10. Wilcox LR, Roskelley C, Sutton T: The relationship of root canal enlargement to finger-spreader induced vertical root fracture, *J Endod* 23(8):533, 1997.
11. Kuttler Y: Microscopic investigation of root apexes, *J Am Dent Assoc* 50(5):544, 1955.
12. Dummer PMH, McGinn JH, Rees DG: The position and topography of the apical canal constriction and apical foramen, *Int Endod J* 17(4):192, 1984.
13. Gutierrez JH, Aguayo P: Apical foraminal openings in human teeth, *Oral Surg Oral Med Oral Pathol Oral Radiol Endod* 79(6):769, 1995.
14. Malueg LA, Wilcox LR, Johnson W: Examination of external apical root resorption with scanning electron microscopy, *Oral Surg Oral Med Oral Pathol Oral Radiol Endod* 82(1):89, 1996.
15. Farzaneh M, Abitbol S, Friedman S: Treatment outcome in endodontics: the Toronto study, Phases I and II: orthograde retreatment, *J Endod* 30(9):627, 2004.
16. de Chevigny C, Dao TT, Basrani BR, et al.: Treatment outcome in endodontics: the Toronto study—phase 4: initial treatment, *J Endod* 34(3):258, 2008.
17. Schaeffer MA, White RR, Walton RA: Determining the optimal obturation length: a meta-analysis of literature, *J Endod* 31(4):271, 2005.
18. Wu MK, Wesselink PR, Walton RE: Apical terminus location of root canal treatment procedures, *Oral Surg Oral Med Oral Pathol Oral Radiol Endod* 89(1):99, 2000.
19. Ricucci D, Russo J, Rutberg M, et al.: A prospective cohort study of endodontic treatments of 1,369 root canals: results after 5 years, *Oral Surg Oral Med Oral Pathol Oral Radiol Endod* 112(6):825, 2011.
20. Nair PN: On the causes of persistent apical periodontitis: a review, *Int Endod J* 39(4):249, 2006.
21. Siqueira Jr JF: Aetiology of root canal treatment failure: why well-treated teeth can fail, *Int Endod J* 34(1), 2001.
22. Friedman S: Management of post-treatment endodontic disease: a current concept of case selection, *Aust Endod J* 26(3), 2000.
23. Wu MK, Dummer PM, Wesselink PR: Consequences of and strategies to deal with residual post-treatment root canal infection, *Int Endod J* 39(5), 2006.
24. Eldeeb ME, Boraas JC: The effect of different files on the preparation shape of severely curved canals, *Int Endod J* 18(1):1, 1985.
25. Chow TW: Mechanical effectiveness of root canal irrigation, *J Endod* 9(11):475, 1983.
26. Ram Z: Effectiveness of root canal irrigation, *Oral Surg Oral Med Oral Pathol* 44(2):306, 1977.
27. Salzgeber RM, Brilliant JD: An in vivo evaluation of the penetration of an irrigating solution in root canals, *J Endod* 3(10):394, 1977.
28. Ørstavik D, Kerekes K, Molven O: Effects of extensive apical reaming and calcium hydroxide dressing on bacterial infection during treatment of apical periodontitis: a pilot study, *Int Endod J* 24(1):1, 1991.
29. Dalton BC, Ørstavik D, Phillips C, et al.: Bacterial reduction with nickel-titanium rotary instrumentation, *J Endod* 24(11):763, 1998.
30. Sjögren U, Figdor D, Spångberg L, Sundqvist G: The antimicrobial effect of calcium hydroxide as a short-term intracanal dressing, *Int Endod J* 24(3):119, 1991.
31. Wu YN, Shi JN, Huang LZ, Xu YY: Variables affecting electronic root canal measurement, *Int Endod J* 25(2):88, 1992.
32. Haapasalo M, Shen Y, Qian W, Gao Y: Irrigation in endodontics, *Dent Clin North Am* 54(2), 2010.

33. Sluis LW vd, Versluis M, Wesselink PR: Passive ultrasonic irrigation of the root canal: a review of the literature, *Int Endod J* 40(6):415, 2007.
34. Usman N, Baumgartner JC, Marshall JG: Influence of instrument size on root canal debridement, *J Endod* 30(2):110, 2004.
35. Rollison S, Barnett F, Stevens RH: Efficacy of bacterial removal from instrumented root canals in vitro related to instrumentation technique and size, *Oral Surg Oral Med Oral Pathol Oral Radiol Endod* 94(3):366, 2002.
36. Card SJ, Sigurdsson A, Ørstavik D, Trope M: The effectiveness of increased apical enlargement in reducing intracanal bacteria, *J Endod* 28(11):779, 2002.
37. Pettiette MT, Delano EO, Trope M: Evaluation of success rate of endodontic treatment performed by students with stainless-steel K-files and nickel-titanium hand files, *J Endod* 27(2):124, 2001.
38. Peters OA: Current challenges and concepts in the preparation of root canal systems: a review, *J Endod* 30, 2004.
39. Paqué F, Boessler C, Zehnder M: Accumulated hard tissue debris levels in mesial roots of mandibular molars after sequential irrigation steps, *Int Endod J* 44(2):148, 2011.
40. Love RM, Jenkinson HF: Invasion of dentinal tubules by oral bacteria, *Crit Rev Oral Biol Med* 13(2):171, 2002.
41. Akpata ES: Effect of endodontic procedures on the population of viable microorganisms in the infected root canal, *J Endod* 2(12):369, 1976.
42. Matsuo T, Shirakami T, Ozaki K, et al.: An immunohistological study of the localization of bacteria invading root pulpal walls of teeth with periapical lesions, *J Endod* 29(3):194, 2003.
43. Peters LB, Wesselink PR, Buijs JF, van Winkelhoff AJ: Viable bacteria in root dentinal tubules of teeth with apical periodontitis, *J Endod* 27(2):76, 2001.
44. Bird DC, Chambers D, Peters OA: Usage parameters of nickel-titanium rotary instruments: a survey of endodontists in the United States, *J Endod* 35(9):1193, 2009.
45. Parashos P, Messer HH: Uptake of rotary NiTi technology within Australia, *Aust Dent J* 50(4):251, 2005.
46. Bjørndal L, Reit C: The adoption of new endodontic technology amongst Danish general dental practitioners, *Int Endod J* 38(1):52, 2005.
47. Waltimo T, Trope M, Haapasalo M, Ørstavik D: Clinical efficacy of treatment procedures in endodontic infection control and one year follow-up of periapical healing, *J Endod* 31(12):863, 2005.
48. Shuping GB, Ørstavik D, Sigurdsson A, Trope M: Reduction of intracanal bacteria using nickel-titanium rotary instrumentation and various medications, *J Endod* 26(12):751, 2000.
49. Siqueira JF, Lima KC, Magalhaes FAC, et al.: Mechanical reduction of the bacterial population in the root canal by three instrumentation techniques, *J Endod* 25(5):332, 1999.
50. Siqueira Jr JF, Rocas IN, Santos SR, et al.: Efficacy of instrumentation techniques and irrigation regimens in reducing the bacterial population within root canals, *J Endod* 28(3):181, 2002.
51. de Gregorio C, Arias A, Navarrete N, et al.: Differences in disinfection protocols for root canal treatments between general dentists and endodontists: a Web-based survey, *J Am Dent Assoc* 146(7), 2015.
52. Tanomaru Filho M, Leonardo MR, da Silva LA: Effect of irrigating solution and calcium hydroxide root canal dressing on the repair of apical and periapical tissues of teeth with periapical lesion, *J Endod* 28(4):295, 2002.
53. Ørstavik D, Haapasalo M: Disinfection by endodontic irrigants and dressings of experimentally infected dentinal tubules, *Endod Dent Traumatol* 6(4):142, 1990.
54. Gernhardt CR, Eppendorf K, Kozlowski A, Brandt M: Toxicity of concentrated sodium hypochlorite used as an endodontic irrigant, *Int Endod J* 37(4):272, 2004.
55. Pashley EL, Birdsong NL, Bowman K, Pashley DH: Cytotoxic effects of NaOCl on vital tissue, *J Endod* 11(12):525, 1985.
56. Reeh ES, Messer HH: Long-term paresthesia following inadvertent forcing of sodium hypochlorite through perforation in maxillary incisor, *Endod Dent Traumatol* 5(4):200, 1989.
57. Witton R, Brennan PA: Severe tissue damage and neurological deficit following extravasation of sodium hypochlorite solution during routine endodontic treatment, *Br Dent J* 198(12):749, 2005.
58. Brown DC, Moore BK, Brown Jr CE, Newton CW: An in vitro study of apical extrusion of sodium hypochlorite during endodontic canal preparation, *J Endod* 21(12):587, 1995.
59. Hülsmann M, Hahn W: Complications during root canal irrigation-literature review and case reports, *Int Endod J* 33(3):186, 2000.
60. Yamada RS, Armas A, Goldman M, Lin PS: A scanning electron microscopic comparison of a high volume final flush with several irrigating solutions: part 3, *J Endod* 9(4):137, 1983.
61. Lambrianidis T, Tosounidou E, Tzoanopoulou M: The effect of maintaining apical patency on periapical extrusion, *J Endod* 27(11):696, 2001.
62. Holland R, Sant'Anna Junior A, Souza V, et al.: Influence of apical patency and filling material on healing process of dogs' teeth with vital pulp after root canal therapy, *Braz Dent J* 16(1), 2005.
63. Izu KH, Thomas SJ, Zhang P, et al.: Effectiveness of sodium hypochlorite in preventing inoculation of periapical tissue with contaminated patency files, *J Endod* 30(2):92, 2004.
64. Vera J, Arias A, Romero M: Dynamic movement of intracanal gas bubbles during cleaning and shaping procedures: the effect of maintaining apical patency on their presence in the middle and cervical thirds of human root canals-an in vivo study, *J Endod* 38(2):200, 2012.
65. Cailleteau JG, Mullaney TP: Prevalence of teaching apical patency and various instrumentation and obturation techniques in United States dental schools, *J Endod* 23(6), 1997.
66. Flanders DH: Endodontic patency. How to get it. How to keep it. Why it is so important, *N Y State Dent J* 68(3), 2002.
67. Buchanan LS: Management of the curved root canal, *J Calif Dent Assoc* 17(4), 1989.
68. Carr GB, Schwartz RS, Schaudinn C, et al.: Ultrastructural examination of failed molar retreatment with secondary apical periodontitis: an examination of endodontic biofilms in an endodontic retreatment failure, *J Endod* 35(9):1303, 2009.
69. Zhu WC, Gyamfi J, Niu LN, et al.: Anatomy of sodium hypochlorite accidents involving facial ecchymosis - a review, *J Dent* 41(11), 2013.
70. Yaylali IE, Demirci GK, Kurnaz S, et al.: Does maintaining apical patency during instrumentation increase postoperative pain or flare-up rate after non-surgical root canal treatment? A systematic review of randomized controlled trials, *J Endod* epub ahead of print, 2018.
71. AAE: *Endodontic case difficulty assessment form and guidelines*. In AAE, editor. Chicago, IL, 2010, American Association of Endodontics.
72. Peters OA, Paqué F: Current developments in rotary root canal instrument technology and clinical use: a review, *Quintessence Int* 41(6):479, 2010.
73. Walia H, Brantley WA, Gerstein H: An initial investigation of the bending and torsional properties of nitinol root canal files, *J Endod* 14(7):346, 1988.
74. Peters OA, Schönenberger K, Laib A: Effects of four NiTi preparation techniques on root canal geometry assessed by micro computed tomography, *Int Endod J* 34, 2001.
75. McSpadden JT, Bonaccorso A, Tocchio C, et al.: The zone technique, *ENDO (Lond Engl)* 2(1):33, 2008.
76. Clark D, Khademi JA: Case studies in modern molar endodontic access and directed dentin conservation, *Dent Clin North Am* 54(2), 2010.
77. Bonessio N, Arias A, Lomiento G, Peters OA: Effect of root canal treatment procedures with a novel rotary nickel titanium instrument (TRUShape) on stress in mandibular molars: a comparative finite element analysis, *Odontology* 105(1), 2017.

78. Peters OA: The guidebook to molar endodontics, 2016. Heidelberg, Germany, pp. 2016.
79. Pruett JP, Clement DJ, Carnes DL: Cyclic fatigue testing of nickel-titanium endodontic instruments, *J Endod* 23(2):77, 1997.
80. Zuolo ML, Walton RE: Instrument deterioration with usage: nickel-titanium versus stainless steel, *Quintessence Int* 28(6):397, 1997.
81. Torabinejad M, Handysides R, Khademi AA, Bakland LK: Clinical implications of the smear layer in endodontics: a review, *Oral Surg Oral Med Oral Pathol Oral Radiol Endod* 94(6):658, 2002.
82. McComb D, Smith DC: A preliminary scanning electron microscopic study of root canals after endodontic procedures, *J Endod* 1(7):238, 1975.
83. Sen BH, Piskin B, Baran N: The effect of tubular penetration of root canal sealers on dye microleakage, *Int Endod J* 29(1):23, 1996.
84. Chailertvanitkul P, Saunders WP, MacKenzie D: The effect of smear layer on microbial coronal leakage of gutta-percha root fillings, *Int Endod J* 29(4):242, 1996.
85. Clark-Holke D, Drake D, Walton R, et al.: Bacterial penetration through canals of endodontically treated teeth in the presence or absence of the smear layer, *J Dent* 31(4):275, 2003.
86. Oksan T, Aktener BO, Sen BH, Tezel H: The penetration of root canal sealers into dentinal tubules. A scanning electron microscopic study, *Int Endod J* 26(5):301, 1993.
87. Wennberg A, Ørstavik D: Adhesion of root canal sealers to bovine dentine and gutta-percha, *Int Endod J* 23(1):13, 1990.
88. Leonard JE, Gutmann JL, Guo IY: Apical and coronal seal of roots obturated with a dentine bonding agent and resin, *Int Endod J* 29(2):76, 1996.
89. Kokkas AB, Boutsioukis A, Vassiliades LP, Stavrianos CK: The influence of the smear layer on dentinal tubule penetration depth by three different root canal sealers: an in vitro study, *J Endod* 30(2):100, 2004.
90. Cobankara FK, Adanr N, Belli S: Evaluation of the influence of smear layer on the apical and coronal sealing ability of two sealers, *J Endod* 30(6):406, 2004.
91. Siqueira Jr JF, Araujo MC, Garcia PF, et al.: Histological evaluation of the effectiveness of five instrumentation techniques for cleaning the apical third of root canals, *J Endod* 23(8), 1997.
92. Wu MK, Wesselink PR: Efficacy of three techniques in cleaning the apical portion of curved root canals, *Oral Surg Oral Med Oral Pathol Oral Radiol Endod* 79(4):492, 1995.
93. Tan BT, Messer HH: The quality of apical canal preparation using hand and rotary instruments with specific criteria for enlargement based on initial apical file size, *J Endod* 28(9):658, 2002.
94. Rosenfeld EF, James GA, Burch BS: Vital pulp tissue response to sodium hypochlorite, *J Endod* 4(5):140, 1978.
95. Svec TA, Harrison JW: Chemomechanical removal of pulpal and dentinal debris with sodium hypochlorite and hydrogen peroxide vs normal saline solution, *J Endod* 3(2):49, 1977.
96. Peters OA, Boessler C, Zehnder M: Effect of liquid and paste-type lubricants on torque values during simulated rotary root canal instrumentation, *Int Endod J* 38(1):223, 2005.
97. Jungbluth H, Peters C, Peters OA, Zehnder M: Physicochemical and pulp tissue dissolution properties of some household bleach brands compared with a dental sodium hypochlorite solution, *J Endod* 38(3):372, 2012.
98. Zehnder M: Root canal irrigants, *J Endod* 32(5):389, 2006.
99. Zehnder M, Kosicki D, Luder H, et al.: Tissue-dissolving capacity and antibacterial effect of buffered and unbuffered hypochlorite solutions, *Oral Surg Oral Med Oral Pathol Oral Radiol Endod* 94(6), 2002.
100. Berutti E, Marini R: A scanning electron microscopic evaluation of the debridement capability of sodium hypochlorite at different temperatures, *J Endod* 22(9):467, 1996.
101. Gambarini G, De Luca M, Gerosa R: Chemical stability of heated sodium hypochlorite endodontic irrigants, *J Endod* 24(6):432, 1998.
102. Oncag O, Hosgor M, Hilmioglu S, et al.: Comparison of antibacterial and toxic effects of various root canal irrigants, *Int Endod J* 36(6):423, 2003.
103. Abou-Rass M, Piccinino MV: The effectiveness of four clinical irrigation methods on the removal of root canal debris, *Oral Surg Oral Med Oral Pathol* 54(3):323, 1982.
104. Ballal NV, Mala K, Bhat KS: Effect of maleic acid and ethylenediaminetetraacetic acid on the dissolution of human pulp tissue—an in vitro study, *Int Endod J* 44(4), 2011.
105. Hülsmann M, Heckendorff M, Lennon A: Chelating agents in root canal treatment: mode of action and indications for their use, *Int Endod J* 36(12):810, 2003.
106. Rossi-Fedele G, Dogramaci EJ, Guastalli AR, et al.: Antagonistic interactions between sodium hypochlorite, chlorhexidine, EDTA, and citric acid, *J Endod* 38(4), 2012.
107. Zehnder M, Schmidlin P, Sener B, Waltimo T: Chelation in root canal therapy reconsidered, *J Endod* 31(11), 2005.
108. Baumgartner JC, Mader CL: A scanning electron microscope evaluation of four root canal irrigation regimes, *J Endod* 13(4):147, 1987.
109. Mai S, Kim YK, Arola DD, et al.: Differential aggressiveness of ethylenediamine tetraacetic acid in causing canal wall erosion in the presence of sodium hypochlorite, *J Dent* 38(3):201, 2010.
110. Guignes P, Faure J, Maurette A: Relationship between endodontic preparations and human dentin permeability measured in situ, *J Endod* 22(2):60, 1996.
111. Hottel TL, El-Rafai NY, Jones JJ: A comparison of the effects of three chelating agents on the root canals of extracted human teeth, *J Endod* 25(11):716, 1999.
112. Lim TS, Wee TY, Choi MY, et al.: Light and scanning electron microscopic evaluation of Glyde File Prep in smear layer removal, *Int Endod J* 36(5):336, 2003.
113. Krell KV, Johnson RJ: Irrigation patterns of ultrasonic endodontic files. Part II. Diamond coated files, *J Endod* 14(2):535, 1988.
114. Mjør IA, Smith MR, Ferrari M, Mannocci F: The structure of dentine in the apical region of human teeth, *Int Endod J* 34(5):346, 2001.
115. Paqué F, Luder HU, Sener B, Zehnder M: Tubular sclerosis rather than the smear layer impedes dye penetration into the dentine of endodontically instrumented root canals, *Int Endod J* 39(1):18, 2006.
116. Scelza MF, Teixeira AM, Scelza P: Decalcifying effect of EDTA-T, 10% citric acid, and 17% EDTA on root canal dentin, *Oral Surg Oral Med Oral Pathol Oral Radiol Endod* 95(2):234, 2003.
117. Calt S, Serper A: Smear layer removal by EGTA, *J Endod* 26(8):459, 2000.
118. Haznedaroglu F: Efficacy of various concentrations of citric acid at different pH values for smear layer removal, *Oral Surg Oral Med Oral Pathol Oral Radiol Endod* 96(3):340, 2003.
119. Baumgartner JC, Brown CM, Mader CL, et al.: A scanning electron microscopic evaluation of root canal debridement using saline, sodium hypochlorite, and citric acid, *J Endod* 10(11):525, 1984.
120. Rosenthal S, Spångberg L, Safavi K: Chlorhexidine substantivity in root canal dentin, *Oral Surg Oral Med Oral Pathol Oral Radiol Endod* 98(4):488, 2004.
121. Jeansonne MJ, White RR: A comparison of 2.0% chlorhexidine gluconate and 5.25% sodium hypochlorite as antimicrobial endodontic irrigants, *J Endod* 20(6):276, 1994.
122. Kuruvilla JR, Kamath MP: Antimicrobial activity of 2.5% sodium hypochlorite and 0.2% chlorhexidine gluconate separately and combined, as endodontic irrigants, *J Endod* 24(7):472, 1998.
123. Vahdaty A, Pitt Ford TR, Wilson RF: Efficacy of chlorhexidine in disinfecting dentinal tubules in vitro, *Endod Dent Traumatol* 9(6):243, 1993.
124. White RR, Hays GL, Janer LR: Residual antimicrobial activity after canal irrigation with chlorhexidine, *J Endod* 23(4):229, 1997.
125. Basrani BR, Manek S, Sodhi RN, et al.: Interaction between sodium hypochlorite and chlorhexidine gluconate, *J Endod* 33(8), 2007.

126. Torabinejad M, Khademi AA, Babagoli J, et al.: A new solution for the removal of the smear layer, *J Endod* 29(3):170, 2003.
127. Torabinejad M, Cho Y, Khademi AA, et al.: The effect of various concentrations of sodium hypochlorite on the ability of MTAD to remove the smear layer, *J Endod* 29(4):233, 2003.
128. Shabahang S, Pouresmail M, Torabinejad M: In vitro antimicrobial efficacy of MTAD and sodium hypochlorite, *J Endod* 29(7):450, 2003.
129. Shabahang S, Torabinejad M: Effect of MTAD on *Enterococcus faecalis*-contaminated root canals of extracted human teeth, *J Endod* 29(9):576, 2003.
130. Zhang B, Alysandratos KD, Angelidou A, et al.: Human mast cell degranulation and preformed TNF secretion require mitochondrial translocation to exocytosis sites: relevance to atopic dermatitis, *J Allergy Clin Immunol* 127(6):1522, 2011.
131. Machnick TK, Torabinejad M, Munoz CA, Shabahang S: Effect of MTAD on the bond strength to enamel and dentin, *J Endod* 29(12):818, 2003.
132. Malkhassian G, Manzur AJ, Legner M, et al.: Antibacterial efficacy of MTAD final rinse and two percent chlorhexidine gel medication in teeth with apical periodontitis: a randomized double-blinded clinical trial, *J Endod* 35(11):1483, 2009.
133. Stojic S, Shen Y, Qian W, et al.: Antibacterial and smear layer removal ability of a novel irrigant, QMiX, *J Endod* 45(4), 2012.
134. Dai L, Khechen K, Khan S, et al.: The effect of QMix, an experimental antibacterial root canal irrigant, on removal of canal wall smear layer and debris, *J Endod* 37(1):80, 2011.
135. Wang Z, Shen Y, Haapasalo M: Effectiveness of endodontic disinfecting solutions against young and old *Enterococcus faecalis* biofilms in dentin canals, *J Endod* 38(10):1376, 2012.
136. Morgental RD, Singh A, Sappal H, et al.: Dentin inhibits the antibacterial effect of new and conventional endodontic irrigants, *J Endod* 39 (in press), 2013.
137. Ordinola-Zapata R, Bramante CM, Brandao Garcia R, et al.: The antimicrobial effect of new and conventional endodontic irrigants on intra-orally infected dentin, *Acta Odont Scand epub ahead of print*, 2012.
138. Vera J, Ochoa J, Romero M, et al.: Intracanal cryotherapy reduces postoperative pain in teeth with symptomatic apical periodontitis: a randomized multicenter clinical trial, *J Endod* 44(1), 2018.
139. Gundogdu EC, Arslan H: Effects of various cryotherapy applications on postoperative pain in molar teeth with symptomatic apical periodontitis: a preliminary randomized prospective clinical trial, *J Endod* 44(3), 2018.
140. Plotino G, Pameijer CH, Grande NM, Somma F: Ultrasonics in endodontics: a review of the literature, *J Endod* 33(2), 2007.
141. Cymerman JJ, Jerome LA, Moodnik RM: A scanning electron microscope study comparing the efficacy of hand instrumentation with ultrasonic instrumentation of the root canal, *J Endod* 9(8):327, 1983.
142. Schulz-Bongert U, Weine FS, Schulz-Bongert J: Preparation of curved canals using a combined hand-filing, ultrasonic technique, *Comp Cont Educ Dent* 16(3):270, 1995.
143. Chenail BL, Teplitsky PE: Endosonics in curved root canals. Part II, *J Endod* 14(5):214, 1988.
144. Gutarts R, Nusstein J, Reader A, Beck M: In vivo debridement efficacy of ultrasonic irrigation following hand-rotary instrumentation in human mandibular molars, *J Endod* 31(3), 2005.
145. Cheung GS, Stock CJ: In vitro cleaning ability of root canal irrigants with and without endosonics, *Int Endod J* 26(6), 1993.
146. Nielsen BA, Craig Baumgartner J: Comparison of the EndoVac system to needle irrigation of root canals, *J Endod* 33(5), 2007.
147. Ahmad M, Pitt Ford TJ, Crum LA: Ultrasonic debridement of root canals: acoustic streaming and its possible role, *J Endod* 13(10):490, 1987.
148. Cameron JA: The use of ultrasonics in the removal of the smear layer: a scanning electron microscope study, *J Endod* 9(7):289, 1983.
149. Archer R, Reader A, Nist R, et al.: An in vivo evaluation of the efficacy of ultrasound after step-back preparation in mandibular molars, *J Endod* 18(11):549, 1992.
150. Weller RN, Brady JM, Bernier WE: Efficacy of ultrasonic cleaning, *J Endod* 6(9):740, 1980.
151. Buchanan LS: The standardized-taper root canal preparation—part 6. GT file technique in abruptly curved canals, *Int Endod J* 34(3), 2001.
152. Steinberg D, Abid-el-Raziq D, Heling I: In vitro antibacterial effect of RC-Prep components on *Streptococcus sobrinus*, *Endod Dent Traumatol* 15(4):171, 1999.
153. Zehnder M, Schmidlin PR, Sener B, Waltimo TM: Chelation in root canal therapy reconsidered, *J Endod* 31(11):817, 2005.
154. Cehreli ZC, Onur MA, Tasman F, et al.: Effects of current and potential dental etchants on nerve compound action potentials, *J Endod* 28(3):149, 2002.
155. Goldberg F, Abramovich A: Analysis of the effect of EDTAC on the dentinal walls of the root canal, *J Endod* 3(3):101, 1977.
156. Powell SE, Wong PD, Simon JH: A comparison of the effect of modified and nonmodified instrument tips on apical canal configuration. Part II, *J Endod* 14(5):224, 1988.
157. Parashos P, Messer HH: Rotary NiTi instrument fracture and its consequences, *J Endod* 32(11):1031, 2006.
158. Degerness RA, Bowles WR: Dimension, anatomy and morphology of the mesiobuccal root canal system in maxillary molars, *J Endod* 36(6):985, 2010.
159. Sjögren U, Hagglund B, Sundqvist G, Wing K: Factors affecting the long-term results of endodontic treatment, *J Endod* 16(10):498, 1990.
160. Wu MK, Sluis LW vd, Wesselink PR: The capability of two hand instrumentation techniques to remove the inner layer of dentine in oval canals, *Int Endod J* 36(3):218, 2003.
161. Paqué F, Balmer M, Attin T, Peters OA: Preparation of oval-shaped root canals in mandibular molars using nickel-titanium rotary instruments: a micro-computed tomography study, *J Endod* 36(4):703, 2010.
162. Ingle JI: A standardized endodontic technique using newly development instruments and filling materials, *Oral Surg Oral Med Oral Pathol* 14(1):83, 1961.
163. Weine FS, Kelly RF, Lio PJ: The effect of preparation procedures on original canal shape and on apical foramen shape, *J Endod* 1(8):255–262, 1975.
164. Walton RE: Histologic evaluation of different methods of enlarging the pulp canal space, *J Endod* 2(10):304, 1976.
165. Morgan LF, Montgomery S: An evaluation of the crown-down pressureless technique, *J Endod* 10(10):491, 1984.
166. Torabinejad M: Passive step-back technique, *Oral Surg Oral Med Oral Pathol* 77(4):398, 1994.
167. Roane JB, Sabala CL, Duncanson Jr MG: The "balanced force" concept for instrumentation of curved canals, *J Endod* 11(5):203, 1985.
168. AAE: *AAE: Rotary instrumentation: an endodontic perspective*, Chicago, IL, 2008, American Association of Endodontics.
169. Bardsley S, Peters CI, Peters OA: The effect of three rotational speed settings on torque and apical force with vortex rotary instruments in vitro, *J Endod* 37(6):860, 2011.
170. Patino PV, Biedma BM, Liebana CR, et al.: The influence of a manual glide path on the separation rate of NiTi rotary instruments, *J Endod* 31(2):114, 2005.
171. Stabholz A, Rotstein I, Torabinejad M: Effect of preflaring on tactile detection of the apical constriction, *J Endod* 21(2):92, 1995.
172. Pecora JD, Capelli A, Guersoli A, et al.: Influence of cervical preflaring on apical file size determination, *Int Endod J* 38(7):430, 2005.
173. Schrader C, Peters OA: Analysis of torque and force with differently tapered rotary endodontic instruments in vitro, *J Endod* 31(2):120, 2005.
174. Paqué F, Zehnder M, Marending M: Apical fit of initial K-files in maxillary molars assessed by micro-computed tomography, *Int Endod J* 43(4):328, 2010.

175. Saini HR, Tewari S, Sangwan P, et al.: Effect of different apical preparation sizes on outcome of primary endodontic treatment: a randomized controlled trial, *J Endod* 38(10):1309, 2012.
176. Arias A, Paque F, Shyn S, et al.: Effect of canal preparation with TRUShape and Vortex rotary instruments on three-dimensional geometry of oval root canals, *Aust Endod J* 44(1), 2018.
177. Peters OA, Arias A, Paque F: A micro-computed tomographic assessment of root canal preparation with a novel instrument, TRUShape, in mesial roots of mandibular molars, *J Endod* 41(9), 2015.
178. Ferreira Murgel CA, Walton RE, Rittman B, Pecora JD: A comparison of techniques for cleaning endodontic files after usage: a quantitative scanning electron microscopic study, *J Endod* 16(5):214, 1990.
179. Sathorn C, Parashos P, Messer HH: Effectiveness of single- versus multiple-visit endodontic treatment of teeth with apical periodontitis: a systematic review and meta-analysis, *Int Endod J* 38(6):347, 2005.
180. Nair PN, Henry S, Cano V, Vera J: Microbial status of apical root canal system of human mandibular first molars with primary apical periodontitis after "one-visit" endodontic treatment, *Oral Surg Oral Med Oral Pathol Oral Radiol Endod* 99(2), 2005.
181. Vera J, Siqueira JF, Ricucci D, et al.: One- versus two-visit endodontic treatment of teeth with apical periodontitis: a histobacteriologic study, *J Endod* 38(8):1040, 2012.
182. Law A, Messer H: An evidence-based analysis of the antibacterial effectiveness of intracanal medicaments, *J Endod* 30(10):689, 2004.
183. Yang SF, Rivera EM, Baumgardner KR, et al.: Anaerobic tissue-dissolving abilities of calcium hydroxide and sodium hypochlorite, *J Endod* 21(12):613, 1995.
184. Safavi KE, Nichols FC: Effect of calcium hydroxide on bacterial lipopolysaccharide, *J Endod* 19(2):76, 1993.
185. Safavi KE, Nichols FC: Alteration of biological properties of bacterial lipopolysaccharide by calcium hydroxide treatment, *J Endod* 20(3):127, 1994.
186. Walton RE, Holton IFJ, Michelich R: Calcium hydroxide as an intracanal medication: effect on posttreatment pain, *J Endod* 29(10):627, 2003.
187. Rivera EM, Williams K: Placement of calcium hydroxide in simulated canals: comparison of glycerin versus water, *J Endod* 20(9):445, 1994.
188. Sigurdsson A, Stancill R, Madison S: Intracanal placement of $Ca(OH)_2$: a comparison of techniques, *J Endod* 18(8):367, 1992.
189. Torres CP, Apicella MJ, Yancich PP, Parker MH: Intracanal placement of calcium hydroxide: a comparison of techniques, revisited, *J Endod* 30(4):225, 2004.
190. Lambrianidis T, Kosti E, Boutsioukis C, Mazinis M: Removal efficacy of various calcium hydroxide/chlorhexidine medicaments from the root canal, *Int Endod J* 39(1):55, 2006.
191. Chang YC, Tai KW, Chou LS, Chou MY: Effects of camphorated parachlorophenol on human periodontal ligament cells in vitro, *J Endod* 25(12):779, 1999.
192. Spångberg L: Cellular reaction to intracanal medicaments, *Trans Int Conf Endod* 5(0):108, 1973.
193. Spångberg L, Rutberg M, Rydinge E: Biologic effects of endodontic antimicrobial agents, *J Endod* 5(6):166, 1979.
194. Harrison JW, Bellizzi R, Osetek EM: The clinical toxicity of endodontic medicaments, *J Endod* 5(2):42, 1979.
195. Thoden van Velzen SK, Feltkamp-Vroom TM: Immunologic consequences of formaldehyde fixation of autologous tissue implants, *J Endod* 3(5):179, 1977.
196. Walton RE, Langeland K: Migration of materials in the dental pulp of monkeys, *J Endod* 4(6):167, 1978.
197. Myers DR, Shoaf HK, Dirksen TR, et al.: Distribution of 14C-formaldehyde after pulpotomy with formocresol, *J Am Dent Assoc* 96(5):805, 1978.
198. Doran MG, Radtke PK: A review of endodontic medicaments, *Gen Dent* 46(5):484, 1998.
199. Harrison JW, Baumgartner JC, Svec TA: Incidence of pain associated with clinical factors during and after root canal therapy. Part 1. Interappointment pain, *J Endod* 9(9):384, 1983.
200. Byström A, Claesson R, Sundqvist G: The antibacterial effect of camphorated paramonochlorophenol, camphorated phenol and calcium hydroxide in the treatment of infected root canals, *Endod Dent Traumatol* 1(5):170, 1985.
201. Walton RE: Intracanal medicaments, *Dent Clin North Am* 28(4):783, 1984.
202. Harrison JW, Baumgartner CJ, Zielke DR: Analysis of interappointment pain associated with the combined use of endodontic irrigants and medicaments, *J Endod* 7(6):272, 1981.
203. Maddox DL, Walton RE, Davis CO: Incidence of post-treatment endodontic pain related to medicaments and other factors, *J Endod* 3(12):447, 1977.
204. Kleier DJ, Mullaney TP: Effects of formocresol on posttreatment pain of endodontic origin in vital molars, *J Endod* 6(5):566, 1980.
205. Torabinejad M, Kettering JD, McGraw JC, et al.: Factors associated with endodontic interappointment emergencies of teeth with necrotic pulps, *J Endod* 14(5):261, 1988.
206. Trope M: Relationship of intracanal medicaments to endodontic flare-ups, *Endod Dent Traumatol* 6(5):226, 1990.
207. Ehrmann EH, Messer HH, Adams GG: The relationship of intracanal medicaments to postoperative pain in endodontics, *Int Endod J* 36(12):868, 2003.
208. Chance K, Lin L, Shovlin FE, Skribner J: Clinical trial of intracanal corticosteroid in root canal therapy, *J Endod* 13(9):466, 1987.
209. Chance KB, Lin L, Skribner JE: Corticosteroid use in acute apical periodontitis: a review with clinical implications, *Clin Prev Dent* 10(1):7, 1988.
210. Dametto FR, Ferraz CCR, Paula B, et al.: In vitro assessment of the immediate and prolonged antimicrobial action of chlorhexidine gel as an endodontic irrigant against Enterococcus faecalis, *Oral Surg Oral Med Oral Pathol Oral Radiol Endod* 99(6):768, 2005.
211. Dammaschke T, Schneider U, Stratmann U, et al.: Effect of root canal dressings on the regeneration of inflamed periapical tissue, *Acta Odont Scand* 63(3):143, 2005.
212. Gomes BPFD, Vianna ME, Sena NT, et al.: In vitro evaluation of the antimicrobial activity of calcium hydroxide combined with chlorhexidine gel used as intracanal medicament, *Oral Surg Oral Med Oral Pathol Oral Radiol Endod* 102(4):544, 2006.
213. De Rossi A, Silva LAB, Leonardo MR, et al.: Effect of rotary or manual instrumentation, with or without a calcium hydroxide/1% chlorhexidine intracanal dressing, on the healing of experimentally induced chronic periapical lesions, *Oral Surg Oral Med Oral Pathol Oral Radiol Endod* 99(5):628, 2005.

15

Obturation and Temporization

NATASHA M. FLAKE AND JAMES D. JOHNSON

CHAPTER OUTLINE

LEARNING OBJECTIVES

After reading this chapter, the student will be able to:

1. Explain the objectives of root canal obturation.
2. Explain the rationale for single-visit versus multi-visit endodontic treatment and identify cases when each approach would be indicated.
3. Explain the rationale for smear layer removal.
4. List the ideal properties of an obturation material.
5. Identify obturation materials that have been used historically and explain why these materials are no longer used.
6. Describe the properties, advantages, and disadvantages of gutta-percha.
7. List the ideal properties of a root canal sealer.
8. Identify types of sealers available on the market and describe their properties.
9. Explain how to perform different obturation techniques using gutta-percha as an obturation material.
10. Explain the advantages and disadvantages of different obturation techniques used with gutta-percha.
11. Describe how obturation materials and techniques are evaluated through research studies.
12. Describe how the results of obturation are clinically evaluated and the impact of obturation on treatment outcomes.
13. Explain the rationale for intraorifice barriers and identify materials used as barriers.
14. Explain the importance of restoration following endodontic treatment and list materials used for temporization.

Objectives of Obturation

Success in endodontic therapy is dependent on adequate instrumentation, disinfection, and obturation of the root canal system. The objective of obturation is to create a watertight seal along the length of the root canal system from the orifice to the apical termination. Obturation prevents leakage of microorganisms and their byproducts into the root canal system from a coronal direction and leakage of periapical tissue fluids into the root canal system from an apical direction. This seal allows for prevention and healing of apical periodontitis (Question 15.1). After adequate obturation, an adequate coronal restoration is also necessary and significantly affects the healing of apical periodontitis and the success of root canal therapy.[1]

Interestingly, a periapical lesion may heal at least temporarily after root canal débridement without obturation.[2] Research has shown that when bacteria are eliminated from the root canal system before obturation, healing of a periapical lesion occurs regardless of the quality of obturation.[3] However, if bacteria remain before obturation, healing is related to the quality of obturation.[3] Although failure to obturate or poor obturation are not desirable treatment options, these results demonstrate the important concept that what is removed from the root canal system is more important than how it is filled.

When to Obturate

One versus Two Visits

The endodontic community has long debated the number of visits in which root canal therapy should be completed. Should a tooth be obturated during the same visit when it is instrumented? Factors influencing the answer to this question include the pulpal and periapical diagnoses, the radiographic presentation, the patient's signs and symptoms, the degree of difficulty, patient management issues, and logistic concerns. In some cases, the degree of difficulty of the case dictates that the treatment be completed in more than one visit, for example, very calcified cases when additional time is needed to locate and instrument canals. Patient management or medical issues may also dictate that treatment be completed in more than one visit, for example, a patient who cannot recline for an extended period of time. Finally, logistic issues may dictate that treatment be completed in more than one visit, for example, a patient presents on an emergency basis, and the dentist has limited time in their schedule to treat the patient.

Opinions vary regarding the advantages and disadvantages of single- versus multiple-visit endodontic treatment when it comes to pulpal and periapical diagnoses, radiographic presentation, and patient signs and symptoms. Consensus exists that a tooth with a vital pulp may have root canal therapy completed in one visit (if time permits), because the canals are not infected. Cases with a vital pulp include those with a pulpal diagnosis of symptomatic irreversible pulpitis, asymptomatic irreversible pulpitis, reversible pulpitis, or a normal pulp. When root canal therapy is performed using proper infection control and disinfection protocols, completing treatment in one visit further precludes the possibility of recontamination of the root canal system caused by coronal leakage between visits. Consensus also generally exists that root canal therapy should not be completed in one visit when the patient has swelling associated with an acute apical abscess, or when the canal cannot be dried as a result of exudate draining from the periapical tissues. In these cases, the clinician should wait until the swelling has resolved and the canal can be dried completely before obturation.

There is disagreement on whether teeth with a necrotic pulp and asymptomatic apical periodontitis, symptomatic apical periodontitis, or a chronic apical abscess should be treated with single- or multiple-visit root canal therapy. The debate centers on the importance of disinfection of the root canal system. The rationale for completing treatment in two visits is that the intracanal medicament placed between visits facilitates disinfection of the root canal system (Question 15.2). This approach is supported by evidence from clinical studies looking at microbial sampling of the root canal system. In a study investigating the role of infection at the time of obturation in teeth that were treated in one visit, teeth were sampled for bacteria before obturation, and all teeth were treated in one visit.[4] After 5 years, complete healing occurred in 94% of cases with a negative culture and in 68% of cases with a positive culture before obturation. These results highlight the importance of completely eliminating bacteria from the root canal system before obturation, which may be aided by an intracanal medicament between visits.

Despite the microbiologic rationale for completing root canal therapy of necrotic teeth in multiple visits using an intracanal medicament, the available outcomes studies do not support an improved prognosis with two-visit treatment. Multiple systematic reviews have found no significant difference in radiologic success of root canal therapy between single- and multiple-visit treatment.[5,6] However, there is some evidence that patients having single-visit root canal therapy may be more likely to experience pain or flare-up and use analgesics in the short-term after treatment.[5,6] Unfortunately, the overall quality of the evidence is poor, because many studies have limitations including low power and risk of bias.[5-7] Thus the debate is ongoing, and the decision to treat in one visit or two is ultimately at the discretion of the clinician for each individual case.

Smear Layer Removal

The smear layer is a combination of organic and inorganic debris present on the root canal walls after instrumentation. When viewed under scanning electron microscope, the smear layer has an amorphous, irregular appearance that represents dentinal shavings, tissue debris, odontoblastic processes, and bacteria and their byproducts.[8] Historically, whether or not to remove the smear layer has been debated; though there is now generalized agreement that the smear layer should be removed before obturation. This is because the smear layer may contain microbes and their byproducts, which would remain in the canal if not removed, and because the smear layer may inhibit adhesion of filling materials to the dentin walls and penetration into dentinal tubules, thereby compromising the seal (Question 15.3). The smear layer is typically removed by irrigation with ethylenediaminetetraacetic acid, which serves as a chelating agent. Proprietary formulations may also be used (e.g., MTAD, SmearClear, QMix).[9]

Obturation Materials

Ideal Properties of an Obturation Material

Grossman suggested the ideal properties of an obturation material[10] (Box 15.1). Currently, no material or combination of materials satisfies all of these criteria.

Core Obturating Materials

Core obturating materials are the primary materials used in obturation and occupy the bulk of the space within the root canal system. Core obturating materials are classified as either solid or semisolid. Solid materials are introduced into the canal as a solid, and they require a sealer to completely seal the canal. Semisolid materials are introduced into the canal in a liquid, paste, or softened form, and then set up within the canal.

Gutta-Percha

Gutta-percha has been used as a root canal filling material for over 160 years.[11,12] It is by far the most popular core obturation material.

Composition

Commercial gutta-percha contains the following ingredients: zinc oxide 59% to 76%, gutta-percha 18% to 22%, waxes and resins 1% to 4%, and metal sulfates 1% to 18%.[13] The gutta-percha is the matrix, and the zinc oxide is the filler. The waxes and resins are the plasticizers, and the metal sulfates, such as barium sulfate, provide the necessary radiopacity.

The stereochemical structure of gutta-percha is 1,4 *trans* polyisoprene, whereas the stereochemical structure of natural rubber is 1,4 *cis* polyisoprene.[14,15] Even though gutta-percha and natural rubber have similar stereochemical structures, studies have shown that there is no cross-reactivity of gutta-percha and natural rubber latex in individuals who have a latex allergy.[16,17]

• BOX 15.1 Desirable Properties of Obturating Materials

Grossman suggested that the ideal obturation material would have the following properties:

- Be easily introduced into the canal
- Seal the canal laterally and apically
- Not shrink after insertion
- Be impervious to moisture
- Be bactericidal, or at least not promote bacterial growth
- Be radiopaque
- Not stain tooth structure
- Not irritate periapical tissues or affect tooth structure
- Be sterile or easily sterilized
- Be easily removed from the root canal

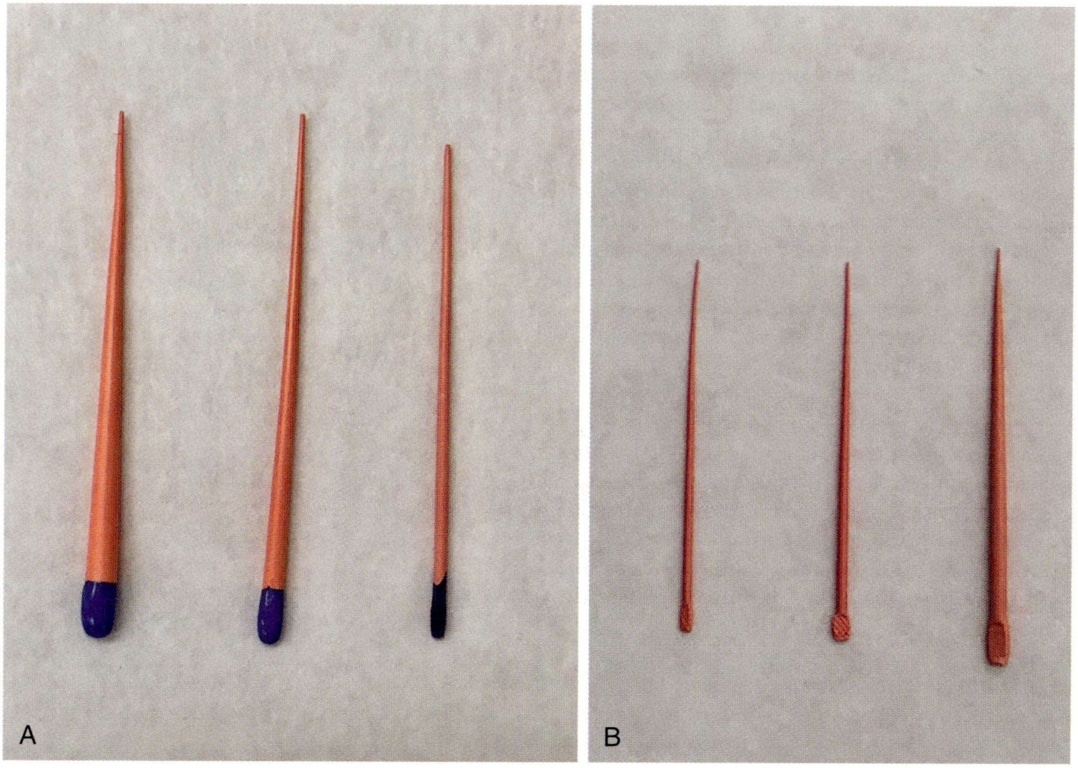

• **Fig. 15.1** Gutta-percha cones are available in a variety of tip sizes and tapers. **(A)** International Organization for Standardization size 30 tip size gutta-percha cones of tapers of 0.02, 0.04, and 0.06. **(B)** Nonstandardized gutta-percha cones with feathered tips.

Gutta-percha has two crystalline forms, alpha and beta.[14,18] Depending on the temperature, gutta-percha can be in different crystalline forms and exhibit different physical characteristics. Commercial gutta-percha comes in the beta crystalline form at room temperature. When the beta form is heated to 42°C to 49°C, it transitions into the alpha phase. When alpha phase gutta-percha is heated above 53°C to 59°C, it transitions into the amorphous phase. This is important when the clinician needs the amorphous form of gutta-percha to flow into all parts of the root canal system utilizing thermoplastic techniques.[19-22]

Shapes

Gutta-percha is formed into either standard or nonstandard cones of different tip sizes and tapers (Fig. 15.1). Standardized cones conform to the requirements of the International Organization for Standardization (ISO) or the American Dental Association/American National Standards Institute (ADA/ANSI). Nonstandardized (conventional) gutta-percha cones do not conform to the standards set by ISO or ADA/ANSI. Standardized gutta-percha cones are manufactured to have the same tip size and taper as the corresponding endodontic instruments used in the preparation of the root canal system. The original specifications called for gutta-percha to have a taper of .02 mm per millimeter increase in length. With the advent of various tapers in endodontic files, gutta-percha cones now come in various tapers, including .04, .06, and so on. Nonstandardized gutta-percha cones end in a feathered tip. Gutta-percha used with thermoplasticizing devices is manufactured as pellets or contained in cartridges (Fig. 15.2). The pellets or cartridges are inserted into a thermoplasticized gutta-percha injection system, and the gutta-percha is heated before dispensing.

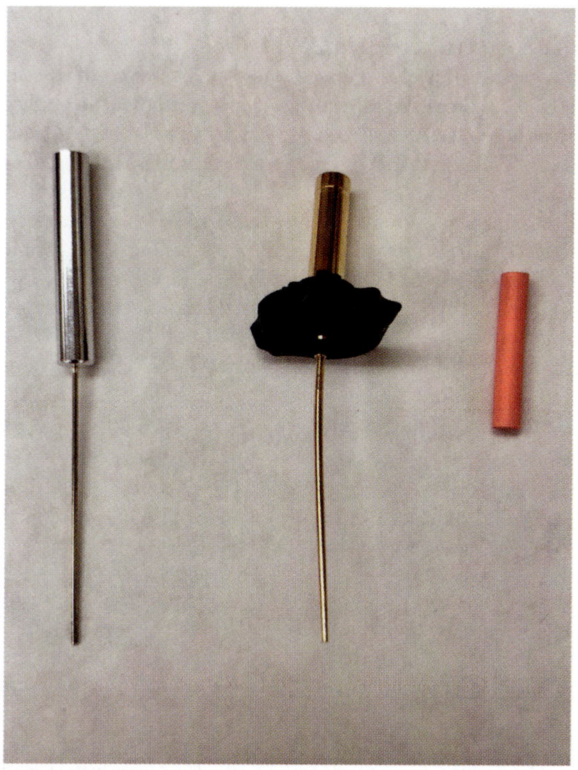

• **Fig. 15.2** Gutta-percha for use in thermoplasticized injection systems is manufactured in cartridges and pellets that fit into their corresponding injection systems.

Advantages

Gutta-percha is by far the most popular and widely accepted root canal filling material. Although it does not meet all of the criteria for an ideal filling material, it satisfies most of them. Gutta-percha has a number of advantages. First, because of its plasticity, gutta-percha adapts well when compacted into prepared root canals, especially when thermoplasticized. Second, gutta-percha has good handling characteristics and is easy to manipulate with multiple obturation techniques. It is relatively stiff and easily placed into canals. Third, gutta-percha is relatively easy to remove from the root canal system, either to create post space or for retreatment. Fourth, gutta-percha is regarded as a very acceptable material with good biocompatibility with the periapical tissues (Question 15.4).

Sealability

To produce an adequate seal, gutta-percha must be used with a sealer.[10] Gutta-percha does not adhere to canal walls, so the space between the gutta-percha and the canal wall must be sealed with a root canal sealer. Additionally, the application of heat or solvents to gutta-percha during different obturation techniques can cause gutta-percha to shrink, further increasing the space between the canal wall and gutta-percha core.

Other Additives to Gutta-Percha

Other ingredients have been added to some brands of gutta-percha to increase its antibacterial properties. Calcium hydroxide has been added to gutta-percha points by Coltene/Whaledent (Langenau, Germany). Activ Point (Coltene/Whaledent, Langenau, Germany) contains chlorhexidine. Other gutta-percha has been introduced that contains iodine-polyvinylpyrrolidone. Although these additives to gutta-percha have been shown to be effective against various bacteria,[23-27] long term clinical studies have not been conducted.

Carrier-Based Gutta-Percha

Several brands of carrier-based gutta-percha are on the market (Fig. 15.3). Carrier-based obturators are composed of gutta-percha surrounding a carrier that is heated and then placed into the canal. The handle of the carrier is cut off and removed, leaving the gutta-percha and carrier in the canal. Many obturators are designed to fit corresponding file systems. Several carrier-based obturators are marketed by Dentsply Sirona (York, PA), including GuttaCore, GuttaCore for WaveOne Gold, WaveOne Gold Obturators, ProTaper Next Obturators, ProTaper Universal Obturators, Thermafil Plus Obturators, Vortex Obturators, GT Obturators, and GT Series X Obturators. Soft-Core is a similar carrier-based obturator marketed by Kerr Endodontics (Orange, CA). SimpliFill (Kerr Endodontics) is a 5-mm apical plug of gutta-percha on the end of a metal carrier. It has the advantage of not leaving the carrier in the canal, as the carrier is twisted off and removed, leaving only the apical plug of gutta-percha. SuccessFil is a carrier-based gutta-percha system that is combined with the UltraFil thermoplasticizied injection system to create what is marketed as the Trifecta System (Coltene/Whaledent, Langenau, Germany). JS Quick-Fill (JS Dental Manufacturing, Inc, Ridgefield, CT) is an alpha phase gutta-percha coated titanium core in ISO sizes 15 to 60. The carrier-based material is spun into the canal at low speed, and the core may be left in the canal or slowly removed.

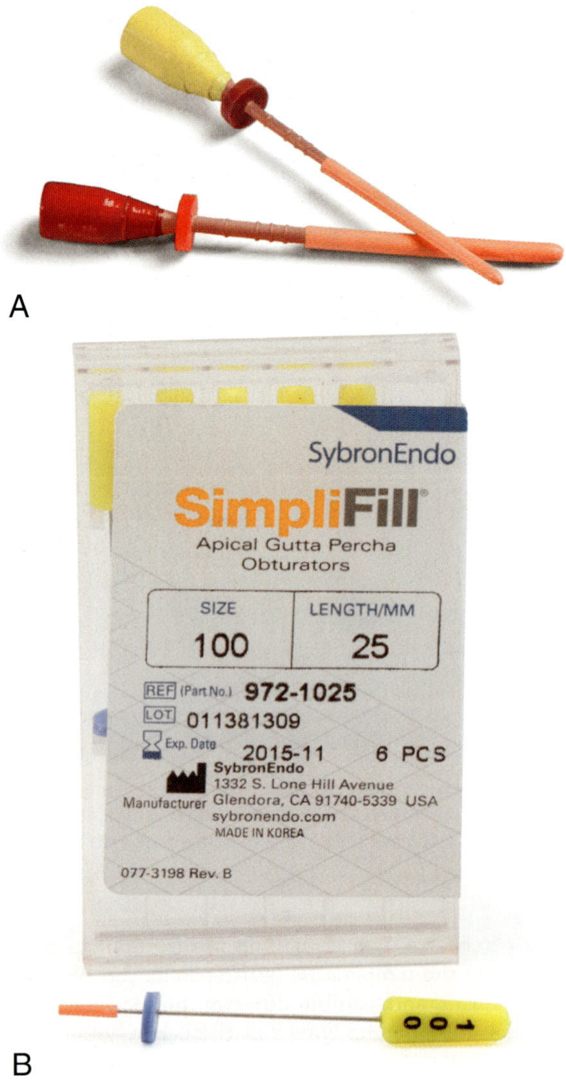

• **Fig. 15.3** Most obturators consist of a carrier core surrounded by gutta-percha. The obturator is warmed and inserted into the canal. **(A)** GuttaCore obturators. (Courtesy Dentsply Sirona.) **(B)** SimpliFill is a type of carrier-based obturator that is not heated. The metal carrier is twisted off, leaving only an apical plug of gutta-percha. SimpliFill is available in large apical sizes. (Courtesy Kerr Endodontics.)

Mineral Trioxide Aggregate

Mineral trioxide aggregate (MTA) is a bioactive calcium silicate material that has many clinical applications in endodontics, including vital pulp therapy, perforation repairs, and root end surgery.[28,29] MTA is used as an obturation material in cases of immature or open apices[29] (Fig. 15.4). Attributes of MTA include biocompatibility, sealability, and a history of documented positive clinical outcomes. Similar to MTA, some of the more recently introduced bioceramic materials can also be used as obturation materials in this fashion. Teeth with open apices where obturation with MTA or other bioceramic material would be indicated are considered moderate or high level of difficulty cases, and referral to a specialist is typically recommended.[30,31]

Silver Points

Silver points were used historically in the mid-1900s and were manufactured to match the size and taper of endodontic hand files used in canal preparation at that time (Fig. 15.5). Thus silver points had a 0.02 taper. Silver points fulfilled some of Grossman's requirements of an ideal obturation material. They were easy to insert and had good length control. However, they did not seal well laterally or apically as a result of their lack of

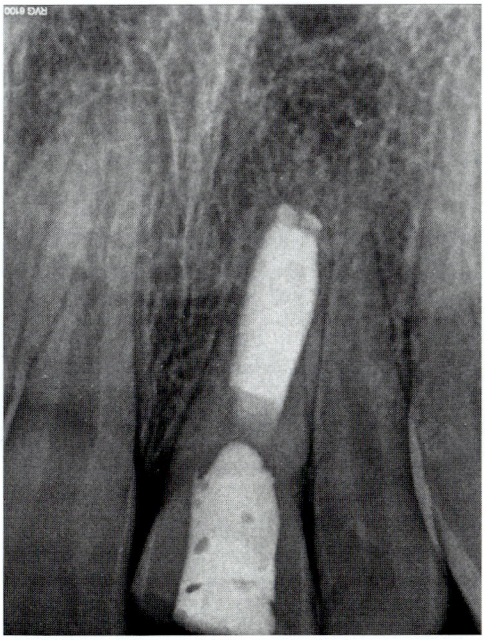

• **Fig. 15.4** Four-year follow-up radiograph of tooth #9 that was obturated with MTA when the patient was 7 years old. The patient experienced trauma, and the tooth became necrotic before the apex had fully matured.

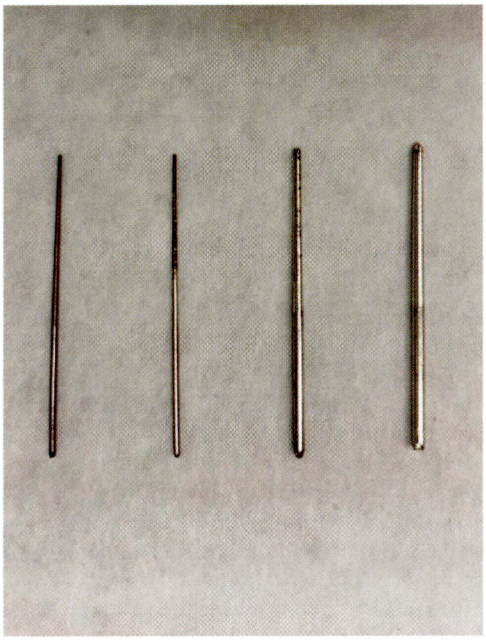

• **Fig. 15.5** Silver points had a 0.02 taper and were manufactured in a variety of tip sizes to match endodontic hand files.

plasticity. Silver points did not adequately fill all of the canal space and could not be compacted into voids within the root canal system. The shape of silver points remained round after insertion, and canals are rarely prepared to a perfectly round shape. The remaining space was filled with sealer, leading to leakage. This leakage allowed for corrosion of the silver points and the formation of silver salts, which were found to be cytotoxic.[32-36] With modern techniques, instrumentation and obturation of smaller canals with gutta-percha is predictable, so the use of silver points declined as a result of their disadvantages. Silver points are not recommended for use in modern endodontic therapy.[37] The characteristic appearance of silver points make them easily identifiable on patients' periapical radiographs (Fig. 15.6). These teeth may require retreatment if pathosis is present or post space is needed; however, prophylactic retreatment of teeth obturated with silver points is not indicated.[37]

Resin

Resin-based obturation materials were used in the early 2000s. Resilon and RealSeal were composed of a polycaprolactone core material with difunctional methacrylate resin, bioactive glass, bismuth and barium salts as fillers, and pigments. These products were used with a resin sealer (Epiphany or RealSeal) that was packaged with the core filling material. The rationale for the product was to create a "monoblock," consisting of a resin sealer with resin tags that enter and bond to dentinal tubules on the canal wall, and which also adhesively bonds to the core material. The product was light cured and sealed coronally as well. The system consisted of a primer, a sealer, and synthetic polymer points or pellets. Research has shown no advantage of these materials over gutta-percha,[38-44] and resin-based obturating materials are no longer on the market.

Pastes (Semisolids)

Pastes are a type of semisolid material that have been used as a core filling material. Zinc oxide is a major component of most paste materials. Because of the solubility of zinc oxide, these pastes do not make effective core filling materials. Other disadvantages of pastes include difficult length control, shrinkage of the material, voids in obturation, and toxic ingredients in some pastes.

One paste filling material is a resorcin-formaldehyde paste, which is a type of phenol-formaldehyde or Bakelite resin.[45,46] Because this material has been widely used in Eastern European countries, and because it stains teeth a characteristic dark red color, it is commonly referred to as *Russian Red* (Fig. 15.7). This material has the advantage of being very antimicrobial, but has the disadvantage of shrinkage once placed in the canal. Additionally, retreatments can be very difficult if the resin sets completely and there is sufficient bulk to the material[46] (Fig. 15.8).

Paraformaldehyde-based pastes are another type of paste fill. The rationale for adding paraformaldehyde to pastes is to provide antimicrobial and mummifying effects. However, paraformaldehyde has severe toxicity to host tissues, and this negates the benefit of any antimicrobial effects it may possess in endodontic materials. These pastes are known as N2 (Indrag-Agsa, Losone, Switzerland), Sargenti, or RC2B, and are made of a liquid and powder. The powder contains zinc oxide, bismuth nitrate, bismuth carbonate, paraformaldehyde, and titanium oxide. The liquid consists of eugenol, peanut oil, and rose oil.[47] N2 has changed in response to studies identifying toxic substances, such as lead oxide, and organic mercury.[48] However, it still contains 4% to 8% paraformaldehyde.[49] N2 is extremely toxic,[50,51] and because it is used as a paste, the extrusion of this material has caused permanent damage in many cases. The material affects bone and soft tissue and can cause permanent neurologic damage resulting in paresthesia, dysesthesia, and pain. Because of the toxicity, risks to patients, legal issues, and the fact that there are numerous other acceptable obturating materials available that provide a better outcome, the use of these materials in modern day endodontics is not acceptable. The Food and Drug Administration lists N2 as an unapproved drug that is not legally imported or shipped across interstate lines, and the ADA does not approve of its use.[52,53] In summary, use

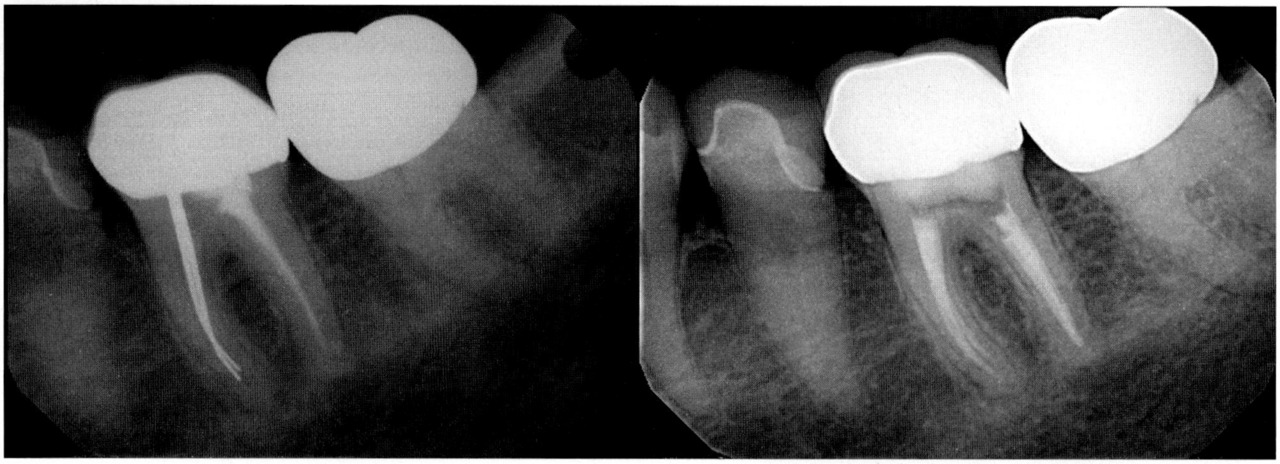

• **Fig. 15.6** The mandibular left first molar was initially obturated with silver points, and the tooth was retreated decades later when the patient presented with symptomatic apical periodontitis. Note the characteristic appearance of the silver points in the mesiobuccal and mesiolingual canals of the preoperative radiograph on the left. The postoperative radiograph on the right is the tooth after retreatment and filling with gutta-percha. (Courtesy Dr. Patrick Mullally.)

of paraformaldehyde-containing endodontic filling materials and sealers is below standard of care, as they have been shown to be both unsafe and ineffective.[54]

Sealers

Sealer is used in conjunction with a core obturating material and is necessary to fulfill the objective of creating a watertight seal in the root canal system (Question 15.5). In addition to the basic requirements for core filling materials, Grossman also identified the ideal requirements for a root canal sealer (Box 15.2).[10] As with core obturation materials, no sealer currently satisfies all of these criteria.

Additionally, the following two requirements could be added to Grossman's original basic requirements: it should not provoke an immune response in periradicular tissues,[55-58] and it should be neither mutagenic nor carcinogenic. [59,60]

Types of Sealers

The primary sealers in use today are those based on zinc oxide eugenol (ZOE), resin, calcium hydroxide, or bioceramics.

Zinc Oxide Eugenol Sealers

Zinc oxide eugenol (ZOE)-containing sealers have been widely used with success for many years. There are many formulations and brands of sealers with zinc oxide as the primary ingredient, differing only by other added components. ZOE sealers allow for the addition of chemicals, such as paraformaldehyde, rosin, Canada balsam, and others, all of which may increase the toxicity of that particular sealer.[49] Grossman's original formula contained zinc oxide, hydrogenated or Staybelite resin, bismuth subcarbonate, barium sulfate, and sodium borate (anhydrous), with eugenol as the liquid component.[61] It has been marketed as Proco-sol sealer (StarDental, Lancaster, PA), as well as other product names. Roth's 801 and 811 sealers (Roth's International LTD, Chicago, IL) were essentially the same as Grossman's original formulation, with the substitution of bismuth subnitrate for bismuth subcarbonate. Despite its popularity, production of Roth's sealer recently ceased.

Rickert's was one of the first zinc oxide sealers. The powder contains zinc oxide, silver, resins, and thymol iodide. The liquid is eugenol, and Canada balsam. One disadvantage is that the silver used to provide radiopacity can also cause staining of tooth structure. Another disadvantage is its rapid setting time in areas of high humidity and heat. Rickert's sealer is marketed as Kerr Pulp Canal Sealer (Kerr Endodontics, Orange, CA), which has traditionally been popular with clinicians who use the warm vertical obturation technique. Pulp Canal Sealer Extended Working Time (EWT) (Kerr Endodontics, Orange, CA), with a working time of 6 hours, was introduced to lengthen the setting time over Kerr Pulp Canal Sealer.[62]

Tubli-Seal (Kerr Endodontics, Orange, CA) was developed as a nonstaining alternative to the silver containing Pulp Canal Sealer. Tubli-Seal comes as two separate tubes. One tube contains a zinc oxide-base paste with barium sulfate for radiopacity, mineral oil, cornstarch, and lecithin. The catalyst tube contains polypale resin, eugenol, and thymol iodide. Tubli-Seal is easy to mix and has a short setting time.[62] Tubli-Seal EWT was developed to provide extended working time.

Wach's cement is made up of a powder of zinc oxide, bismuth subnitrate, bismuth subiodide, magnesium oxide, and calcium phosphate. The liquid consists of oil of cloves, eucalyptol, Canada balsam, and beechwood creosote. Wach's cement has a distinctive odor of an old-time dental office.[62] It has a smooth consistency, and the Canada balsam makes the sealer tacky. Medicated Canal Sealer (Medidenta, Woodside, NY) contains iodoform for antibacterial purposes and is to be used with MGP gutta-percha, which also contains 10% iodoform.[63]

Calcium Hydroxide Sealers

Sealapex (Kerr Endodontics, Orange, CA) is a noneugenol polymeric sealer that contains calcium hydroxide. It is packaged in two tubes, one of which is a base, and the other a catalyst. Sealapex has zinc oxide in the base plus calcium hydroxide. It also contains butyl benzene, sulfonamide, and zinc stearate. The catalyst tube has barium sulfate and titanium dioxide for radiopacity, and a proprietary resin, isobutyl salicylate, and AEROSIL R792.[62] Sealapex has similar sealing ability as Tubli-Seal.[64] Apexit

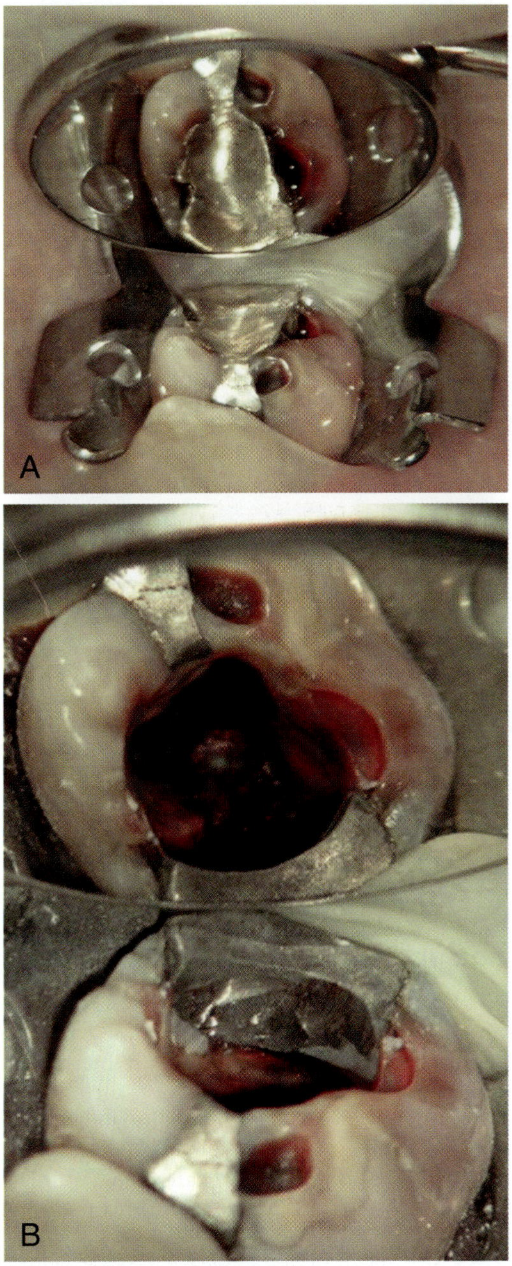

• **Fig. 15.7** This mandibular molar was treated with a resorcinol-formaldehyde resin paste. Dark red-stained dentin can be seen both through the occlusal surface and upon access. The dentin is solid.

(Ivoclar Vivadent, Schaan, Liechtenstein) is a calcium hydroxide sealer with salicylates also incorporated into the formula. CRCS (Calciobiotic Root Canal Sealer, Coltene/Whaledent, Mahwah, NJ) is a calcium hydroxide-containing sealer that has a zinc oxide-eugenol and eucalyptol base. CRCS is a rather slow-setting sealer, especially in dry or in humid climates. It may require up to 3 days to fully set.[62] The set sealer is quite stable, which improves its sealing qualities, but may mean that calcium hydroxide is not as readily released and the stimulation of cementum and bone formation may be severely limited.

Resin Sealers

Epoxy resin sealers have been used in endodontics for some time, including AH26, and its successor AH Plus (Dentsply Sirona, York, PA). AH26 is a sealer that has been used for many years. It is a bisphenol epoxy resin sealer that uses hexamethylenetetramine (methenamine) for polymerization.[45,65] A major disadvantage of AH26 was that the methenamine gave off formaldehyde as it set. It would also stain tooth structure and had an extended working time. One advantage of AH26 is it was not affected by moisture.[62] AH Plus and ThermaSeal Plus (Dentsply Sirona, York, PA) are formulated with a mixture of amines that allows for polymerization without the unwanted formation of formaldehyde.[65,66] They have the advantages of AH26, which include increased radiopacity, low solubility, slight amount of shrinkage, and tissue computability. AH Plus is an bisphenol epoxy resin that also contains adamantine.[45] AH Plus comes in a two paste system, unlike the liquid-powder system of AH26, and has a working time of 4 hours and a setting time of 8 hours. Additional improvements of AH Plus over AH26 include thinner film thickness and decreased solubility.

Bioceramic Sealers

Mineral trioxide aggregate (MTA) is a calcium silicate bioceramic material, which has many applications in endodontics. MTA has been a very successful material because of its biologic and physical characteristics. MTA is extremely biocompatible and provides a good seal. Because of these biologic and physical attributes, several bioceramic sealers are now on the market. ProRoot Endo Sealer (Dentsply Sirona, York, PA) is an MTA-based sealer manufactured in a powder and gel form. The powder is MTA with enhanced radiopacity, which contains tricalcium silicate, dicalcium silicate, calcium sulfate, bismuth oxide, and a small amount of tricalcium aluminate. The gel is a viscous aqueous solution of a water soluble polymer. MTAFillapex (Angelus, Londrina, PR, Brazil) is a dual paste system. It contains salicylate resin, diluent resin, natural resin, bismuth oxide, nanoparticulate silica, MTA, and pigments. Endosequence BC Sealer (Root SP) (Brasseler USA, Savannah, GA) is a calcium silicate based sealer manufactured as a single paste system. It contains zirconium oxide, calcium silicates, calcium phosphate monobasic ($CaH_2P_2O_8$), calcium hydroxide, filler, and thickening agents. iRoot SP (Innovative BioCeramix Inc., Vancouver, Canada) is another calcium silicate based sealer that contains zirconium oxide, calcium silicates, calcium phosphate, calcium hydroxide, filler, and thickening agents.

Silicone Based Sealers

Silicone based sealers provide adhesion, a moisture resistant seal, and stability.[45] Lee Endo-Fill (Lee Pharmaceuticals, El Monte, CA) is a silicone based root canal sealer. RoekoSeal (Coltene/Whaledent, Langenau, Germany) is a polyvinylsiloxane that is a white paste-like sealer and will polymerize without shrinkage, which results in less leakage.[45,67] It utilizes platinum as a catalyzing agent.[45] GuttaFlow (Coltene/Whaledent, Langenau, Germany) is a polyvinylsiloxane that has finely milled gutta-percha particles added to the RoekoSeal sealer. GuttaFlow additionally contains silicone oil, paraffin oil, platin catalyst, zirconium dioxide, nano-silver as a preservative, and a coloring agent. It does not contain eugenol. GuttaFlow is a cold flowable gutta-percha filling system for the obturation of root canals. GuttaFlow is triturated in its cannula and passively injected into the canal and then used with single or multiple gutta-percha points.

Urethane Methacrylate Sealers

EndoREZ (Ultradent, South Jordon, UT) is a hydrophilic urethane dimethacrylate (UDMA) resin sealer that reportedly has

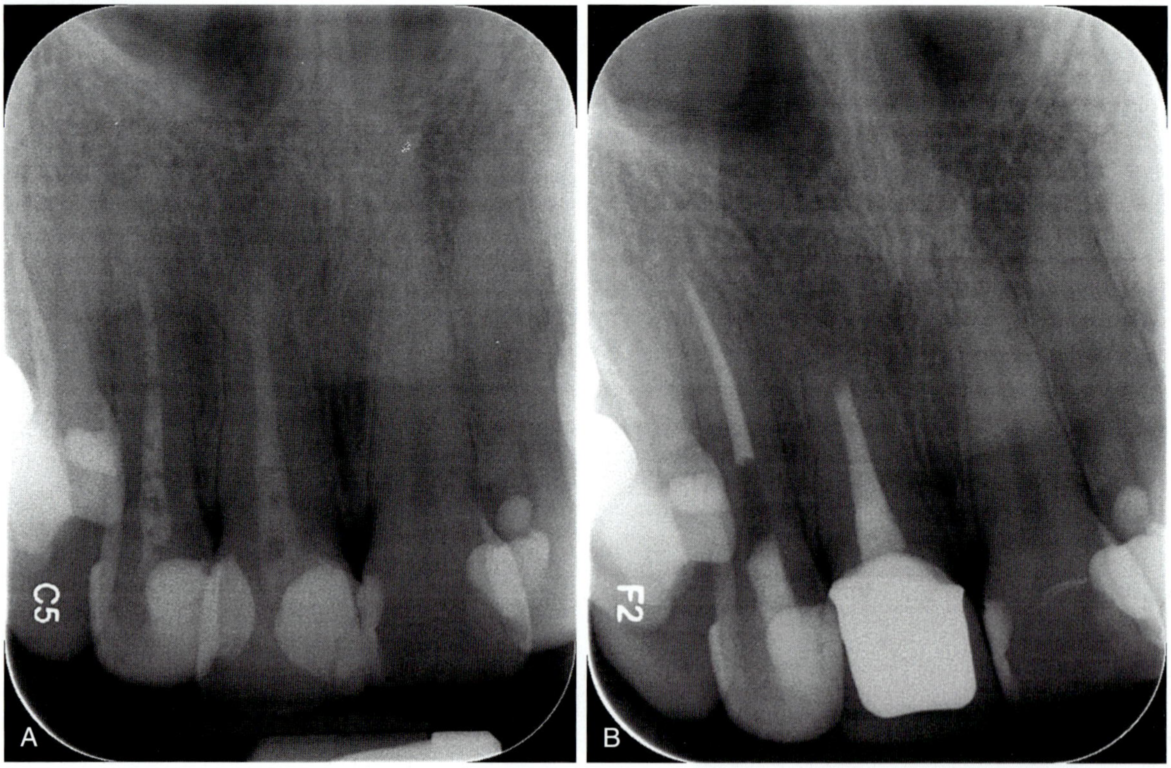

• **Fig. 15.8** The maxillary right lateral and central incisor were treated with a resorcinol-formaldehyde resin paste. **(A)** The teeth have characteristic voids visible radiographically in the obturation, especially tooth #7, as seen in this preoperative radiograph. All of the paste could not be removed during nonsurgical retreatment of tooth #8, so root-end surgery was performed. **(B)** Tooth #7 was later successfully retreated nonsurgically, as shown in this postoperative radiograph.

• **BOX 15.2 Requirements for an Ideal Root Canal Sealing Material**

1. It should be tacky when mixed to provide good adhesion between it and the canal wall when set.
2. It should make a hermetic [sic] seal.
3. It should be radiopaque so that it can be visualized on the radiograph.
4. The particles of powder should be very fine so that they can mix easily with the liquid.
5. It should not shrink upon setting.
6. It should not stain tooth structure.
7. It should be bacteriostatic or at least not encourage bacterial growth.
8. It should set slowly.
9. It should be insoluble in tissue fluids.
10. It should be tissue tolerant, that is, nonirritating to periapical tissues.
11. It should be soluble in a common solvent, if it is necessary to remove the root canal filling.

good canal wetting and flow into dentinal tubules.[67] The hydrophilic property improves its sealing abilities if some moisture is still in the canal at obturation.[45] EndoREZ is introduced into the canal with a narrow 30-gauge NaviTip needle (Ultradent). A single gutta-percha point, or the lateral compaction obturation technique, may be utilized. EZ Fill (Essential Dental Systems, South Hackensack, NJ) is a noneugenol epoxy resin sealer that is placed with a bidirectional spiral rotating in a hand piece. It may be used with a single gutta-percha point technique. It is nonshrinking on setting and is hydrophobic, rendering it resistant to fluid degradation.

Evaluation and Comparison of Sealers

Orstavik[45,68] has listed the various evaluation parameters for testing endodontic sealers. They include technologic tests that have been standardized by the ISO and ADA/ANSI internationally and in the United States. These technological tests include flow, working time, setting time, radiopacity, solubility and disintegration, and dimensional change after setting. Additionally, biologic tests, usage testing, and antibacterial testing are useful. Clinical testing should be included to establish outcomes of treatment.

Study Questions

1. What is the primary objective of obturation?
2. What is the rationale for completing root canal therapy in two visits versus one visit?
3. Why is the smear layer removed before obturation?
4. What are the advantages of gutta-percha as a core obturation material?
5. Why must a sealer be used when obturating with gutta-percha?

Obturation Techniques with Gutta-Percha

Gutta-percha is the most widely used and clinically acceptable obturation material, thus the techniques described in this chapter will focus on the use of this material. Gutta-percha is available in many different forms and sizes, both gutta-percha cones and gutta-percha for thermoplasticized injection systems (see Figs. 15.1 and 15.2). The choice of obturation method is primarily based on clinician training and preference, as well as the specific anatomy of each

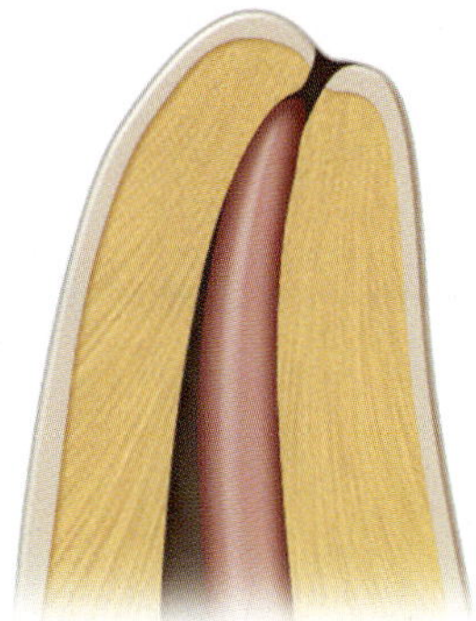

• **Fig. 15.9** The master cone should have slight frictional fit in the most apical portion of the canal.

case. There are attributes and limitations of each technique, but no significant difference in outcomes has been demonstrated between contemporary obturation techniques using gutta-percha.[69,70]

Cold Lateral Condensation

Cold lateral condensation (commonly referred to as lateral condensation or lateral compaction) is the most common obturation technique taught to predoctoral dental students.[71] Advantages of lateral condensation are that it can be used in a wide variety of cases, does not require specialized equipment, and has a track record of clinical success. In addition, lateral condensation is safe and simple to learn for novice clinicians; it is less technique-sensitive than other methods and has predictable length control (less likely to overfill). A disadvantage of lateral condensation is that it requires more time than some filling techniques.[72] In addition, it is challenging to use in some clinical cases (e.g., very curved canals, internal resorption, wide open apices, or other anomalous canal anatomy) (Question 15.6). However, these cases are considered "high difficulty" and are typically referred to a specialist for treatment.[30,31]

The technique for lateral condensation, and all obturation techniques, varies slightly from clinician to clinician. The following is a description of a traditional lateral condensation technique.

1. The canal is dried. A paper point placed to working length should come out of the canal dry, with no irrigant, blood, or exudate on it.
2. A master gutta-percha cone is selected. Gutta-percha cones should be handled using cotton pliers (locking are preferred), and measured using a millimeter ruler. In classic cold lateral condensation, the master cone is a 0.02 taper cone and has a tip size that matches the master apical file size to which the canal has been prepared. The selected cone should seat to working length, not be able to be pushed beyond working length, and exhibit a sensation of slight resistance when removing the cone from the canal. This resistance (referred to as *tug-back*) indicates that the cone is binding the walls of the canal (Fig. 15.9). A master cone that does not seat all the way to working length is too large (i.e., it is binding short of working length). A master cone that can be pushed beyond working length is too small (i.e., it is not binding at working length and overfilling will result). A master cone that does not display any resistance upon removal is also too small (i.e., it is not snug at working length), though this sensation can be difficult to detect. Careful inspection should catch any cone that buckles when placed to working length and removed; this indicates that the cone does not fit well. A cone that buckles near the tip may be too small (Fig. 15.10). A cone that buckles more coronally may be too large (it will appear that the cone is seating to working length because the cotton pliers seat to the reference point, but the cone will be short as a result of the buckling). Variations of selecting a master cone preferred by some clinicians include using a 0.04 taper cone or a nonstandardized cone with the tip cut to a custom diameter. Specialized instruments are available on the market to help cut the tip of gutta-percha cones to a specific diameter (Fig. 15.11). Often the clinician may try multiple master cones, even of the same size, before selecting the master cone they want to use for obturation of a canal. As a result of manufacturing variations, there will be variations in gutta-percha cone actual sizes, even among those labeled as the same ISO size and taper.[73]
3. Sealer is placed in the canal. Different methods have been used to apply sealer to the walls of the canal. These include using a hand file place to length and spinning counterclockwise, using a lentulo spiral drill, and using the master cone (Fig. 15.12). The goal is to have a thin layer of sealer on all walls of the canal. In most cases, sealer is placed both in the canal before seating the master cone, and on the master cone itself before seating it. The choice of sealer type is up to the discretion of the clinician.

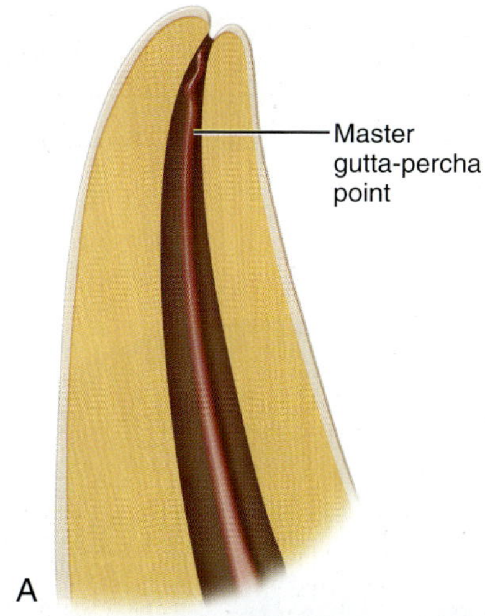

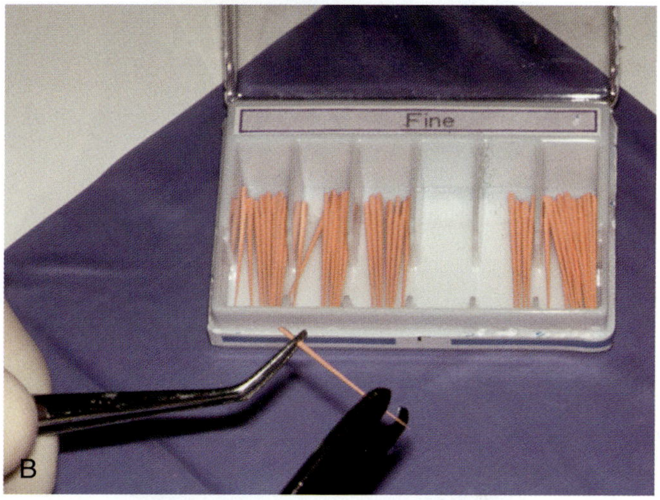

• **Fig. 15.10** **(A)** A master cone that buckles near the tip when inserted into the canal is too small. **(B)** A larger cone should be selected or clipped to form a larger size at the tip.

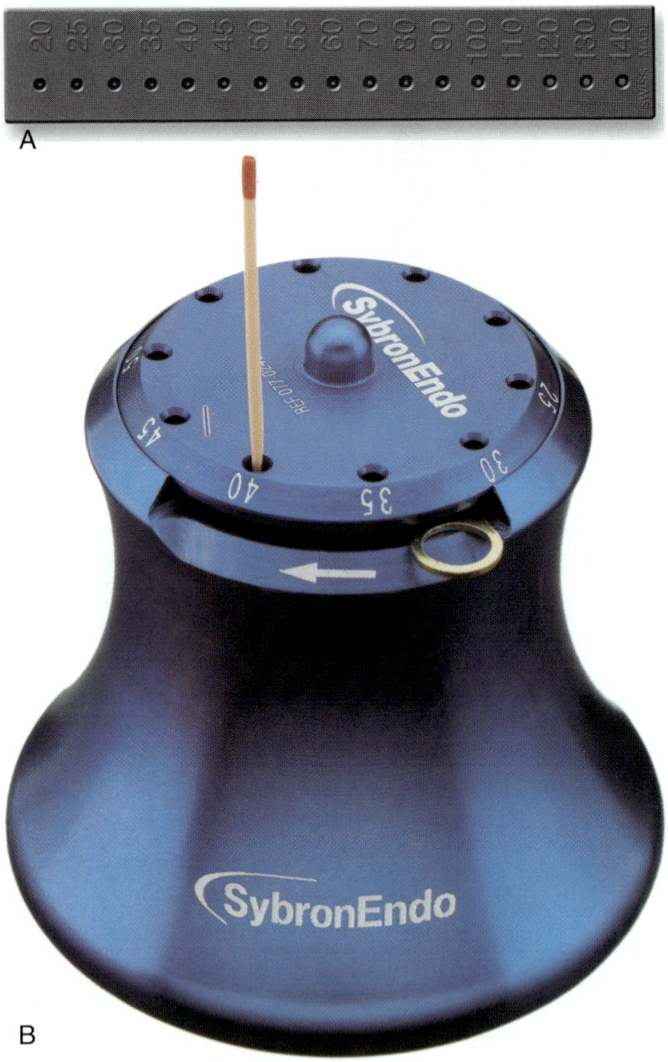

• **Fig. 15.11** Specialized instruments for cutting gutta-percha cones to a customized International Organization for Standardization tip size are commercially available. **(A)** Gutta Gauge. (Courtesy Dentsply Sirona.) **(B)** Tip Snip. (Courtesy Kerr Endodontics.)

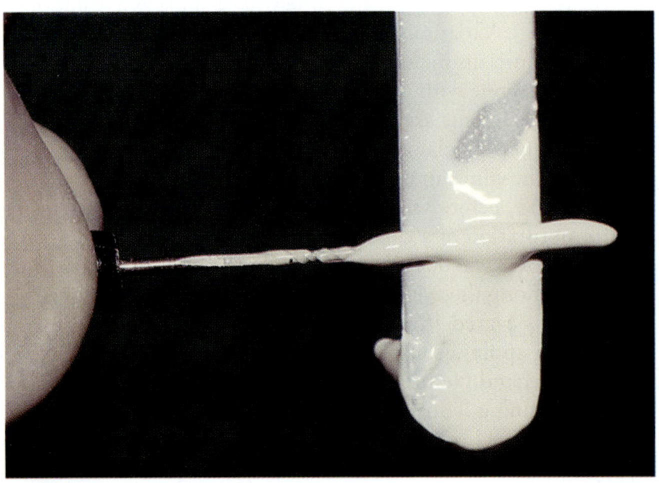

• **Fig. 15.12** A simple, effective method of sealer application. A hand file covered with sealer is inserted into the canal and spun counterclockwise to coat the canal walls.

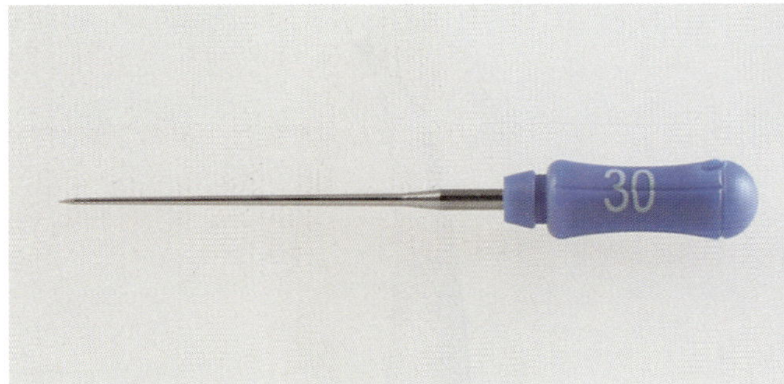

• **Fig. 15.13** Size 30 finger spreader. (Courtesy Dentsply Sirona.)

4. Sealer is placed on the master cone, and the master cone is seated in the canal to working length. The cone is seated using gentle, continuous pressure. If the cone does not seat to length on the first attempt, it should be pulled out a few millimeters and slowly reseated. The master cone may need to be gently "pumped" up and down a few times to get the cone to seat to the desired working length.
5. A spreader is selected for use in lateral condensation. The length, size, and degree of taper varies between spreaders. Nickel-titanium finger spreaders or stainless steel hand spreaders may be used (Fig. 15.13). Nickel-titanium finger spreaders have the advantages of being able to be inserted into the canal to a greater depth while exerting less force on the canal walls[74-76] (Fig. 15.14). Finger spreaders also are preferred by many because they are gripped and used in a fashion similar to finger files, and they may be easier to access difficult areas of the mouth. The chosen spreader should be able to be placed in the canal to within approximately 1 to 2 mm of the working length.
6. The spreader is placed into the canal and rotated using a back-and-forth motion, keeping the long axis of the spreader in the same plane, to create lateral space within the canal. Moderate pressure is applied in an apical direction, while rotating the handle through an arc of approximately 30 degrees. The apical force is kept on the long axis of the spreader. The spreader will feel looser as it is moved in this motion. The spreader is removed from the canal also using a back-and-forth motion. During removal of the spreader, it is recommended to hold the tip of the cone(s) that have already been seated in the canal, to prevent the master cone and any accessory cones from being dislodged from working length.
7. Accessory cones are added in the space created by the spreader (Fig. 15.15). Different types of accessory cones may be used, and the cones are matched to the spreader size. Commonly, nonstandardized cones or size 25, 0.02 taper standardized cones are used as accessory cones. In very large canals, larger accessory cones and a larger size spreader may be used. Caution must be exercised during lateral condensation not to use too much force in the canal during the condensation process (this same caution should be used during other techniques as well). It is recommended that the force used should be no more than 2.5 lbs, in order to avoid vertical root fracture[77,78] (Fig. 15.16).
8. Most clinicians choose to expose a radiograph after the master cone is seated in the canal. The purpose for the "master cone radiograph" is to check that the gutta-percha is seated to the desired working length (not short and not long). Alternatively, the clinician may choose to add one to two

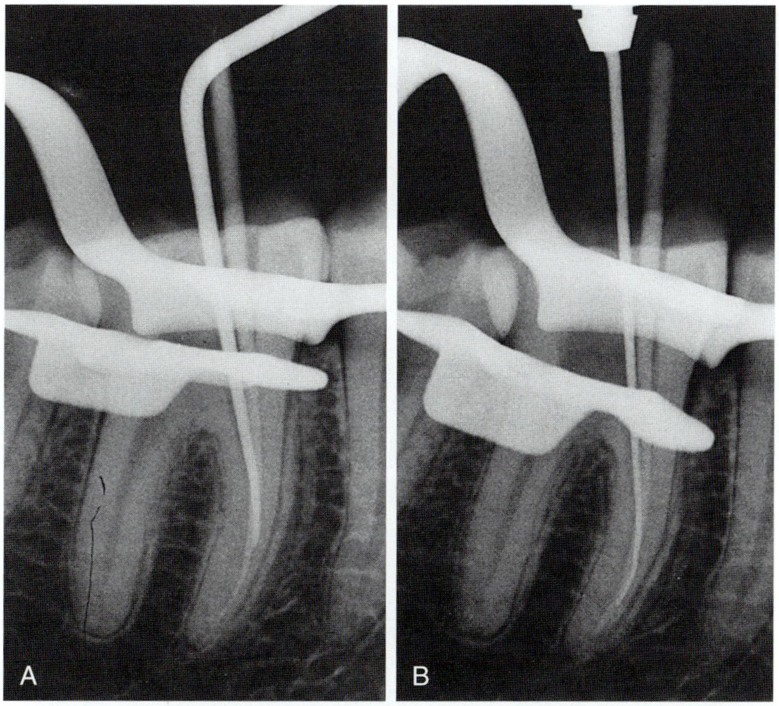

• **Fig. 15.14** Comparison of hand spreader with finger spreader. **(A)** The stiff, more tapered hand spreader will not negotiate the curve. **(B)** The smaller, more flexible finger spreader permits deeper penetration and produces less force on the canal wall.

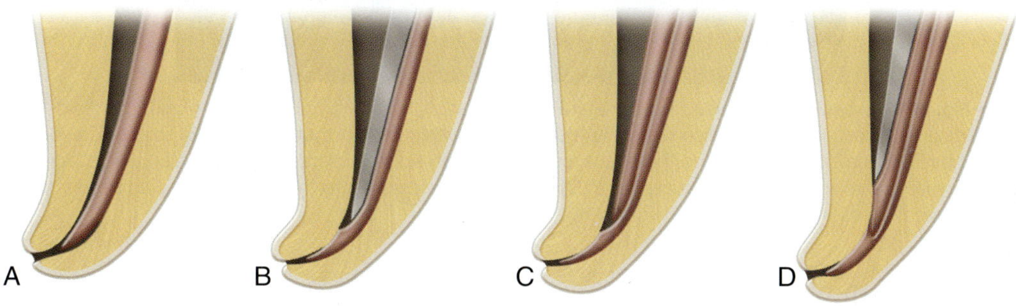

• **Fig. 15.15** The steps of lateral condensation. **(A)** The master cone is fit. **(B)** A spreader is inserted, ideally to 1 to 2 mm from working length. **(C)** The spreader is rotated and removed, and an accessory cone is placed in the space created. **(D)** The process is repeated.

accessory cones before exposing the radiograph. This "initial condensation radiograph" is used to check the length of the gutta-percha, that the master cone is not dislodged during the initial condensation, and that no voids are present in the apical third of the canal. If an error is detected on the master cone or initial condensation radiograph, it is still possible to easily remove the cone(s) from the canal, before they have been seared off, and correct the error or chose a new master cone. Cones are removed by slowly pulling the gutta-percha from the canal.

9. If the master cone or initial condensation radiograph is acceptable, then lateral condensation continues (Fig. 15.17). The spreader is used, and subsequent accessory cones are also coated in sealer before placement in the canal. As more accessory cones are added, the spreader will seat less and less deep in the canal. Condensation should continue until the spreader can no longer be placed more than approximately 4 mm below the level of the orifice (Fig. 15.18).
10. When the appropriate level of obturation is reached, the gutta-percha cones are seared off at the desired level. An electrically heated plugger can be used to sear off the cones (Fig. 15.19). Historically, a Bunsen burner or alcohol torch with a hand plugger were used and may be used if an electrically heater plugger is not available. A cold hand plugger is used to plug the remaining gutta-percha vertically, filling any coronal voids and creating a smooth surface of gutta-percha in the coronal aspect of the canal (Fig. 15.20). If an intraorifice barrier is to be placed, the desired level of gutta-percha is 1 to 2 mm apical to the level of the facial cemento-enamel junction (CEJ) or the pulp chamber floor (in a molar). The 1 to 2 mm space is then filled with the intraorifice barrier material. If an intraorifice barrier is not placed, then the gutta-percha is brought to the level of the facial CEJ or the pulp chamber floor. If post space is needed, additional gutta-percha may be removed to a level as appropriate for the post space.

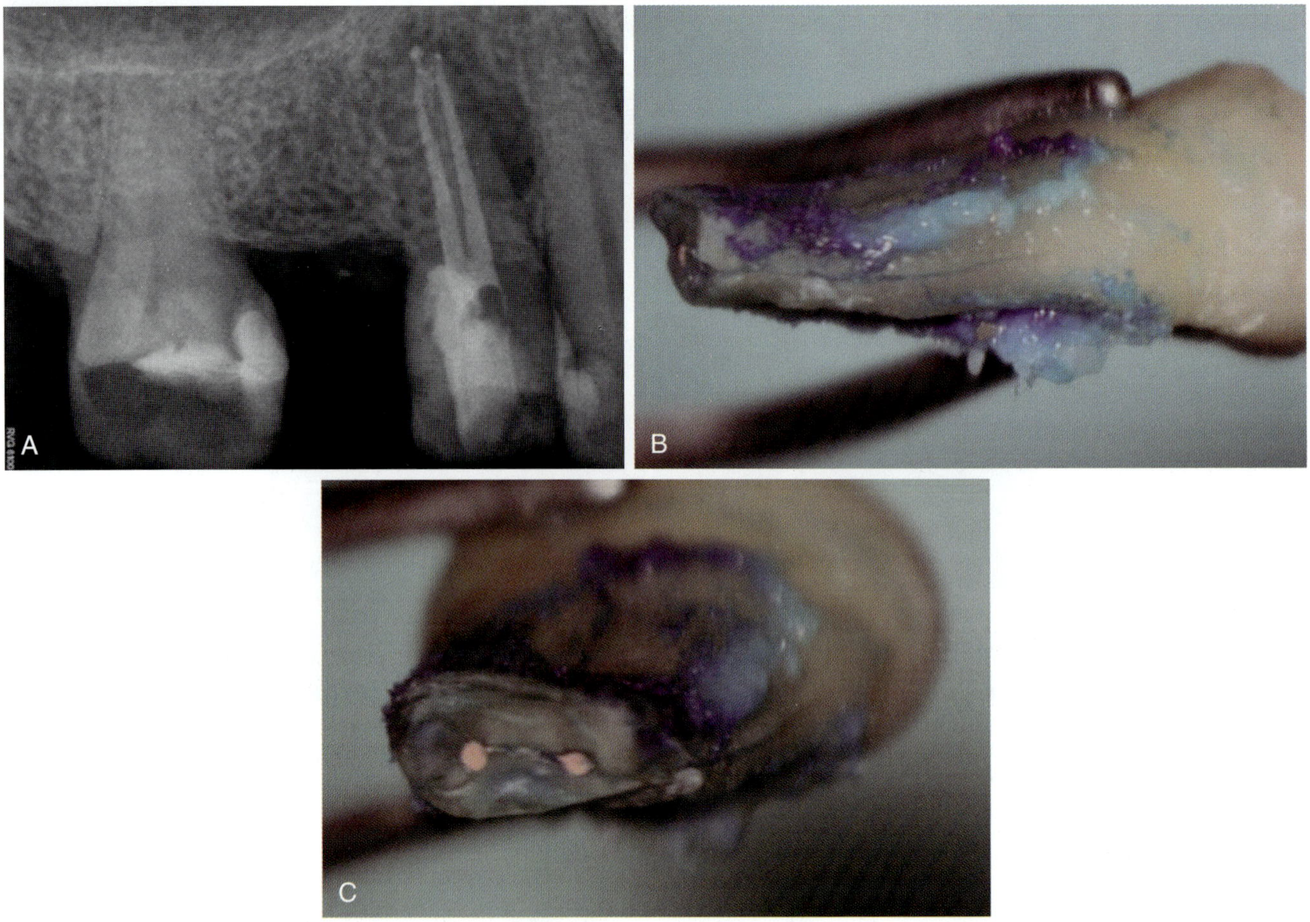

• **Fig. 15.16** Excessive force used during lateral condensation, or any obturation technique, can lead to vertical root fracture. **(A)** Periapical radiograph of tooth #4 with a vertical root fracture. **(B)** The vertical root fracture is visualized extending up the buccal surface from an apical direction. The root has been stained with methylene blue for better visualization. **(C)** The fracture extends into the buccal canal, as seen from the apical direction. (Courtesy Dr. Alex Hanley.)

Warm Vertical Condensation

Warm vertical condensation (also known as warm vertical compaction or the Schilder technique) is another widely used obturation method. The technique is commonly credited to Dr. Herb Schilder,[79,80] although modifications have been made to the original technique over the years as technology has advanced. The main advantage of warm vertical condensation is that warmed gutta-percha can be adapted to the canal walls, which is particularly desirable in irregularly shaped canals, such as cases of internal resorption. Disadvantages of warm vertical condensation compared with lateral condensation are that it is more technique-sensitive, and length control is particularly difficult (higher risk of overfilling).[70,81] Warm vertical condensation also requires additional instruments and equipment, and it is difficult to visualize the level of gutta-percha in the canal unless a dental operating microscope is used during treatment (Question 15.7).

As with lateral condensation, the technique used for warm vertical condensation varies slightly from clinician to clinician. A basic tenet for warm vertical condensation is that the preparation should be a continuously tapering funnel with the apical foramen kept as small as possible. A description of a basic warm vertical condensation follows, starting with a dried canal.

1. A master gutta-percha cone is selected. The cone usually replicates the canal taper (e.g., if a canal is prepared to a 0.04 taper, a 0.04 taper master cone is chosen). The cone should seat short of the desired working length, up to 2 mm short. The warm vertical condensation technique is expected to push the gutta-percha apically to the desired working length during condensation. Some clinicians opt to select a master cone that seats snugly at working length.
2. Sealer is applied and the master cone is seated.
3. The coronal portion of the cone is seared off at the orifice level using an electrically heated plugger.
4. The remaining gutta-percha is plugged apically in the canal, using a prefit cold hand plugger. The plugger should not bind the sides of the canal during condensation. If the plugger is too large, it will bind the walls of the canal, creating excess force on the walls and risking vertical root fracture. If the plugger is too small, it will poke indentations in the mass of gutta-percha, rather than compacting it in an apical direction. The plugger is used to circumferentially plug the gutta-percha in the canal.
5. The gutta-percha mass is seared off again, at a deeper level in the canal, and a "bite" of gutta-percha is removed from the canal by inserting the heat source a few millimeters into the gutta-percha. The gutta-percha mass is plugged apically again using a cold hand plugger.
6. This process is repeated until the apical portion of the canal is filled with an "apical plug" to a level 4 to 6 mm from working length. As the gutta-percha is plugged apically, the mass of

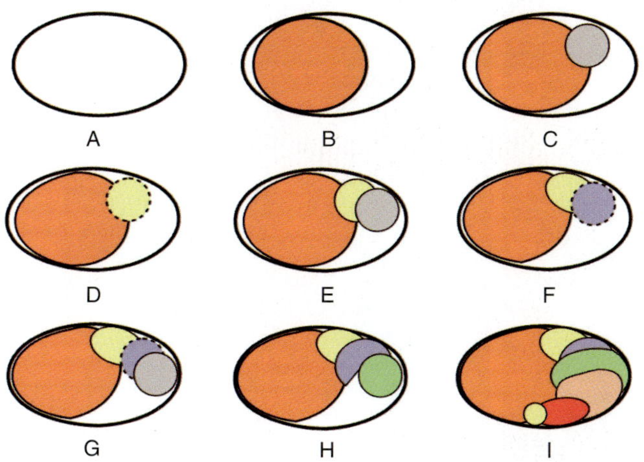

A. Prepared canal
B. Master cone inserted
C. Spreader placed
D. Placement of accessory cone (shown as dashed circle)
E-H. Continuation of lateral compaction
I. Completion of obturation

• **Fig. 15.17** Schematic of the steps of lateral condensation. Each insertion of the spreader to its most apical extent laterally compacts the gutta-percha cone toward the opposing wall. At the completion of obturation, the canal is filled with a series of cones that have been cold-welded together with sealer. (Courtesy Dr. J. Schweitzer.)

gutta-percha is pushed to working length and into any canal irregularities. Note that caution must be exercised when using an electrically heated plugger in the canal to avoid transmitting dangerous levels of heat to the periodontal ligament.[82,83]

7. The remainder of the canal is then backfilled with thermoplasticized gutta-percha from an injection system (Fig. 15.21). The warm injection tip is first placed in contact with the apical plug of gutta-percha, to warm the existing gutta-percha before more is added to the canal. Thermoplasticized gutta-percha is then injected, as the instrument is "backed out" of the canal. The injected gutta-percha is plugged apically with a cold plugger, with apical pressure being applied as the gutta-percha cools, to minimize shrinkage. The backfill may be accomplished in one or more segments, depending on the length of the canal. Before thermoplasticized gutta-percha injection systems were commercially available, small segments of gutta-percha were added back to the canal, heated, and condensed.
8. The backfilled gutta-percha is seared off at the desired level, as with lateral condensation. The backfill may be stopped short, or not completed at all, if post space is desired.

Continuous Wave

The continuous wave of condensation is a variation of warm vertical compaction.[84] Continuous wave primarily differs from warm vertical in the down pack procedure (*down pack* may refer to both the procedure for removing coronal gutta-percha from the canal, and the apical plug of gutta-percha that results). Classic warm vertical obturation accomplishes the down pack in multiple steps of heating, removing gutta-percha, and plugging vertically. In contrast, the continuous wave technique employs one continuous motion for the down pack. Once the master cone is seated, a prefit plugger is chosen. Electrically heated plugger tips that match the taper of the canal are used (Fig. 15.22). The warmed plugger is moved apically through the gutta-percha in one motion over 1 to 2 seconds, until the desired level of the down pack is achieved. The heat plugger is inactivated, and pressure is applied apically for 5 to 10 seconds, to reduce shrinkage of the cooling gutta-percha. A burst of heat is then applied, as the plugger is moved side-to-side, to separate the plugger from the apical gutta-percha. The plugger is then removed from the canal, and any excess gutta-percha coronal to the down pack level should be removed from the canal on the plugger. The apical portion of gutta-percha is plugged apically with a cold plugger, and the canal is backfilled, as in warm vertical condensation. The advantage of the continuous wave technique is the reduced amount of time needed to obturate.[72] A disadvantage is that the method is quite technique-sensitive: the down pack of apical gutta-percha may be removed with the plugger, or the coronal gutta-percha may not be removed with the plugger. As with warm vertical compaction, length control is more difficult with the continuous wave technique versus cold lateral condensation.

Formed Cones

The use of a custom formed master cone is a variation used in obturation. Formed cones are most commonly employed in conjunction with cold lateral condensation but may also be used with warm vertical techniques. The technique involves selecting a gutta-percha cone that is larger than the apical preparation of the canal, then softening the tip of the cone in chloroform so that an "impression" of the apical few millimeters of the prepared canal is created. Chloroform softens the outer skin of the gutta-percha. The cone is then reseated after sealer has been placed in the canal.

Some clinicians choose to use the formed cone technique on every case. Others employ it only in specific cases. Cases where the formed cone would be indicated include those with a large apical foramen, an irregularly shaped apical preparation, lack of an apical stop, or as a trouble-shooting technique when the master cone is not seating to working length (Question 15.8). The formed cone should fit like a key in a lock when root canal sealer is applied and the cone is placed back into the canal in the same orientation in which it was removed after making the impression. As condensation continues, the use of a spreader and/or plugger will cause the softened gutta-percha to move into irregularities in the root canal system. The disadvantages of any gutta-percha solvent technique are the time needed to form the cone and the potential for shrinkage of the gutta-percha as the chloroform evaporates. In vitro testing suggests the possibility of shrinkage after use of chloroform, but no clinical studies have shown shrinkage to be a clinically significant problem.

The formed cone technique is as follows:

1. An oversized gutta-percha master cone (that does not seat to working length) is selected. This is most commonly a 0.02 taper cone but could be a larger taper cone depending on the case and clinician preference. The cone should seat approximately 1 mm short of working length when placed in the canal with gentle pressure. This is typically a cone that is one to two sizes larger than the master apical file size.
2. The cone is grasped with a locking cotton plier at the appropriate working length. The apical 3 to 4 mm of the cone is quickly dipped into chloroform (for approximately 1 second). Other solvents may also be used.
3. The cone is seated with gentle but continuous pressure. The cone is pulled out a few millimeters and gently reseated in the canal to mold or adapt the apical portion. The cone should seat to working length.
4. Measure to confirm that the cone seats to working length. If the cone is short of working length, the cone may be dipped again in

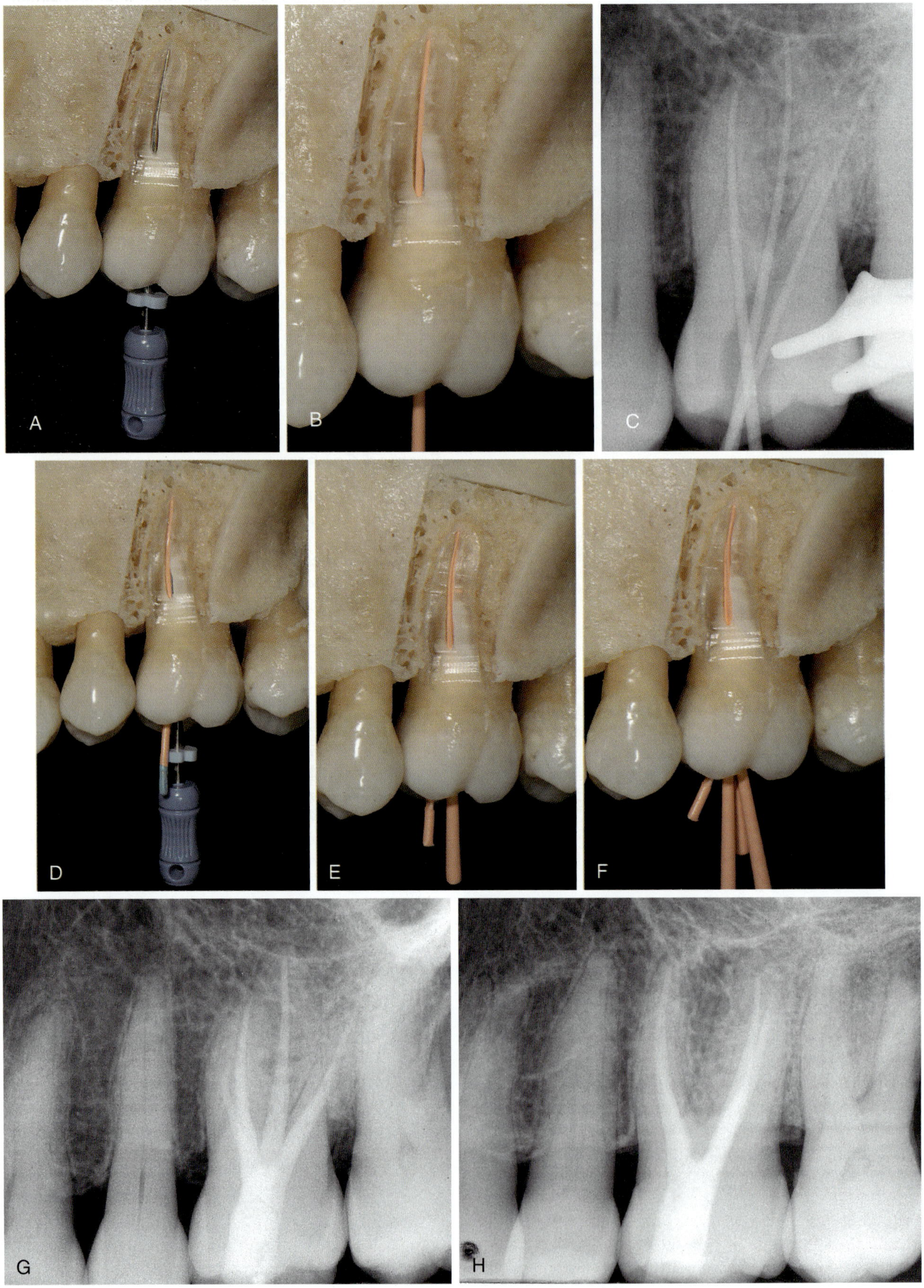

• **Fig. 15.18** Lateral condensation. **(A)** A hand file matching the size of the master apical file is inserted to ensure it seats to working length. **(B)** Standardized gutta-percha cones are seated to working length. **(C)** The position of the cones is verified radiographically. **(D)** Once the sealer has been placed and the cone seated to length, the spreader is inserted along the side of the cemented cone (here, in the mesiobuccal canal). **(E)** An accessory cone is placed in the space created by the spreader. **(F)** The process is repeated (i.e., reinsertion of the spreader, followed by placement of another accessory cone) until the spreader does not penetrate beyond the middle third of the canal. The cones are removed at the orifice with heat, and the coronal mass then is vertically compacted. **(G)** The remaining canals are obturated in the same manner. **(H)** The final radiograph demonstrates four canals properly obturated. (Courtesy Dr. W. Johnson.)

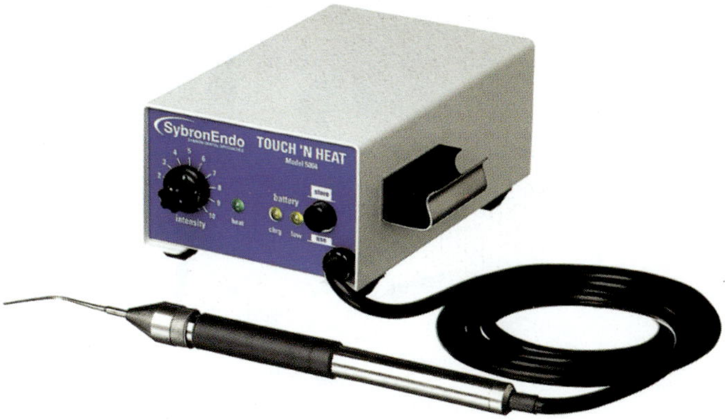

• **Fig. 15.19** An electrically heated plugger can be used to sear off gutta-percha during obturation with lateral condensation, as well as carry heat into the canal to remove gutta-percha during warm obturation techniques. The Touch 'n Heat was the first mass marketed electrically heated plugger, and is still on the market today. (Courtesy Kerr Endodontics.)

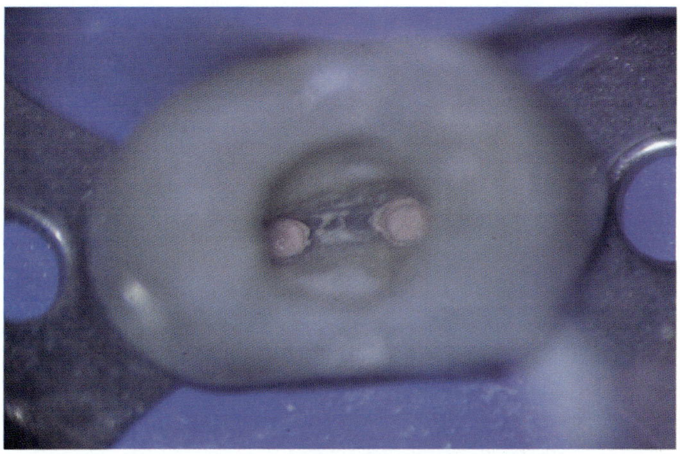

• **Fig. 15.20** The gutta-percha has been seared off and vertically compacted with a cold hand plugger at the level of the orifice in this maxillary premolar. (Courtesy Dr. Kyle Countryman.)

chloroform and reseated using gentle continuous pressure, or a new cone may be used. If the cone buckles, it should be discarded.

5. The tip of the cone is examined to make certain that the cone has adapted to the apical canal (Fig. 15.23). If the cone has properly formed, "skid marks" will be visible where the softened cone has touched the canal wall. Smooth, uninterrupted areas that look like the fresh cone are an indication that the cone is too small and is not contacting the canal in all dimensions. If this occurs, a new, larger cone should be formed, or the tip of the softened cone should be trimmed and reformed.
6. After the master cone is formed, sealer is applied, and obturation is completed using the preferred technique.

Carrier-Based Obturation

Carrier-based obturation utilizes an "obturator" composed of a core carrier material surrounded by a gutta-percha coating that is used to fill the root canal system. The earliest version of an obturator had a metal core, but later versions have utilized plastic as the core material. The most recently introduced core material is a crosslinked version of gutta-percha (see Fig. 15.3, *A*). Obturators are available in standardized sizes designed to match a designated master apical file size, and some endodontic rotary files are marketed with corresponding carriers as a "system."

When the canal is ready to obturate, it is dried and sealer is applied. The obturator is heated using a time- and temperature-controlled oven, which softens the gutta-percha surrounding the carrier (Fig. 15.24). The obturator is inserted into the canal to the appropriate working length. The carrier portion of the obturator is rigid enough to carry the gutta-percha to working length but flexible enough to be placed around common canal curvatures. The handle of the carrier must then be removed, typically using a long-shank round bur, and the coronal gutta-percha is smoothed using a plugger.

The advantages of carrier-based obturation are time efficiency and the ability of warmed gutta-percha to fill canal irregularities.[85] Disadvantages include length control (overfilling is a risk), and stripping of the gutta-percha off the carrier during seating.[86] As such, carrier-based obturation can be technique-sensitive. In addition, post space preparation and retreatment are difficult, as retrieving the carrier from the canal may be challenging or impossible in some cases (Question 15.9).

A variation on carrier-based obturation uses a metal carrier with an apical plug of gutta-percha attached (see Fig. 15.3, *B*). After the gutta-percha is seated to working length, the metal carrier is twisted off and removed from the canal, leaving an apical plug of gutta-percha. This type of carrier is not heated.

Single Cone Obturation

Growing attention has been given in recent years to the use of a "single-cone" obturation technique. In this technique, the canal is obturated with a single gutta-percha cone that is designed to match the size and taper of the canal preparation. For example, a canal prepared to a master apical file of size 40/.04 would be obturated with a single gutta-percha master cone of size 40/.04. Some clinicians advocate using a master cone one size smaller than the master apical file size. The advantages of this technique are time efficiency and length control. The main disadvantage is that the gutta-percha does not adapt to an irregularly shaped canal and voids may be present along the length of the canal. The sealer is expected to fill any irregularities in the canal. The technique has been popularized in recent years in conjunction with the use of a bioceramic sealer. Despite the growing popularity of the single-cone technique, there is little clinical research published evaluating its use.[87]

Evaluation of Obturation

How Obturation Materials and Techniques Are Evaluated in Research

Obturation materials and techniques are commonly evaluated in research using in vitro studies.[88] The quality or density of fill created by different obturation methods can be compared by filling extracted or artificial teeth using different methods. The teeth are then sectioned at different levels of the root, and the cross-sectional areas filled by gutta-percha, sealer, or voids are measured.[72,81] Microcomputed tomography imaging may be used in similar studies, where three-dimensional volumetric measurements can be made both before and after obturation of the root canal system; the volume of filled space can then be measured.[89] Benchtop studies may also be used to investigate the fracture resistance of teeth or the presence of dentin microcracks after obturation with different methods or materials.[90] In vitro studies are also employed to assess the sealability of obturation techniques

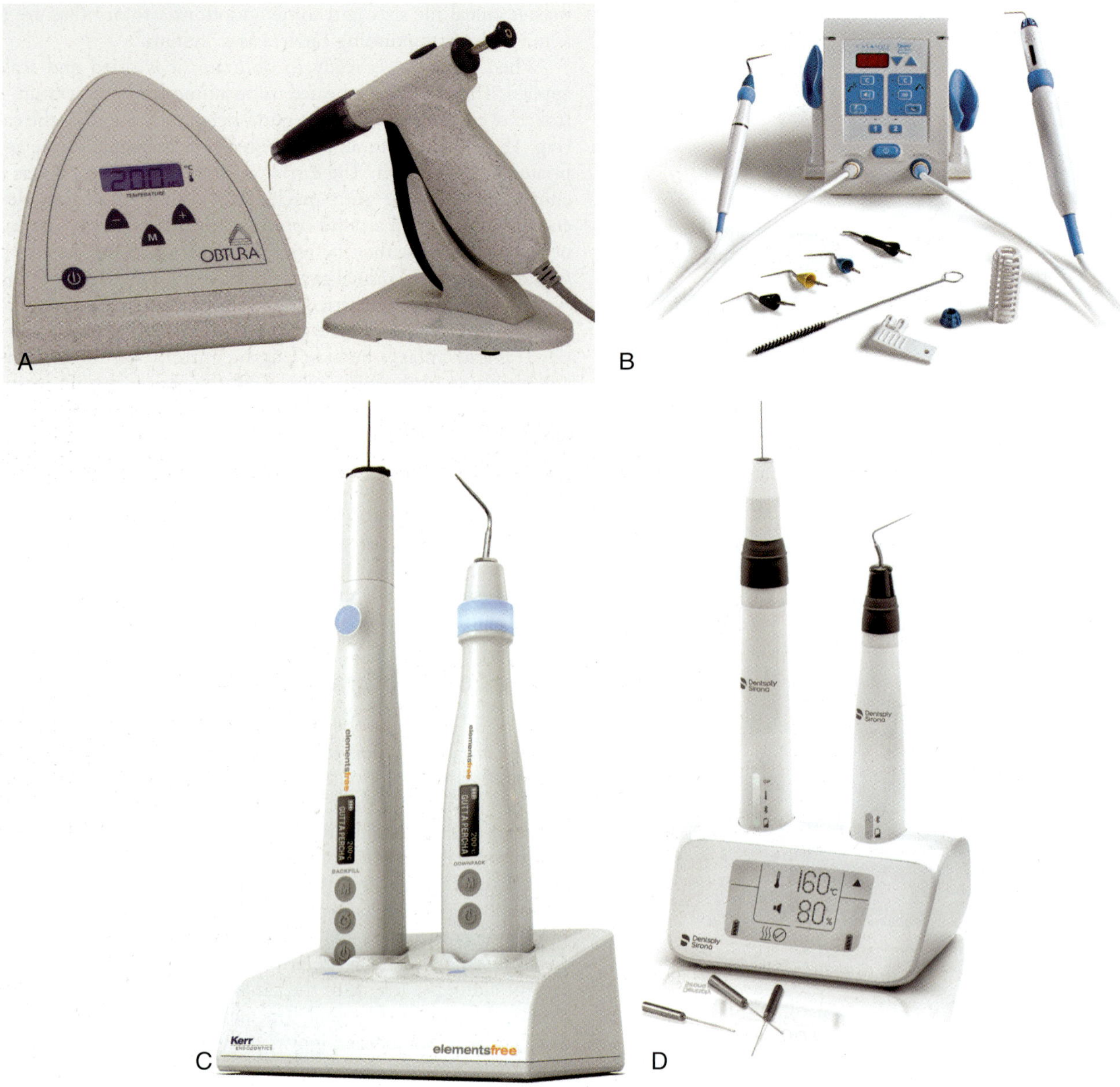

• **Fig. 15.21** Thermoplasticized gutta-percha injection systems. **(A)** The Obtura system uses pellets of gutta-percha, similar to a glue gun. (Courtesy Obtura Spartan.) **(B)** The Calamus Dual has both a heat source and a gutta-percha injection hand piece on one console. The gutta-percha handpiece utilizes cartridges of gutta-percha made to specifically fit in the handpiece. (Courtesy Dentsply Sirona.) **(C and D)** The Elements Free and Gutta Smart systems are cordless, and each has both a heat source handpiece and a gutta-percha injection handpiece with corresponding cartridges of gutta-percha made to fit each product. Both cordless hand pieces share a charging base in each system. (Courtesy Kerr Endodontics and Dentsply Sirona.)

or materials, where ability of bacteria to penetrate an obturated canal is measured.[91] Further, biocompatibility and antimicrobial effectiveness of obturation materials are also tested by in vitro cell culture and microbiologic research assays.[92-94]

How Obturation Is Evaluated Clinically—Radiographic Evaluation

In clinical cases, obturation is commonly evaluated using periapical radiographs. The length, taper, and density of obturation are assessed. Radiographic evidence of errors include obturation short or beyond the desired working length and voids in the obturation. Radiographic evaluation of a previously treated tooth may provide information about not only the quality of the previous treatment (e.g., presence of voids) but the type of filling material used (e.g., silver points have a different radiographic appearance compared with gutta-percha) (see Fig. 15.6). Cone beam computed tomography (CBCT) is not usually a helpful method to evaluate voids in obturation, as a result of the scatter produced by the obturation materials. However, the obturation observed on a CBCT image may show important information, such as when a canal has been missed or transported (Fig. 15.25).

It is important to understand that the obturation as assessed on a postoperative periapical radiograph may also reflect the quality

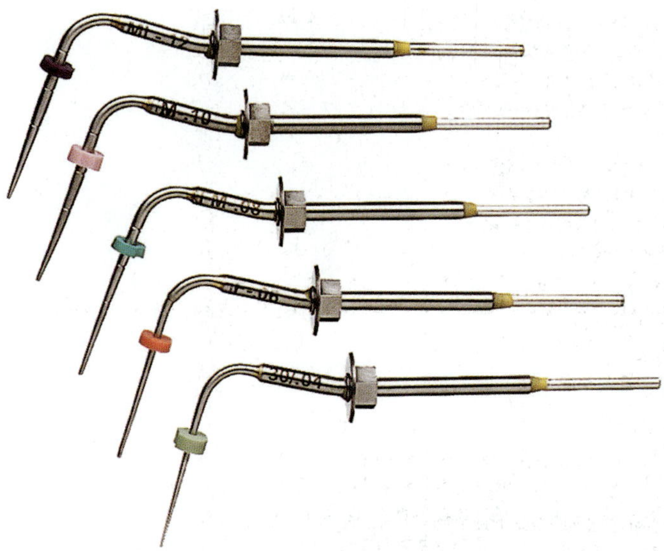

• **Fig. 15.22** Specialized heated pluggers available in a variety of tapers are advocated for use in the continuous wave of condensation technique. (Courtesy Kerr Endodontics.)

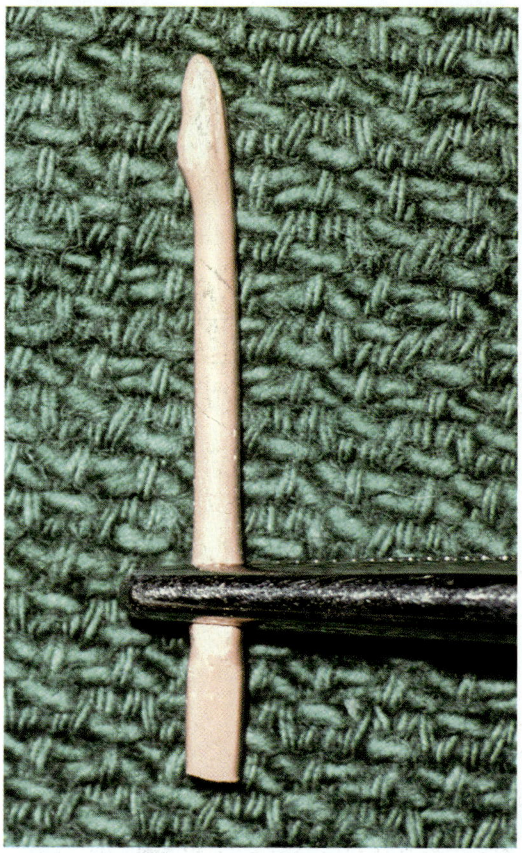

• **Fig. 15.23** The chloroform-dipped master gutta-percha cone is seated to working length and removed. The cone should show an impression of the apical preparation of the canal.

of instrumentation. That is, inadequate instrumentation will be manifest radiographically as inadequate obturation (e.g., a canal that has been instrumented short will also be filled short). In some cases, serial radiographs can be used to troubleshoot if an error occurred during instrumentation or obturation. For example, if a master cone radiograph shows the cone short of working length,

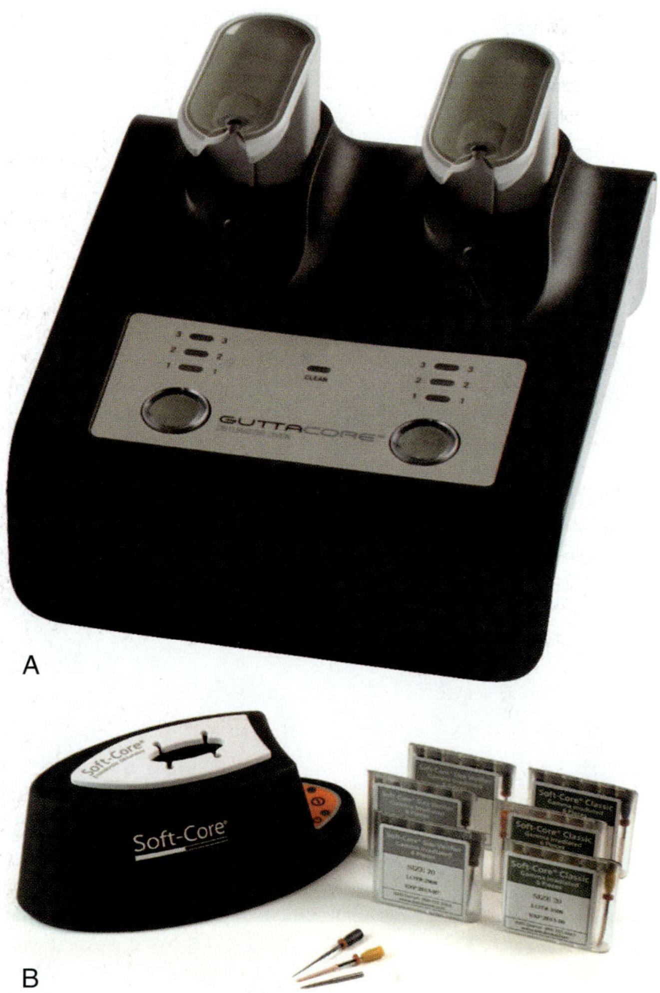

• **Fig. 15.24** Specialized ovens are used to heat obturators, softening the gutta-percha surrounding the core. **(A)** The GuttaCore oven is marketed for use with GuttaCore obturators and has two arms that are pressed down to move the obturator into the heating chamber. (Courtesy Dentsply Sirona.) **(B)** The Soft-Core Heater is marketed for use with Soft-Core obturators and holds up to four obturators at once. (Courtesy Kerr Endodontics.)

but the master apical file radiograph shows the master file to the correct working length, this indicates an obturation error. However, if the master apical file radiograph also shows the file short of working length, this indicates an instrumentation error.

The ideal research design to compare obturation techniques or materials would be a prospective, randomized clinical trial evaluating the outcomes of endodontic treatment after the use of two different techniques or materials. Unfortunately, such outcomes studies do not exist in the endodontic literature and are unlikely to be conducted. The feasibility of such research is poor as a result of the very large sample size needed to have adequate power to detect small differences in outcomes and poor recall rates, especially long-term recall rates needed to obtain valuable data. The outcomes studies available in the literature largely report outcomes of a specific technique, or show no significant difference between contemporary obturation techniques.[69,70,87]

Length of Obturation—Outcomes Studies

The ideal length to which canals should obturated has long been a subject of debate in endodontics.[95] The level of obturation should

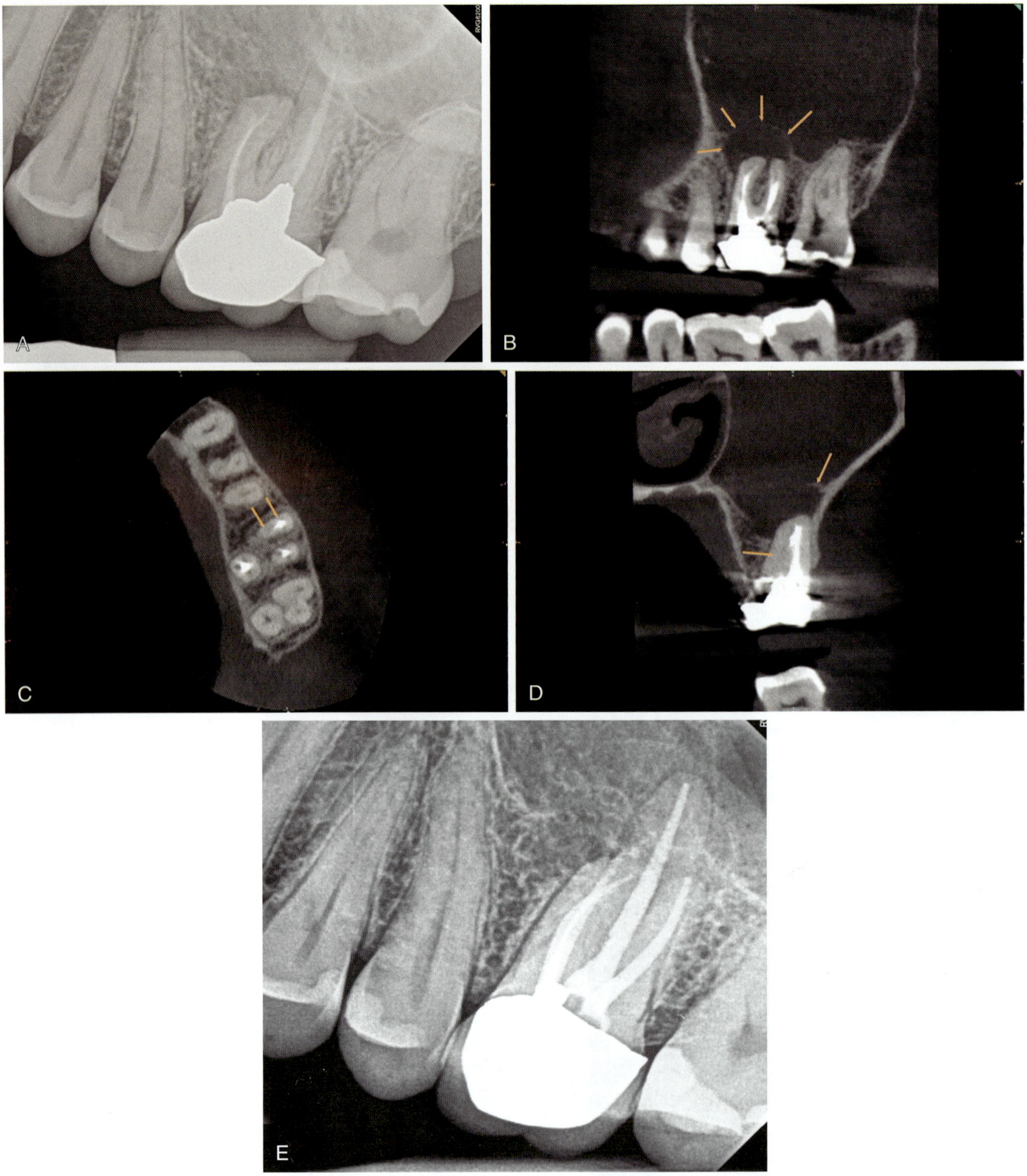

• **Fig. 15.25** This patient presented with pain in the maxillary left posterior and percussion sensitivity on tooth #14. **(A)** The preoperative periapical radiograph shows that tooth #14 has been previously endodontically treated, and the obturation of the MB root appears short. **(B)** The sagittal view of the CBCT image shows a large periapical radiolucency. **(C and D)** Both the axial and coronal views show a missed MB2 canal. **(E)** The postoperative radiograph after nonsurgical retreatment shows two canals treated in the MB root. *MB*, Mesiobuccal; *CBCT*, cone beam computed tomography. (Courtesy Dr. Randy Ball.)

be consistent with the level of instrumentation. Clinicians' preferences vary between treating to the radiographic apex or the "foramen" reading on an electronic apex locator, or 0.5 to 1 mm short of one of these levels. The rationale for instrumenting and obturating to a longer length is to ensure that the most apical extent of the canal has been cleaned. The rationale for instrumenting and obturating to a shorter length is to preserve the integrity of the periapical tissues and avoid debris extrusion or overfilling the canal.

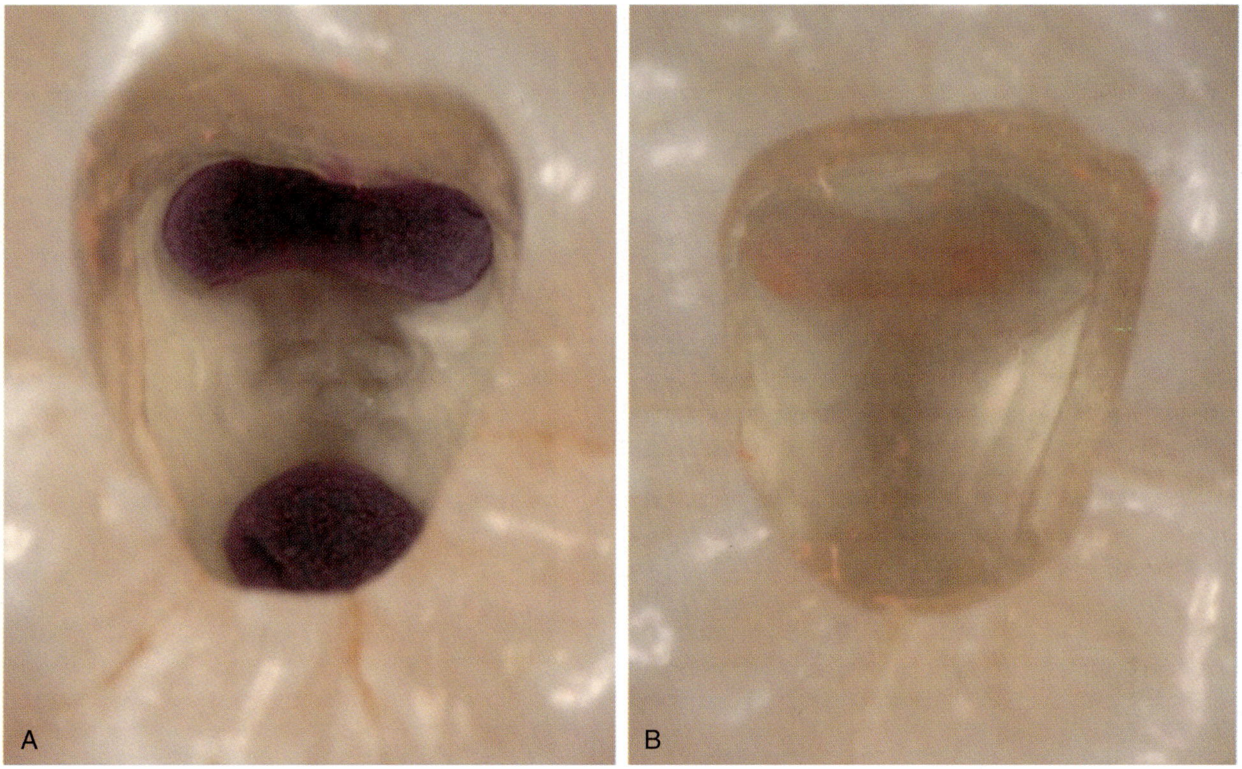

• **Fig. 15.26** Intraorifice barrier materials are placed in the coronal 1 to 2 mm of the canal. **(A)** PermaFlo Purple flowable composite orifice barrier. The purple color is easily distinguished from dentin. **(B)** Vitrebond glass ionomer intraorifice barrier. (Courtesy Dr. Scott Starley.)

Several outcomes studies have investigated the influence of the level of obturation on treatment success. Research supports improved outcomes of root canal therapy when the canal is filled 0 to 2 mm from the radiographic apex.[96-98] In a prospective study of the factors affecting outcomes of nonsurgical root canal treatment, the extension of canal cleaning as close as possible to the apical terminus significantly improved periapical healing.[69] In a systematic review, root filling extending to within 2 mm of the radiographic apex significantly improved the outcome of root canal treatment.[99] These studies do not assess obturation level in more detail than the 0 to 2 mm range, and debate still exists as to the ideal instrumentation and obturation length within that range.

Temporization

Intraorifice Barriers

The success of endodontic therapy depends on removal of bacteria from the root canal system and preventing recontamination. Coronal leakage occurs when microorganisms enter the root canal from a coronal direction and is a major cause of failure of endodontic treatment.[1] Bacteria and their byproducts may then permeate the root canal system and extend into the periradicular tissues, resulting in sequelae that include symptomatic or asymptomatic apical periodontitis, acute or chronic apical abscess formation, and/or pain. Further treatment is then needed (retreatment, endodontic surgery, or extraction). Recontamination of the root canal system after endodontic therapy may occur if there is a delay in placing the permanent restoration, breakdown of the temporary restoration seal, recurrent caries, leaky margins, and/or fracture or loss of the restoration or tooth structure. Research has shown that leakage can occur through the obturated root canal system in a relatively short amount of time[100-103] (Question 15.10).

To prevent coronal leakage and subsequent failure of the root canal treatment, intraorifice barriers (also referred to as orifice barriers) are often placed coronal to the root canal filling material.[104] Many dental materials have been investigated as intraorifice barriers, but glass ionomer and flowable composite resin are the most widely used in clinical practice. As obturation is completed, the gutta-percha is removed to a level 1 to 2 mm apical to the facial cementoenamel junction or the floor of the chamber in a molar. Any excess sealer and debris is removed from the chamber, typically using alcohol-soaked cotton pellets. The chamber is dried. The intraorifice barrier material is applied in the coronal 1 to 2 mm of the canal using the recommended instructions for the chosen material (Fig. 15.26). In some cases, the chamber floor is also covered (Fig. 15.27).

Temporary Filling Materials

As stated previously, prevention of coronal leakage is an important factor in successful endodontic outcomes. The choice of an interim restoration material to seal the access preparation, either between endodontic appointments or between completion of root canal therapy and the definitive restoration, is an integral part of a successful endodontic outcome. Temporization may be relatively straightforward, as in the case of a single-surface occlusal or lingual access preparation. Temporization may also be more challenging and time-consuming, as in the case of a tooth with extensive caries and/or defective restorations that must be removed before endodontic treatment. If one or more proximal surfaces of the tooth are missing after removal of caries and/or

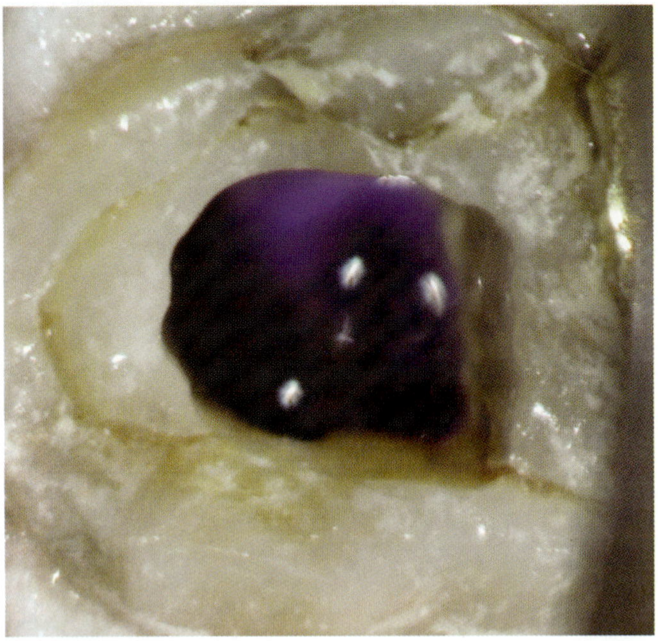

• **Fig. 15.27** Intraorifice barrier that covers the entire pulp chamber floor in a molar. This approach would seal the root canals and any furcation canals against leakage.

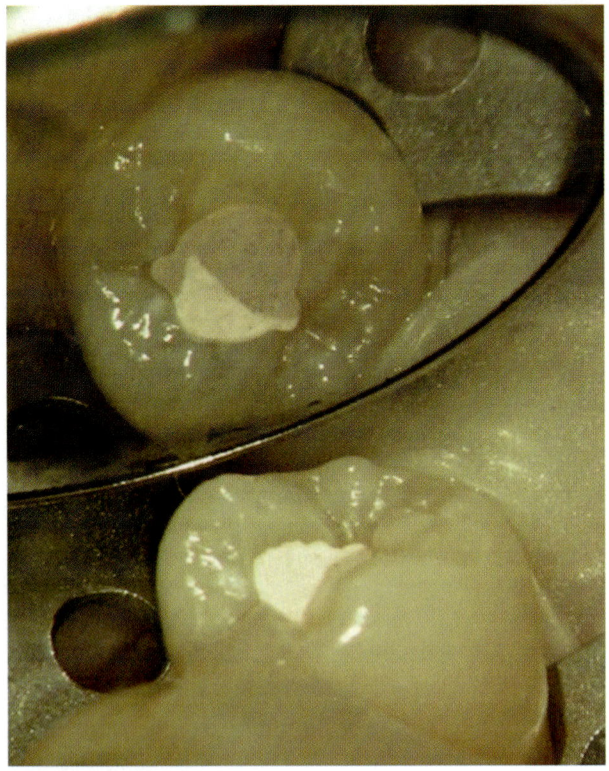

• **Fig. 15.28** Occlusal access cavity filled with Cavit as a temporary restoration on a mandibular premolar.

defective restorations, it may be necessary to restore the tooth with a temporary buildup material, either at the start of treatment or at the end of the appointment. If adequate isolation is not achievable after caries removal, then the tooth must be built up before continuing with root canal therapy. This allows for easier isolation of the tooth and prevention of salivary contamination when the caries are deep. It also allows for the ideal access preparation to create a reservoir to contain irrigant during treatment. The decision to wait until the end of the appointment to build up the missing walls has the advantage of saving time at the beginning of the appointment. This approach may also allow more light into the access for better visibility, and in some cases, it may make it easier for the clinician to insert files into the tooth during treatment (e.g., in the case of a missing mesial wall of a maxillary molar).

Cavit (ESPE, Seefeld, Germany) is a very popular temporary filling material that has been found to prevent leakage in numerous studies when used to close endodontic access preparations.[105-112] Cavit is premixed and is easily introduced into the access cavity, as well as easy to remove from the access cavity at the subsequent appointment (Fig. 15.28). Cavit contains zinc oxide, calcium sulfate, zinc sulfate, glycol acetate, polyvinyl acetate resin, polyvinylchloride-acetate, triethanolamine, and red pigment.[105] The calcium sulfate is hydrophilic, causing the hydroscopic expansion of the material. This absorption of moisture and expansion causes the Cavit to seal very well as it sets in a moist environment. A depth of at least 3.5 mm of Cavit is needed to adequately seal an access preparation.[113]

TERM (Dentsply Sirona, York, PA/L.D. Caulk Division, Milford, DE) is a composite resin interim restorative material for endodontics. It is a visible light cured resin containing urethane dimethacrylate polymers, inorganic radiopaque filler, pigments, and initiators.[105] If 3.5 mm of space does not exist for a temporary filling material, TERM may provide a superior temporary restoration to Cavit. TERM provides an adequate seal at 1, 2, 3, and 4 mm.[114] REVOTEK LC (GC Corporation, Tokyo, Japan), Tempit (Centrix, Milford, CT), and Systemp inlay (Vivadent, Schaan, Liechtenstein) are also temporary filling materials that have been reported to have good antibacterial and sealing qualities[115] (Fig. 15.29).

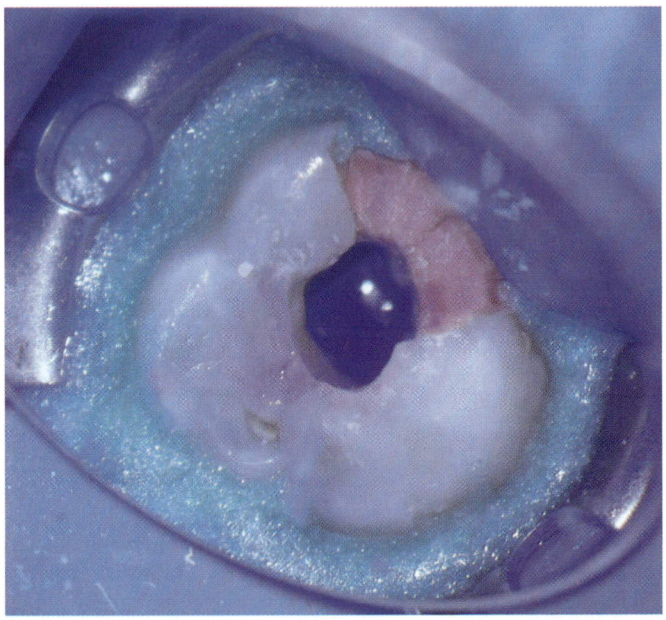

• **Fig. 15.29** Tooth #15 was diagnosed with symptomatic irreversible pulpitis and symptomatic apical periodontitis. The tooth had deep mesial recurrent caries, which needed to be removed before root canal therapy. A temporary buildup was completed using Fuji TRIAGE glass ionomer, to facilitate isolation during root canal therapy. PermaFlo Purple covers the pulp chamber floor as an intraorifice barrier after the completion of obturation. (Courtesy Dr. Kyle Countryman.)

Study Questions

6. What are the advantages and disadvantages of lateral condensation as an obturation technique?
7. What are the advantages and disadvantages of warm vertical condensation as an obturation technique?
8. In what cases would a custom formed gutta-percha master cone be indicated?
9. What are the advantages and disadvantages of carrier-based obturation?
10. Why must coronal leakage be prevented after root canal therapy?

ANSWERS

Answer Box 15

1 a. The objective of obturation is to create a seal along the length of the root canal system to prevent leakage of microorganisms and their byproducts into the root canal system

2 a. The rationale for completing root canal therapy in two visits is to allow time for an intracanal medicament to aid disinfection of the root canal system between visits.

3 a. The smear layer is removed because it may contain microorganisms and their byproducts and because it may prevent adhesion of filling materials to the dentin walls.

4 a. Advantages of gutta-percha include its biocompatibility, plasticity, handling characteristics, and ability to be removed from the root canal system if needed

5 a. Sealer is used with gutta-percha to help create an adequate seal in the root canal system

6 a. Advantages of lateral condensation are that it is appropriate for use by novice clinicians in a variety of cases. Lateral condensation also is less technique-sensitive than some techniques, has predictable length control, does not require specialized equipment, and has a track record of clinical success. Disadvantages of lateral condensation are that it requires more time than some filling techniques and is difficult to use in some cases with challenging anatomye

7 a. An advantage of warm vertical condensation is that warmed gutta-percha is adapted to the canal walls, which is particularly useful in some irregularly-shaped canals. Disadvantages of warm vertical condensation are that it is more technique-sensitive than some techniques, has less predictable length control, requires additional equipment, and is difficult to visualize within the canal without adequate magnification and lighting

8 a. A formed gutta-percha master cone is useful in cases with a large apical foramen, an irregularly shaped apical preparation, lack of an apical stop, or as a trouble-shooting technique when the master cone is not seating as expected.

9 a. Advantages of carrier-based obturation are time efficiency and the ability of warmed gutta-percha to fill canal irregularities. Disadvantages of carrier-based obturation are length control, stripping gutta-percha off the carrier during seating, and difficult post space preparation and retreatment

10 c. Coronal leakage must be prevented because it allows recontamination of the root canal system with microorganisms and is a major cause of endodontic treatment failure.

References

1. Gillen BM, Looney SW, Gu LS, et al.: Impact of the quality of coronal restoration versus the quality of root canal fillings on success of root canal treatment: a systematic review and meta-analysis, *J Endod* 37(7):895–902, 2011.
2. Klevant FJ, Eggink CO: The effect of canal preparation on periapical disease, *Int Endodontic J* 16(2):68–75, 1983.
3. Fabricius L, Dahlen G, Sundqvist G, Happonen RP, Moller AJ: Influence of residual bacteria on periapical tissue healing after chemomechanical treatment and root filling of experimentally infected monkey teeth, *Eur J Oral Sci* 114(4):278–285, 2006.
4. Sjogren U, Figdor D, Persson S, Sundqvist G: Influence of infection at the time of root filling on the outcome of endodontic treatment of teeth with apical periodontitis, *Int Endodontic J* 30(5):297–306, 1997.
5. Manfredi M, Figini L, Gagliani M, Lodi G: Single versus multiple visits for endodontic treatment of permanent teeth, *Cochrane Database Syst Rev* 12:CD005296, 2016.
6. Schwendicke F, Gostemeyer G: Single-visit or multiple-visit root canal treatment: systematic review, meta-analysis and trial sequential analysis, *BMJ Open* 7(2):e013115, 2017.
7. De-Deus G, Canabarro A: Strength of recommendation for single-visit root canal treatment: grading the body of the evidence using a patient-centred approach, *Int Endodontic J* 50(3):251–259, 2017.
8. Violich DR, Chandler NP: The smear layer in endodontics - a review, *Int Endodontic J* 43(1):2–15, 2010.
9. Haapasalo M, Shen Y, Wang Z, Gao Y: Irrigation in endodontics, *Br Dent J* 216(6):299–303, 2014.
10. Grossman LI, Oliet S, Del Rio CE: *Endodontic practice*, Philadelphia, 1988, Lea & Febiger.
11. Grossman LI: Endodontics 1776-1976: a bicentennial history against the background of general dentistry, *J Am Dent Assoc* 93:78–87, 1976.
12. Keane HC: *A century of service to dentistry*, Philadelphia, 1944, S.S. White Dental Manufacturing Co.
13. Friedman CM, Sandrik JL, Heuer MA, Rapp GW: Composition and mechanical properties of gutta-percha endodontic points, *J Dent Res* 54(5):921–925, 1975.
14. Bunn CW: Molecular structure of rubber-like elasticity. Part I: the crystal structure of gutta-percha, rubber and polychloroprene, *Proc R Soc Lond (Biol)* 80:40, 1942.
15. Marciano J, Michailesco P, Abadie MJ: Stereochemical structure characterization of dental gutta-percha, *J Endod* 19(1):31–34, 1993.
16. Costa GE, Johnson JD, Hamilton RG: Cross-reactivity studies of gutta-percha, gutta-balata, and natural rubber latex (Hevea brasiliensis), *J Endod* 27(9):584–587, 2001.
17. Hamann C, Rodgers PA, Alenius H, Halsey JF, Sullivan K: Cross-reactivity between gutta-percha and natural latex: assumption vs. reality, *J Am Dent Assoc* 133:1357–1367, 2002.
18. Marciano J, Michailesco P, Charpentier E, Carrera LC, Abadie MJ: Thermomechanical analysis of dental gutta-percha, *J Endod* 18(6):263–270, 1992.
19. Schilder H, Goodman A, Aldrich W: The thermomechanical properties of gutta-percha. I. The compressibility of gutta-percha, *Oral Surg Oral Med Oral Pathol* 37(6):946–953, 1974.
20. Goodman A, Schilder H, Aldrich W: The thermomechanical properties of gutta-percha. II. The history and molecular chemistry of gutta-percha, *Oral Surg Oral Med Oral Pathol* 37(6):954–961, 1974.
21. Schilder H, Goodman A, Aldrich W: The thermomechanical properties of gutta-percha. III. Determination of phase transition temperatures for gutta-percha, *Oral Surg Oral Med Oral Pathol* 38(1):109–114, 1974.
22. Schilder H, Goodman A, Aldrich W: The thermomechanical properties of gutta-percha. Part V. Volume changes in bulk gutta-percha as a function of temperature and its relationship to molecular phase transformation, *Oral Surg Oral Med Oral Pathol* 59(3):285–296, 1985.
23. Chogle S, Mickel AK, Huffaker SK, Neibaur B: An in vitro assessment of iodoform gutta-percha, *J Endod* 31:814–816, 2005.
24. Holland R, Murata SS, Dezan E, Garlipp O: Apical leakage after root canal filling with an experimental calcium hydroxide gutta-percha point, *J Endod* 22:71–73, 1996.

25. Lin S, Levin L, Weiss EI, Peled M, Fuss Z: In vitro antibacterial efficacy of a new chlorhexidine slow-release device, *Quintessence Int* 37(5):391–394, 2006.
26. Podbielski A, Boeckh C, Haller B: Growth inhibitory activity of gutta-percha points containing root canal medications on common endodontic bacterial pathogens as determined by an optimized in vitro assay, *J Endod* 26:398–403, 2000.
27. Melker KB, Vertucci FJ, Rojas MF, Progulske-Fox A, Belanger M: Antimicrobial efficacy of medicated root canal filling materials, *J Endod* 32(2):148–151, 2006.
28. Parirokh M, Torabinejad M, Dummer PMH: Mineral trioxide aggregate and other bioactive endodontic cements: an updated overview - part I: vital pulp therapy, *Int Endodontic J* 51(2):177–205, 2018.
29. Torabinejad M, Parirokh M, Dummer PMH: Mineral trioxide aggregate and other bioactive endodontic cements: an updated overview - part II: other clinical applications and complications, *Int Endodontic J* 51(3):284–317, 2018.
30. American Association of Endodontists: *Endodontic case difficulty assessment form and guidelines*. Available from www.aae.org.
31. American Association of Endodontists: *Endodontic case difficulty assessment and referral. endodontics: colleagues for excellence*, Chicago, IL, 2005, American Association of Endodontists.
32. Seltzer S, Green DB, Weiner N, DeRensis F: A scanning EM examination of silver cones removed from endodontically treated teeth, *Oral Surg* 33:589–605, 1972.
33. Brady JM, Del Rio CE: Corrosion of endodontic silver cones in humans: a scanning electron microscope and X-ray microprobe study, *J Endod* 1(6):205–210, 1975.
34. Goldberg F: Relationship between corroded silver points and endodontic failure, *J Endod* 7:224–227, 1981.
35. Gutierrez JH, Villena F, Gigoux C, Mujica F: Microscope and scanning electron microscope examination of silver points corrosion caused by endodontic materials, *J Endod* 8:301–311, 1982.
36. Kehoe JC: Intracanal corrosion of a silver cone producing localized argyria, *J Endod* 10:199–201, 1984.
37. American Association of Endodontists: *Use of silver points: AAE position statement*. Available from https://www.aae.org/specialty/wp-content/uploads/sites/2/2017/06/silverpointsstatement.pdf 2017.
38. Tay FR, Pashley DH, Yiu CK, et al.: Susceptibility of a polycaprolactone-based root canal filling material to degradation. II. Gravimetric evaluation of enzymatic hydrolysis, *J Endod* 31:737–741, 2005.
39. Tay FR, Pashley DH, Williams MC, et al.: Susceptibility of a polycaprolactone-based root canal filling material to degradation. I. Alkaline hydrolysis, *J Endod* 31(8):593–598, 2005.
40. Tay FR, Loushine RJ, Weller RN, et al.: Ultrastructural evaluation of the apical seal in roots filled with a polycaprolactone-based root canal filling material, *J Endod* 31:514–519, 2005.
41. Tay FR, Loushine RJ, Monticelli F, et al.: Effectiveness of resin-coated gutta-percha cones and a dual-cured, hydrophilic methacrylate resin-based sealer in obturating root canals, *J Endod* 31:659–664, 2005.
42. Tay FR, Hiraishi N, Pashley DH, et al.: Bondability of Resilon to a methacrylate-based root canal sealer, *J Endod* 32(2):133–137, 2006.
43. Gesi A, Raffaelli O, Goracci C, Pashley DH, Tay FR, Ferrari M: Interfacial strength of Resilon and gutta-percha to intraradicular dentin, *J Endod* 31:809–813, 2005.
44. Barborka BJ, Woodmansey KF, Glickman GN, Schneiderman E, He J: Long-term clinical outcome of teeth obturated with Resilon, *J Endod* 43(4):556–560, 2017.
45. Orstavik D: Materials used for root canal obturation: technical, biological and clinical testing, *Endod Topics* 12:25–38, 2005.
46. Schwandt NW, Gound TG: Resourcinol-formaldehyde resin "Russian Red" endodontic therapy, *J Endod* 29:435–437, 2003.
47. Huang FM, Tai K-W, Chou M-Y, Chang Y-C: Cytotoxicity of resin-, zinc oxide-eugenol, and calcium hydroxide-based root canal sealers on human periodontal ligament cells and permanent V79 cells, *Int Endod J* 35:153–158, 2002.
48. England MC, West NM, Safavi K, Green DB: Tissue lead levels in dogs with RC-2B root canal fillings, *J Endod* 6:728–730, 1980.
49. Hauman CH, Love RM: Biocompatibility of dental materials used in contemporary endodontic therapy: a review. Part 2. Root canal filling materials, *Int Endod J* 36(3):147–160, 2003.
50. Spangberg LS: Biologic effects of root-canal-filling materials. The effect on bone tissue of two formaldehyde-containing root canal pastes: N2 and Riebler's paste, *Oral Surg Oral Med Oral Pathol* 38:934–944, 1974.
51. Spangberg LS, Langeland K: Biologic effects of dental materials. I. Toxicity of root-canal-filling materials on HeLa cells *in vitro*, *Oral Surg Oral Med Oral Pathol* 35:402–414, 1973.
52. FDA explains status of N2 material, *J Am Dent Assoc* 123(7):236–237, 1992.
53. Council on Dental Therapeutics ADA: The use of root canal filling materials containing paraformaldehyde: a status report, *J Am Dent Assoc* 114:95, 1987.
54. American Association of Endodontists: *Concerning paraformaldehyde-containing endodontic filling materials and sealers: AAE position statement*. Available from https://www.aae.org/specialty/wp-content/uploads/sites/2/2017/06/paraformaldehydefillingmaterials.pdf 2017.
55. Block RM, Lewis RD, Sheats JB, Burke SH: Antibody formation to dog pulp tissue altered by N2-type paste within the root canal, *J Endod* 8:309–315, 1977.
56. Block RM, Sheats JB, Lewis RD, Fawley J: Cell-mediated response to dog pulp tissue altered by N2 paste within the root canal, *Oral Surg Oral Med Oral Pathol* 45:131–142, 1978.
57. Block RM, Lewis RB, Sheats JB, Fawley J: Cell-mediated immune response to dog pulp tissue altered by Kerr (Rickert's) sealer via the root canal, *J Endod* 4:110–116, 1978.
58. Torabinejad M, Kettering JD, Bakland LK: Evaluation of systemic immunological reactions to AH-26 root canal sealer, *J Endod* 5:196–200, 1979.
59. Harnden DG: Tests for carcinogenicity and mutagenicity, *Int Endod J* 14:35–40, 1981.
60. Lewis BB, Chestner SB: Formaldehyde in dentistry: a review of the mutagenic and carcinogenic potential, *J Am Dent Assoc* 103:429–434, 1981.
61. Grossman LI: *Endodontic practice*, ed 10, Philadelphia, 1982, Lea & Febiger, p 297.
62. Ingle JI, Newton CW, West JD, et al.: Obturation of the radicular space. In Ingle JI, Bakland LK, editors: *Endodontics*, ed 5, Hamilton, London BC, 2002, Decker Inc.
63. Martin H, Martin TR: Iodoform gutta-percha: MGP a new endodontic paradigm, *Dent Today* 18:76, 1999.
64. Sleder FS, Lumley PJ, Bohacek JR: Long-term sealing ability of a calcium hydroxide sealer, *J Endod* 17:541–543, 1991.
65. Spangberg LS, Barbosa SV, Lavigne GD: AH 26 releases formaldehyde, *J Endod* 19:596–598, 1993.
66. Leonardo MR, da Silva LAB, Filho MT, da Silva RS: Release of formaldehyde by 4 endodontic sealers, *Oral Surg Oral Med Oral Pathol Oral Radiol Endod* 88:221–225, 1999.
67. Whitworth J: Methods of filling root canals: principles and practices, *Endod Topics* 12:2–24, 2005.
68. Orstavik D: Physical properties of root canal sealers: measurement of flow, working time, and compressive strength, *Int Endod J* 16(3):99–107, 1983.
69. Ng YL, Mann V, Gulabivala K: A prospective study of the factors affecting outcomes of nonsurgical root canal treatment: part 1: periapical health, *Int Endodontic J* 44(7):583–609, 2011.
70. Peng L, Ye L, Tan H, Zhou X: Outcome of root canal obturation by warm gutta-percha versus cold lateral condensation: a meta-analysis, *J Endod* 33(2):106–109, 2007.
71. American Association of Endodontists Predoctoral Directors Workshop. Unpublished data. Chicago, IL, 2012.
72. Kececi AD, Unal GC, Sen BH: Comparison of cold lateral compaction and continuous wave of obturation techniques following manual or rotary instrumentation, *Int Endodontic J* 38(6):381–388, 2005.

73. American Dental Association: *Revised American National Standard/ American Dental Association Standard No. 78 Dental Obturating Cones*, 2013.
74. Wilson BL, Baumgartner JC: Comparison of spreader penetration during lateral compaction of .04 and .02 tapered gutta-percha, *J Endod* 29(12):828–831, 2003.
75. Lertchirakarn V, Palamara JEA, Messer HH: Load and strain during lateral condensation and vertical root fracture, *J Endodont* 25(2):99–104, 1999.
76. Schmidt KJ, Walker TL, Johnson JD, Nicoll BK: Comparison of nickel-titanium and stainless-steel spreader penetration and accessory cone fit in curved canals, *J Endod* 26(1):42–44, 2000.
77. Holcomb JQ, Pitts DL, Nicholls JI: Further investigation of spreader loads required to cause vertical root fracture during lateral condensation, *J Endod* 13(6):277–284, 1987.
78. Pitts DL, Matheny HE, Nicholls JI: An in vitro study of spreader loads required to cause vertical root fracture during lateral condensation, *J Endod* 9(12):544–550, 1983.
79. Schilder H: Filling root canals in three dimensions, *Dent Clin North Am*723–744, 1967.
80. Schilder H: Filling root canals in three dimensions, *J Endod* 32(4):281–290, 2006.
81. Peters CI, Sonntag D, Peters OA: Homogeneity of root canal fillings performed by undergraduate students with warm vertical and cold lateral techniques, *Oral Surg Oral Med Oral Pathol Oral Radiol Endod* 110(3):e41–e49, 2010.
82. Lee FS, Van Cura JE, BeGole E: A comparison of root surface temperatures using different obturation heat sources, *J Endod* 24(9):617–620, 1998.
83. Lipski M: Root surface temperature rises during root canal obturation, in vitro, by the continuous wave of condensation technique using System B HeatSource, *Oral Surg Oral Med Oral Pathol Oral Radiol Endod* 99(4):505–510, 2005.
84. Buchanan LS: Continuous wave of condensation technique, *Endod Prac* 1(4):7–10, 1998. 13–16, 18 passim.
85. Mirfendereski M, Roth K, Fan B, et al.: Technique acquisition in the use of two thermoplasticized root filling methods by inexperienced dental students: a microcomputed tomography analysis, *J Endod* 35(11):1512–1517, 2009.
86. Wong AW, Zhang S, Li SK, Zhang C, Chu CH: Clinical studies on core-carrier obturation: a systematic review and meta-analysis, *BMC Oral Health* 17(1):167, 2017.
87. Chybowski EA, Glickman GN, Patel Y, Fleury A, Solomon E, He J: Clinical outcome of non-surgical root canal treatment using a single-cone technique with endosequence bioceramic sealer: a retrospective analysis, *J Endod* 44(6):941–945, 2018.
88. Silva Almeida LH, Moraes RR, Morgental RD, Pappen FG: Are premixed calcium silicate-based endodontic sealers comparable to conventional materials? A systematic review of in vitro studies, *J Endod* 43(4):527–535, 2017.
89. Keles A, Alcin H, Kamalak A, Versiani MA: Micro-CT evaluation of root filling quality in oval-shaped canals, *Int Endodontic J* 47(12):1177–1184, 2014.
90. De-Deus G, Belladonna FG, Silva E, et al.: Micro-CT assessment of dentinal micro-cracks after root canal filling procedures, *Int Endodontic J* 50(9):895–901, 2017.
91. Tasdemir T, Er K, Yildirim T, et al.: Comparison of the sealing ability of three filling techniques in canals shaped with two different rotary systems: a bacterial leakage study, *Oral Surg Oral Med Oral Pathol Oral Radiol Endod* 108(3):e129–e134, 2009.
92. Poggio C, Riva P, Chiesa M, Colombo M, Pietrocola G: Comparative cytotoxicity evaluation of eight root canal sealers, *J Clin Exp Dent* 9(4):e574–e578, 2017.
93. Collado-Gonzalez M, Garcia-Bernal D, Onate-Sanchez RE, et al.: Biocompatibility of three new calcium silicate-based endodontic sealers on human periodontal ligament stem cells, *Int Endodontic J* 50(9):875–884, 2017.
94. Kapralos V, Koutroulis A, Orstavik D, Sunde PT, Rukke HV: Antibacterial activity of endodontic sealers against planktonic bacteria and bacteria in biofilms, *J Endod* 44(1):149–154, 2018.
95. Mounce RE: Mothers, pulp lovers, and apical barbarians, *Dent Today* 22(8):58–60, 2003.
96. Orstavik D, Qvist V, Stoltze K: A multivariate analysis of the outcome of endodontic treatment, *Eur J Oral Sci* 112(3):224–230, 2004.
97. Sjogren U, Hagglund B, Sundqvist G, Wing K: Factors affecting the long-term results of endodontic treatment, *J Endod* 16(10):498–504, 1990.
98. Peak JD, Hayes SJ, Bryant ST, Dummer PM: The outcome of root canal treatment. A retrospective study within the armed forces (Royal Air Force), *Br Dental J* 190(3):140–144, 2001.
99. Ng YL, Mann V, Rahbaran S, Lewsey J, Gulabivala K: Outcome of primary root canal treatment: systematic review of the literature — Part 2. Influence of clinical factors, *Int Endod J* 41(1):6–31, 2008.
100. Swanson K, Madison S: An evaluation of coronal microleakage in endodontically treated teeth. Part I. Time periods, *J Endod* 13:56–59, 1987.
101. Torabinejad M, Ung B, Kettering JD: In vitro bacterial penetration of coronally unsealed endodontically treated teeth, *J Endod* 16:556–559, 1990.
102. Magura ME, Kafrawy AH, Brown CE, Newton CW: Human saliva coronal microleakage in obturated root canals: an in vitro study, *J Endod* 17:324–331, 1991.
103. Khayat A, Lee SJ, Torabinejad M: Human saliva penetration of coronally unsealed obturated root canals, *J Endod* 19:458–461, 1993.
104. Wolcott JF, Hicks ML, Himel VT: Evaluation of pigmented intraorifice barriers in endodontically treated teeth, *J Endod* 25(9):589–592, 1999.
105. Barkhordar RA, Stark MM: Sealing ability of intermediate restorations and cavity design used in endodontics, *Oral Surg Oral Med Oral Pathol* 69(1):99–101, 1990.
106. Beach CW, Calhoun JC, Bramwell JD, Hutter JW, Miller GA: Clinical evaluation of bacterial leakage of endodontic temporary filling materials, *J Endod* 22(9):459–462, 1996.
107. Balto H: An assessment of microbial coronal leakage of temporary filling materials in endodontically treated teeth, *J Endod* 28:762–764, 2002.
108. Lee YC, Yang SF, Hwang YF, Chueh LH, Chung KH: Microleakage of endodontic temporary restorative materials, *J Endod* 19(10):516–520, 1993.
109. Noguera AP, McDonald NJ: A comparative in vitro coronal microleakage study of new endodontic restorative materials, *J Endod* 16:523–527, 1990.
110. Kazemi RB, Safavi KE, Spangberg LS: Assessment of marginal stability and permeability of an interim restorative endodontic material, *Oral Surg Oral Med Oral Pathol* 78(6):788–796, 1994.
111. Mayer T, Eickholz P: Microleakage of temporary restorations after thermocycling and mechanical loading, *J Endod* 23(5):320–322, 1997.
112. Teplitsky PE, Meimaris IT: Sealing ability of Cavit and TERM as intermediate restorative materials, *J Endod* 14:278–282, 1988.
113. Webber RT, del Rio CE, Brady JM, Segall RO: Sealing quality of a temporary filling material, *Oral Surg Oral Med Oral Pathol* 46(1):123–130, 1978.
114. Hansen SR, Montgomery S: Effect of restoration thickness on the sealing ability of TERM, *J Endod* 19(9):448–452, 1993.
115. Slutzky H, Slutzky-Goldberg I, Weiss EI, Matalon S: Antibacterial properties of temporary filling materials, *J Endod* 32(3):214–217, 2006.

16 Restoration of Endodontically Treated Teeth

BRIAN J. GOODACRE, SHANE N. WHITE, AND CHARLES J. GOODACRE

CHAPTER OUTLINE

LEARNING OBJECTIVES

After reading this chapter, the student should be able to:

1. Describe the main factors involved in the survival of root-filled teeth.
2. Summarize factors contributing to loss of tooth strength and describe the structural importance of remaining tooth tissue.
3. Explain the importance of a coronal seal and how it is achieved.
4. Describe the requirements of an adequate restoration.
5. Outline postoperative risks to the unrestored tooth.
6. Discuss the rationale for immediate restoration.
7. Identify restorative options before root canal treatment is started.
8. Discuss the advantages and disadvantages of direct and indirect restorations.
9. Outline indications for post placement in anterior and posterior teeth.
10. Describe common post systems and the advantages and disadvantages of each.
11. Describe core materials and their placement.
12. Describe techniques for restoring an access opening through an existing restoration.

Endodontic therapy is predictable. However, for success the teeth need to be restored to their previous form and function. Before endodontic therapy, restorability must be determined; this involves careful evaluation of the existing tooth structure, including removal of all caries along with any existing restorations, both to reduce the risk of marginal leakage during treatment[1] and to reveal the amount of sound tooth structure.[2] Specific restorative options must be evaluated based on functional demand and remaining tooth structure.[2,3] This chapter will discuss the considerations needed to properly restore endodontically treated teeth.

Criteria for a Restorable Tooth

A tooth must retain sufficient sound tooth structure after root canal therapy to allow predictable restoration. Evaluation of a tooth requires clinical, radiographic, and esthetic evaluation. The first step is to remove any existing caries and restorative materials. This process allows clear visualization of the remaining tooth structure and removes bacteria. A periodontal probe can be used to measure the height of the remaining tooth structure that will provide a ferrule; measure pocket depths, which can reveal periodontal status and possible signs of root fracture; and map the subgingival root morphology. A bitewing radiograph should be used to evaluate the remaining tooth structure, pulp chamber, and bone levels; and periapical radiographs should be used to evaluate tooth length and root morphology.

Amount of Remaining Coronal Tooth Structure

Most teeth requiring root canal treatment have been structurally compromised by caries and subsequent restorative procedures. Additional loss of tooth structure occurs during endodontic access, leading to further weakening of the tooth. When the access cavity

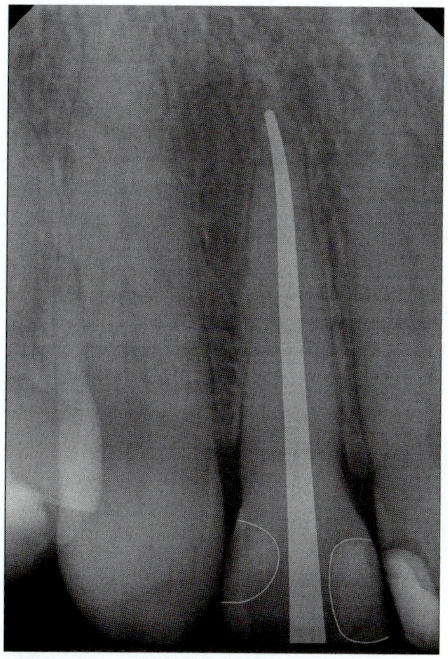

• **Fig. 16.1** Teeth requiring root canal treatment have commonly been structurally compromised by caries and restorative procedures. Endodontic access further compromises the tooth.

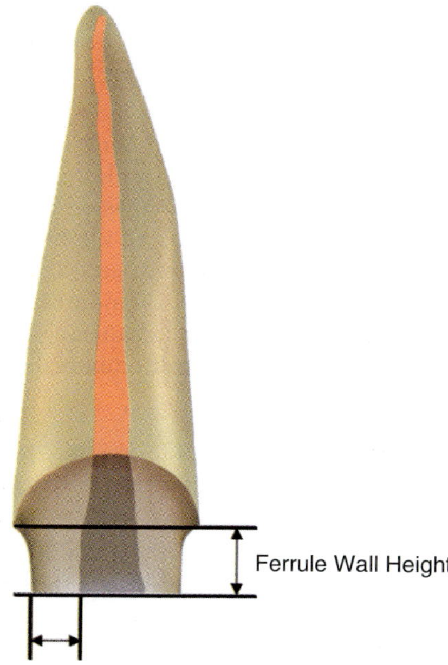

• **Fig. 16.2** Ferrule refers to the amount of cervical tooth structure available to resist tooth fracture and does not include any build-up material.

is surrounded by walls of dentin, it only has a minor weakening effect.[4] In a tooth already seriously compromised by caries, trauma, or large restorations, access preparation is more significant, particularly if some marginal ridges have been lost (Fig. 16.1).[5,6] Excessive coronal flaring of the access preparation also results in greater susceptibility to fracture.[7]

The formation of a ferrule around the remaining coronal tooth structure is important to prevent tooth fracture in endodontically treated teeth. Ferrule refers to the amount of cervical tooth structure, or the height of the remaining tooth structure under a crown, that is available to resist tooth fracture (Fig. 16.2). The more tooth structure present, the more resistant the tooth will be to fracture.

Ferrule Wall Height

The ferrule wall height is simply measured from the tooth preparation finish line to the coronal aspect of the remaining tooth structure.

The types of margin preparation or bevels on the remaining tooth structure are unimportant; the total height of the tooth structure is key.[8-12] The exact crown ferrule height required for success has been debated for many years; recommendations range from 1.0 mm to 3.0 mm heights.[10-14] We suggest that at least a 1.5 to 2.0 mm high circumferential wall of tooth structure be present above the crown finish line to ensure adequate fracture resistance and enhance the coronal seal provided by the final restoration (Fig. 16.3).

Ferrule Wall Thickness

Endodontic therapy requires the removal of tooth structure to gain access to the root canal system. The ferrule wall width refers to the amount of tooth structure remaining from the pulp chamber and/or access preparation to the external surface of the tooth. The amount of remaining ferrule wall thickness may be jeopardized by crown preparation. Decay and prior restoration may leave minimal ferrule wall thickness. The ability of a tooth to resist

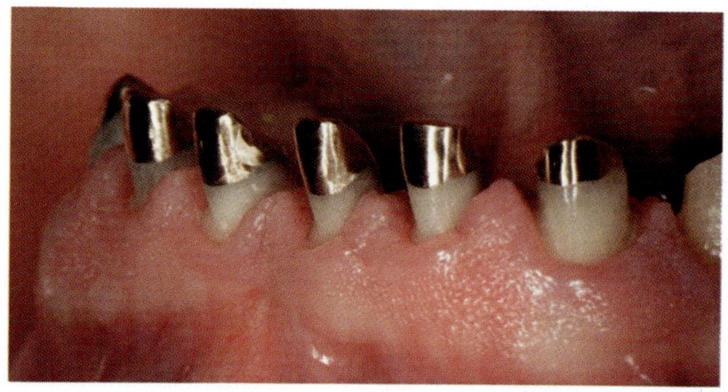

• **Fig. 16.3** Root canal–treated mandibular anterior teeth with a ferrule extending 2 mm beyond the core for optimal resistance to tooth fracture.

lateral forces is directly proportional to the thickness of remaining dentin.[15] More than 1.0 mm of dentin thickness around the root canal is needed for adequate resistance to fracture.[16-19]

Re-Establishing Coronal Tooth Structure

In a clinical situation where minimal tooth structure remains, the establishment of an adequate ferrule height can be challenging. In such situations, two factors are important to ensure success. First, it is important to reestablish a 1.5 mm to 2.0 mm ferrule and second to maintain the patient's biologic width. Biologic width refers to the junctional epithelium and connective tissue attachment present from the alveolar bone crest to the depth of the periodontal sulcus. It is suggested that the average biologic width is around 2 mm;[20] commonly the sulcus depth is also included in this measurement, resulting in a suggested measurement of 3 mm. However, the exact biologic width will vary from patient to patient. This suggests that approximately 5 mm of tooth height should remain coronal to the alveolar bone. When this is not available, height can be reestablished by means of surgical crown lengthening or orthodontic extrusion (see Chapter 21).

Surgical Crown Lengthening

Crown lengthening is a way to reestablish a ferrule by removing supporting periodontal structures to expose additional tooth structure. However, if a tooth has reduced bone support, short roots, a poor crown-to-root ratio, or if it could lead to an unacceptable esthetic result, crown lengthening would be contraindicated. [21] Additionally, the apical relocation of the finish line to a narrower part of the root exposes less cross-sectional area, predisposing to a weaker tooth[22] and potentially to furcation involvement. Therefore the ideal tooth for crown lengthening is a periodontally healthy, long, single rooted tooth, with minimal root taper.

Orthodontic Extrusion

Orthodontic extrusion involves the forced eruption of a tooth. The eruption must be performed using rapid orthodontic extrusion allowing only the movement of the tooth. If slow orthodontic extrusion is performed, coronal migration of the bone and gingiva occurs, thereby not allowing the formation of the desired ferrule. It is also suggested to perform supracrestal fiberotomy and root planning to help minimize the coronal migration of bone and gingival tissues when rapidly extruding a tooth.[23] Rapid orthodontic extrusion involves 1 to 3 weeks of activation followed by 8 to 12 weeks of retention of the tooth before starting restoration.[24] However, when extruding a tooth with tapered roots, not only is the bone support reduced, the cross-sectional area is reduced, making an esthetic and structurally sound restoration more difficult.

Complications Associated with Endodontically Treated Teeth

Although root canal treated teeth are at greater risk of extraction than vital teeth,[25] their long-term survival rate is very high. Numerous studies investigating the survival of endodontically treated teeth have documented that at most 1% to 2% are lost per year,[26-29] and one very large study of almost 1.5 million cases reported that only 2.9% were lost after 8 years.[28] A recent meta-analysis showed a mean tooth survival of 87% after 8 to 10 years.[26] Factors that affect the survival of root-filled teeth include:

1. *Caries and periodontal disease.* Caries and periodontal disease are responsible for up to half of all extractions of root-filled teeth.[30-32] Emerging evidence suggests that root-filled teeth may be more susceptible to caries than vital teeth, though the reasons are unknown.[33,34]
2. *Lack of definitive restoration.* A surprisingly high percentage of teeth are not appropriately restored after root canal treatment.[27,31,35] In one study of U.S. insurance data,[6] almost 30% of teeth had not been restored 2 years after root canal treatment, and 11% of these teeth were extracted.
3. *Inadequate restoration.* Lack of coronal coverage for posterior teeth is a major restorative factor in their loss after root canal treatment.[26-28,36] A lack of cuspal protection, coronal coverage predisposes the tooth to unrestorable crown or root fracture. Direct restorations do not provide adequate protection for posterior teeth unless the access opening is very conservative.
4. *Occlusal stresses.* Teeth serving as abutments for fixed or removable prostheses are at significantly increased risk of loss, as are teeth lacking mesial and distal proximal support from adjacent teeth.[26,27,37]
5. *Endodontic factors.* Typically only about 10% of extractions of root canal treated teeth result from endodontic causes, such as persistent pain.[30-32,38] Endodontic pathology (development or persistence of a periapical lesion) is generally amenable to further management rather than extraction; likewise procedural complications, including perforation, may be managed.

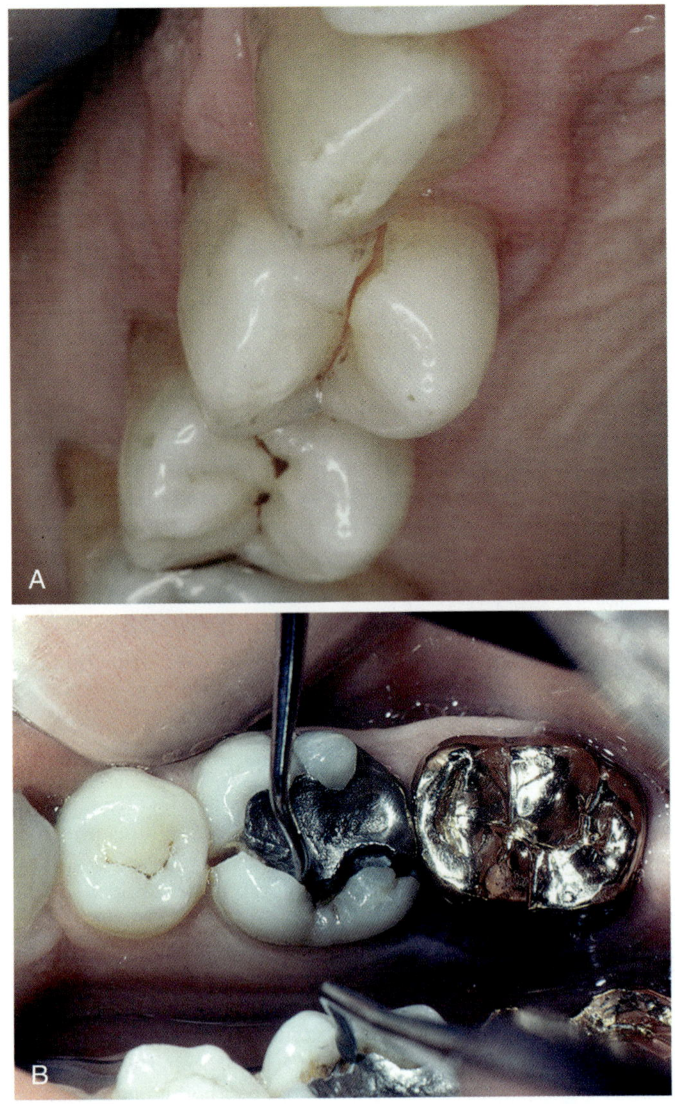

• **Fig. 16.4** **(A)** Root fracture of a maxillary premolar without any existing restorations. **(B)** Crown-root fracture (split tooth) of a root canal–treated tooth restored with amalgam but lacking protection of undermined, weakened cusps. (Courtesy Dr. H. Colman.)

Structural, Esthetic, and Restorative Considerations

Teeth function in a challenging environment, with heavy occlusal forces and repeated loading at a frequency of more than 1 million cycles per year for many decades. Caries, restorative procedures, and occlusal stresses add to the risk of serious damage to teeth during normal function, and root canal treated teeth are at greater risk than intact teeth (Fig. 16.4). As noted previously, unrestorable crown fracture is a common sequel to inadequately protected root canal treated teeth.[36,39] It is important to understand the basis for this fracture susceptibility when planning the restoration.

Structural Changes in Dentin

It is now generally recognized that many mechanical properties of the dentin of endodontically treated teeth differ only to a minor extent from those of the dentin of vital teeth (strength, hardness, modulus of elasticity).[40,41] Prior studies were generally confounded by drying of studied teeth after extraction.[42-45]

Biomechanical Factors

Normal function generates large stresses that are capable of causing cusp fracture and even vertical root fracture in intact vital teeth.[46] Repeated functional loading and cyclic mechanical fatigue have the potential to weaken teeth over time, particularly after tooth structure has been lost to caries, restoration, and access preparation, which places even more stress upon the remaining diminished tooth structure.[4-6] The distribution of masticatory stresses in the restored root canal treated tooth is markedly and adversely changed from those in the intact, vital tooth.[44] Hence, the restoration must be designed to minimize and to protect against fracture.

Esthetic Considerations

Increasingly, patients wish to enhance the esthetic appearance of restorations; for endodontically treated teeth this often involves the use of crowns. Crown preparation necessitates further tooth reduction to provide adequate thickness of the ceramic material to provide a more natural appearance. The amount of required tooth reduction varies based on the material being used. Dark stained teeth may require additional tooth reduction to mask discoloration when translucent all-ceramic crowns are used, further weakening the tooth.

Requirements for an Adequate Restoration

The definitive restoration should (1) preserve as much tooth structure as possible, but not forget the appropriate thickness of the restorative material; (2) protect remaining tooth structure, cuspal coverage protecting posterior teeth; (3) satisfy function and esthetics; (4) provide a coronal seal; and (5) be completed in a timely manner. Care must be taken to ensure that esthetic demands do not lead to the weakening of teeth by excessive removal of remaining tooth structure.

Coronal Seal

Coronal leakage is a major cause of endodontic failure.[47,48] Even a well-obturated canal does not provide an enduring barrier to bacterial penetration[49]; we rely on the restoration for long-term integrity of the coronal seal. The restoration may provide the coronal seal either as a separate step (e.g., placing a barrier over canal orifices)[50,51] or, more commonly, as an integral part of the restoration. For direct restoration of a small access cavity, a bonded restoration provides the most reliable seal.[52] Experimental leakage studies consistently demonstrate that leakage occurs around posts, regardless of the type of post or luting cement.[53] However, a crown with an adequate ferrule and sound core foundation provides an effective barrier against coronal leakage.[54,55]

A frequently asked question with regard to lost or leaking restorations is, "How long can a root filling be exposed to oral fluids before it should be retreated?" The question has no clear answer. Experimental studies suggest that complete leakage along the length of the root filling occurs rapidly, within days or weeks.[56,57] A recent review, however, concluded that coronal leakage may be clinically less significant than is suggested by experimental laboratory leakage studies.[58] Clinically, bacterial invasion is often limited to the coronal third of the canal, and periapical lesions may take several years to develop.[59,60] One commonly accepted guideline is that the root canal should be retreated if it is exposed to oral fluids for more than 2 to 3 months.[47] Others suggest 2 to 3 weeks.[48] However, if the root filling has been performed to a high technical standard and periapical pathology is absent, it may be sufficient to replace the lost or leaking restoration rather than provide endodontic retreatment.[59] Of course, retreatment can be provided after pathology has eventually become evident, but the earlier bacteria are removed, the better the endodontic prognosis.

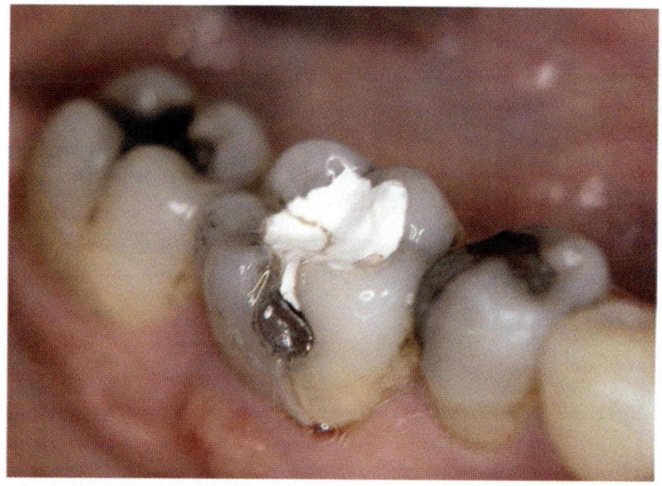

• **Fig. 16.5** Unrestorable fracture during root canal treatment. The lack of cuspal protection combined with deep anatomic grooves led to fracture within days of endodontic access.

Restoration Timing

Unless there are specific reasons for delay, definitive restoration is completed as soon as practical.[47,53,61,62] The core restoration should be placed at the time of obturation, before the rubber dam is removed.

If placement of the core restoration is to be delayed, orifice barriers can be placed at the time of obturation using composite resin[63] or glass ionomer or an adhesive cement. The gutta-percha is removed from the canal orifice 1 mm below the pulpal floor or 1 mm below the level of the cementoenamel junction (CEJ), creating a small depression. The tooth is etched and primer placed for composite resin or the tooth is conditioned for glass ionomer. One option is to seal the orifice with clear composite resin to allow easy visualization of the canal and gutta-percha should reentry into the canal ever be needed; another is to use an opaque white material so that it can easily be distinguished from natural tooth structure.

Most provisional restorative materials commonly used to seal the endodontic access opening allow substantial occlusal wear and loss of the coronal seal within weeks. The tooth has been weakened by access preparation and remains at risk until definitive restoration has been completed. The provisional restoration does not provide protection against masticatory forces, even when the

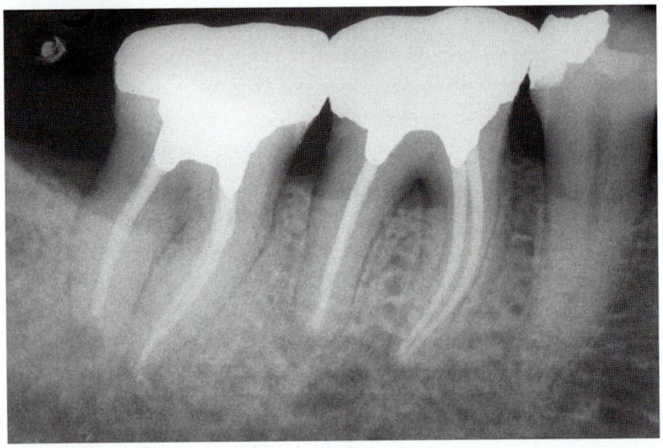

• **Fig. 16.6** Chamber and canal orifices retain an amalgam core, taking advantage of natural undercuts. The teeth can be prepared for crowns without removing the amalcore, or the amalgams may be definitive restorations if the cusps are adequately protected. (Courtesy D.P. Parashos.)

tooth is out of occlusion. Because nonrestorable fracture during or soon after treatment is all too common (Fig. 16.5), protection can be provided in the form of a well-made provisional crown.

For most teeth, it is both unnecessary and unwise to wait for radiographic evidence of healing before the definitive restoration is placed. Prompt restoration will improve the prognosis because it provides better protection against fracture and loss of the coronal seal.

When definitive restoration of the tooth is delayed, the provisional restoration must be durable and must protect, seal, and meet functional and esthetic demands. Provisional materials such as Cavit are inadequate.[64] For posterior teeth, some form of cuspal protection is desirable, even with provisional restorations.[65] A good long-term posterior provisional restoration will cover weakened cusps, thus providing functional and sealing protection. The definitive crown preparation can be completed later without removing the core (Fig. 16.6). Comparable anterior restorations are more challenging owing to esthetic demands and difficulties with the coronal seal.[53] A one-piece provisional postcrown is at risk of dislodgment, thereby compromising an adequate seal.[66] It is preferable to place a definitive post and core immediately after obturation when a provisional crown is indicated.[62,67]

Restoration Design

Guiding Principles

1. *Conservation of tooth structure.* Most anterior root canal treated teeth should be restored simply and conservatively using composite resin rather than with a more radical crown or a crown combined with a post and core.[68,69] Some data even indicate that molars that are intact (except for endodontic access openings) can be restored using only composite resin.[70] However, most root canal treated posterior teeth require crown placement so that the cusps and remaining tooth structure can be encompassed, minimizing the potential for tooth fracture.[36,39] The antiquated and unsound processes used by some practitioners of routinely creating a very large access preparation or decoronating an endodontically treated tooth and then rebuilding it are neither desirable nor in keeping with contemporary knowledge.
2. *Retention and resistance.* The definitive coronal restoration of a root canal treated tooth may consist only of a restorative filling in the endodontic access opening when it is retained by surrounding tooth structure. When the tooth is structurally compromised a crown is needed. It is retained by remaining dentin and a restorative material core that replaces missing tooth structure. Only if the core cannot be adequately retained by the remaining coronal tooth structure should a post be placed into the root canal to provide retention and resistance for the core. Because posts weaken teeth[71-75] and may produce root fracture or lead to root perforation during preparation of the root canal,[76] they should be used only when the core cannot be retained by any other means, such as mechanical and chemical bonding of a restorative material.[77,78]
3. *Protection of remaining tooth structure.* In posterior teeth, this applies to protecting weakened cusps by minimizing undue flexure and preventing fracture. The restoration is designed to encompass the cusps, thereby splinting the tooth and minimizing the chance of tooth fracture.

Planning the Definitive Restoration

A tooth that is intact except for the access preparation can simply be restored using amalgam or composite. All of the provisional restorative materials must be removed along with any cotton or foam pellet, the pulpal floor cleaned of any sealer or gutta-percha, and the round or oval obturations be clearly visualized, so that there will be no void between restoration and the pulpal floor or obturation.

When the tooth requires a crown, the type of definitive treatment can be determined only after the existing restoration (or restorations) have been removed, to ensure that there is no caries present and to expose the remaining sound tooth structure. Therefore the specific crown material will be determined based on esthetic and functional demands.

Anterior Teeth

Whenever possible, direct restoration of the endodontic access opening (e.g., etched and bonded composite resin) is used. Further esthetic issues can be addressed conservatively through internal bleaching and the use of porcelain veneers. For grossly damaged anterior teeth, complete coronal coverage using a crown, or a crown retained by a post, may be necessary.

Either a prefabricated post with direct core buildup (see Fig. 16.7) or a cast post and core (see Fig. 16.8) can be used for anterior teeth. In esthetically demanding situations, discoloration of the crown by a metal post and core can be concerning. To prevent discoloration one can use prefabricated metal posts that are coated with a thin layer of opaque resin along with a tooth colored composite resin core. Alternatively, a cast post can be fabricated using a metal ceramic alloy that allows the application of opaque porcelain to mask the metallic color, thereby achieving better esthetic outcomes (Fig. 16.9). Tooth colored fiber or ceramic posts may also be considered.

Anterior root canal treated teeth must withstand tipping and lateral forces from mandibular excursive movements which, if transmitted excessively via a post, can fracture the root. Consideration should be given to the occlusal scheme. Where possible, the excursive load should be limited, with more force being borne by adjacent, more structurally sound teeth.

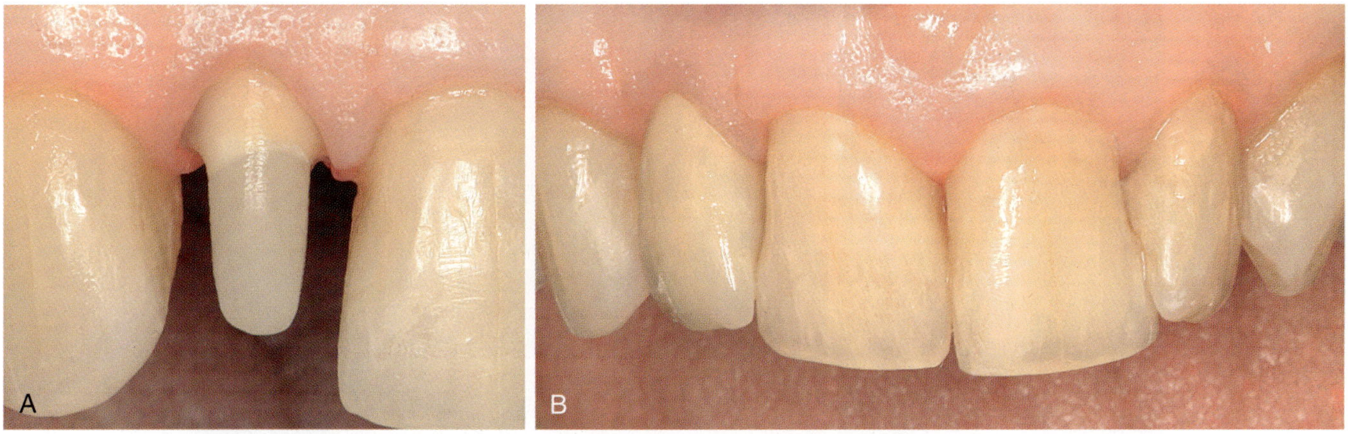

• **Fig. 16.7 (A)** Composite resin core buildup, with a ferrule incorporated into the preparation so that the crown can grasp the tooth structure cervical to the core. **(B)** The metal-ceramic crown as the definitive restoration.

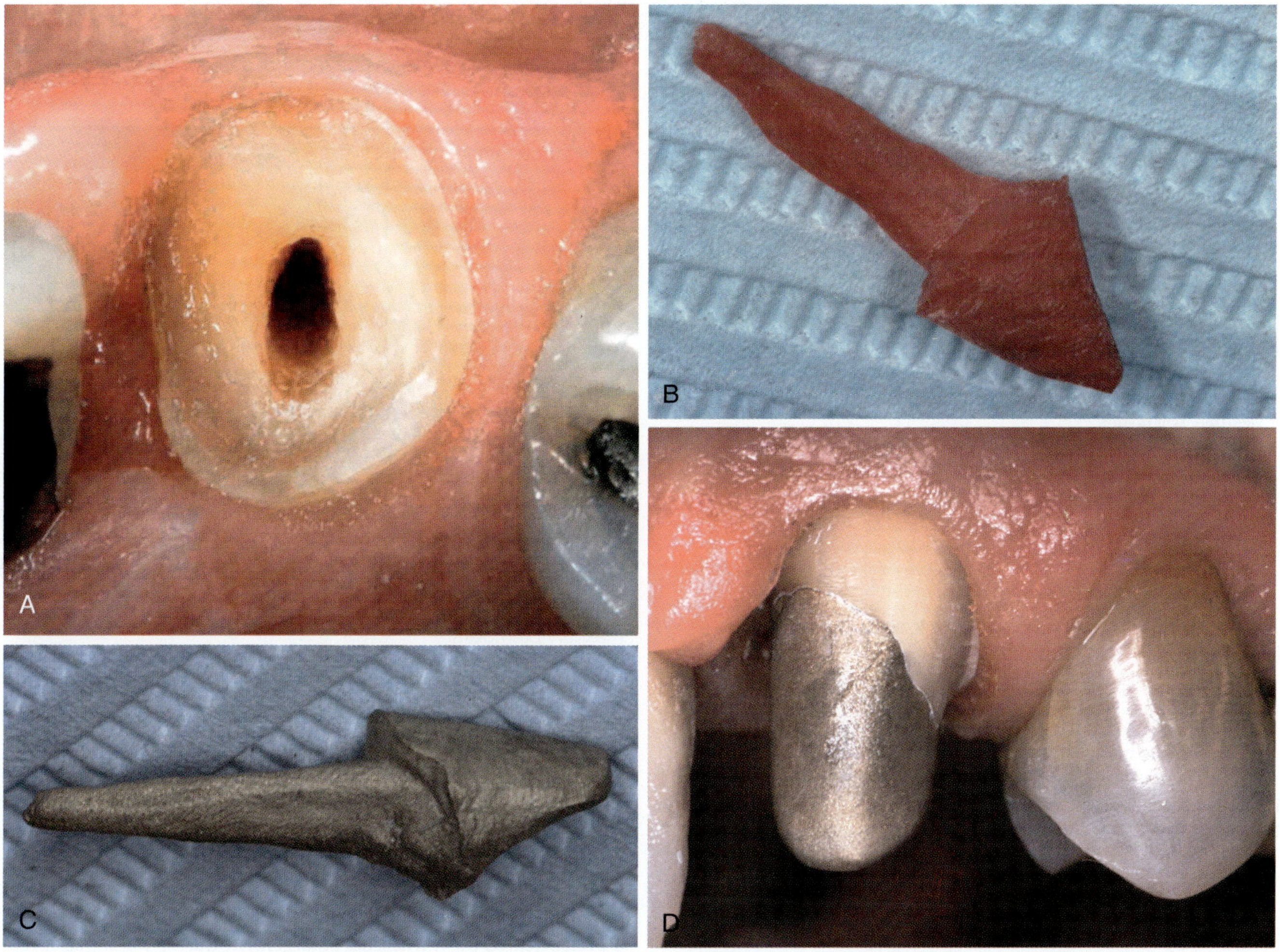

• **Fig. 16.8 (A)** Maxillary canine with oval root canal. This tooth is not morphologically suited for a prefabricated post because the post would contact only a small portion of the mesial and distal walls, or the tooth would have to be extensively prepared to a round form, weakening the tooth or possibly perforating it where the proximal root depressions are present. **(B)** A resin pattern was made directly in the tooth. **(C)** The pattern was invested and cast. **(D)** The cast post and core are cemented, and the tooth is ready for final preparation. (Courtesy Dr. J. Kan.)

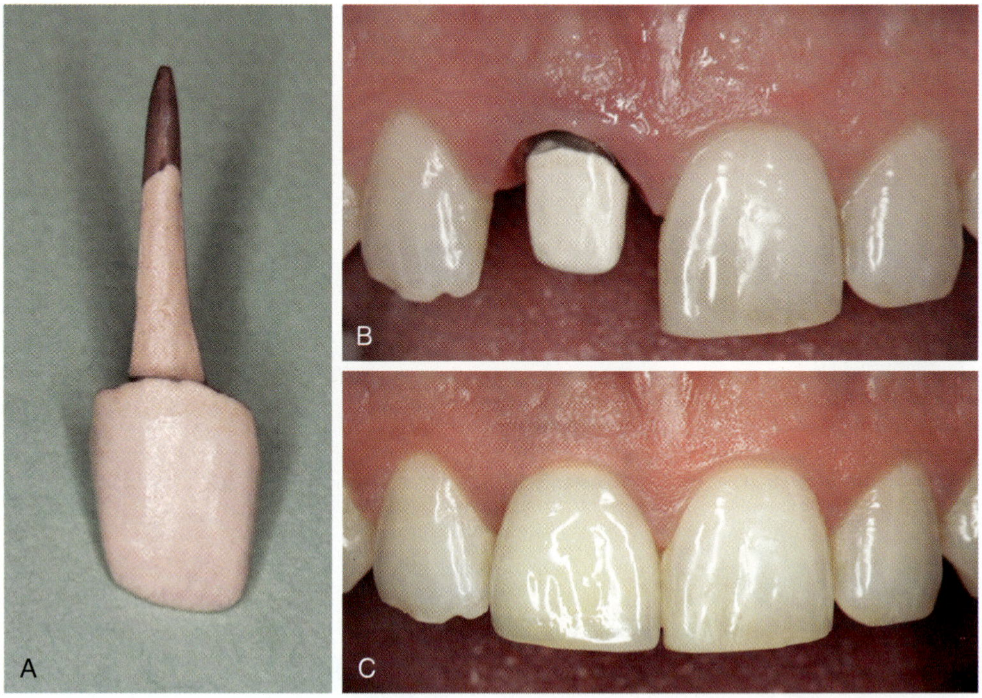

• **Fig. 16.9** **(A)** Cast post and core fabricated using metal ceramic alloy with porcelain opaque layer applied. **(B)** Cast post and core cemented on central incisor. **(C)** Final restoration.

Study Questions

1. What is the most important determination before endodontic therapy?
   a. Length of root
   b. Curvature of root
   c. Restorability of tooth
   d. Location of tooth
2. Which of the following are criteria of a restorable tooth?
   a. Amount of remaining coronal tooth structure
   b. Ferrule wall height
   c. Ferrule wall thickness
   d. All of the above
3. What is the minimally suggested ferrule wall height?
   a. 1.0mm
   b. 2.0mm
   c. 3.0mm
   d. 4.0mm
4. Which of the following are contraindications to surgical crown lengthening?
   a. Reduced bone support
   b. Short roots
   c. Poor crown-to-root ratio
   d. Poor esthetic results
   d. All of the above
5. Which complications associated with endodontically treated teeth is the most comm?
   a. Caries and periodontal disease
   b. Lack of definitive restoration
   c. Inadequate restoration
   d. Occlusal stresses
   e. Endodontic factors
6. When restoring an anterior tooth with a conservative endodontic access and no existing restorations, the ideal restoration is a bonded composite
   a. True
   b. False

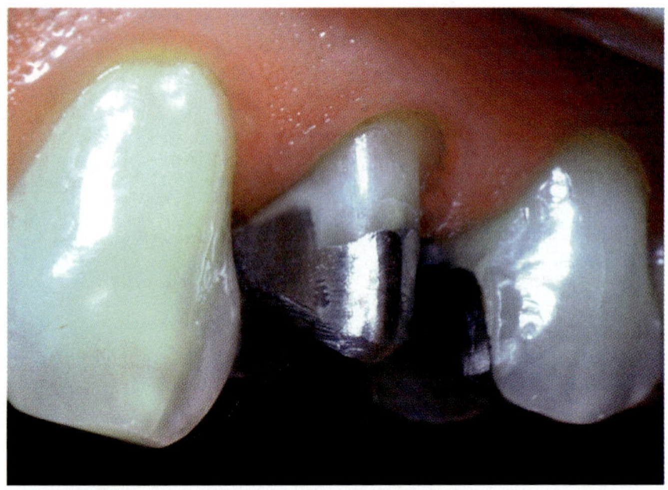

• **Fig. 16.10** A cast post and core provides the best foundation for restoring maxillary premolars.

Posterior Teeth

Premolars with substantial loss of coronal structure, missing buccal or palatal cusps, particularly maxillary premolars, often necessitate a cast post and core (Fig. 16.10). Premolar roots present many risks to post placement. Narrow mesiodistal root width and large developmental root concavities, coupled with tapered roots, may result in excessive removal of root structure or perforation when the tooth is prepared for a prefabricated post. Additionally, the mesiodistal thinness of the tooth may not permit adequate core thickness to allow strength when using a prefabricated post. Minimal enlargement during post space preparation is essential to preserve sufficient dentin thickness.[79] In maxillary premolars with two roots, the palatal canal is generally used for the post because the buccal root can frequently have a concavity on its furcal aspect.[79,80] A small, short (2 mm to 3 mm) post in the buccal canal can be used to provide some retention, resistance, and antirotation. As a rule of thumb, when a root canal is circular (Fig. 16.11) a

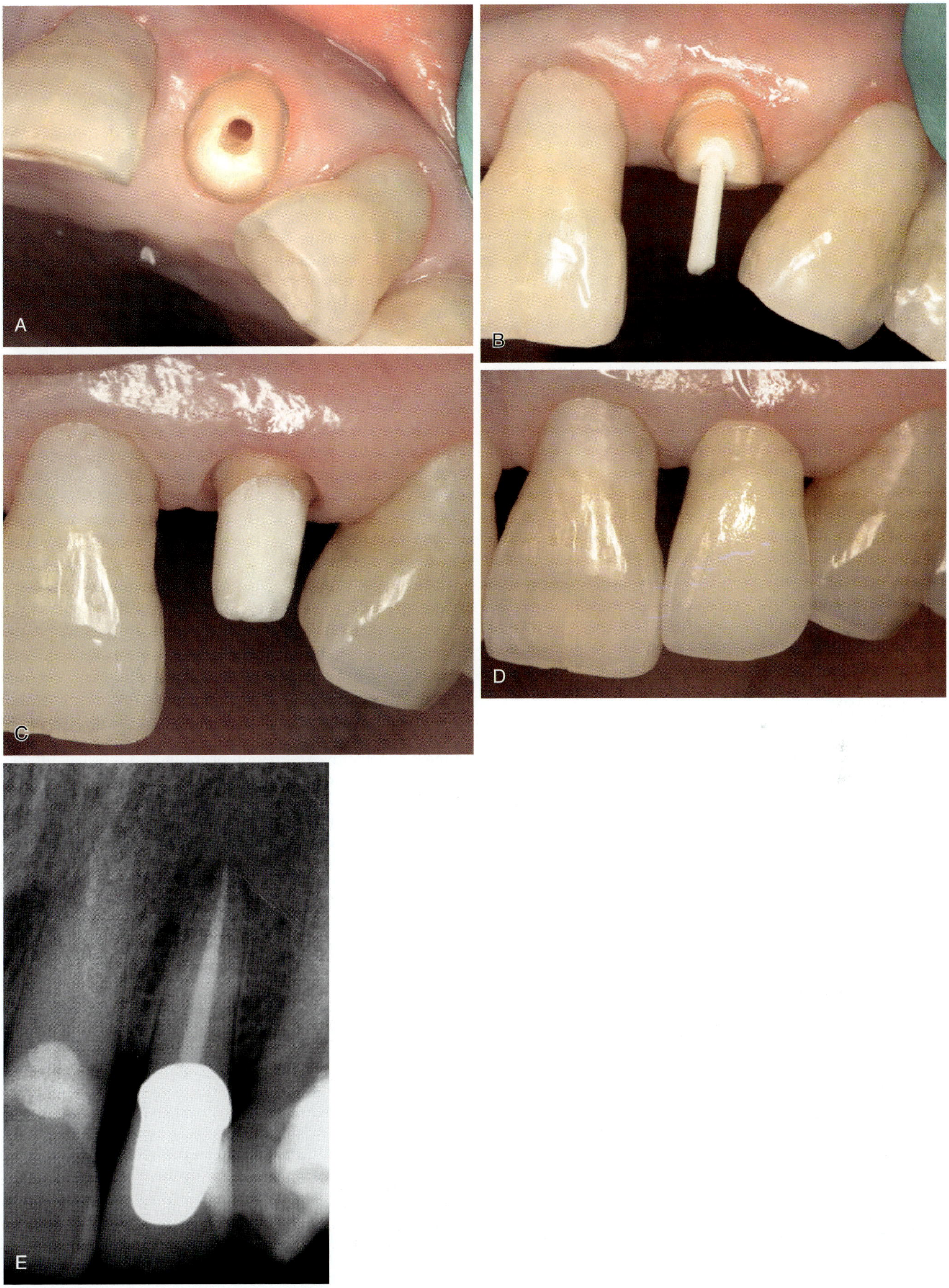

• **Fig. 16.11** **(A)** Maxillary lateral incisor with a circular canal is prepared for glass fiber post. **(B)** Fiber post bonded into prepared root canal. **(C)** Composite resin core and completed tooth preparation. **(D)** Cemented crown. **(E)** Radiograph showing the zirconia core with porcelain veneer and slightly radiopaque fiber post.

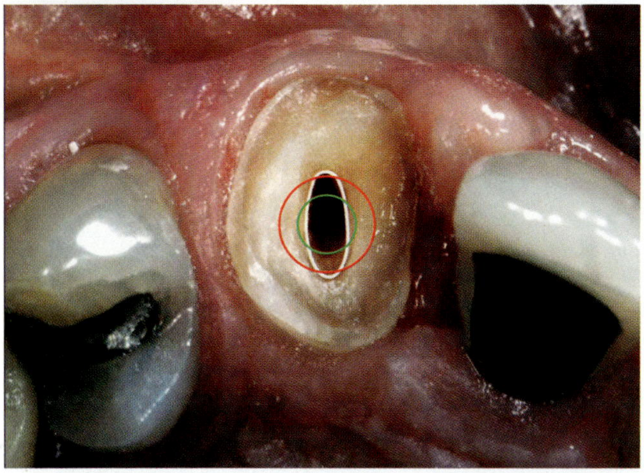

• **Fig. 16.12** An ovoid canal is prepared for a cast post and core (*white outline*), providing the best foundation for restoring maxillary premolars. If a prefabricated post space was created (*green outline*) the post would have minimal contact with the tooth, being retained primarily by cement. If a larger post space was created (*red outline*) the tooth would be structurally compromised, leading to perforation or fracture.

prefabricated post may be used. However, if the root canal is ovoid, a prefabricated post would be in close proximity to the mesial and distal walls of the canal whereas the facial and lingual areas would be filled with cement (Fig. 16.12). Therefore if the root canal is ovoid or ribbon shaped a custom cast post is suggested.

Most molars can be restored with a direct core foundation, gaining retention and resistance form from their relatively large pulp chambers, without the need of a post (Fig. 16.13). Additional core resistance and retention form is gained by extending the core material 1 mm to 2 mm into the canal orifices (see Figs. 16.6 and 16.13).[82] With fast-setting amalgam, the tooth may be prepared for the crown at the same visit, although preparation is easier when the material has fully hardened. A widely used alternative to amalgam is composite resin, which has a fracture resistance comparable to that of amalgam and produces more favorable tooth fracture patterns if failure occurs.[83,84] Composite resin has the advantage of allowing immediate crown preparation.[83] Glass ionomer does not have sufficient compressive strength for use as a core material. However, when minimal remaining coronal tooth structure is present and a small pulp chamber will not provide sufficient core retention, a post may occasionally be needed to provide retention for molar cores. The longest and straightest canal is preferred for the post, typically the palatal canal of maxillary molars and a distal canal in mandibular molars.[81] Even these roots can be hazardous; the palatal root typically curves toward the buccal, and the distal root of lower molars typically has large mesial and distal concavities. Other molar canals are generally even more problematic and generally should be avoided.

Considerations for Direct Restorations

Anterior teeth should generally be restored with direct restorations. Posterior teeth may be restored with direct restorations when they are largely intact, most of the marginal ridges remaining, along with a conservative access cavity and minimal overall loss of tooth structure.

Posterior teeth with substantial tooth structure loss may be restored with amalgam if it is esthetically acceptable and if unsupported cusps are adequately protected by the amalgam.[85] Some cuspal coverage amalgams have lasted for many years (Fig. 16.14), whereas others have fractured as a result of the presence of heavy occlusal forces. Assessment of occlusal forces and functional activity helps determine whether a cuspal coverage amalgam is a suitable restoration. A conventional Class II amalgam without cuspal coverage does not provide cuspal protection and ordinarily should not be used.[86] At a minimum, cusps adjacent to a lost marginal ridge should be onlayed with sufficient thickness of amalgam (at least 2.0 mm)[87] to resist occlusal forces (see Fig. 16.14). The amalgam should extend into the pulp chamber and canal orifices to aid retention. The amalgam may subsequently serve as a core for an indirectly fabricated restoration if indicated (see Fig. 16.13). Bonded amalgams have also been used, but their clinical performance in root-filled teeth has not been well documented, and bond failure is likely to be catastrophic in the presence of weakened, unprotected cusps.

The need for a tooth-colored restoration warrants the use of bonded composite resin restorations. The use of bonding continues to improve as materials and techniques improve, and good results have been reported in a long-term prospective clinical study of composite resin restorations.[88] Proximal leakage and recurrent proximal caries remain a concern, particularly when the restorations have subgingival margins and were placed without the use of a rubber dam. However, the ability to replace the missing tooth structure with a tooth colored, bonded restoration offers many benefits that should not be overlooked.

Considerations for Indirect Restorations

All-metal cast restorations (onlays and three-quarter and complete crowns) provide excellent occlusal protection and are optimal when the loss of tooth structure requires coronal coverage. The attractiveness of onlays is that the tooth preparation design is more conservative than complete coverage preparations, yet provides good cuspal coverage. The strength and toughness of gold allows conservative tooth reduction, with a reverse bevel providing effective cuspal coverage. Complete coverage all-metal crowns are used when there is insufficient coronal tooth structure present for a more conservative restoration or if functional or parafunctional stresses require the protective effect of complete coronal coverage.

When a tooth is prepared for a crown, the coronal access opening should be restored and sealed with an amalgam or a bonded composite resin as part of the core foundation for the crown. Glass ionomer can also be used to restore the access opening, as long as its purpose is to seal the opening and it is not forming a substantial portion of the axial walls that will be used for retention of the crown.

The esthetic requirements of many patients prevent the use of all-metal crowns. Metal-ceramic and all-ceramic crowns have become frequently used materials for root canal-treated teeth. Although all-ceramic crowns provide enhanced esthetics, metal-ceramic crowns can also be esthetic and they provide a reliable, strong restoration that protects against root fracture (Fig. 16.15).[78,89-92] However, root canal treatment may have required substantial tooth structure removal and that, coupled with the reduction needed for a crown, can necessitate placement of a core restoration and sometimes a post to retain the core.

To plan the core shape there must be complete exposure of the tooth's perimeter. Gingival retraction cord and sometimes soft tissue removal through electrosurgery or use of a laser are beneficial methods that help prevent undersized cores being made because of incomplete visualization of the tooth preparation finish line. When a core is used as a foundation for the crown without the use of a post, the material must be well retained into remaining tooth structure and must be of sufficient thickness so that the material will not fracture during function, resulting in crown failure (Fig. 16.16).

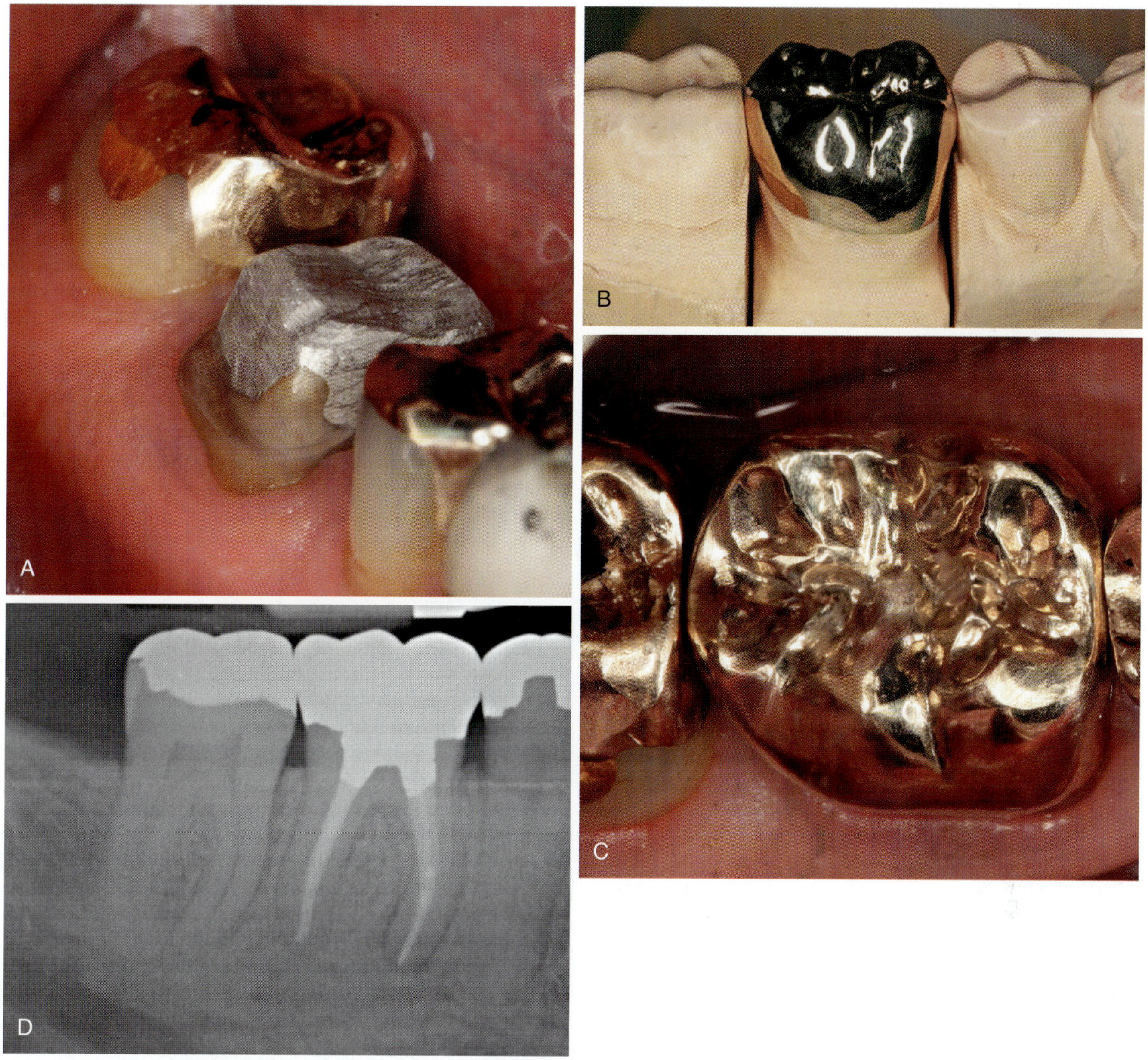

• **Fig. 16.13** **(A)** Amalgam core that covered the cusps has been prepared for a complete gold crown. **(B)** Complete crown on the working cast. **(C)** Occlusal view of the cemented crown. **(D)** Periapical radiograph of the cemented crown showing the amalgam core extended into the pulp chamber.

Posts

Coronal Tooth Preparation

Caries and prior restorations must be removed. Thin delicate spurs of tooth structure may be removed, but there is no need to make a flat uniform occlusal or incisal surface; the height of the remaining tooth structure should be maintained.

Ferrule

The use of a cervical ferrule that encompasses the tooth structure is the key to preventing tooth fracture and restoration loss (Fig. 16.17). Ferrules formed by a crown that extends cervically to engage the tooth structure apical to the core help teeth resist fracture, whereas ferrules created by the core overlapping the coronal tooth structure are generally not effective.[9-12] Crown ferrules that encompass more than 1 mm of tooth structure are the most effective in helping teeth resist fracture.[10] Ferrules that encompass 2 mm of tooth structure around the entire circumference of a tooth produce higher fracture resistance than ferrules that engage only part of the tooth circumference (see Fig. 16.10).[11,12]

Post Selection

A post is used to retain the core and provide resistance to lateral or tipping forces. The need for a post is dictated by the amount of remaining coronal tooth structure available to retain the core. A major disadvantage of posts is that they weaken teeth by additional removal of dentin and by creating stresses that predispose

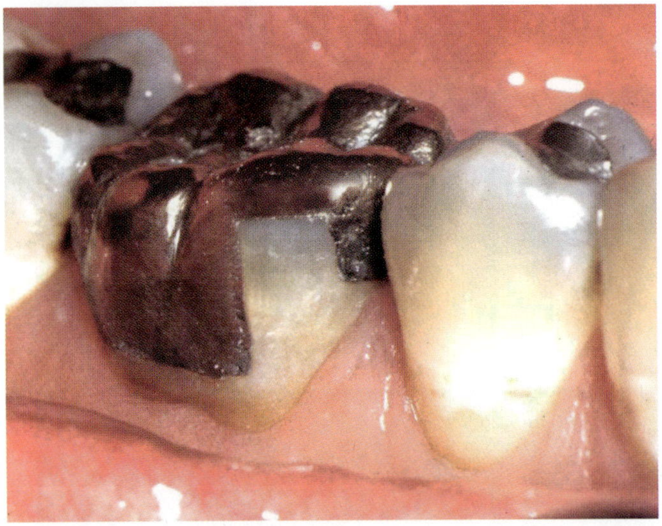

• **Fig. 16.14** Amalgam restoration replaced multiple cusps while also protecting mesiobuccal and lingual cusps with 2 mm of amalgam. It functioned well for more than 10 years, at which point the patient requested a crown on the tooth.

to root fracture.[77,78,83,93,94] Therefore posts are only used when the core cannot be retained in the tooth by any other means.

The tooth should not be prepared and adapted to the post system; rather, the post system and preparation design should be selected as appropriate to the tooth and its morphology. Therefore custom-cast posts and cores are preferred for roots that have very tapered root canals. Also, roots with substantial root concavities are best served by using cast posts and cores made to fit the existing morphology after root canal treatment rather than removing tooth structure to make the root fit the form of a prefabricated post. Prefabricated round posts may be particularly problematic in mandibular incisors, mandibular molars, maxillary first premolars, and all canals that are oval to ribbon-shaped (see Fig. 16.12).

Conservative round prefabricated round posts are well-suited for use in teeth that have round roots and round root canals because slight removal of some root structure to adapt the tooth to the post usually does not result in substantial weakening. A wide variety of passively seated prefabricated posts are available. Parallel-sided posts provide more retention than tapered posts. However, they require more apical post space preparation than tapered posts or cast posts

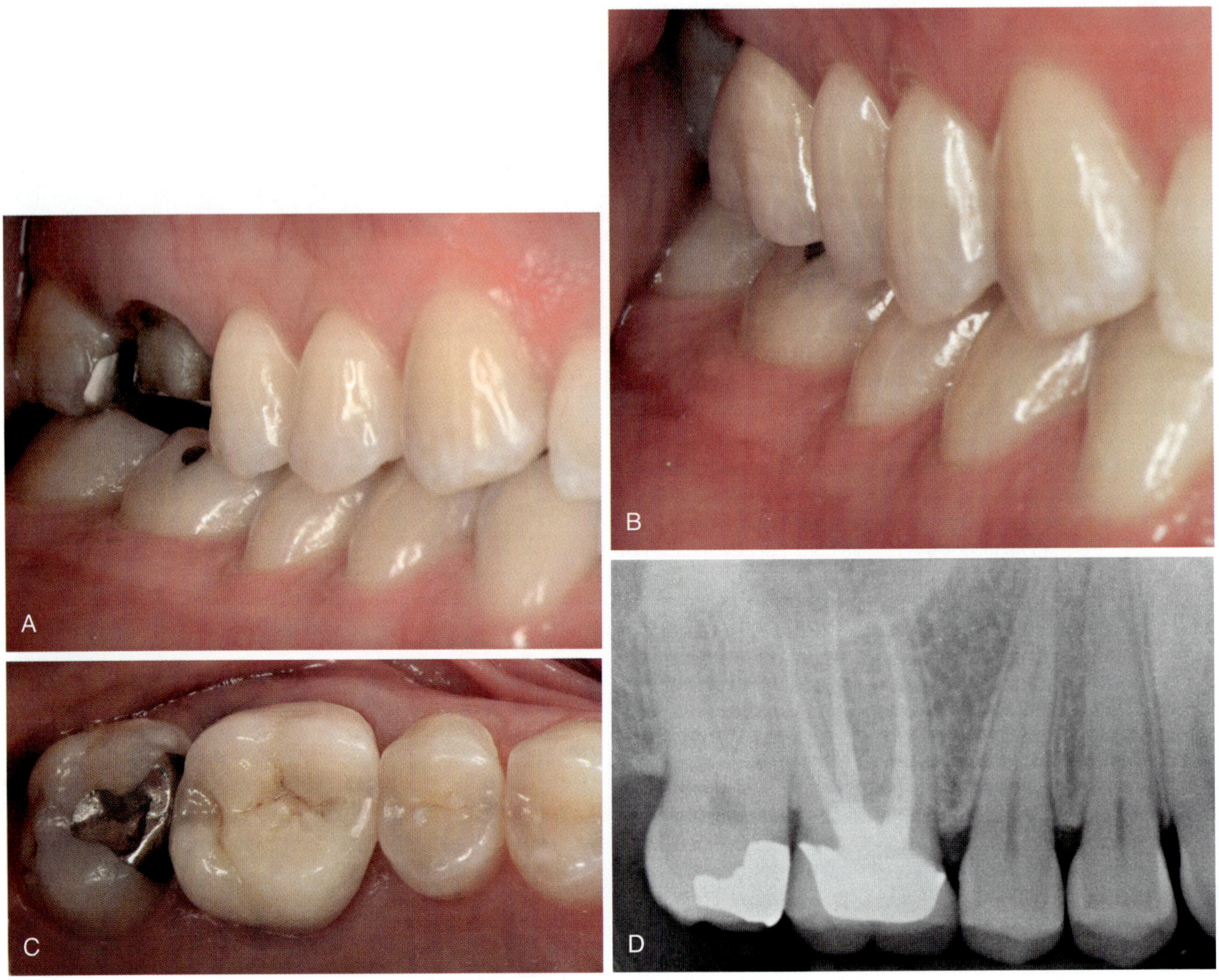

• **Fig. 16.15** **(A)** Endodontically treated maxillary first molar with amalgam core prepared for metal-ceramic crown. **(B)** Cemented crown. **(C)** Occlusal view of the crown. **(D)** Periapical radiograph showing the cemented crown and amalgam core.

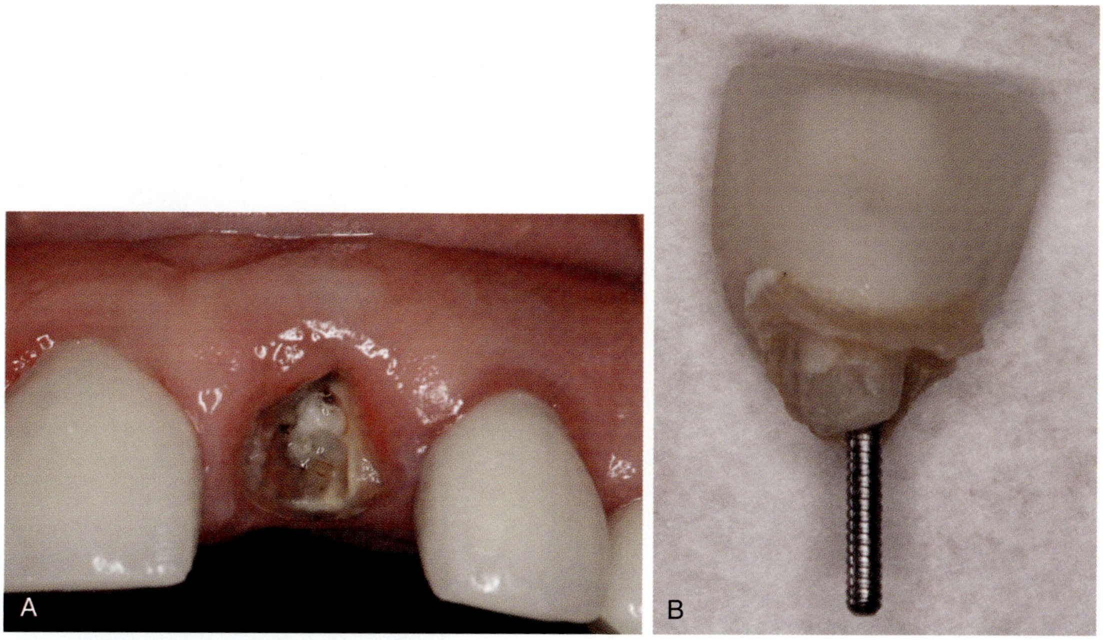

• **Fig. 16.16** **(A)** The patient presented with crown failure caused by a lack of tooth ferrule. **(B)** The prefabricated post and composite core had minimal tooth structure with primarily cement retaining the entire crown. This was no match for the forces applied to anterior teeth.

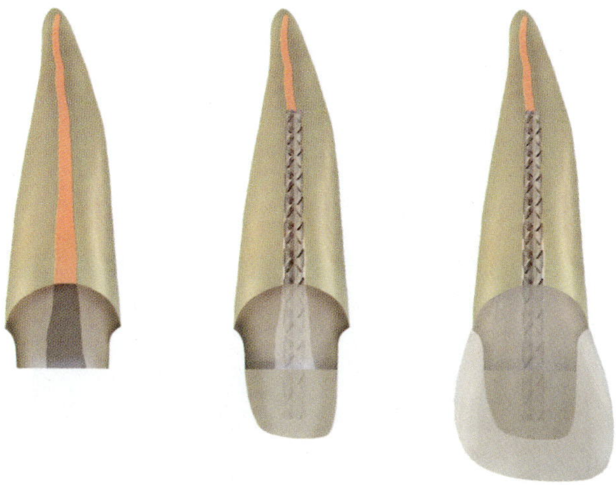

• **Fig. 16.17** (*Left*) Root canal-treated tooth with adequate ferrule. (*Middle*) Post space has been created, post cemented (note white cement between post and canal walls), and composite core build-up. (*Right*) Outline of the final crown and components of a root canal-treated tooth restored with a prefabricated post and core.

and cores; matching post size to canal size is important to minimize dentin removal and cement thickness. The post should closely approximate the root canal walls without binding, but it need not contact dentin throughout its entire length. Threaded, active, posts should be avoided; passive posts are preferred.[94,116,117] Serrations and vents allow the post to be seated without undue pressure and the set cement to grip the post.

There has been a debate regarding how the post should interact with the tooth under load and whether the post material should be similar in stiffness to root dentin (quartz fiber), somewhat stiffer (carbon fiber, titanium, and gold), or much stiffer (zirconia, stainless steel, and cobalt-chromium alloys).[95] Stiff posts have been successfully used for decades, help to protect restorations, but they may lead to a slightly increased risk of tooth fracture, whereas the more flexible posts deform with the tooth and may tend to fail more frequently but without fracturing the tooth.[96] Long-term clinical trials are needed to determine how posts should interact with teeth and what degree of stiffness functions best.

Tooth-colored post and core materials are needed beneath all-ceramic crowns to prevent discoloration and to allow some light transmission through the crown and tooth; this situation has created increased interest in fiber posts (see Fig. 16.11). The desire to have posts flex in concert with tooth structure has also raised interest in fiber posts. Quartz fiber posts appear to be advantageous with regard to root fracture potential.[97-112] However, these types of posts were less retentive than metal posts in laboratory tests,[113] indicating the need for optimal post length. Clinical results with fiber posts have been mixed; many studies have reported high levels of success, but other, longer term studies[103,111,112] have reported higher failure rates.[103,110,112] Post loosening, post fracture, and even root fracture have been reported. Hence, it is proposed that fiber posts be used cautiously when post length is less than optimal (Fig. 16.18), when peripheral walls are missing (Fig. 16.19),[114] or when heavy occlusal forces or parafunctional habits are present.[115]

Post Space Length

When a post is required for core retention, the minimum post space (length, diameter, and taper) should be prepared under rubber dam. Preparation consists of removing gutta-percha to the required length, followed by the least amount of enlargement and shaping needed to receive the post (see

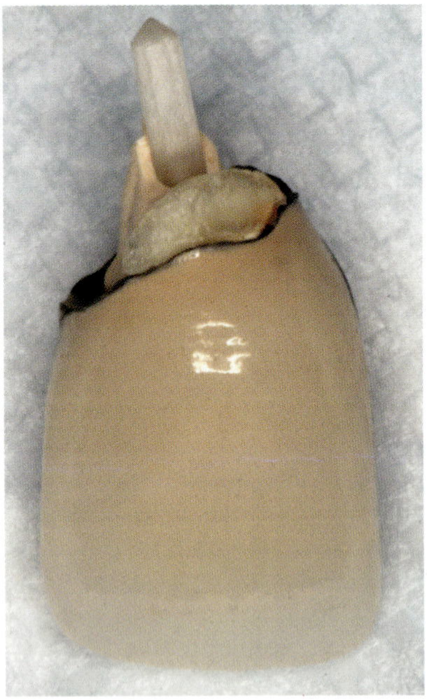

• **Fig. 16.18** Excessively short fiber post that rapidly failed and resulted in fracture of the remaining facial tooth structure, visible inside the crown. (Courtesy Dr. N. Baba.)

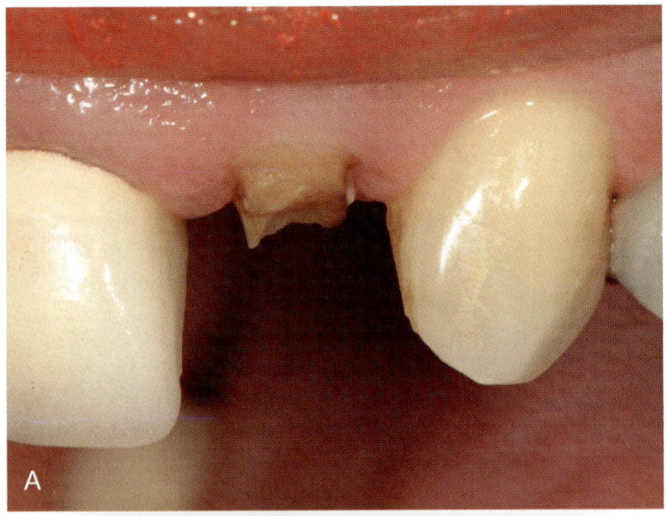

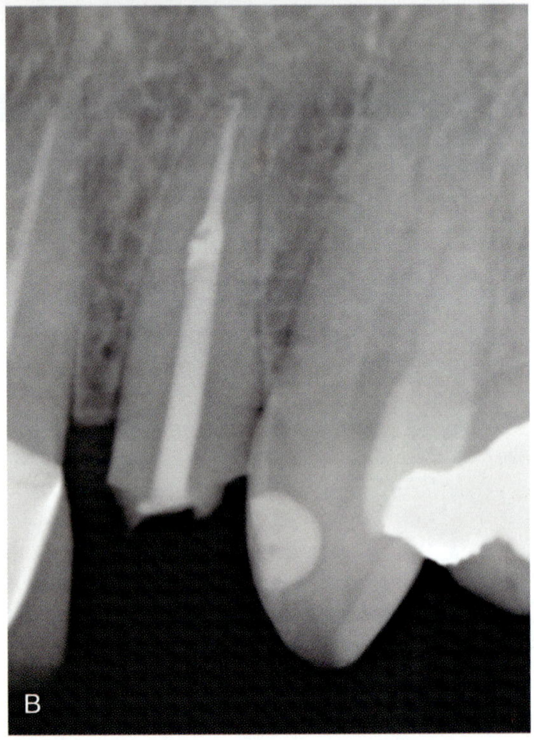

• **Fig. 16.19** **(A)** Fiber post that fractured. Note the lack of peripheral walls to help support the post. **(B)** Radiograph showing the fractured fiber post. (Courtesy Dr. N. Baba.)

Fig. 16.17). Caution is required because excessive removal of gutta-percha results in a defective apical seal.[118,119] Because there is evidence that longer posts are more retentive[119,120] and have less potential to cause root fracture than do short posts,[120-124] optimizing post length is appropriate as long as the apical seal is not compromised.

In order to protect the apical seal it is recommended that at least 5.0 mm of apical gutta-percha be retained and the post extended to that level (see Fig. 16.17). For molars, the length is determined by the potential for root thinning or perforation and root curvature.[125] Posts should be extended only 5.0 mm into the root canal and only in the straightest widest molar root (distal root of the mandibular molars and palatal root of the maxillary molars) (Fig. 16.20).

Radiographs may be deceptive as a guide to root curvature and diameter by disguising root concavities and curves in the faciolingual plane; off-angle radiographs are helpful in understanding faciolingual curvature.[81] As a general rule, the post diameter should be minimal, particularly apically, and not more than one quarter to one third of the root diameter (see Fig. 16.20).[79] Tapered post preparations minimize the amount of tooth structure removed apically and thereby reduce the amount of tooth structure removed. However, tapered posts have been shown to be less retentive and cause more stress on the tooth as a result of a wedging effect.[126,127]

Removal of Gutta-Percha

Whenever possible, gutta-percha is removed under rubber dam isolation immediately after obturation, and the tooth is robustly provisionalized before rubber dam removal, to ensure apical and coronal sealing.[128] At this stage, the dentist is most familiar with the canal features, including shape, length, size, and curvature. Gutta-percha is removed to the desired length using a hot instrument. The remaining gutta-percha is then vertically condensed before the sealer has set. A radiograph confirms that sufficient gutta-percha remains (5 mm) for the apical seal.[128,129]

Gutta-percha removal at a subsequent appointment is also an appropriate process.[128-130] A safe procedure is the use of a heated instrument. Gutta-percha is removed in increments to the desired length using a heated plugger that has sufficient heat capacity. Solvents should not be used for removing gutta-percha to create a post space because of messiness and unpredictable depth of penetration. Rotary instruments may be used, but caution is required, because they can create a channel that does not follow the root canal, causing root thinning or, worse yet, perforation. Gates-Glidden drills are less likely to go off track or perforate than Peeso reamers. Rotary instruments may also "grab" and displace the apical gutta-percha. Nickel-titanium rotary instruments specially designed for preparing post spaces are available; these have a noncutting tip.

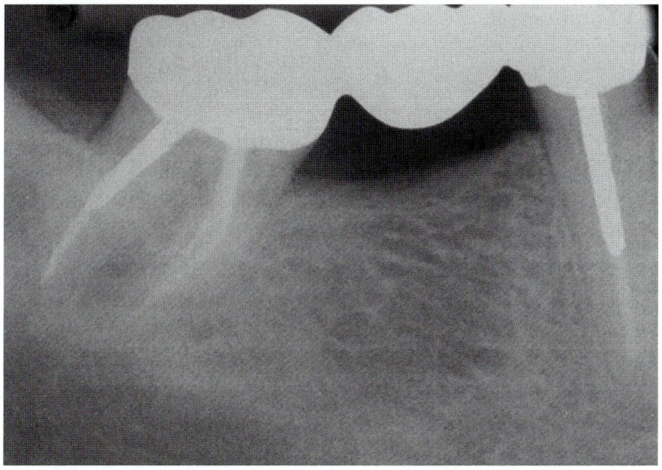

• **Fig. 16.20** Molar abutment for fixed partial denture has a post in the distal root that extends 5 mm beyond the base of the pulp chamber into the root canal. The post was prepared with a tapered form to minimize tooth reduction. In the premolar abutment, a parallel-wall post was used because of the more favorable root morphology and dimensions.

They can be effective[131] and pose low risks of ledging or canal transportation.[132,133]

Completing the Post Space Preparation

After the post length and diameter have been established, the post space may need further refinement to eliminate small undercuts. After gutta-percha has been removed, rotary instruments can be used for final post space shaping; however, as stated previously, they should be used carefully to avoid excessive tooth removal that weakens the root or causes a perforation. Post spaces for prefabricated posts should be finished using the manufacturer's recommended drill. Final shaping can also be performed using hand manipulation of the rotary instruments because only small amounts of tooth need to be removed in most situations. After a post space has been made, a robust provisional restoration must be used to exclude oral bacteria, and a calcium hydroxide intracanal medicament will provide further protection until the post has been cemented.

Post Cementation

Proper post cementation is vital; the recommended procedures are:

1. Rubber dam isolation is needed before removal of the provisional restoration and intracanal medicament.
2. The post should be fitted to the canal and the seating verified radiographically. Custom cast posts can be adjusted to achieve a passive fit using a silicone disclosing medium (e.g., Fit Checker), then air particle abraded using 50-µm aluminum oxide, before being cleaned.
3. The walls of the post space should be disinfected using sodium hypochlorite; the smear layer removed using ethylenediaminetetraacetic acid (EDTA); rinsed with water; and dried using paper points, not by blowing air.
4. After referring to the cement procedural instructions, properly mix or activate the cement and place cement in the canal system. Depending on the specific cement used, a slow-speed handpiece and lentulo spiral turning clockwise may be used to uniformly disperse the cement throughout the canal system. Some cements preclude the use of a lentulo spiral because it speeds up their setting time.

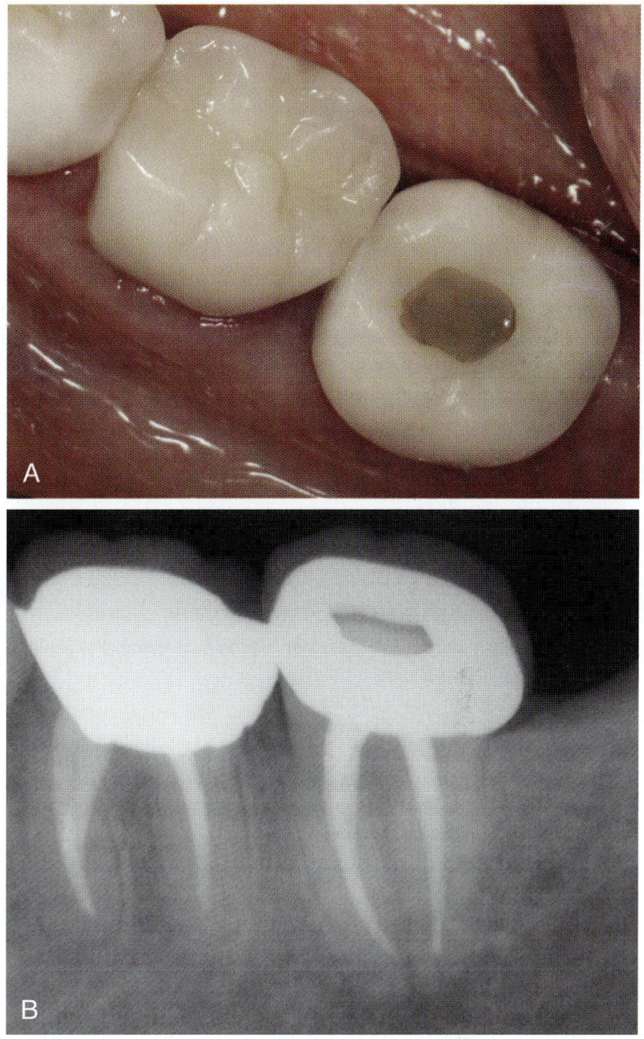

• **Fig. 16.21** **(A)** Access through existing crown that has been sealed with composite. **(B)** Radiograph showing root canal treatment through crown.

5. Place cement onto the post and carefully seat the post. Remove excess cement once it has set enough for the cement to come off in solid pieces.
6. Allow complete setting of the cement before using any rotary instruments to shape or refine finish lines to avoid potential weakening of the cemented post caused by vibration. Depending on the cement used this may require provisional restoration of the tooth and returning at another appointment to refine the interface between post and tooth.
7. Build-up of the core is performed for the prefabricated posts using a definitive restorative material (composite resin, amalgam). The tooth with core build-up is then refined for the final restoration and an impression made, or the prepared tooth scanned.

Restoring Access Through an Existing Restoration

Occasionally, pulps undergo irreversible pulpitis or necrosis after placement of a crown, requiring root canal treatment (Fig. 16.21).[76,93,134] Access through the restoration, with subsequent definitive repair of the opening, is preferable to making a new crown.

For the restoration to remain functional, four conditions must be met: (1) The restoration must be proved to be without leakage, preferably recently placed; (2) the interface between the restoration and the repair material must provide a good coronal seal; (3) retention of the crown must not be compromised; and (4) the final core structure must support the restoration against functional or minor traumatic stresses. Access, particularly if overextended, may leave only a thin shell of axial dentin, especially in anterior teeth and premolars. Retention then depends almost entirely on the repair material. Fortunately, the chamber and canal are available to create a core that provides adequate retention and support in many instances. Placement of a post through an access opening in an existing crown into the root canal adds little additional support and retention and is rarely indicated.

The repair material should have high compressive and shear strength. Amalgam is an excellent material that maintains (and even improves) its seal with time and is easily condensed into the entire chamber and access opening as a single unit. Composite resins are usually the material of choice in tooth-colored crowns.[83] Glass ionomer and other cements do not have the required shear, tensile, or compressive strength.

Essential Precepts

Key points in retaining and restoring all root canal-treated teeth by any method include:

1. Careful preoperative assessment regarding the amount of remaining tooth structure and planning for the definitive restoration;
2. Conservation of tooth structure during access preparation and restorative procedures;
3. Use of rubber dam isolation until after a definitive core restoration or post has been placed;
4. Use of coronal coverage to bind the cusps together on most posterior teeth;
5. Avoidance of crowns on anterior teeth, unless absolutely necessary;
6. Avoidance of posts unless there is no other way to provide resistance or retention for the final restoration;
7. Prompt restoration without delay.

Study Questions

7. When restoring a mandibular molar with a large pulp chamber which of the following is the preferred technique?
   a. Post cemented in the distal root
   b. Direct core placed in pulp chamber and crown
   c. Occlusal composite filling
   d. Cast post and core with crown
8. Posterior endodontically treated teeth should primarily be restored with what type of definitive restoration?
   a. Crown
   b. Direct composite filling
   c. Direct amalgam filling
   d. Inlay
9. What is the primary purpose of a post?
   a. Strengthen the tooth
   b. Retain the core build-up
   c. Compensate for minimal ferrule
   d. Improve esthetics
10. What is the minimum amount of gutta percha required to maintain an apical seal?
    a. 3.0mm
    b. 4.0mm
    c. 5.0mm
    d. 6.0mm
11. Which of the following are key elements that an existing crown must display prior to accessing through an existing restoration?
    a. The restoration must be proven to be without leakage
    b. The interface between the restoration and the repair material must provide good coronal seal
    c. Retention of the crown must not be compromised
    d. The final core structure must support the restoration against functional or minor traumatic stresses
    e. All of the above

ANSWERS

Answer Box 16

1 c. Restorability of tooth
2 d. All of the above
3 b. 2.0mm
4 e. All of the above
5 a. Caries and periodontal disease
6 a. True
8 b. Direct core placed in pulp chamber and crown
7 a. Crown
9 b. Retain the core build-up
10 c. 5.0mm
11 e. All of the above

References

1. Abbott PV: Assessing restored teeth with pulp and periapical diseases for the presence of cracks, caries and marginal breakdown, *Aust Dent J* 49:33–39, 2004.
2. McDonald AV, Setchell D: Developing a tooth restorability index, *Dent Update* 32:343–344, 2005.
3. Bandlish RB, McDonald AV, Setchell DJ: Assessment of the amount of remaining coronal dentine in root-treated teeth, *J Dent* 34:699–708, 2006.
4. Reeh ES, Messer HH, Douglas WH: Reduction in tooth stiffness as a result of endodontic and restorative procedures, *J Endod* 15:512–516, 1989.
5. Hood JAA: Biomechanics of the intact, prepared and restored tooth: some clinical implications, *Int Dent J* 41:25–32, 1991.
6. Panitvisai P, Messer HH: Cuspal deflection in molars in relation to endodontic and restorative procedures, *J Endod* 21:57–61, 1995.
7. Hansen EK, Asmussen E: Cusp fracture of endodontically treated posterior teeth restored with amalgam: teeth restored in Denmark before 1975 versus after 1979, *Acta Odontol Scand* 51:73–77, 1993.
8. Nicholls JI: The dental ferrule and the endodontically compromised tooth, *Quintessence Int* 32(2):171–173, 2001 Feb.
9. Sorensen JA, Engelman MJ: Ferrule design and fracture resistance of endodontically treated teeth, *J Prosthet Dent* 63:529–536, 1990.
10. Libman WJ, Nicholls JI: Load fatigue of teeth restored with cast posts and cores and complete crowns, *Int J Prosthodont* 8:155–161, 1995.

11. Tan PL, Aquilino SA, Gratton DG, et al.: In vitro fracture resistance of endodontically treated central incisors with varying ferrule heights and configurations, *J Prosthet Dent* 93:331–336, 2005.
12. Ng CC, Dumbrigue HB, Al-Bayat MI, et al.: Influence of remaining coronal tooth structure location on the fracture resistance of restored endodontically treated anterior teeth, *J Prosthet Dent* 95:290–296, 2006.
13. Hoag EP, Dwyer TG: A comparative evaluation of three post and core techniques, *J Prosthet Dent* 47:177–181, 1982.
14. Pereira JR, de Ornelas F, Conti PC, do Valle AL: Effect of a crown ferrule on the fracture resistance of endodontically treated teeth restored with prefabricated posts, *J Prosthet Dent* 95:50–54, 2006.
15. Assif D, Gorfil C: Biomechanical considerations in restoring endodontically treated teeth, *J Prosthet Dent* 71:565–567, 1994.
16. Caputo AA, Standlee JP: Pins and Posts – Why, When and How, *Dent Clin North Am* 20:299–311, 1976.
17. Tjan AH, Whang SB: Resistance to root fracture of dowel channels with various thicknesses of buccal dentin walls, *J Prosthet Dent* 53:496–500, 1985.
18. Sedgley CM, Messer HH: Are endodontically treated teeth more brittle? *J Endod* 18:332–335, 1992.
19. Pilo R, Shapenco E, Lewinstein I: Residual dentin thickness in bifurcated maxillary first premolars after root canal and post space preparation with parallel-side drills, *J Prosthet Dent* 99:267–273, 2008.
20. Gargiulo AW, Wentz FM, Orban B: Dimensions and relations of the dentogingival junction in humans, *J Periodontol*261–267, 1961.
21. Pontoriero R, Carnevale G: Surgical crown lengthening: a 12-month clinical wound healing study, *J Periodontol* 72:841–848, 2001.
22. Gegauff A: Effect of crown lengthening and ferrule placement on static load failure of cemented cast post-cores and crowns, *J Proshet Dent* 84:169–179, 2000.
23. Carvalho CV, Bauer FP, Romito GA, Pannuti CM, De Micheli G: Orthodontic extrusion with or without circumferential supracrestal fiberotomy and root planning, *Int J Periodontics Restorative Dent* 26:87–93, 2006.
24. Simon JH, Kelly WH, Gordon DG, Ericksen GW: Extrusion of endodontically treated teeth, *J Am Dent Assoc* 97:17–23, 1978.
25. Caplan DJ, Cai J, Yin G, et al.: Root canal filled versus non-root canal filled teeth: a retrospective comparison of survival times, *J Public Health Dent* 65:90–96, 2005.
26. Ng Y-L, Mann V, Gulabivala K: Tooth survival following non-surgical root canal treatment: a systematic review of the literature, *Int Endod J* 43:171–189, 2010.
27. Lazarski MP, Walker WA, Flores CM, et al.: Epidemiological evaluation of the outcomes of nonsurgical root canal treatment in a large cohort of insured dental patients, *J Endod* 27:791–796, 2001.
28. Salehrabi R, Rotstein I: Endodontic treatment outcomes in a large patient population in the USA: an epidemiological study, *J Endod* 30:846–850, 2004.
29. Chen SC, Chueh LH, Hsaio CK, et al.: An epidemiological study of tooth retention after non-surgical endodontic treatment in a large population in Taiwan, *J Endod* 33:226–229, 2007.
30. Chen SC, Chueh LH, Hsaio CK, et al.: First untoward events and reasons for tooth extraction after non-surgical endodontic treatment in Taiwan, *J Endod* 34:671–674, 2008.
31. Zadik Y, Sandler V, Bechor R, et al.: Analysis of factors related to tooth extraction of endodontically treated teeth, *Oral Surg Oral Med Oral Pathol Oral Radiol Endod* 106:e31–e35, 2008.
32. Touré B, Faye B, Kane AW, et al.: Analysis of reasons for extraction of endodontically treated teeth: a prospective study, *J Endod* 37:1512–1515, 2011.
33. Merdad K, Sonbul H, Bukhary S, et al.: Caries susceptibility of endodontically versus nonendodontically treated teeth, *J Endod* 37:139–142, 2011.
34. Frisk F, Merdad K, Reit C, et al.: Root-filled teeth and recurrent caries: a study of three repeated cross-sectional samples from the city of Jönköping, Sweden, *Acta Odontol Scand* 69:401–405, 2011.
35. Lynch CD, Burke FM, Ni Riordáin R, et al.: The influence of coronal restoration type on the survival of endodontically treated teeth, *Eur J Prosthodont Restor Dent* 12:171–176, 2004.
36. Aquilino SA, Caplan DJ: Relationship between crown placement and the survival of endodontically treated teeth, *J Prosthet Dent* 87:256–263, 2002.
37. Alley BS, Kitchens GG, Alley LW, et al.: A comparison of survival of teeth following endodontic treatment performed by general dentists or by specialists, *Oral Surg Oral Med Oral Pathol Oral Radiol Endod* 98:115–118, 2004.
38. Ng Y-L, Mann V, Gulabivala K: A prospective study of the factors affecting outcomes of non-surgical root canal treatment. Part 2. Tooth survival, *Int Endod J* 44:610–625, 2011.
39. Vire DE: Failure of endodontically treated teeth: classification and evaluation, *J Endod* 17:338–342, 1991.
40. Huang T-JG, Schilder H, Nathanson D: Effects of moisture content and endodontic treatment on some mechanical properties of human dentin, *J Endod* 18:209–215, 1992.
41. Sedgley CM, Messer HH: Are endodontically treated teeth more brittle? *J Endod* 18:332–335, 1992.
42. Papa J, Cain C, Messer HH: Moisture content of endodontically treated vs vital teeth, *Endod Dent Traumatol* 10:91–93, 1994.
43. 1017 Helfer AR, Melnick S, Schilder H: Determination of the moisture content of vital and pulpless teeth, *Oral Surg Oral Med Oral Pathol* 34:661–670, 1972.
44. Kishen A: Mechanisms and risk factors for fracture predilection in endodontically treated teeth, *Endod Topics* 13:57–83, 2006.
45. Kahler B, Swain MV, Moule A: Fracture toughening mechanisms responsible for differences in work to fracture of hydrated and dehydrated dentine, *J Biomech* 36:229–237, 2003.
46. Chan CP, Lin CP, Tseng SC, et al.: Vertical root fracture in endodontically versus non-endodontically treated teeth: a survey of 315 cases in Chinese patients, *Oral Surg Oral Med Oral Pathol Oral Radiol Endod* 87:504–507, 1999.
47. Slutzky-Goldberg I, Slutzky H, Gorfil C, et al.: Restoration of endodontically treated teeth: review and treatment recommendations, *Int J Dent* 2009(150251):1–9, 2009, https://doi.org/10.1155/2009/150251. Epub 2010 Jan 26.
48. Heling I, Gorfil C, Slutzky C, et al.: Endodontic failure caused by inadequate restorative procedures: review and treatment recommendations, *J Prosthet Dent* 87(6):674–678, 2002.
49. Nair PNR: On the causes of persistent apical periodontitis: a review, *Int Endod J* 39:249–281, 2006.
50. Gillen BM, Looney SW, Gu L-S, et al.: Impact of the quality of coronal restoration versus the quality of root canal fillings on success of root canal treatment: a systematic review and meta-analysis, *J Endod* 37:895–902, 2011.
51. Guerra JA, Skribner JE, Lin LM: Influence of base on coronal microleakage of post-prepared teeth, *J Endod* 20:589–591, 1994.
52. Jenkins S, Kulild J, Williams K, et al.: Sealing ability of three materials in the orifices of root canal systems obturated with gutta-percha, *J Endod* 32:225–227, 2006.
53. Schwartz RS, Fransman R: Adhesive dentistry and endodontics: materials, clinical strategies and procedures for restoration of access cavities: a review, *J Endod* 31:151–165, 2005.
54. Wu MK, Pehlivan Y, Kontakiotis EG, et al.: Microleakage along apical root fillings and cemented posts, *J Prosthet Dent* 79:264–269, 1998.
55. Nissan J, Rosner O, Gross O, et al.: Coronal leakage in endodontically treated teeth restored with posts and complete crowns using different luting agent combinations, *Quintessence Int* 42:317–322, 2011.
56. Schmid-Schwap M, Graf A, Preinerstorfer A, et al.: Microleakage after thermocycling of cemented crowns: a meta-analysis, *Dent Mater* 27:855–869, 2011.
57. Magura ME, Kafrawy AH, Brown Jr CE, et al.: Human saliva coronal microleakage in obturated root canals: an in vitro study, *J Endod* 17:324–331, 1991.
58. Khayat A, Lee SJ, Torabinejad M: Human saliva penetration of coronally unsealed obturated root canals, *J Endod* 19:458–461, 1993.
59. Kainan D, Moshonov J, Smidt A: Is endodontic re-treatment mandatory for every relatively old temporary restoration? A narrative review, *J Am Dent Assoc* 142:391–396, 2011.

60. Ricucci D, Gröndahl K, Bergenholtz G: Periapical status of root-filled teeth exposed to the oral environment by loss of restoration or caries, *Oral Surg Oral Med Oral Pathol Oral Radiol Endod* 90:354–359, 2000.
61. Ricucci D, Bergenholtz G: Bacterial status in root-filled teeth exposed to the oral environment by loss of restoration and fracture or caries: a histopathological study of treated cases, *Int Endod J* 36:787–802, 2003.
62. Tang W, Wu Y, Smales RJ: Identifying and reducing risks for potential fractures in endodontically treated teeth, *J Endod* 36:609–617, 2010.
63. Wolanek GA, Loushine RJ, Weller RN, Kimbrough WF, Volkmann KR: In vitro bacterial penetration endodontically treated teeth coronally sealed with a dentin bonding agent, *J Endod* 27:354–357, 2001.
64. Friedman S, Shani J, Stabholz A, et al.: Comparative sealing ability of temporary filling materials evaluated by leakage of radiosodium, *Int Endod J* 19:187–193, 1986.
65. Pane ES, Palamara JE, Messer HH: Stainless steel bands in endodontics: effects on cuspal flexure and fracture resistance, *Int Endod J* 35:467–471, 2002.
66. Fox K, Gutteridge DL: An in vitro study of coronal microleakage in root canal–treated teeth restored by the post and core technique, *Int Endod J* 30:361–368, 1997.
67. Demarchi MGA, Sato EFL: Leakage of interim post and cores used during laboratory fabrication of custom posts, *J Endod* 28:328–329, 2002.
68. Gluskin AH, Radke RA, Frost SL, et al.: The mandibular incisor: rethinking guidelines for post and core design, *J Endod* 21:33–37, 1995.
69. Pontius O, Hutter JW: Survival rate and fracture strength of incisors restored with different post and core systems and endodontically treated incisors without coronoradicular reinforcement, *J Endod* 28:710–715, 2002.
70. Nagasiri R, Chitmongkolsuk S: Long-term survival of endodontically treated molars without crown coverage: a retrospective cohort study, *J Prosthet Dent* 93:164–170, 2005.
71. Lovdahl PE, Nicholls JI: Pin-retained amalgam cores vs cast-gold dowel-cores, *J Prosthet Dent* 38:507–514, 1977.
72. Guzy GE, Nicholls JI: In vitro comparison of intact endodontically treated teeth with and without endo-post reinforcement, *J Prosthet Dent* 42:39–44, 1979.
73. Leary JM, Aquilino SA, Svare CW: An evaluation of post length within the elastic limits of dentin, *J Prosthet Dent* 57:277–281, 1987.
74. Trope M, Maltz DO, Tronstad L: Resistance to fracture of restored endodontically treated teeth, *Endod Dent Traumatol* 1:108–111, 1985.
75. McDonald AV, King PA, Setchell DJ: In vitro study to compare impact fracture resistance of intact root-treated teeth, *Int Endod J* 23:304–312, 1990.
76. Goodacre CJ, Bernal G, Rungcharassaeng K, et al.: Clinical complications in fixed prosthodontics, *J Prosthet Dent* 90:31–41, 2003.
77. Gutmann JL: The dentin-root complex: anatomic and biologic considerations in restoring endodontically treated teeth, *J Prosthet Dent* 67:458–467, 1992.
78. Assif D, Nissan J, Gafni Y, et al.: Assessment of the resistance to fracture of endodontically treated molars restored with amalgam, *J Prosthet Dent* 89:462–465, 2003.
79. Raiden G, Costa L, Koss S, et al.: Residual thickness of root in first maxillary premolars with post space preparation, *J Endod* 25:502–505, 1999.
80. Tamse A, Katz A, Pilo R: Furcation groove of buccal root of maxillary first premolars: a morphometric study, *J Endod* 26:359–363, 2000.
81. Perez E, Zillich R, Yaman P: Root curvature localizations as indicators of post length in various tooth groups, *Endod Dent Traumatol* 2:58–61, 1986.
82. Nayyar A, Walton RE, Leonard LA: An amalgam coronal-radicular dowel and core technique for endodontically treated posterior teeth, *J Prosthet Dent* 43:511–515, 1980.
83. Schwartz RS, Robbins JW: Post placement and restoration of endodontically treated teeth: a literature review, *J Endod* 30:289–301, 2004.
84. Pilo R, Cardash HS, Levin E, et al.: Effect of core stiffness on the in vitro fracture of crowned, endodontically treated teeth, *J Prosthet Dent* 88:302–306, 2002.
85. Plasmans PJ, Creugers NH, Mulder J: Long-term survival of extensive amalgam restorations, *J Dent Res* 77:453–460, 1998.
86. Linn J, Messer HH: Effect of restorative procedures on the strength of endodontically treated molars, *J Endod* 20:479–485, 1994.
87. Summit JB, Burgess JO, Berry TG, et al.: The performance of bonded vs pin-retained complex amalgam restorations, *J Am Dent Assoc* 132:923–931, 2001.
88. Mannocci F, Qualtrough AJ, Worthington HV, et al.: Randomized clinical comparison of endodontically treated teeth restored with amalgam or with fiber posts and resin composite: five-year results, *Oper Dent* 30:9–15, 2005.
89. Sorensen JA, Martinoff JT: Intracoronal reinforcement and coronal coverage: a study of endodontically treated teeth, *J Prosthet Dent* 51:780–784, 1984.
90. Valderhaug J, Jokstad A, Ambjornsen E, et al.: Assessment of the periapical and clinical status of crowned teeth over 25 years, *J Dent* 25:97–105, 1997.
91. Monaco C, Llukacej A, Baldissara P, Arena A, Scotti R: Zirconia-based versus metal-based single crowns veneered with overpressing ceramic for restoration of posterior endodontically treated teeth: 5-year results of a randomized controlled clinical study, *J Dent* 65:56–63, 2017.
92. Reich S, Schierz O: Chair-side generated posterior lithium disilicate crowns after 4 years, *Clin Oral Investig* 17:1765–1772, 2013.
93. Goodacre CJ, Spolnik KJ: The prosthodontic management of endodontically treated teeth: a literature review. I. Success and failure data, treatment concepts, *J Prosthodont* 3:243–250, 1994.
94. Obermayr G, Walton RE, Leary JM, et al.: Vertical root fracture and relative deformation during obturation and post cementation, *J Prosthet Dent* 66:181–187, 1991.
95. Asmussen E, Peutzfeldt A, Sahafi A: Finite element analysis of stresses in endodontically treated, dowel-restored teeth, *J Prosthet Dent* 94:321–329, 2005.
96. Sirimai S, Riis DN, Morgano SM: An in vitro study of the fracture resistance and the incidence of vertical root fracture of pulpless teeth restored with six post-and-core systems, *J Prosthet Dent* 81:262–269, 1999.
97. Akkayan B, Gulmez T: Resistance to fracture of endodontically treated teeth restored with different post systems, *J Prosthet Dent* 87:431–437, 2002.
98. Newman MP, Yaman P, Dennison J, et al.: Fracture resistance of endodontically treated teeth restored with composite posts, *J Prosthet Dent* 89:360–367, 2003.
99. Fredriksson M, Astback J, Pamenius M, et al.: A retrospective study of 236 patients with teeth restored by carbon fiber–reinforced epoxy resin posts, *J Prosthet Dent* 80:151–157, 1998.
100. Glazer B: Restoration of endodontically treated teeth with carbon fiber posts: a prospective study, *J Can Dent Assoc* 66:613–618, 2000.
101. Malferrari S, Monaco C, Scotti R: Clinical evaluation of teeth restored with quartz fiber–reinforced epoxy resin posts, *Int J Prosthodont* 16:39–44, 2003.
102. Monticelli F, Grandini S, Goracci C, et al.: Clinical behavior of translucent-fiber posts: a 2-year prospective study, *Int J Prosthodont* 16:593–596, 2003.
103. King PA, Setchell DJ, Rees JS: Clinical evaluation of a carbon fiber reinforced endodontic post, *J Oral Rehabil* 30:785–789, 2003.
104. Tidehag P, Lundström J, Larsson B, et al.: A 7-year retrospective study of Composipost root canal posts (abstract 4080), *J Dent Res* 83, 2004 (Special Issue A).
105. Grandini S, Goracci C, Tay FR, et al.: Clinical evaluation of the use of fiber posts and direct resin restorations for endodontically treated teeth, *Int J Prosthodont* 18:399–404, 2005.
106. Mannocci F, Qualtrough AJ, Worthington HV, et al.: Randomized clinical comparison of endodontically treated teeth restored with amalgam or with fiber posts and resin composite: five-year results, *Oper Dent* 30:9–15, 2005.

107. Cagidiaco MC, Radovic I, Simonetti M, et al.: Clinical performance of fiber post restorations in endodontically treated teeth: 2-year results, *Int J Prosthodont* 20:293–298, 2007.
108. Turker SB, Alkumru HN, Evren B: Prospective clinical trial of polyethelene fiber ribbon–reinforced, resin composite post-core build-up restorations, *Int J Prosthodont* 20:55–56, 2007.
109. Wennström J: The C-Post system, *Compend Contin Educ Dent* 20(Suppl):S80–S85, 1996.
110. Naumann M, Blankenstein F, Dietrich T: Survival of glass fiber–reinforced composite post restorations after 2 years: an observational clinical study, *J Dent* 33:305–312, 2005.
111. Segerstrom S, Astback J, Ekstrand KD: A retrospective long term study of teeth restored with prefabricated carbon fiber reinforced epoxy resin posts, *Swed Dent J* 30:1–8, 2006.
112. Ferrari M, Cagidiaco MC, Goracci C, et al.: Long-term retrospective study of the clinical performance of fiber posts, *Am J Dent* 20:287–291, 2007.
113. Gallo JR, Miller T, Xu X, et al.: In vitro evaluation of the retention of composite fiber and stainless steel posts, *J Prosthodont* 11:25–29, 2002.
114. Signore A, Kaitsas V, Ravera G, et al.: Clinical evaluation of an oval-shaped prefabricated glass fiber post in endodontically treated premolars presenting an oval canal cross-section: a retrospective cohort study, *Int J Prosthodont* 24:255–263, 2011.
115. Mehta SB, Millar BJ: A comparison of the survival of fibre posts cemented with two different composite resin systems, *Br Dent J* 205:1–8, 2008 (Online: E23.DOI:10.1038/sj.bdj. 2008.1036).
116. Henry PJ: Photoelastic analysis of post core restorations, *Aust Dent J* 22:157–159, 1977.
117. Creugers NH, Mentink AG, Kayser AF: An analysis of durability data on post and core restorations, *J Dent* 21:281–284, 1993.
118. Kvist T, Rydin E, Reit C: The relative frequency of periapical lesions in teeth with root canal–retained posts, *J Endod* 15:578–580, 1989.
119. Pappen AF, Bravo M, Gonzalez-Lopez S, et al.: An in vitro study of coronal leakage after intraradicular preparation of cast-dowel space, *J Prosthet Dent* 94:214–218, 2005.
120. Colley IT, Hampson EL, Lehman ML: Retention of post crowns: an assessment of the relative efficiency of posts of different shapes and sizes, *Br Dent J* 124:63–69, 1968.
121. Johnson JK, Sakumura JS: Dowel form and tensile form, *J Prosthet Dent* 40:645–649, 1978.
122. Standlee JP, Caputo AA, Collard EW, et al.: Analysis of stress distribution by endodontic posts, *Oral Surg Oral Med Oral Pathol Oral Radiol Endod* 33:952–960, 1972.
123. Trabert KC, Caputo AA, Abou-Rass M: Tooth fracture: a comparison of endodontic and restorative treatments, *J Endod* 4:341–345, 1978.
124. Hunter AJ, Feiglin B, Williams JF: Effects of post placement on endodontically treated teeth, *J Prosthet Dent* 62:166–172, 1989.
125. Abou-Rass M, Jann JM, Jobe D, et al.: Preparation of space for posting: effect of thickness of canal walls and incidence of perforation in molars, *J Am Dent Assoc* 104:834–837, 1982.
126. Standlee JP, Caputo AA, Hanson EC: Retention of endodontic dowels: effects of cement, dowel length, diameter, and design, *J Prosthet Dent* 39:400–405, 1978.
127. Sorensen JA, Martinoff JT: Clinically significant factors in dowel design, *J Prosthet Dent* 52:28–35, 1984.
128. Fan B, Wu MK, Wesselink PR: Coronal leakage along apical root fillings after immediate and delayed post space preparation, *Endod Dent Traumatol* 15:124–126, 1999.
129. Goodacre CJ, Spolnik KJ: The prosthodontic management of endodontically treated teeth: a literature review. II. Maintaining the apical seal, *J Prosthodont* 4:51–53, 1995.
130. Abramovitz I, Tagger M, Tamse A, et al.: The effect of immediate vs delayed post space preparation on the apical seal of a root canal filling: a study in an increased-sensitivity pressure-driven system, *J Endod* 26:435–439, 2000.
131. Coniglio I, Magni E, Goracci C, et al.: Post space cleaning using a new nickel titanium endodontic drill combined with different cleaning regimens, *J Endod* 34:83–86, 2008.
132. Rödig T, Hülsmann M, Kahlmeier C: Comparison of root canal preparation with two rotary NiTi instruments: ProFile .04 and GT Rotary, *Int Endo J* 40:553–562, 2007.
133. Cheung GS, Liu CS: A retrospective study of endodontic treatment outcome between nickel-titanium rotary and stainless steel hand filing techniques, *J Endod* 35:938–943, 2009.
134. Cheung GS, Lai SC, Ng RP: Fate of vital pulps beneath a metal-ceramic crown or a bridge retainer, *Int Endod J* 38:521–530, 2005.

17 Bleaching Discolored Nonvital Teeth

ILAN ROTSTEIN AND TORY SILVESTRIN

CHAPTER OUTLINE

LEARNING OBJECTIVES

After reading this chapter, the student should be able to:

1. Identify the causes and nature of tooth discoloration.
2. Describe means of preventing tooth discolorations.
3. Differentiate between dentin and enamel discolorations.
4. Evaluate both the short-term and long-term prognoses of bleaching treatments.
5. Explain the mechanism of tooth bleaching.
6. Select the bleaching agent and technique according to the cause of discoloration.
7. Describe each step of the internal "walking bleach" technique.
8. Select the appropriate method to restore the access cavity after tooth bleaching.
9. Describe how bleaching agents may alter tooth structures.
10. Recognize the potential adverse effects of tooth bleaching and discuss means of prevention.

Bleaching discolored teeth may be internal (within the pulp chamber) or external (on the enamel surface) and involve various approaches. The objectives of treatment are to reduce or eliminate discoloration, improve the degree of coronal translucency, and alleviate present and prevent future clinical signs and symptoms.

To better understand bleaching procedures, you should know the techniques involved, understand the causes of discoloration, recognize the location of the discoloring agent, and apply the correct treatment modality. Also important is the ability to predict the outcome of treatment (i.e., how successfully various discolorations can be treated and how long the esthetic result will last). Therefore before attempting to correct discoloration, there must be a diagnosis (to determine the cause and location of the discoloration), a treatment plan (to select the appropriate bleaching material and technique), and a prognosis (to anticipated short- and long-term success). Patients must be informed of these factors before undergoing the procedure; any discoloration treatment is tempered by the explanation that bleaching bears a certain degree of unpredictability in matching the esthetics of the tooth involved fully and that substantial improvement may or may not occur. However, with proper recognition of the causes of discoloration and careful treatment protocol, no irreversible damage to the crown or root occurs.

Causes of Discoloration

Tooth discolorations may occur during or after enamel and dentin formation. Some discolorations appear after tooth eruption, and others are the result of dental procedures. *Acquired* (natural) discolorations may be superficial and located on the surface of the tooth or may be embedded and be physically incorporated into tooth hard tissues. Sometimes they result from flaws in enamel formation and structure or a traumatic injury. *Inflicted* (iatrogenic) discolorations, resulting from certain dental procedures, are usually incorporated into tooth structure and are largely preventable.

Acquired (Natural) Discolorations

Pulp Necrosis

Although microorganisms are the main cause of pulpal injury, mechanical or chemical irritation of the pulp may also result in

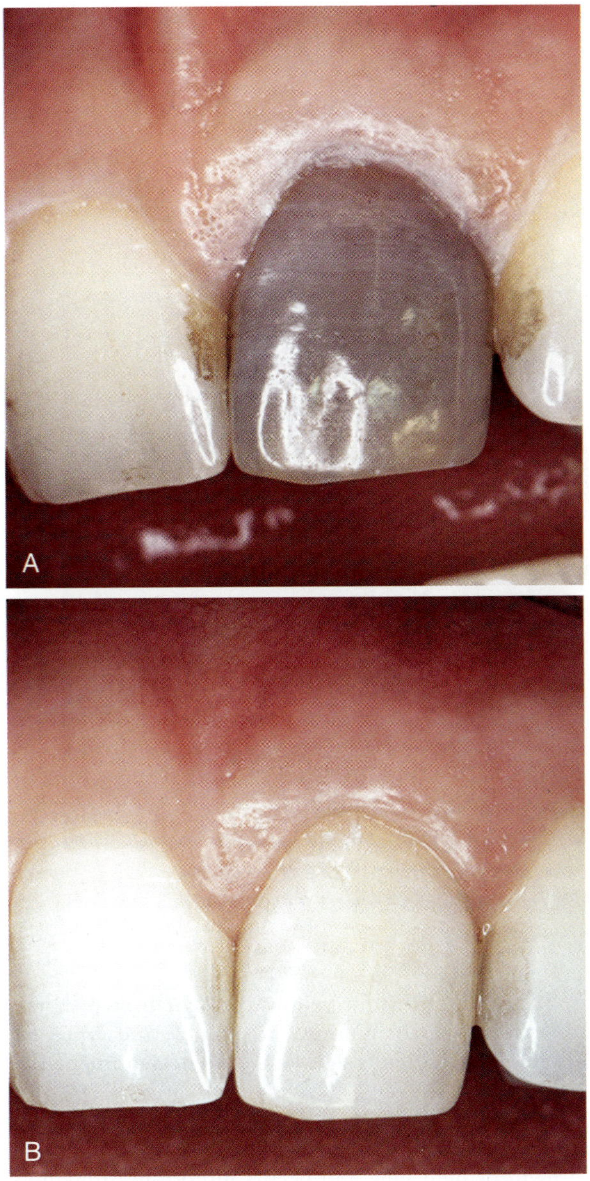

• **Fig. 17.1** **(A)** Discoloration as a result of a traumatic injury followed by pulp necrosis. **(B)** After root canal treatment, a paste of sodium perborate and water mixed to a consistency of wet sand was sealed in the pulp chamber. After 21 days of walking bleach, the tooth regained its original shade. (Courtesy of Dr. A. Claisse).

tissue necrosis. Pulp necrosis can occur via stagnation of the vasculature and formation of microabscesses. Red blood cells stagnated in the vasculature will lyse and lead to accumulation of hemoglobin and other pulp breakdown byproducts. These tissue disintegration byproducts are colored compounds that may permeate tubules to stain surrounding dentin. The degree of discoloration is likely related to how long the pulp has been necrotic.[1,2] The longer the discoloration compounds are present in the pulp chamber, the greater the discoloration. This type of discoloration can be bleached internally, usually with both short- and long-term success (Fig. 17.1).

Intrapulpal Hemorrhage

Intrapulpal hemorrhage is usually associated with an impact injury to a tooth that results in disrupted coronal blood vessels, hemorrhage into the pulp space, stasis of this extravasated material, and lysis of erythrocytes. Erythrocyte lysis leads to an accumulation of disintegration products, such as iron sulfides. These iron sulfides may permeate dentinal tubules to stain surrounding dentin. Discoloration tends to increase with time.

If the pulp becomes necrotic, the discoloration usually remains. If the pulp survives, the discoloration may resolve and the tooth regains its original shade. Sometimes, mainly in young individuals, a discolored tooth can respond unpredictably to vitality tests. Therefore you should not rely on a single clinical test to establish your diagnosis of the case. If intracoronal discoloration remains despite diagnostic testing indicating presence of a healthy pulp and normal periapex, a porcelain veneer can be considered. Although more invasive, sometimes significantly darker stain may necessitate consideration for elective root canal therapy to remove stain that would not be effectively hidden under a coronal esthetic restoration.

Internal bleaching of discoloration after intrapulpal hemorrhage is usually successful both short term and long term.[1-4]

Calcific Metamorphosis

Calcific metamorphosis, also known as *pulp canal obliteration*, is extensive formation of tertiary dentin in the pulp chamber that causes circumferential narrowing of the pulp chamber and root canal. This phenomenon usually follows an impact injury that did not result in pulp necrosis. There is likely temporary disruption of the blood supply with partial destruction of odontoblasts. Odontoblasts are usually replaced by cells that rapidly form irregular dentin on the walls of the pulp chamber and root canal space. As a result, the crowns take on a "flat" and yellow or yellow-brown discolored appearance as they gradually decrease in translucency (Fig. 17.2). The pulp usually remains vital and does not require root canal treatment. However, routine follow-up is recommended as a result of potential of pulp necrosis after a traumatic injury.[5]

If the patient desires color correction, external bleaching should be attempted first. If this is unsuccessful, root canal treatment can be performed, and internal bleaching done. The esthetic prognosis for such treatment is not always predictable. The unpredictability of this procedure results from the bleaching agent addressing discolored pigmentation in the regular structure of the dentinal tubules but not in the bulk of irregular dentin from the aberrant calcification.

Age

In older patients, color changes in the crown occur physiologically as a result of extensive dentin apposition and thinning of and optical changes in the enamel. Food and beverages also have a cumulative discoloring effect because of the inevitable cracking and other changes on the enamel surface and in the underlying dentin. In addition, previously applied restorations that degrade over time cause further discoloration. Bleaching is usually external because the discoloration is primarily on the enamel surface. Success may vary, depending on the causal factor of discoloration.

Location

The most commonly bleached teeth are the maxillary incisors. Maxillary central incisors comprise 69% of internally bleached teeth, whereas maxillary lateral incisors comprise 20% of bleached teeth.[5]

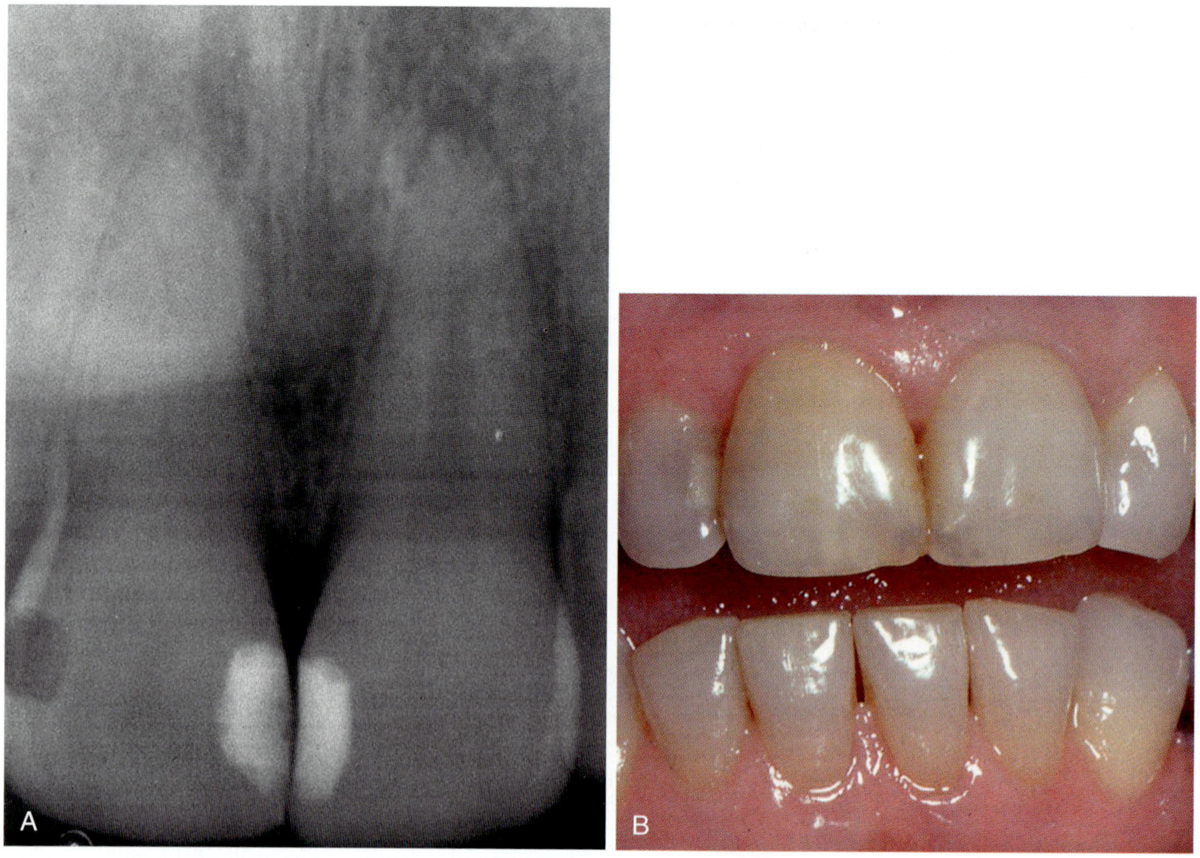

• **Fig. 17.2** Calcific metamorphosis. Impact trauma resulted in reversible pulp damage in one of the central incisors **(A)** with extensive tertiary dentin formation **(B).** These teeth may present difficulties with root canal treatment and internal bleaching.

Developmental Defects

Discolorations may also result from developmental defects or from substances incorporated into enamel or dentin during tooth formation.

Endemic Fluorosis

Ingestion of excessive amounts of fluoride during tooth formation produces defects in mineralized structures, particularly enamel matrix, with resultant hypoplasia. The severity and degree of subsequent staining generally depend on the degree of hypoplasia, which depends in turn on the patient's age and the amount of fluoride ingested during odontogenesis.[6] The teeth are not discolored on eruption but may appear chalky. Their surface, however, is porous and gradually absorbs stains from chemicals in the oral cavity.

Because the discoloration is in the porous enamel, such teeth are treated externally. Esthetic success depends mainly on the degree and duration of the discoloration. Some regression and recurrence of discoloration tend to happen but can be corrected with future rebleaching.

Systemic Drugs

Administration or ingestion of certain drugs or chemicals (many of which have not yet been identified) during tooth formation may cause discoloration, which is occasionally severe.[7]

The most common and most dramatic discoloration of this type occurs after tetracycline ingestion, usually in children. Discoloration is bilateral, affecting multiple teeth in both arches. It may range from yellow through brownish to dark gray, depending on the amount, frequency, and type of tetracycline, and the patient's age (stage of development) during administration.

Tetracycline discoloration has been classified into three groups according to severity.[8] First-degree discoloration is light yellow, light brown, or light gray and occurs uniformly throughout the crown without banding. Second-degree discoloration is more intense and is also without banding. Third-degree discoloration is very intense, and the clinical crown exhibits horizontal color banding. This type of discoloration usually predominates in the cervical region.[8] The location of the band correlates to the part of the dentin that was undergoing formation at the time of systemic tetracycline ingestion. It is therefore recommended to limit systemic tetracycline use in patients with active permanent tooth development.

Tetracycline binds to calcium, which then is incorporated into the hydroxyapatite crystal in both enamel and dentin. Most of the tetracycline, however, is found in dentin. Chronic sun exposure of teeth with the incorporated drug may cause formation of a reddish purple tetracycline oxidation byproduct, resulting in further discoloration of permanent teeth.

A phenomenon of adult-onset tetracycline discoloration has also been reported.[9] It occurs occasionally in mature teeth in patients receiving long-term minocycline therapy, which is usually given for control of cystic acne. The discoloration is gradual because of incorporation of minocycline in continuously forming dentin.[7] Staining generally is not severe.

Two approaches have been used for bleaching tetracycline discoloration. The first, which involves bleaching the external enamel surface, is limited to lighter, yellowish discoloration and requires multiple appointments to achieve a satisfactory result.[10] The second, root canal treatment followed by internal bleaching, is a predictable procedure, is useful for all degrees of discoloration severity (especially linear-band type discoloration), and has proved successful in both the short term and long term.[11]

Defects in Tooth Formation

Defects in tooth formation are confined to the enamel and are either hypocalcific or hypoplastic. Enamel hypocalcification is common, appearing as a distinct brownish or whitish area, often on the facial aspect of a crown. The enamel is well formed and intact on the surface and feels hard to the explorer. Both the whitish and the brownish spots are amenable to correction externally with good results.

Enamel hypoplasia differs from hypocalcification in that the enamel in the former is defective and porous. This condition may be hereditary (amelogenesis imperfecta) or may result from environmental factors. In the hereditary type, both deciduous and permanent dentitions are involved. Defects caused by environmental factors may involve only one or several teeth. Presumably during tooth formation the matrix is altered and does not mineralize properly. The porous enamel readily acquires stains from the oral cavity. Depending on the severity and extent of hypoplasia and the nature of the stain, these teeth may be bleached externally with some degree of success.

Blood Dyscrasias and Other Factors

Various systemic conditions may cause massive lysis of erythrocytes.[2] If this occurs in the pulp at an early age, blood disintegration products are incorporated into the forming dentin causing discoloration. An example of this phenomenon is the severe discoloration of primary teeth that usually follows erythroblastosis fetalis. This disease in the fetus, or newborn, results from Rh incompatibility factors that lead to massive systemic lysis of erythrocytes. Large amounts of hemosiderin pigment then stain the forming dentin of the primary teeth. This discoloration is not correctable by bleaching. However, this type of lysis is now uncommon because of new preventive measures.

High fever during tooth formation may result in linear defined hypoplasia. This condition, known as *chronologic hypoplasia,* is a temporary disruption in enamel formation that results in a banding type of surface defect that acquires stain. Hyperbilirubinemia, thalassemia, and sickle cell anemia may cause intrinsic bluish, brown, or green discolorations. Amelogenesis imperfecta may result in yellowish or brownish discolorations. Dentinogenesis imperfecta can cause brownish violet, yellowish, or gray discoloration. Porphyria, a metabolic disease, may cause deciduous and permanent teeth to show a red or brownish discoloration. These conditions are also not amenable to bleaching and should be corrected by minimally invasive restorative means.

Other staining factors related to systemic conditions or ingested drugs are rare and may not be identifiable.[2]

Inflicted (Iatrogenic) Discolorations

Discolorations caused by various chemicals and materials used in dentistry are usually avoidable. Many of these discolorations

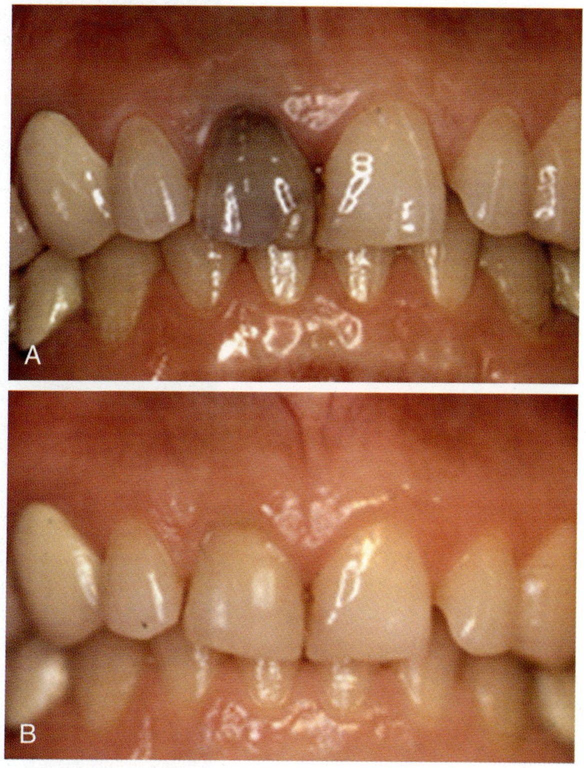

• **Fig. 17.3** **(A)** Discoloration as a result of trauma and subsequent treatment. The patient was involved in an accident that caused a coronal fracture. Root canal treatment was performed, but gutta-percha and sealer were not completely removed from the pulp chamber. An additional discoloration factor was the defective leaking restoration. **(B)** Two appointments of walking bleach and placement of a new, well-sealed composite restored esthetics. (Courtesy of Dr. M. Israel.)

respond well to bleaching, but some are more difficult to correct by bleaching alone.

Endodontically Related Discolorations

Obturating Materials

Obturating materials are the most common and severe cause of single tooth discoloration. Incomplete removal of materials from the pulp chamber upon completion of treatment often results in dark discoloration (Figs. 17.3 and 17.4). Removing all obturation materials to a level just cervical to the gingival margin can prevent such discoloration. Sometimes, removal of the obturating material 1 to 2 mm further apically is required. Common obturating materials that can lead to stain are sealer remnants, whether of the zinc oxide–eugenol type or resins. These materials may also darken with time.[12-15] Sealer remnants gradually cause progressive coronal discoloration.[15] The prognosis of bleaching in such cases depends on the components of the sealer. Sealers with metallic components often do not bleach well, and the bleaching effect tends to regress with time.

Remnants of Pulpal Tissue

Pulp fragments remaining in the crown, usually in pulp horns, can cause gradual discoloration. Pulp horns must be exposed

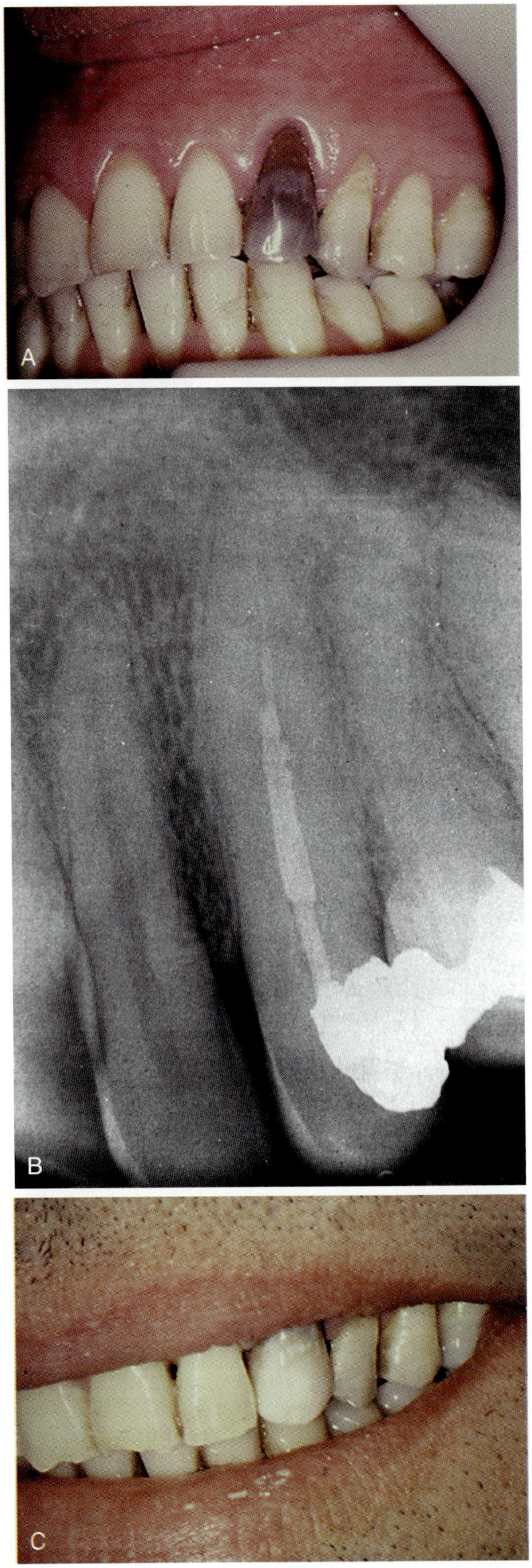

• **Fig. 17.4 (A)** Severely discolored canine. **(B)** Poor root canal treatment, in which material extended into the pulp chamber, caused some of the discoloration. **(C)** After retreatment and three appointments of walking bleach, esthetics have markedly improved. Although some cervical discoloration remains, it is largely hidden by the upper lip. (Courtesy of Dr. H. Libfeld.)

and cleaned during access preparation to ensure removal of pulpal remnants and to prevent retention of sealer at a later stage. Internal bleaching in such cases is usually successful.

Intracanal Medicaments

Several medicaments have the potential to cause internal discoloration of the dentin.[1,2,16,17] These intracanal medications, sealed in the root canal space, are in direct contact with dentin, sometimes for long periods, allowing penetration to dentin tubules and oxidization. These compounds have a tendency to discolor the dentin gradually. Most such discolorations are not marked and are readily and permanently corrected by bleaching. However, discoloration by intracanal medication containing iodoform tends to be more severe.

Coronal Restorations

Restorations are generally metallic or composite. The reasons for discoloration (and therefore the appropriate correction) are quite different.

Metallic Restorations

Amalgam is the worst offender because its dark metallic elements may turn dentin dark gray. If used to restore an access preparation, amalgam often discolors the crown (Figs. 17.4 and 17.5).

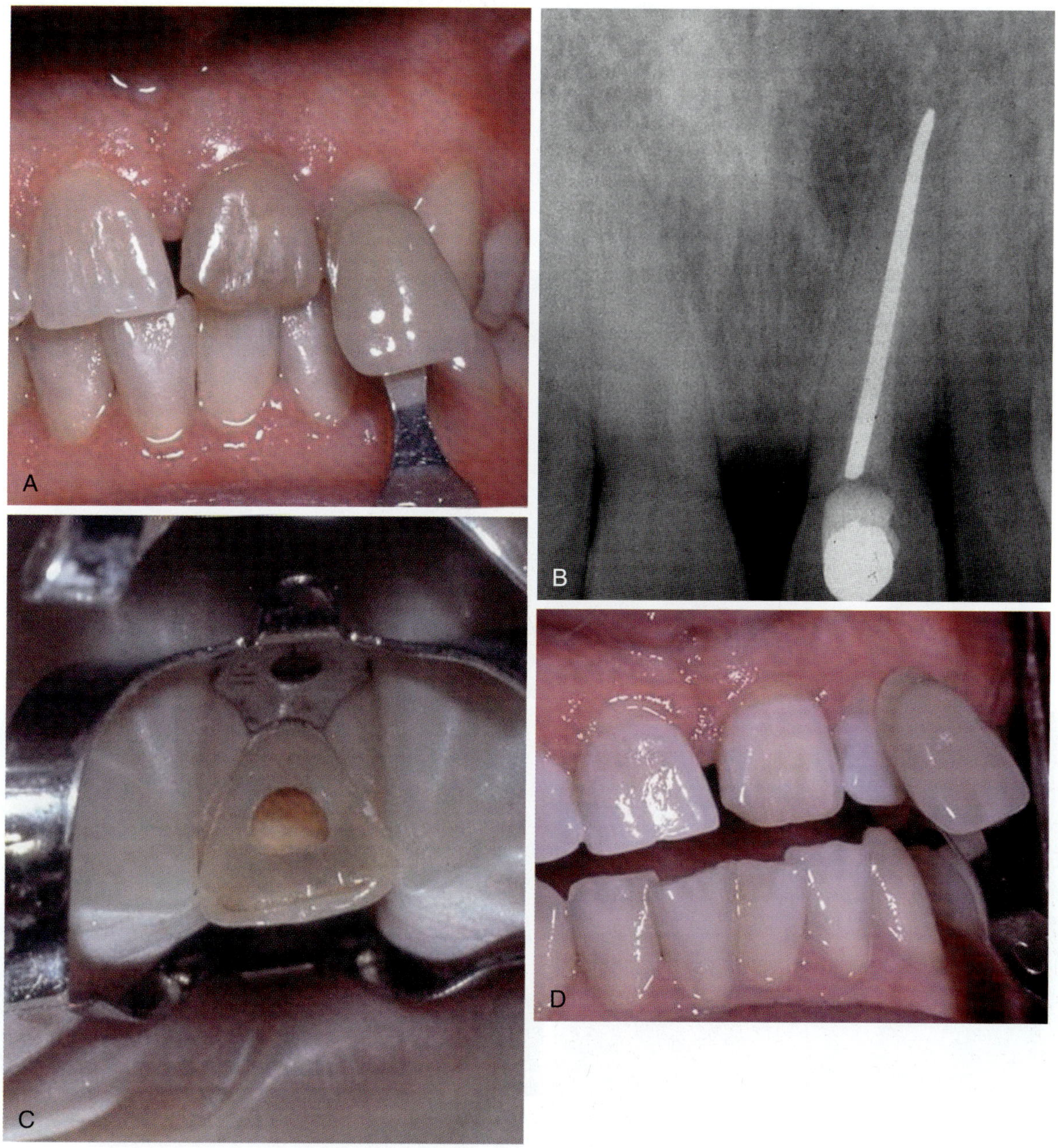

• **Fig. 17.5** **(A)** Discoloration of endodontically treated maxillary central incisor. **(B)** The presence of a silver cone in the canal, failure to remove all remnants of pulpal tissue from the chamber, and amalgam placed in the access cavity appear to be the causes of discoloration. **(C)** Removal of amalgam and refinement of the access cavity. The silver cone was removed, and endodontic retreatment was performed. **(D)** Internal bleaching, followed by placement of a new composite, restored esthetics.)

Such discolorations are difficult to bleach and tend to recur with time. However, bleaching them is worth a try. The result may be an improvement that satisfies the patient. The use of amalgam for tooth restoration is gradually decreasing in many parts of the world.

Discoloration from inappropriately placed metal pins and prefabricated posts in anterior teeth may sometimes occur. This is caused by metal that is visible through the composite or tooth structure. Occasionally, discoloration from amalgam is also caused by visibility of the restoration through translucent tooth structure. In such cases, replacement of old metallic material with an esthetically pleasing restoration will suffice.

Composite Restorations

Microleakage of composites causes discoloration. Open margins may permit chemicals to permeate gaps between the restoration and tooth structure to stain the underlying dentin. In addition, composites may become discolored with time and alter the shade of the crown. These conditions can sometimes be corrected by replacing the old composite with a new, well-sealed esthetic restoration. In many cases, internal bleaching is carried out first with good results (Fig. 17.6).

Bleaching Materials

Bleaching chemicals may act as either oxidizing or reducing agents. Most bleaching agents are oxidizers, and many preparations are available. Commonly used agents are solutions of hydrogen peroxide of different strengths, sodium perborate, and carbamide peroxide. Sodium perborate and carbamide peroxide are chemical compounds that are gradually degraded to release low levels of hydrogen peroxide. Hydrogen peroxide and carbamide peroxide are mainly indicated for external bleaching, whereas sodium perborate is mostly used for internal bleaching. All have proved effective.

Hydrogen Peroxide

Hydrogen peroxide is a powerful oxidizer that is available in various strengths, but 30% to 35% stabilized solutions (Superoxyl, Perhydrol) are the most common. These high-concentration solutions must be handled with care because they are unstable, lose oxygen quickly, and may explode unless they are refrigerated and stored in a dark container. Also, these are caustic chemicals and will burn tissue on contact.

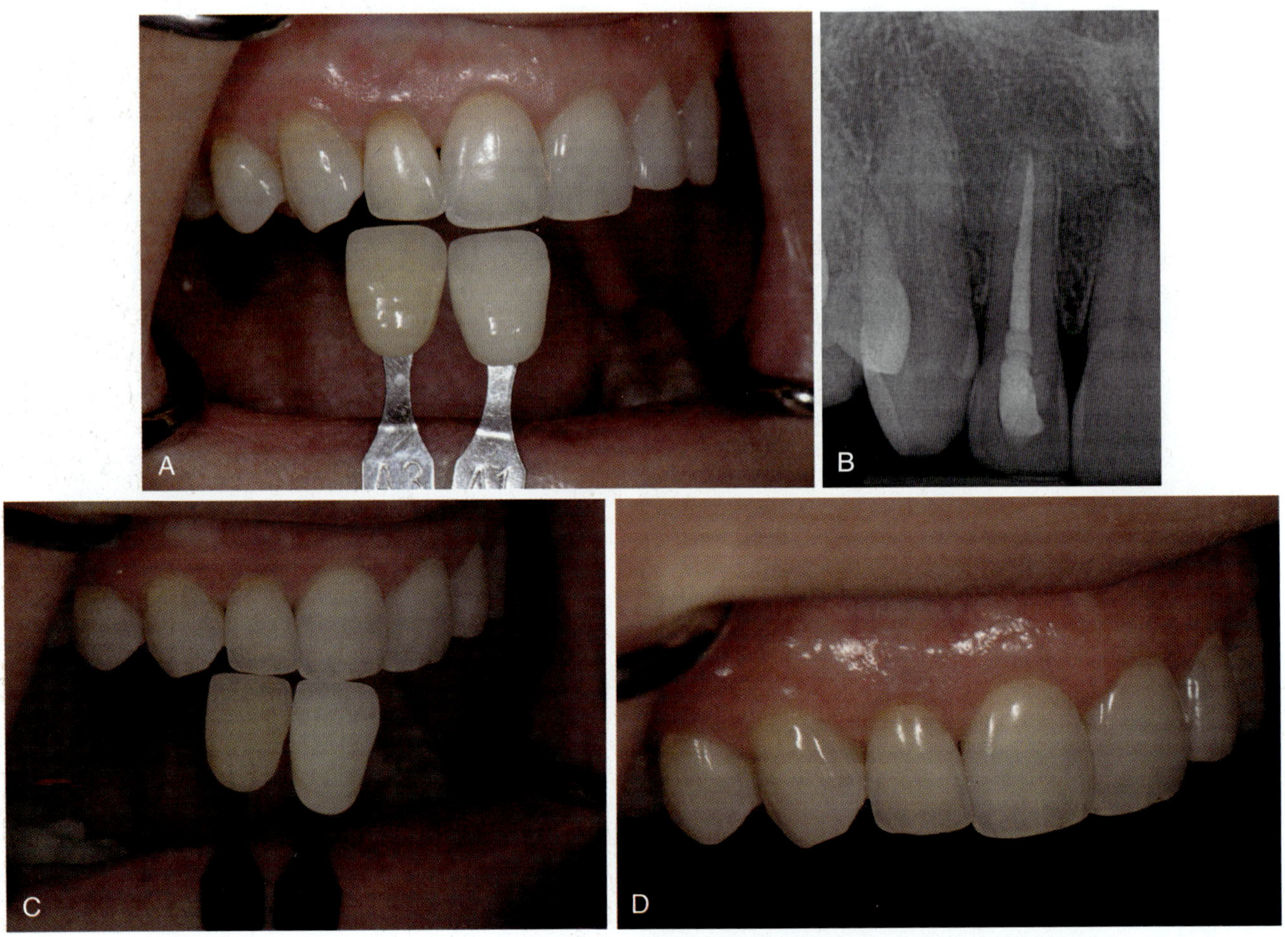

• **Fig. 17.6** **(A)** Discoloration of an endodontically treated maxillary lateral incisor in a 61-year-old female. Note the difference in coronal shade between the lateral incisor and the adjacent central incisor. Probable cause of discoloration is coronal microleakage. **(B)** Preoperative radiograph. **(C)** Immediate postoperative results after internal bleaching. The coronal shade of the treated tooth has improved and is now matching the shade of the adjacent central incisor. **(D)** Fifteen-month follow-up appointment. The treated tooth maintains pleasing esthetic results. (Courtesy of Dr. A. Sameni.)

Although highly concentrated hydrogen peroxide bleaches quickly, other chemicals that release much lower levels of peroxide are available; usually they bleach effectively with longer application periods.[18]

Sodium Perborate

Sodium perborate is available in powder form or in various commercial proprietary combinations.[19,20] When fresh, it contains about 95% perborate, corresponding to 9.9% available oxygen. Sodium perborate is stable when dry, but in the presence of acid, warm air, or water, it decomposes to form sodium metaborate, hydrogen peroxide, and nascent oxygen. Various types of sodium perborate preparations are available: monohydrate, trihydrate, and tetrahydrate. They differ in oxygen content, which determines their bleaching efficacy.[20] Commonly used sodium perborate preparations are alkaline; their pH depends on the amount of hydrogen peroxide released and the residual sodium metaborate.[21]

Sodium perborate is more easily controlled and safer than concentrated hydrogen peroxide solutions.[2,3,4,19,22,23] Therefore in most cases, it should be the material of choice for internal bleaching.

Carbamide Peroxide

Carbamide peroxide is usually available in concentrations varying between 3% and 15%. Popular commercial preparations contain about 10% carbamide peroxide and have an average pH of 5 to 6.5. They usually also include glycerin or propylene glycol, sodium stannate, phosphoric or citric acid, and flavor. In some preparations, Carbopol, a water-soluble resin, is added to prolong the release of active peroxide and to improve shelf life. Ten percent carbamide peroxide breaks down into urea, ammonia, carbon dioxide, and approximately 3.5% hydrogen peroxide.

Carbamide peroxide and hydrogen peroxide–based systems are mostly used for external bleaching and have been associated with varying degrees of alterations to dental hard tissues and surrounding mucosa.[24,25] They may adversely affect the bond strength of composite resins and their marginal seal.[24-28] Therefore these materials must be used with caution and usually under strict supervision of the dentist.

Other Agents

In the past, a preparation of sodium peroxyborate monohydrate (Amosan), which releases more oxygen than does sodium perborate, was recommended for internal bleaching. Today, this product is not available in all countries, and its clinical use is less common.

Sodium hypochlorite is a common root canal irrigant that is commonly available commercially as a 3% to 8% household bleach. Although used as a household bleaching agent, it does not release enough oxidizer to be effective and is not commonly used for routine tooth bleaching.

Other nonperoxide bleaching agents have also been suggested for clinical use; however, these have not been significantly more effective than traditional agents.[29,30]

Study Questions

1. Tooth discoloration under existing composites occurs because of:
   a. Open margins of the restoration allowing leakage
   b. Discoloration of the composite itself over time
   c. Excess bonding agent becoming more opaque with time
   d. All of the above
   e. A and B only
2. In order to prevent discoloration from remaining pulpal tissue, the operator should:
   a. Access the entire pulp chamber and pulp horns to completely débride the tissue
   b. Rely primarily on chemical débridement
   c. Ensure that sealer does not contact any tissue remnants, as sealer will only discolor if in contact with pulp tissue remnants
   d. All of the above
   e. A and B only
3. The condition caused by a temporary disruption in enamel formation resulting in a banding type of surface defect acquiring stain is known as:
   a. Progressive dentinal hypoplasticity
   b. Chromatic chronologic dimorphism
   c. Chronologic hypoplasia
   d. Acute progressive chromatism
   e. All of the above
4. When considering internal bleaching of a tooth with pulp necrosis, which of the following is correct:
   a. Tissue disintegration products leach into dentinal tubules to cause stain
   b. The degree of discoloration is related to the duration of pulp necrosis
   c. Dark discolorations have only short-term success when bleached
   d. All of the above
   e. A and B only
5. What is the current recommended bleaching material used for the "walking bleach" technique?
   a. 5.25% sodium hypochlorite
   b. 30% hydrogen peroxide
   c. Sodium perborate
   d. Iodoform
   e. A and B only

Mechanism of Tooth Bleaching

Tooth bleaching is a dynamic process that involves diffusion of the bleaching material into the dental hard tissues. It is initiated by movement of bleaching agent into the tooth structure, to interact with the stain molecules. Consequently, micromorphologic alterations and changes within the dental structures occur that affect their optical properties and perception.[31]

The mechanism resulting in changed perception of tooth color can be divided into three phases: (1) movement of the bleaching agent into the tooth structures; (2) interaction of the bleaching agent with the stain molecules; and (3) alteration of the tooth structures to reflect light differently. The outcome of this sequence of events results in the final color change of the tooth.[31]

It is theorized that the mechanism of tooth bleaching involves interaction of oxidizing agent with organic chromophores.[32] Chromophores are the parts of molecules responsible for demonstrating color. Bleaching works by an oxidation process removing electrons that allows large pigmented organic molecules to be dissolved into smaller, less pigmented constituents.[32] The altered chromophores are still present, but their size is significantly reduced and not as visible by the human eye.

Internal (Nonvital) Bleaching Techniques

The methods most commonly used to bleach teeth in conjunction with root canal treatment are the *thermocatalytic* technique and the so-called *walking bleach* technique.[1,2,19,33] These techniques are somewhat different but produce similar results.[3,4,19] The walking bleach technique (described later in the chapter) is preferred because it requires the least chair time and is more comfortable and safer for the patient. Whatever technique is used, the active ingredient is the oxidizer, which is available in different chemical forms. The least potent form is preferred.

Indications for internal bleaching technique are: (1) discolorations of pulp chamber origin; (2) dentin discolorations; and (3) discolorations that are not amenable to external bleaching. Contraindications are: (1) superficial enamel discolorations; (2) defective enamel formation; (3) severe dentin loss; (4) presence of caries; and (5) discolored proximal composites (unless they are replaced after bleaching).

Thermocatalytic Technique

The thermocatalytic technique involves placing the oxidizing agent in the pulp chamber and then applying heat. Heat may be supplied by heat lamps, light or laser, flamed instruments, or electrical heating devices, which are manufactured specifically to bleach teeth.[33]

Potential damage from the thermocatalytic approach includes the possibility of external cervical root resorption because of irritation to cementum and the periodontal ligament, possibly from the oxidizing agent in combination with heat.[34,35] Therefore the application of heat during internal bleaching is contraindicated. Also, the thermocatalytic technique has not proved more effective long term than other methods and is not recommended for routine internal bleaching.

A thermocatalytic variation is ultraviolet photo-oxidation. A 30% to 35% hydrogen peroxide solution is placed in the pulp chamber on a cotton pellet, followed by a 2-minute exposure to ultraviolet light applied to the coronal labial surface of the tooth. Supposedly this causes the release of oxygen similar to that seen in other thermocatalytic bleaching techniques.[36,37] It is probably no more effective than the walking bleach technique and requires more chair time. Because of toxicity considerations with concentrated hydrogen peroxide, this technique is not recommended for internal bleaching of nonvital teeth.

Walking Bleach

The walking bleach technique should be used in all situations requiring internal bleaching. Not only is it as effective as the techniques previously described, but it also is the safest and has the shortest chair time requirement.[19,38] The technique is described step-by-step in Fig. 17.7 and Box 17.1.

It is often thought that "overbleaching" is desirable because of future recurrence of discoloration. However, bleaching a tooth to a lighter shade than its neighbors should be performed with caution because the overbleached tooth may not discolor to match the shade of adjacent teeth. A tooth that is too light may be as unesthetic as one that is too dark.

Treatments at subsequent visits are similar. If early bleaching appointments do not provide satisfactory results, the following additional procedures may be attempted: (1) a thin layer of stained facial dentin is removed with a small round bur (see Box 17.1, step 7); and (2) the walking bleach paste is strengthened by mixing the sodium perborate with hydrogen peroxide (start with 3% hydrogen peroxide and increase the concentration gradually, only if necessary) instead of water. Heat is not used. The more potent oxidizer may enhance the bleaching effect but may increase the risk of subsequent root damage.[34,35,39]

Carbamide peroxide has also been suggested for internal bleaching.[40] This agent, however, is probably not superior to sodium perborate.

Although usually the final results are excellent, occasionally only partial lightening is achieved. Surprisingly, the patient often is very pleased and satisfied with a modest improvement and does not expect perfection. Therefore internal bleaching is worth the attempt.

The number of applications varies based on the degree of discoloration and its cause.[5] On average, most discolorations (75%) can be handled in one to two appointments, but sometimes more appointments and reapplications are necessary.[5,38,41]

Final Restoration

Proper tooth restoration is essential for long-term successful internal bleaching results.[42-44] The pulp chamber and access cavity are restored at the final visit (see Fig. 17.7, *E*). Although it has been proposed that substances such as acrylic monomer or silicones be placed in the chamber to fill the dentinal tubules, this is not beneficial. Furthermore, these substances may themselves lead to discoloration with time. However, it is important to restore the chamber carefully and to seal the lingual access to enhance the new shade and prevent leakage. The ideal method for filling the chamber after tooth bleaching has not been determined. However, the chamber must not be filled totally with composite; this may cause a loss of translucency of the tooth.[43]

It is easy and effective to fill the chamber with a light-colored gutta-percha temporary stopping, glass ionomer, or a light shade of zinc phosphate cement and then to restore the lingual access with a light-cured, acid-etched composite.[44] Composite resins have different levels of color and contrast ratio.[45] Awareness of such optical properties aids in material selection. An adequate depth of composite should be ensured to seal the cavity and provide some incisal support. Light curing from the labial, rather than the lingual, surface is recommended because this results in shrinkage of the composite resin toward the axial walls, reducing the rate of microleakage.[46] Coronal microleakage of lingual access restorations is a problem.[47] A leaky restoration may lead to recurrence of discoloration.

Residual peroxides of bleaching agents, mainly hydrogen peroxide and carbamide peroxide, may affect the bonding strength of composites to the tooth.[27,48-50] Sodium perborate mixed with water can result in much less loss of bond strength than does concentrated hydrogen peroxide.[50] Therefore it is not recommended that the tooth be restored with composite immediately after bleaching but only after an interval of a few days. The use of catalase and other agents has also been proposed for fast elimination of residual peroxides from the access cavity and for protection against potential hazardous effects[51-54]; this merits further studies.

It has been suggested that packing calcium hydroxide paste in the chamber for a few weeks before the final restoration is placed would reverse the acidity caused by bleaching agents and prevent resorption; however, this procedure is ineffective and unnecessary.[21,38]

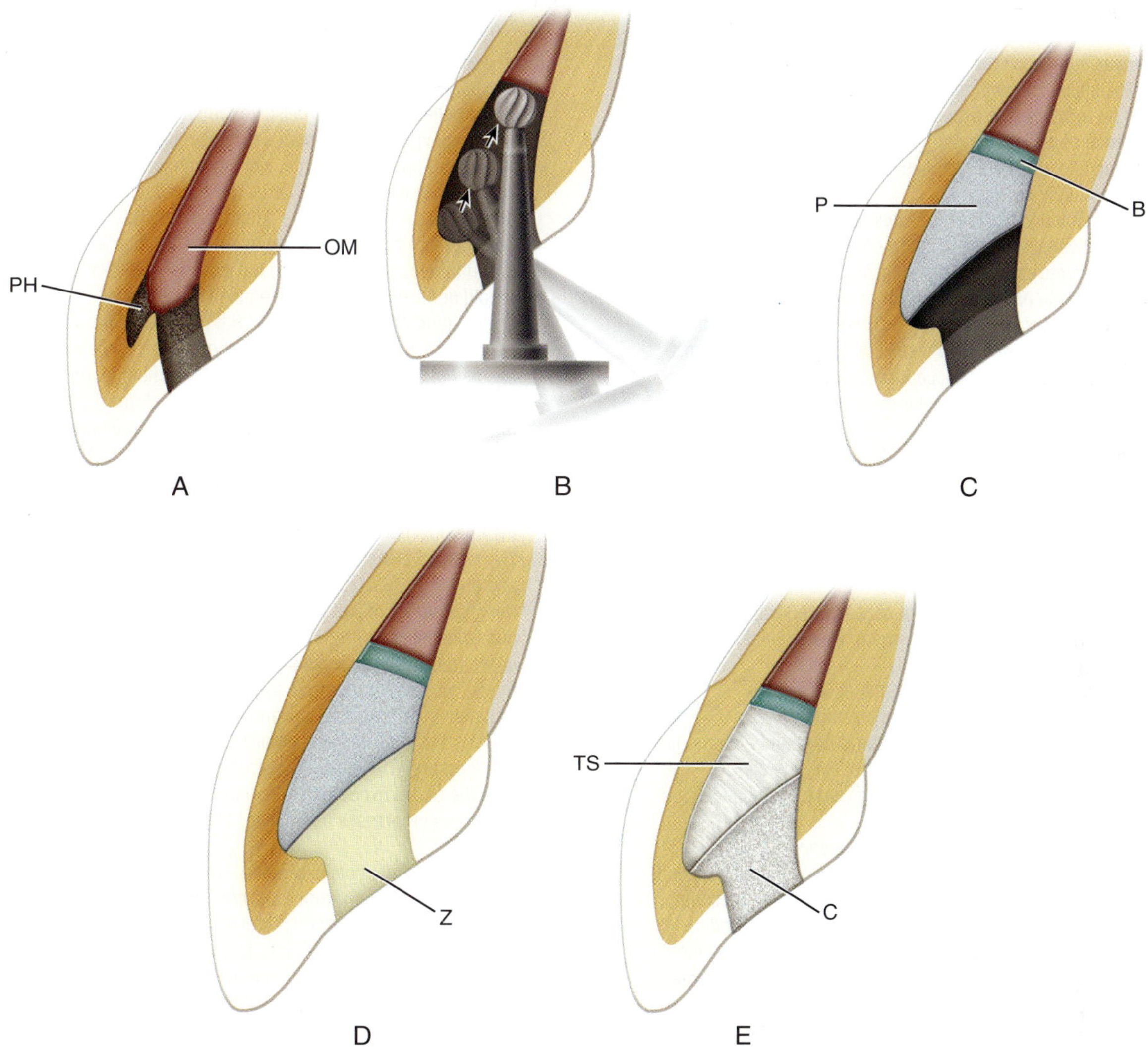

• **Fig. 17.7** Walking bleach. **(A)** Internal staining of dentin caused by remnants of obturating materials *(OM)* in the pulp chamber and by materials and tissue debris in the pulp horns *(PH)*. **(B)** Coronal restoration is removed completely, access preparation is improved, and gutta-percha is removed apically to just below the cervical margin. Next, the pulp horns are cleaned with a round bur. (Shaving a thin layer of dentin from the facial wall is optional and may be attempted at later appointments if discoloration persists.) **(C)** An optional protective cement base *(B)* is placed over the gutta-percha, not extending above the cervical margin. After the removal of sealer remnants and materials from the chamber with solvents, a paste *(P)* composed of sodium perborate and water (mixed to the consistency of wet sand) is placed. The incisal area is undercut to retain the temporary restoration. **(D)** A thick mixture of a zinc oxide–eugenol–type temporary filling *(Z)* seals the access. **(E)** At a subsequent appointment, when the desired shade has been reached, a permanent restoration is placed. A suggested method is to fill the chamber with white temporary stopping *(TS)* or with light polycarboxylate or zinc phosphate base. Acid-etched composite *(C)* restores lingual access and extends into the pulp horns for retention and to support the incisal edge. (From Walton RE: Bleaching procedures for teeth with vital and nonvital pulps. In Levine N, editor: *Current treatment in dental practice,* Philadelphia, 1986, Saunders.)

Other agents have been proposed to enhance the bleaching effect or to open tubules; none have been shown to be significantly effective.[55,56]

Future Rediscoloration

Although initial bleaching is successful, many of these teeth may rediscolor after several years.[57,58] Patients must be informed of this possible occurrence and that rebleaching usually will be successful.

When to Bleach

Internal bleaching may be performed at various intervals after root canal treatment (see Figs. 17.1 and 17.5). The appearance of the discolored tooth may be improved soon after treatment. However, the walking bleach technique may be initiated at the same appointment as the obturation. In fact, this may motivate the patient to accept bleaching because the appearance of the discolored tooth may be improved soon after treatment. Bleaching may also be attempted successfully many years after

• BOX 17.1 Walking Bleach Technique

The steps of the walking bleach technique are as follows (see Fig. 17.7).

1. The patient is familiarized with the probable causes of discoloration, the procedure to be followed, the expected outcome, and the possibility of future recurrence of discoloration (regression). To avoid disappointment or misunderstanding, effective communication before, during, and after treatment is absolutely necessary.
2. Radiographs are made to assess the status of the periapical tissues and the quality of root canal treatment. Treatment failure or questionable obturation requires retreatment before bleaching.
3. The quality and shade of any restoration present are assessed. If defective, the restoration is replaced. Often tooth discoloration results from leaking or discolored restorations. Also, the patient is informed that the bleaching procedure may temporarily (or permanently) affect the seal and color match of the restoration, requiring its replacement.
4. Tooth color is evaluated with a shade guide, and clinical photographs are taken at the beginning of and throughout the procedure. These provide a point of reference for future comparison by both dentist and patient.
5. The tooth is isolated with a dental dam. Interproximal wedges may also be used for better isolation. If hydrogen peroxide is used, a protective cream (e.g., petroleum jelly, Orabase, or cocoa butter) must be applied to the gingival tissues before dam placement. This protection is not required with sodium perborate use.
6. The restorative material is removed from the access cavity (see Fig. 17.7, *B*). Refinement of access and removal of all old obturating and restorative materials from the pulp chamber comprise the most important stage in the bleaching process. The clinician must check that pulp horns or other "hidden" areas have been opened and are free of pulp tissue remnants.
   A chamber totally filled with composite resin presents a clinical problem. First, this material is resistant to cutting with burs. Second, its shade is often indistinct from that of dentin. However, all composite must be removed to allow the bleaching agent to contact and penetrate the dentin. Care must be taken during restoration removal to avoid inadvertent cutting of sound dentin. The operating microscope or magnifying loupes are beneficial.
7. (Optional). This step may be necessary if the discoloration seems to be of metallic origin or if, on the second or third appointment, bleaching alone does not seem to be sufficient. A thin layer of stained dentin is carefully removed toward the facial aspect of the chamber with a round bur in a slow-speed handpiece. This removes much of the discoloration (which is concentrated in the pulpal surface area). It may also open the dentinal tubules for better penetration by the bleaching agents.
8. All materials should be removed to a level just apical to the gingival margin. Appropriate solvents (e.g., orange solvent, or chloroform, on a cotton pellet) are used to dissolve remnants of the common sealers.
9. If hydrogen peroxide is used, a sufficient layer of protective cement barrier (e.g., polycarboxylate, zinc phosphate, glass ionomer, intermediate restorative material [IRM], or Cavit at least 2 mm thick) is applied as a barrier on the obturating material. This is essential to minimize leakage of bleaching agents.[53] The barrier should protect the dentin tubules and conform to the external epithelial attachment.[54] It should not extend incisal to the gingival margin (see Fig. 17.7, *C*). Acid etching of dentin internally with phosphoric (or other) acid to remove the smear layer and open the tubules is not necessary.[55,56] The use of any caustic chemical in the chamber is unwarranted because periodontal ligament irritation or external root resorption may result.[56] The same reservation applies to solvents such as ether or acetone before application of the bleaching agent. The application of concentrated hydrogen peroxide with heat (thermocatalytic) has been suggested as the next step. This may not be more effective and also may be questionable from a safety standpoint.
10. The walking bleach paste is prepared by mixing sodium perborate and an inert liquid, such as water, saline, or anesthetic solution, to the consistency of wet sand (approximately 2 g/mL). Although sodium perborate mixed with 30% hydrogen peroxide bleaches faster, in most cases the long-term results are similar to those of sodium perborate mixed with water; therefore the former mixture should not be used routinely.[3,4,19,38] Another advantage of sodium perborate and inert liquid is that a protective cement barrier and gingival protection are unnecessary. With a plastic instrument, the pulp chamber is packed with the paste. Excess liquid is removed by tamping with a cotton pellet. This also compresses and pushes the paste into the recesses (see Fig. 17.7, *C*).
11. Excess oxidizing paste is removed from undercuts in the pulp horns and gingival area with an explorer. A cotton pellet is not used, but a thick mix of zinc oxide–eugenol (preferably IRM) or Cavit is packed carefully to a thickness of at least 3 mm to ensure a good seal (see Fig. 17.7, *D*).
12. The dental dam is removed. The patient is informed that the bleaching agent works slowly and that significant lightening may not be evident for 2 or more weeks. It is common to see no change initially, but dramatic results occur in successive days or weeks or after a future reapplication.
13. The patient is scheduled to return approximately 2 to 4 weeks later, and the procedure is repeated. If at any future appointment (third or fourth) progressive lightening is not evident, further walking bleach treatments with sodium perborate and water solution may not prove beneficial.[38]

discoloration has occurred (see Figs. 17.3 and 17.4), even with porcelain veneer restorations (Fig. 17.8). Such teeth show no markedly greater tendency for recurrence of discoloration than teeth stained for shorter discoloration periods.[57] However, it is probable that a shorter discoloration period tends to improve the chances for successful bleaching and reduce the likelihood of recurrence of discoloration.[58]

Other factors that may influence long-term success have also been evaluated clinically. The patient's age and the rate of discoloration have no major effect on the long-term stability of bleaching.[57]

Complications and Safety

Patient safety is always the major concern in any procedure. Some possible adverse effects produced by chemicals and bleaching procedures are discussed in the following sections.

External Root Resorption

Clinical reports[35,59] and histologic studies[34,39] have shown that internal bleaching may induce external root resorption. The oxidizing agent, particularly 30% hydrogen peroxide, and heat may be the culprits. However, the exact mechanism by which periodontium or cementum is damaged has not been fully elucidated. Presumably, the irritating chemical diffuses through the dentinal tubules[60] and reaches the periodontium through defects in the cementoenamel junction.[61] Chemicals combined with heat are likely to cause necrosis of the cementum, inflammation of the periodontal ligament, and subsequent root resorption.[34,39] The process is liable to be enhanced in the presence of bacteria.[62] Previous traumatic injury and young age may also act as predisposing factors.[1,2] Therefore injurious chemicals and procedures should be avoided if they are not essential for bleaching. Again, sodium perborate mixed with water should be preferred over 35% hydrogen

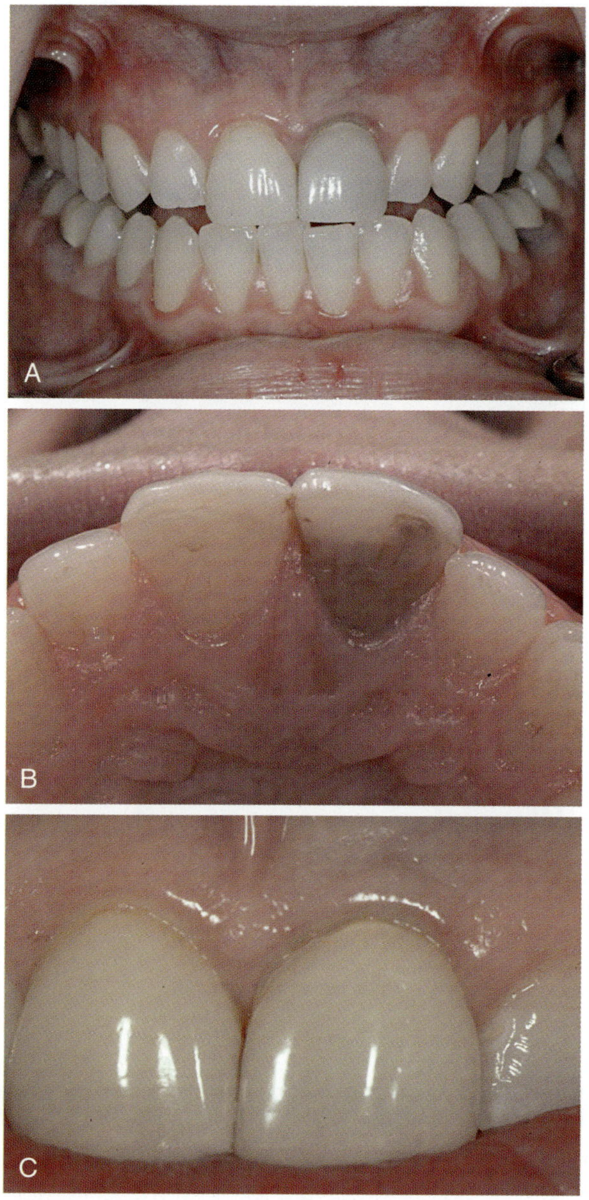

• **Fig. 17.8 (A)** Discoloration of endodontically treated incisor restored with a porcelain veneer. Discoloration is reflected through the veneer and is most evident at the cervical area. **(B)** Lingual view reveals extensive discoloration of the dentin and composite that was used to restore the access cavity. **(C)** Removal of discolored composite, internal bleaching, and placement of a new, well-sealed composite restored tooth esthetics. (Courtesy of Dr. A. Sameni.)

peroxide.[38,63] Also, apical to the cervical margin, oxidizing agents should not be exposed to more of the pulp space and dentin than is absolutely necessary to obtain a satisfactory esthetic clinical result.

Coronal Fracture

Slightly increased brittleness of the coronal tooth structure, particularly when heat is applied, is also thought to result from certain bleaching procedures. This supposedly is a result of either desiccation or alterations to the physicochemical characteristics of the dentin and enamel.[64-67] It appears that bleached teeth are no more susceptible to fracture if properly restored.[68]

Chemical Burns

As mentioned earlier, sodium perborate is safe; however, 30% hydrogen peroxide is caustic and can cause chemical burns and sloughing of the gingiva. When this strong chemical is used, the soft tissues should be coated with an isolation cream such as petroleum jelly, Orabase, or cocoa butter. Animal studies suggest that catalase applied to oral tissues before hydrogen peroxide treatment fully prevents the associated tissue damage.[69]

Intrinsic Discolorations

Intrinsic discolorations are those incorporated into tooth structure during tooth formation.[70] Significantly, most of these discolorations are in dentin and are relatively difficult to treat externally. A good example is staining from tetracycline that is incorporated into the mineral structure of the developing tooth. The incorporated tetracycline imparts its color to the dentin.

Tetracycline

Both external and internal bleaching techniques have been advocated as a means of improving the appearance of tetracycline-discolored teeth. As noted earlier, the internal technique is more effective and has a very good long-term prognosis.[11,70] However, the best resolution for tetracycline discolorations is prevention.

The technique involves root canal treatment followed by an internal walking bleach technique, as outlined earlier in this chapter. If the procedure is explained to patients, they may accept this approach, with gratifying results (Fig. 17.9). However, this procedure is not for every patient. Many will prefer to keep their pulps intact and opt to external bleaching.

Other Intrinsic Discolorations

Other drugs or ingested chemicals are incorporated into teeth that are forming and cause discoloration. There are no reports of attempts to bleach these teeth. Presumably, attempts to lighten teeth with dentinal discolorations by the external application of bleaching agents would be only marginally effective.

Extrinsic Discolorations

Extrinsic discolorations are more superficial and are obviously more amenable to external bleaching. The success of bleaching, however, depends more on the depth of the stain in the enamel rather than on the color of the stain itself. These discolorations are not treated by internal bleaching.

When and What to Refer

The demand for tooth bleaching has been steadily increasing in the last decade.[31,71] It has been proven to be safe and effective when done by a trained dental professional. Most bleaching procedures can be performed by general dentists, particularly if the cause of the discoloration is diagnosed. If the general practitioner cannot make this identification, referral to a specialist should be considered.

The practitioner may also wish to refer patients whose tooth discoloration does not respond to conventional methods of bleaching. Unidentified factors may be preventing the bleaching chemicals from effectively reaching the stain. The specialist may be able to identify and correct these factors.

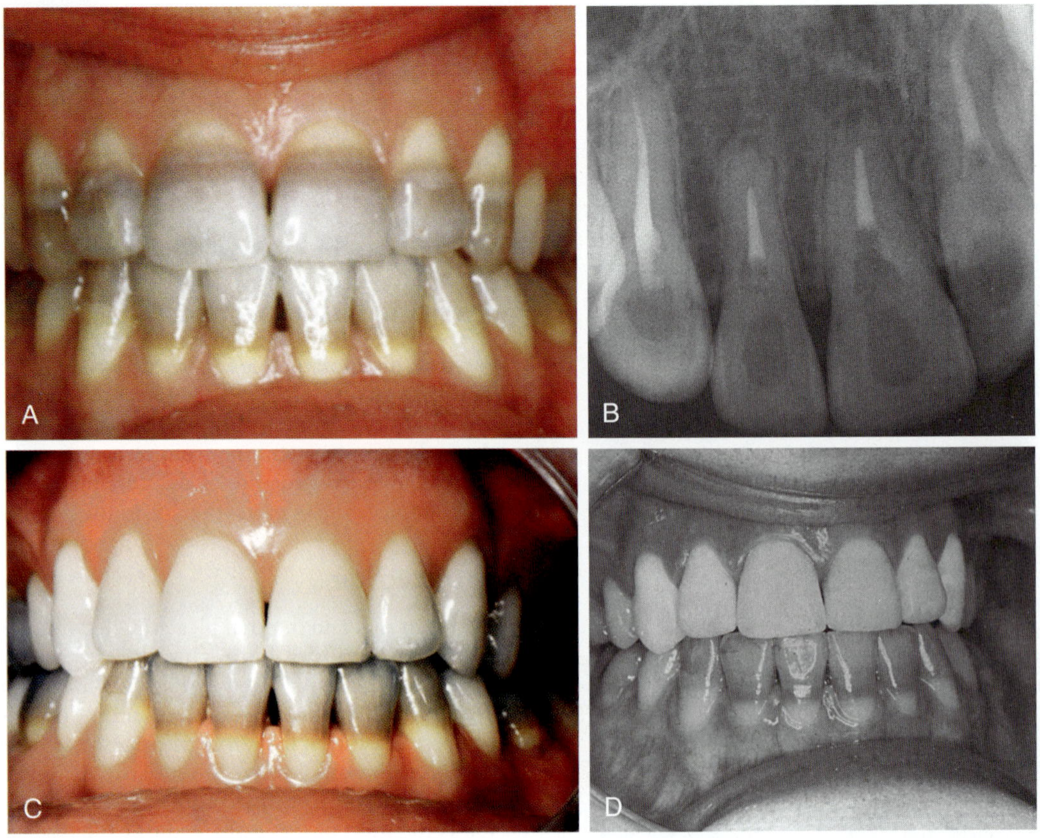

• **Fig. 17.9** **(A)** Characteristic grayish discoloration and banding of tetracycline discolorations. Cervical regions on maxillary and mandibular teeth show no discoloration; tetracycline was not administered during those periods of tooth development. **(B)** Root canal treatment has been completed on the maxillary anterior teeth, with subsequent walking bleach procedures. **(C)** After the necessary number of bleaching appointments, the teeth are restored permanently. Note the marked contrast with the mandibular incisors, which remain untreated. **(D)** At the 4-year follow-up, no regression and no recurrence of discoloration are seen. (Courtesy of Dr. H. Wayne Mohorn.)

Study Questions

6. Carbamide peroxide:
   a. Is used mainly for external bleaching
   b. Improves composite bond strength
   c. Does not cause any mucosal tissue damage
   d. All of the above
   e. B and C only
7. The mechanism of bleaching is most correctly summarized by the following:
   a. Bleaching proceeds by washing out the pigment of molecules and leaving behind only their unstained external structure.
   b. Reactive oxygen species cause the breakdown of larger pigmented molecules into smaller less visibly pigmented molecules.
   c. Bleaching occurs via alteration of trans bonds to a cis fashion that allows kinked structures to be better aligned and thus creates less visible pigmentation in the visible light spectrum.
   d. Chromophores attack the bonds of other molecules, leading to dissolution of the reactive oxygen species (which otherwise contribute to pigmentation of molecules).
   e. B and C
8. In case internal bleaching procedure requires more than two attempts, it is recommended to:
   a. Remove the coronal aspect of the obturation material and place the orifice barrier more apically.
   b. Place less concentrated hydrogen peroxide containing bleaching material.
   c. Continue replacement of the bleaching agent via the same procedure until the desired shade is reached.
   d. Use a slow speed round bur to hollow out the dentin in the pulp chamber in a deliberate fashion that allows better light transmission.
   e. A and D
9. Which of the following is correct when considering restoration of endodontically treated teeth that have recently undergone internal bleaching?
   a. Acrylic monomer or silicones should be placed as a liner to occlude the dentinal tubules before final restoration of the tooth.
   b. The pulp chamber should not be filled completely with composite resin because it could decrease the natural translucency of the tooth.
   c. Placement of calcium hydroxide for 1 to 2 weeks after bleaching is recommended to increase the pH of the dentin before placement of a restoration.
   d. When curing the access composite, it is recommended to cure from the lingual aspect rather than from the labial.
   e. B and D

Study Questions—cont'd

10. Which of the following statements about internal bleaching is correct?
    a. Long-standing discolorations that are bleached internally are always more prone to rediscoloration than short-term discolorations.
    b. Patient age plays a critical role in the success of internal bleaching procedures.
    c. Although the exact mechanism is not fully clear, it is presumed that the etiology of bleaching related root resorption may be caused by leaching of hydrogen peroxide through dentinal tubules and defects in the CEJ and root surface causing irritation to the periodontium.
    d. Internally bleached teeth are shown to be more brittle and more prone to fracture.
    e. All of the above

ANSWERS

Answer Box 17

1 e. A and B only.
2 a. Access the entire pulp chamber and pulp horns to completely débride the tissue.
3 c. Chronologic hypoplasia.
4 e. A and B only.
5 c. Sodium perborate.
6 a. Is used mainly for external bleaching.
7 b. Reactive oxygen species cause the breakdown of larger pigmented molecules into smaller less visibly pigmented molecules.
8 a. Remove the coronal aspect of the obturation material and place the orifice barrier more apically.
9 b. The pulp chamber should not be filled completely with composite resin because it could decrease the natural translucency of the tooth.
10 c. Although the exact mechanism is not fully clear, it is presumed that the etiology of bleaching related root resorption may be due to leaching of hydrogen peroxide through dentinal tubules and defects in the CEJ and root surface causing irritation to the periodontium.

References

1. Rotstein I: Intracoronal bleaching of nonvital teeth. In Greenwall L, editor: *Tooth whitening techniques*, ed 2, Boca Raton, 2017, CRC Press, p 143.
2. Rotstein I, Walton R: Bleaching discolored teeth. In Torabinejad M, Walton RE, Fouad AF, editors: *Endodontics: principles and practice*, ed 5, St Louis, 2015, Elsevier/Saunders, p 428.
3. Rotstein I, Zalkind M, Mor C, et al.: In vitro efficacy of sodium perborate preparations used for intracoronal bleaching of discolored non-vital teeth, *Endod Dent Traumatol* 7:177, 1991.
4. Rotstein I, Mor C, Friedman S: Prognosis of intracoronal bleaching with sodium perborate preparation in vitro: 1-year study, *J Endod* 19:10, 1993.
5. Abott P, Heah SY: Internal bleaching of teeth: an analysis of 225 teeth, *Aust Dent J* 54:326, 2009.
6. Driscoll WS, Horowitz HS, Meyers RJ, et al.: Prevalence of dental caries and dental fluorosis in areas with optimal and above-optimal water fluoride concentrations, *J Am Dent Assoc* 107:42, 1983.
7. Tredwin CJ, Scully C, Bagan-Sebastian JV: Drug-induced disorders of teeth, *J Dent Res* 84:596, 2005.
8. Jordan RE, Boksman L: Conservative vital bleaching treatment of discolored dentition, *Compend Contin Educ Dent* 5:803, 1984.
9. Chiappinelli JA, Walton RE: Tooth discoloration resulting from long-term tetracycline therapy: a case report, *Quintessence Int* 23:539, 1992.
10. Botelho MG, Chan AWK, Newsome PRH, et al.: A randomized controlled trial of home bleaching of tetracycline-stained teeth, *J Dent* 67:29, 2017.
11. Walton RE, O'Dell NL, Lake FT, et al.: Internal bleaching of tetracycline-stained teeth in dogs, *J Endod* 9:416, 1983.
12. Davis MC, Walton RE, Rivera EM: Sealer distribution in coronal dentin, *J Endod* 28:464, 2002.
13. Thomson AD, Athanassiadis B, Kahler B, et al.: Tooth discoloration: staining effects of various sealers and medicaments, *Aust Endod J* 38:2, 2012.
14. Lenherr P, Allgayer N, Weiger R, et al.: Tooth discoloration induced by endodontic materials: a laboratory study, *Int Endod J* 45:942, 2012.
15. Parsons JR, Walton RE, Ricks-Williamson L: In vitro longitudinal assessment of coronal discoloration from endodontic sealers, *J Endod* 27:699, 2001.
16. Kim JH, Kim Y, Shin SJ, et al.: Tooth discoloration of immature permanent incisor associated with triple antibiotic therapy: a case report, *J Endod* 36:1086, 2010.
17. Kirchhoff AL, Raldi DP, Salles AC, et al.: Tooth discolouration and internal bleaching after the use of triple antibiotic paste, *Int Endod J* 48:1181, 2015.
18. Lim MY, Lum SO, Poh RS, et al.: An in vitro comparison of the bleaching efficacy of 35% carbamide peroxide with established intracoronal bleaching agents, *Int Endod J* 37:483, 2004.
19. Spasser H: A simple bleaching technique using sodium perborate, *NY State Dent J* 27:332, 1961.
20. Weiger R, Kuhn A, Lost C: In vitro comparison of various types of sodium perborate used for intracoronal bleaching of discolored teeth, *J Endod* 20:338, 1994.
21. Rotstein I, Friedman S: pH variation among materials used for intracoronal bleaching, *J Endod* 17:376, 1991.
22. Asfora KK, Santos C, Montes MA, et al.: Evaluation of biocompatibility of sodium perborate and 30% hydrogen peroxide using the analysis of the adherence capacity and morphology of macrophages, *J Dent* 33:155, 2005.
23. Maleknejad F, Ameri H, Kianfar I: Effect of intracoronal bleaching agents on ultrastructure and mineral content of dentin, *J Conserv Dent* 15:174, 2012.
24. Majeed A, Farooq I, Grobler SR, et al.: Tooth bleaching: a review of the efficacy and adverse effects of various tooth whitening products, *J Coll Physicians Surg Pak* 25:891, 2015.
25. Goldberg M, Grootveld M, Lynch E: Undesirable and adverse effects of tooth-whitening products: a review, *Clin Oral Investig* 14:1, 2010.
26. Crim GA: Post-operative bleaching: effect on microleakage, *Am J Dent* 5:109, 1992.
27. Titley KC, Torneck CD, Ruse ND: The effect of carbamide-peroxide gel on the shear bond strength of a microfill resin to bovine enamel, *J Dent Res* 71:20, 1992.
28. Moosavi H, Ghavamnasiri M, Manari V: Effect of postoperative bleaching on marginal leakage of resin composite and resin-modified glass ionomer restorations at different delayed periods of exposure to carbamide peroxide, *J Contemp Dent Pract* 10:e009, 2009.
29. Marin PD, Heithersay GS, Bridges TE: A quantitative comparison of traditional and non-peroxide bleaching agents, *Endod Dent Traumatol* 14:64, 1998.

30. Kaneko J, Inoue S, Kawakami S, et al.: Bleaching effect of sodium percarbonate on discolored pulpless teeth in vitro, *J Endod* 26:25, 2000.
31. Kwon SR, Wertz PW: Review of the mechanism of tooth whitening, *J Esthet Restor Dent* 27:240, 2015.
32. Plotino G, Buono L, Grande MN, et al.: Nonvital tooth bleaching: a review of the literature and clinical procedures, *J Endod* 34:394, 2008.
33. Buchalla W, Attin T: External bleaching therapy with activation by heat, light or laser: a systematic review, *Dent Mater* 23:586, 2007.
34. Madison S, Walton R: Cervical root resorption following bleaching of endodontically treated teeth, *J Endod* 16:570, 1990.
35. Friedman S, Rotstein I, Libfeld H, et al.: Incidence of external root resorption and esthetic results in 58 bleached pulpless teeth, *Endod Dent Traumatol* 4:23, 1988.
36. Howell RA: Bleaching discoloured root-filled teeth, *Br Dent J* 148:159, 1980.
37. Lin LC, Pitts DL, Burgess Jr LW: An investigation into the feasibility of photobleaching tetracycline-stained teeth, *J Endod* 14:293, 1988.
38. Holmstrup G, Palm AM, Lambjerg-Hansen H: Bleaching of discoloured root-filled teeth, *Endod Dent Traumatol* 4:197, 1988.
39. Rotstein I, Friedman S, Mor C, et al.: Histological characterization of bleaching-induced external root resorption in dogs, *J Endod* 17:436, 1991.
40. Devji T: Walking bleach technique of endodontically treated teeth with 35% hydrogen peroxide and 37% carbamide peroxide may result in similar improvements in tooth color and patient satisfaction, *J Am Dent Assoc* 149:e113, 2018.
41. Attin T, Paque F, Ajam F, et al.: Review of the current status of tooth whitening with the walking bleach technique, *Int Endod J* 36:313, 2003.
42. Deliperi S: Clinical evaluation of nonvital tooth whitening and composite resin restorations: five-year results, *Eur J Esthet Dent* 3:148, 2008.
43. Freccia WF, Peters DD, Lorton L: An evaluation of various permanent restorative materials' effect on the shade of bleached teeth, *J Endod* 8:265, 1982.
44. Rivera EM, Vargas M, Ricks-Williamson L: Considerations for the aesthetic restoration of endodontically treated anterior teeth following intracoronal bleaching, *Pract Periodont Aesthet Dent* 9:117, 1997.
45. de Costa J, Vargas M, Swift EJ, et al.: Color and contrast ratio of resin composites for whitened teeth, *J Dent* 1:e27, 2009.
46. Lemon RR: Bleaching and restoring endodontically treated teeth, *Curr Opin Dent* 1:754, 1991.
47. Wilcox LR, Diaz-Arnold A: Coronal microleakage of permanent lingual access restorations in endodontically treated anterior teeth, *J Endod* 15:584, 1989.
48. Titley KC, Torneck CD, Ruse ND, et al.: Adhesion of a resin composite to bleached and unbleached human enamel, *J Endod* 19:112, 1993.
49. Sundfeld RH, Briso AL, De Sa PM, et al.: Effect of time interval between bleaching and bonding on tag formation, *Bull Tokyo Dent Coll* 46:1, 2005.
50. Timpawat S, Nipattamanon C, Kijsamanmith K, et al.: Effect of bleaching agents on bonding to pulp chamber dentine, *Int Endod J* 38:211, 2005.
51. Rotstein I: Role of catalase in the elimination of residual hydrogen peroxide following tooth bleaching, *J Endod* 19:567, 1993.
52. Lima AF, Lessa FC, Mancini MN, et al.: Transdentinal protective role of sodium ascorbate against the cytopathic effects of H_2O_2 released from bleaching agents, *Oral Surg Oral Med Oral Pathol Oral Radiol Endod* 109:e70, 2010.
53. Rotstein I, Zyskind D, Lewinstein I, et al.: Effect of different protective base materials on hydrogen peroxide leakage during intracoronal bleaching in vitro, *J Endod* 18:114, 1992.
54. Steiner DR, West JD: A method to determine the location and shape of an intracoronal bleach barrier, *J Endod* 20:304, 1994.
55. Casey LJ, Schindler WG, Murata SM, et al.: The use of dentinal etching with endodontic bleaching procedures, *J Endod* 15:535, 1989.
56. Camps J, Pommel L, Aubut V, et al.: Influence of acid etching on hydrogen peroxide diffusion through human dentin, *Am J Dent* 23:168, 2010.
57. Dahl JE, Pallesen U: Tooth bleaching: a critical review of the biological aspects, *Crit Rev Oral Biol Med* 14:292, 2003.
58. Brown G: Factors influencing successful bleaching of the discolored root-filled tooth, *Oral Surg Oral Med Oral Pathol* 20:238, 1965.
59. Heithersay GS, Dahlstrom SW, Marin PD: Incidence of invasive cervical resorption in bleached root-filled teeth, *Aust Dent J* 39:82, 1994.
60. Rotstein I, Torek Y, Misgav R: Effect of cementum defects on radicular penetration of 30% H_2O_2 during intracoronal bleaching, *J Endod* 17:230, 1991.
61. Neuvald L, Consolaro A: Cementoenamel junction: microscopic analysis and external cervical resorption, *J Endod* 26:503, 2000.
62. Heling I, Parson A, Rotstein I: Effect of bleaching agents on dentin permeability to *Streptococcus faecalis*, *J Endod* 21:540, 1995.
63. Rokaya ME, Beshr K, Hashem Mahram A, et al.: Evaluation of extraradicular diffusion of hydrogen peroxide during intracoronal bleaching using different bleaching agents, *Int J Dent* 2015:493795, 2015.
64. Rotstein I, Lehr Z, Gedalia I: Effect of bleaching agents on inorganic components of human dentin and cementum, *J Endod* 18:290, 1992.
65. Lewinstein I, Hirschfeld Z, Stabholz A, et al.: Effect of hydrogen peroxide and sodium perborate on the microhardness of human enamel and dentin, *J Endod* 20:61, 1994.
66. Chng HK, Ramli HN, Yap AU, et al.: Effect of hydrogen peroxide on intertubular dentine, *J Dent* 33:363, 2005.
67. Eimar H, Siciliano R, Abdallah MN, et al.: Hydrogen peroxide whitens teeth by oxidizing the organic structure, *J Dent* 40(suppl 2):e25, 2012.
68. Roberto AR, Sousa-Neto MD, Viapiana R, et al.: Effect of different restorative procedures on the fracture resistance of teeth submitted to internal bleaching, *Braz Oral Res* 26:77, 2012.
69. Rotstein I, Wesselink PR, Bab I: Catalase protection against hydrogen peroxide–induced injury in rat oral mucosa, *Oral Surg Oral Med Oral Pathol* 75:744, 1993.
70. Lake FT, O'Dell NL, Walton RE: The effect of internal bleaching on tetracycline in dentin, *J Endod* 11:415, 1985.
71. Joiner A, Luo W: Tooth colour and whiteness: a review, *J Dent* 67S:S3, 2017.

18 Procedural Accidents

ALI NOSRAT, YOSHITSUGU TERAUCHI, AND MAHMOUD TORABINEJAD

CHAPTER OUTLINE

LEARNING OBJECTIVES

After reading this chapter, the student should be able to recognize procedural accidents and describe the causes, prevention, and treatment of the following:

1. Pulp chamber perforation during access preparation
2. Ledging
3. Dental materials or dentin shavings obstructing the canal
4. Coronal or radicular perforation
5. Separated instrument
6. Obturation short of prepared working length
7. Obturation materials extended beyond apex
8. Incomplete obturation
9. Post space preparation mishaps
10. Accidental injections

Introduction

Like other complex disciplines of dentistry, root canal therapy can present unwanted or unforeseen challenges that can affect the prognosis. These mishaps are collectively termed *procedural accidents*. However, fear of procedural accidents should not deter a practitioner from performing root canal treatment if proper case selection and competency issues are observed.

Knowledge of the etiologic factors involved in procedural accidents is essential for their prevention. In addition, methods of recognition and treatment, as well as the effects of such accidents on prognosis, must be learned. Most problems can be avoided by adhering to the basic principles of diagnosis, case selection, treatment planning, access preparation, cleaning and shaping, obturation, and post space preparation.

Examples of procedural accidents include swallowed or aspirated endodontic instruments, crown or root perforation, ledge formation, separated instruments, underfilled or overfilled canals, and vertically fractured roots. A good practitioner uses knowledge, dexterity, intuition, patience, and awareness of personal limitations to minimize these accidents. When an accident occurs during root canal treatment, the patient should be informed about (1) the incident, (2) procedures necessary for correction, (3) alternative treatment modalities, and (4) the effect of this accident on prognosis. Proper medical-legal documentation is mandatory. A successful practitioner learns from past experiences and applies them to future challenges. In addition, the practitioner who knows her/his own limitations will recognize potentially difficult cases and will refer the patient to an endodontist. The beneficiary will be the patient, who will receive the best care.

This chapter discusses the causes, prevention, and treatment of several types of procedural accidents that may occur at different phases of root canal treatment. The effect of these accidents on short- and long-term prognoses will be also described.

Perforations During Access Cavity Preparation

The prime objective of an access cavity is to provide an unobstructed or straight-line pathway to the apical foramen (Fig. 18.1). Accidents, such as excess removal of tooth structure or perforation, may occur during attempts to locate canals. Failure to achieve straight-line access is often the main etiologic factor for other types of intracanal accidents.

Causes

Despite anatomic variations in the configuration of various teeth, the pulp chamber, in most cases, is located in the center of the anatomic crown. The pulp system is located in the long axis of the tooth. Lack of attention to the degree of axial inclination of a tooth

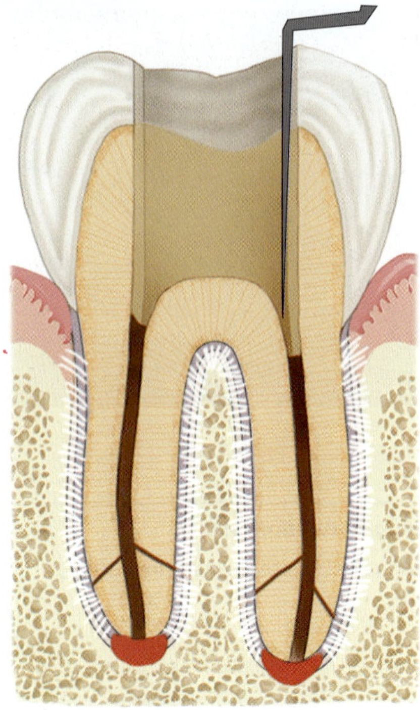

• **Fig. 18.1** Making an unobstructed and straight-line pathway to the apical foramen of root canals prevents accidental procedures.

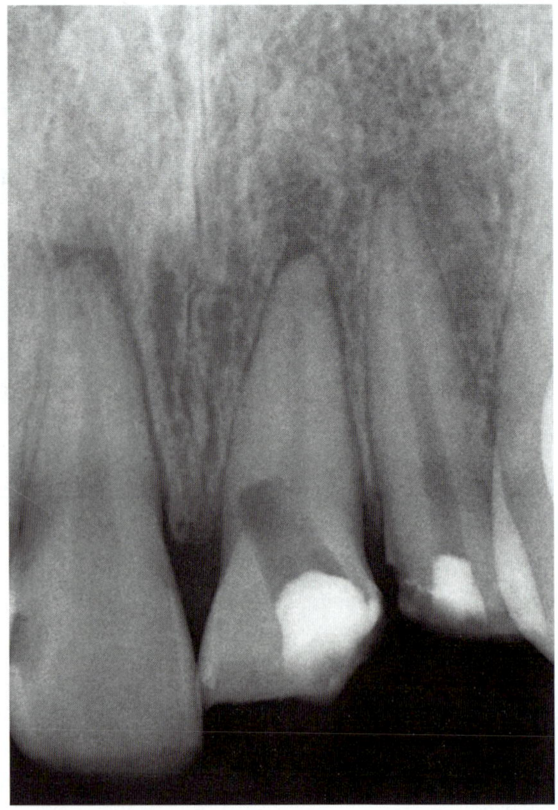

• **Fig. 18.2** Lack of attention to the degree of axial inclination of central incisor in relation to adjacent teeth and to alveolar bone resulted in severe gouging and near perforation in an otherwise simple access preparation.

in relation to adjacent teeth and to alveolar bone may result in either gouging or perforation of the crown or the root at various levels (Fig. 18.2). After establishing the proper access outline form, failure to direct the bur parallel to the long axis of a tooth will cause gouging or perforation of the crown or root. This problem often occurs when the dentist must use the reflected image from an intraoral mirror to make the access preparation. In these situations, the natural tendency is to direct the bur away from the long axis of the root to improve vision through the mirror. Another reason that can cause failure in directing the bur parallel to the long axis of the root is access cavity preparation under higher magnifications. The clinician may lose "depth perception" when using the microscope at higher magnifications, which can cause deviation from the long axis. Failure to check the orientation of the access opening during preparation may result in a perforation. The dentist should stop periodically to review the bur-tooth relationship. Aids for evaluating progress include transillumination, magnification, and radiographs. Bite-wing radiographs taken during access cavity preparation are useful to adjust the mesiodistal orientation. Shifted periapical radiographs are useful to adjust the buccolingual orientation.

Searching for the pulp chamber or orifices of canals through an underprepared access cavity may also result in accidents. Failing to recognize when the bur passes through a small or flattened (disk-like) pulp chamber in a multirooted tooth may also result in gouging or perforation of the furcation (Fig. 18.3, *A*).

A cast crown often is not aligned in the long axis of the tooth; directing the bur along the misaligned casting may result in a coronal or radicular perforation.

Prevention

Clinical Examination

Thorough knowledge of tooth morphology, including both surface and internal anatomy and their relationship, is mandatory to prevent pulp chamber perforations. Next, location and angulation of the tooth must be related to adjacent teeth and alveolar bone to avoid a misaligned access preparation. In addition, radiographs of teeth from different angles provide information about the size and extent of the pulp chamber and the presence of internal changes such as calcification or resorption. The radiograph is a two-dimensional projection of a three-dimensional object. Varying the horizontal exposure angle will provide at least a distorted view of the third dimension and may be helpful in supplying additional anatomic information. Cone beam computed tomography (CBCT) can also provide invaluable information in cases with severe calcification or unusual canal anatomy. In complex cases, referral to an endodontist may be indicated.

Operative Procedures

Use of a rubber dam (Fig. 18.4) during root canal treatment is usually indicated.[1,2] However, in situations in which problems are anticipated in locating pulp chambers (e.g., tilted teeth, misoriented castings, or calcified chambers), initiating access without a rubber dam is preferred because it allows better crown-root alignment. However, when access is made without rubber dam placement, no intracanal instruments, such as files, reamers, or broaches, should be used unless they are secured by a piece of floss[6] and a throat pack is placed. Constricted chambers or canals must be sought patiently, with small amounts of dentin removed at a time.

Failure to recognize when the bur passes through the roof of the pulp chamber, if the chamber is calcified, may result in gouging or perforation of the furcation. After penetration of the roof of

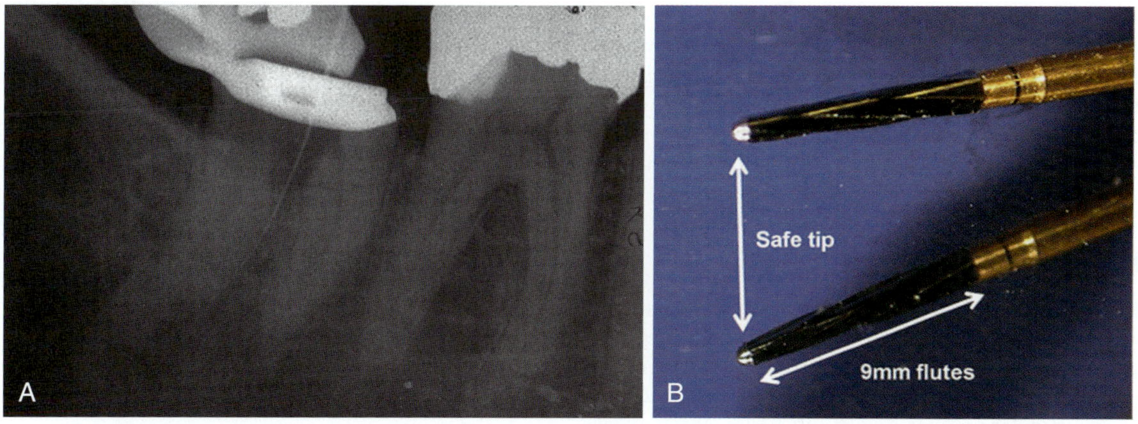

• **Fig. 18.3** **(A)** Failure to recognize when the bur passes through the roof of the pulp chamber in a calcified pulp chamber may result in gouging or perforation of the furcation. The use of apex locators and angled radiographs is necessary for early perforation detection. Early detection reduces damage and improves repair. **(B)** Use of a "safe-ended" access bur will prevent perforation of the chamber floor.

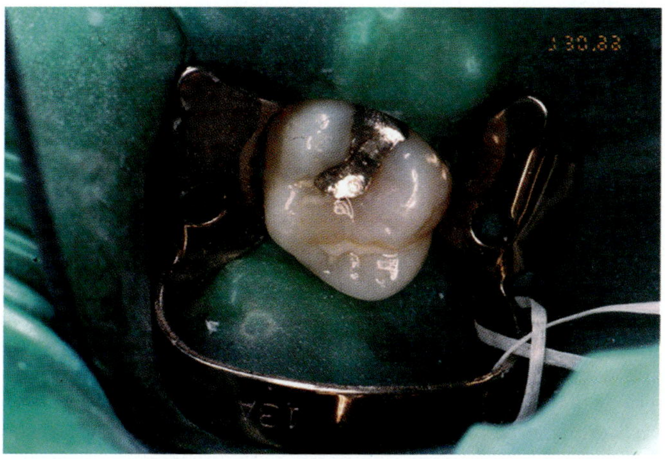

• **Fig. 18.4** Rubber dam must be applied in the anterior and posterior teeth. It provides isolation of the target tooth and prevents procedural accidents.

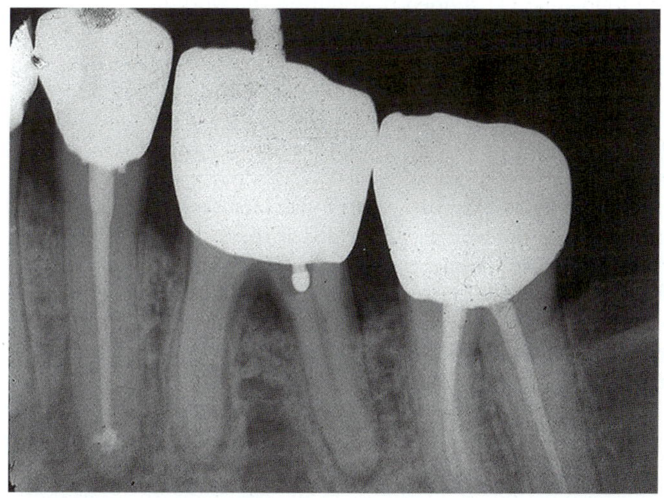

• **Fig. 18.5** A small bur is placed during access preparation when orientation is a problem. This provides information about angulation and depth of bur penetration.

the chamber, using a "safe-ended" access bur, such as the Endo Z (Dentsply/Maillefer, Tulsa, OK) or a pulp shaper bur (Dentsply/Tulsa Dental, Tulsa, OK), will prevent perforation of the chamber floor (Fig. 18.3, *B*).

The use of apex locators and angled radiographs is necessary for early perforation detection. Early detection reduces damage caused by continued treatment (irrigation, cleaning, and shaping) and improves the prognosis for nonsurgical repair.

Another useful method of providing isolation and visualizing the crown-root alignment is the use of a "split" dam. This dam can be applied in the anterior region without a rubber dam clamp (see Chapter 13) or in posterior regions by quadrant isolation if a distal tooth can be clamped. Also, elimination of the metal clamp from the field of operation allows radiographic orientation of coronal access preparation.

To orient the access, a bur may be placed in the preparation hole (secured with cotton pellets) and then radiographed (Fig. 18.5). This provides information about depth of access in relation to canal location. Remember, a single canal is located in the center of the root. A direct facial radiograph will show the mesiodistal relationship; a mesial- or distal-angled film will show the faciolingual location. This procedure is helpful for locating small canals.

Use of a fiberoptic light during access preparation may assist in locating canals. This strong light illuminates the cavity when the beam is directed through the access opening (reflected light) and illuminates the pulp chamber floor (transmitted light). In the latter case, a canal orifice appears as a dark spot. Using magnifying glasses or an operative microscope[3-7] will also aid in locating a small orifice. Magnification loupes (2.5 or greater) are useful especially when combined with transillumination. The ultimate aid in canal location is the operating microscope. Patients with problems requiring significant magnification for canal location should be referred to an endodontist who has this specialized equipment.

CBCT imaging is a useful tool to locate and negotiate the canals, specifically in teeth with complicated or calcified internal anatomy.[8-10] CBCT can be used before and, if needed, during the treatment to prevent perforation and to locate the canals in teeth with calcified pulp chamber. Limited field of view images are preferred over large field of view images as they provide accurate images with higher resolution. The axial cross-sections at the cementoenamel junction (CEJ) level can show the position of the calcified pulp chamber relative to the external surface of the crown. If the clinician cannot find the canals after the access cavity preparation is started, the CBCT can be taken to help locating the canals. The clinician can adjust the depth of troughing as well as the mesiodistal and buccolingual position of the bur using axial, sagittal, and coronal cross-sections, respectively.

Recognition and Treatment

Perforation into the periodontal ligament (PDL) or bone usually (but not always) results in immediate and continuous hemorrhage. The canal or chamber is difficult to dry, and placement of a paper point or cotton pellet may increase or renew the bleeding. Bone is relatively avascular compared with soft tissue. Mechanical perforation may initially produce only hemorrhage equal to that of pulp tissue.

Perforations must be recognized early to avoid subsequent damage to the periodontal tissues with intracanal instruments and irrigants. Early signs of perforation may include one or more of the following: (1) sudden pain during the working length determination when local anesthesia was adequate during access preparation; (2) sudden appearance of hemorrhage; (3) burning pain or a bad taste during irrigation with sodium hypochlorite; or (4) other signs, including a radiographically malpositioned file or a PDL reading from an apex locator that is short of the working length on an initial file entry.

Unusually severe postoperative pain may result from cleaning and shaping procedures performed through an undetected perforation. At a subsequent appointment, the perforation site will be hemorrhagic because of the inflammation of the surrounding tissues. The overall prognosis of the tooth must be evaluated with respect to the strategic value of the tooth, the location and size of the defect, and the potential for repair.

Perforation into the PDL at any location will have a negative effect on long-term prognosis.[11] The dentist must inform the patient of the questionable prognosis[12] and closely monitor the long-term periodontal response to any treatment. In addition, the patient must know what signs or symptoms indicate failure and, if failure occurs, what the subsequent treatment will be.

Perforations during access cavity preparation present a variety of problems. When a perforation occurs or is strongly suspected, the patient should be considered for referral to an endodontist. In general, a specialist is better equipped to manage these patients (Fig. 18.6, *A–C*). Also, after long-term evaluation, other procedures, such as surgery, may be necessary if future failure occurs.

Lateral Root Perforation

The location and size of the perforation during access are important factors in a lateral perforation. If the defect is located above the height of crestal bone, the prognosis for perforation repair is favorable.[13] These defects can be easily "exteriorized" and repaired with standard restorative material such as amalgam, glass ionomer, or composite. Periodontal curettage or a flap procedure is occasionally required to place, remove, or smooth excess repair material. In some cases, the best repair is placement of a full crown with the margin extended apically to cover the defect.

Teeth with perforations at or below the crestal bone in the coronal third of the root generally have the poorest prognosis.[12,13] Attachment often recedes and a periodontal pocket forms, with attachment loss extending apically to at least the depth of the defect. The treatment goal is to position the apical portion of the defect above the crestal bone. Orthodontic root extrusion is generally the procedure of choice for teeth in the esthetic zone.[14] Surgical crown lengthening may be considered when the esthetic result will not be compromised or when adjacent teeth require surgical periodontal therapy. Internal repair of these perforations by mineral trioxide aggregate (MTA) has been shown to provide an adequate seal compared with other materials.[15] Ideally, repair of these perforations should be done as soon as it happens to prevent the damage to the periodontium. Generally, repair of perforations in the coronal third after attachment loss and pocket formation has a very poor prognosis. However, a recent case report showed calcium-silicate–based materials might have the potential to induce healing in the periodontium even when perforation repair is done after pocket formation.[16]

Furcation Perforation

A perforation of the furcation is generally one of two types: the "direct" or the "stripping" type. Each is created and managed differently, and the prognoses vary. The direct perforation usually occurs during a search for a canal orifice. It is more of a "punched-out" defect into the furcation with a bur and is usually accessible, may be small, and may have walls. This type of perforation should be immediately (if possible) repaired with MTA (Fig. 18.7). If proper conditions exist (dryness), glass ionomer or composite can be used to seal the defect. Prognosis is usually good if the defect is sealed immediately.

A stripping perforation involves the furcation side of the coronal root surface and results from excessive flaring with files or drills. Whereas direct perforations are usually accessible and therefore can be repaired nonsurgically, stripping perforations are generally inaccessible, requiring more elaborate approaches. The usual consequences of untreated stripping perforations are inflammation followed by development of a periodontal pocket. Long-term failure results from leakage of the repair material, which produces periodontal breakdown with attachment loss. Skillful use of MTA has significantly improved the prognosis of nonsurgical repair of stripping perforations compared with other repair materials (Fig. 18.8, *A–C*).

Nonsurgical Treatment

If feasible, nonsurgical repair (Fig. 18.9) of furcation perforations is preferred over surgical intervention as a result of difficult access and possibility of further damage to the periodontium during the surgery. Traditionally, materials such as amalgam, gutta-percha, zinc oxide–eugenol, Cavit, calcium hydroxide, freeze-dried bone, and indium foil have been used clinically and experimentally to seal these defects.[17,18] Repair is difficult because of potential problems with visibility, hemorrhage control, and management and sealing ability of the repair materials. In general, perforations occurring during access preparation should be sealed immediately, but the patency of the canals must be protected. Immediate repair of the perforations with bioactive materials (i.e., MTA and MTA-like materials[19]) offers the best results for perforation repair.[12,20-23]

Surgical Treatment

Surgery requires more complex restorative procedures and more demanding oral hygiene from the patient.[24] Surgical alternatives include repair of the perforation with MTA if accessible by a surgical approach. The exact location and size of the perforation, and also the accessibility of the perforation, can be assessed using CBCT images.[25] If the perforation is not repairable or accessible by a surgical approach, hemisection, bicuspidization,

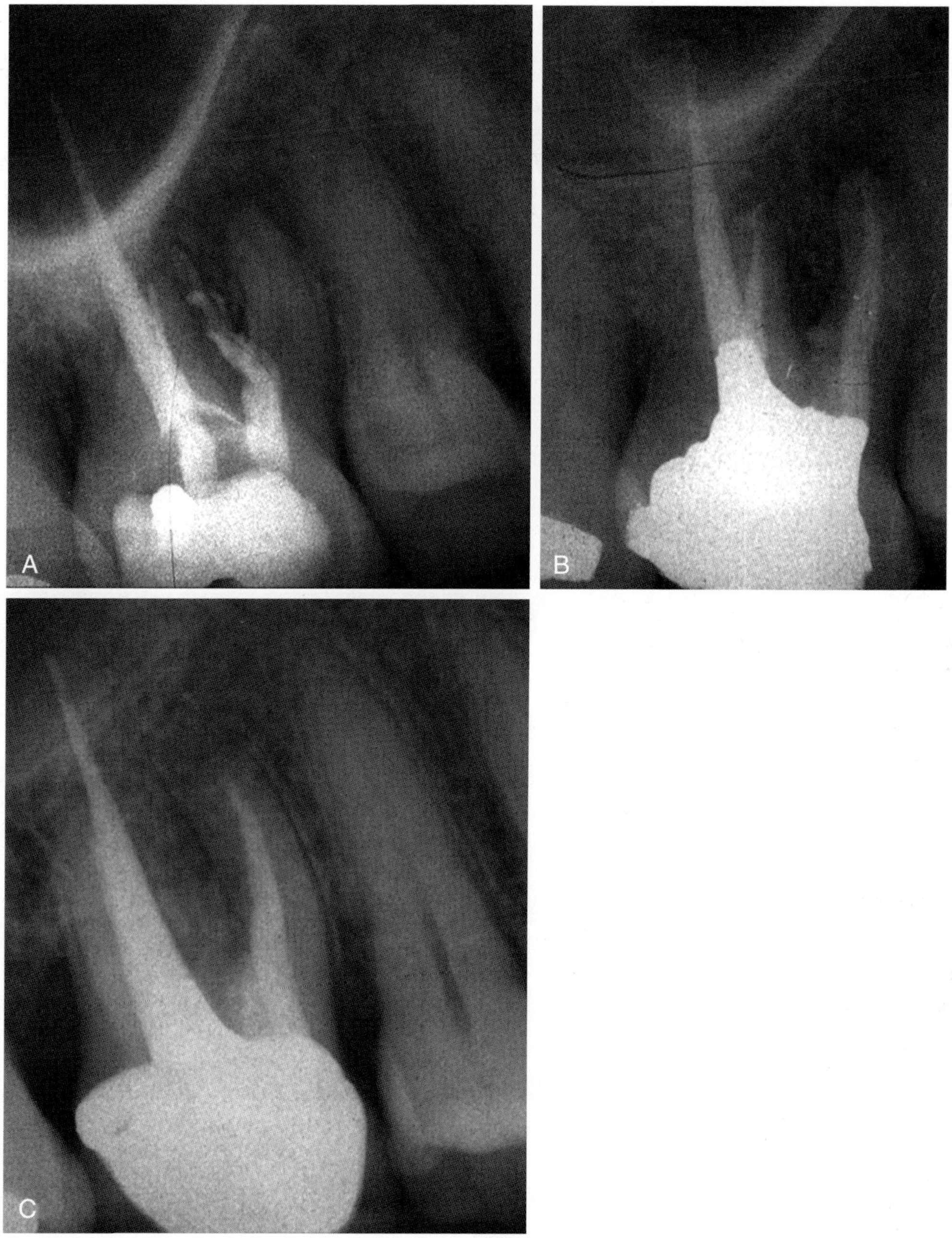

• **Fig. 18.6** **(A)** A search for the MB canal in a partially calcified chamber resulted in a furcation perforation and extrusion of filling materials into the periapical tissues. An apex locator reading, or an angled radiograph, would have detected this type of error. **(B)** The initial treatment was redone and the perforation was sealed with mineral trioxide aggregate (MTA). **(C)** Radiograph (3 years later) shows no evidence of pathosis in the repaired area. (Courtesy Dr. George Bogen.)

root amputation, or intentional replantation should be considered. Teeth with divergent roots and bone levels that allow preparation of adequate crown margins are suitable for either hemisection or bicuspidization (Fig. 18.10). Intentional replantation is indicated when the defect is inaccessible or when multiple problems exist, such as a perforation combined with a separated instrument, or when the prognosis with other surgical procedures is poor. Both the dentist and the patient must recognize that the prognosis for treatment of surgically altered teeth is questionable because of the increased technical difficulty associated with restorative procedures and demanding oral hygiene requirements. The remaining roots are prone to caries, periodontal disease, and vertical root fracture. Treatment planning options, including extraction, should be discussed with the patient when the prognosis is poor.

Prognosis

Factors affecting the long-term prognosis of teeth after perforation repair include the location of the defect in relation to the crestal bone, length of the root trunk, accessibility for repair, size of the defect, presence or absence of a periodontal communication to the

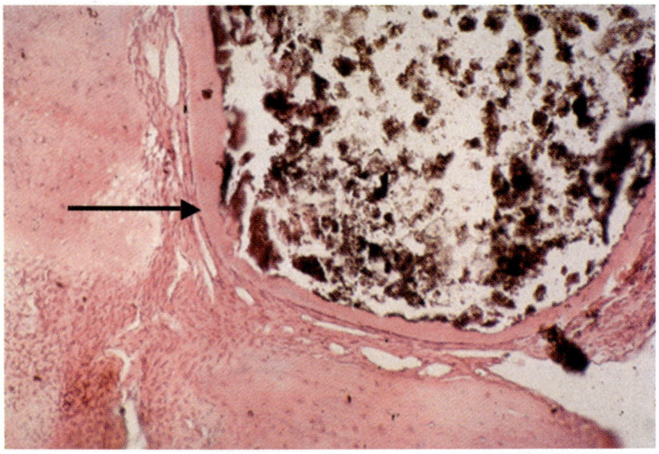

• **Fig. 18.7** Immediate repair of a perforation in the furcation of a dog premolar with mineral trioxide aggregate (MTA) results in the formation of cementum (*arrow*) adjacent to the material.

defect, time lapse between perforation and repair, sealing ability of restorative material, and subjective factors such as the technical competence of the dentist and the attitude and oral hygiene of the patient.[13] Early recognition and repair will improve the prognosis by minimizing damage to the periodontal tissues by bacteria, files, and irrigants. Additionally, a small perforation (less than 1 mm) causes less tissue destruction and is more amenable to repair than a larger perforation. Electronic apex locators or angled radiographs with files in place aid in early detection. Another useful tool to diagnose and locate the perforations is CBCT. CBCT images can help clinicians to understand the spatial position of the perforation and determine a realistic treatment plan (surgical or nonsurgical) to repair the perforation.[26]

An unrecognized or untreated perforation in the furcation usually results in a periodontal defect that communicates through the gingival sulcus within weeks or sometimes days. A preexisting periodontal communication caused by perforation worsens the prognosis; the time between perforation and repair should be as short as possible.[27,28] Immediate sealing of the defect reduces

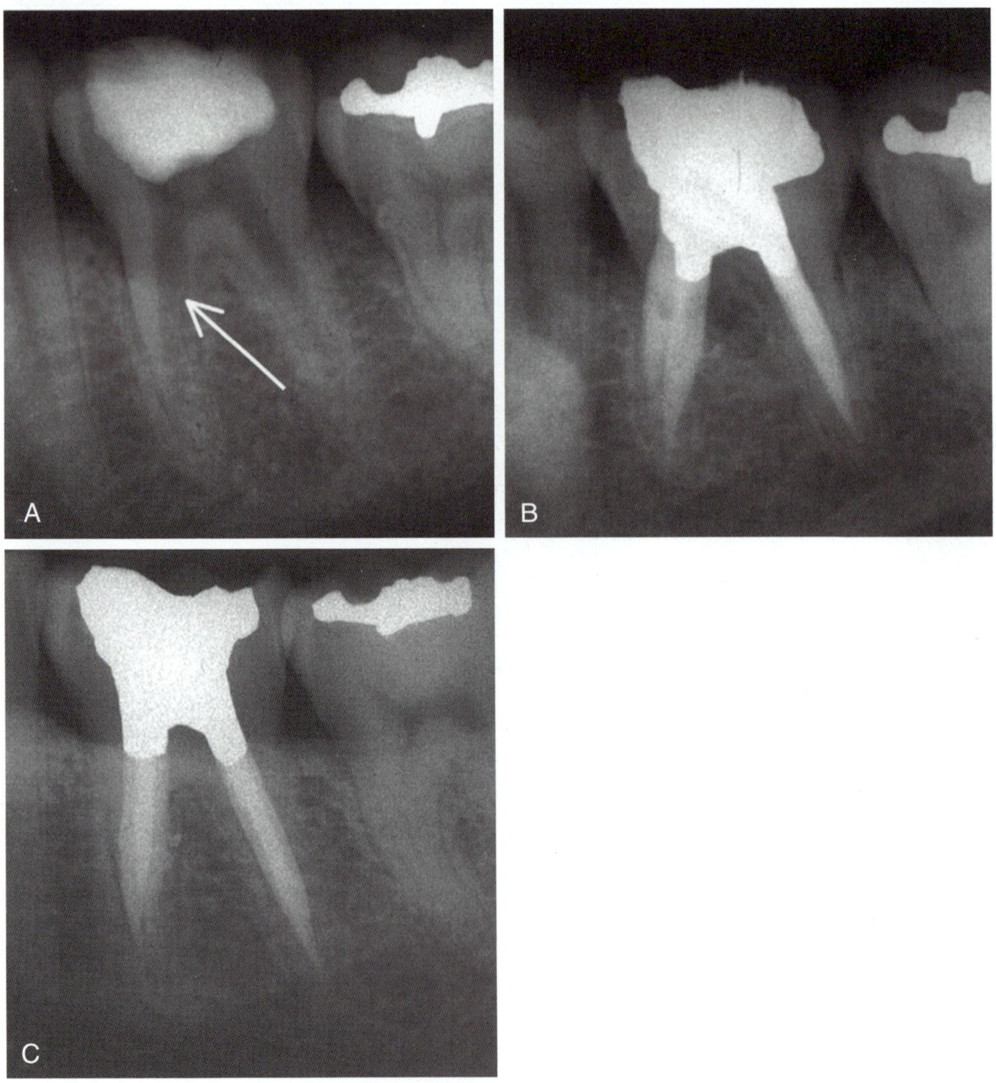

• **Fig. 18.8 (A)** Radiograph shows stripping perforation (*arrow*) in the mesiobuccal root of the first mandibular molar. **(B)** The mesial roots were filled with mineral trioxide aggregate (MTA) and the distal root with gutta-percha and root canal sealer. **(C)** A radiograph taken 1 year later shows no periradicular pathosis.

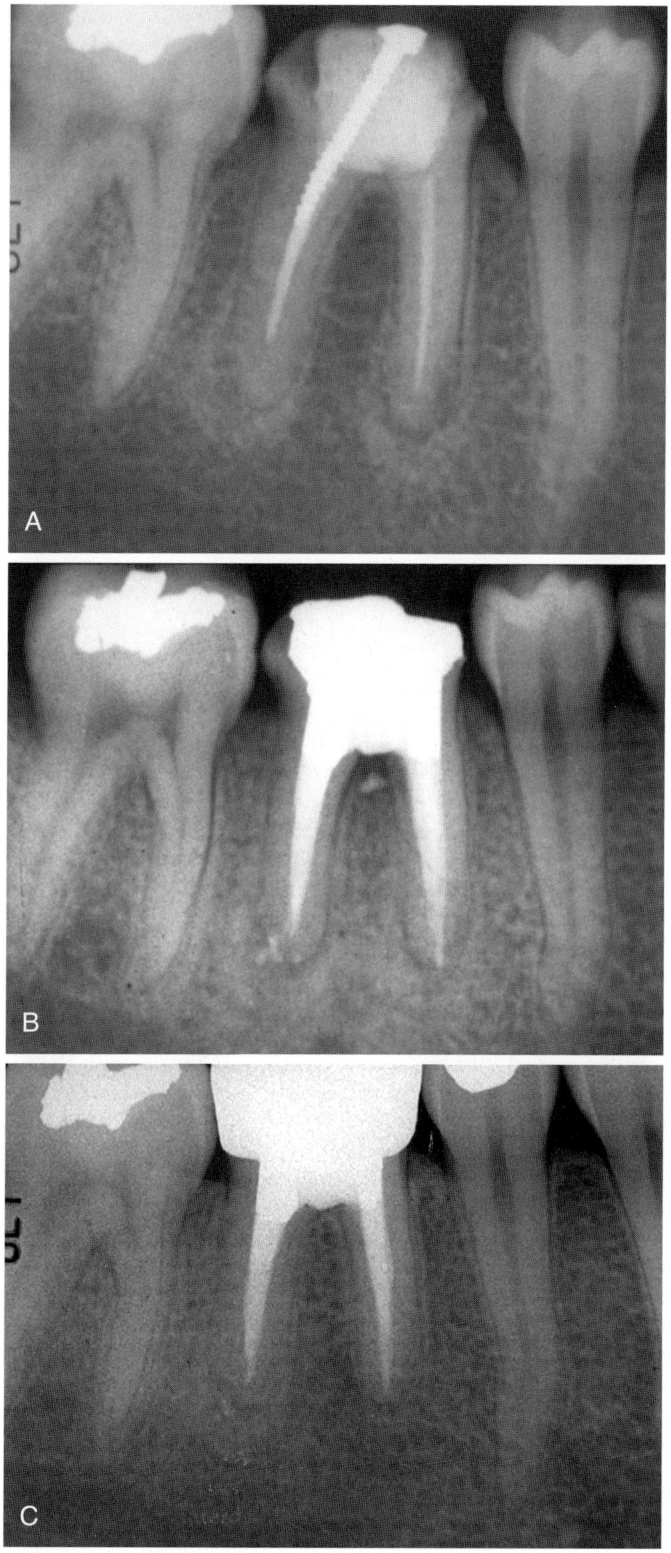

• **Fig. 18.9** **(A)** Periapical radiograph shows presence of a furcation perforation in the first mandibular molar. **(B)** The root canal was retreated and the perforation was repaired with mineral trioxide aggregate (MTA). **(C)** Radiograph taken 26 months later shows evidence of osseous healing in the furcation.

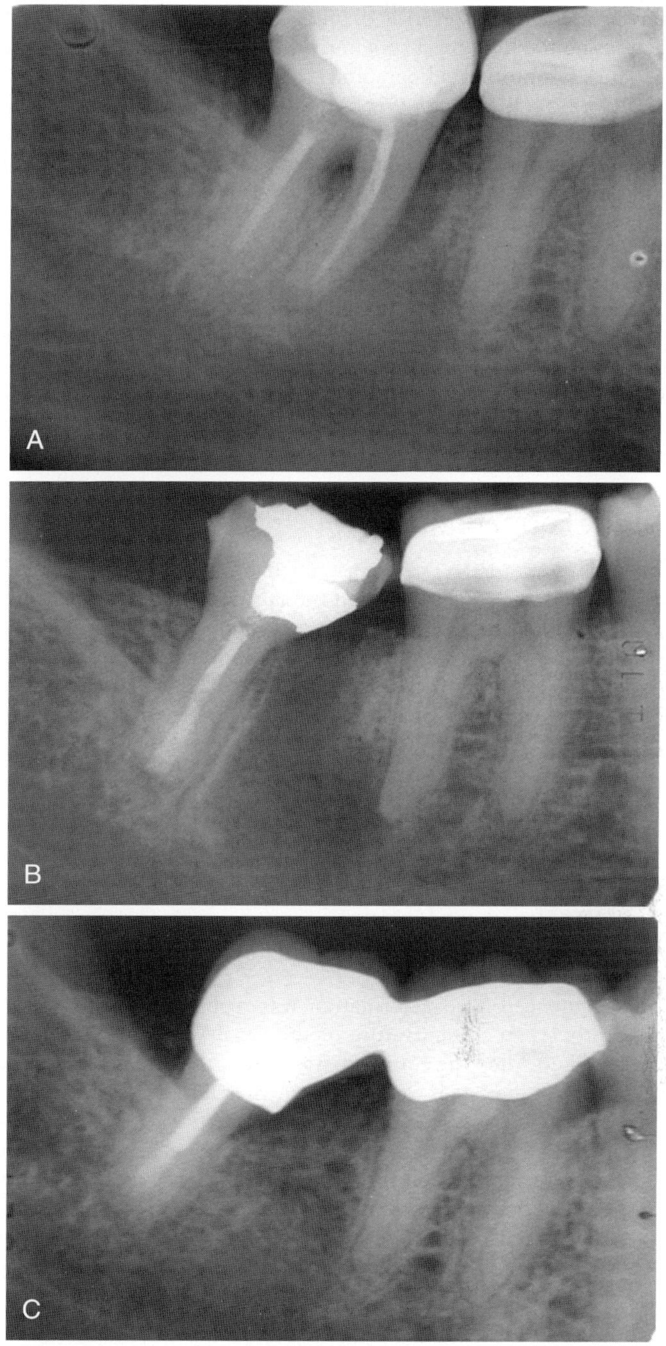

• **Fig. 18.10** **(A)** Postoperative radiograph of a 58-year-old female after endodontic treatment. The patient is percussion-sensitive, and periapical lesions are present. A 7-mm periodontal pocket exists on the mesiobuccal aspect of the mesial root of the second molar. A fracture is suspected, and extract-replant was performed for diagnostic reasons. The tooth was extracted, and a fracture was noted on the mesial root. **(B)** The mesial root was resected and the tooth was replanted after retrofilling of the distal root with mineral trioxide aggregate (MTA). **(C)** Radiograph 1 year later shows osseous repair and restoration of this tooth. The periodontal pocket healed.

the incidence and severity of periodontal breakdown. To best determine the long-term prognosis, the dentist must monitor the patient's symptoms, radiographic changes, and, most importantly, periodontal status. Radiographs and periodontal probing during recall examination are the best measures of success or failure of the repair procedure. Formation of a periodontal pocket adjacent to the site of perforation is a definitive sign for failure.

Accidents During Cleaning and Shaping

The most common procedural accidents during cleaning and shaping of the root canal system are ledge formation, artificial canal creation, root perforation, instrument separation, and extrusion of irrigating solution periapically. Correction of these accidents is usually difficult, and the patient should be referred to an endodontist.

Ledge Formation

By definition, a ledge has been created when the working length can no longer be negotiated and the original patency of the canal is lost. The major causes of ledge formation include (1) inadequate straight-line access into the canal, (2) failure to precurve the files, (3) forcing large files into curved canals, (4) inadequate irrigation or lubrication, and (5) packing of debris in the apical portion of the canal.

Prevention of a Ledge

Preoperative Evaluation

Prevention of ledging begins with examination of preoperative radiographs taken from different angles and CBCT images for curvatures, length, and initial size.

Curvatures

The incidence of ledge formation was reported to increase significantly when the curvature of the canal was greater than 20 degrees, and when the curvature was greater than 30 degrees more than 50% of the canals were ledged.[29] Most important is the coronal third of the root canal. Severe coronal curvature predisposes the apical canal to ledging. Straight-line access to the orifice of the canal can be achieved during access preparation, but accessibility to the apical third of the canal is achieved only with coronal flaring and using precurved files. Severe apical curvatures require a proper sequence of cleaning and shaping procedures to maintain patency (see Chapter 14).

Length

Longer canals are more prone to ledge formation compared with shorter and larger diameter canals. Careful attention to maintaining patency is required to prevent ledging.

Initial Size

Smaller-diameter canals are more easily ledged than larger-diameter canals.

In summary, the canals most prone to ledging are small, curved, and long. Radiographs are two-dimensional and cannot provide accurate information about the actual shape and curvature of the root canal system. All root canals have some degree of curvature, including faciolingual curves, which may not be apparent on straight facial exposures (Fig. 18.11). CBCT images are the most accurate tools for understanding the presence and degree of curvatures.[8]

Instruments

Instruments with more flexibility cause less apical transportation, resulting in a ledge formation. The flexibility of the instruments depends on several interrelated factors such as the cross-sectional design, core diameter, pitch, metallurgical properties, surface treatment of the instruments, heat treatment, the type of kinematics (continuous rotation, reciprocation, and adaptive motion), the number of contact points with the canal walls, and the type of the alloys used for the instruments (conventional, R-phase, M-Wire, CM-wire, MaxWire, and GOLD Wire).[30,31] The most common way to increase file flexibility is to decrease the metal mass of the file by increasing the number of flutes per unit length; increasing the depth of the flutes; and decreasing the helix angle, the taper, size, and/or core diameter of the file. Thus an increased taper results in the increased cross-sectional area and decreased flexibility.[32] The tip design may also affect the incidence of ledge formation. Instruments with pyramidal tips were reported to form ledges.[33] Flexible files (nickel-titanium) with noncutting tips reduce the chances for ledge formation. Failing to use the instruments in sequential order may also lead to ledge formation.

Technical Procedures

Determination of working length in the cleaning and shaping process is a continuation of the access preparation. Optimum straight-line access to the apical third is not achieved until cleaning and shaping have been completed. An accurate working length measurement is a requirement because cleaning and shaping short of the ideal length is a prelude to ledge formation. Frequent recapitulation and irrigation, along with the use of lubricants, are mandatory. Sodium hypochlorite may be used initially for hemorrhage control and removal of debris. However, this agent alone may not be adequate to provide maximum lubrication.

Silicone, glycerine, and wax-based lubricants are commercially available for canal lubrication. Because these materials are viscous, they are carried into the apical regions of the canal with the file. Enhanced lubrication permits easier file insertion, reduces stress to the file, and assists with removal of debris. The lubricant is easily removed with sodium hypochlorite irrigation. Overusing ethylenediaminetetraacetic acid (EDTA)-based lubricants can increase the risk of ledge formation.

Passive step-back and balanced force techniques are two beneficial methods of canal preparation that reduce the chances of ledge formation. Each file is used in sequence with circumferential filing to remove any irregularities before a larger diameter file is placed. The effective use of circumferential filing ensures smoothness of the canal walls and flaring toward the apical end of the canal, which will help to prevent the formation of ledges.

Canals with a severe coronal curvature require a passive step-back cleaning and shaping technique (see Chapter 14). A No. 15 file is used at working length. With maximum irrigation or lubrication, the canal is passively and progressively flared in a step-back fashion. The No. 15 file is recapitulated many times to maintain patency. This preflaring technique reduces the coronal curvature and enlarges the canal. Better control of the files is gained for enlarging and cleaning the apical third of the canal as the last step (see section on Apical Clearing in Chapter 14). Using this technique, the chances of ledge formation are reduced. Rotary files with increased taper will blend and join the shape into a tapering funnel.

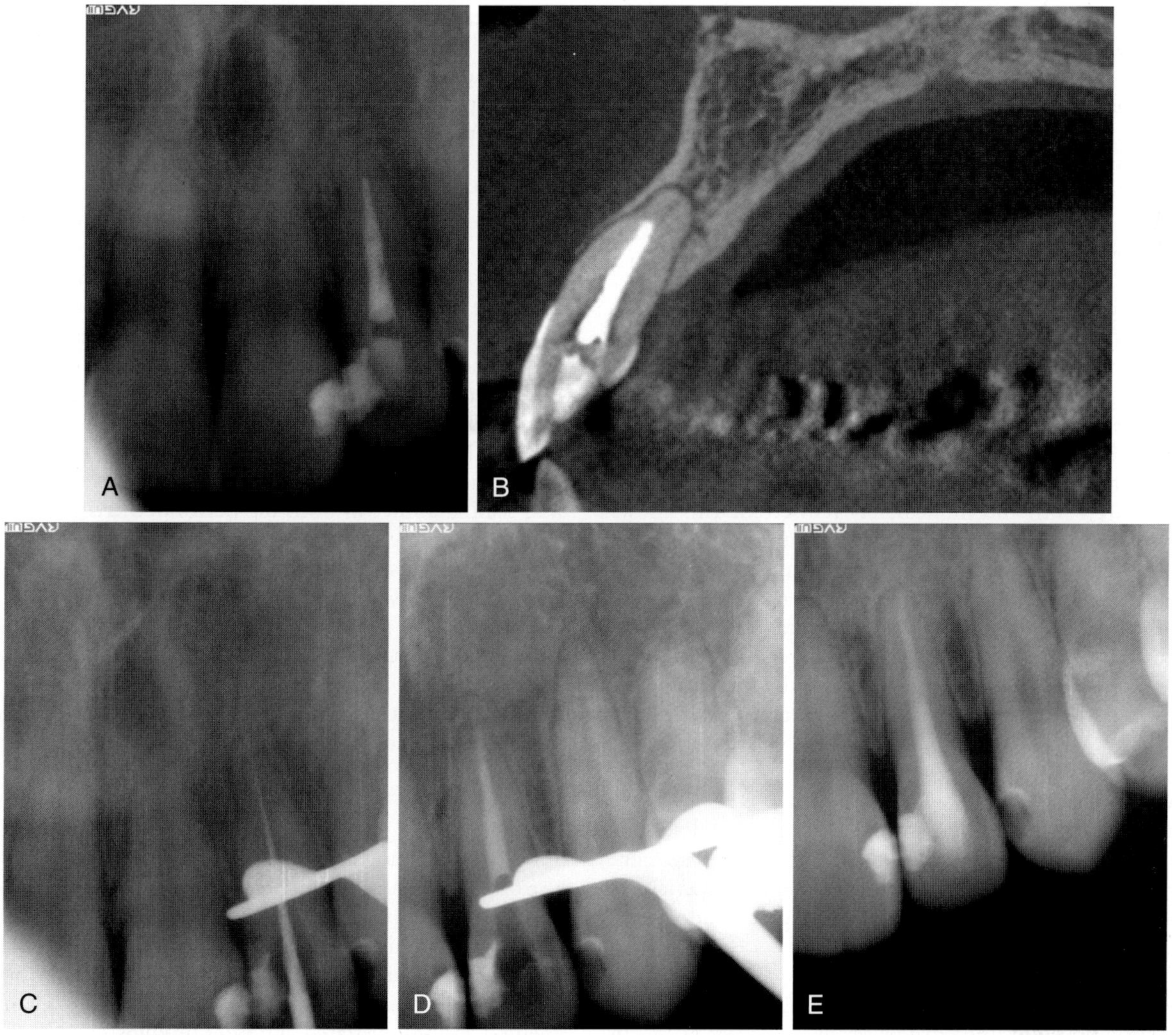

• **Fig. 18.11** **(A)** Preoperative radiograph shows the maxillary left lateral incisor is underfilled and the presence of the canal apical to the end of the root filling is present. **(B)** Sagittal view of cone beam computed tomography (CBCT) imaging shows the presence of the ledge formation in relation to the apical one third of the canal with a small sized lesion. **(C)** Ledge was bypassed, and the apical patency was established. **(D)** Mineral trioxide aggregate (MTA) was obturated into the canal. **(E)** Three-month postoperative radiograph showing apical healing.

Management of a Ledge

Once created, a ledge is difficult to correct. If possible, both the original canal and the ledge must be located under the microscope and with the help of CBCT imaging. If the ledge is not clearly located, the canal should be enlarged to the ledge in an anticurvature direction with a No. 3 Gates-Glidden (GG) bur in a brushing motion as a ledge often forms in a straight line. Then the attempt should be made to bypass the ledge and instrument the canal using one of the following techniques: "Hand instruments," "Ultrasonic tips," "Rotary instruments," and "Surgical approach."

Hand Instruments

A small K file such as a No. 10 K file is the key instrument used in bypassing a ledged canal. The file tip (2 to 3 mm) is sharply bent and worked in the canal in the direction of the canal curvature. A "pecking" motion is used to attempt to feel the catch of the original canal space, which is slightly short of the apical extent of the ledge. A microfile designed to be used under the microscope such as the micro-Opener with #10/.06 taper (Dentsply Sirona, Switzerland) and the microexplorer (Dental Engineering laboratories, Seattle, WA) is best to place in the original canal when the original canal is visible under the microscope. Once the file has been placed in the original canal, a short up-and-down movement is repeated to enlarge the entrance to the original canal (see Fig. 18.11). Then a larger file is subsequently placed in the canal until the ledge is reduced to allow any file to be smoothly inserted to working length.

Ultrasonic Tips

The small diameter ultrasonic tips will help improve visibility with the added benefit of reducing the need for sacrificing sound dentin in bypassing or removing the ledge. The use of longer ultrasonic tips may also facilitate bypassing or reducing the ledge in the apical third under the microscope. First, the entrance to the original canal is located under the microscope. Then the ultrasonic tip to be used should be sharpened with a metal polishing bur and precurved to the original canal. The precurved ultrasonic tip is placed is in the original canal and activated to enlarge the entrance to it. Once the entrance to the original pathway has been enlarged for file insertion, negotiating files should be placed into the canal to establish patency and to smooth out the irregularities on the canal walls that may have been created with ultrasonics. Root canal preparation with nickle-titanium (NiTi) rotary or hand files will be followed (see Fig. 18.11).

Rotary Instruments

If a rotary file is used to bypass a ledge, it should be a less tapered instrument such as a #13 PathFile with .02 taper (Dentsply Sirona, Switzerland) or a Race International Organization for Standardization (ISO) 10 with .02 taper (FKG, Switzerland). First the apical portion, "the apical 2 to 3 mm," of the .02 taper rotary file is precurved to 30 to 45 degrees and is rotated at 100 rpm or slower, brought into the canal, and moved apically. If a ledge or sharp apical curvature is encountered, the instrument is withdrawn about 1 mm and immediately reinserted. This allows the precurved tip to move to a different orientation in the canal when reinserted. This may require several withdrawals and reinsertions as the clinician cannot anticipate when to get into the original pathway before fully negotiating the canal. This procedure is followed in sequence by a larger diameter file to preliminarily enlarge the original pathway and reduce the ledge until the root canal preparation with conventional NiTi rotary instruments becomes possible.

Surgical Approach

If a ledge cannot be bypassed with any of the techniques described previously and the periapical lesion persists, then the treatment options are limited to surgical intervention such as periapical surgery and intentional replantation with retrograde endodontic treatment.

Prognosis

Ledge formation does not immediately result in surgery or loss of the tooth. The presence of ledges may affect the prognosis depending on whether the canal apical to the ledge can be adequately cleaned or not. In general, short and cleaned apical ledges have good prognoses. Teeth with vital pulp tissue apical to a ledge, in general, have a better prognosis than teeth with necrotic infected tissues apical to a ledge that has not been previously cleaned before the formation of the ledge. The patient must be informed of the prognosis, the importance of the recall examination, and what signs indicate failure. Future appearance of clinical symptoms or radiographic evidence of failure may require referral for apical surgery or retreatment.

Creating an Artificial Canal

Cause and Prevention

Deviation from the original pathway of the root canal system and creation of an artificial canal cause an exaggerated ledge; it is initiated by the factors that cause ledge formation and transportation. Therefore the recommendations for preventing ledge formation should be followed to avoid creating artificial canals. The unfortunate sequence is as follows: A ledge is created and the proper working length is lost. The operator, eager to regain that length, "bores" apically with each file, thus creating an artificial canal. Used persistently, the file eventually perforates the root surface. Aggressive use of stainless-steel files is the most common cause of this problem. Creation of an artificial canal can be prevented by taking an intraoperative radiograph with the negotiating file placed in the canal as soon as the working length is lost, negotiating the canal under the microscope to locate the original pathway, and using a precurved small file oriented to the original pathway.

Management

Negotiating the original canal with the exaggerated ledge is usually very difficult. However, if the original pathway can be located in the CBCT images and under the microscope, negotiating the original canal should not be as difficult. If a perforation exists in the artificial canal, it needs to be evaluated to manage the artificial canal. If the size of perforation at the apical extent of the artificial canal is larger than 0.5 mm in diameter, it should be sealed with MTA before negotiating the original canal (Fig. 18.12). This allows for easier negotiation of the main canal. The prognosis of the tooth with perforation depends on débridement and sealing ability of both the perforated artificial canal and the original canal.[27,34] For the canal with a perforation sized smaller than 0.5 mm in diameter, both canals should be cleaned, shaped, and obturated with MTA at the same time. If nonsurgical management of the perforation repair is difficult, surgical intervention should be considered (see the section Root Perforations in this chapter).

To obturate the canal without perforation, the original canal should be located, negotiated, cleaned, and shaped along with the artificial canal.

Prognosis

Prognosis depends on the ability of the operator to renegotiate the original canal and the remaining uninstrumented and unfilled portion of the main canal. Unless a perforation exists, teeth in which the original canal can be renegotiated and obturated have a prognosis similar to those without procedural complications. In contrast, when a large portion of the main canal is uninstrumented and unobturated, a poorer prognosis exists, and the tooth must be examined periodically. Perforations at the crestal bone level have the worst prognosis as a result of damage to the periodontal attachment and pocket formation. Failure usually means surgery will be required to resect the uninstrumented and unobturated root.

Root Perforations

Roots may be perforated at different levels during cleaning and shaping. Location (apical, middle, or cervical) of the perforation and the stage of treatment affect prognosis.[27] The periodontal response to the injury is affected by the level and size of the perforation. Also, perforations at the early stages of cleaning and shaping affect prognosis significantly.

Apical Perforations

Apical perforations occur through the apical foramen (overinstrumentation or transportation at the level of apical foramen) or through the body of the root (perforated new canal).

Etiology and Indicators

Instrumentation of the canal beyond the apical constriction results in perforation. Incorrect working length or inability to maintain proper working length causes "zipping"[4] or "blowing out" of the apical foramen. The appearance of fresh hemorrhage in the canal or on instruments, pain during canal preparation

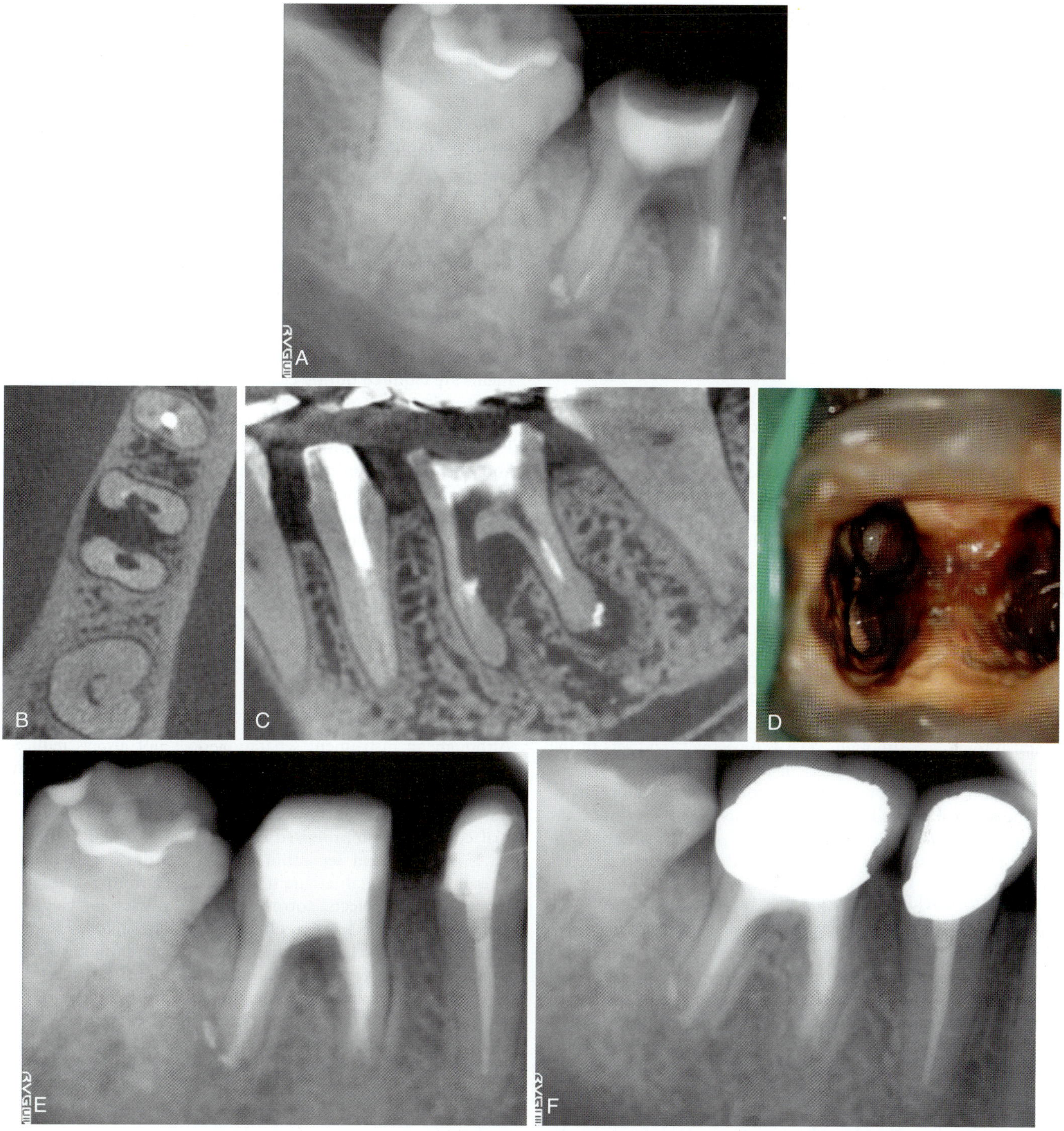

• **Fig. 18.12** **(A)** Preoperative radiograph showing periapical and furcal lesions. **(B)** Axial view of cone beam computed tomography (CBCT) imaging shows a large furcal perforation in the MB canal causing furcal lesions. **(C)** Sagittal view of CBCT imaging shows the MB canal perforated on the distal wall into the furcation and periapical lesions associated with both the mesial and the distal roots. **(D)** Perforation on the distal wall in the MB canal (*arrow pointing*). **(E)** Three-month postoperative radiograph after obturation showing reduced size periapical and furcal lesions. **(F)** Six-month postoperative radiograph showing furcal and periapical healing.

in a previously asymptomatic tooth, and sudden loss of the apical stop are indicators of perforation through apical foramen. Extension of the largest (final) file beyond the radiographic apex is also a sign. An electronic apex locator may also confirm this procedural accident.

Prevention

To prevent apical perforation, proper working lengths must be established and maintained throughout the procedure. In curved canals, the flexibility of files with respect to size and taper must be considered. Cleaning and shaping procedures straighten the canal somewhat and effectively decrease the working length by as much as 1 to 2 mm, thereby requiring compensation. To prevent apical perforation, the working length should be verified with an apex locator before and after completion of cleaning and shaping steps. Using an electrical motor for rotary files with a built-in apex locator is another option.

Treatment

Treatment includes establishing a new working length, creating an apical seat (taper), and obturating the canal to its new length. Depending on the size and location of the apical foramen, a new working length 1 to 2 mm short of the point of perforation should be established. The canal is then cleaned, shaped, and obturated to the new working length. The master cone must have a positive apical stop at the working length before obturation. Placement of MTA as an apical barrier can prevent extrusion of obturation materials.

MTA can also be used for filling the canal and repairing the perforation at the same time. The apical diameter is measured with a series of K files. Then a NiTi rotary file that is one or two sizes smaller than the apical diameter is selected. The selected NiTi rotary file is connected to an apex locator, followed by MTA compaction into the canal as well as the perforation site using the file manually. The working length should be reached once or twice with the NiTi rotary file rotating counterclockwise manually to further condense MTA into the canal space.

Prognosis

The prognosis depends primarily on the size, shape, and location of the defect as well as the material used for perforation repair.[20] An open apex or reverse funnel should be sealed with MTA as it provides adequate seal even when the material is extruded beyond the apical foramen. Although MTA is bioactive[19] and sets in the presence of blood and moisture,[35] it is recommended to prevent the extrusion of MTA[36] and any types of root canal filling material. The surgical accessibility of perforations also are important variables for long-term success. Repair of apical perforations in anterior teeth is easier and more practical than in posterior teeth.

Lateral (Midroot) Perforations

Etiology and Treatment

Lateral (midroot) perforations happen as a result of continued efforts in reaching the working length in an artificial canal that is not diagnosed by the clinician. The reader is referred to the topic of "Creating an Artificial Canal" to find information about causes, prevention, and treatment of the lateral (midroot) perforations.

Prognosis

The prognosis of teeth with midroot perforations depends on the effectiveness of débridement of the canal, control of hemorrhage, and the ability to obturate the canal apical to the perforation. MTA is the material of choice not only for perforation repair. It can also be used as the obturation material when there is a midroot perforation. Teeth with perforations close to the apex after complete or partial débridement of the canal have a better prognosis than those with perforations that occur earlier. In general, small perforations are easier to seal than large ones.

On recall, both radiographic and periodontal examinations for signs and symptoms are performed. Failure generally requires surgery or other approaches. These approaches depend on the severity of perforation, the strategic importance of the tooth, and the location and accessibility of the perforation. Corrective techniques include repair of the perforation site, root resection to the level of the perforation, root amputation, hemisection, replantation, and extraction.

Coronal Root Perforations

Etiology and Indicators

Coronal root perforations can occur by over-enlarging canals in the cervical portion of a canal by files, GG drills, Orifice openers, or Peeso reamers. Using the methods described earlier in this chapter can minimize perforations during access preparation. Removal of restorations when possible, use of fiberoptic lights for illumination, magnification, CBCT imaging, straight-line access to the orifice of the canals, and cautious exploration for the canal orifice can prevent most problems during access preparation. Careful flaring (step-back) and conservative use of flaring instruments are required during cleaning and shaping procedures.

Treatment and Prognosis

Preventing the communication between the perforation site and the gingival sulcus is very critical in prognosis of teeth with coronal root perforations. Repair of a strip perforation in the coronal third of the root, especially when the perforation is coronal to the crestal bone, has the worst prognosis because of quick periodontal attachment loss. The canal apical to the perforation should be filled with MTA first and subsequently the defect should be repaired with the same material for the optimal seal and healing.

Instrument Separation

Etiology

Although an instrument separation does not always reduce the prognosis, it might affect the outcome of endodontic treatment. Studies showed that instrument separation negatively affects the outcome of endodontic treatments only in cases where microbial control is compromised or periapical lesions preexist[37](Fig. 18.13). Instrument separation in endodontics occurs mainly as a result of the metal fatigue (cyclic fatigue and torsional fatigue), manufacturing defects, corrosion of the instrument in the presence of NaOCl,[38,39] or a combination of these factors. Despite the high flexibility, NiTi instruments in general are more susceptible to fracture at a lower force than stainless steel instruments.[40] Other factors associated with instrument separation are as follows: operator experience,[41,42] rotational speed,[43] canal curvature (radius),[44] instrument design and technique,[45] torque setting,[46] manufacturing process,[47] the type of NiTi alloys used,[48] the type of rotational motion (continuous rotations or reciprocating motions),[49] the type of tooth,[50,51] and absence of glide path.[52]

Recognition

A shortened file with a blunt tip and subsequent loss of patency to the original length are the main clues for the presence of a separated instrument. A radiograph is essential for confirmation. It is imperative that the patient be informed of the accident and its effect on prognosis.[1] As with other procedural accidents, detailed documentation is also necessary for medical-legal considerations.

Prevention

Recognition of the physical properties and stress limitations of files is critical. Continual lubrication with either irrigating

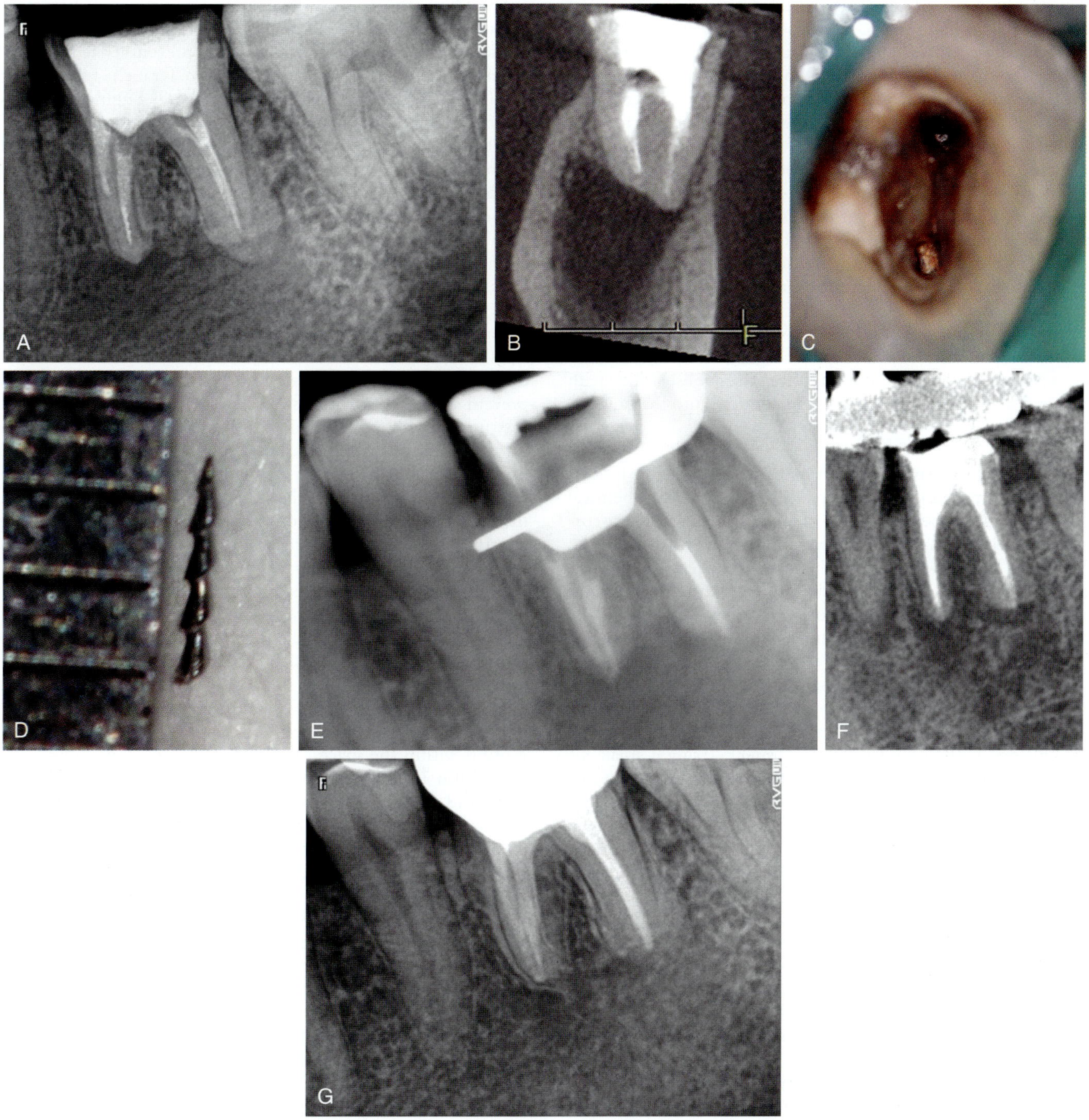

• **Fig. 18.13** **(A)** Preoperative radiograph showing a fractured instrument in the apical one third of the mesiobuccal canal with large periapical lesions associated with the mesial and distal roots. **(B)** Preoperative coronal view of cone beam computed tomography (CBCT) imaging showing the fractured instrument in the MB canal with a large periapical lesion. **(C)** Magnified view showing the fractured instrument in the MB canal (*arrow*). (D) Retrieved instrument measuring 2.5 mm. **(E)** Postoperative radiograph mineral trioxide aggregate (MTA) filling in mesial canals, gutta-percha obturation in distal canals. **(F)** Six-month postoperative sagittal view of CBCT imaging showing healing of the periapical lesion. **(G)** Twelve-month postoperative radiograph showing periapical healed.

solution or lubricants is required. Each instrument is examined before use. If an unwound or twisted file is rotated and viewed, reflections from the chairside light will magnify fluting distortions. Rotation of a file with a large diameter in a curved canal increases cyclic fatigue compared with a file with a smaller diameter. To reduce cyclic fatigue of an instrument in a curved canal, a file with a smaller diameter should be used with reduced rotational speed. In the meantime, rotating a small diameter file in a tight canal makes it more susceptible to fracture because of torsional fatigue. To reduce torsional fatigue of an instrument, the rotational speed should be increased, and the file should be used with light apical pressure.

The fatigue life of NiTi instruments is longer in liquid media than in air, which indicates the effect of temperature and environment on the risk of instrument separation.[53] An aqueous medium may be able to serve as an effective heat sink to reduce the risk of instrument separation.

The use of reciprocal motions is reported to extend the lifespan of an instrument[54] and increase cyclic fatigue resistance compared with continuous rotation.[49] It is important to establish a glide path with hand files before rotary files are introduced into the canal.

Treatment

Nonsurgical management of fractured instruments can be categorized into mechanical and chemical methods. The chemical method includes the use of chemical solvents for instrument corrosion and electrochemical process for instrument dissolution, which may be time-consuming because the chemical solvents can only contact the exposed surface of the fractured instrument in the canal to corrode the whole instrument. Therefore the mechanical method for instrument retrieval is solely discussed in this chapter.

There are three approaches to managing an intracanal fractured instrument: (1) attempt to remove the instrument nonsurgically or surgically, (2) attempt to bypass it, or (3) prepare and obturate the canal with the fractured instrument. Using a small file and following the guidelines described for negotiating a ledge, the operator should attempt to bypass the separated instrument. After bypassing the separated instrument, ultrasonic files[55] or Hedstrom files are used to remove the segment. If removal of the separated piece is unsuccessful, the canal is cleaned, shaped, and obturated to its new working length.

First, a diagnosis and a treatment plan for instrument retrieval should be made by using periapical radiography and CBCT imaging. With CBCT imaging, accurate procedural information about the removal of the separated instrument such as the length of the separated instrument, the degrees of the curve, the thickness of the canal walls, the presence of perforation, and the presence of preoperative lesions, can be obtained.

The great majority of NiTi rotary instruments fracture in the apical third of the canals.[56] When a fractured instrument is beyond the curve and extruded mostly beyond the apical foramen, a surgical approach should be considered. A nonsurgical approach should be performed if the amount of dentin removal is minimal and reasonable and does not impose the risk of ledging or perforations.

Predictable instrument retrieval requires precise preparations. First, the canal needs to be enlarged to the level of fractured instrument with a #3 GG bur without the pilot tip (#3 modified GG bur). Then the microtrephine bur (Dental Engineering laboratories, Santa Barbara, CA) is inserted into the canal and rotated counterclockwise at 600 rpm to both loosen the fractured instrument and expose the coronal 1 mm portion of the separated instrument. If the separated instrument is around the curve or beyond the curve, a large diameter NiTi rotary file approximately three sizes larger than the estimated diameter of the separated instrument should be used instead of the GG bur without using the microtrephine bur to prevent ledge formation. Then a sharp ultrasonic tip, such as the Terauchi File Retrieval Kit (TFRK)-12/6 and the TFRK-S (Dental Engineering Laboratories, Santa Barbara, CA), is used to create a thin space in the gap between the fractured instrument and the inner wall or the surrounding wall in the straight portion of the canal where the dentin wall thickness is the largest. When the fractured instrument is ultrasonically oscillated from the inner wall of a curved canal, it will be shifted coronally, whereas ultrasonic oscillation from the outer wall will result in pushing it more apically. The ultrasonic tip used in preparation must be small enough to not only slip into the gap on the inner wall, but also allow for proper visualization in the canal under the microscope. The ultrasonic tip should be activated intermittently (on and off) at the lowest power setting that allows minimal dentin removal to both prevent the temperature rise[57,58] and breakage of the fractured instrument or the ultrasonic tip. The thin space to be created on the inner wall with ultrasonics should be at least longer than one third of the fractured instrument and more than 180 degrees semicircular around it on the inner wall to loosen the fractured instrument. The preparation for instrument retrieval should continue by deepening the space or extending the semicircular space until the fractured instrument is seen moving or "dancing." A longer NiTi fractured instrument tends to be flexing with ultrasonics, which is often misinterpreted as moving or "dancing" under the microscope. After the separated file is loosened, the retrieval process should be attempted. During retrieval by ultrasonics the root canal space should be filled with EDTA. When the sharp ultrasonic tip is placed in the space created on the inner wall and activated continuously in an up-and-down motion within the space, the fractured instrument should come out within 10 seconds. The space between the fractured instrument and the canal wall must be wider than the diameter of the fractured instrument to allow it to flow out of the canal. If the loop device is used to retrieve the fractured instrument, the minimum space required for the placement of the loop is 0.4 mm wide and 0.5 mm long on the side of the coronal portion of the fractured instrument. A #40 plugger should be introduced into the space to see if the space is wide enough to place the loop. The loop size must be adjusted to the size of the fractured instrument with a DG-16 endodontic explorer. The loop should be bent to 45 degrees to facilitate the placement of the loop. Then the loop is placed over the fractured instrument, tightened around it with minimum force, and gently pulled out of the canal as the fractured instrument is already dislodged from the canal walls. If the resistance is felt from pulling the fractured instrument up with the loop, gently swing the loop in several lateral and coronal directions (Fig. 18.14).

If the instrument is separated in an apical curved portion of the canal beyond the straight section of the canal, the use of a staging platform should not be attempted as ledging, perforation, or excessive loss of dentin may result.[59]

If the instrument cannot be bypassed or removed, preparation and obturation should be performed to the coronal level of the fragment.

For most cases involving fractured instruments, the patient should be referred to an endodontist for management.

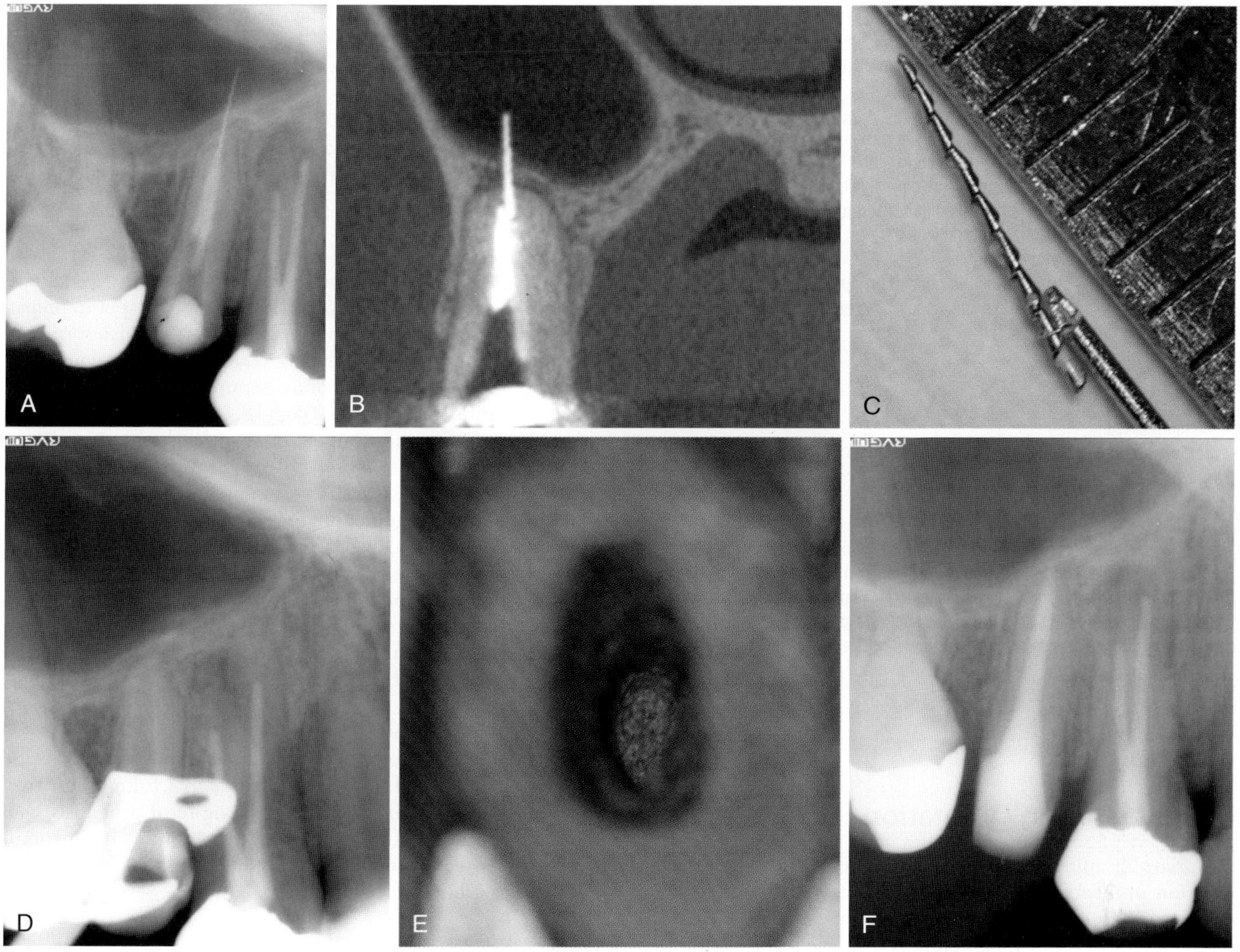

• **Fig. 18.14** **(A)** Preoperative radiograph showing a fractured file in the root canal with the apical portion extruded into the maxillary sinus. **(B)** Preoperative coronal view of cone beam computed tomography (CBCT) image showing the position of the fractured file. **(C)** Retrieved fractured file measuring 6 mm. **(D)** Radiograph taken immediately after the retrieval. **(E)** Microscopic image showing mineral trioxide aggregate (MTA) obturation. **(F)** Postoperative radiograph showing MTA obturation well adapted to the root canal.

Prognosis

The prognosis is best when separation of a large instrument occurs in the later stages of preparation close to the working length. Prognosis is worse for teeth with undébrided canals in which a small instrument is separated short of the apex early in preparation. For medical-legal reasons, the patient must be informed (with documentation in the record) of an instrument separation. Despite the concern of both the patient and the dentist, clinical reports indicate that the prognosis in most procedures involving fractured instruments is favorable.[60] The most important prognostic factor for teeth with retained fractured instruments is the presence of periapical lesion. The prognosis of endodontically treated teeth with retained instruments remains unchanged.[37,60]

If the tooth remains symptomatic or there is a subsequent failure, the tooth can be treated surgically. Accessible roots are resected with placement of a root-end filling material. Accessibility of the root apex for surgical intervention is critical to the outcome.

Role of 3D Imaging in Prevention

CBCT provides the clinician with a three-dimensional view of the internal anatomy, which helps the clinician to prevent most of the procedural accidents. For instance, if CBCT imaging shows an abrupt apical curvature and an apical foramen on the distal side of the mesial root of a mandibular molar, ledge formation, perforation, and instrument fracture can be prevented during instrumentation directed to the apex of the root. Axial slices typically show the number of canals and the thickness of the canal wall in relation to the long axis of the root to prevent perforation during the access preparation and instrumentation. Sagittal and coronal slices reveal canal curvature in relation to the coronal access to the root canal and the long axis of the root to prevent formation of ledges and instrument fracture. CBCT images reveal periapical lesions better than periapical radiographs, which gives the clinician a better understanding of the prognosis if a procedural accident happens.[61] On the other hand, studies showed that CBCT imaging has no advantage over periapical radiographs in detecting the fractured instruments in root-filled teeth.[62]

Study Questions

1. What type of canal is prone to ledge formation during instrumentation?
   a. Short and curved canal
   b. Short canal with small diameter
   c. Long canal with small diameter and curvature
   d. Long canal with large diameter and curvature
2. What kind of instrument is less likely to ledge the canal?
   a. Large diameter instrument with an increased taper
   b. Small diameter instrument with minimal taper
   c. NiTi instrument with a cutting tip
   d. Stainless steel instrument with a noncutting tip
3. Which side of the canal should a thin space be created with ultrasonics in preparation for instrument retrieval?
   a. Outer wall
   b. Inner wall
   c. Thickest wall
   d. Thinnest wall
4. What is the objective of the root canal preparation for instrument retrieval?
   a. To visualize the fractured instrument
   b. To loosen the fractured instrument
   c. To expose the coronal portion of the fractured instrument
   d. To create a semicircular space in the space on the inner wall
5. What does the axial view of CBCT image show to prevent perforation during the access cavity preparation and instrumentation?
   a. The number of canals and the thickness of the canal wall
   b. Canal curvature and the long axis of the root
   c. The presence of periapical lesions
   d. The presence of a ledge

Accidents During Obturation

Appropriate cleaning and shaping are the keys to preventing obturation problems because these accidents usually result from improper canal preparation. In general, adequately prepared canals are obturated without mishap. However, problems do occur. The quality of obturation reflects the quality of canal preparation.

Underfilling

Etiology

Some causes of underfilling include a natural barrier in the canal, a ledge created during preparation, insufficient flaring, a poorly adapted master cone, and inadequate condensation pressure. Bypassing (if possible) any natural or artificial barrier to create a smooth funnel is one key to avoiding an underfill. The advent of NiTi rotary files of increased taper has greatly improved the predictability of proper funnel and taper.

Treatment and Prognosis

Removal of underfilled gutta-percha and retreatment is preferred. The focus of the retreatment should be on the cause of underfilling. In other words, the clinician should first determine what caused the underfill and then address this issue during retreatment. Forcing gutta-percha apically by increased spreader or plugger pressure is not a solution and can fracture the root. If lateral condensation is the method of obturation, the master cone should be marked to indicate the working length. If displacement of the master cone during condensation is suspected, a radiograph is made before excess gutta-percha is removed. Removal can then be accomplished by pulling the cones in the reverse order of placement. Removal of gutta-percha in canals obturated with lateral condensation is easier than removal with other obturation techniques.

Overfilling

Extruded obturation material causes tissue damage and inflammation. Postoperative discomfort (mastication sensitivity) usually lasts for a few days or weeks.

Etiology

Overfilling is usually the consequence of overinstrumentation through the apical constriction or lack of proper taper in prepared canals. When the apex is open naturally by apical resorption or its constriction is removed during cleaning and shaping, there is no matrix against which to condense; uncontrolled condensation forces extrusion of materials (Fig. 18.15). Other causes include inflammatory resorption and incomplete development of the root.

Prevention

To avoid overfilling, guidelines for preventing apical foramen perforation should be followed. Tapered preparation with an apical "matrix" usually prevents overfill. The largest file and master cone at working length should have a positive stop. If overfilling is suspected, a radiograph should be made before excess gutta-percha is removed. As with underfilling, the gutta-percha mass may be removed if the sealer has not set.

Treatment and Prognosis

When signs or symptoms of endodontic failure appear, apical surgery may be required to remove the material from apical tissues and place root-end filling material. Long-term prognosis is dictated by the quality of the apical seal, the amount and biocompatibility of extruded material, host response, and toxicity and sealing ability of the root-end filling material.

Vertical Root Fracture

Complete vertical root fracture causes untreatable failure. Aspects of vertical root fracture are described in more detail in Chapter 4.

Etiology

Causative factors include root canal treatment procedures and associated factors such as post placement. A main cause of vertical root fracture is post cementation. The secondary cause is overzealous application of condensation forces to obturate an underprepared or overprepared canal.[63] A study showed that vertical root fracture is associated with two canals in a root, presence of isthmus between the canals in a root, and condensation forces during obturation.[64]

Prevention

As related to root canal treatment procedures, the best means of preventing vertical root fractures are appropriate canal preparation and use of balanced pressure during obturation. A major reason for flaring canals is to provide space for condensation instruments. Finger spreaders produce less stress and distortion of the root than their hand counterparts.[65] Furthermore, NiTi finger spreaders produce less stress during compaction than stainless-steel finger spreaders.[66]

Indicators

Long-standing vertical root fractures are often associated with a narrow and deep periodontal pocket with or without a sinus

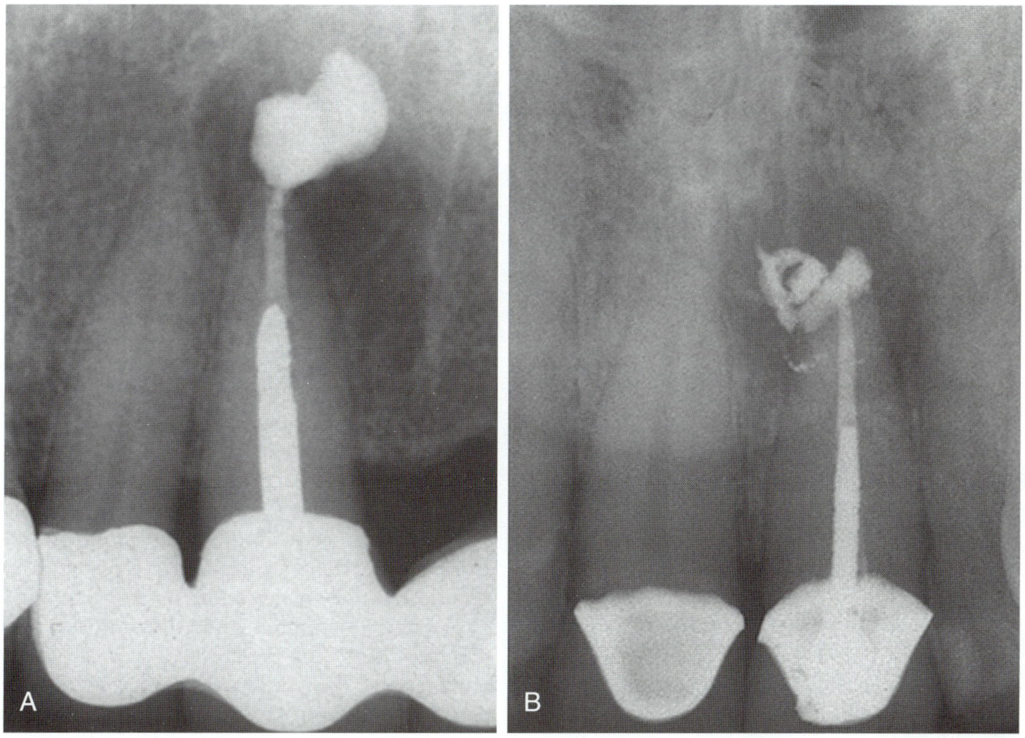

• **Fig. 18.15** **(A)** Lack of proper length measurements can result in overfilling with root canal sealer or **(B)** sealer and gutta-percha.

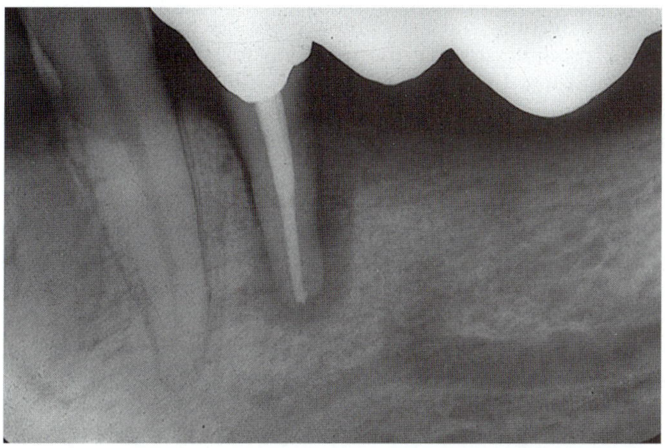

• **Fig. 18.16** A "tear-drop" lateral radiolucency and a narrow probing defect extend to the apex of a tooth with vertical fracture.

tract stoma, as well as a lateral or a J-shaped radiolucency (Fig. 18.16) extending to the apical portion of the vertical fracture.[67] To confirm the diagnosis, a vertical fracture must be visualized. Exploratory surgery or removal of the restoration is usually necessary to visualize this mishap. More recently, CBCT has been used to confirm or rule out vertical root fractures. However, scatter from posts or root canal filling materials may make interpretation of vertical root fractures difficult in CBCT images.[68]

Prognosis and Treatment

Complete vertical root fracture predicts an unfavorable prognosis. Treatment is removal of the involved root in multirooted teeth or extraction of single-rooted teeth.

Accidents During Post Space Preparation

To prevent root perforation, gutta-percha may be removed to the desired level with heated pluggers or electronic heating devices, such as the "Touch N Heat" or System B (SybronEndo, Orange, CA). This "pilot" post space provides a path of least resistance for the post drills. Attempting to remove gutta-percha with a drill can only result in perforation. When a canal is prepared to receive a post, drills should be used sequentially, starting with a size that fits passively to the desired level. Miscalculation and incorrect preparation may result in perforation at any level. Knowledge of root anatomy is necessary for determining the size and depth of posts.

Indicators

Appearance of fresh blood during post space preparation is an indication for the presence of a root perforation. The presence of a sinus tract stoma or probing defects extending to the base of a post is often a sign of root fracture or perforation. Radiographs often show a lateral radiolucency along the root or perforation site.

Treatment and Prognosis

As outlined earlier, the prognosis of teeth with root perforation during post space preparation depends on the root size, location relative to epithelial attachment, and accessibility for repair. Management of the post perforation generally is surgical if the post cannot be removed. If the post can be removed, nonsurgical repair is preferred (Fig. 18.17). Ideally, repair of the perforation should be done immediately after the perforation is diagnosed (Fig. 18.18). Teeth with small root perforations that are in the apical region and are accessible for surgical repair have a better prognosis

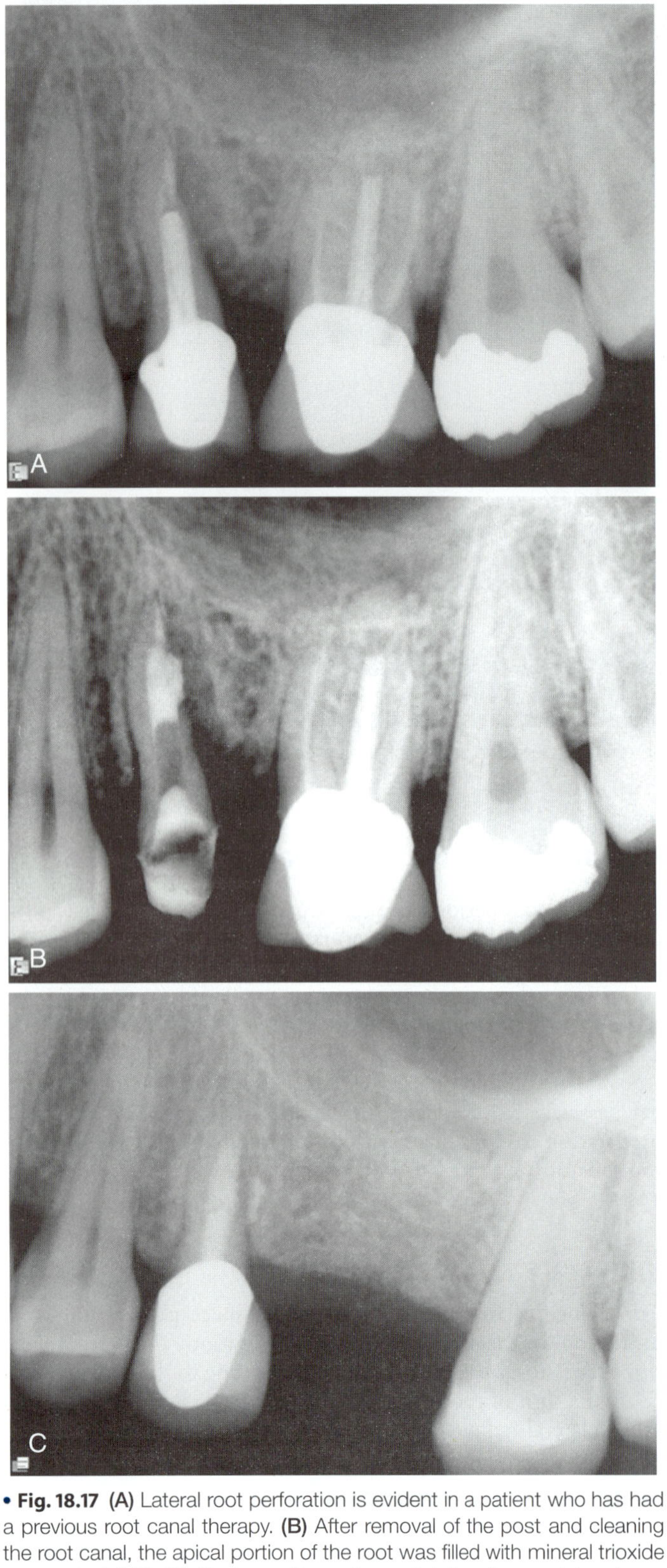

• **Fig. 18.17** **(A)** Lateral root perforation is evident in a patient who has had a previous root canal therapy. **(B)** After removal of the post and cleaning the root canal, the apical portion of the root was filled with mineral trioxide aggregate (MTA). **(C)** Postoperative radiograph taken 9 years later shows absence of any periradicular pathosis.

than those that have large perforations, are close to the gingival sulcus, or are inaccessible. Because of the complexity of diagnosis, surgical techniques, and follow-up evaluation, patients with post perforations should be referred to an endodontist for evaluation and treatment.

Other Accidents

Aspiration or Ingestion

Aspiration or ingestion of instruments is a serious event but is easily avoided with proper precautions. Use of the rubber dam is the standard of care to prevent such ingestion or aspiration and subsequent lawsuits.

The disappearance of an instrument that has slipped from the dentist's fingers followed by violent coughing or gagging by the patient and radiographic confirmation of a file in the alimentary tract or airway are the chief signs. These patients require immediate referral to a medical service for appropriate diagnosis and treatment. According to a survey by Grossman, 87% of these instruments are swallowed and the rest are aspirated.[69] Surgical removal is required for some swallowed (Fig. 18.19) and nearly all aspirated instruments.

Extrusion of Irrigant

Wedging of a needle in the canal (or particularly out of a perforation) with forceful expression of irrigant (usually sodium hypochlorite) causes penetration of irrigants into the periradicular tissues and inflammation and discomfort for patients.[70] Extrusion of NaOCl into the periapical tissues can cause a life-threatening emergency.[71] This situation is called *sodium hypochlorite accident*. A survey of the Board-Certified Endodontists in the United States showed that about one third of the endodontists have experienced an NaOCl accident.[72] NaOCl accidents happened more commonly in maxillary posterior teeth diagnosed with pulp necrosis and periapical lesion.[72] Loose placement of irrigation needles and careful irrigation with light pressure and use of a side-perforated needle precludes forcing the irrigating solution into the periradicular tissues. In addition, it is recommended to place a rubber stop on the irrigation needle, shorter than working length, to stay away from apical foramen during irrigation. Up-down movement of the needle during irrigation also helps to prevent locking needle inside the canal. Sudden prolonged and sharp pain during irrigation followed by rapid diffuse swelling (the "sodium hypochlorite accident") usually indicates penetration of solution into the periradicular tissues. The acute episode will subside spontaneously with time (Fig. 18.20). In teeth with open apices, the use of less concentrated irrigants, or saline, will prevent the possibility of irrigation accidents.

Initially, there is no reason to prescribe antibiotics. If there is a visible swelling an incision and drainage is recommended to reduce the pressure.[70] Treatment is palliative. Analgesics and steroids are prescribed, and the patient is reassured. Because the outcome is so dramatic, evaluation is performed frequently to follow progress.

Accidental Injections

In dentistry, local anesthesia, saline, sodium hypochlorite, chloroform, hydrogen peroxide, formalin, and alcohol are frequently used. They are all clear, transparent solutions and each has specific indications for use. Accidental injection occurs when a clear solution like sodium hypochlorite, chloroform, or formalin is loaded into an empty local anesthetic cartridge. A recent review study showed that the following solutions were injected inadvertently: sodium hypochlorite, formalin, formocresol, chlorhexidine, benzalkonium chloride (zephiran), 1:1000 adrenaline, and lighter fuel.[73] In all incidents, the patients felt immediate severe pain in the area of injection. Overall, long-term consequences were more devastating when the accidental injection was an inferior alveolar nerve block compared with local infiltrations.[73]

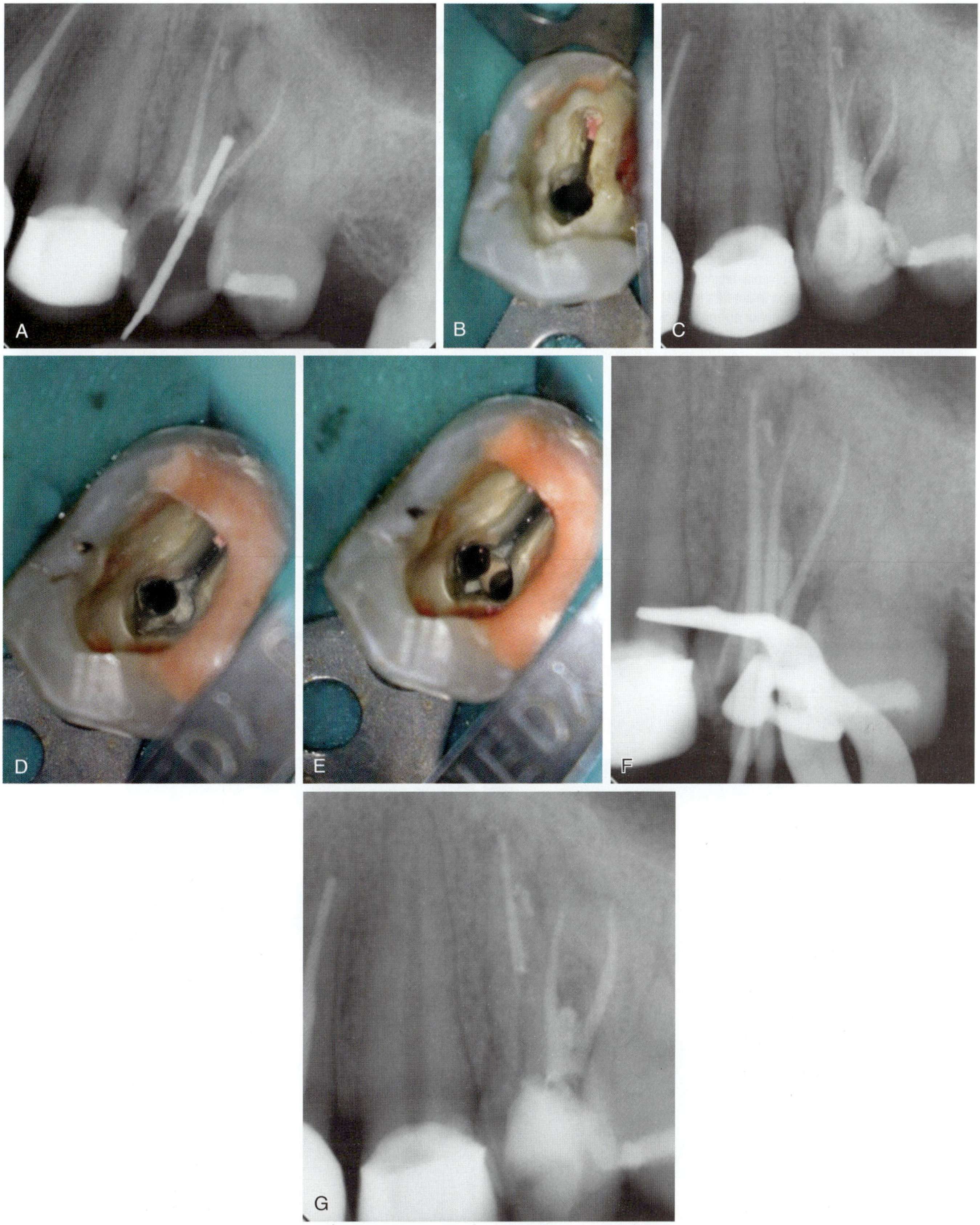

• **Fig. 18.18** **(A)** Perforation during post space preparation in tooth #12. The periapical radiograph shows a missed MB canal. **(B)** After locating and preparing the MB canal. The image shows the orifice of MB below the level of furcation perforation. **(C)** Perforation repaired with mineral trioxide aggregate (MTA) and the pathway of MB was kept patent using a single cone of gutta-percha. **(D)** After MTA setting, the cone in MB was removed. **(E)** The retreatment continued in DB and P canals. The image shows pulp chamber floor built up with MTA. **(F)** Radiograph with master cones in all three canals. **(G)** Final radiograph showing adequate root canal treatment in all three canals, perforation in the pulp chamber floor repaired, and a post space prepared in the P canal.

Study Questions

6. Which perforation has the worst prognosis?
   a. Perforation at the apical third
   b. Perforation at the middle third
   c. Perforation at the crestal bone level without pocket formation
   d. Perforation at the crestal bone level with pocket formation
7. Which one is the main reason for overfilling?
   a. Lack of apical stop caused by overinstrumentation
   b. Apical resorption
   c. Inadequate taper
   d. All of the above
8. Which accidental injection can have the most devastating effects?
   a. NaOCl injected as inferior alveolar block
   b. NaOCl injected as infiltration in anterior maxilla
   c. Normal saline injected as inferior alveolar block
   d. Normal saline injected as buccal infiltration
9. In which of the following is the risk of NaOCl accident higher?
   a. Maxillary posterior teeth
   b. Maxillary anterior teeth
   c. Mandibular posterior teeth
   d. Mandibular anterior teeth
10. In what pulpal/periapical condition is the risk of NaOCl accident the highest?
    a. Irreversible pulpitis with symptomatic apical periodontitis
    b. Pulp necrosis with periapical lesion
    c. Pulp necrosis with normal periapex
    d. Irreversible pulpitis with normal periapex

ANSWERS

Answers Box 18

1 c. Long canal with small diameter and curvature
2 b. Small diameter instrument with minimal taper
3 b. Inner wall
4 b. To loosen the fractured instrument
5 a. The number of canals and the thickness of the canal wall
6 d. Perforation at the crestal bone level with pocket formation
7 d. All of the above
8 a. NaOCl injected as inferior alveolar block
9 a. Maxillary posterior teeth
10 b. Pulp necrosis with periapical lesion

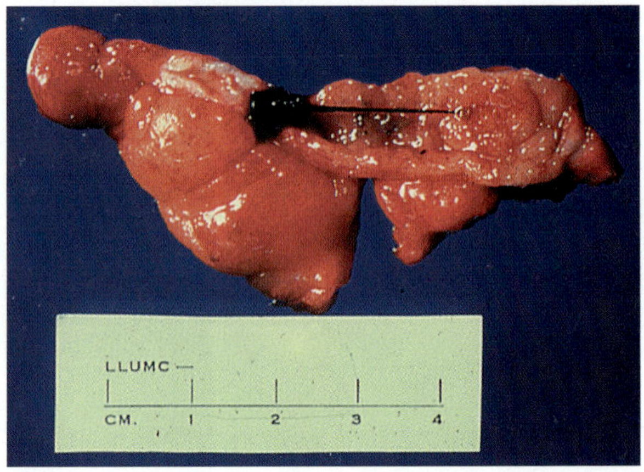

• **Fig. 18.19** A swallowed broach resulted in removal of a patient's appendix and a subsequent lawsuit against a dentist who did not use a rubber dam during root canal therapy. (Courtesy Dr. L. Thompsen.)

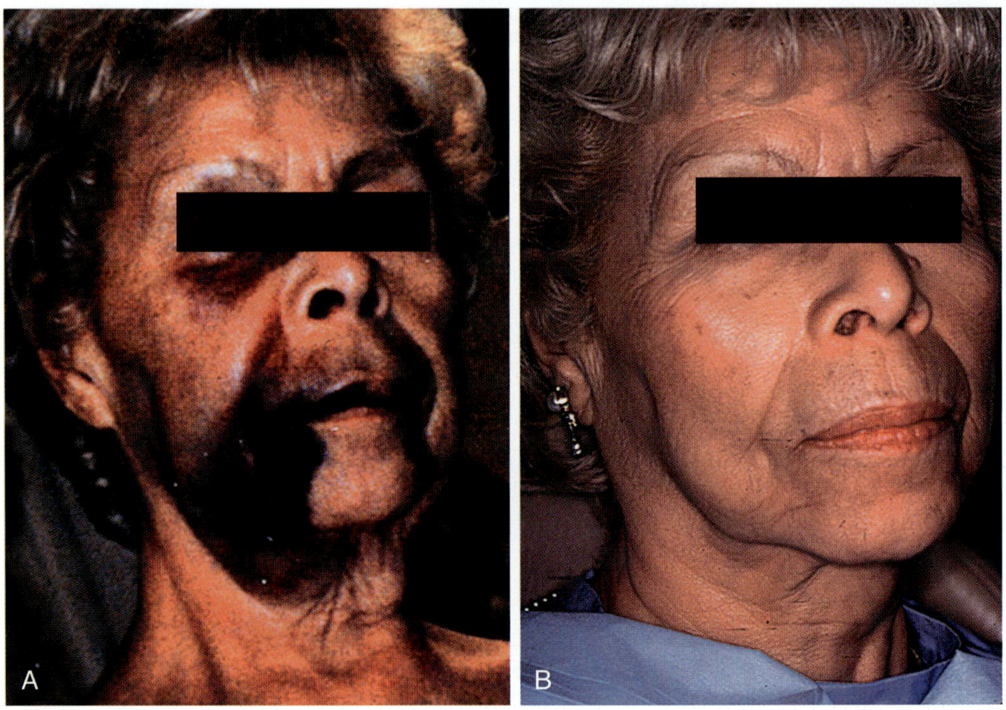

• **Fig. 18.20** **(A)** NaOCl was inadvertently expressed through an apical perforation in a maxillary cuspid during irrigation. Hemorrhagic reaction was rapid and diffuse. **(B)** No treatment was necessary; the swelling and hematoma disappeared within a few weeks. (Courtesy Dr. James Stick.)

References

1. Lambrianidis T, Beltes P: Accidental swallowing of endodontic instruments, *Endod Dent Traumatol* 12(6):301–304, 1996.
2. Fishelberg G, Hook D: Patient safety during endodontic therapy using current technology: a case report, *J Endod* 29(10):683–684, 2003.
3. Nosrat A, Verma P, Hicks ML, et al.: Variations of palatal canal morphology in maxillary molars: a case series and literature review, *J Endod* 43(11):1888–1896, 2017.
4. Gorduysus MO, Gorduysus M, Friedman S: Operating microscope improves negotiation of second mesiobuccal canals in maxillary molars, *J Endod* 27(11):683–686, 2001.
5. Karapinar-Kazandag M, Basrani BR, Friedman S: The operating microscope enhances detection and negotiation of accessory mesial canals in mandibular molars, *J Endod* 36(8):1289–1294, 2010.
6. Nosrat A, Deschenes RJ, Tordik PA, Hicks ML, Fouad AF: Middle mesial canals in mandibular molars: incidence and related factors, *J Endod* 41(1):28–32, 2015.
7. Baldassari-Cruz LA, Lilly JP, Rivera EM: The influence of dental operating microscope in locating the mesiolingual canal orifice, *Oral Surg Oral Med Oral Pathol Oral Radiol Endod* 93(2):190–194, 2002.
8. Nosrat A, Schneider SC: Endodontic management of a maxillary lateral incisor with 4 root canals and a dens invaginatus tract, *J Endod* 41(7):1167–1171, 2015.
9. Blattner TC, George N, Lee CC, Kumar V, Yelton CD: Efficacy of cone-beam computed tomography as a modality to accurately identify the presence of second mesiobuccal canals in maxillary first and second molars: a pilot study, *J Endod* 36(5):867–870, 2010.
10. Tahmasbi M, Jalali P, Nair MK, Barghan S, Nair UP: Prevalence of middle mesial canals and isthmi in the mesial root of mandibular molars: an in vivo cone-beam computed tomographic study, *J Endod* 43(7):1080–1083, 2017.
11. Farzaneh M, Abitbol S, Friedman S: Treatment outcome in endodontics: the Toronto study. Phases I and II: orthograde retreatment, *J Endod* 30(9):627–633, 2004.
12. Tsesis I, Rosenberg E, Faivishevsky V, et al.: Prevalence and associated periodontal status of teeth with root perforation: a retrospective study of 2,002 patients' medical records, *J Endod* 36(5):797–800, 2010.
13. Tsesis I, Fuss Z: Diagnosis and treatment of accidental root perforations, *Endodontic Topics* 13:95–107, 2006.
14. Lemon RR: Simplified esthetic root extrusion techniques, *Oral Surg Oral Med Oral Pathol* 54(1):93–99, 1982.
15. Lee SJ, Monsef M, Torabinejad M: Sealing ability of a mineral trioxide aggregate for repair of lateral root perforations, *J Endod* 19(11):541–544, 1993.
16. Asgary S, Verma P, Nosrat A: Periodontal healing following nonsurgical repair of an old perforation with pocket formation and oral communication, *Restor Dent Endod* 43(2):e17, 2018.
17. Sinai IH: Endodontic perforations: their prognosis and treatment, *J Am Dent Assoc* 95(1):90–95, 1977.
18. Hartwell GR, England MC: Healing of furcation perforations in primate teeth after repair with decalcified freeze-dried bone: a longitudinal study, *J Endod* 19(7):357–361, 1993.
19. Kim JR, Nosrat A, Fouad AF: Interfacial characteristics of Biodentine and MTA with dentine in simulated body fluid, *J Dent* 43(2):241–247, 2015.
20. Siew K, Lee AH, Cheung GS: Treatment outcome of repaired root perforation: a systematic review and meta-analysis, *J Endod* 41(11):1795–1804, 2015.
21. Samiee M, Eghbal M, Parirokh M, Abbas F, Asgary S: Repair of furcal perforation using a new endodontic cement, *Clin Oral Investig* 14(6):653–658, 2010.
22. Parirokh M, Torabinejad M: Mineral trioxide aggregate: a comprehensive literature review—Part III: clinical applications, drawbacks, and mechanism of action, *J Endod* 36(3):400–413, 2010.
23. Asgary S, Nosrat A: Conservative management of class 4 invasive cervical root resorption using calcium-enriched mixture cement, *J Endod* 42(8):1291–1294, 2016.
24. Lemon RR: Nonsurgical repair of perforation defects. Internal matrix concept, *Dent Clin North Am* 36(2):439–457, 1992.
25. Venskutonis T, Plotino G, Juodzbalys G, Mickeviciene L: The importance of cone-beam computed tomography in the management of endodontic problems: a review of the literature, *J Endod* 40(12):1895–1901, 2014.
26. AAE and AAOMR Joint Position Statement: use of cone beam computed tomography in endodontics 2015 update, *J Endod* 41(9):1393–1396, 2015.
27. Fuss Z, Trope M: Root perforations: classification and treatment choices based on prognostic factors, *Endod Dent Traumatol* 12(6):255–264, 1996.
28. Ford TR, Torabinejad M, McKendry DJ, Hong CU, Kariyawasam SP: Use of mineral trioxide aggregate for repair of furcal perforations, *Oral Surg Oral Med Oral Pathol Oral Radiol Endod* 79(6):756–763, 1995.
29. Greene KJ, Krell KV: Clinical factors associated with ledged canals in maxillary and mandibular molars, *Oral Surg Oral Med Oral Pathol* 70(4):490–497, 1990.
30. Capar ID, Ertas H, Ok E, Arslan H, Ertas ET: Comparative study of different novel nickel-titanium rotary systems for root canal preparation in severely curved root canals, *J Endod* 40(6):852–856, 2014.
31. Schafer E, Florek H: Efficiency of rotary nickel-titanium K3 instruments compared with stainless steel hand K-Flexofile. Part 1. Shaping ability in simulated curved canals, *Int Endod J* 36(3):199–207, 2003.
32. Javaheri HH, Javaheri GH: A comparison of three Ni-Ti rotary instruments in apical transportation, *J Endod* 33(3):284–286, 2007.
33. Ponce de Leon Del Bello T, Wang N, Roane JB: Crown-down tip design and shaping, *J Endod* 29(8):513–518, 2003.
34. Seltzer S, Sinai I, August D: Periodontal effects of root perforations before and during endodontic procedures, *J Dent Res* 49(2):332–339, 1970.
35. Oloomi K, Saberi E, Mokhtari H, et al.: Evaluation of the effect of blood contamination on the compressive strength of MTA modified with hydration accelerators, *Restor Dent Endod* 38(3):128–133, 2013.
36. Nosrat A, Nekoofar MH, Bolhari B, Dummer PM: Unintentional extrusion of mineral trioxide aggregate: a report of three cases, *Int Endod J* 45(12):1165–1176, 2012.
37. Spili P, Parashos P, Messer HH: The impact of instrument fracture on outcome of endodontic treatment, *J Endod* 31(12):845–850, 2005.
38. Peters OA, Roehlike JO, Baumann MA: Effect of immersion in sodium hypochlorite on torque and fatigue resistance of nickel-titanium instruments, *J Endod* 33(5):589–593, 2007.
39. Berutti E, Angelini E, Rigolone M, Migliaretti G, Pasqualini D: Influence of sodium hypochlorite on fracture properties and corrosion of ProTaper Rotary instruments, *Int Endod J* 39(9):693–699, 2006.
40. Powers J, Sakaguchi R: *Craig's restorative dental materials*, ed 12, St Louis, 2006, Mosby.
41. Parashos P, Gordon I, Messer HH: Factors influencing defects of rotary nickel-titanium endodontic instruments after clinical use, *J Endod* 30(10):722–725, 2004.
42. Terauchi Y, O'Leary L, Kikuchi I, et al.: Evaluation of the efficiency of a new file removal system in comparison with two conventional systems, *J Endod* 33(5):585–588, 2007.
43. Lopes HP, Ferreira AA, Elias CN, et al.: Influence of rotational speed on the cyclic fatigue of rotary nickel-titanium endodontic instruments, *J Endod* 35(7):1013–1016, 2009.
44. Lopes HP, Moreira EJ, Elias CN, de Almeida RA, Neves MS: Cyclic fatigue of ProTaper instruments, *J Endod* 33(1):55–57, 2007.

45. Kosti E, Zinelis S, Lambrianidis T, Margelos J: A comparative study of crack development in stainless-steel Hedstrom files used with step-back or crown-down techniques, *J Endod* 30(1):38–41, 2004.
46. Gambarini G: Rationale for the use of low-torque endodontic motors in root canal instrumentation, *Endod Dent Traumatol* 16(3):95–100, 2000.
47. Alapati SB, Brantley WA, Svec TA, et al.: SEM observations of nickel-titanium rotary endodontic instruments that fractured during clinical use, *J Endod* 31(1):40–43, 2005.
48. Gao Y, Shotton V, Wilkinson K, Phillips G, Johnson WB: Effects of raw material and rotational speed on the cyclic fatigue of ProFile Vortex rotary instruments, *J Endod* 36(7):1205–1209, 2010.
49. Pedulla E, Grande NM, Plotino G, Gambarini G, Rapisarda E: Influence of continuous or reciprocating motion on cyclic fatigue resistance of 4 different nickel-titanium rotary instruments, *J Endod* 39(2):258–261, 2013.
50. Cuje J, Bargholz C, Hulsmann M: The outcome of retained instrument removal in a specialist practice, *Int Endod J* 43(7):545–554, 2010.
51. Shen Y, Peng B, Cheung GS: Factors associated with the removal of fractured NiTi instruments from root canal systems, *Oral Surg Oral Med Oral Pathol Oral Radiol Endod* 98(5):605–610, 2004.
52. Patino PV, Biedma BM, Liebana CR, Cantatore G, Bahillo JG: The influence of a manual glide path on the separation rate of NiTi rotary instruments, *J Endod* 31(2):114–116, 2005.
53. Shen Y, Qian W, Abtin H, Gao Y, Haapasalo M: Effect of environment on fatigue failure of controlled memory wire nickel-titanium rotary instruments, *J Endod* 38(3):376–380, 2012.
54. You SY, Bae KS, Baek SH, et al.: Lifespan of one nickel-titanium rotary file with reciprocating motion in curved root canals, *J Endod* 36(12):1991–1994, 2010.
55. Suter B, Lussi A, Sequeira P: Probability of removing fractured instruments from root canals, *Int Endod J* 38(2):112–123, 2005.
56. Wu J, Lei G, Yan M, et al.: Instrument separation analysis of multi-used ProTaper Universal rotary system during root canal therapy, *J Endod* 37(6):758–763, 2011.
57. Ettrich CA, Labossiere PE, Pitts DL, Johnson JD: An investigation of the heat induced during ultrasonic post removal, *J Endod* 33(10):1222–1226, 2007.
58. Madarati AA, Qualtrough AJ, Watts DC: Efficiency of a newly designed ultrasonic unit and tips in reducing temperature rise on root surface during the removal of fractured files, *J Endod* 35(6):896–899, 2009.
59. Ward JR, Parashos P, Messer HH: Evaluation of an ultrasonic technique to remove fractured rotary nickel-titanium endodontic instruments from root canals: an experimental study, *J Endod* 29(11):756–763, 2003.
60. Panitvisai P, Parunnit P, Sathorn C, Messer HH: Impact of a retained instrument on treatment outcome: a systematic review and meta-analysis, *J Endod* 36(5):775–780, 2010.
61. Uraba S, Ebihara A, Komatsu K, Ohbayashi N, Okiji T: Ability of cone-beam computed tomography to detect periapical lesions that were not detected by periapical radiography: a retrospective assessment according to tooth group, *J Endod* 42(8):1186–1190, 2016.
62. Rosen E, Venezia NB, Azizi H, et al.: A comparison of cone-beam computed tomography with periapical radiography in the detection of separated instruments retained in the apical third of root canal-filled teeth, *J Endod* 42(7):1035–1039, 2016.
63. Obermayr G, Walton RE, Leary JM, Krell KV: Vertical root fracture and relative deformation during obturation and post cementation, *J Prosthet Dent* 66(2):181–187, 1991.
64. Chai H, Tamse A: The effect of isthmus on vertical root fracture in endodontically treated teeth, *J Endod* 41(9):1515–1519, 2015.
65. Dang DA, Walton RE: Vertical root fracture and root distortion: effect of spreader design, *J Endod* 15(7):294–301, 1989.
66. Gharai SR, Thorpe JR, Strother JM, McClanahan SB: Comparison of generated forces and apical microleakage using nickel-titanium and stainless steel finger spreaders in curved canals, *J Endod* 31(3):198–200, 2005.
67. Tamse A, Kaffe I, Lustig J, Ganor Y, Fuss Z: Radiographic features of vertically fractured endodontically treated mesial roots of mandibular molars, *Oral Surg Oral Med Oral Pathol Oral Radiol Endod* 101(6):797–802, 2006.
68. Hassan B, Metska ME, Ozok AR, van der Stelt P, Wesselink PR: Detection of vertical root fractures in endodontically treated teeth by a cone beam computed tomography scan, *J Endod* 35(5):719–722, 2009.
69. Grossman LI: Prevention in endodontic practice, *J Am Dent Assoc* 82(2):395–396, 1971.
70. Guivarc'h M, Ordioni U, Ahmed HM, et al.: Sodium hypochlorite accident: a systematic review, *J Endod* 43(1):16–24, 2017.
71. Bowden JR, Ethunandan M, Brennan PA: Life-threatening airway obstruction secondary to hypochlorite extrusion during root canal treatment, *Oral Surg Oral Med Oral Pathol Oral Radiol Endod* 101(3):402–404, 2006.
72. Kleier DJ, Averbach RE, Mehdipour O: The sodium hypochlorite accident: experience of diplomates of the American Board of Endodontics, *J Endod* 34(11):1346–1350, 2008.
73. Verma P, Tordik P, Nosrat A: Hazards of improper dispensary: literature review and report of an accidental chloroform injection, *J Endod* 44(6):1042–1047, 2018.

19 Nonsurgical Retreatment

YOSHITSUGU TERAUCHI, MASOUD PARIROKH, AND ROBERT HANDYSIDES

CHAPTER OUTLINE

LEARNING OBJECTIVES

After reading this chapter, the student should be able to:

1. Recognize causes of the initial root canal therapy failure that require nonsurgical endodontic retreatment.
2. Identify if an initial root canal therapy requires additional treatment
3. Identify the treatment options available for teeth that need endodontic retreatment.
4. State the indications and contraindications for nonsurgical endodontic retreatment.
5. Describe how an accurate diagnosis should be made for nonsurgical endodontic retreatment.
6. Discuss the treatment plans for nonsurgical endodontic retreatment.
7. Describe the risks and benefits of nonsurgical endodontic retreatment.
8. Describe techniques and materials used in nonsurgical endodontic retreatment.
9. Discuss restorative options and follow-up care.
10. Discuss the prognosis and outcomes for nonsurgical endodontic retreatment.

Introduction

When providing root canal treatment using today's techniques the clinician expects excellent success rates. Modern methodologies and materials have demonstrated this in studies looking at maintaining tooth function and retention.[1,2] Initial root canal therapy, however, does not always result in healing for a multitude of reasons. Failure to adequately disinfect the root canal system may result in nonhealing. Bacteria may persist after initial treatment as a result of areas that were inaccessible to instrumentation and irrigation.[3-6] Causes of treatment failure may include lack of tooth isolation; inadequate cleaning, shaping, and irrigation; and incomplete obturation (Fig. 19.1). In addition to complex anatomic variations in the root canal anatomy, root canal obstructions, including calcifications, can also be a problem[3-5] The reestablishment of root canal infection after initial treatment may also lead to progression of disease.[7-9] This reintroduction of microorganisms is primarily caused by coronal microleakage and recurrent decay.[3,4,9,10] Furthermore, initial treatment may be compromised by long-term use of temporary materials before placement of definitive restorations.[12-14]

Nonhealing after initial nonsurgical root canal therapy may also be related to procedural errors or the presence of biofilms.[11] Procedural errors include perforations, canal transportation, fractured instruments, and ledge formations, all of which can negatively affect the treatment outcome.[3,6]

It is also important to recognize that vertical root fractures (VRF) may sometimes appear as nonhealing lesions. These are longitudinal fractures that occur after root canal treatment and may be related to the weakening of roots from excessive dentin removal or simply from the stresses on teeth from normal function.[15-17]

Causes of Nonhealing of Initial Root Canal Treatment

A significant reduction or elimination of bacteria in the root canal system after initial endodontic treatment should reduce the presence of periapical periodontitis. The causes of the initial endodontic treatment failure can include inability of the procedure to eradicate bacteria, introduced intraradicular microorganism,[18] extraradicular infection,[19] foreign body reaction,[20] accidental procedures,[21] and nonendodontic related events such as VRF, traumatic injuries, and periodontal disease.[22] Most studies on the unfavorable outcomes of endodontic treatment reported that microorganisms in the root canals or periradicular lesions play a major role in the persistence of apical periodontitis (Fig. 19.2).[8,22-24]

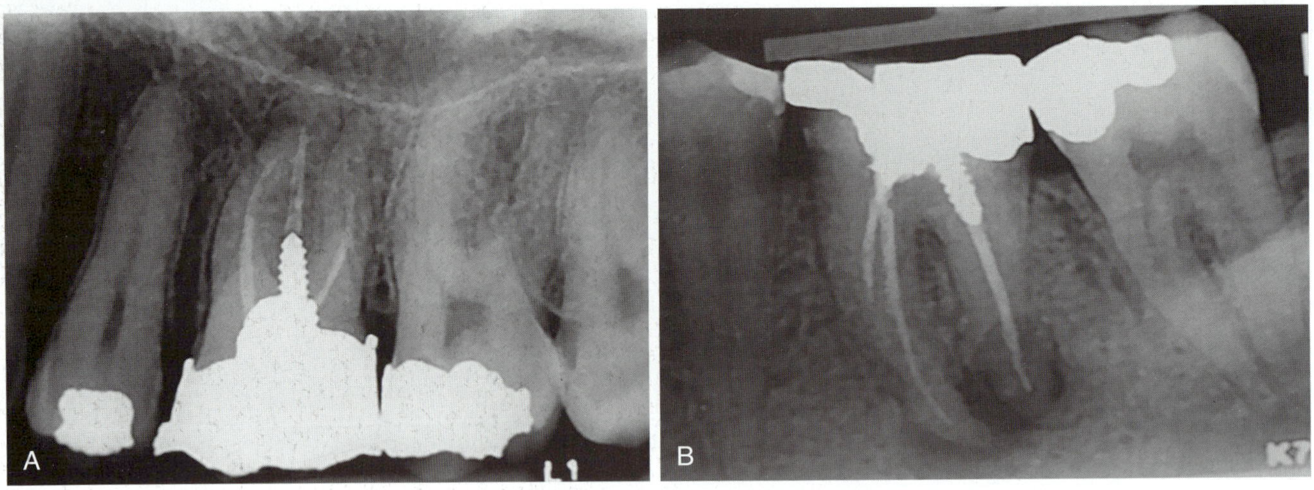

• **Fig. 19.1** **(A)** A patient has had sensitivity to palpation and percussion. Review of the periapical radiograph of the maxillary left first molar is showing the presence of apical pathosis. **(B)** Periapical radiograph of the mandibular left first molar is showing incomplete obturation and large periapical pathosis. The tooth restoration has been fractured and needs a full coverage restoration.

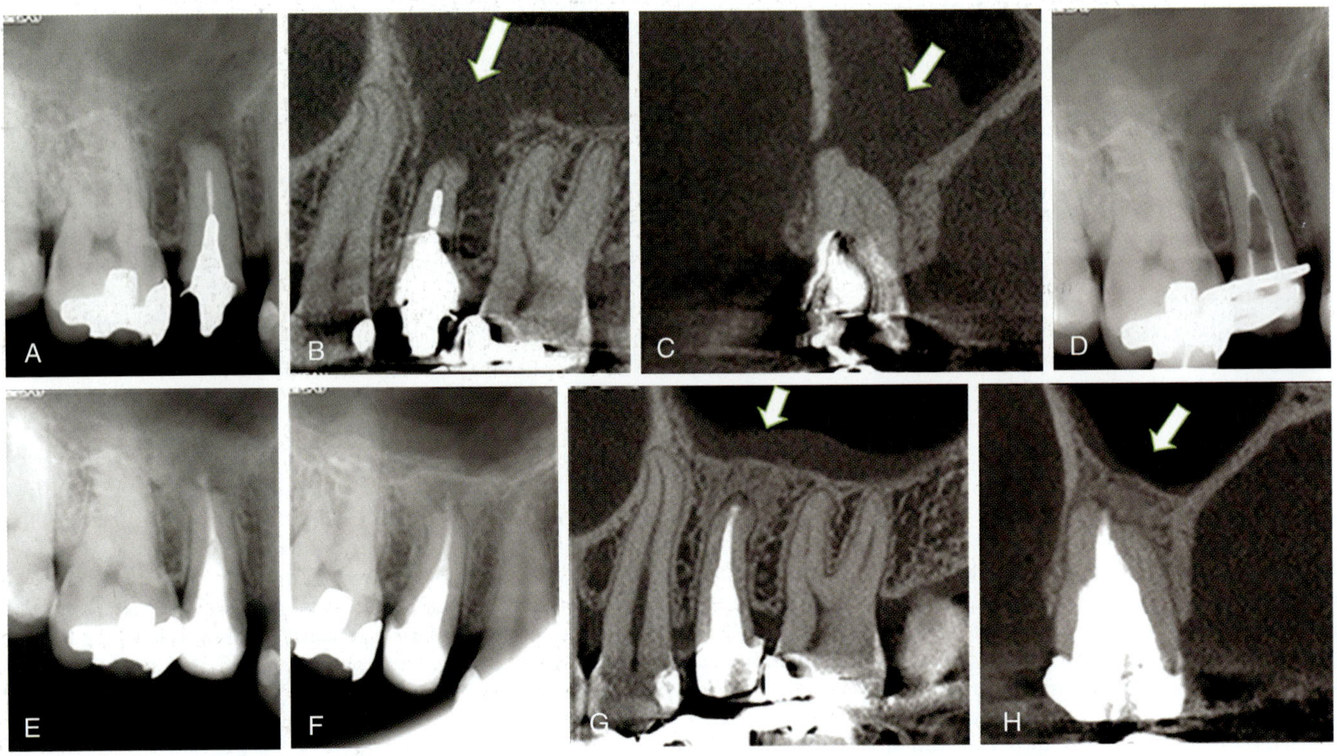

• **Fig. 19.2** **(A)** Preoperative radiograph of the maxillary right second premolar showing a large periapical lesion. **(B)** Sagittal view of CBCT imaging reveals an unfilled canal space apical to the root filling and the periapical lesion extending to the maxillary sinus cavity (*arrow*). **(C)** Coronal view of CBCT imaging reveals complete resorption of maxillary sinus floor on the root (*arrow*). **(D)** Postoperative radiograph showing root canal fillings with MTA. **(E)** Three-month postoperative radiograph showing a reduced periapical lesion. **(F)** Six-month postoperative radiograph showing nice periapical healing. **(G)** Six-month postoperative sagittal view of CBCT imaging reveals both periapical healing and reformation of the maxillary sinus floor (*arrow*). **(H)** Six-month postoperative coronal view of CBCT imaging reveals complete reformation of the maxillary sinus floor (*arrow*).

Diagnosis and Retreatment Options

Diagnosis of a tooth in need of endodontic retreatment should be based on clinical signs and symptoms, radiographic and, when necessary, tomographic interpretations.

Periapical radiographs should be taken in two different horizontal angles to evaluate the quality of obturation, crestal bone level, presence of missed root canals, procedural errors, resorptions, and lateral or periapical radiolucent lesions (Fig. 19.3).

Introduction of cone beam computed tomography (CBCT) to endodontics has had a considerable and positive effect on the diagnosis and treatment planning. However, CBCT images reveal more periapical lesions compared with the two-dimensional conventional radiographic techniques.[25,26] An investigation by Torabinejad et al.

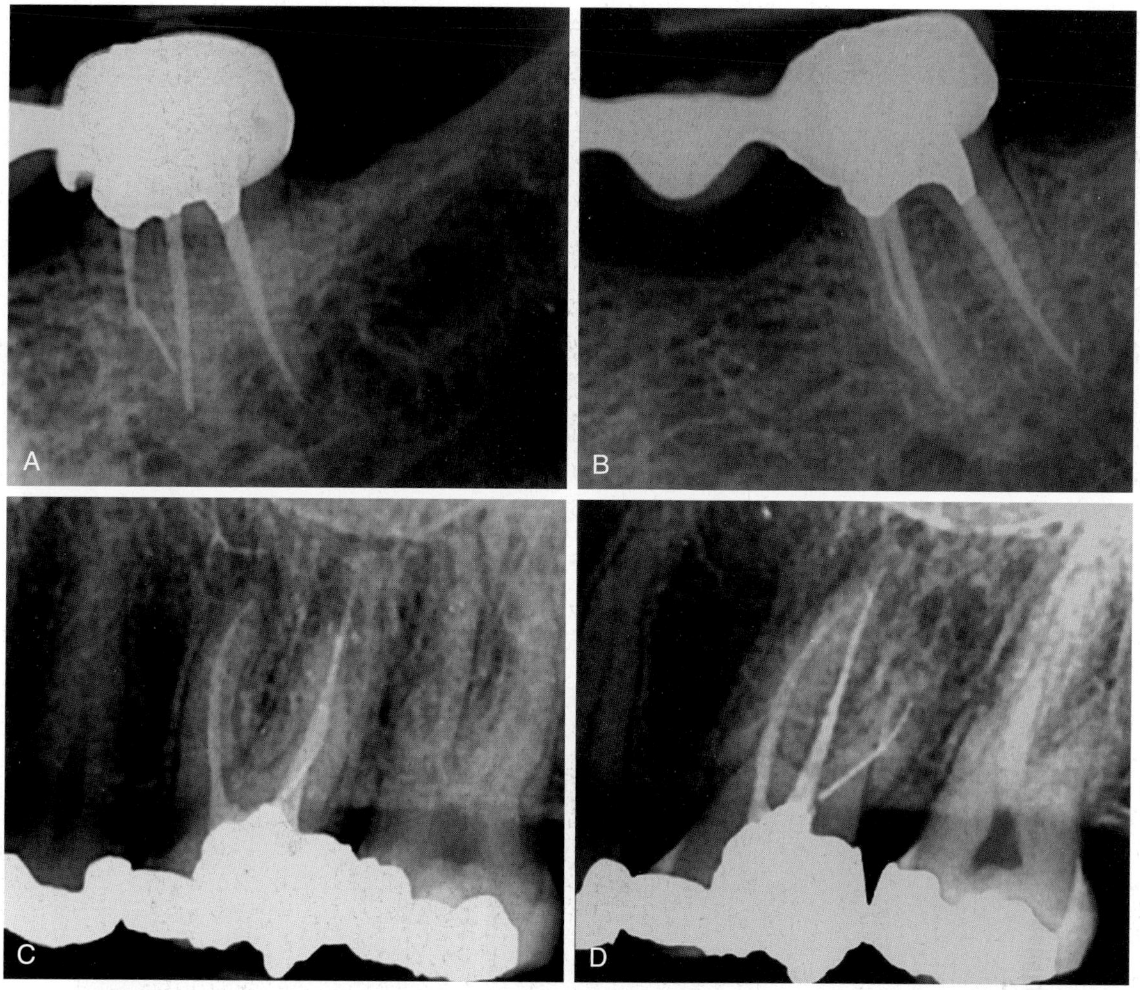

• **Fig. 19.3** Importance of taking preoperative periapical radiograph with different angles. **(A)** Mandibular left second molar shows broken instruments in one of the mesial root canals. **(B)** Different horizontal angle of the same tooth shows a possibility of root canal transportation as well as perforation in the same root. **(C)** Periapical radiography of the maxillary left first molar when taken from distal resulted in superimposition of the distobuccal root over the palatal root. **(D)** Taking the radiograph with a different horizontal angle shows broken instrument in the distobuccal root.

showed that 20% of the teeth with a history of root canal therapy that had no visible radiographic periapical lesions exhibited periapical radiolucencies >1 mm in size when evaluated by CBCT. They cautioned clinicians not to consider all these lesions as treatment failures because the radiolucency might be a previous lesion in its healing phase, persistent periapical disease, or even fibrous scar tissue.[27] They recommended further follow-up as well as a work-up of the case to determine the true nature of these radiolucencies (Fig. 19.4).

Both intraradicular and extraradicular infections might result in nonhealing of root canal treatment. If a periapical radiograph shows adequate root canal therapy, presence of extraradicular infection should also be considered as a reason for failure.[28]

The reason a tooth requires endodontic retreatment should always be confirmed. In addition to performing endodontic retreatment for the failed cases, in some instances, as a result of the fracture of the preexisting restoration, leakage, or unacceptable esthetics, endodontic retreatment should be performed for teeth with inadequate root canal therapy despite the absence of clinical signs or symptoms and radiographic pathosis (Fig. 19.5).

In some cases, dental practitioners might not have a similar treatment plan to manage a tooth with previously failed root canal therapy.[29] Factors such as the practitioners' personal experience, skill, available armamentarium, patients' attitude, and demands for receiving endodontic retreatment might influence the treatment plan. Therefore a dentist would help patients participate in a shared decision-making process through full description of all the treatment options, their risks and benefits, as well as economic advantages and disadvantages. Patients usually attend a dental office when they are in pain and discomfort, need to repair a preexisting restoration, have fractured or traumatized teeth, or need treatment as a result of dental caries. Occasionally, making decisions may be difficult because of conditions that could be genuinely complicated. It would be wise to precisely evaluate each case by clinical and radiographic examinations and, if necessary, refer the patient to a periodontist or a prosthodontist to make sure that the tooth is restorable and maintainable after endodontic retreatment. It is critically important to describe all information in a simple language that is easily understood by the patients.[30] Therefore patients' age, first/second language, and educational background should be considered for better communication.[31,32]

The treatment options in endodontics, when previous root canal therapy is showing signs of failure or when the tooth needs a new permanent restoration, would include nonsurgical root canal

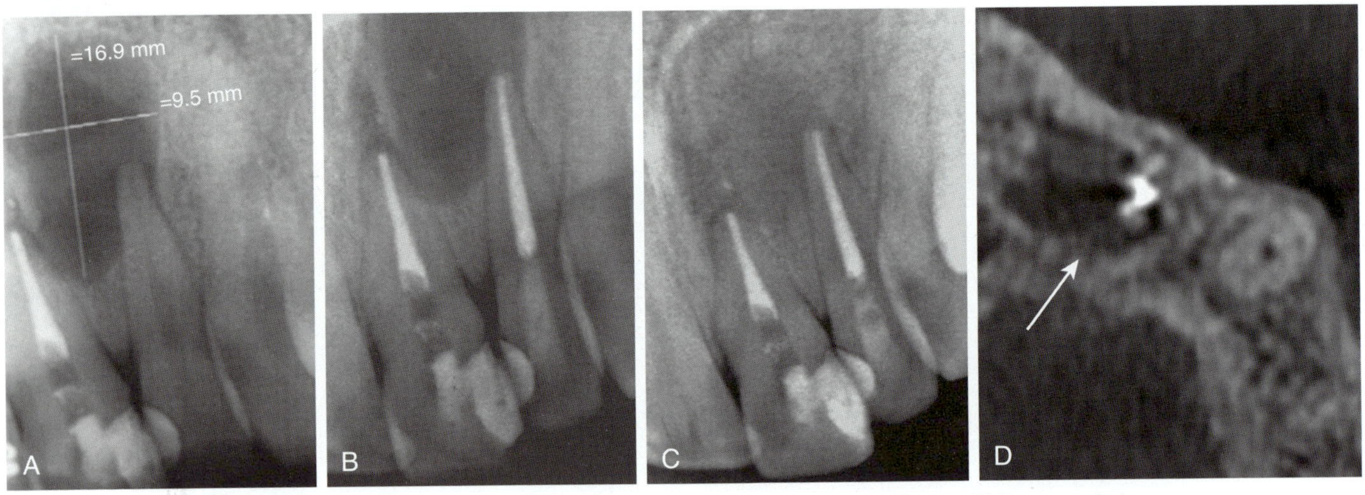

• **Fig. 19.4** An example of working up a case that shows periapical lesion in CBCT image. **(A)** Presence of a large periapical lesion around the maxillary left lateral incisor. **(B)** Root canal treatment of the lateral incisor. **(C)** Periapical healing 2 years after the treatment. **(D)** Presence of a radiolucency around the maxillary lateral incisor in axial view of the tooth that was treated 2 years ago (*white arrow*). No treatment should be performed for this case because the patient is symptom free and the follow-up radiograph showed healing compared with the preoperative radiograph.

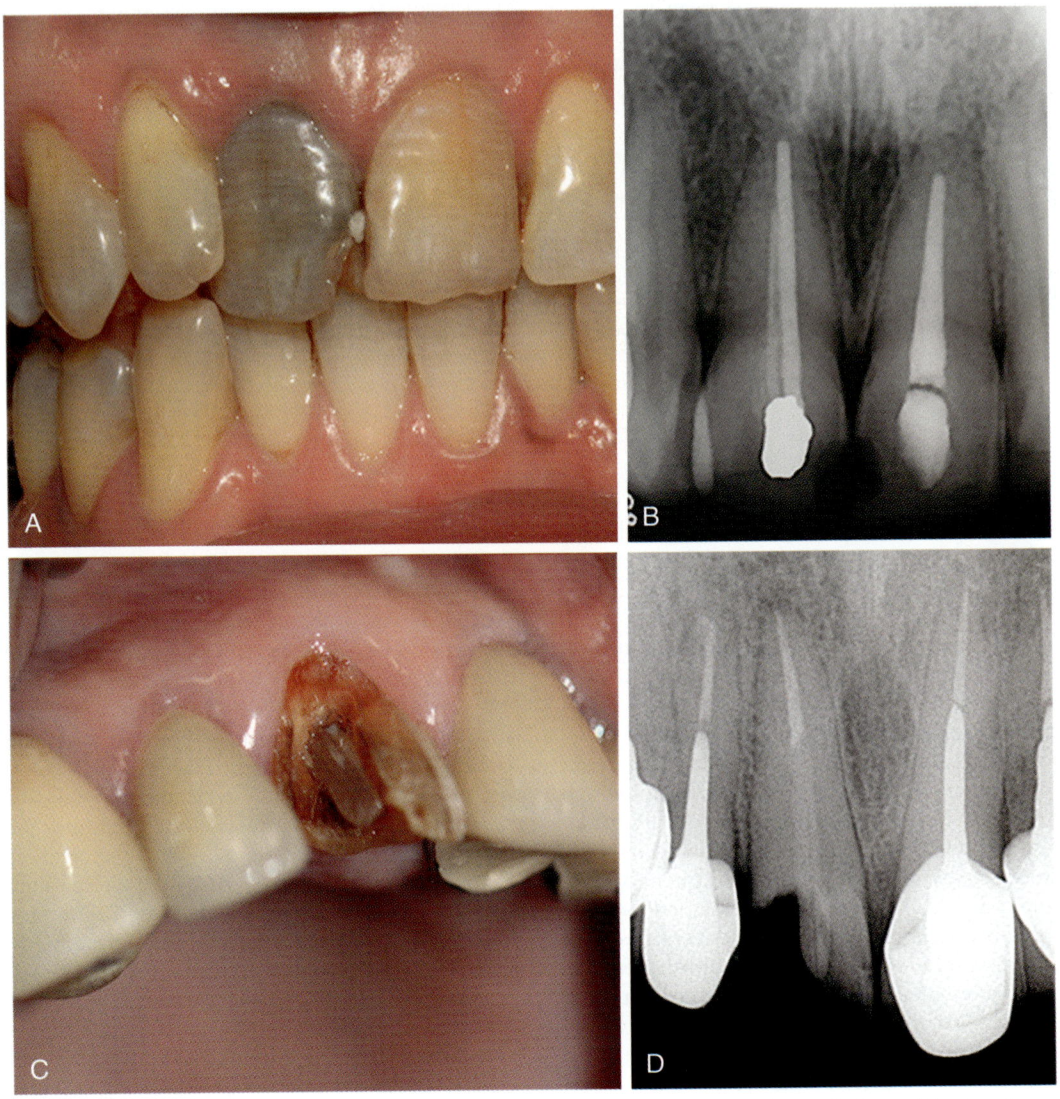

• **Fig. 19.5 (A-D)** Endodontic retreatment is needed as a result of unacceptable esthetic and fractured crown in maxillary right central incisors.

retreatment, surgical retreatment, replantation, transplantation, and possible extraction followed by placement of an implant.[33]

Indications for Nonsurgical Endodontic Retreatment

Retreatment is considered the primary procedural option when the tooth exhibits inadequate initial root canal treatment, has palpation and percussion sensitivity, localized swelling, recurrent caries, leaky provisional restorations, and substandard or missing coronal restorations. Radiographic evaluation may show the presence of untreated canals, poor canal obturation with voids, separated instruments, recurrent caries not located during clinical examination, or defective restorations with open margins that can potentially contribute to nonhealing. Any combination of clinical symptoms, radiographic evidence, and other clinical findings may indicate that nonhealing is evident but may also arise without any contribution of the aforementioned conditions.

Contraindications for Nonsurgical Endodontic Retreatment

A major factor to determine the requirement for nonsurgical retreatment is the restorability of the tooth after the necessary removal of preexisting restorative materials. Additional tooth structure may be lost during caries elimination and removal of post and core materials. The restorability decision often requires comprehensive disassembly of preexisting restorations and evaluation of the remaining root canal system. Other factors include the presence of extensive periodontal involvement that weakens tooth support and/or the presence of problematic coronal or radicular fractures. Patients who are not motivated to save the natural tooth are poor candidates for retreatment.

Treatment Planning for Nonsurgical Retreatment

In most instances, nonsurgical root canal retreatment is the first treatment of choice for either overcoming a nonhealing outcome of a previous root canal treatment or correcting a previous inadequate endodontic treatment with no clinical and radiographic signs of failure (Fig. 19.6).[33,34] Moreover, nonsurgical endodontic retreatment is usually preferred to other treatment options because the procedure is less invasive than surgical endodontics, replantation, transplantation, and extraction and replacement with implant.[2]

In addition to the technical challenge of performing endodontic retreatment, other aspects of the treatment should also be considered.[35] Important factors in this respect include cost-effectiveness of the treatment, periodontal status, the remaining tooth structure after removing all caries and preexisting restorations, restorability of the tooth, the total cost of treatment, the need for crown lengthening in order to place a suitable full-coverage restoration, and esthetic and functional conditions.

Cost-effectiveness of a treatment might affect decision-making when there are different treatment options. Both microsurgical endodontic retreatment or nonsurgical endodontic retreatment with a crown are more cost-effective treatments compared with extraction and placement of an implant.[36]

The practitioner should always evaluate periodontal status, restorability, and function of the tooth during the examination visit. The occlusal contacts of the tooth should also be evaluated, particularly if during the previous treatment the occlusal surface of the tooth has been reduced for a long time (Fig. 19.7).

An important aid in treatment planning is to order CBCT before commencing endodontic retreatment.[37] Practitioners should only request CBCT after taking relevant courses and gaining experience and knowledge on interpretation of CBCT images and their limitations.[25] The European Academy of DentoMaxilloFacial Radiology has recommended incorporating courses on CBCT into both undergraduate and postgraduate curricula as well as continuing education programs for dentists and endodontists in order to improve their skills in relation to the interpretation of the tomographic images used in their clinical practice.[38]

Although CBCT could be an important aid for the practitioner, it does not mean it should be ordered for all the endodontic retreatment cases.[39,40] For endodontic retreatment purposes CBCT could be ordered if[25,40,41]:

- Conventional two-dimensional radiography (periapical) did not provide enough information regarding the reason(s) for failure in a tooth that previously received endodontic treatment (Fig. 19.8).
- Conventional two-dimensional radiography (periapical) shows the possibility of complex root canal anatomy in a tooth with a history of endodontic therapy (Fig. 19.9).
- There is possibility of mishaps and overlooked root canal(s) that are not adequately detected by conventional two-dimensional radiography (Figs. 19.9 and 19.10).

Based on standards of care, the dentist should choose whether conventional radiography is sufficient for commencing endodontic retreatment or there is need for more information by ordering CBCT. The practitioner should discuss the risks and benefits of requesting CBCT with the patient and both arrive at a decision either to order the tomography or to only use conventional radiography during treatment planning. Higher radiation dose, higher cost, and lower resolution are disadvantages of CBCT compared with periapical radiography.[42]

There is no unique treatment plan for all the teeth with a history of endodontic therapy and nonhealing periapical lesions.[30] Each case should be evaluated individually and decisions on the treatment plan should be made based on patients' preference, possibility of rendering ideal treatment, and considering the prognosis. Most patients are interested in being active or collaborative in making a decision when teeth have apical periodontitis.[43] Variables should be discussed with patients and a final shared decision should be made.[44]

Risks and Benefits of Retreatment

Like any dental treatment, the risks, benefits, alternative treatments, and the subsequent consequences of choices must always be discussed with the patient. This conversation occurs before commencing treatment and includes an explanation of what the treatment entails, expected treatment time, prognosis, and costs.[36]

Nonsurgical root canal retreatment procedures have numerous potential risks. These include fracture of a porcelain crown during the access procedure, fracture of the root during post removal procedures, and dislodgment of the crown, which may necessitate replacement. In addition, iatrogenic challenges may arise such as extensive removal of tooth structure, canal transportation, creation of ledges, or even perforations.[5,6,45] The separation of an instrument is also possible, which may impede the ability to completely remove obturation materials. These complications potentially affect the retreatment outcome. The benefits of retreatment include the preservation and retention of the patient's natural tooth and the avoidance of more extensive clinical treatment and costs.

Study Questions

1. Nonhealing of root canal therapy may be caused by:
   a. Inadequate tooth isolation
   b. Inadequate instrumentation
   c. Inadequate obturation
   d. All of the above
2. Radiographic "apical lesions" after root canal therapy may be a result of:
   a. Nonhealing after treatment
   b. Reestablishment of disease
   c. Vertical root fracture
   d. All of the above
3. When should risks benefits and alternatives to treatment be given to a patient?
   a. Before treatment
   b. During treatment
   c. After treatment
4. Which of the following describes a disadvantage of CBCT compared with the conventional radiography?
   a. Higher radiation dose
   b. Higher cost
   c. Lower resolution
   d. All of the above
5. Which of the following is a contraindication for endodontic retreatment?
   a. Absence of coronal restoration
   b. None–restorable crown
   c. Tooth discoloration
   d. A history of soft tissue swelling

Endodontic Retreatment Procedures

Access Through Full-Coverage or Preexisting Restorations

The decision to remove all the existing restorations during endo-dontic retreatment depends on several factors. In most cases, the practitioner should remove all the existing restorations before commencing the endodontic retreatment procedure because of the possibility of leakage and presence of recurrent caries. In addition, it is reasonable to remove a previous restoration as well as caries before performing endodontic retreatment to determine whether future restoration is possible or not.[46] However, in some instances, the patient might have recently received a suitable restoration and removing it would increase the cost of the treatment. In such a case, providing access cavity through the previous restoration might be recommended (Fig. 19.11). Preserving a crown restoration could also help to improve dental dam isolation and maintain occlusion, with the least alteration in esthetics. However, it might restrict the practitioners' ability to observe cracks, missed root canal(s), and recurrent caries. If a prior restoration of the retreated tooth is amalgam, there would always be a chance of inadvertent pushing of amalgam fragments (induced during access cavity preparation) into the root canal space and blocking the root canal negotiation.

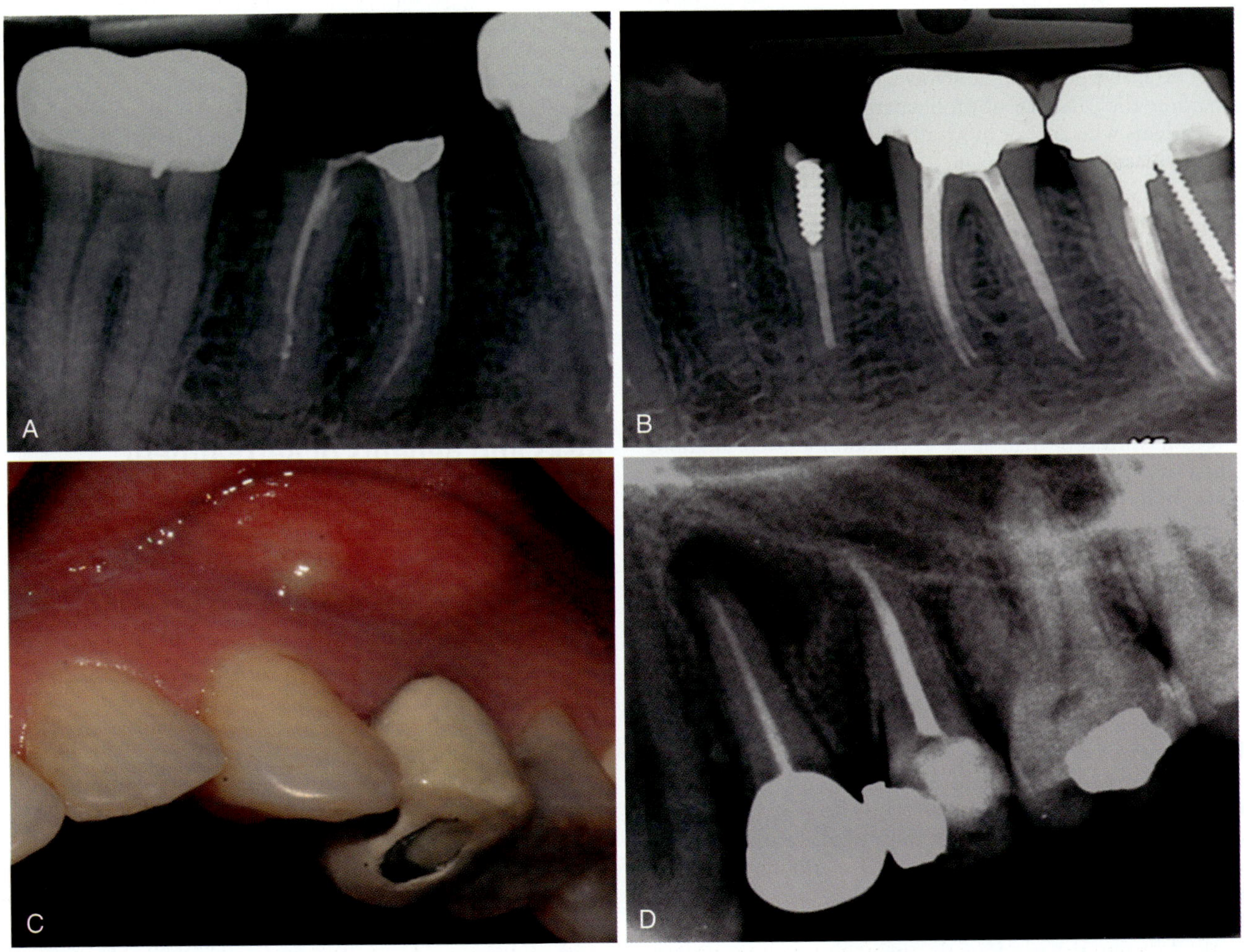

• **Fig. 19.6** Typical cases that need endodontic retreatment because of various reasons. **(A** and **B)** The teeth need endodontic retreatment as a result of fracture of their restorations. **(C** and **D)** Maxillary left first premolar needs endodontic retreatment as a result of failure of the previous root canal therapy.

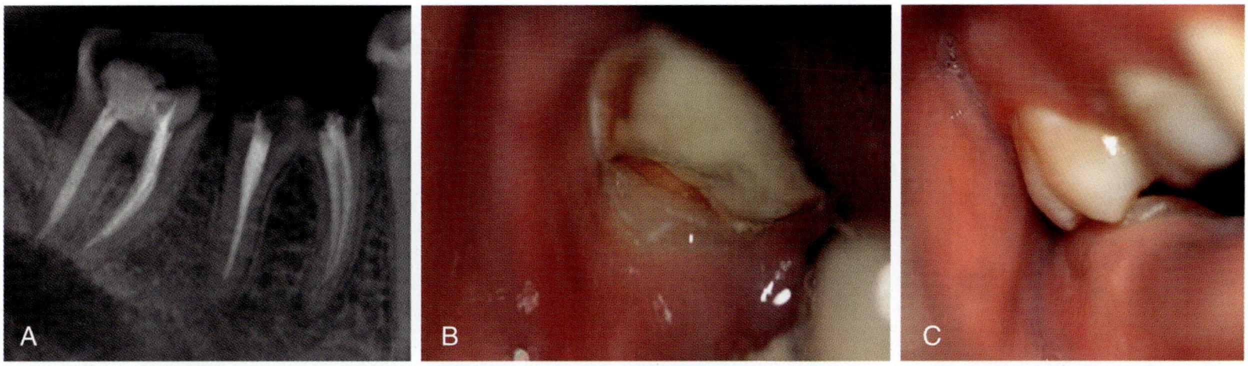

• **Fig. 19.7** **(A)** Occlusal surface of the mandibular right second molar has been reduced after the previous root canal treatment. **(B)** Occlusal view of the tooth that needs reconstruction. **(C)** No space for placing a full coverage restoration over the tooth.

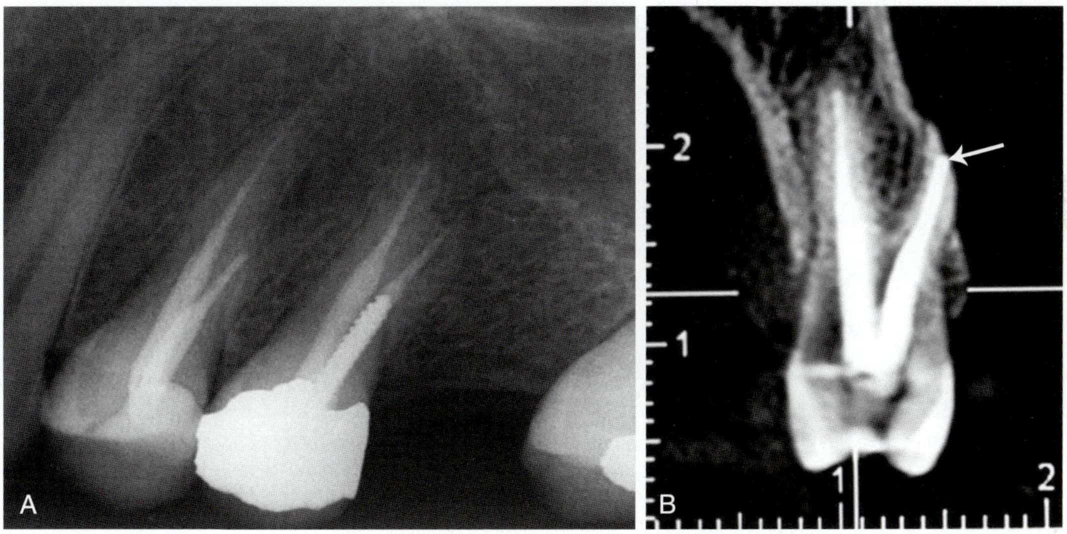

• **Fig. 19.8** **(A)** Maxillary left second premolar received root canal therapy 2 years ago; however, the patient complained of pain and sensitivity on percussion and palpation since the treatment visit. **(B)** The CBCT image in coronal view showed apical perforation in the buccal root (*white arrow*).

Based on the American Association of Endodontists (AAE) difficulty assessment form,[47] root canal retreatment has been categorized as highly difficult. If the tooth has received a full-coverage crown or is an abutment for a bridge and needs to receive endodontic retreatment, it will definitely increase the difficulty, and it may be wiser to refer the patient to an endodontist. For more information on the subject, the reader should refer to Chapter 6 of this book.

If either a prefabricated or a cast post is present even in a tooth that recently received a restoration, removal of all the existing restorations is highly recommended.

Removal of Existing Restorations

Endodontic treatment outcomes may depend more on the marginal adaptation of the restoration than the quality of root canal fillings.[48,49] Hence, because of the possibility of coronally induced bacterial ingress into the canals, it is essential to remove the preexisting coronal restorations and evaluate the presence of secondary caries and root canal contamination (Fig. 19.12). When a tooth presents with a full coverage restoration, composite resin, or amalgam restoration with recurrent caries, open margins, or loss of marginal integrity, complete removal of the restoration is indicated. In the majority of cases, removal of the full coverage restoration is necessary to see if there is any undetected bacterial contamination.[5,6,50] Disassembly of the preexisting restorations allows inspection for possible recurrent caries and fractures and evaluation of the tooth's restorability.[6,50,51] If coronally induced bacterial ingress is evident, the entire remaining tooth structure should be inspected, including the canals and the pulpal floor. When the remaining coronal structure is assessed as being inadequate, orthodontic extrusion of the root should be considered (see Chapter 21).

Removal of Canal Obstructions

Canal obstructions usually prevent successful negotiation of the root canal system during nonsurgical root canal treatment. Surgical treatment may need to be included to manage these treatment challenges.

Canal obstructions include posts and cores, calcifications of the root canal system, iatrogenic ledges, dentinal debris in the root canal system, fractured instruments, silver points or metallic debris, and some paste materials.[3,5,6] Removals of canal

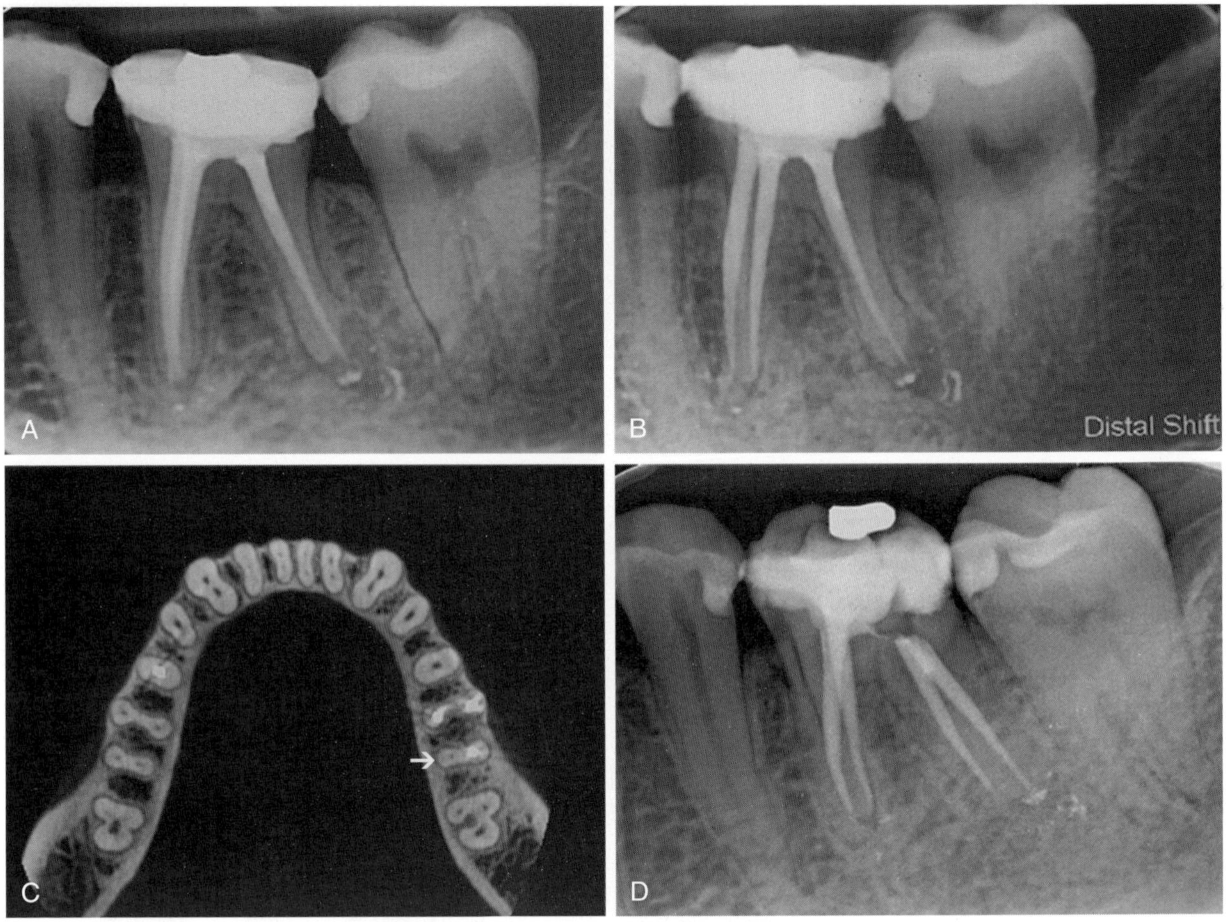

• **Fig. 19.9** **(A** and **B)** Periapical radiography showed possibility of a complex root canal anatomy in mandibular left first molar. **(C)** CBCT image in axial view showed that the distolingual root had been overlooked *(white arrow)*. **(D)** The tooth received endodontic retreatment.

obstructions are typically complex treatment situations that frequently require extensive operator training and experience to manage. For the benefit of the patient, referral to an endodontist should be considered and offered.[52]

There are basically three approaches to managing intracanal fractured instruments: (1) attempting to remove the instrument nonsurgically or surgically,[53] (2) attempting to bypass the instrument, or (3) preparing and obturating the canal with the fractured instrument.

First, a diagnosis and a treatment plan for instrument retrieval should be made with periapical radiography and CBCT imaging (see Chapter 18).

As discussed in Chapter 18, the majority of nickel-titanium (NiTi) rotary instruments fracture in the apical one third of the canals.[54] When a fractured instrument is lodged beyond the curve and extrudes primarily beyond the apical foramen, a surgical approach should be considered because removal sacrifices less valuable structure compared with the nonsurgical approach. A nonsurgical procedure should be initiated if the amount of tooth structure removal after surgery is expected to be greater than a nonsurgical approach.

Bypassing a fractured instrument may not be as successful as removal with ultrasonics,[55,56] and attempts to bypass the instrument may lead to iatrogenic accidents such as ledge formation, perforations, and transportations, particularly in curved canals.[57] In general, bypassing a broken instrument is a technique-sensitive procedure requiring experience, tactile sense, and perseverance by the clinician.[58-68]

When an instrument fractures in the apical one third of the canal in a later stage of canal instrumentation and if an excessive amount of tooth structure must be sacrificed to retrieve it, the separate file should be incorporated as part of the filling material and scheduled for periodic review.[69-72] The sealing ability of the obturation material is not compromised by the presence of a fractured file or other metallic debris.[73]

The use of ultrasonics can effectively remove a fractured instrument when performed under high magnification and illumination.[74-78]

Ledge formation during root canal preparations can be analogous to broken instruments because they can also limit instrumentation in an apical direction. Ledges are typically generated on the outer canal wall when preparation of the curved canal is not maintained (Fig. 19.13).[68] These canal problems typically occur when stainless steel files are not properly precurved to match the canal curvature. Traditional stainless steel files have aggressive cutting tips (pyramidal tips) compared with NiTi files and are apt to straighten canals unless properly precurved, resulting in ledge formation. Root canal transportation and ledging can also occur during preparation if debris accumulation is not consistently removed. It is important to keep the canal wet and constantly irrigate the canal with an irrigation needle smaller than the root canal diameter during instrumentation to avoid debris blockage. Recognition and

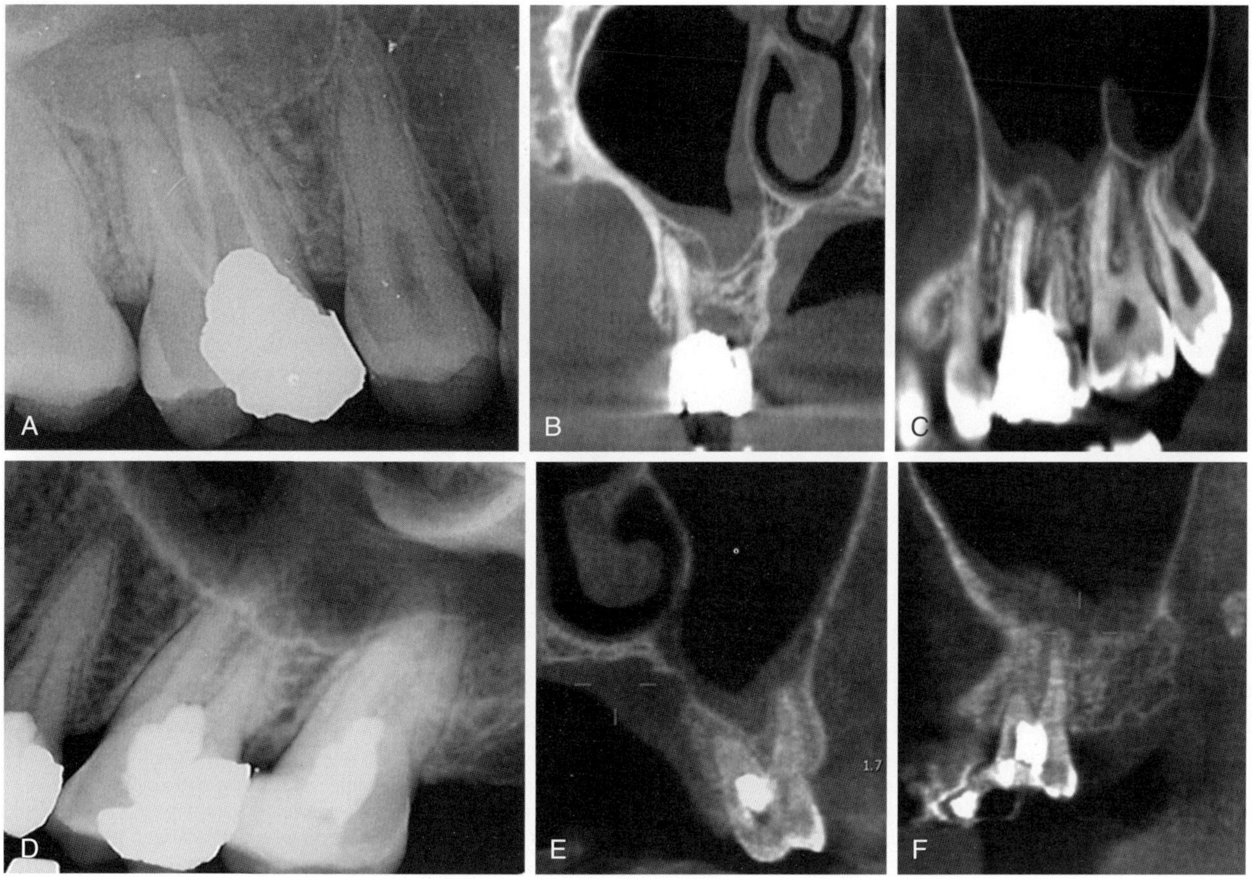

• **Fig. 19.10** **(A)** The maxillary right first molar with inadequate root canal therapy showed a possibility of mishap during access cavity preparation. Both CBCT images in coronal **(B)** and sagittal **(C)** views showed trifurcation perforation. **(D)** Maxillary left first and second molars showed the possibility of trifurcation perforation of a previous pulpotomy. No sign of trifurcation perforation was observed on CBCT images in coronal **(E)** and sagittal **(F)** views.

visualization of canal ledges is essential for avoiding perforations and other procedural errors. Studies have shown flexible nonlanded NiTi instruments with noncutting tips produce significantly less apical transportation than landed NiTi instruments or NiTi instruments with cutting tips.[69,70] For more information regarding the ledge management, readers should refer to Chapter 18 of this book.

Post and Core Removal

Successful removal of posts and cores during retreatment depends on multiple factors. They include the operator's level of skill, experience, training, and instrumentation selection. Small-diameter long shank carbide burs and ultrasonic systems used in conjunction with the dental operating microscope (DOM) facilitate predictable treatment. Other outcome considerations include the type of core material (cast versus resin or amalgam); the length and diameter of the prefabricated or cast post, post location, post material type (metallic or nonmetallic); and variety of cement or bonding system used to secure the post and core system.[6,45,50] Any number of methods used to remove posts can compromise the existing tooth structure.[45] Some posts may be difficult to remove if they are long, well fitted, or cemented with bonding systems or resin cements (Fig. 19.14). Most posts are essentially straight and can be usually managed using small-diameter long shank carbide burs under the DOM. However, nonmetallic posts such as tooth colored zirconia or fiber posts may be difficult to differentiate from the tooth structure. The small-diameter burs partnered with the DOM allow conservative post removal without sacrificing additional tooth structure (see Fig. 19.14).

In preparation for post removal, the coronal core material must be carefully sectioned and removed incrementally with diamond, zirconia-diamond, transmetal, or carbide burs, and ultrasonic tips to preserve the portion of the post that extrudes coronally from the root canal to facilitate removal of various core materials.[6,45,50]

This procedure is best performed using illumination and magnification to help preserve adjacent tooth structure during the procedure. After core removal, any visible cement surrounding the post can be circumferentially removed using fine ultrasonic tips or flame-tipped diamond burs.[6,71] Loosening of the post should be observed as the ultrasonic activation progresses.

Screw posts can usually be loosened with ultrasonics applied to them in a counterclockwise rotation and picked up with various-sized hemostats or small-tipped forceps or pliers. However, this procedure must be executed with caution because it rapidly generates extremely high temperatures without water coolant. In addition, ultrasonic energy should be delivered in different locations around the exposed portion of the post at intervals lasting no longer than 15 seconds.[6,53,72,73] Ultrasonic tips used without water coolant and placed in contact with posts generate temperature increases of 10°C within 1 minute on the external root surface.[74] If this threshold temperature is reached, heat generation can cause necrosis of periodontal tissues, with possible loss of the tooth and supporting bone.

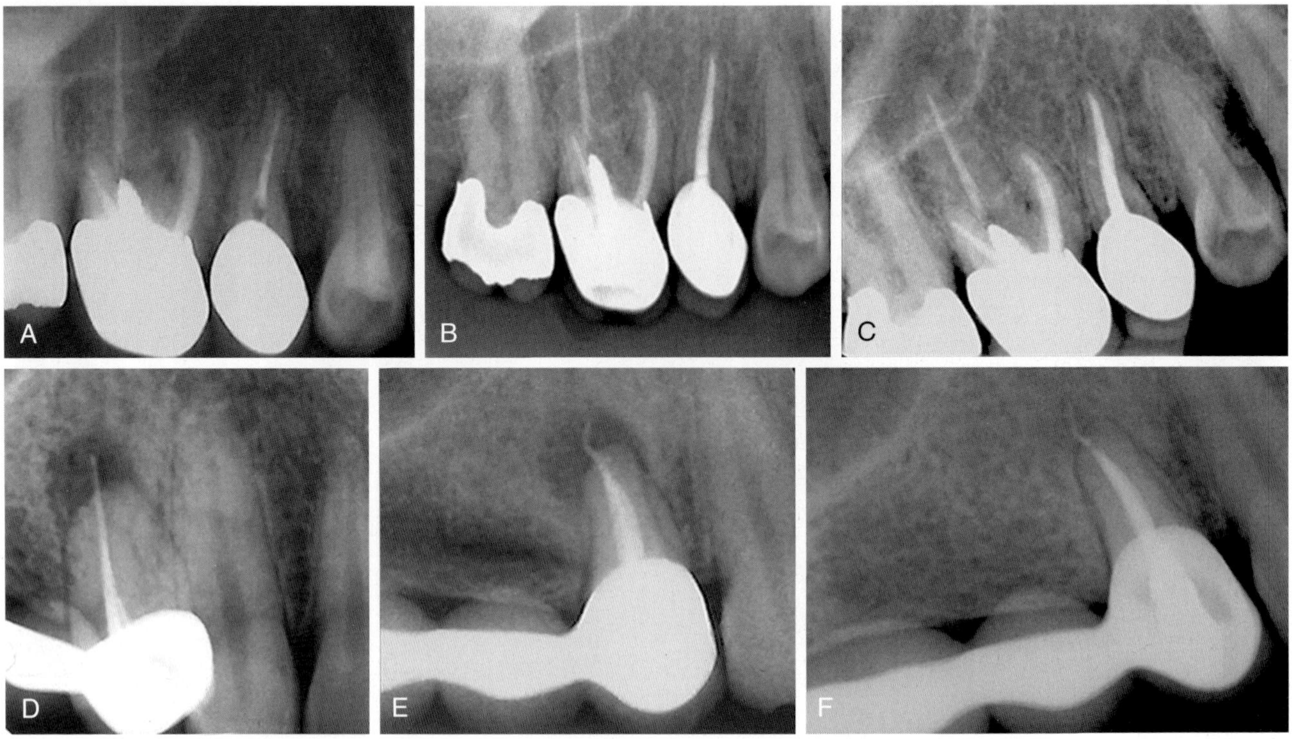

• **Fig. 19.11** Examples of access cavity preparation with and without preexisting restoration. **(A)** A maxillary right second premolar with a history of recently placed porcelain fused to metal crown being clinically symptomatic. **(B)** The access cavity was prepared through the crown. **(C)** Follow-up radiography 1 year after the treatment showed successful outcome and the tooth was clinically symptom free. **(D)** Maxillary right first premolar was an abutment of a bridge. Because of suitable marginal adaptation of the bridge and favorable esthetic, endodontic retreatment was performed through the full coverage restoration. **(E)** The missed root canal was located. **(F)** Despite unsuccessful effort for removing overextended gutta-percha, periapical radiograph showed that the radiolucent lesion healed 18 months later.

Posts cemented with resin cements and fiber posts are difficult to loosen and remove with ultrasonics.[50] Therefore those posts should be ground down with small-diameter carbide burs under the DOM.

After post removal, any excess cement can be removed using a combination of solvents, rotary or hand instruments, or ultrasonic tips.[6,45,50]

Removal of Gutta-Percha

Gutta-percha is the universally and most commonly used obturation material. Therefore it requires removal more frequently during endodontic retreatment than other materials in order to better prepare a root canal space or improve a canal with an inadequate filling during retreatment. Because biofilms are the primary cause of chronic and recurrent endodontic infections, removal of gutta-percha is essential to successfully retreat the root canal system.[74] This can be accomplished using hand and rotary instruments, ultrasonic instruments, heat systems, or solvents and generally requires a combination of these methods.

The use of Gates-Glidden burs should probably be limited to the coronal portion of the canal, and excessive force must not be used because of the possible presence of apical root resorption or poorly adapted gutta-percha root fillings, which may result in the material extrusion (Fig. 19.15).[75,76] The most efficient way to remove gutta-percha root fillings is to use ultrasonic and hand instruments under the DOM, followed by rotary instruments (Fig. 19.16). Moreover, chloroform has been reported to be capable of reducing the intracanal levels of *Enterococcus faecalis,* a common microbe detected in endodontic failures.[7,77] However, if chloroform is used during the early stages of gutta-percha removal, more filling material will most likely remain in the canal and may contribute to excess extrusion beyond the apical foramen.[78,79] Xylene, halothane, eucalyptol, eucalyptus oil, carbon disulfide, benzene, and orange oil can also be used for this purpose. Even though they have been shown to be less effective at softening gutta-percha than chloroform, the majority of those solvents do not pose a significant health risk to patients.[80-82] One investigation measured the amount of residual chloroform, halothane, and xylene expressed through the apical foramen during retreatment procedures.[81] It was determined that the amount of each solvent expressed was below the levels that may pose a health concern to patients.

Removal of Carrier-Based Gutta-Percha Obturators

A popular method of obturation utilizes carrier-based gutta-percha obturators. These devices have a central core of plastic, metal, or other dense material that is coated with gutta-percha. During nonsurgical root canal retreatment, these obturators can be removed using a combination of techniques similar to those for removing posts, silver points, and gutta-percha. Treatment begins by creating a pathway adjacent to the central core to allow an instrument to engage the carrier. Soften the gutta-percha on the surface of the carrier with a heat source or solvent.[83-88] When heat is used to soften the gutta-percha, a thermostatically controlled device, plugger, or endodontic heat carrier heated over an open flame is effective.[87] As increased temperature can damage the surrounding periapical tissues; care should be taken to avoid placing

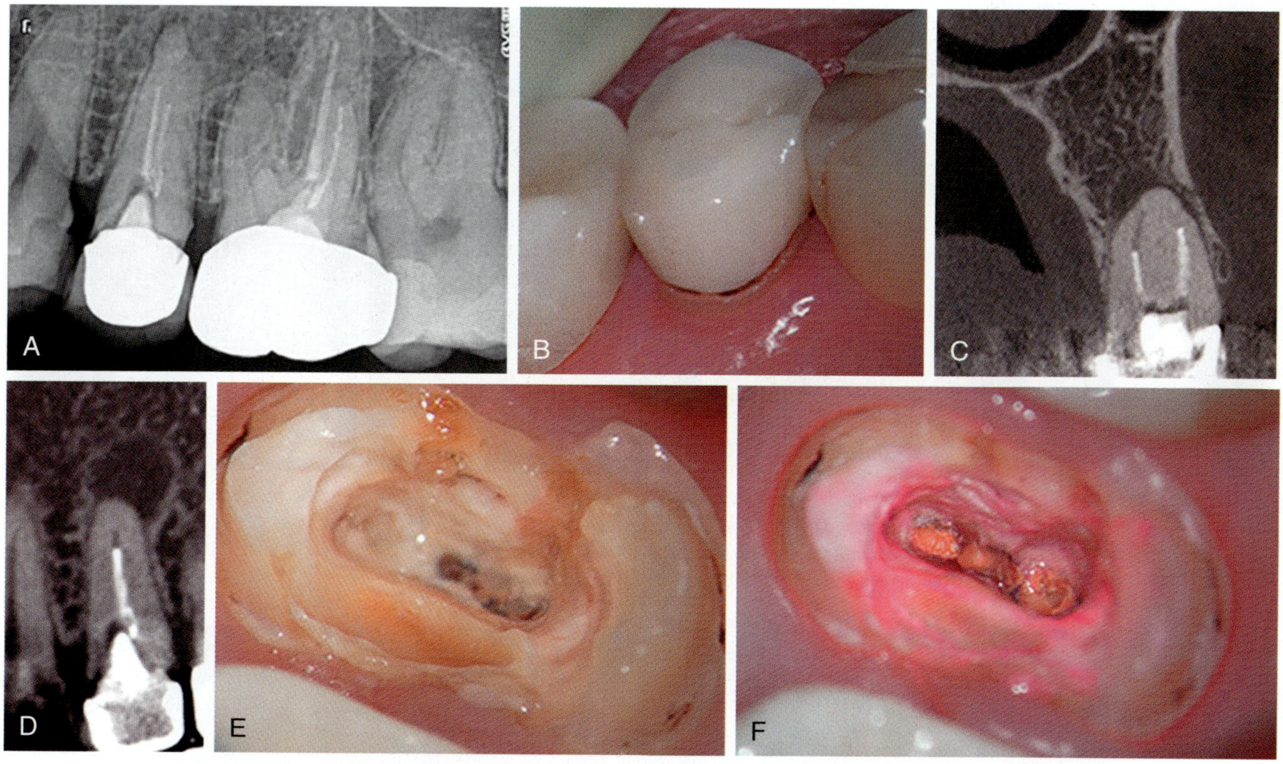

• **Fig. 19.12** **(A)** Preoperative radiograph showing a wide gap between the coronal restoration and the root with a periapical lesion. **(B)** Intraoral photograph showing poor marginal adaptation of the crown. **(C)** Coronal view of CBCT imaging shows a wide space between the two root canals and the core with a periapical lesion associated with the root. **(D)** Sagittal view of CBCT imaging also shows spaces between the two root canals and the coronal. **(E)** Extensive carious lesions discovered under the coronal restoration. **(F)** Dentin stained with carious detector dye reveals deep carious lesions into the two canals.

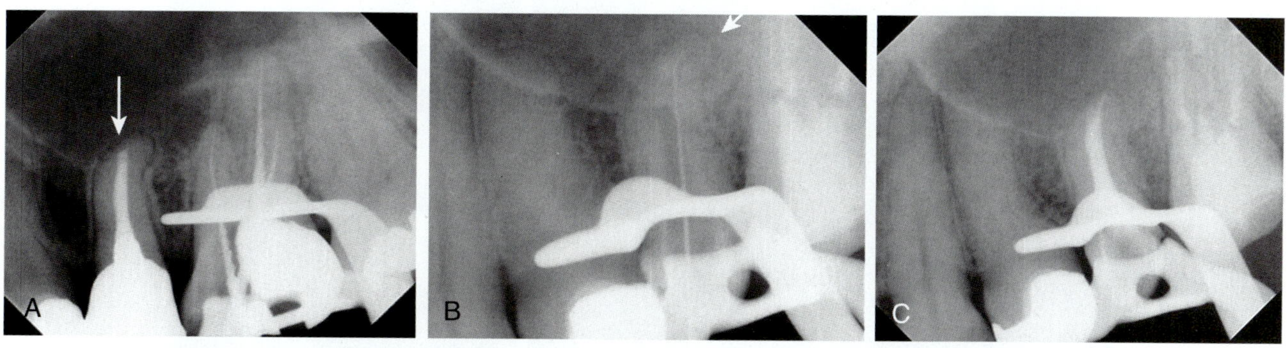

• **Fig. 19.13** **(A)** Preoperative radiograph showing a ledge formation on the outer canal wall in relation to the canal curvature *(white arrow)*. **(B)** Intraoperative radiograph showing a precurved #10 K file in the original pathway after filling the ledged space with MTA *(white arrow)*. **(C)** Postoperative radiograph showing the root filling in the original canal beyond the ledge.

the heated tip in contact with the dentin wall for long periods.[88] Gutta-percha can also be softened using rotary instrumentation at higher speeds (1500 to 2500 rpm), but use of these instruments should be limited to straight canals because the possibility of instrument fracture in a curved canal is high.[89,90]

Once a pathway has been created, single or multiple Hedstrom files can be used to engage and remove the carrier.[83,84,86,87] Rotary files may also be used to engage and remove plastic-based carriers. These strategies work better for plastic carriers than for metal-based carriers because of the difficulty of engaging the metal surface with files. Metal carriers are more easily removed using techniques used to remove silver points such as the braided file technique or using modified hemostats, pliers, and ultrasonic instruments. After successful removal of the carriers and gutta-percha, canal preparation and obturation can be completed.

Removal of Silver Cones (Points)

Silver points are commonly embedded in the build-up core material. Illumination and magnification with the DOM are essential adjuncts during core removal to ensure preservation of the coronal aspect of the silver point.[50,91,92] After removal of the core material, solvents, ultrasonic instruments, or hand files are used to create a

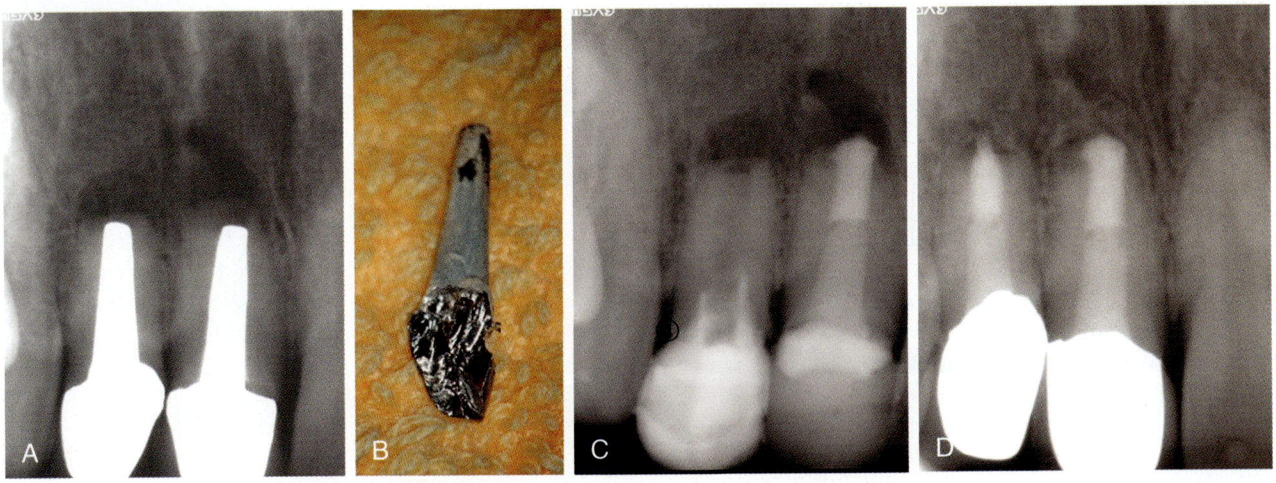

• **Fig. 19.14** **(A)** Preoperative radiograph showing a long cast post placed in the canal of the maxillary right incisor with periapical lesions. **(B)** Removed cast post showing the metal portion that was in the canal looks intact. **(C)** Radiograph taken immediately after the removal of the post shows the untouched dentin wall. **(D)** Twelve-month postoperative radiograph showing periapical healing.

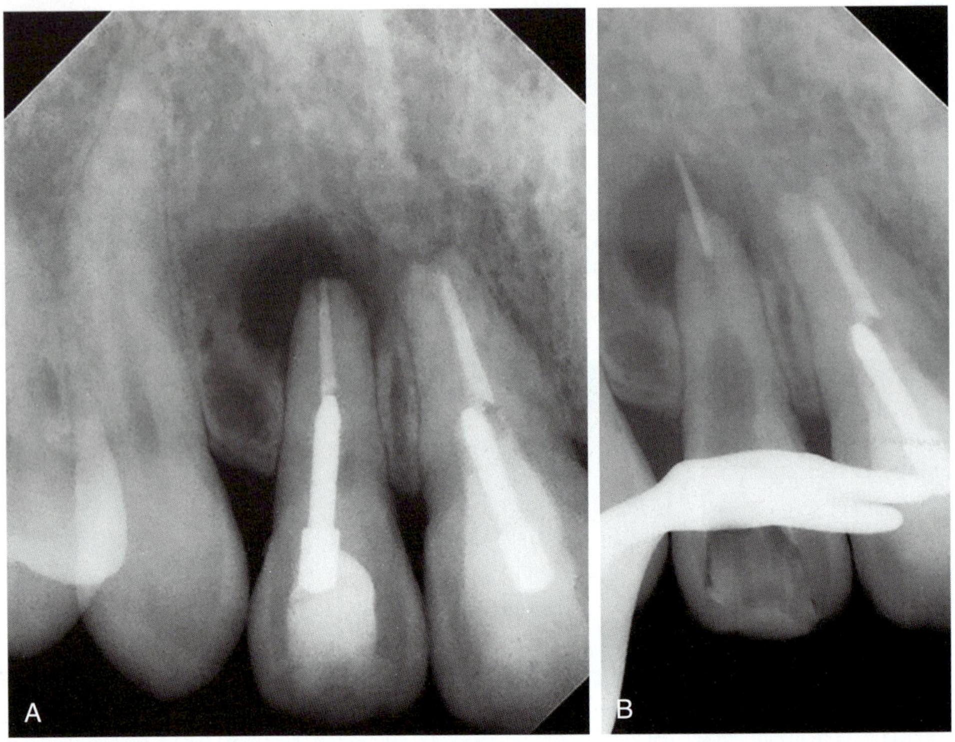

• **Fig. 19.15** **(A)** Preoperative radiograph showing a large periapical lesion. **(B)** Intraoperative radiograph showing the old gutta-percha root filling pushed into the periapical tissues by a #2 GG bur.

space around the exposed silver point.[92-94] Silver points are soft, and contact with ultrasonic tips or burs can easily cut through them.

The key in removing the silver points is breaking the seal around the silver point. A method for achieving this is by engaging and braiding one or two files around the cone, then applying a force such as ultrasonic energy or leveraging with a hemostat. This energy application facilitates cone removal by rapidly breaking down the cement seal.

The coronal portion of a loosened cone extending from the pulp chamber can then be grasped and pulled from the canal with a variety of devices. These include various types of specialized hemostats, modified or regular Steiglitz forceps, needle holders, gold foil pliers, Caufield silver point retrievers, or splinter forceps.[45,93,94] If the coronal portion of the cone is not present or is accidentally removed during removal of the core material, one or more hand files can be used to engage and extract the cone.[45,80] An alternative method to remove cones in this situation includes flexible metal tubes or needle-sleeve devices that grasp the cone with a file or wire, or bond the cone head using cyanoacrylate glue. [45,80,91,95] These techniques require the use of a trepan bur to trough an access area for the devices. After successful removal of the silver point, cleaning and shaping procedures can proceed (Fig. 19.17). Silver points that cannot be removed may necessitate surgical intervention.

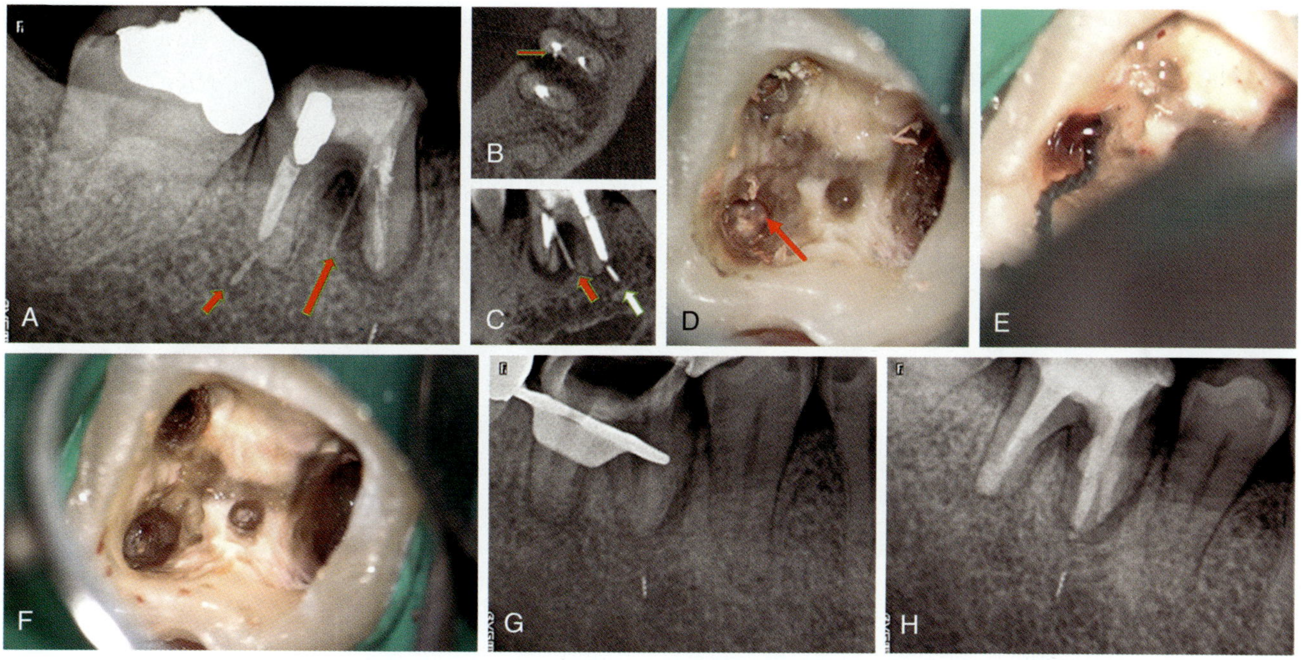

• **Fig. 19.16** **(A)** Preoperative radiograph showing root fillings extruded into the periapical tissues with periapical lesions (*arrows*). **(B)** Preoperative axial view of CBCT imaging showing the root fillings extruded from the perforation in the mesiobuccal canal (*arrow*). **(C)** Preoperative sagittal view of CBCT imaging showing the root fillings extruded from the perforation in the mesiobuccal canal (*red arrow*) and from the distal canal (*white arrow*). **(D)** Microscopic view showing the perforation in the mesiobuccal canal (*arrow*), which is identical to the axial view of CBCT imaging. **(E)** Microscopic view showing removal of gutta-percha extruded into the periapical tissues from the perforation site with the XP-3D shaper. **(F)** Microscopic view showing removal of all the root fillings was completed. **(G)** Intraoperative radiograph confirms the removal of the root fillings from both the root canals and the periapical tissues. **(H)** Postoperative radiograph showing MTA obturation in all the canals.

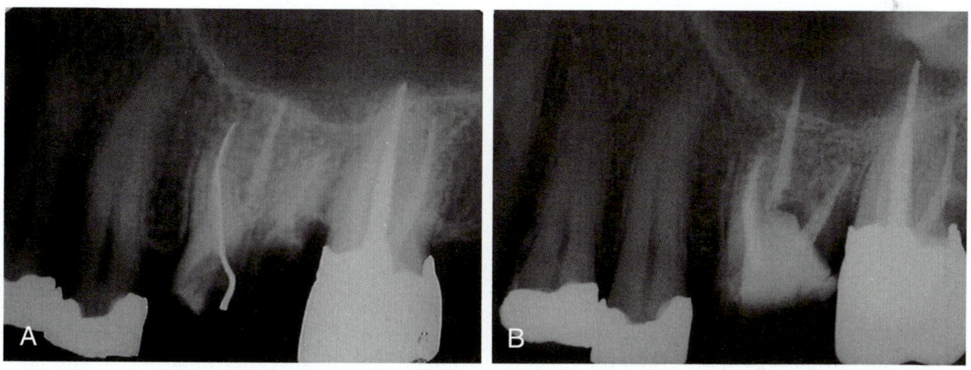

• **Fig. 19.17** **(A)** Mesiobuccal root of a maxillary left first molar has been obturated with a silver cone, whereas the other root canal was filled with gutta-percha. As a result of extensive caries the tooth needed endodontic retreatment. **(B)** The silver point was removed by grasping with Steiglitz forceps and gutta-percha was removed by chloroform and Hedstrom file. All root canals were obturated with gutta-percha and AH26 root canal sealer.

Removal of Soft and Hard Pastes

Soft pastes are easily removed utilizing hand or rotary instruments.[80] Copious irrigation and a crown-down preparation technique are recommended when removing soft materials from the canal system to minimize postoperative flare ups[80] (Fig. 19.18).

Hard-setting pastes are far more challenging to remove. As much of the coronal aspect of the hard paste is removed first with a bur or ultrasonic tip.[50,80,96] If this does not result in an opening up of a canal system, one strategy is to remove 4 mm from the tip of a K-file, creating a sharp edge at the tip so as to better cut into and remove the hardened material.[97] Dental companies now manufacture files with hardened sharp points that can be used to initially penetrate these materials. Perforation and the creation of ledges are potential problems when attempting to remove hardened cements in the root canals, especially if the canals are curved.[80]

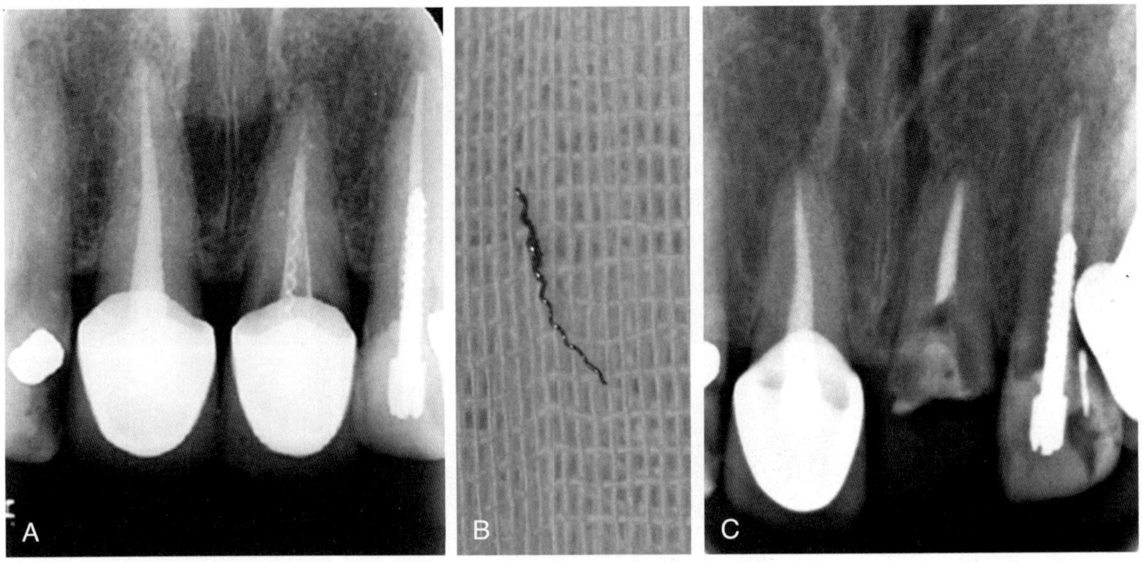

• **Fig. 19.18** **(A)** Preoperative radiographic image of a maxillary left central incisor showed a fractured lentulo spiral during placement of paste inside the root canal. **(B)** The lentulo spiral has been removed. **(C)** Root canal obturation after paste and the lentulo spiral removal.

Various endodontic solvents have been investigated for their efficacy in softening hard obturation pastes to facilitate their removal. Although one investigation reported sodium hypochlorite (NaOCl) to be effective in softening a resorcinol-formalin paste (Russian Red), a follow-up study comparing six different solvents, including NaOCl, found none to be more effective than water, which was used as the control (Fig. 19.19).[98,99] Mechanical instrumentation remains the most predictable means of hard paste removal. If removal of the hard paste is not successful, the option of surgery should be considered for tooth retention.

Removal of Calcifications

Root canal calcifications are often noted radiographically before treatment. Clinical management and internal visualization of these calcifications inside the access is greatly aided by magnification and illumination using the DOM. Other obstructions must be removed before exploring the calcified area. Once accessed and appropriately visualized, calcifications are managed using a combination of chelating agents, stiff hand files (e.g., C and C+ files), and ultrasonic tips or Mueller-type burs to remove the calcified tissue and locate the root canal system apical to the calcification. Use of ultrasonic instrumentation and Mueller type burs is restricted to the coronal/straight portion of the root canal. When the canal is located with the aid of microexplorers and the DOM, a small bend can be placed on stiff, small-diameter hand files, and the curved portion of the canal can be carefully negotiated using various chelating agents and lubricants. The canal may be enlarged, using the crown-down technique, with a combination of hand files and NiTi rotary file systems. If the canal cannot be negotiated as a result of extensive calcification, surgical intervention must be considered.

Management of Biofilms

Unattached microorganisms in the root canal space might aggregate, attach, and colonize the surface of root canal walls, producing bacterial biofilms. Bacterial biofilms can form not only within the root canal space but also over the root surface, resulting in nonhealing apical periodontitis despite adequate root canal therapy.[28,100,101]

Apical periodontitis around the root(s) of a tooth with a history of root canal therapy could be either persistent, recurrent, or the result of secondary infection. A tooth with apical periodontitis at the time of initial root canal therapy that does not resolve after the treatment has persistent infection. Secondary infection occurs if the practitioner cannot completely isolate the tooth during root canal therapy or when there is coronal microleakage after treatment. An example for the recurrent infection is a tooth with apical periodontitis at the time of initial endodontic therapy that recovered after treatment, exhibiting recurrent disease at a later stage.[102-104]

There is a higher possibility of biofilm formation over the root canal walls of teeth in need of nonsurgical endodontic retreatment as a result of the presence of persistent, recurrent, or secondary infections. Therefore the practitioner should always consider strategies to remove biofilms during root canal cleaning and shaping in retreatment cases.

Most investigations have confirmed the ability of NaOCl as an irrigant to disrupt biofilm formed by *Enterococcus faecalis* or other microorganisms, such as *Streptococcus mutans, Streptococcus oralis,* and *Actinomyces oris*.[105,106]

Compared with 5.25% NaOCl, 2% chlorhexidine could not effectively dissolve biofilms.[105,107] The concentration of NaOCl is an important variable for dissolving biofilms. Concentrations of 2.5% and 5.25% of NaOCl were significantly more effective on old and young *E. faecalis* biofilms compared with 1% NaOCl, which was only effective on young biofilms.[108]

If NaOCl is used as an irrigant during endodontic retreatment, the contact time of the solution is also an important variable for dissolving biofilms. When 1% or 2.5% NaOCl is used as an irrigant, the minimum contact time of 30 minutes should be considered, particularly if the practitioner is focusing on cleaning the apical third of the root canal.[107]

NaOCl is the best irrigant for dissolving organic tissues within the root canal space; however, because of its inability to remove inorganic debris, a chelating agent is also recommended. Both NaOCl and ethylenediaminetetraacetic acid (EDTA) could affect various types of biofilms via dissolving biofilm matrix

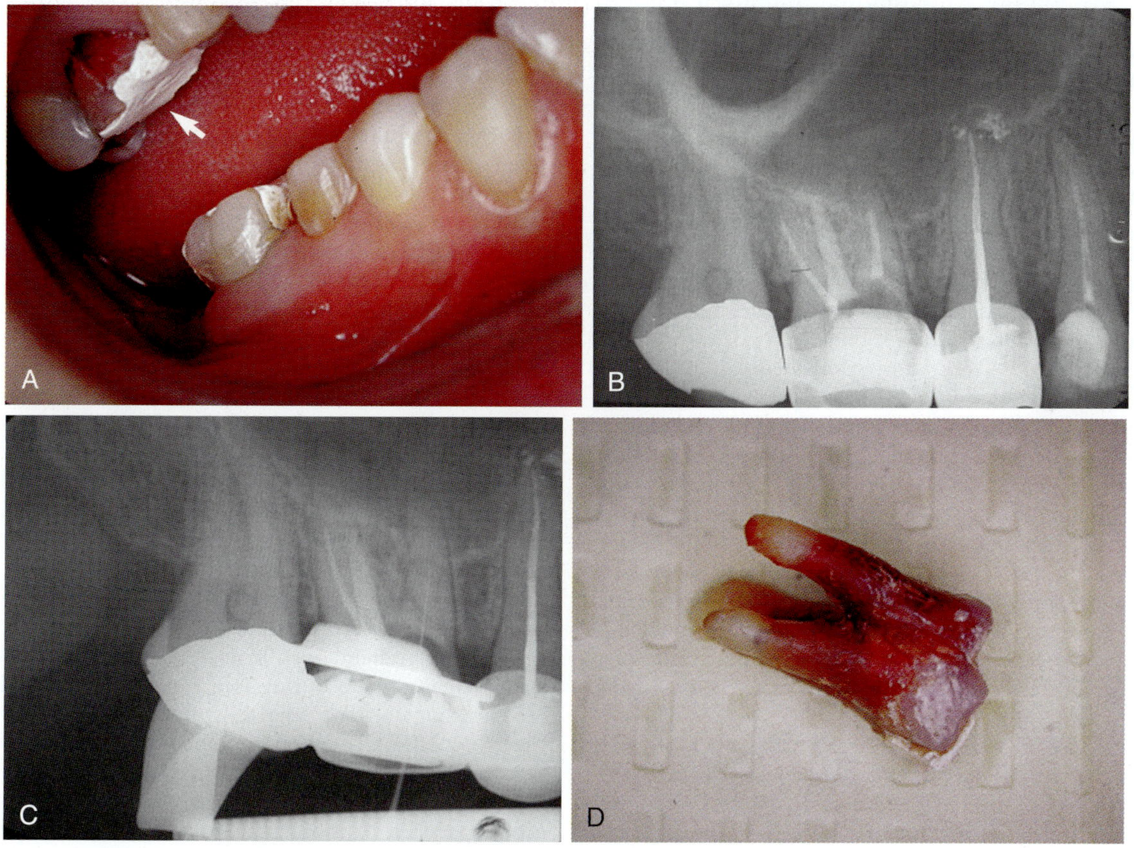

• **Fig. 19.19** **(A)** Tooth (*arrow*) exhibits red discoloration of the crown as a result of root canal obturation with a hard resorcinol paste material. **(B)** The resorcinol obturations are short of ideal length in all three canals of tooth #3. Resorcinol paste was also present in the premolars. **(C)** The resorcinol material was successfully removed from the coronal portion of the mesiobuccal canal, but the canal was calcified apical to the level of the previous obturation. A root perforation occurred during attempts to remove the material from the palatal canal. The treatment plan was altered, and the tooth was extracted and replaced as part of a bridge. **(D)** Note that the red discoloration of the roots extends to the level of the previous resorcinol obturations.

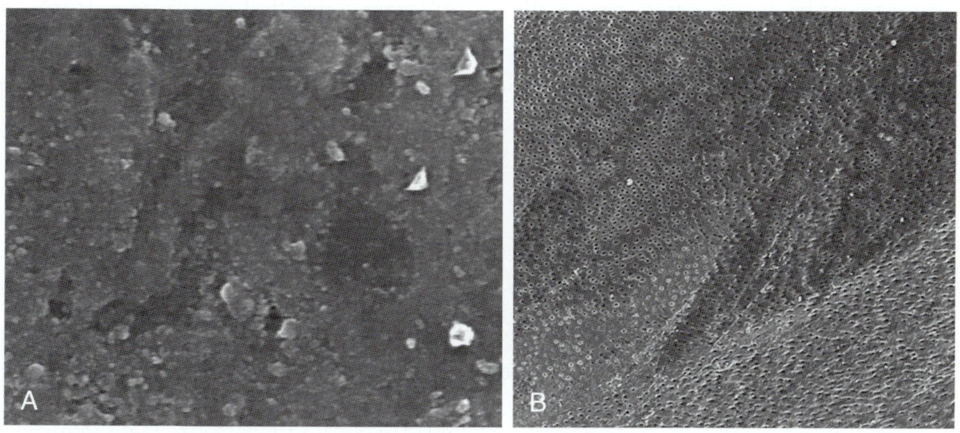

• **Fig. 19.20** **(A)** A scanning electron microscopic image shows presence of biofilm over the root canal wall. **(B)** After root canal preparation and irrigation with 5.25% NaOCl followed by ethylenediaminetetraacetic acid (EDTA), root canal wall was clean and dentinal tubules could be observed.

polysaccharides.[105] Therefore use of NaOCl as an irrigant and removal of the smear layer with EDTA or MTAD should be considered in endodontically treated teeth that require endodontic retreatment (Fig. 19.20, *A–B*).

In addition to the concentration of the irrigation solution and contact time, the needle penetration depth is another important factor that might affect biofilm removal. Needle penetration depth up to 2 mm short of the working length was more effective in removing biofilms.[109] However, irrigation should be performed with caution to prevent NaOCl accidents. To review methods used to avoid NaOCl accidents during root canal irrigation, the reader is referred to Chapter 18 of this book.

Root Canal Preparation in Retreatment

Root canal preparation technique in nonsurgical endodontic retreatment mostly focuses on removing preexisting root canal filling materials. This allows effective operation of instruments and irrigants on dentinal tubules that are covered with the fragments of these materials. Therefore root canal preparation could reduce microorganisms and debris associated with persistent, secondary, or recurrent apical periodontitis. Hand, rotary, and reciprocating instruments have been introduced for removing root canal filling materials; however, none of the instrumentation techniques can completely remove all the filling materials from the root canal space.[110-112]

There are variables that might have some effect on root canal preparation of the teeth in need of endodontic retreatment. These variables include the outline of the access cavity, cross-sectional shape of the root canal, instrumentation technique, motion during the preparation technique, working length estimation, apical preparation size, root canal anatomy, and the type of root canal filling material.

The outline of the access cavity might affect removal of filling materials from the root canal space. Contracted access cavities in oval-shaped root canals result in higher volume of residual filling materials after endodontic retreatment.[110] Therefore a standard outline of access cavity should be provided for endodontic retreatment, particularly in teeth with oval-shaped root canals.

Crown-down preparation is the instrumentation method of choice for endodontic retreatment because it minimizes apically extruded debris during root canal preparation.[113]

Oval-shaped root canals provide more challenges during endodontic retreatment because there is a higher possibility that the root canal walls will remain untouched during removal of the obturating materials.[114]

If the practitioner is going to use engine-driven instruments during retreatment, an endodontic motor with the capacity of adaptive motion (SybronEndo, Orange, CA) is recommended because of its significantly higher ability to remove more root canal filling materials compared with the reciprocating motion,[115] particularly in oval-shaped root canals.[116] Endodontic motors with adaptive motions have been designed to have both rotational and reciprocal motions based on the stresses exerted on the instrument. With no or low stress, the instrument's motion would consist of 600 degrees clockwise rotation, a complete stop, and then followed by restarting another clockwise motion. However, when the instrument engages with either the root canal wall or the filling materials, the motor will switch to reciprocating motion.

In relation to the time needed for removing root canal filling materials, hand instruments require significantly more time compared with the rotary instruments.[117] Thus from the clinical standpoint the time here is not very valuable because irrigants need a minimum contact time for root canal disinfection, and the short time spent on removing root canal filling materials and root canal preparation have not shown any advantages over the use of rotary instruments.[107,118] In addition, the possibility of iatrogenic accidents is significantly higher, particularly broken instruments, when rotary instruments are used to remove root canal filling materials.[117]

One of the most important steps in root canal instrumentation of retreatment cases is to determine the working length. Presence of obturating materials within the root canal could affect root canal impedance, therefore affecting estimation accuracy of electronic apex locators (EAL).[119] Relying on EAL without considering periapical radiography might result in overinstrumentation or underestimation of the working length; therefore both EAL and periapical radiography should be used at this step to prevent further complications.[120,121]

Feeling lower or no digital tactile sense is one of the disadvantages of rotary instruments during root canal preparation. Use of hand instruments between activation of rotary instruments would allow the clinician to use his/her digital tactile sense during root canal preparation and, in combination with the information collected from EAL and periapical radiography, it may prevent further overinstrumentation. In fact, digital tactile sense would be a supplementary aid during root canal preparation. If a clinician believes that the root canal instrument might penetrate beyond the length estimated by EAL and periapical radiography, it may be best to reconsider the working length measurement.[122]

Another important factor that should be considered during preparation of root canal space is obtaining apical terminus patency to increase the success rate of retreatment procedures.[123]

Larger preparation size results in lower residual root canal filling material,[117] which significantly improves bacterial reduction in teeth that have apical periodontitis with a history of previous endodontic therapy.[124] However, it should be kept in mind that larger preparation size does not mean that the dentist should ignore the risk of root canal transportation and sacrifice dentinal structure, making the tooth prone to VRF. Therefore the practitioner should also consider several factors such as the bulk of the root, root canal configuration as well as curvature, presence of danger zones, and root surface depressions during root canal preparation in order to avoid further mishaps.

Another important point is the fact that removing root canal filling materials from teeth with complicated root canal anatomy is more difficult than from those with straight root canals.[117] In cases with complicated root canal anatomy, it is highly recommended that the patient be referred to an endodontist.

The type of root canal filling materials is also another variable that might affect root canal preparation in endodontic retreatment. Several bioactive endodontic sealers have been introduced to the market.[125] Retreatment of teeth filled with gutta-percha and these sealers might be very difficult. The type of the bioactive root canal sealer, type of the solvent, and the root canal configuration are variables that might affect successful removal of root canal filling materials during endodontic retreatment.[126] In most situations, the practitioner usually does not know the type of root canal sealer used in the obturation of a tooth designated for endodontic retreatment.

Shaping of root canal space in retreated cases depends on the root canal preparation during the initial endodontic treatment. If the root canals have not been prepared well and single-cone gutta-percha is observed in the periapical radiography, cleaning and shaping during retreatment should be performed like routine

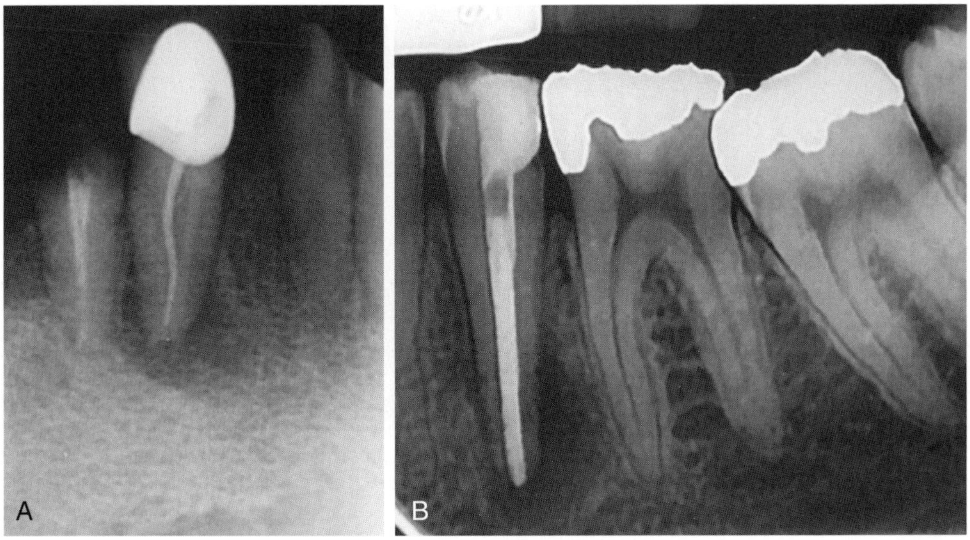

• **Fig. 19.21** **(A)** A swimming gutta-percha cone in a mandibular right canine tooth. Root canal preparation during endodontic retreatment in this tooth should be performed similar to a routine primary root canal therapy. **(B)** Endodontic retreatment for the mandibular left second premolar should be focused on removing preexisting root canal filling materials and using irrigants for root canal disinfection.

primary root canal therapy (Fig. 19.21, *A*). However, if the previous endodontic treatment shows either well-shaped or overenlarged root canal(s), more emphasis on reshaping the root canal space might make the tooth susceptible to future fracture. In this case the practitioner is advised to focus on removing all preexisting obturating materials and using irrigants to clean the root canal space as much as possible with conservative reshaping of the root canal(s) (Fig. 19.21, *B*).

There is no general agreement on performing endodontic retreatment in a single visit or in multiple visits. The advantage of endodontic retreatment in more than one visit is the benefit of antibacterial activity of the medicaments placed within the root canal between the appointments. However, there is not sufficient evidence of significantly higher success rates when retreatment is performed in more than one visit.[127] Several investigations have posed the question whether endodontic treatment in nonvital infected cases should be performed in more than one visit to achieve a higher success rate.[128-131] Single-visit root canal therapy has some advantages, including better cost-effectiveness and less time needed for both the patient and practitioner.[131] Therefore in certain cases with no contraindications for completing the retreatment process (i.e., no wiping exudate or no symptomatic apical periodontitis), endodontic retreatment can be performed in one visit to prevent further recontamination of the root canal space that can occur between the appointments.

Irrigation in Retreatment

If all canals of the tooth are found and cleaned, a high success rate can be achieved. However, it has been shown that there are always some areas within the root canal space that remain untouched by various instrumentation techniques.[132] An important aid during endodontic retreatment is the use of chemical solutions to remove necrotic tissues, as well as bacteria and their byproducts from the root canal space.

NaOCl is the most popular irrigation solution among the members of the AAE and U.S. dentists.[133,134] All the concentrations of NaOCl provide significant reductions in microorganisms in the root canal space; however, they exhibit differences in their ability to remove biofilms.[108]

The results of a systematic review and meta-analysis on laboratory studies showed that use of intracanal activation techniques (passive ultrasonic irrigation, apical negative pressure, sonic irrigation) are superior to conventional passive form of placing a needle within the root canal and irrigating to remove debris and the smear layer.[135]

Sealing ability of root filling materials can significantly be improved by removing the smear layer before root canal obturation.[136] Smear layer removal using a combination of NaOCl and EDTA results in a marginally significant effect on the success rate of initial root canal therapy; however, in endodontic retreatment, it can significantly increase the number of healed cases.[123] Removing the smear layer may also help NaOCl better penetrate the dentinal tubules and dissolve biofilms (Fig. 19.22).

The advantages of the use of 5.25% NaOCl compared with the lower concentrations of the same solution include less postoperative pain,[137] short time needed for removing biofilms,[107] and greater efficacy against old biofilms.[108]

Obturation After Retreatment

Endodontic retreatment procedures might induce cracks during removal of preexisting root canal filling materials.[138] The method of root canal obturation during initial endodontic treatment may also affect induction of cracks and tooth vulnerability to VRF after removal of filling materials after preparation of the root canal space. The teeth initially obturated by warm vertical compaction exhibit more cracks after retreatment compared with the teeth that received cold lateral condensation as the initial obturation technique.[139]

Most often, the practitioner does not know which type of obturation technique was previously used in teeth requiring endodontic retreatment; therefore, the practitioner should always consider preparation and obturation techniques that apply lower pressure on the root canal wall. For example, use of NiTi spreaders for cold lateral compaction has been recommended as a result of lower risk of inducing cracks compared with stainless steel spreaders.[140,141] Moreover, Thermafil also exhibited promising long-term outcomes as a root canal obturation technique after endodontic retreatment.[142]

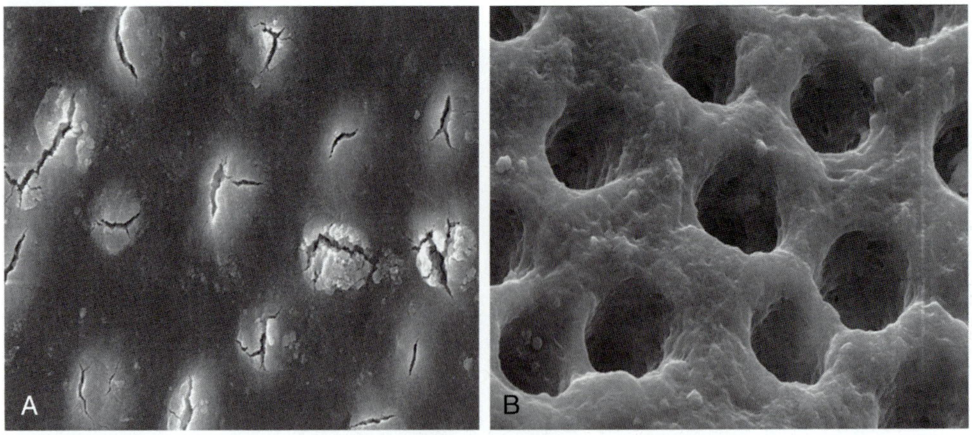

• **Fig. 19.22** **(A)** If the root canal wall is only irrigated with NaOCl, smear layer would cover dentinal tubules. **(B)** Irrigation with 17% ethylenediaminetetraacetic acid (EDTA) followed by NaOCl could successfully remove the smear layer.

Single-cone obturation technique with bioactive endodontic sealers has been introduced as an option for obturating root canals after endodontic retreatment; however, supporting investigations do not currently share high levels of evidence.[143,144]

Restorative Options

The literature shows the quality of the endodontic treatment, the presence of coronal restoration, and apical extension of root canal filling were significantly associated with healthy periapical tissues.[145] Therefore it is essential to consider a proper restoration on an endodontically treated tooth for the long-term success as the coronal restoration works as a "barrier" not only to prevent reinfection of the root canal system after endodontic treatment but also to protect the tooth from root fracture. Hence, the amount of coronal tooth structure, the presence of an adequate dentin ferrule, careful selection of luting agents for post cementation, and the type of coronal restoration are all important factors that affect endodontic treatment outcomes.[146-150] The presence of fiber posts may also contribute to the long-term success of endodontically treated teeth as fiber-reinforced, resin-based composite posts with a modulus of elasticity similar to dentin can reduce the risk of VRF.[151,152] One recent study on long-term clinical outcomes of endodontically treated teeth demonstrated that teeth restored with fiber posts yielded significantly less tooth loss than teeth restored without a post, regardless of the presence or absence of a full-coverage crown.[153] The primary reasons for VRF of endodontically treated teeth are closely related to restorative procedures and include the absence of adequate remaining tooth structure[154] and excessive occlusal forces.[155] Although endodontically treated teeth restored with crowns show a higher resistance against fracture than resin-based composites, teeth with one or two tooth surface losses and two proximal contacts restored with resin composite exhibit a more favorable distribution of occlusal forces and, hence, a survival rate comparable with full-coverage restorations.[156-158] In addition to the requirement of protecting the endodontically treated tooth with a proper cuspal coverage restoration, it is also important to place a definitive restoration as soon as possible to prevent coronal microleakage, avoid propagation of existing coronal infractions if present, conserve remaining tooth structure, and prevent the need for additional retreatment or surgical procedures. Long-term provisional restorations can lead to recontamination of the filling material, which may lead to tooth extraction and its consequences.[13]

Follow-Up Care and Posttreatment Complications

Follow-up visits are important for monitoring symptoms and ensuring that healing occurs. An initial follow-up visit usually takes place at 6 months post-retreatment, and then yearly. The first follow-up visit may be sooner than 6 months if there are extenuating circumstances requiring it. In addition to a radiographic examination, follow-up visits should include a clinical evaluation of mobility, periodontal probing, and palpation and percussion testing.

Some studies have indicated posttreatment flare-ups occur more frequently in nonsurgical root canal retreatment cases, compared with initial root canal therapy.[159-161]An explanation for this increase in flare-ups may be that retreatment procedures may result in a greater extrusion of bacteria and other irritants into the apical tissues.[9] The crown-down technique, paired with frequent use of irrigants injected with side-venting needles, promotes debris removal in a coronal direction and helps minimize this complication.

Prognosis

Nonsurgical endodontic retreatment has favorable outcomes when the cause of previous failure has been diagnosed and corrected by using contemporary technologies[162] (Fig. 19.23). In addition to successful outcomes, the teeth receiving endodontic retreatment have exhibited high survival rates.[2]

In general, nonsurgical endodontic retreatment has a lower success rate compared with primary root canal therapy. However, retreatment can have a high successful outcome that is comparable with primary root canal therapy if the apical foramen can be negotiated and the cause of failure overcome. Negotiating the entire root canal length should help eradicate microorganisms, debris, and previous filling materials from the root canal space.[123,163]

For more information on predictors of the outcome of endodontic treatments, the reader is referred to Chapter 22 of this book.

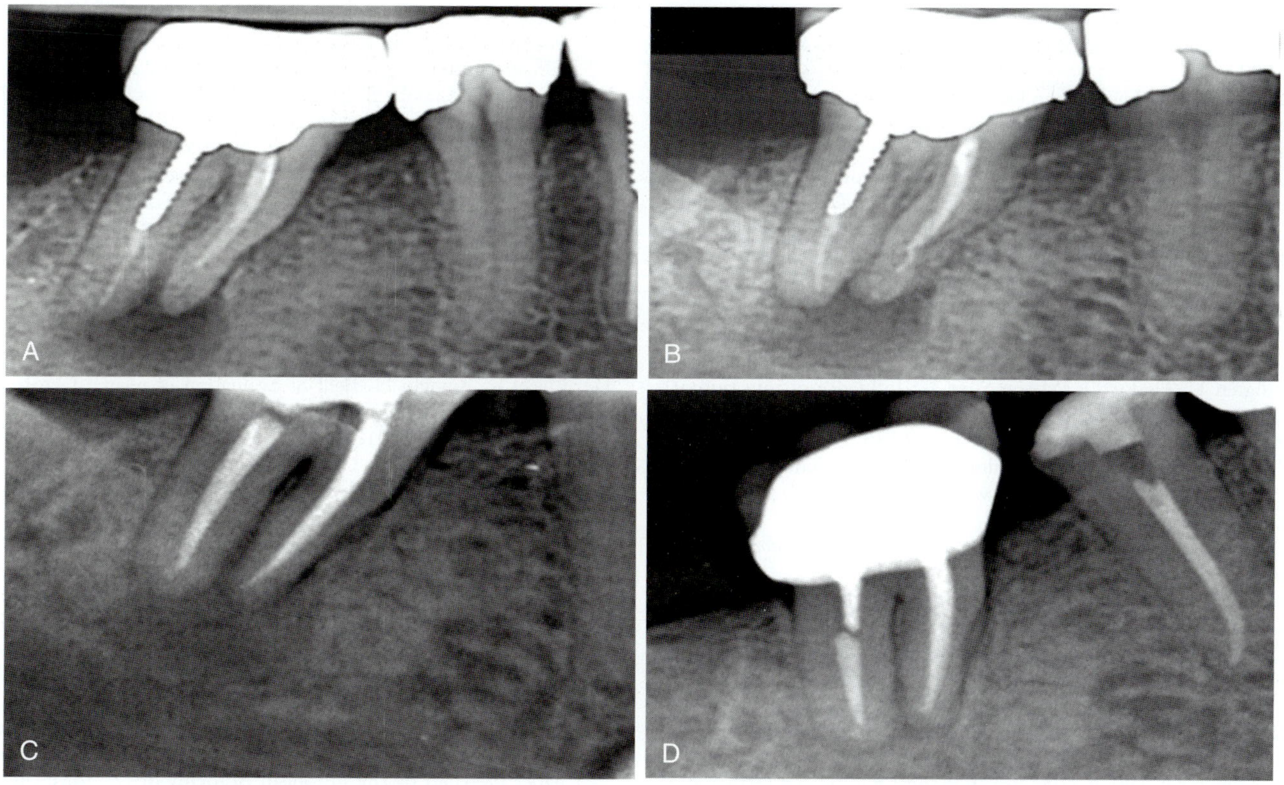

• **Fig. 19.23** **(A** and **B)** Mandibular right second molar with inadequate root canal therapy and periapical lesion. **(C)** Endodontic retreatment was performed. **(D)** Periapical lesion healed 2 years later.

Study Questions

6. What is the most predictable way to remove hard pastes?
   a. Use of solvents
   b. Use of mechanical instrumentation
   c. There is no predictable way to remove hard pastes
7. Which of the following are among the disadvantages of preparing the access cavity without removing the previous coronal restoration during endodontic retreatment?
   a. Difficulty in tooth isolation and irrigation
   b. Limitation for negotiating apical foramen
   c. Restricts the clinician from observing possible cracks
   d. Increases the possibility of electronic apex locator errors
8. The most important aspect to removing silver points successfully is:
   a. Use of solvents
   b. Use of illumination and magnification
   c. Use of ultrasonic energy
9. When would retreatment have a comparable successful outcome to primary root canal treatment?
   a. No foul odor after removing coronal restoration
   b. Using rotary instruments for root canal preparation
   c. The apical foramen of all root canals could be negotiated
   d. The tooth had no coronal discoloration before the treatment
10. A 36-year-old male with a history of previous root canal treatment for tooth number 20 presents with pain when chewing. Periapical radiograph shows a radiolucent lesion around the mesial root of the tooth. His record shows that the tooth was vital at the time of root canal treatment. Which is the type of infection most expected for that tooth?
    a. Persistent
    b. Secondary
    c. Recurrent
    d. Extraradicular

ANSWERS

Answer Box 19

1 d. All of the above
2 d. All of the above
3 a. Before treatment
4 d. All of the above
5 c. None–restorable crown
6 b. Use of mechanical instrumentation
8 b. Use of illumination and magnification
7 c. Restricts the clinician from observing possible cracks
9 c. The apical foramen of all root canals could be negotiated
10 b. Secondary

Acknowledgment

The authors wish to thank Dr. George Bogen for editing the chapter and making invaluable comments.

References

1. Alley BS, Kitchens GG, Alley LW, et al.: A comparison of survival of teeth following endodontic treatment performed by general dentists or by specialists, *Oral Surg Oral Med Oral Pathol Oral Radiol Endod* 98:115–118, 2004.
2. Salehrabi R, Rotstein I: Epidemiologic evaluation of the outcomes of orthograde endodontic retreatment, *J Endod* 36:790–792, 2010.
3. Allen RK, Newton CW, Brown Jr CE: A statistical analysis of surgical and nonsurgical endodontic retreatment cases, *J Endod* 15:261–266, 1989.

4. Hoen MM, Pink FE: Contemporary endodontic retreatments: an analysis based on clinical treatment findings, *J Endod* 28:834–836, 2002.
5. Friedman S, Stabholz A: Endodontic retreatment-case selection and technique. Part 1. Criteria for case selection, *J Endod* 12:28–33, 1986.
6. Ruddle CJ: Nonsurgical retreatment, *J Endod* 30:827–845, 2004.
7. Molander A, Reit C, Dahlen G, et al.: Microbiological status of root-filled teeth with apical periodontitis, *Int Endod J* 31:1–7, 1998.
8. Sundqvist G, Figdor D, Persson S, et al.: Microbiologic analysis of teeth with failed endodontic treatment and the outcome of conservative re-treatment, *Oral Surg Oral Med Oral Pathol Oral Radiol Endod* 85:86–93, 1998.
9. Siqueira Jr JF: Microbial causes of endodontic flare-ups, *Int Endod J* 36:453–463, 2003.
10. Sjögren U, Figdor D, Persson S, et al.: Influence of infection at the time of root filling on the outcome of endodontic treatment of teeth with apical periodontitis, *Int Endod J* 30:297–306, 1997.
11. Ricucci D, Siqueira Jr JF: Biofilms and apical periodontitis: study of prevalence and association with clinical and histopathologic findings, *J Endod* 36:1277–1288, 2010.
12. Chong BS: Coronal leakage and treatment failure, *J Endod* 21:159, 1995.
13. Begotka BA, Hartwell GR: The importance of the coronal seal following root canal treatment, *Va Dent J* 73:8–10, 1996.
14. Hartwell GR, Loucks CA, Reavley BA: Bacterial leakage of provisional restorative materials used in endodontics, *Quintessence Int* 41:335–339, 2010.
15. Tamse A: Iatrogenic vertical root fractures in endodontically treated teeth, *Endod Dent Traumatol* 4:190–196, 1988.
16. Sedgley CM, Messer HH: Are endodontically treated teeth more brittle? *J Endod* 18:332, 1992.
17. Fuss Z, Lustig J, Katz A, et al.: An evaluation of endodontically treated vertically fractured roots: impact of operative procedures, *J Endod* 1:46–48, 2001.
18. Friedman S, Abitbol S, Lawrence HP: Treatment outcome in endodontics: the Toronto Study—phase 1: initial treatment, *J Endod* 29:787–793, 2003.
19. Setzer FC, Boyer KR, Jeppson JR, et al.: Long-term prognosis of endodontically treated teeth: a retrospective analysis of preoperative factors in molars, *J Endod* 37:21–25, 2011.
20. Barbizam JV, Fariniuk LF, Marchesan MA, et al.: Effectiveness of manual and rotary instrumentation techniques for cleaning flattened root canals, *J Endod* 28:365–366, 2002.
21. De Cleen MJ, Schuurs AH, Wesselink PR, Wu MK: Periapical status and prevalence of endodontic treatment in an adult Dutch population, *Int Endod J* 26:112–119, 1993.
22. Gomes BPFA, Pinheiro ET, Jacinto RC, et al.: Microbial analysis of canals of root-filled teeth with periapical lesions using polymerase chain reaction, *J Endod* 34:537–540, 2008.
23. Lin LM, Skribner JE, Gaengler P: Factors associated with endodontic treatment failures, *J Endod* 18:625–627, 1992.
24. Lin LM, Rosenberg PA, Lin J: Do procedural errors cause endo-dontic treatment failure?, *J Am Dent Assoc* 136: 187–193. quiz 231, 2005.
25. Patel S, Brown J, Semper M, Abella F, Mannocci F: European Society of Endodontology position statement: Use of cone beam computed tomography in Endodontics: European Society of Endodontology (ESE) developed by. *Int Endod J* 52:1675–1678, 2019.
26. Kruse C, Spin-Neto R, Wenzel A, et al.: Impact of cone beam computed tomography on periapical assessment and treatment planning five to eleven years after surgical endodontic retreatment, *Int Endod J* 51:729–737, 2018.
27. Torabinejad M, Rice DD, Maktabi O, et al.: Incidence and size of periapical radiolucencies using cone-beam computed tomography in teeth without apparent intraoral radiographic lesions: a new periapical index with a clinical recommendation, *J Endod* 44:389–394, 2018.
28. Pereira RS, Rodrigues VAA, Furtado WT, et al.: Microbial analysis of root canal and periradicular lesion associated to teeth with endodontic failure, *Anaerobe* 48:12–18, 2017.
29. Burns LE, Visbal LD, Kohli MR, et al.: Long-term evaluation of treatment planning decisions for nonhealing endodontic cases by different groups of practitioners, *J Endod* 44:226–232, 2018.
30. Hamedy R, Shakiba B, Fayazi S, et al.: Patient-centered endodontic outcomes: a narrative review, *Iran Endod J* 8:197–204, 2013.
31. Jawale BA, Bendgude V, Husain N, et al.: Soft skill appraisal for dentistry: a tool for positive practice management, *J Contemp Dent Pract* 12:475–478, 2011.
32. Riley 3rd JL, Gilbert GH, Heft MW: Orofacial pain-related communication patterns: sex and residential setting differences among community-dwelling adults, *Pain* 99:415–422, 2002.
33. Torabinejad M, White SN: Endodontic treatment options after unsuccessful initial root canal treatment: alternatives to single-tooth implants, *J Am Dent Assoc* 147:214–220, 2016.
34. Olcay K, Ataoglu H, Belli S: Evaluation of related factors in the failure of endodontically treated teeth: a cross-sectional study, *J Endod* 44:38–45, 2018.
35. Wenteler GL, Sathorn C, Parashos P: Factors influencing root canal retreatment strategies by general practitioners and specialists in Australia, *Int Endod J* 48:417–427, 2015.
36. Kim SG, Solomon C: Cost-effectiveness of endodontic molar retreatment compared with fixed partial dentures and single-tooth implant alternatives, *J Endod* 37:321–325, 2011.
37. Rodríguez G, Patel S, Durán-Sindreu F, et al.: Influence of Cone-beam computed tomography on endodontic retreatment strategies among general dental practitioners and endodontists, *J Endod* 43:1433–1437, 2017.
38. Brown J, Jacobs R, Levring Jäghagen E, et al.: Basic training requirements for the use of dental CBCT by dentists: a position paper prepared by the European Academy of DentoMaxilloFacial Radiology, *Dentomaxillofac Radiol* 43:20130291, 2014.
39. Special Committee to Revise the Joint AAE/AAOMR Position Statement on use of CBCT in Endodontics. AAE and AAOMR joint position statement: use of cone beam computed tomography in endodontics 2015 update, *Oral Surg Oral Med Oral Pathol Oral Radiol* 120:508–512, 2015.
40. European Society of Endodontology, Patel S, Durack C, et al.: European Society of Endodontology position statement: the use of CBCT in endodontics, *Int Endod J* 47:502–504, 2014.
41. Weissman J, Johnson JD, Anderson M, et al.: Association between the presence of apical periodontitis and clinical symptoms in endodontic patients using cone-beam computed tomography and periapical radiographs, *J Endod* 41:1824–1829, 2015.
42. Mahasneh SA, Horner K, Cunliffe J, et al.: Guidelines on radiographic imaging as part of root canal treatment: a systematic review with a focus on review imaging after treatment, *Int Endod J* 51:e238–e249, 2018.
43. Azarpazhooh A, Dao T, Ungar WJ, et al.: Clinical decision making for a tooth with apical periodontitis: the patients' preferred level of participation, *J Endod* 40:784–789, 2014.
44. Azarpazhooh A, Dao T, Ungar WJ, et al.: Patients' values related to treatment options for teeth with apical periodontitis, *J Endod* 42:365–370, 2016.
45. Hülsmann M: Methods for removing metal obstructions from the root canal, *Endod Dent Traumatol* 9:223–237, 1993.
46. Jensen AL, Abbott PV, Castro Salgado J: Interim and temporary restoration of teeth during endodontic treatment, *Aust Dent J* 52: S83–99, 2007.
47. https://www.semanticscholar.org/paper/AAE-Endodontic-Case-Difficulty-Assessment-Form-and/5c8c17ad-d6120eecef28321d325f6351ba079970 (accessed: 12/25/2019).
48. Ray HA, Trope M: Periapical status of endodontically treated teeth in relation to the technical quality of the root filling and the coronal restoration, *Int Endod J* 28:12–18, 1995.
49. Gillen BM, Looney SW, Gu LS, et al.: Impact of the quality of coronal restoration versus the quality of root canal fillings on success of root canal treatment: a systematic review and meta-analysis, *J Endod* 37:895–902, 2011.

50. Stabholz A, Friedman S: Endodontic retreatment: case selection and technique. Part 2. Treatment planning for retreatment, *J Endod* 14:607–614, 1988.
51. Taschieri S, Machtou P, Rosano G, et al.: The influence of previous non-surgical re-treatment on the outcome of endodontic surgery, *Minerva Stomatol* 59:625–632, 2010.
52. Selbst AG: Understanding informed consent and its relationship to the incidence of adverse treatment events in conventional endodontic therapy, *J Endod* 16:387–390, 1990.
53. Dixon EB, Kaczkowski PJ, Nicholls JI, et al.: Comparison of two ultrasonic instruments for post removal, *J Endod* 28:111–115, 2002.
54. Wu J, Lei G, Yan M, et al.: Instrument separation analysis of multi-used protaper universal rotary system during root canal therapy, *J Endod* 37:758–763, 2011.
55. Nevares G, Cunha RS, Zuolo ML, da Silveira Bueno CE: Success rates for removing or bypassing fractured instruments: a prospective clinical study, *J Endod* 38:442–444, 2012.
56. Hulsmann M, Schinkel I: Influence of several factors on the success or failure of removal of fractured instruments from the root canal, *Endod Dent Traumatol* 15:252–258, 1999.
57. Weine FS, Kelly RF, Lio PJ: The effect of preparation procedures on original canal shape and on apical foramen shape, *J Endod* 1:255–262, 1975.
58. Ramirez-Salomon M, Soler-Bientz R, de la Garza-Gonzalez R, et al.: Incidence of Lightspeed separation and the potential for bypassing, *J Endod* 23:586–587, 1997.
59. Feldman G, Solomon C, Notaro P, Moskowitz E: Retrieving broken endodontic instruments, *J Am Dent Assoc* 88:588–591, 1974.
60. Souyave LC, Inglis AT, Alcalay M: Removal of fractured endodontic instruments using ultrasonics, *Br Dent J* 159:251–253, 1985.
61. Fox J, Moodnik RM, Greenfield E, Atkinson JS: Filling root canals with files: radiographic evaluation of 304 cases, *NY State Dent J* 38:154–157, 1972.
62. Saunders JL, Eleazer PD, Zhang P, Michalek S: Effect of a fractured instrument on bacterial penetration of obturated root canals, *J Endod* 30:177–179, 2004.
63. Suter B, Lussi A, Sequiera P: Probability of removing fractured instruments from root canals, *Int Endod J* 38:112–123, 2005.
64. Ruddle CJ: Nonsurgical retreatment. In Cohen S, Burns RC, editors: *Pathways of the pulp*, ed 8, St. Louis, MO, 2002, CV Mosby, pp 875–929.
65. Nagai O, Tani N, Kayaba Y, et al.: Ultrasonic removal of fractured instruments in root canals, *Int Endod J* 19:298–304, 1986.
66. Chenail BL, Teplitsky PE: Orthograde ultrasonic retrieval of root canal obstructions, *J Endod* 13:186–190, 1987.
67. Ward JR, Parashos P, Messer HH: Evaluation of an ultrasonic technique to remove fractured rotary nickel-titanium endodontic instruments from root canals: an experimental study, *J Endod* 29:756–763, 2003.
68. Jafarzadeh H: Ledge formation: review of a great challenge in endodontics, *J Endod* 33:1155–62, 2007.
69. García M, Duran-Sindreu F, Mercadé M, et al.: A comparison of apical transportation between profile and RaCe rotary instruments, *J Endod* 38:990–992, 2012.
70. Ponce de Leon Del Bello T, Wang N, Roane JB: Crown-down tip design and shaping, *J Endod* 29:513–518, 2003.
71. Machtou P, Sarfati P, Cohen AG: Post removal prior to retreatment, *J Endod* 15:552–554, 1989.
72. Smith BJ: Removal of fractured posts using ultrasonic vibration: an in vivo study, *J Endod* 27:632–634, 2001.
73. Dominici JT, Clark S, Scheetz J, et al.: Analysis of heat generation using ultrasonic vibration for post removal, *J Endod* 31:301–303, 2005.
74. Tronstad L, Sunde PT: The evolving new understanding of endodontic infections, *Endodontic Topics* 6:57–77, 2003.
75. Laux M, Abbott PV, Pajarola G, et al.: Apical inflammatory root resorption: a correlative radiographic and histological assessment, *Int Endod J* 33:483–493, 2000.
76. Vier FV, Figueiredo JA: Prevalence of different periapical lesions associated with human teeth and their correlation with the presence and extension of apical external root resorption, *Int Endod J* 35:710–719, 2002.
77. Edgar SW, Marshall JG, Baumgartner JC: The antimicrobial effect of chloroform on enterococcus faecalis after gutta-percha removal, *J Endod* 32:1185–1187, 2006.
78. Huang X, Ling J, Gu L: Quantitative evaluation of debris extruded apically by using ProTaper Universal Tulsa Rotare System in endodontic retreatment, *J Endod* 33:1102–1105, 2007.
79. Ma J, Al-Ashaw AJ, Shen Y, et al.: Efficacy of ProTaper Universal Rotary Retreatment System for gutta-percha removal from oval root canals: a micro-computed tomography study, *J Endod* 38:1516–1520, 2012.
80. Friedman S, Stabholz A, Tamse A: Endodontic retreatment: case selection and technique. Part 3. Retreatment techniques, *J Endod* 16:543–549, 1990.
81. Chutich MJ, Kaminski EJ, Miller DA, Lautenschlager EP: Risk assessment of the toxicity of solvents of gutta-percha used in endodontic retreatment, *J Endod* 24:213–216, 1998.
82. Hansen MG: Relative efficiency of solvents used in endodontics, *J Endod* 24:38–40, 1998.
83. Ibarrola JL, Knowles KI, Ludlow MO: Retrievability of Thermafil plastic cores using organic solvents, *J Endod* 19:417–418, 1993.
84. Imura N, Zuolo ML, Kherlakian D: Comparison of endodontic retreatment of laterally condensed gutta-percha and Thermafil with plastic carriers, *J Endod* 19:609–612, 1993.
85. Wilcox LR: Thermafil retreatment with and without chloroform solvent, *J Endod* 19:563–566, 1993.
86. Zuolo ML, Imura N, Ferreira MO: Endodontic retreatment of Thermafil or lateral condensation obturations in post space prepared teeth, *J Endod* 20:9–12, 1994.
87. Wolcott JF, Himel VT, Hicks ML: Thermafil retreatment using a new "System B" technique or a solvent, *J Endod* 25:761–764, 1999.
88. Lipski M, Wozniak K: In vitro infrared thermographic assessment of root surface temperature rises during Thermafil retreatment using system B, *J Endod* 29:413–415, 2003.
89. Fishelberg G, Pawluk JW: Nickel-titanium rotary-file canal preparation and intracanal file separation, *Compend Contin Educ Dent* 25:17–18, 2004.
90. Rödig T, Hausdörfer T, Konietschke F, et al.: Efficacy of D-RaCe and ProTaper universal retreatment NiTi instruments and hand files in removing gutta-percha from curved root canals: a micro-computed tomography study, *Int Endod J* 45:580–589, 2012.
91. Krell KV, Fuller MW, Scott GL: The conservative retrieval of silver cones in difficult cases, *J Endod* 10:269–273, 1984.
92. Suter B: A new method for retrieving silver points and separated instruments from root canals, *J Endod* 24:446–448, 1998.
93. Plack 3rd WF, Vire DE: Retrieval of endodontic silver points, *Gen Dent* 32:124–127, 1984.
94. Friedman S: Considerations and concepts of case selection in the management of post-treatment endodontic disease, *Endo Topics* 1:54–78, 2002.
95. Spriggs K, Gettleman B, Messer HH: Evaluation of a new method for silver point removal, *J Endod* 16:335–338, 1990.
96. Fachin EV, Wenckus CS, Aun CE: Retreatment using a modified-tip instrument, *J Endod* 21:425–428, 1995.
97. Jeng HW, ElDeeb ME: Removal of hard paste fillings from the root canal by ultrasonic instrumentation, *J Endod* 13:295–298, 1987.
98. Vranas RN, Hartwell GR, Moon PC: The effect of endodontic solutions on resorcinol-formalin paste, *J Endod* 29:69–72, 2003.
99. Gambrel MG, Hartwell GR, Moon PC, et al.: The effect of endodontic solutions on resorcinol-formalin paste in teeth, *J Endod* 31:25–29, 2005.
100. Tennert C, Feldmann K, Haamann E, et al.: Effect of photodynamic therapy (PDT) on Enterococcus faecalis biofilm in experimental primary and secondary endodontic infections, *BMC Oral Health* 14:132, 2014.

101. Del Fabbro M, Samaranayake LP, Lolato A, et al.: Analysis of the secondary endodontic lesions focusing on the extraradicular microorganisms: an overview, *J Investig Clin Dent* 5:245–254, 2014.
102. Nair PN: On the causes of persistent apical periodontitis: a review, *Int Endod J* 39:249–281, 2006.
103. Ricucci D, Siqueira Jr JF: Recurrent apical periodontitis and late endodontic treatment failure related to coronal leakage: a case report, *J Endod* 37:1171–1175, 2011.
104. Siqueira Jr JF: Rôças IN, Ricucci D, Hülsmann M: Causes and management of post-treatment apical periodontitis, *Br Dent J* 216:305–312, 2014.
105. Tawakoli PN, Ragnarsson KT, Rechenberg DK, Mohn D, Zehnder M: Effect of endodontic irrigants on biofilm matrix polysaccharides, *Int Endod J* 50:153–160, 2017.
106. Rodrigues CT, de Andrade FB, de Vasconcelos LRSM, et al.: Antibacterial properties of silver nanoparticles as a root canal irrigant against Enterococcus faecalis biofilm and infected dentinal tubules, *Int Endod J* 51:901–911, 2018.
107. Del Carpio-Perochena AE, Bramante CM, Duarte MA, et al.: Biofilm dissolution and cleaning ability of different irrigant solutions on intraorally infected dentin, *J Endod* 37:1134–1138, 2011.
108. Forough Reyhani M, Rezagholizadeh Y, Narimani MR, et al.: Antibacterial effect of different concentrations of sodium hypochlorite on *Enterococcus faecalis* biofilms in root canals, *J Dent Res Dent Clin Dent Prospects* 11:215–221, 2017.
109. Mohmmed SA, Vianna ME, Penny MR, et al.: The effect of sodium hypochlorite concentration and irrigation needle extension on biofilm removal from a simulated root canal model, *Aust Endod J* 43:102–109, 2017.
110. Niemi TK, Marchesan MA, Lloyd A, Seltzer RJ: Effect of instrument design and access outlines on the removal of root canal obturation materials in oval-shaped canals, *J Endod* 42:1550–1554, 2016.
111. Martins MP, Duarte MA, Cavenago BC, et al.: Effectiveness of the protaper next and reciproc systems in removing root canal filling material with sonic or ultrasonic irrigation: a micro-computed tomographic study, *J Endod* 43:467–471, 2017.
112. Yılmaz F, Koç C, Kamburoğlu K, et al.: Evaluation of 3 different retreatment techniques in maxillary molar teeth by using micro-computed tomography, *J Endod* 44:480–484, 2018.
113. al-Omari MA, Dummer PM: Canal blockage and debris extrusion with eight preparation techniques, *J Endod* 21:154–158, 1995.
114. Rechenberg DK, Paqué F: Impact of cross-sectional root canal shape on filled canal volume and remaining root filling material after retreatment, *Int Endod J* 46:547–555, 2013.
115. Capar ID, Arslan H, Ertas H, et al.: Effectiveness of ProTaper Universal retreatment instruments used with rotary or reciprocating adaptive motion in the removal of root canal filling material, *Int Endod J* 48:79–83, 2015.
116. Crozeta BM, Silva-Sousa YT, Leoni GB, et al.: Micro-computed tomography study of filling material removal from oval-shaped canals by using rotary, reciprocating, and adaptive motion systems, *J Endod* 42:793–797, 2016.
117. Rossi-Fedele G, Ahmed HM: Assessment of root canal filling removal effectiveness using micro-computed tomography: a systematic review, *J Endod* 43:520–526, 2017.
118. Retamozo B, Shabahang S, Johnson N, et al.: Minimum contact time and concentration of sodium hypochlorite required to eliminate *Enterococcus faecalis*, *J Endod* 36:520–523, 2010.
119. Al-bulushi A, Levinkind M, Flanagan M, et al.: Effect of canal preparation and residual root filling material on root impedance, *Int Endod J* 41:892–904, 2008.
120. Er O, Uzun O, Ustun Y, et al.: Effect of solvents on the accuracy of the Mini Root ZX apex locator, *Int Endod J* 46:1088–1095, 2013.
121. Mancini M, Palopoli P, Iorio L, et al.: Accuracy of an electronic apex locator in the retreatment of teeth obturated with plastic or cross-linked gutta-percha carrier-based materials: an ex vivo study, *J Endod* 40:2061–2065, 2014.
122. Mandlik J, Shah N, Pawar K, et al.: An in vivo evaluation of different methods of working length determination, *J Contemp Dent Pract* 14:644–648, 2013.
123. Ng YL, Mann V, Gulabivala K: A prospective study of the factors affecting outcomes of nonsurgical root canal treatment: part 1: periapical health, *Int Endod J* 44:583–609, 2011.
124. Rodrigues RCV, Zandi H, Kristoffersen AK, et al.: Influence of the apical preparation size and the irrigant type on bacterial reduction in root canal-treated teeth with apical periodontitis, *J Endod* 43:1058–1063, 2017.
125. Parirokh M, Torabinejad M: Mineral trioxide aggregate: a comprehensive literature review—Part I: chemical, physical, and antibacterial properties, *J Endod* 36:16–27, 2010.
126. Parirokh M, Torabinejad M, Dummer PMH: Mineral trioxide aggregate and other bioactive endodontic cements: an updated overview - part I: vital pulp therapy, *Int Endod J* 51:177–205, 2018.
127. Manfredi M, Figini L, Gagliani M, Lodi G: Single versus multiple visits for endodontic treatment of permanent teeth, *Cochrane Database Syst Rev* 12:CD005296, 2016.
128. Molander A, Warfvinge J, Reit C, Kvist T: Clinical and radiographic evaluation of one- and two-visit endodontic treatment of asymptomatic necrotic teeth with apical periodontitis: a randomized clinical Trial, *J Endod* 33:1145–1148, 2007.
129. Sathorn C, Parashos P, Messer H: Antibacterial efficacy of calcium hydroxide intracanal dressing: a systematic review and meta-analysis, *Int Endod J* 40:2–10, 2007.
130. Su Y, Wang C, Ye L: Healing rate and post-obturation pain of single- versus multiple-visit endodontic treatment for infected root canals: a systematic review, *J Endod* 37:125–132, 2011.
131. Almeida DO, Chaves SC, Souza RA, Soares FF: Outcome of single- vs multiple-visit endodontic therapy of nonvital teeth: a meta-analysis, *J Contemp Dent Pract* 18:330–336, 2017. 1.
132. Lopes RMV, Marins FC, Belladonna FG, et al.: Untouched canal areas and debris accumulation after root canal preparation with rotary and adaptive systems, *Aust Endod J*, 44:260–266, 2018.
133. Dutner J, Mines P, Anderson A: Irrigation trends among American Association of Endodontists members: a web-based survey, *J Endod* 38:37–40, 2012.
134. Savani GM, Sabbah W, Sedgley CM, Whitten B: Current trends in endodontic treatment by general dental practitioners: report of a United States national survey, *J Endod* 40:618–624, 2014.
135. Virdee SS, Seymour DW, Farnell D, et al.: Efficacy of irrigant activation techniques in removing intracanal smear layer and debris from mature permanent teeth: a systematic review and meta-analysis, *Int Endod J* 51:605–621, 2018.
136. Shahravan A, Haghdoost AA, Adl A, et al.: Effect of smear layer on sealing ability of canal obturation: a systematic review and meta-analysis, *J Endod* 33:96–105, 2007.
137. Farzaneh S, Parirokh M, Nakhaee N, Abbott PV: Effect of two different concentrations of sodium hypochlorite on postoperative pain following single-visit root canal treatment: a triple-blind randomized clinical trial, *Int Endod J* 51:e2–e11, 2018.
138. Shemesh H, Roeleveld AC, Wesselink PR, Wu MK: Damage to root dentin during retreatment procedures, *J Endod* 37:63–66, 2011.
139. Capar ID, Saygili G, Ergun H, et al.: Effects of root canal preparation, various filling techniques and retreatment after filling on vertical root fracture and crack formation, *Dent Traumatol* 31:302–307, 2015.
140. Berry KA, Loushine RJ, Primack PD, Runyan DA: Nickel-titanium versus stainless-steel finger spreaders in curved canals, *J Endod* 24:752–754, 1998.
141. Gharai SR, Thorpe JR, Strother JM, McClanahan SB: Comparison of generated forces and apical microleakage using nickel-titanium and stainless steel finger spreaders in curved canals, *J Endod* 31:198–200, 2005.

142. Pirani C, Iacono F, Gatto MR, et al.: Outcome of secondary root canal treatment filled with Thermafil: a 5-year follow-up of retrospective cohort study, *Clin Oral Investig* 22:1363–1373, 2018.
143. Chybowski EA, Glickman GN, Patel Y, et al.: Clinical outcome of non-surgical root canal treatment using a single-cone technique with endosequence bioceramic sealer: a retrospective analysis, *J Endod* 44:941–945, 2018.
144. Torabinejad M, Parirokh M, Dummer PMH: Mineral trioxide aggregate and other bioactive endodontic cements: an updated overview - part II: other clinical applications and complications, *Int Endod J* 51:284–317, 2018.
145. Gomes AC, Nejaim Y, et al.: Influence of endodontic treatment and coronal restoration on status of periapical tissues: a cone-beam computed tomographic study, *J Endod* 41:1614–1618, 2015.
146. Cheung GS, Chan TK: Long-term survival of primary root canal treatment carried out in a dental teaching hospital, *Int Endod J* 36:117–128, 2003.
147. Cagidiaco MC, Goracci C, Garcia-Godoy F, Ferrari M: Clinical studies of fiber posts: a literature review, *Int J Prosthodont* 21:328–336, 2008.
148. Sterzenbach G, Franke A, Naumann M: Rigid versus flexible dentine-like endodontic posts–clinical testing of a biomechanical concept: seven-year results of a randomized controlled clinical pilot trial on endodontically treated abutment teeth with severe hard tissue loss, *J Endod* 38:1557–1563, 2012.
149. Dejak B, Motkowski A: 3D-Finite element analysis of molars restored with endocrowns and posts during masticatory simulation, *Dent Mater* 29:e309–e317, 2013.
150. Verıssimo C, Simamoto Junior PC, Soares CJ, et al.: Effect of the crown, post, and remaining coronal dentin on the biomechanical behavior of endodontically treated maxillary central incisors, *J Prosthet Dent* 111:234–246, 2014.
151. Ferrari M, Vichi A, Fadda GM, et al.: A randomized controlled trial of endodontically treated and restored premolars, *J Dent Res* 91: 72S–78S. 2012.
152. Ferrari M, Cagidiaco MC, Grandini S, et al.: Post placement affects survival of endodontically treated premolars, *J Dent Res* 86:729–734, 2007.
153. Guldener KA, Lanzrein CL, et al.: Long-term clinical outcomes of endodontically treated teeth restored with or without fiber post-retained single-unit restorations, *J Endod* 43:188–193, 2017.
154. Shemesh H, Wesselink PR, Wu MK: Incidence of dentinal defects after root canal filling procedures, *Int Endod J* 43:995–1000, 2010.
155. Randow K, Glantz PO: On cantilever loading of vital and non-vital teeth. An experimental clinical study, *Acta Odontol Scand* 44:271–277, 1986.
156. Suksaphar W, Banomyong D, et al.: Survival rates from fracture of endodontically treated premolars restored with full-coverage crowns or direct resin composite restorations: a retrospective study, *J Endod* 44:233–238, 2018.
157. Aquilino SA, Caplan DJ: Relationship between crown placement and the survival of endodontically treated teeth, *J Prosthet Dent* 87:256–263, 2002.
158. Caplan DJ, Weintraub JA: Factors related to loss of root canal filled teeth, *J Public Health Dent* 57:31–39, 1997.
159. Torabinejad M, Kettering JD, McGraw JC, et al.: Factors associated with endodontic interappointment emergencies of teeth with necrotic pulps, *J Endod* 14:261–266, 1988.
160. Trope M: Flare-up rate of single-visit endodontics, *Int Endod J* 24:24–26, 1991.
161. Walton R, Fouad A: Endodontic interappointment flare-ups: a prospective study of incidence and related factors, *J Endod* 18:172–177, 1992.
162. He J, White RK, White CA, et al.: Clinical and patient-centered outcomes of nonsurgical root canal retreatment in first molars using contemporary techniques, *J Endod* 43:231–237, 2017.
163. Al-Nuaimi N, Patel S, Davies A, et al.: Pooled analysis of 1-year recall data from three root canal treatment outcome studies undertaken using cone beam computed tomography, *Int Endod J* 51:e216–e226, 2018.

20
Apical Microsurgery

RICHARD RUBINSTEIN, MOHAMED I. FAYAD, AND MAHMOUD TORABINEJAD

CHAPTER OUTLINE

LEARNING OBJECTIVES

After reading this chapter, the student should be able to:

1. Discuss the role of endodontic surgery in treatment planning for a patient.
2. Recognize situations in which surgery is the treatment of choice.
3. Define the terms incision for drainage, apical curettage, root-end resection, root-end preparation, root-end filling, grafting, and suturing.
4. Briefly describe the step-by-step procedures involved in periapical surgery, including those for incision and reflection, access to the apex, apical curettage, root-end resection, root-end preparation and filling, flap replacement, and suturing.
5. State the different flap designs.
6. Diagram the various flap designs and describe the indications, advantages, and disadvantages of each.
7. List the more common root-end filling materials.
8. Review the different materials for grafting.
9. Review the basic principles of suturing.
10. Write out instructions to be given to the patient concerning postoperative care after endodontic surgery.
11. Review the outcome of apical microsurgery.

A Brief History

Systematic reviews with meta-analysis, studies with large sample sizes, and practice-based research networks studies all indicate extremely high medium-term and long-term survival rates for nonsurgical endodontically treated teeth without intervention.[1-9] If a nonsurgical endodontically treated tooth fails and cannot be retreated nonsurgically, and it is determined that the reason for failure is not periodontal, traumatic, or restorative in nature, apical surgery (AS) is often the treatment of choice.

Although the origins of AS can be traced to pre-Colombian times,[10,11] contemporary endodontic surgery began its journey in the early 1960s along with the recognition of endodontics as a specialty in the United States in 1964.[12,13]

The main purpose of AS is to save a natural tooth. This is accomplished by removing a portion of a root with anatomic complexities laden with tissue debris and microorganisms and/or sealing the canal when a complete seal cannot be accomplished through nonsurgical procedures.[5] Significant advances in the use of magnification and illumination, specifically the introduction of the surgical operating microscope (SOM) in the late 1980s and the supportive armamentarium and materials that followed, have benefited treatment protocols in AS such that teeth that might otherwise have been extracted now have a predictable chance for retention. AS is now considered a microsurgical procedure in the truest sense.[14] The purpose of this chapter is to discuss indications and contraindications for apical microsurgery, procedures involved in apical microsurgery, including those for incision and reflection, access to the apex, apical curettage, root-end resection, root-end preparation and filling, flap replacement, and suturing as well as instructions to be given to the patient concerning postoperative care after endodontic surgery.

Indications for Apical Surgery

The main indications for AS are failing root canal treatments, procedural accidents, irretrievable materials in the root canal or periapical tissues, anatomic complexity of the root canal system that prevents complete cleaning, shaping, and obturation of the root canal system through the coronal

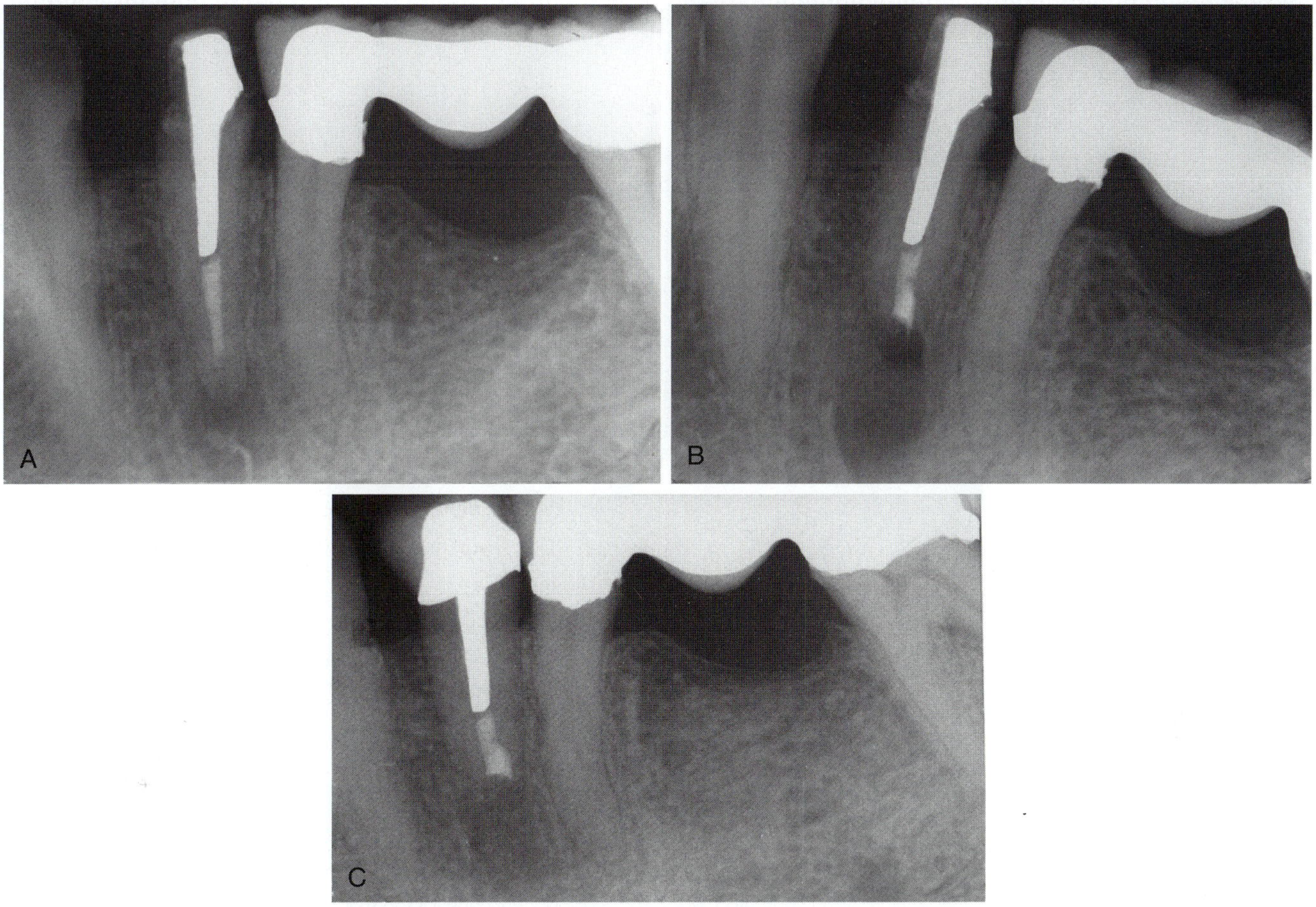

• **Fig. 20.1** **(A)** An inadequate root canal treatment, a large post, and patient's discomfort led to a decision to perform a periapical surgery on the mandibular first premolar. **(B)** Postoperative radiograph after endodontic surgery. Mineral trioxide aggregate (MTA) was used as a root-end filling material. **(C)** Periapical radiograph taken four and half years later shows complete healing and a functional tooth.

access, symptomatic cases, adjunctive surgeries, and exploratory surgery.

Failing Root Canal Treatments

When previous nonsurgical root canal treatment cannot be improved or performed because regaining access to the canal or removing posts would risk a perforation or root fracture and/or create a restorative problem, surgical endodontics is indicated (Fig. 20.1).

Procedural Accidents

Most procedural accidents can be corrected nonsurgically (see Chapter 18). However, when nonsurgical correction of these accidents is not feasible or practical, AS is indicated to save these teeth. Procedural accidents that may require AS include ledge formation, root perforation, separated instruments, and underfilled or overfilled canals (Fig. 20.2).

Irretrievable Filling Materials

When obturation materials cannot be removed nonsurgically or are beyond the root canal space and cause problems, AS is indicated to save the tooth (Fig. 20.3).

Anatomic Complexity of the Root Canal System

Complex anatomy, severe curvature, and canal calcifications that cannot be treated nonsurgically are indications for surgical endodontics (Fig. 20.4).

Symptomatic Cases

When nonsurgical retreatment does not provide relief of pain and discomfort and nonsurgical retreatment is not possible, AS should be considered to reduce pain and discomfort for the patient (Fig. 20.5).

Adjunctive Surgeries

Adjunctive surgical procedures include root resection, hemisection, crown lengthening, tooth replantation, and transplantation (see Chapter 21).

Exploratory Surgery

There are some radiolucencies that are not caused by root canal infection and may mimic periapical lesions of endodontic origin. Suspicious and nonhealing lesions require exploratory surgery and the taking of a biopsy for histologic examination (see Chapter 5).

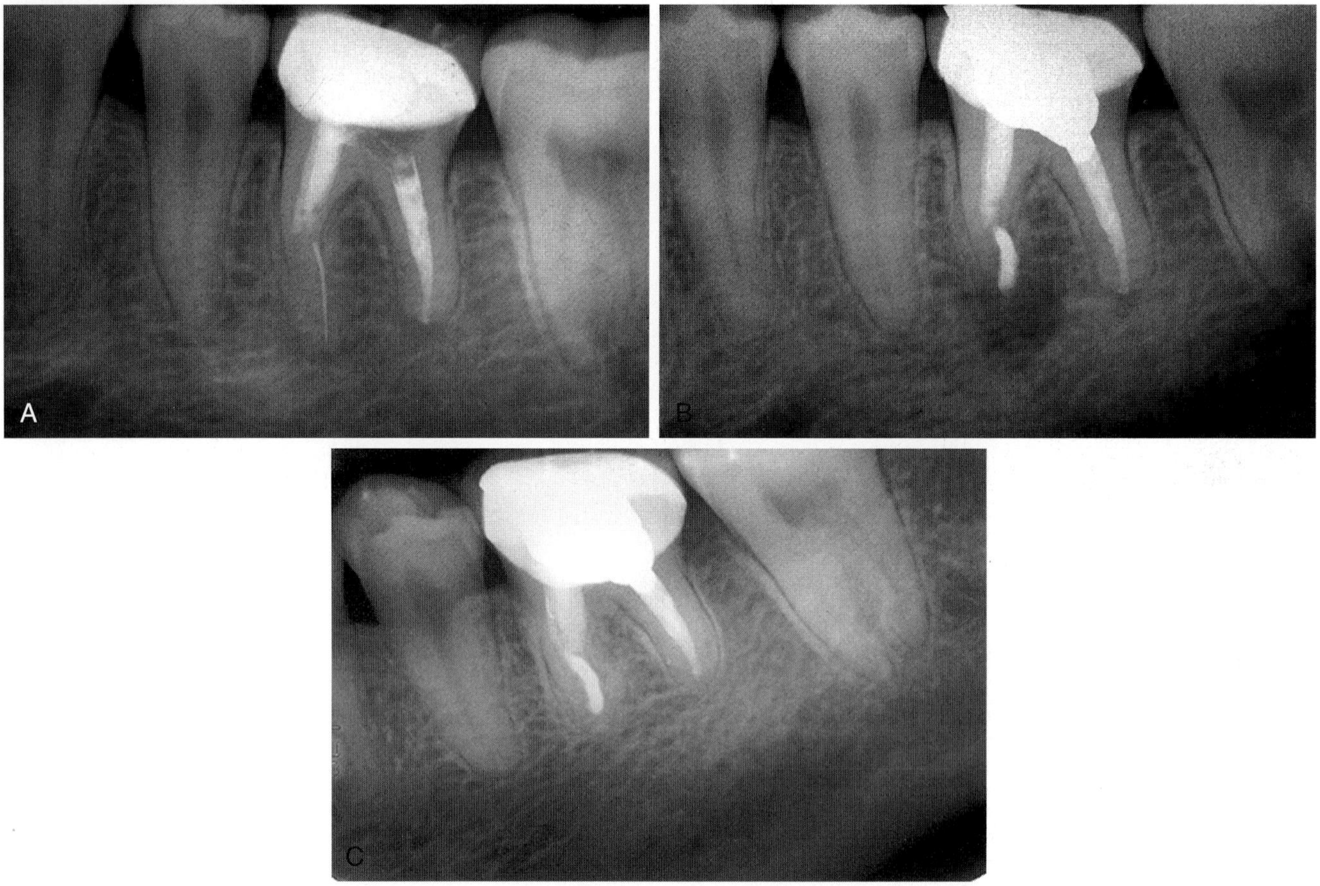

• **Fig. 20.2** **(A)** Nickel-titanium file is separated inside the mesiobuccal canal of the mandibular first molar. **(B)** Because of the patient's discomfort, a periapical surgery was performed. Mineral trioxide aggregate (MTA) was used as a root-end filling material. **(C)** Periapical radiograph taken 32 months later shows complete healing.

Contraindications for Apical Surgery

Contraindications for AS include (1) medical or systemic complications; (2) indiscriminate use of periapical surgery; (3) anatomic factors; and (4) an unidentified cause of treatment failure.

Case Selection and Contemporary Treatment Planning

One of the most important caveats in performing apical microsurgery is in knowing when to perform apical microsurgery. Case selection will heavily affect treatment outcomes, which then influences future treatment choices and long-term success rates. The most important diagnostic tool to this end has been the introduction of cone beam computed tomography (CBCT; see Chapter 3). In addition, an appropriate armamentarium and strategic approaches can be prepared well in advance of the actual surgery.

CBCT examination can help us plan treatment by locating the exact position of the apical periodontitis.

Apical Microsurgery

Although general practitioners may not perform microsurgical procedures, it is incumbent upon them to understand the armamentarium, materials, and methods so that the best treatment possible can be provided for their patients. In order to understand the objectives of apical microsurgery and the application of armamentaria, materials, and methods, it is helpful to divide the subject into multiple stages or sections.

Flap Design

The first step in AS is designing a flap that allows adequate exposure of the site of the surgery. The following general guidelines and principles should be used during flap design.

1. The flap should be designed for maximal access to the site of surgery.
2. An adequate blood supply to the reflected tissue is maintained with a wide flap base.
3. Incisions over bony defects or over the periradicular lesion should be avoided; these might cause postsurgical soft tissue fenestrations or nonunion of the incision.
4. The actual bony defect is larger than the size observed radiographically.
5. A minimal flap, which should include at least one tooth on either side of the intended tooth, should be used.
6. Acute angles in the flap must be avoided. Sharp corners are difficult to reposition and suture and may become ischemic and slough, resulting in delayed healing and possibly scar formation.
7. Incisions and reflections include periosteum as part of the flap. Any remaining pieces or tags of cellular nonreflected periosteum will hemorrhage, compromising visibility.
8. The interdental papilla must not be split (incised through) and should be either fully included or excluded from the flap.

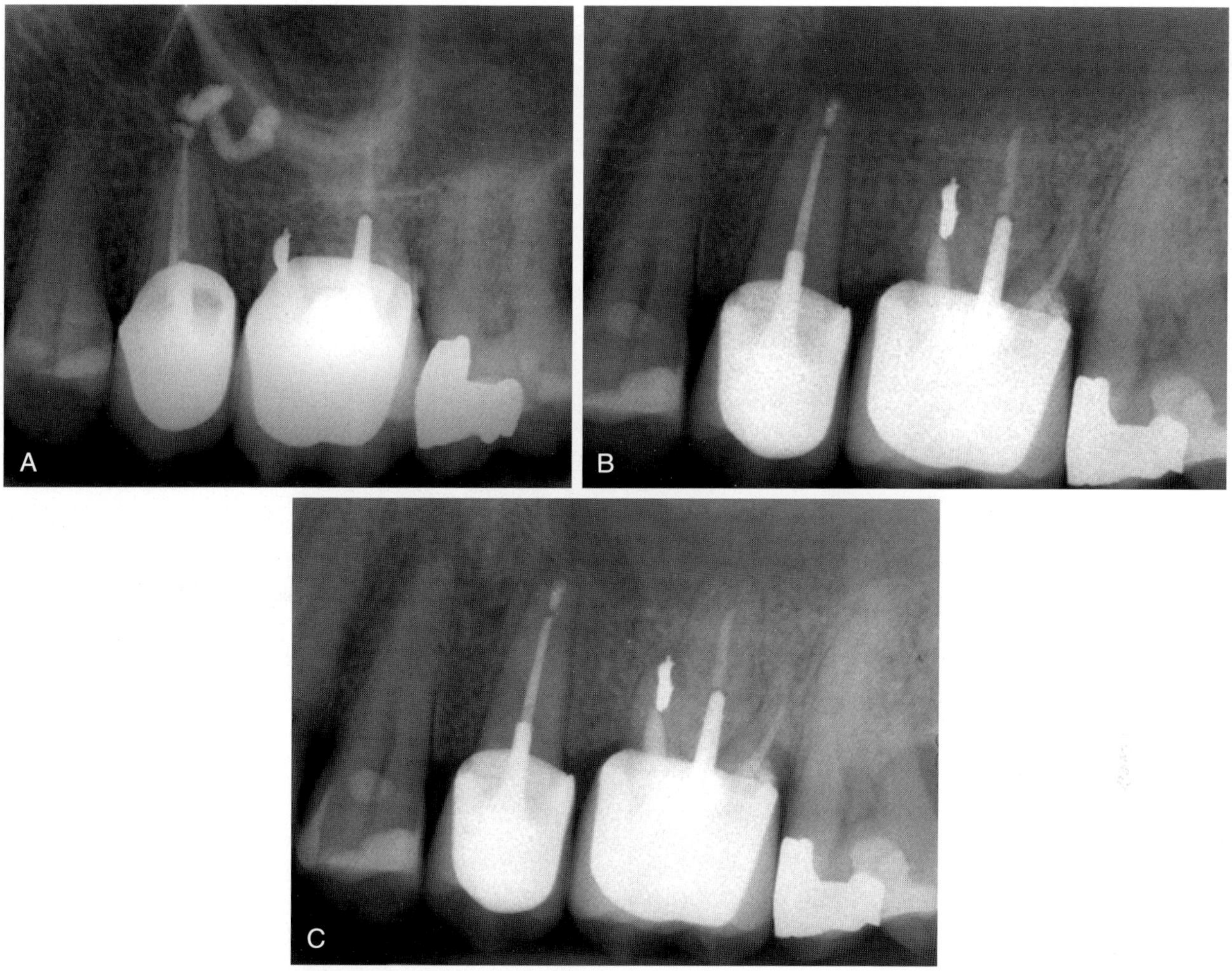

• **Fig. 20.3** **(A)** Preoperative radiograph shows presence of extruded filling materials into the periapical tissues of the maxillary left bicuspid tooth. **(B)** Because of the patient's discomfort, a periapical surgery was performed. Mineral trioxide aggregate (MTA) was used as a root-end filling material. **(C)** Postoperative radiograph taken 18 months later shows healing of the periapical tissues.

9. Vertical incisions must be extended to allow the retractor to rest on bone and not crush portions of the flap.

Although there are numerous flap designs, two meet most AS needs: the full mucoperiosteal flap (triangular or rectangular) and the submarginal flap (triangular or rectangular).

Submarginal Curved Flap

The submarginal curved flap is a slightly curved, half-moon-shaped horizontal incision made in the attached gingiva with the convexity nearest the free gingival margin. It is simple and easily reflected and provides access to the apex without impinging on the tissue surrounding the crowns. Its disadvantages include restricted access with limited visibility, tearing of the incision corners if the operator tries to improve access by stretching the tissue, and leaving the incision directly over the lesion if the surgical defect is larger than anticipated. The incision margins of this flap frequently heal with scarring. The submarginal curved flap is limited by the presence of the frenum, muscle attachments, or canine and other bony eminences. Because of its many disadvantages, this design is generally not indicated or used.

Full Mucoperiosteal Flap

The full mucoperiosteal (intrasulcular) flap consists of an incision at the gingival crest with full elevation of the interdental papillae, free gingival margin, attached gingiva, and alveolar mucosa. It may have either one (triangular) or two (rectangular) vertical releasing incisions. It allows maximal access and visibility, precludes incision over a bony defect, and has less of a tendency for hemorrhage. This design permits periodontal curettage, root planing, and bony reshaping, and it heals with minimal scar formation. Its disadvantages include the difficulty of replacing, suturing, and making alterations (height and shape) to the free gingival margin, in addition to possible gingival recession after surgery and exposure of the crown margins.

Submarginal Triangular and Rectangular Flaps

Triangular and rectangular flaps are known as *modified submarginal curved flaps*. A scalloped horizontal incision (Ochsenbein-Luebke) is made in the attached gingiva with one or two accompanying vertical incisions. This flap is used most successfully in maxillary anterior teeth with crowns. An alternative submarginal flap design is the papilla-based incision, in which the interdental papillae are left intact. Prerequisites are 4 mm of attached gingiva, minimal probing depths, and good periodontal health. Disadvantages are possible scarring and hemorrhage from the cut margins to the surgical site. This design also provides less visibility than the full mucoperiosteal flap.

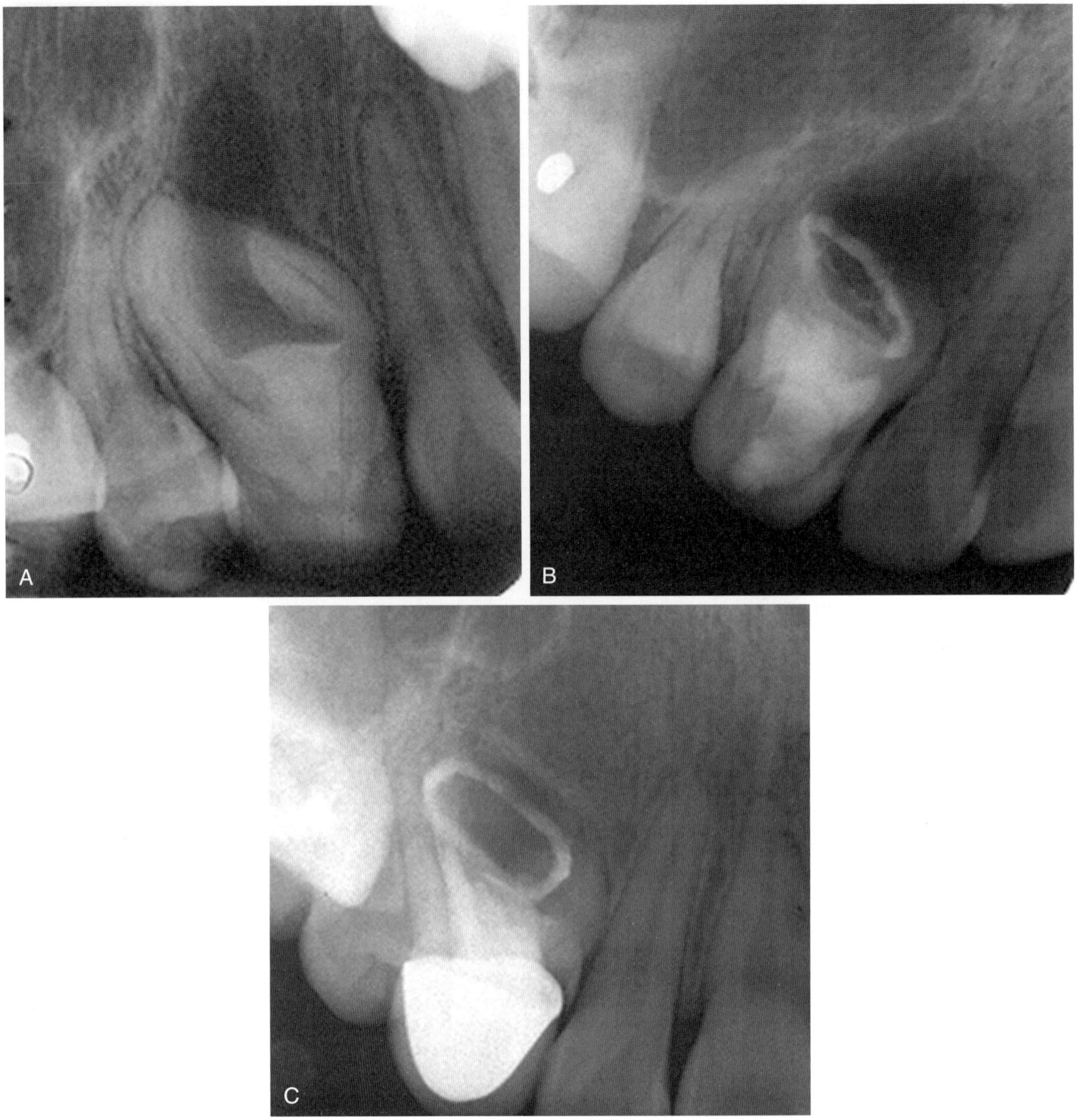

• **Fig. 20.4** **(A)** Preoperative radiograph shows presence of a dens in dente in the maxillary right cuspid tooth. **(B)** Because of inability of the operator to perform nonsurgical root canal treatment, a periapical surgery was performed. **(C)** Postoperative radiograph taken 20 months later shows complete resolution of the lesion in this tooth.

After anesthesia is obtained, and before incising the surgical flap, the oral cavity should be rinsed with a disinfectant solution such as chlorhexidine. A 0.12% chlorhexidine rinse has been shown to significantly reduce the bacterial count in the oral cavity in advance of operative procedures.[15] For a complete discussion of anesthesia see Chapter 8.

Microscalpels (Fig. 20.6) (Kerr Endodontics, Orange, CA) are used in the design of the free gingival margin flap to delicately and atraumatically incise the interdental papillae when full-thickness flaps are required. Feather Microsurgical Blades (Fig. 20.7, *A*) (J. Morita USA, Inc. Irvine, CA) are made of high quality stainless using high precision grinding technology, which produces ultra-sharp cutting edges that work with a variety of handles. These blades allow for a very fine incision and minimize the risk of tissue injury (Fig. 20.7, *B–D*).

Historically flaps have been reflected with a Molt 2-4 curette or variation of the Molt 2-4. The recently introduced periosteal elevator (Fig. 20.8) (G. Hartzell & Son, Concord, CA) has two working ends of 2 mm and 3.5 mm and 2 mm and 7 mm and accomplishes the goals of atraumatic flap reflection.

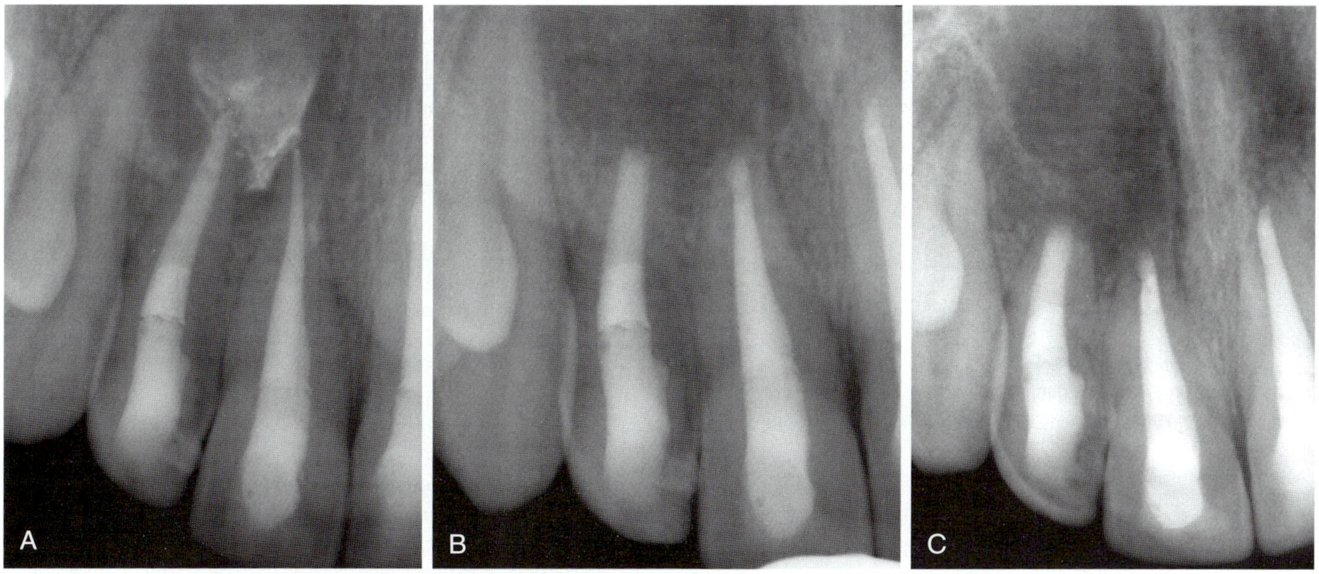

• **Fig. 20.5** **(A)** Preoperative radiograph of the right maxillary region in a young patient shows extrusion of filling materials into the periapical tissues. **(B)** Because of the presence of continued swelling and discomfort, a periapical surgery was performed on both incisors. **(C)** Postoperative radiograph taken 12 months later shows complete resolution of the lesion.

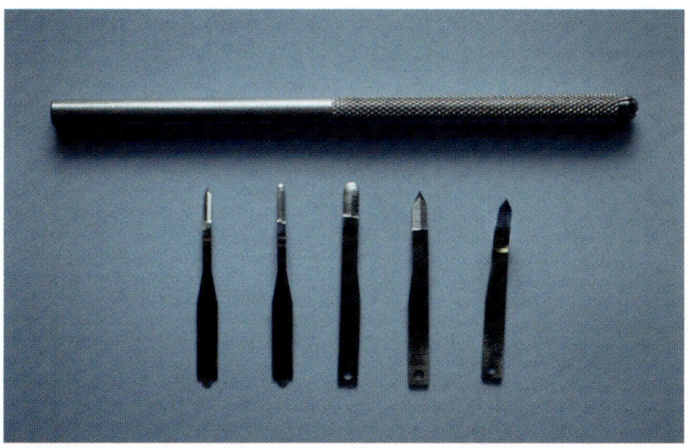

• **Fig. 20.6** A variety of microscalpels sized 1 to 5 used for precise incision.

Osteotomy

Because we can see better with the SOM, bone removal can be more conservative. Handpieces such as the Impact Air 45 (Kerr Endodontics, Orange, CA) introduced by oral surgeons to facilitate sectioning mandibular third molars are also suggested for AS to gain better access to the apices of maxillary and mandibular molars. When using the handpiece, the water spray is aimed directly into the surgical field, but the air stream is ejected out through the back of the handpiece, thus eliminating much of the splatter that occurs with conventional high-speed handpieces. Because there is no pressurized air or water, the chances of producing pyemia and emphysema are significantly reduced.

Burs such as a Lindemann H161 or H162 bone cutter (Brasseler USA, Savannah, GA) are extremely efficient and are recommended for hard tissue removal. They are 9 mm in length and have only four flutes, which result in less clogging. With the use of an SOM and an Impact Air 45, high-speed surgical burs can be placed even in areas of anatomic jeopardy with a high degree of confidence and accuracy (Fig. 20.9). The size of the osteotomy should be as small as practical so that wound healing will not be impaired, yet large enough to allow for complete débridement of the bony crypt and access for root-end procedures that will follow.

Curettage and Biopsy

It goes without saying that if tissue warrants removal, it warrants examination and diagnosis by an oral pathologist. At no time should a surgeon remove tissue and accept the responsibility of its diagnosis based on clinical impression, color, or consistency. In addition, any foreign material present in the bony crypt should be removed as it could cause persistent irritation and may prevent complete healing of the tissues.[16] For further discussion of radiolucent periapical pathosis see Chapter 5.

Apical Resection and Resected Apex Evaluation

There is general agreement that the main cause of failure in conventional endodontic treatment is the clinician's inability to adequately shape, disinfect, and obturate the entire root canal system. [17] The majority of this untreated anatomy is located in the apical 3 mm and for this reason a 3 mm resection is recommended.[18-20] With the introduction of ultrasonics for creating root-end preparations, a second reason for a 3 mm resection has emerged. Several authors have studied the incidence of craze line, cracks, and fractures in the root and cemental surfaces after ultrasonic root-end preparations.[21-25] Although all of these studies showed a statistically significant increase, none have shown any clinical significance as a result of their findings.

Historically, a long bevel was created in order to provide access for a microhead handpiece. With the introduction of periapical ultrasonics, little to no bevel is needed. This results in fewer cut dentinal tubules and less chance of leakage. Recent advancements in electric motor design and straight handpieces afford the clinician opportunities for direct visualization of the root-end while performing root resection and the creation of axial bevels that approximate zero degrees (Figs. 20.10 and 20.11).

After the root-end resection has been completed, the beveled surface of the root can be examined under midrange magnification. Using a small CX-1 microexplorer (Kerr Endodontics, Orange, CA), small microfractures, isthmuses, and portals of exit (POEs) can readily be seen (Figs. 20.12 and 20.13).

Study Questions

1. If a nonsurgical symptomatic endodontically treated tooth fails, and the quality of the root canal treatment is unacceptable, what is the appropriate first line of treatment?
   a. Surgical retreatment
   b. Nonsurgical retreatment
   c. Exploratory surgery
   d. Watch
2. Significant advances in endodontic microsurgery include all of the following except:
   a. Magnification
   b. Ultrasonics
   c. Impact air handpiece
   d. Bioceramic root-end filling materials
3. All of the following are contraindications for apical surgery except:
   a. Medical or systemic complications
   b. Indiscriminate use of periapical surgery
   c. Anatomic factors
   d. Do not have the skills
4. The surgical flap should be designed to be exactly the size of the periapical lesion.
   a. True
   b. False
5. To avoid gingival recession and papillae shrinkage in the esthetic zone, submarginal flap is the flap of choice.
   a. True
   b. False

Apical Preparation

Since the introduction of periapical ultrasonic technology in the early 1990s by Carr, apical preparations have been made with ultrasonic tips.[26] A variety of tips and tip configurations have been introduced to accommodate virtually any access situation (Fig. 20.14). Most ultrasonic tips are .25 mm in diameter and approximately 3 mm in length.

Diamond coated tips are suggested as the last ultrasonic tip to be used in root-end preparation to avoid intradentin and canal cracks.[27] Furthermore, clinical use of diamond tips has shown that they are more efficient at removing gutta-percha compared with stainless steel tips (Figs. 20.15 and 20.16).

Piezosurgery

Piezosurgery is a bone-cutting modality with rapidly increasing indications in different surgical fields, including endodontic surgery. The main advantages of piezosurgery include protection of soft tissues, optimal visualization of the surgical field, decreased blood loss, reduced vibration and noise, increased comfort for the patient, and protection of tooth structures. Some disadvantages of piezosurgery include the initial financial burden associated with the purchase of the device, the long duration of the surgical procedure, and the fact that the instruction manuals of many piezoelectric units discourage use of these devices in patients with implanted cardiac pacemakers.[27] The technology was developed in

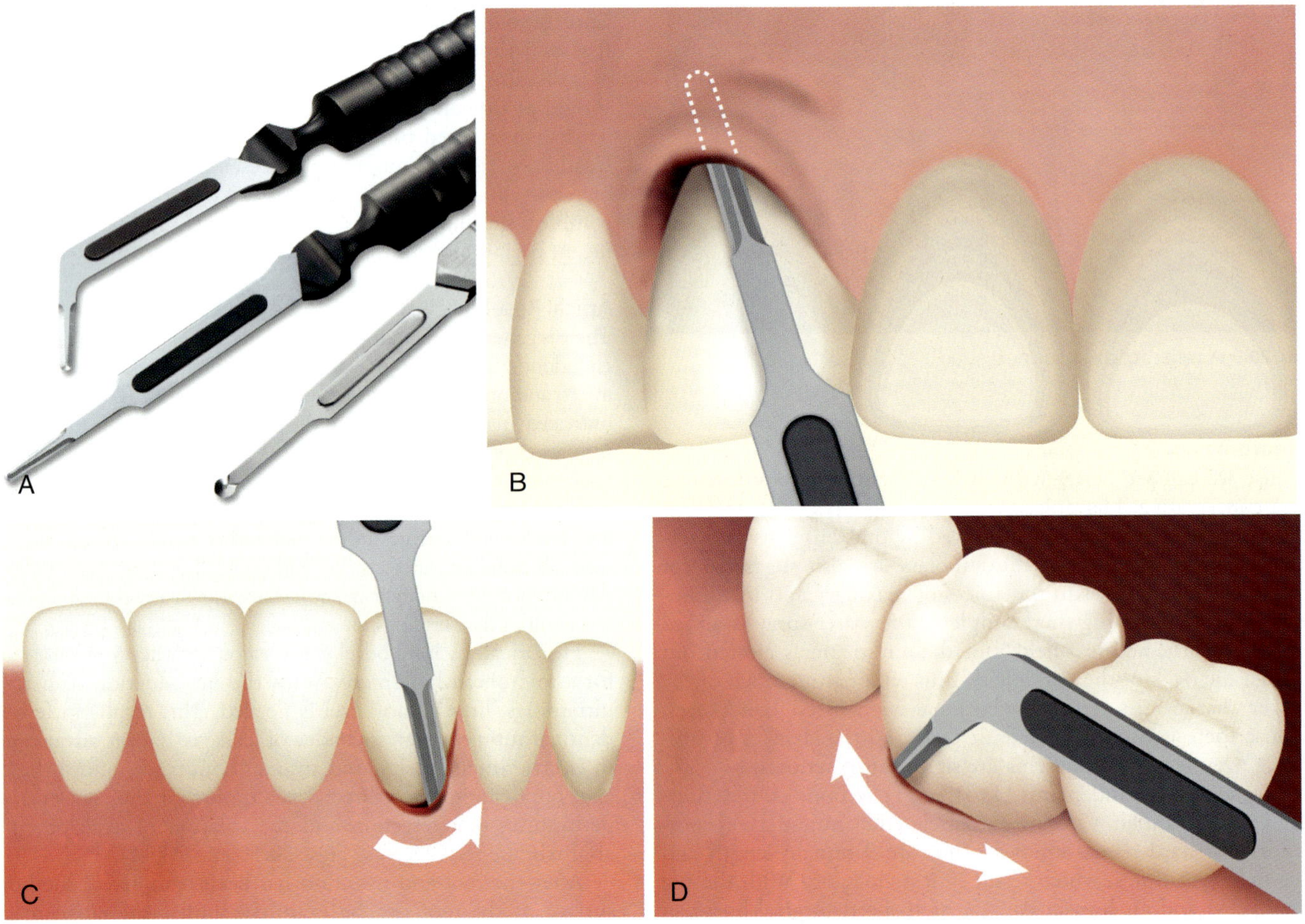

• **Fig. 20.7 (A)** Feather microsurgical blades. (Courtesy of J. Morita.) **(B–D)** Application of Feather microsurgery blades. (Courtesy of J. Morita.)

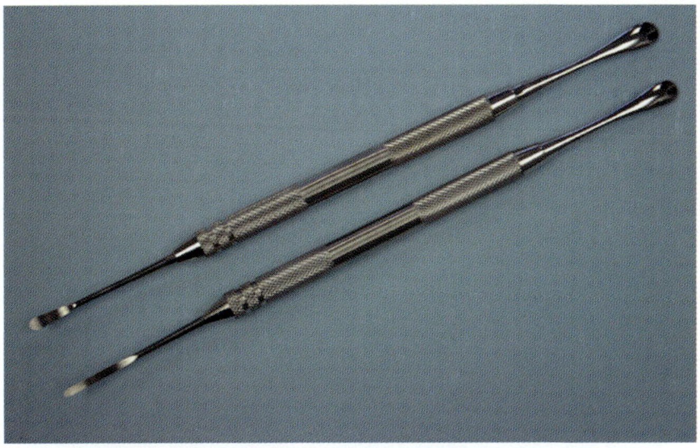

• **Fig. 20.8** PR-1 and PR-2 periosteal elevators.

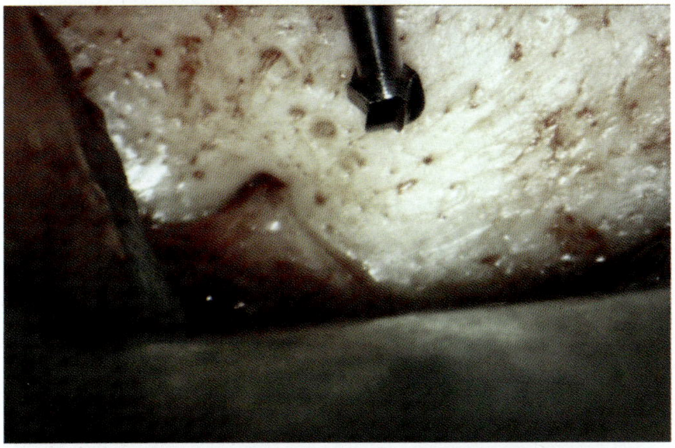

• **Fig. 20.9** Impact Air 45 and surgical length bur in close proximity to the mental nerve 8x.

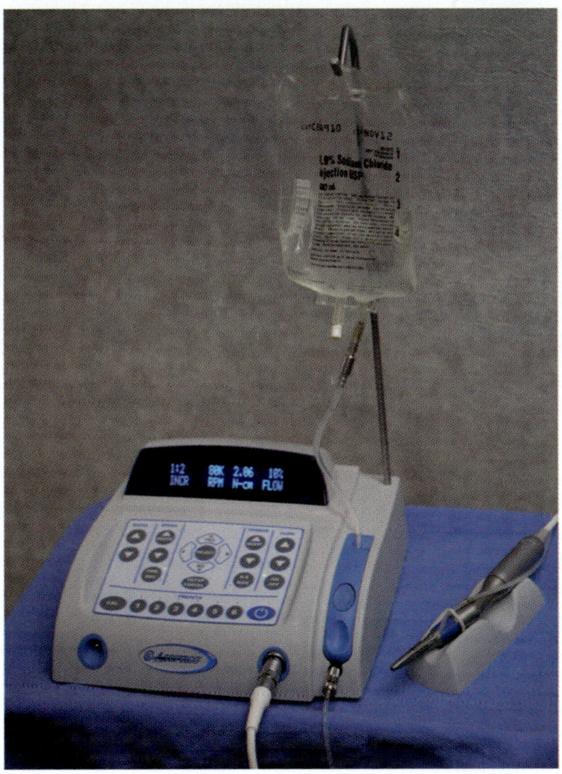

• **Fig. 20.10** Aseptico 7000 motor and NSK 2:1 nose-cone handpiece.

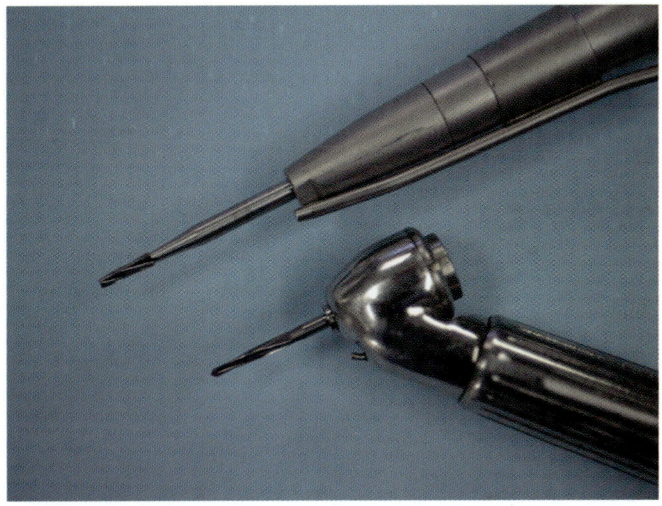

• **Fig. 20.11** A comparison of Impact Air 45 and NSK 2:1 nose-cone handpiece and surgical length burs.

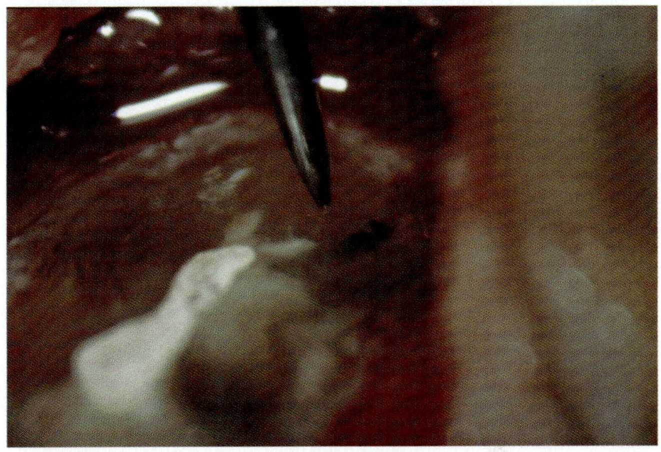

• **Fig. 20.12** CX-1 explorer locating an untreated portal of exit (POE) on the beveled surface of a previously retrofilled root at ×20.

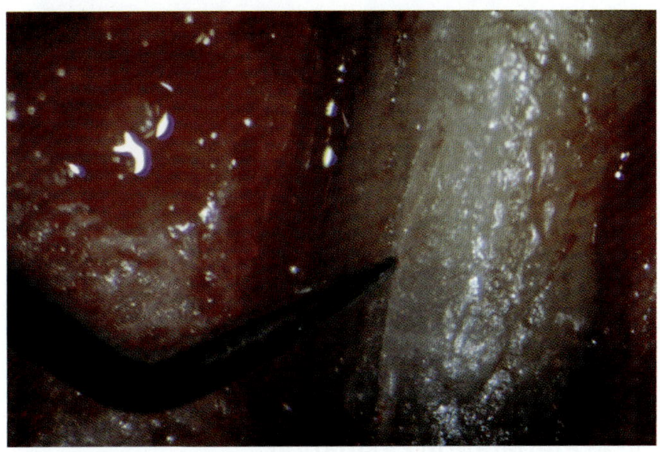

• **Fig. 20.13** CX-1 explorer locating a crack on the facial surface of a root at ×20.

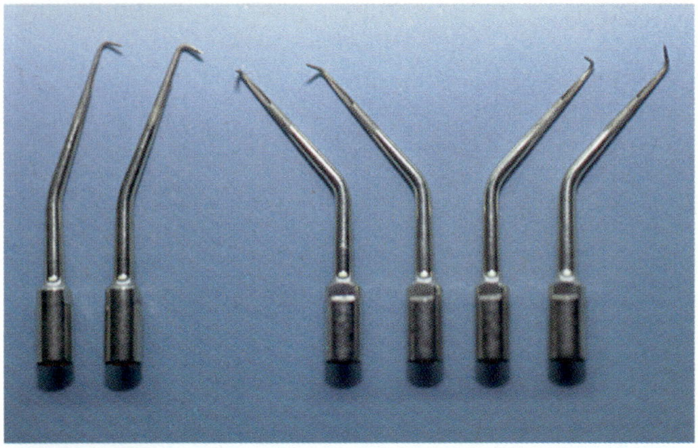

• **Fig. 20.14** Various ultrasonic tips with different shapes and angles.

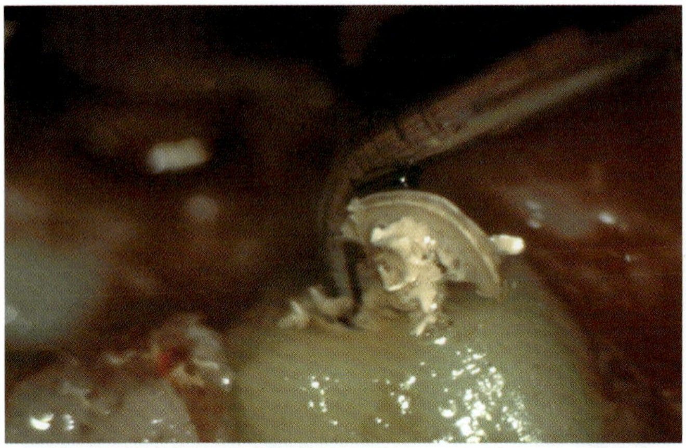

• **Fig. 20.15** Thermoplasticized gutta-percha spinning around a stainless steel tip at ×16.

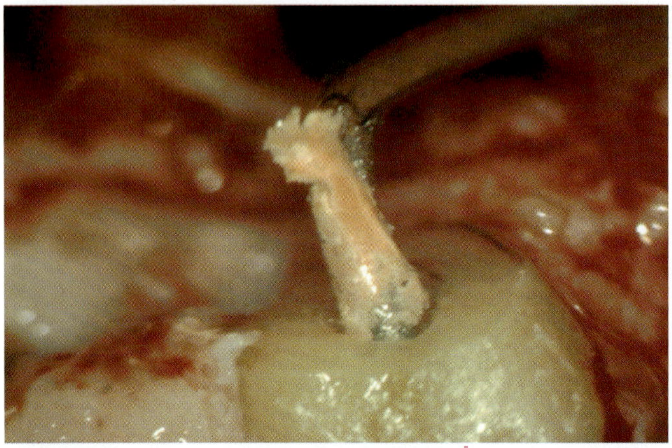

• **Fig. 20.16** Thermoplasticized gutta-percha "walking" out of the preparation at ×16.

1998 by the Italian oral surgeon Tomaso Vercellotti to overcome the limitations of conventional bone surgery[28] (Fig. 20.17).

Apical Preparation Evaluation

Another development in apical microsurgery has been the introduction of the surgical micromirror. Micromirrors come in a variety of shapes and sizes and have diameters ranging from 1 mm to

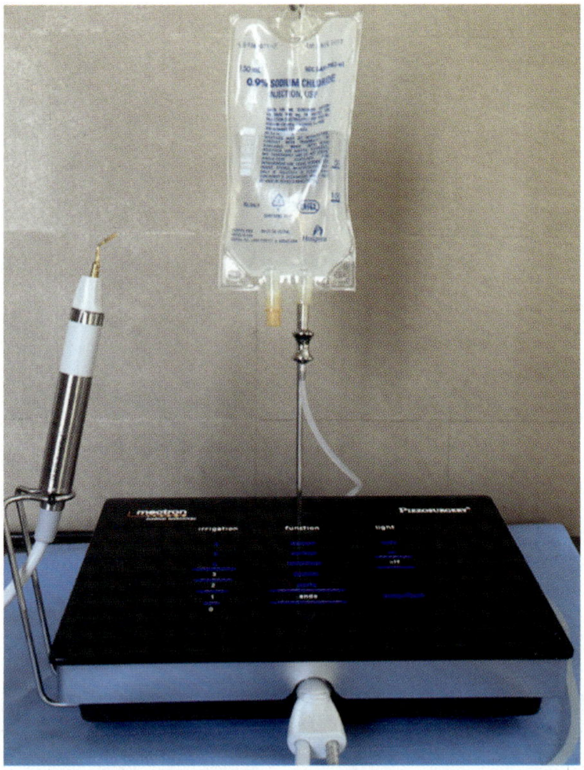

• **Fig. 20.17** Piezosurgery Touch (Mecron, Via Loreta, GE, Italy). The control panel allows the clinician to choose surgical procedure (power) and irrigation types.

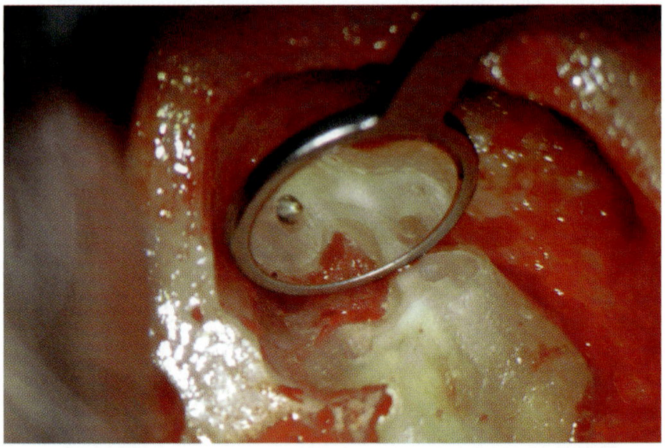

• **Fig. 20.18** Rhodium micromirror view of the beveled surface of the root at ×13.

5 mm. Recently introduced micromirrors utilize a rhodium coating. Rhodium is extremely hard and durable and is unsurpassed in reflectivity, clarity, and brightness. They are front surface, scratch resistant, and autoclavable (JEDMED, St. Louis, MO) (Fig. 20.18). Before using micromirrors, it was impossible to assess the thoroughness of apical preparation. Failure to completely remove old root canal filling material and debris from the facial wall of the apical preparation (Fig. 20.19) may lead to facial wall leakage and eventual failure if not cleaned before placement of an apical seal. Clearly, it is necessary to circumferentially remove all debris from the apical preparation to satisfy the criteria set forth by Gilheany et al. and Ricucci and Siqueira.[29,30]

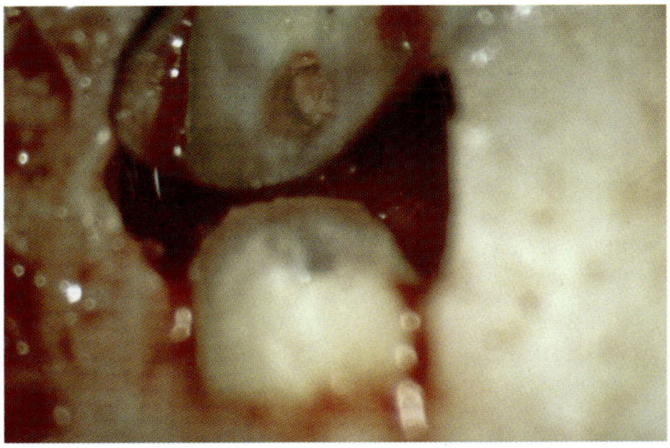

• **Fig. 20.19** Micromirror view of gutta-percha and debris on the facial wall of the apical preparation at ×16.

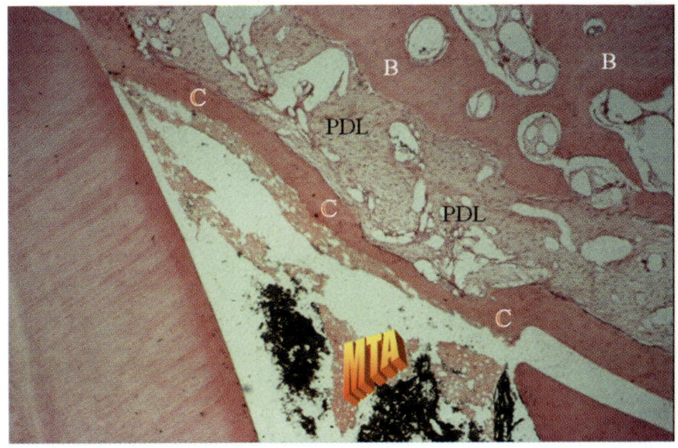

• **Fig. 20.20** Complete regeneration of periapical tissues after using MTA as a root-end filling material in mokkeys. *B*, Bone; *PDL*, periodontal ligament; *C*, cementum; *MTA*, mineral trioxide aggregate.

Hemostasis

Before selecting and placing retrofilling materials, it is essential to have established good hemostasis. Hemostasis begins by obtaining and reviewing the patient's health questionnaire. Consultation with the patient's physician may be necessary. Anesthesia must be profound with an adequate vasoconstrictor. There are many hemostatic materials available. Such a list could include ferric sulfate, aluminum chloride, collagen, hemostatic gauze, racemic epinephrine, or electro-cautery. When selecting hemostatic agents, one should consider their effect on hard and soft tissue and whether their use could compromise healing. For a complete discussion of local anesthesia see Chapter 8.

Selecting Retrofilling Materials

Historically, amalgam was first suggested for retrofillings by Farrar and reported in Dental Cosmos in 1884.[31] In 1978 Oynick and Oynick showed collagen fibers from the periodontal ligament against SuperEBA (Southern Anesthesia and Surgical, West Columbia, SC) retrofills and possibly into the SuperEBA matrix as well and suggested that SuperEBA may promote healing.[32] Bioceramics such as ProRoot mineral trioxide aggregate (MTA) (Dentsply Tulsa Dental, Tulsa, OK), BioAggregate (Innovative Bioceramix, Vancouver, Canada), EndoSequence Root Repair Material (Brasseler USA, Savannah, GA), Grey MTA Plus (Avalon Biomed, Bradenton, FL), and Biodentine (Septodont USA, Louisville, CO) were soon to follow. The class of bioceramics includes alumina and zirconia, bioactive glass, glass ceramics, coatings and composites, calcium silicates, hydroxyapatite, resorbable calcium phosphates, and radiotherapy glasses. The general class is used for joint and tissue replacement and for coating metal implants to improve biocompatibility. They are chemically and physically stable in a biologic environment and they chemically bond to dentin. ProRoot MTA, BioAggregate, EndoSequence Root Repair Material, and Grey MTA Plus all fit this definition.

The question as to whether SuperEBA had different outcomes than ProRoot MTA was studied by Song et al. and reported as a prospective randomized controlled study.[33] They reported that there was no significant difference in the clinical outcomes of endodontic microsurgery when SuperEBA and ProRoot MTA were used as root-end filling materials. However, ProRoot MTA produces complete periapical regeneration histologically whereas SuperEBA is incapable of doing the same thing (Fig. 20.20).

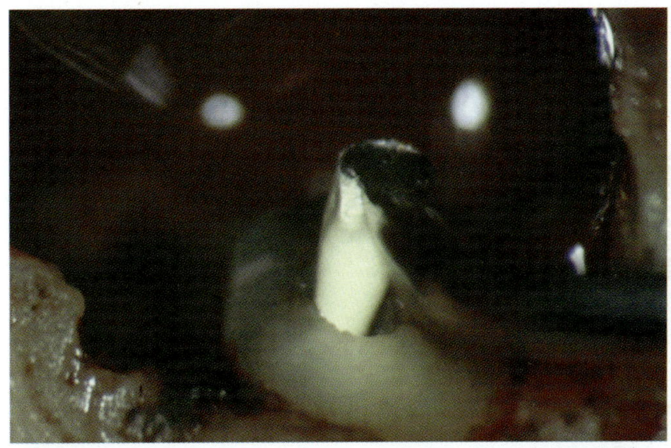

• **Fig. 20.21** Placing SuperEBA into the apical preparation with a #12 spoon excavator at ×16.

Mixing, Placing, Condensing, Carving, and Finishing Retrofilling Materials

Cement consistency retrofilling materials, such as SuperEBA and desiccated intermediate restorative material (IRM), are mixed to a putty consistency and carried to the apical preparation in small truncated cones 1 mm to 2 mm in size on a #12 spoon excavator (Fig. 20.21). Between each aliquot of material, a small plugger (JEDMED Instrument Company, St. Louis, MO) that will fit inside the apical preparation is used to condense the material (Fig. 20.22).

Final examination of the retrofilling is performed after the surface has been dried with a Stropko Irrigator because it is more accurate to check the margins of the preparation when the beveled surface of the root is dry (Fig. 20.23). Materials such as ProRoot MTA are best delivered to the apical preparation with a carrier-based system (Fig. 20.24).

When placing ProRoot MTA, select a carrier that will fit into the apical preparation (Fig. 20.25). This will avoid spilling material into the bony crypt. As ProRoot MTA is cohesive to itself but only slightly adhesive to the walls of the preparation, care must be exerted to avoid pulling the material out of the preparation (Fig. 20.26). ProRoot MTA retrofilling is finished by wiping the beveled surface of the root with a moist cotton pellet (Fig. 20.27).

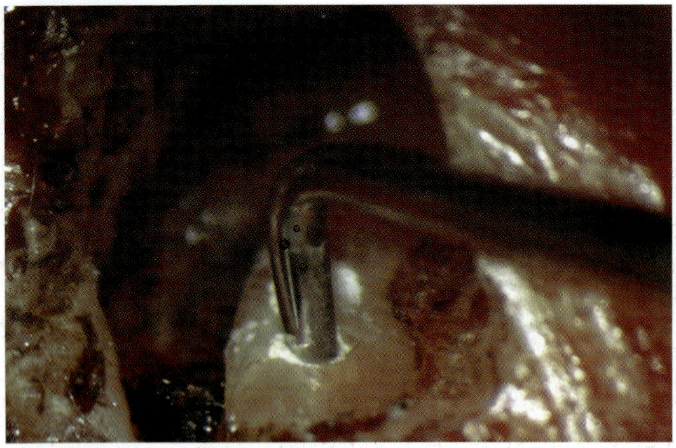

• **Fig. 20.22** Plugging SuperEBA into the apical preparation with a small plugger at ×16.

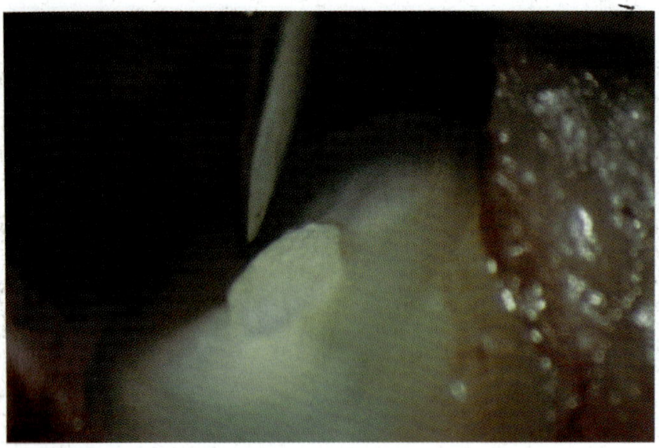

• **Fig. 20.23** Checking for marginal integrity with a CX-1 explorer at ×20.

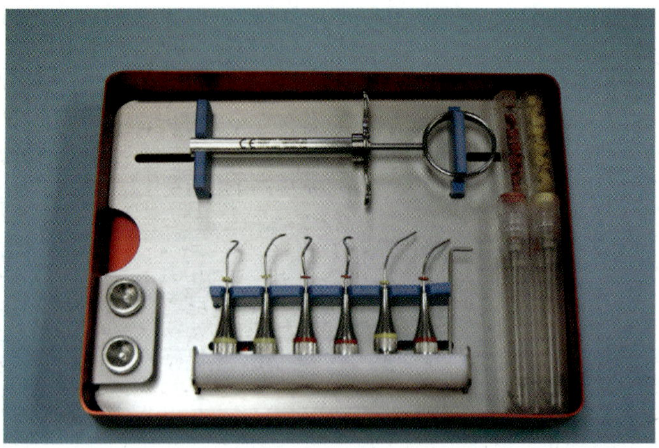

• **Fig. 20.24** Micro Apical Placement System.

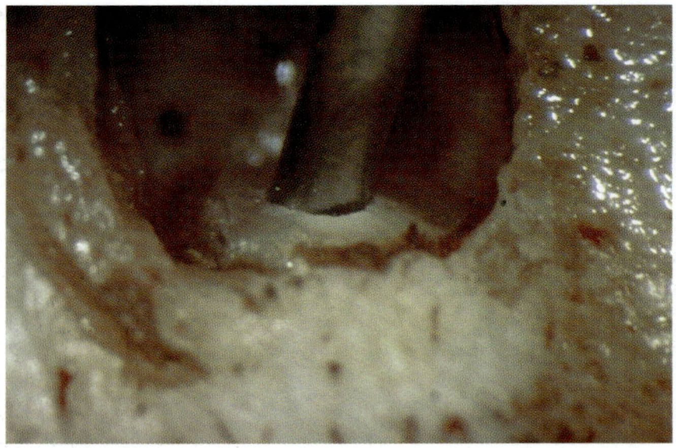

• **Fig. 20.25** MAP carrier placed inside the apical preparation at ×16.

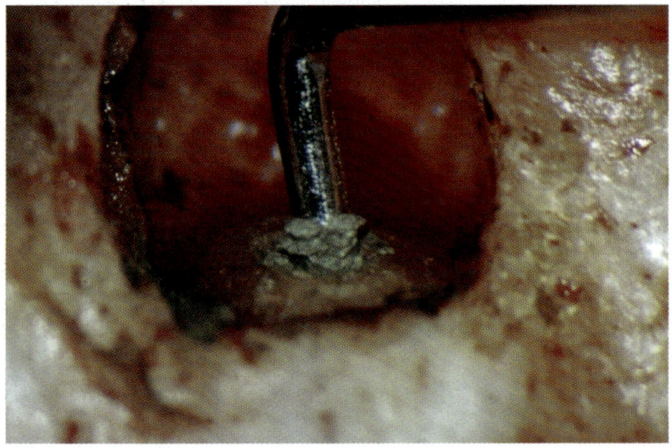

• **Fig. 20.26** ProRoot mineral trioxide aggregate (MTA) being pulled out of the apical preparation at ×16.

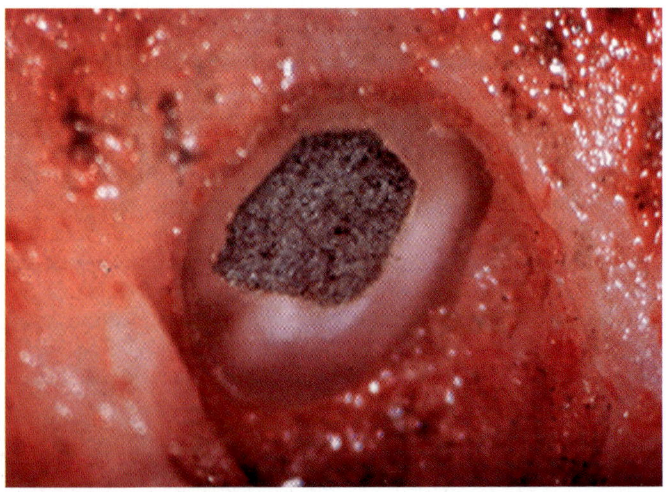

• **Fig. 20.27** Checking the marginal integrity mineral trioxide aggregate (MTA) after its application at ×20.

Placing Bone Grafts and Membranes

A frequently asked question is whether a bone graft should be placed in the bony crypt or a membrane placed over the surgical site as a matter of routine. According to the review paper by Lin et al., biologically a clot is a better space filler than all bone grafting materials as it contains the host's own biologic product to provide an excellent scaffold for wound healing. The best application of membrane barriers in periapical surgery appears to be in combined endodontic-periodontal lesions or large periapical lesions communicating with the alveolar crest. They also concluded that there is no conclusive evidence to demonstrate that the application of membrane barriers in large or through-and-through bony lesions has a better long-term outcome than a control group in periapical surgery. If formation of periradicular scaring is anticipated, a membrane can be placed for cosmetic reasons.

Dahlin et al. showed complete osseous healing of experimentally induced bone defects in rat jaws occurred after 6 weeks when polytetrafluorethylene (PTFE) membranes were placed on both sides of the defect.[34] Pecora and Andreana repeated the Dahlin study with calcium sulfate as a barrier and found the same results.[35] For further discussion of grafting procedures see the section on grafting in Chapter 21.

Flap Closure

The final stage of apical microsurgery is flap closure. Care must be taken to reapproximate the flap in order to promote healing by primary intention. Suturing is a critical part of flap closure. There are several suturing materials available. Parirokh et al. showed significantly more bacterial contamination and physical debris with silk sutures compared with polyvinylidene fluoride (PVDF), a monofilament suture, at 3, 5, and 7 days post placement.[36] However, PVDF is difficult to handle and needs to be pulled several times to erase the stiff memory. In addition, patients often complain that the tag ends of the suture are stiff and irritating to the oral mucosa.

Maxima PTFE (Henry Schein, NY, USA) is a PTFE coated monofilament suture that has handling properties similar to silk but produces less inflammation and contamination.

Although selection of suture material is important, it is also necessary to consider needle design. Reverse cutting needles have their cutting surfaces on the convex surface of the needle, making them ideal for suturing gingiva and oral mucosa. Maxima PTFE sutures are available with a laser cut premium needle that provides a smoother transition between the needle and the suture material, further reducing drag and tissue trauma.

Although the Adson tissue forceps can hold the flap firmly while suturing, newer instruments such as the Corn tissue forceps (Laschal Surgical Inc., Purchase, NY) are designed for precision needle placement (Fig. 20.28). The forceps grasp the tissue and the needle enters the tissue through an opening in the ends of the forceps.

There are a variety of needle holders available for the clinician. The recently introduced Baraquer needle holder (Laschal Surgical Inc., Purchase, NY) (Fig. 20.29) has an additional advantage in that it contains a small scissors that can also cut the suture.

Once the sutures are placed, the flap should be compressed with a saline soaked gauze and firm finger pressure for a minimum of 3 minutes. This will lessen the chance for the formation of a hematoma under the flap.

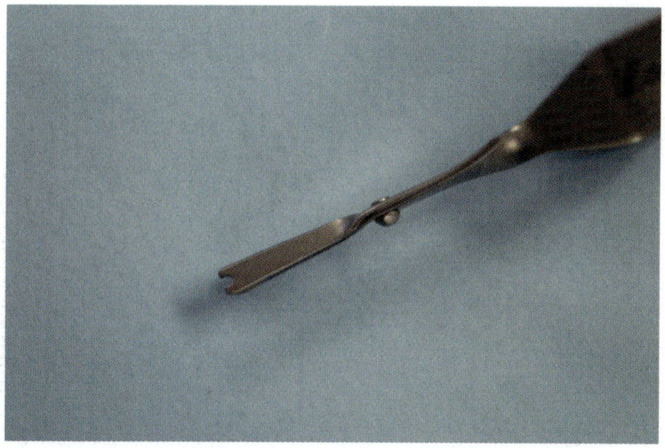

• **Fig. 20.28** Corn tissure forceps.

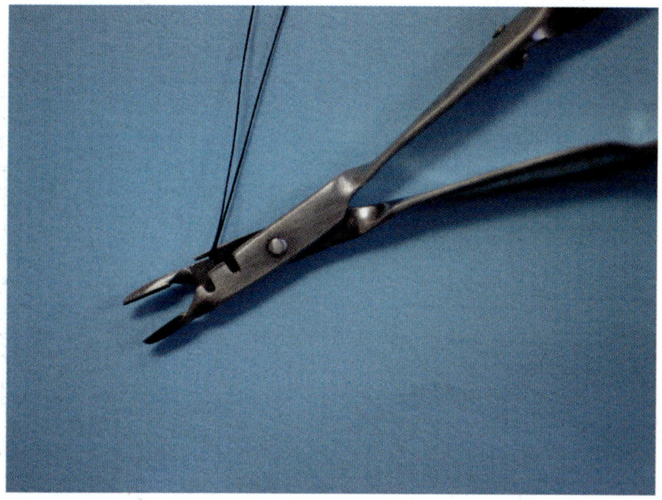

• **Fig. 20.29** Baraquer needle holder/scissors with suture material engaged in the scissor.

Postoperative Instructions

Both oral and written postoperative instructions should be given to the patient. Instructions should be written in simple, straightforward language. They should minimize patient anxiety arising from normal postoperative symptoms by describing how to promote healing and comfort.

A typical list of postoperative instructions is as follows:

1. Some swelling and discoloration are common. Use an ice pack with moderate pressure on the outside of your face (20 minutes on and 5 minutes off) until you go to bed tonight. Application of ice and pressure reduces bleeding and swelling and provides an analgesic effect.
2. Some oozing of blood is normal. If bleeding increases, place a moistened gauze pad or facial tissues over the area and apply finger pressure for 15 minutes. If bleeding continues, call the dentist's office.
3. Do not lift your lip or cheek to look at the area. The stitches are tied, and you may tear them out.
4. Starting tomorrow, dissolve 1 teaspoon of salt in a glass of warm water and gently rinse your mouth three or four times daily. Rinsing with a 0.12% chlorhexidine mouthwash may promote healing. Mouthwashes containing alcohol should be

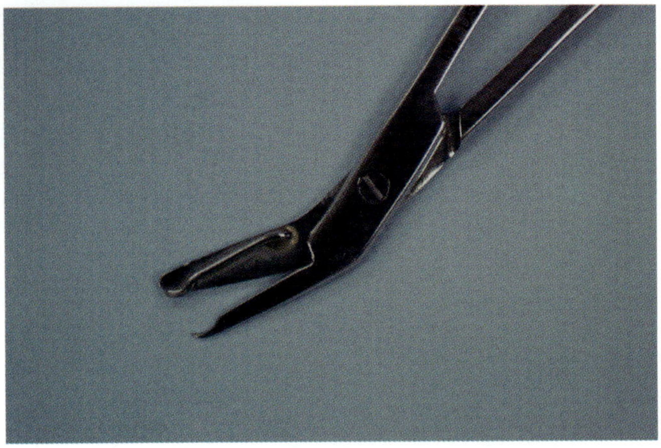

• **Fig. 20.30** Scissors/Forcepts Combo suture removal instrument.

avoided for the first several days after surgery. Careful brushing is important, but vigorous brushing may damage the area of surgery. Tonight you should brush and floss all areas except the surgery site. Tomorrow night you can carefully brush the surgery site.

5. Proper diet and fluid intake are essential after surgery. Eat a soft diet and chew on the opposite side of your mouth. Drink lots of fluids and eat soft foods such as cottage cheese, yogurt, eggs, and ice cream.
6. Pain is usually minimal after AS, and strong analgesics are normally not required. Some discomfort is normal. If pain medication was prescribed, follow the instructions. If no medication was prescribed, take your preferred nonprescription pain remedy if needed. If this is not sufficient, call the dentist's office.
7. If you are a smoker, do not smoke for the first 3 days after the procedure.
8. If you experience excessive swelling or pain or if you run a fever, call the dentist's office immediately.
9. Keep your appointment to have the stitches removed. (Sutures are removed 3 to 7 days after surgery.)
10. Call the dentist's office if you have any concerns or questions.

Suture Removal

The key to suture removal is in the healing of the epithelium. Harrison and Jurosky reported that a thin epithelial seal was established in the horizontal incisional wound at 24 hours and a multilayered epithelial seal was established in the vertical incisional wound between 24 and 48 hours.[37] Most clinicians would agree that sutures could be left in place for up to 7 days without causing significant soft tissue irritation.

Recently introduced for suture removal is the Scissors/Forceps Combo instrument (Fig. 20.30) (Laschal Surgical Inc., Purchase, NY). Safety ended suture scissors (Laschal Surgical Inc., Purchase, NY) have been designed to remove sutures that are buried in edematous or hypertrophic tissue.

Prognosis

Based on the results of several meta-analyses endodontic microsurgery enjoys high success rates ranging from 91.4% to 94.4%[38-53] (see Chapter 22).

Study Questions

6. Apical preparation evaluation was not possible before the introduction of:
   a. Stainless steel periapical ultrasonic tips
   b. Micromirrors
   c. Piezosurgery
   d. Diamond coated periapical ultrasonic tips
7. The most important factor in controlling bleeding is:
   a. The patient's health questionnaire
   b. Ferric sulfate
   c. Hemostatic gauze
   d. Electro-cautery
8. All of the following are bioceramic retrofilling materials except:
   a. ProRoot MTA
   b. EndoSequence Root Repair Material
   c. Amalgam
   d. Grey MTA Plus
9. According to Lin et al. the best material for a bone graft is:
   a. Calcium sulfate
   b. Allograft
   c. The patient's own blood clot
   d. Bioactive glass
10. The key to suture removal is:
   a. Postoperative instructions
   b. The healing of the epithelium
   c. Needle size
   c. The choice of the suture material

ANSWERS

Answers Box 20

1 b. Nonsurgical retreatment
2 c. Impact air handpiece
3 d. Do not have the skills
4 b. False
5 a. True
6 b. Micromirrors
7 a. The patient's health questionnaire
8 c. Amalgam
9 c. The patient's own blood clot
10 b. The healing of the epithelium

References

1. Iqbal MK, Kim S: For teeth requiring endodontic therapy, what are the differences in the outcomes of restored endodontically treated teeth compared to implant-supported restorations? *Int J Oral Maxillofac Implants* 221(Suppl):96–116, 2007.
2. Torabinejad M, Anderson P, Bader J, et al.: The outcomes of endodontic treatment, single implant, fixed partial denture and no tooth replacement: a systematic review, *JPD* 98:285–311, 2007.
3. Ng YL, Mann V, Gulabivala K: Tooth survival following non-surgical root canal treatment: a systematic review of the literature, *Int Endod J* 43:171–189, 2010.
4. Lazarski MP, Walker 3rd WA, Flores CM, et al.: Epidemiological evaluation of the outcomes of nonsurgical root canal treatment in a large cohort of insured dental patients, *J Endod* 27:791, 2001.
5. Salehrabi R, Rotstein I: Endodontic treatment outcomes in a large patient population in the USA: an epidemiological study, *J Endod* 30:846–850, 2004.
6. Chen S, Chueh L, Hsiao CK, et al.: An epidemiologic study of tooth retention after nonsurgical endodontic treatment in a large population in Taiwan, *J Endod* 33:226–229, 2007.

7. Raedel M, Hartmann A, Bohm S, Walter MH: Three-year outcomes of root canal treatment: mining an insurance database, *J Dent* 43(4):412–417, 2015.
8. Bernstein SD, Horowitz AJ, Man M, et al.: Outcomes of endodontic therapy in general practice: a study by the Practitioners Engaged in Applied Research and Learning Network, *J Am Dent Assoc* 143:478–487, 2012.
9. Gilbert GH, Tilashalski KR, Litaker MS, et al.: Outcomes of root canal treatment in Dental Practice-Based Research Network practices, *Gen Dent* 58:28–36, 2010.
10. Saville MH: Pre-Colombian decoration of teeth in Ecuador, *Am Anthropol* 15:377–394, 1913.
11. Andrews RR: Evidence of prehistoric dentistry in Central America, *Trans Pan Am Med Cong* 2:1872–1873, 1893.
12. Frank AL, Glick DH, Patterson SS, Weine FS: Long-term evaluation of surgically placed amalgam fillings, *J Endod* 18(8):391–398, 1992.
13. Gutmann JL, Harrison JW: Surgical endodontics. Boston, 1991, Blackwell.
14. Shabahang S: State of the art and science of endodontics, *J Am Dent Assoc* 136(1):41–52, 2005.
15. Veksler AE, Kayrouz GA, Newman MG: Reduction of salivary bacteria by pre-procedural rinses with chlorhexidine 0.12%, *J Periodontol* 62(11):649–651, 1991.
16. Lin LM, Gaengler P, Langeland K: Periradicular curettage, *Int Endod J* 29(4):220–227, 1996.
17. Nair PN: On the causes of persistent apical periodontitis: a review. *Int Endod J.* 39(4):249–281, 2006.
18. Weller RN, Niemczyk SP, Kim S: Incidence and position of the canal isthmus. Part 1. Mesiobuccal root of the maxillary first molar, *J Endod* 21(7):380–383, 1995.
19. West JD: *The relationship between the three-dimensional endodontic seal and endodontic failures*, Thesis. Boston University Goldman School of Graduate Dentistry, 1975.
20. Kim S PG, Rubinstein R: *Color atlas of microsurgery in endodontics*, Philadelphia, 2001, WB Saunders.
21. Layton CA, Marshall JG, Morgan LA, Baumgartner JC: Evaluation of cracks associated with ultrasonic root-end preparation, *J Endod* 22(4):157–160, 1996.
22. Beling KL, Marshall JG, Morgan LA, Baumgartner JC: Evaluation for cracks associated with ultrasonic root-end preparation of gutta-percha filled canals, *J Endod* 23(5):323–326, 1997.
23. Min MM, Brown Jr CE, Legan JJ, Kafrawy AH: In vitro evaluation of effects of ultrasonic root-end preparation on resected root surfaces, *J Endod* 23(10):624–628, 1997.
24. Morgan LA, Marshall JG: A scanning electron microscopic study of in vivo ultrasonic root-end preparations, *J Endod* 25(8):567–570, 1999.
25. Rainwater A, Jeansonne BG, Sarkar N: Effects of ultrasonic root-end preparation on microcrack formation and leakage, *J Endod* 26(2):72–75, 2000.
26. Carr G: Microscopes in endodontics, *J Calif Dent Assoc* 11:55, 1992.
27. Brent PD, Morgan LA, Marshall JG, Baumgartner JC: Evaluation of diamond-coated ultrasonic instruments for root-end preparation, *J Endod* 25(10):672–675, 1999.
28. Vercellotti T: Technological characteristics and clinical indications of piezoelectric bone surgery, *Minerva Stomatol* 53(5):207–214, 2004.
29. Gilheany PA, Figdor D, Tyas MJ: Apical dentin permeability and microleakage associated with root end resection and retrograde filling, *J Endod* 20(1):22–26, 1994.
30. Ricucci D, Siqueira Jr JF: Biofilms and apical periodontitis: study of prevalence and association with clinical and histopathologic findings, *J Endod* 36(8):1277–1288, 2010.
31. Siqueira JF: Reaction of periradicular tissues to root canal treatment: benefits and drawbacks, *Endodontic Topics* 10:123–147, 2005.
32. Nair PN, Henry S, Cano V, Vera J: Microbial status of apical root canal system of human mandibular first molars with primary apical periodontitis after "one-visit" endodontic treatment, *Oral Surg Oral Med Oral Pathol Oral Radiol Endod* 99(2):231–252, 2005.
33. Teixeira FB, Sano CL, Gomes BP, et al.: A preliminary in vitro study of the incidence and position of the root canal isthmus in maxillary and mandibular first molars, *Int Endod J* 36(4):276–280, 2003.
34. Mannocci F, Peru M, Sherriff M, et al.: The isthmuses of the mesial root of mandibular molars: a micro-computed tomographic study, *Int Endod J* 38(8):558–563, 2005.
35. Degerness R, Bowles W: Anatomic determination of the mesiobuccal root resection level in maxillary molars, *J Endod* 34(10):1182–1186, 2008.
36. Gutarts R, Nusstein J, Reader A, Beck M: In vivo debridement efficacy of ultrasonic irrigation following hand-rotary instrumentation in human mandibular molars, *J Endod* 31(3):166–170, 2005.
37. Abella F, de Ribot J, Doria G, et al.: Applications of piezoelectric surgery in endodontic surgery: a literature review, *J Endod* 40(3):325–332, 2014.
38. Baldi D, Menini M, Pera F, et al.: Sinus floor elevation using osteotomes or piezoelectric surgery, *Int J Oral Maxillofac Surg* 40(5):497–503, 2011.
39. Walmsley AD, Laird WR, Williams AR: Dental plaque removal by cavitational activity during ultrasonic scaling, *J Clin Periodontol* 15(9):539–543, 1988.
40. Farrar JN: Radical and heroic treatment of alveolar abscess by amputation of roots of teeth, with description and application of the cantilever crown, *The Dental Cosmos* 26(3):135–139, 1884.
41. Oynick J, Oynick T: A study of a new material for retrograde fillings, *J Endod* 4(7):203–206, 1978.
42. Song M, Shin SJ, Kim E: Outcomes of endodontic micro-resurgery: a prospective clinical study, *J Endod* 37(3):316–320, 2011.
43. Omnell KA: Electrolytic precipitation of zinc carbonate in the jaw; an unusual complication after root resection, *Oral Surg Oral Med Oral Pathol* 12(7):846–852, 1959.
44. Dahlin C, Linde A, Gottlow J, Nyman S: Healing of bone defects by guided tissue regeneration, *Plast Reconstr Surg* 81(5):672–676, 1988.
45. Pecora G, Andreana S, Margarone 3rd JE, et al.: Bone regeneration with a calcium sulfate barrier, *Oral Surg Oral Med Oral Pathol Oral Radiol Endod* 84(4):424–429, 1997.
46. Parirokh M, Asgary S, Eghbal MJ, et al.: A scanning electron microscope study of plaque accumulation on silk and PVDF suture materials in oral mucosa, *Int Endod J* 37(11):776–781, 2004.
47. Harrison JW, Jurosky KA: Wound healing in the tissues of the periodontium following periradicular surgery. I. The incisional wound, *J Endod* 17(9):425–435, 1991.
48. Setzer FC, Shah S, Kohli M, et al.: Outcome of endodontic surgery: a meta-analysis of the literature—part 1: comparison of traditional root-end surgery and endodontic microsurgery, *J Endod* 36:1757, 2010.
49. Setzer FC, Kohli M, Shah S, et al.: Outcome of endodontic surgery: a meta-analysis of the literature - part 2: comparison of endodontic microsurgical techniques with and without the use of higher magnification, *J Endod* 38:1, 2012.
50. Tsesis I, Rosen E, Taschieri S, et al.: Outcomes of surgical endodontic treatment performed by a modern technique: an updated meta-analysis of the literature, *J Endod* 39:332, 2013.
51. Kohli MR, Berenji H, Setzer FC, et al.: Outcome of endodontic surgery: a meta-analysis of the literature-part 3: comparison of endodontic microsurgical techniques with 2 different root-end filling materials, *J Endod* 44:923, 2018.
52. Torabinejad M, Dinsbach N, Turman M, et al.: Survival of intentionally replanted teeth and implant-supported single crowns: a systemic review, *J Endod* 41:992–998, 2015.
53. Torabinejad M, Landaez M, Milan M, et al.: Tooth retention through endodontic microsurgery or tooth replacement using single implants: a systematic review of treatment outcomes, *J Endod* 41:1–10, 2015.

21 Adjunctive Procedures

MAHMOUD TORABINEJAD AND MOHAMMAD SABETI

CHAPTER OUTLINE

LEARNING OBJECTIVES

After reading this chapter, the student should be able to:

1. Discuss the role of adjunctive endodontic surgery in patient treatment planning.
2. Recognize situations in which adjunctive surgical procedures are the treatments of choice.
3. Define the terms incision and drainage, root resection, hemisection, crown lengthening, tooth replantation, tooth transplantation, and socket preservation.
4. Discuss the indications for each procedure listed in objective 3.
5. Describe in brief the step-by-step procedures involved in objective 3.
6. Discuss the prognosis for each procedure listed in objective 3.

Introduction

Adjunctive surgical procedures are those that are used to treat either pathologic conditions or mishaps that occur during root canal treatment. One of the pathologic conditions that requires an adjunctive procedure is an incision for drainage for acute apical abscesses. As discussed in Chapter 18, most procedural accidents can be corrected nonsurgically. When nonsurgical correction is not feasible or impractical, these conditions are treated surgically, as discussed in Chapter 20. Adjunctive surgical procedures are additional. So it is additional treatment modalities to treatment modalities prevent tooth loss and preserve natural dentition. The purpose of this chapter is to discuss the indications, contraindications, procedures involved, and prognosis for some of these procedures such as incision for drainage, root resection, hemisection, crown lengthening, tooth replantation, and transplantation. In addition, principles and materials for socket preservation after extraction using regenerative techniques and guided bone regeneration (GBR) will be discussed.

Incision for Drainage

The objective of incision for drainage is to remove inflammatory exudates and purulence from a soft tissue swelling. Incision for drainage reduces discomfort resulting from the buildup of pressure and speeds healing.

Indications

The best treatment for swelling originating from an acute apical abscess of pulpal origin is to establish drainage through the offending tooth (Fig. 21.1, *A*). When adequate drainage cannot be accomplished through the tooth itself, drainage is obtained through soft tissue incision. Drainage through the soft tissue is accomplished most effectively when the swelling is fluctuant. A fluctuant swelling is a fluid-containing mass in which a wavelike sensation is felt when pressure is applied (Fig. 21.1, *B*). Incising a fluctuant swelling releases purulence immediately and provides rapid relief. If the swelling is nonfluctuant or firm, incision for drainage often results in drainage of only blood and serous fluids. Incision and drainage of a nonfluctuant abscess reduces pressure and facilitates healing by reducing irritants and increasing circulation in the area.

Contraindications

There are relatively few contraindications to the use of incision for drainage. Patients with prolonged bleeding or clotting times or those who are on bisphosphonates must be approached with caution, and hematologic screening is often indicated. An abscess in or near an anatomic space should be handled very carefully.

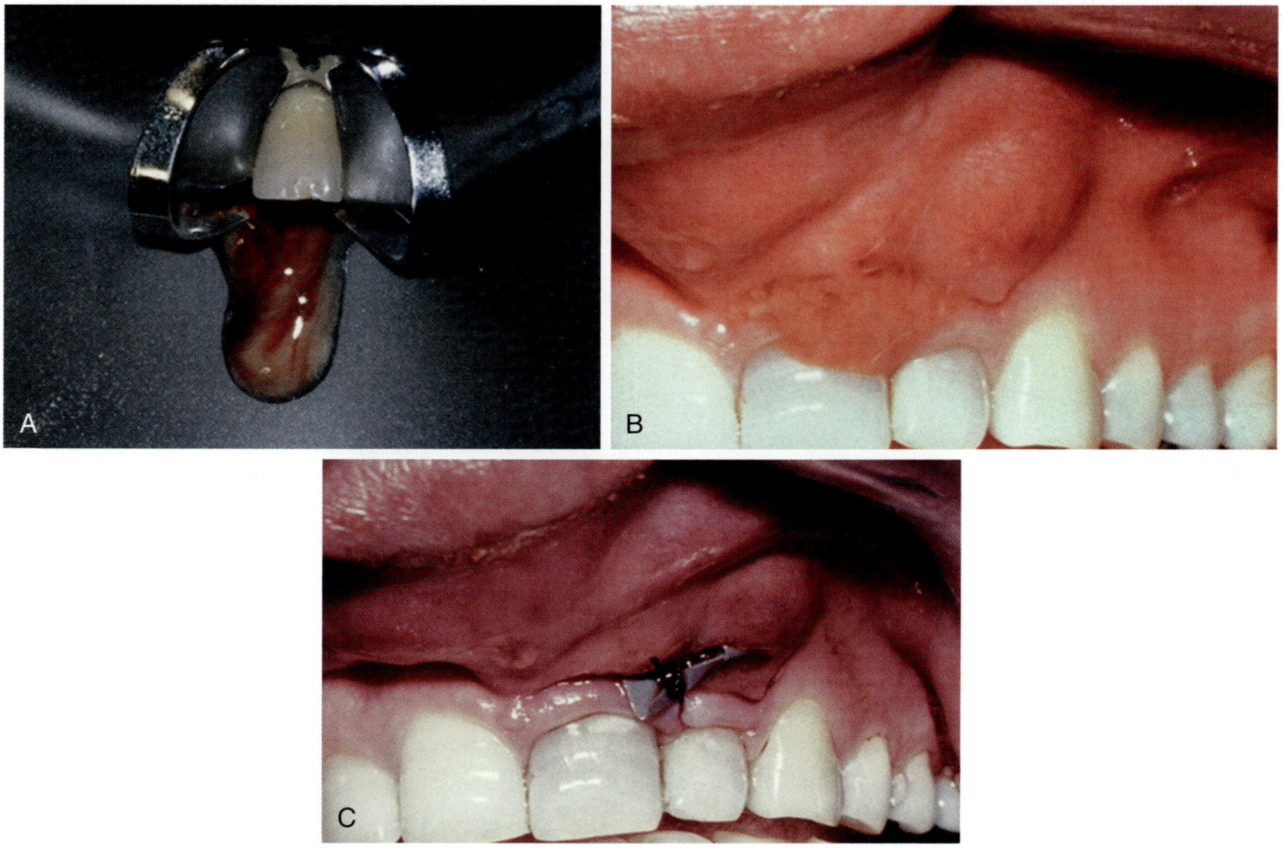

• **Fig. 21.1** **(A)** Establishment of drainage through an offending tooth. **(B)** A fluctuant swelling is present because of the presence of an infection in the right lateral incisor. **(C)** An incision for drainage is performed and a rubber drain is sutured in place to prevent immediate closure of the incision.

Procedures

Anesthesia

Profound anesthesia is sometimes difficult to obtain in the presence of inflammation, swelling, or exudates. Because direct subperiosteal infiltration is ineffective and may be quite painful, regional block anesthetic techniques are preferred. Mandibular blocks for posterior areas, bilateral mental blocks for the anterior mandible, posterior superior alveolar blocks for the posterior maxilla, and infraorbital blocks for the premaxilla area are the preferred choices. These injections may be supplemented by regional infiltration.

In addition to block anesthesia, one of the following methods may also be used. The first technique is infiltration that starts peripheral to the swelling. After the application of topical anesthetic, the solution is injected slowly with limited pressure and depth, and this is followed by additional injections in previously anesthetized tissue, moving progressively closer to the center of the swelling. This procedure results in improved anesthesia without extreme discomfort.

The second technique is the use of topical ethyl chloride. A stream of this solution is directed onto the swelling from a distance, permitting the liquid to volatilize on the tissue surface. Within seconds, the tissue at the site of volatilization turns white. The incision is quickly accomplished with continued ethyl chloride spray. This topical anesthesia is a supplement to block anesthesia when a quick incision is required. If none of these procedures work, nitrous oxide/oxygen sedation or intravenous (IV) sedation can be used for incision and drainage.

Incision

After anesthesia, the incision is made vertically with a No. 11 scalpel (Fig. 9-6C). Vertical incisions are parallel with the major blood vessels and nerves and leave very little scarring. The incision should be made firmly through periosteum to bone. If the swelling is fluctuant, pus usually flows immediately, followed by blood. If the swelling is nonfluctuant, the predominant drainage is blood.

Drainage

After the initial incision, a small closed hemostat may be placed in the incision and then opened to enlarge the draining tract (Fig. 9-6D). This procedure is indicated with more extensive swellings. To maintain a path for drainage, an I-shaped or "Christmas tree" drain cut from a rubber dam or a piece of iodoform gauze can be placed (suturing is optional) in the incision (Fig. 21.1, C). The drain should be removed after 2 to 3 days; if it is not sutured, the patient may remove the drain at home.

Root Resection

Root resection is removal of the whole or part of a root from any multirooted tooth. This operation is usually performed in maxillary molars, but it can also be done in mandibular molars.[1]

Indications

The main indication for root resection is presence of severe bone loss in a periodontally involved root that cannot be treated by periodontal

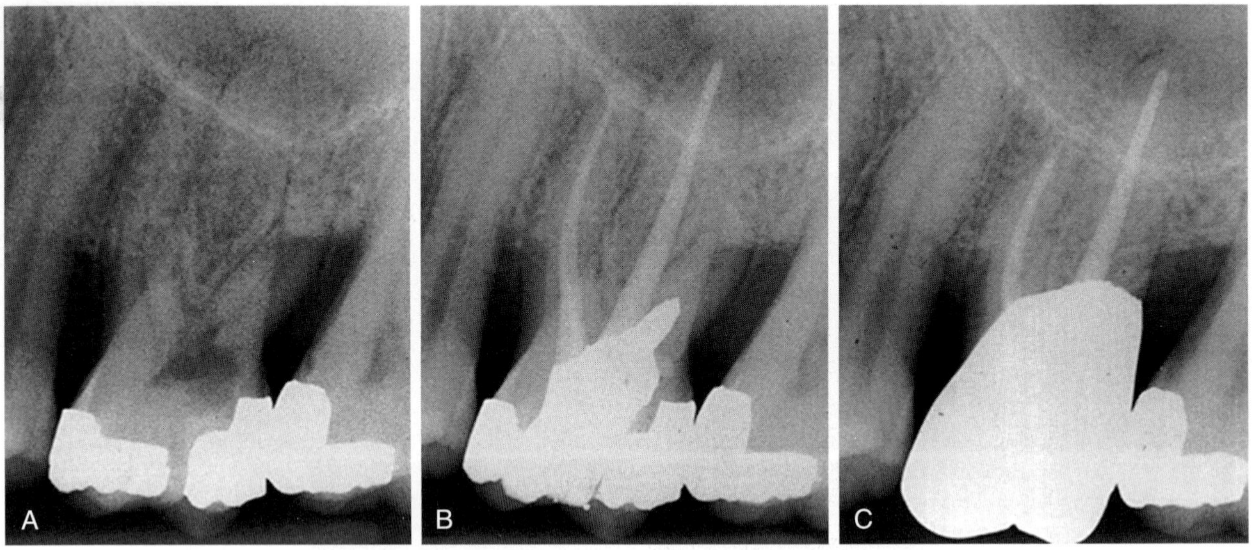

• **Fig. 21.2 (A)** A maxillary molar with severe bone loss around the distobuccal root. **(B)** Root canal treatment was followed by an amalgam core extending 3 to 4 mm into the distobuccal canal. **(C)** The root was amputated, and a crown subsequently placed.

treatment. In addition, root resection is indicated for root(s) of multirooted teeth with severe caries, resorption, vertical root fracture, or untreatable procedural accidents in the furcation of multirooted teeth.

Contraindications

Root resection is contraindicated when there is insufficient bony support for the remaining root(s), patients on bisphosphonates, and in the presence of fused roots.

Procedures

Root resection can be performed with and without a surgical flap. Raising a surgical flap provides better visibility for the operator. After raising a flap, root resection is performed using a fissure bur to cut the involved root and separating it from the crown. The remaining stump should be contoured to the surface of the crown, providing the patient a good hygiene (Fig. 21.2). The prognosis for root resection has been reported as fair to good depending on case selection, patient hygiene, and motivation.[1]

Hemisection

Hemisection is the surgical division of a multirooted tooth into two segments. It is usually performed in mandibular molars and in rare occasions in maxillary molars. The indications and contraindications for hemisection are similar to those for root resection.[2-6]

Procedures

Like in root resection, hemisection can be performed with and without a surgical flap. After raising a flap, a vertical cut is made through the crown into the furcation using a fissure bur. The initial cut should be made close and at the expense of the unsalvageable root. The tooth is sectioned through the bifurcation. The unsalvageable root is then removed. The anatomic crown of the remaining root(s) should then be contoured to the surface of the root without any ledges. This action provides good, smooth margins for the prosthetic crown and adequate access for good hygiene by the patient (Fig. 21.3). The success rates of teeth that have had root amputation or hemisection has been reported to be 70% to 85%.[3,4] Like root resection, the main factors affecting the long-term success of this procedure are case selection and the patient's oral hygiene.[3,5,6]

Crown Lengthening

Although clinicians often prefer supragingival margin placement, some situations like presence of subgingival decay, crown fracture, root perforation, short clinical crown, tooth hypersensitivity, or esthetic demands may dictate subgingival margin for placement of restoration. Placing restoration margins below gingiva can cause persistent gingival inflammation and eventually tooth loss.[7-11] To prevent these complications and establish biological width, crown lengthening can be performed either surgically or nonsurgically. Surgical crown lengthening (SCL) usually consists of removal of soft and/or hard tissues to achieve a longer clinical crown and reestablish the proper biologic width dimensions around a tooth.

Indications

SCL is indicated for teeth with a short natural clinical crown and shortened clinical crown resulting from the presence of pathologic conditions such as extensive decay, resorption, iatrogenic perforation, or crown fracture extending subgingivally.[12-13] SCL is indicated when the operator expects that the final restorative margin will be located less than 3 mm from the alveolar bone crest.

Contraindications

SCL is contraindicated for medical reasons, patients on bisphosphonates, when the procedure could result in exposure of a tooth furcation, or it is near vital anatomic structures such maxillary sinus or mental foramen and for teeth in the esthetic zone, when the procedure results in the presence of a long clinical crown for only one tooth.[13]

Procedures

SCL is typically accomplished by either gingivectomy or placing gingival tissue flap apically with or without bone removal.

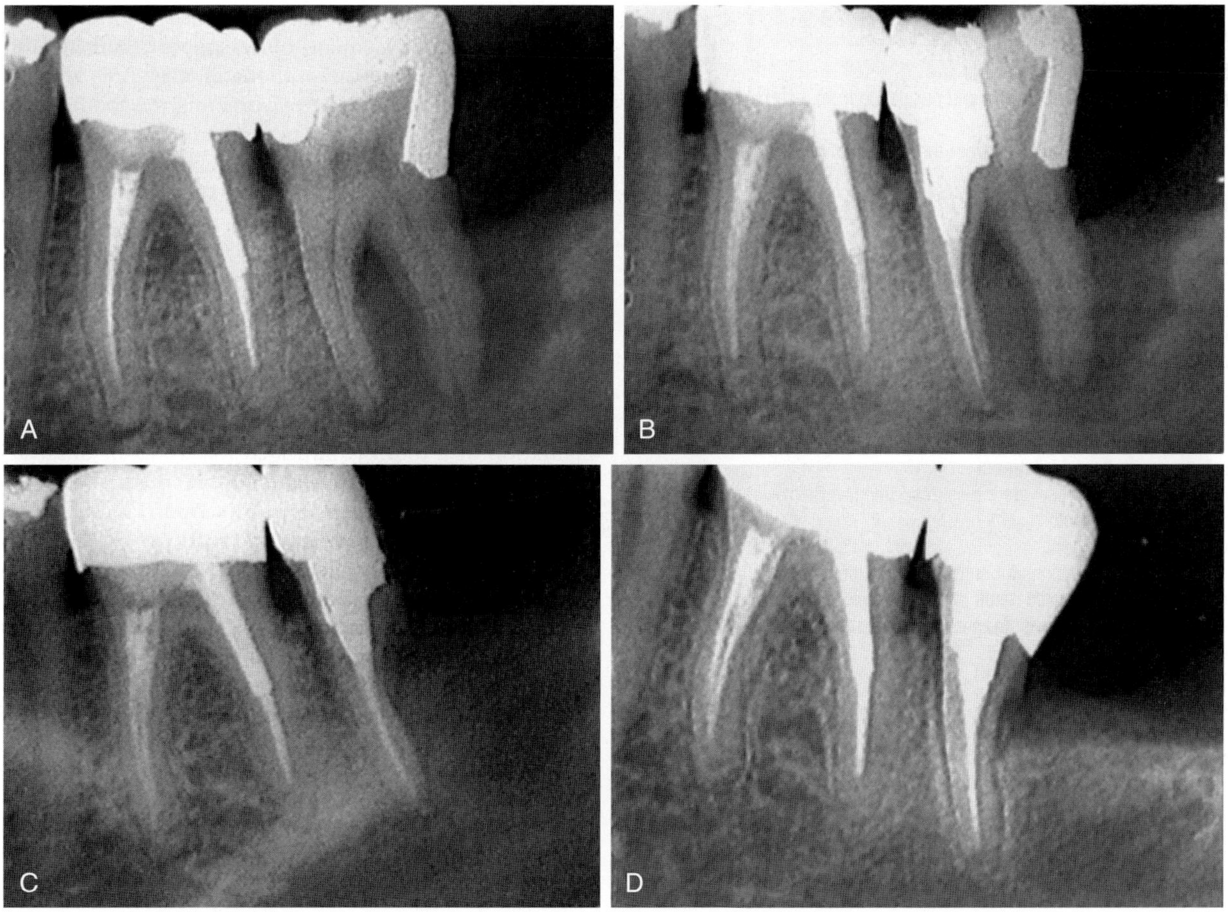

• **Fig. 21.3** **(A)** A mandibular second molar with severe bone loss around distal root. **(B)** A postoperative radiograph after root canal treatment on the mesial roots and placing an amalgam core. **(C)** A postoperative radiograph after performing hemisection. **(D)** A postoperative radiograph 2 years later.

After raising a full-thickness flap, a submarginal incision is performed. Then, soft and hard tissues are removed, and the flap is sutured in the appropriate level to allow reestablishment of the epithelial and connective tissue attachment and for allowance of enough tooth structure for adequate support of the planned restoration (Fig. 21.4). The mean survival rates of SCL procedure have been reported at 83% after 10 years.[14] However, a recent systematic review with limited data concludes that SCL can result in increased crown length and possible gingival margin rebound.[15]

Root Extrusion

An alternative to SCL is orthodontic extrusion or forced eruption.[16,17]

Indications and Contraindications

Root extrusion is indicated for any tooth with horizontal crown or root fractures, decay, resorption, or accidental perforations that extend below the crestal bone 0 to 4 mm.[17] The contraindications for root extrusion are short roots, insufficient space to extrude the root, and periodontal disease.[17]

Procedures

If there is enough tooth structure available after root canal treatment, brackets are placed on the incisal third of the crown of the involved tooth and the adjacent teeth. Vertical force is applied to the involved tooth by placing elastic bands on the adjacent teeth and connecting them to the endodontically treated tooth with inadequate coronal structure (Fig. 21.5). When there is not enough coronal tooth structure available, a paper clip is cemented with intermediate restorative material (IRM) in the coronal portion of the root canal treated tooth. After cementing a horizontal wire on the adjacent teeth, vertical force is applied to the involved tooth by placing elastic bands from the paper clip in the root canal-treated tooth and the horizontal wire. Because of light extrusion forces, the tooth and the entire periodontal attachment apparatus will move coronally. This procedure may take 2 to 4 weeks. After accomplishing adequate extrusion, the tooth must be stabilized for at least 2 months before placing a final restoration[17] (Fig. 21.6). This treatment can also be expedited with fiberotomy. When performed, the marginal bone level will mostly stay in the original position.[18]

The disadvantages of orthodontic root extrusion include esthetic issues during the procedure, required time to accomplish ideal results, and surgical fiberotomy after root extrusion. Because of these disadvantages, surgical extrusion (Fig. 21.7) has been suggested as an alternative to crown lengthening by orthodontic extrusion.[19] The surgical extrusion consists of extraction and stabilization of the extracted tooth for 4 to 6 weeks and its concept is based on information from the dental trauma literature regarding treatment of extrusive luxation.

Study Questions

1. The objectives of incision for drainage are:
   a. Remove inflammatory exudates and purulence from a soft tissue swelling
   b. It reduces discomfort resulting from the buildup of pressure
   c. Speeds healing
   d. Increasing circulation in the area
   e. None of the above
   f. All of the above
2. What are the contraindications for incision and drainage?
   a. Patients with prolonged bleeding or clotting times
   b. An abscess in or near an anatomic space should be handled very carefully
   c. Patient with fluctuant swelling and a fluid-containing mass
   d. A and B
3. What are the main indications for root resection?
   a. Severe bone loss in a periodontally involved root that cannot be treated by periodontal treatment
   b. Multirooted teeth with severe caries, resorption, vertical root fracture
   c. Presence of fused roots
   d. A and B
4. What are the contraindications for surgical crown lengthening?
   a. When the procedure could result in exposure of a tooth furcation
   b. Proximity to vital anatomic structures such as maxillary sinus or mental foramen
   c. None of the above
   d. A and B
5. What are the indications for root extrusion?
   a. Any tooth with horizontal crown or root fractures
   b. Any tooth with decay and resorption
   c. Short roots
   d. A and B

Tooth Replantation

Tooth replantation is the reinsertion of a tooth into its own alveolar socket after performing apical surgery out of the socket.[20] This procedure is indicated when an apical surgery is contraindicated or very difficult to perform and is the last treatment option to save a tooth (Fig. 21.8).

There are several factors that affect the clinical success of intentional replantation. They include: age, sex, type of tooth replanted, presence of fractures, stage of root development, status of surrounding alveolar bone, contamination of the replanted tooth, cleansing procedure, and antibiotic therapy.[21]

The apical size (correlated with age) and the length of time the tooth has been out of the socket are, respectively, two of the most important factors to determine prognosis.[22] The success factor for intentional replantation stems from the ability of the replanted tooth to be integrated back into the body in a timely fashion. The timeliness relates directly to the viability of the surrounding mesenchymal cells around the implanted tooth. Teeth that have been dried out have minimal capability to revascularize or regenerate any of the mesenchymal cells in the periodontal ligament or cementum, which are vital for the success of reimplantation.

The adverse effects of replantation include surface resorption and ankylosis; these signs are typically observed within 12 months after replantation.[23] There is a noticeably higher success rate with implant supported crowns than with intentionally replanted teeth: 97% and 88%, respectively.[24] Although the data show much more predictable results with implants, intentional replantation is still considered a reliable procedure and should be considered as a treatment option to patients for those that are seeking to maintain their dentition.[25]

Tooth replantation is contraindicated for teeth that are not restorable, have inadequate bony support, and are difficult to extract. Patients on bisphosphonates may not be good candidates for this procedure. After extracting the tooth with minimal trauma, the apical surgery is performed outside of the mouth and then the tooth is reinserted into its original socket.[24] Tooth replantation has a long history in dentistry.[26] When properly planned and performed, tooth replantation has been shown to be quite successful (mean survival of 88%).

Transplantation

Transplantation is extraction of an erupted, embedded, or impacted tooth from one part of the mouth into an extraction site or surgically prepared recipient site within the same individual.[20] Transplantation of a tooth is indicated for either an unsalvageable or missing tooth.[27,28] It is contraindicated if the transplanted tooth is not restorable, has inadequate bony support, is difficult to extract, and does not fit the recipient site. Patients on bisphosphonates are not be good candidates for transplantation. Ideally, root canal treatment should be performed on the transplanted tooth before this procedure. After extracting the unsalvageable tooth and preparing the socket for transplantation of a new tooth, the extracted healthy tooth is extracted with minimal trauma and damage to the periodontium. An apical surgery is performed on the extracted tooth outside of the mouth, and then the tooth is reinserted into its new socket (Fig. 21.9). During tooth transplantation, the tooth must be kept in moist gauze to prevent dehydration and necrosis of the periodontal ligament. When appropriately indicated and performed, transplanted teeth have a good prognosis.[28]

Guided Tissue Regeneration and Guided Bone Regeneration in Endodontics

Guided tissue regeneration (GTR), as a technique, follows from observations that the type of tissue that forms the attachment to an exposed root surface is a result of the types of cells that first populate the area.[29] A long junctional epithelium will form from advancing epithelial tissues, root resorption may occur from advancing gingival connective tissue, resorption and ankylosis follows from bone in contact to the root surface and, finally, if periodontal ligament (PDL) cells propagate, a connective tissue attachment may form. As an ideal outcome, PDL cells will lead to an appropriately oriented new connective tissue attachment and subsequent bone formation. Early studies showed that preserved PDL tissues on the extracted teeth of dogs auto-implanted into areas of the jaw promoted healing, and thus a functionally oriented connective tissue attachment. In practice, GTR is often used for cases where periodontitis has led to significant clinical attachment loss. With the addition of bone grafting, GBR can be used in concert with GTR to fill bony defects. Generally, after surgical exposure of the areas of clinical attachment loss with a bony defect and débridement of the exposed root surface, bone grafting material is placed with a barrier to prevent the apical migration of gingival epithelium and the formation of gingival connective tissue, root resorption, or ankylosis. Thus PDL fibers will be allowed to form a proper connective tissue attachment with alveolar bone filling in the space.[30] It is worth noting that epithelial derived cells migrate up to 10 times faster than other periodontally derived cells, thus these types of cells must be prevented from apical migration by use of a barrier to allow the cells with regenerative potential (the PDL cells) to proliferate.[31]

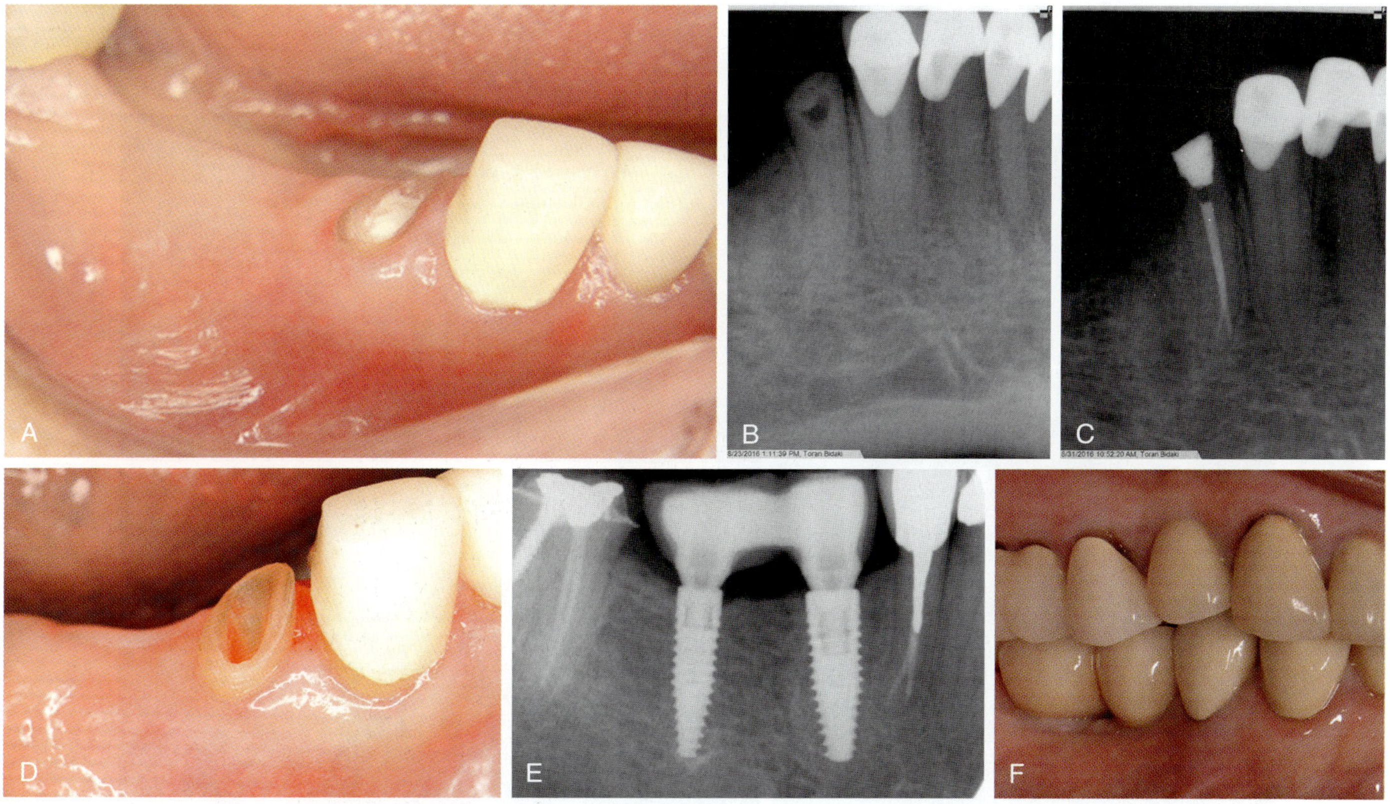

• **Fig. 21.4** **(A)** Clinical appearance of mandibular first premolar tooth requiring crown lengthening surgery. **(B)** A preoperative radiograph of the same tooth showing presence of adequate root canal treatment. **(C)** A postoperative radiograph after root canal treatment. **(D)** A postoperative clinical appearance of the same tooth after crown lengthening procedure. Note increase in supragingival tooth structure compared with **A**. **(E)** Postoperative radiograph after restoration of that tooth with post and a crown and placement of two implants in the edentulous area. **(F)** A postoperative clinical appearance of the region after restoration. (Courtesy of Dr. Brian Goodacre.)

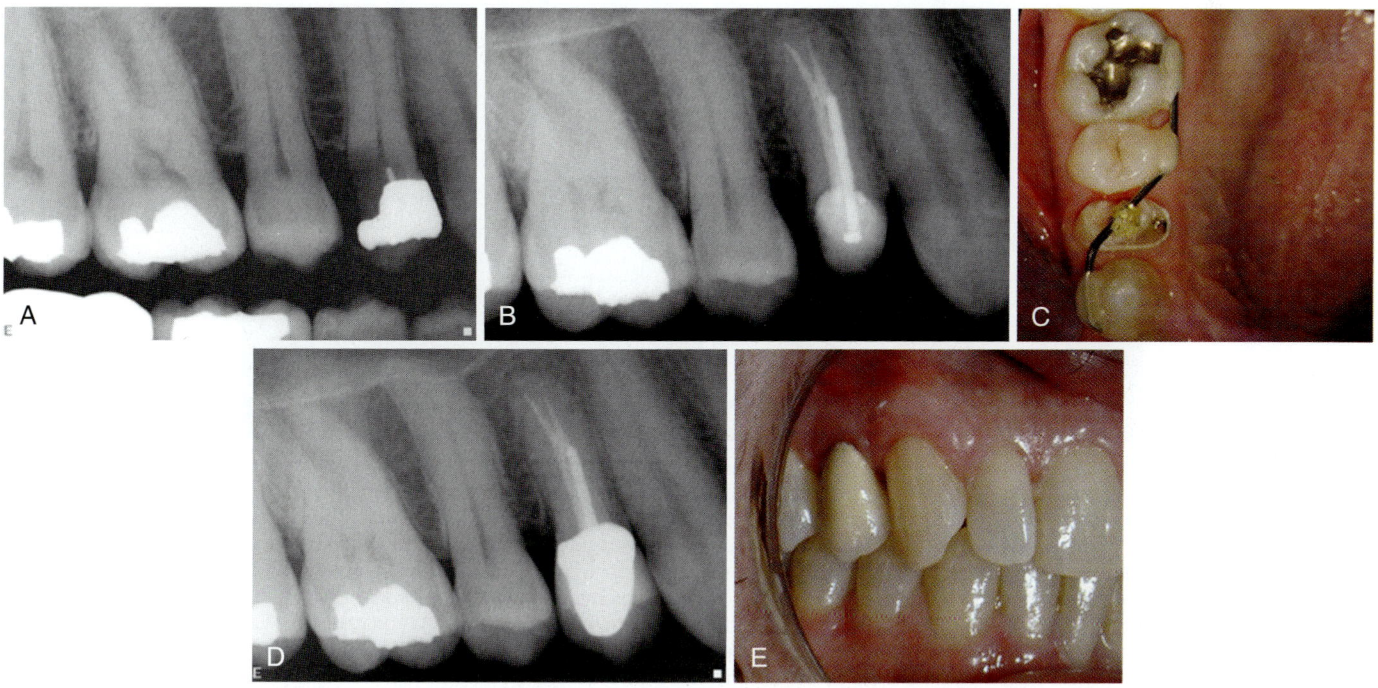

• **Fig. 21.5** **(A)** A preoperative radiograph of a maxillary first premolar with an inadequate clinical crown for restoration. **(B)** A radiograph showing completed root canal treatment on this tooth. **(C)** A clinical photograph of placement of extrusion apparatus to extrude the tooth orthodontically. **(D)** A postoperative radiograph after extrusion of this tooth. **(E)** Postoperative radiograph after root canal treatment, extrusion, and placement of a crown 15 months after completion of the procedures. (Courtesy of Dr. M. Pouresmail.)

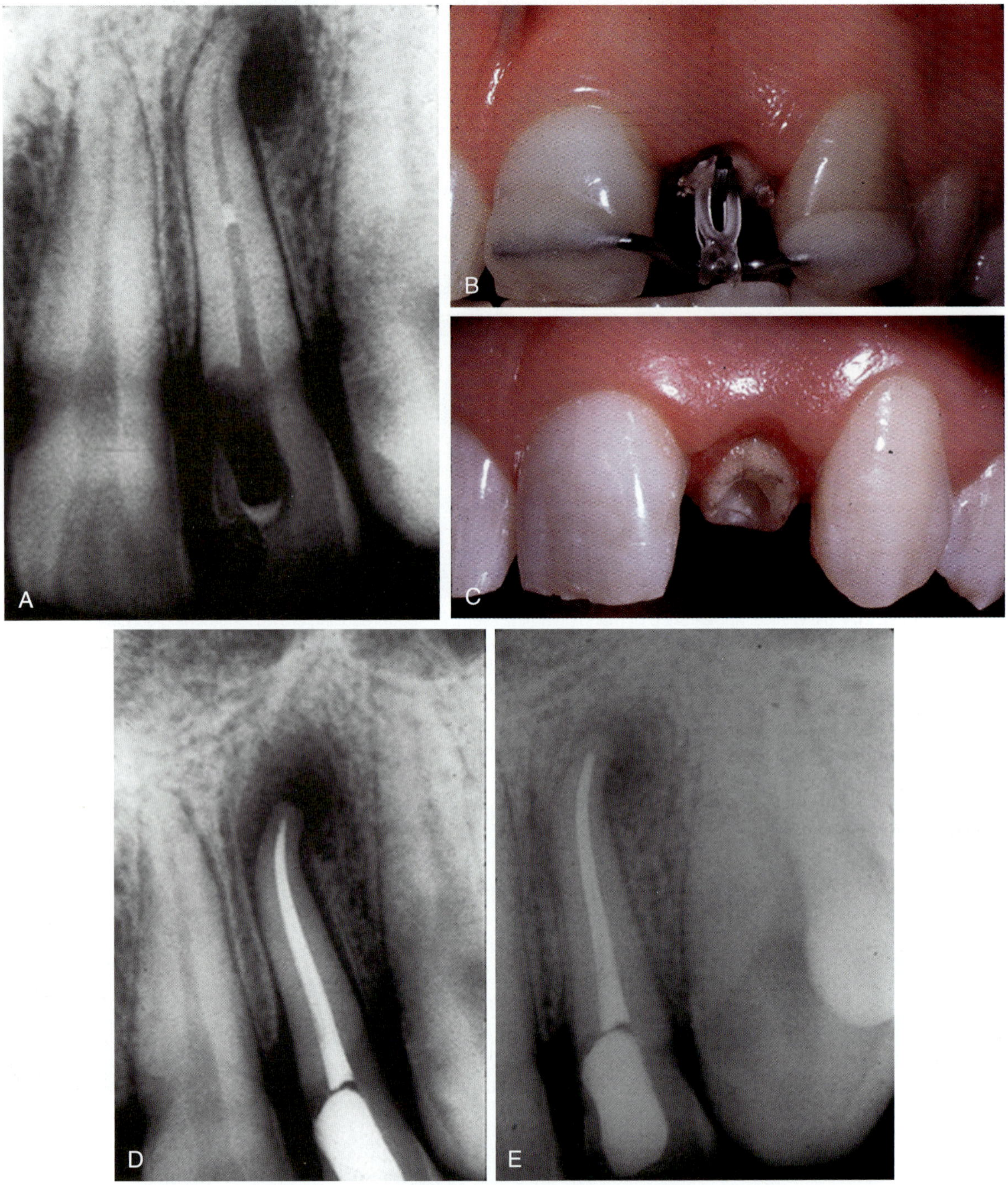

• **Fig. 21.6** **(A)** A preoperative radiograph of a maxillary lateral incisor with severe cervical decay with an inadequate clinical crown for restoration. **(B)** After completing root canal treatment, a paper clip is cemented with intermediate restorative material (IRM) in the coronal portion of the root canal treated tooth. After cementing a horizontal wire on the adjacent teeth, vertical force is applied to the involved tooth by placing elastic bands from the paper clip in the root canal treated tooth and the horizontal wire. **(C)** Because application of light extrusion forces for 4 weeks has resulted in the movement of the tooth and the gingiva, a gingivectomy has been performed to expose the root completely. **(D)** A postoperative radiograph after extrusion of this tooth. **(E)** A postoperative radiograph after root canal treatment, extrusion, and placement of a crown 15 months after completion of the procedures.

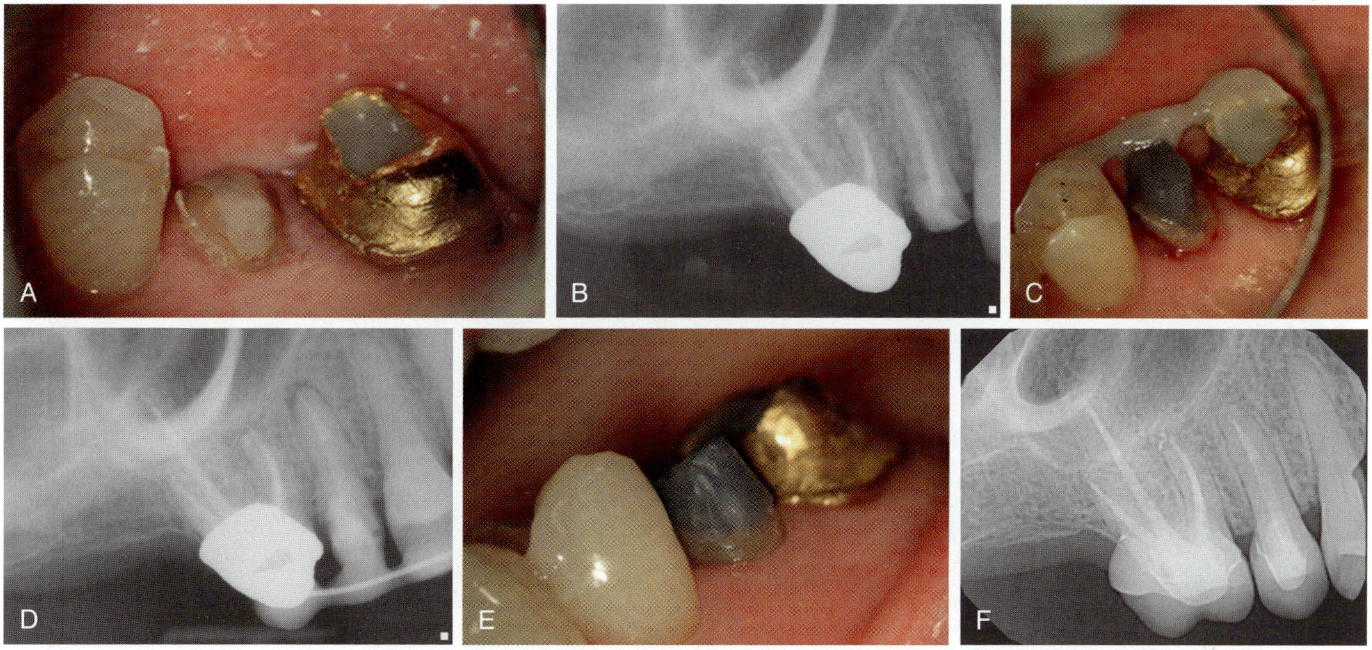

• **Fig. 21.7** **(A)** A preoperative photograph of a maxillary second premolar with an inadequate clinical crown for restoration. **(B)** A radiograph showing this tooth has adequate root canal treatment. **(C)** A clinical photograph of this tooth after surgical extrusion and splinting it to the adjacent teeth. **(D)** A postoperative radiograph after extrusion and splinting of this tooth. **(E)** A clinical photograph of this tooth 3 weeks later. **(F)** A postoperative radiograph after extrusion and placement of a crown 4 months after completion of the procedures. (Courtesy of Dr. Rajiv Patel.)

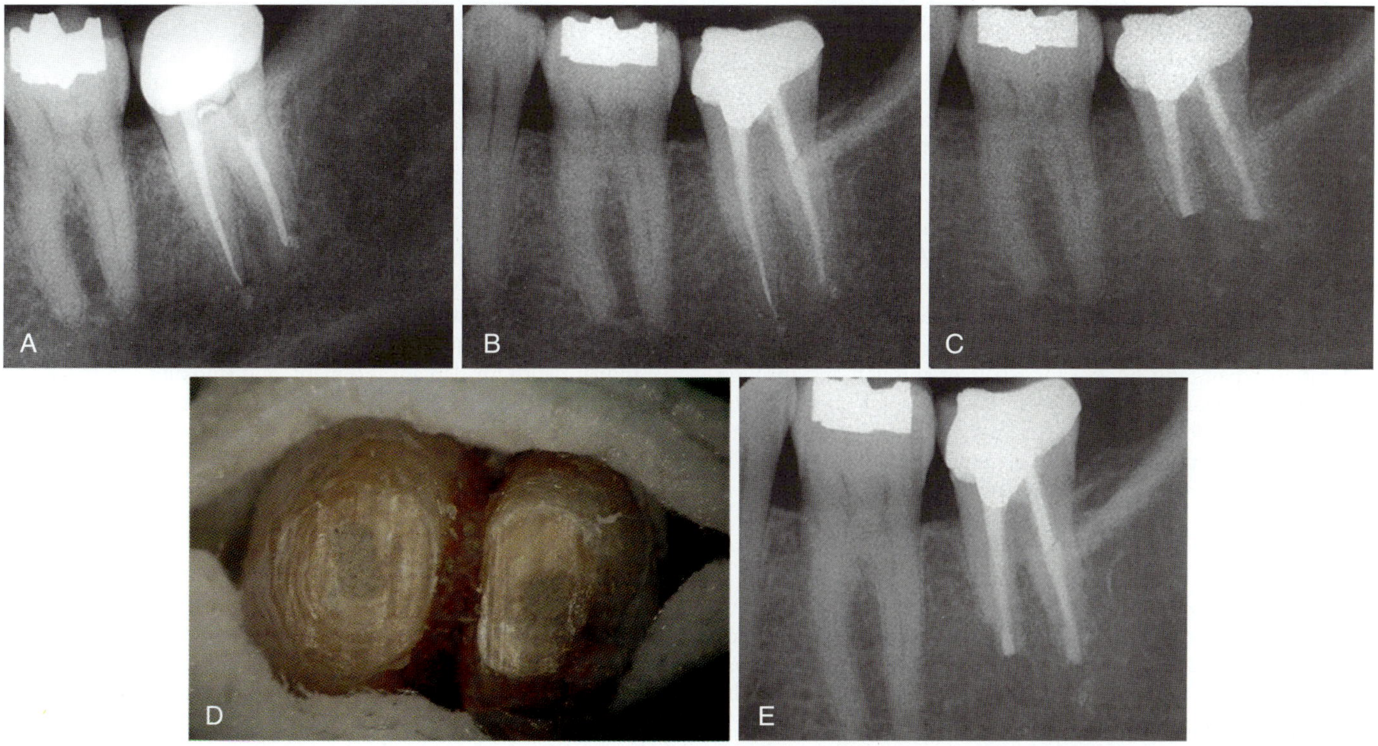

• **Fig. 21.8** **(A)** Preoperative radiograph of a second mandibular molar with a completed root canal treatment with continuous pain. **(B)** A postoperative radiograph after nonsurgical retreatment. The patient remained symptomatic. **(C)** Immediate postoperative radiograph after tooth replantation. **(D)** A postoperative clinical views of the roots after root resection and root end filling with mineral trioxide aggregate (MTA). **(E)** A postoperative radiograph taken 2 years later. The tooth had no clinical symptoms at this time.

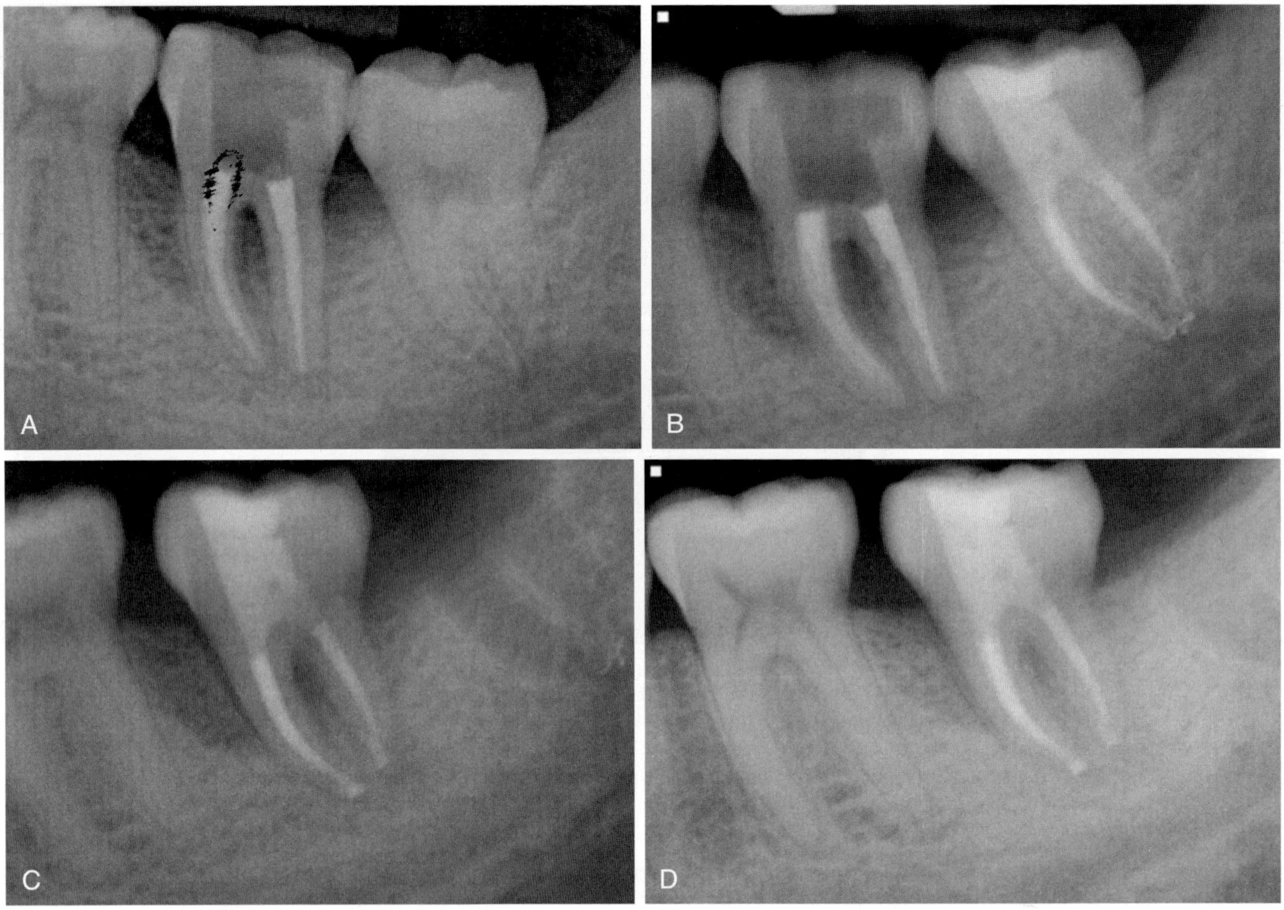

• **Fig. 21.9** **(A)** Preoperative radiograph of a nonrestorable mandibular second mandibular molar with vertical root fractures. Radiographic and clinical examinations showed presence of a third intact tooth suitable for transplantation. **(B)** A postoperative radiograph after completion of root canal treatment on the third molar. **(C)** Immediate postoperative radiograph after tooth transplantation. **(D)** Postoperative radiograph seven and half years later shows excellent healing. The tooth had no clinical symptoms at this time.

Rankow et al. listed endodontic clinical applications where GTR may be beneficial. A survey of members of the American Association of Endodontists in 2011 showed that 10.1% of respondents would use GTR for repair of small (<1 cm) periapical lesions, 62.9% for repair of large (>1 cm) periapical lesions, 63.9% for furcation or root perforation repair, and 88.7% for repair of through-and-through (transosseous) lesions.[30] In a review by Corbella et al., studies using GTR with a barrier membrane for endodontic surgery were categorized based on two classification systems.[32,33] Guidelines for the management of the surgical site when using GTR are available.[34]

Indications

It was noted that GTR used for treatment of large periapical lesions may be of some benefit, as well as for through-and through periapical lesions. The use of resorbable membrane barriers showed more favorable outcomes over nonresorbable membranes or the use of a graft without membrane.

Contraindications

Potential contraindications for endodontic surgery are no different from any elective dental treatment.[34] Case selection should consider the potential for improvement with the proposed treatment versus alternative treatments, evaluation of the patient's medical condition, general oral health, and medication use. Contraindications have been suggested for the use of GTR techniques and include any medical condition incompatible with the procedure, active infection at the site, and poor oral hygiene. Additionally, relative contraindications were suggested for improper interproximal bone level, inadequate tissue thickness, inadequate amount of keratinized gingiva, improper vestibular depth for flap advancement, and smoking.[35] Similar contraindications and relative contraindications were given for GBR techniques used for root coverage in patients with gingival recession.[36] It is important to note that active infection at the site will likely be present when using GTR/GBR techniques during endodontic surgery, but that ideally the source of the infection is removed.

Procedure

In brief: restorable membranes should be used in order to prevent a second surgical procedure to remove the membrane. The membrane should extend 2 to 3 mm past the margins of the bony crypt and supported with the bone graft material. The membrane should be entirely covered when suturing the tissue, and postoperative compression is contraindicated. Additionally, smoking should be avoided as it has been shown to significantly affect a positive outcome.

Prognosis

Prognosis of endodontic surgery on Classes A to C is very good, as studies have shown positive outcomes above 96%. Classes D to

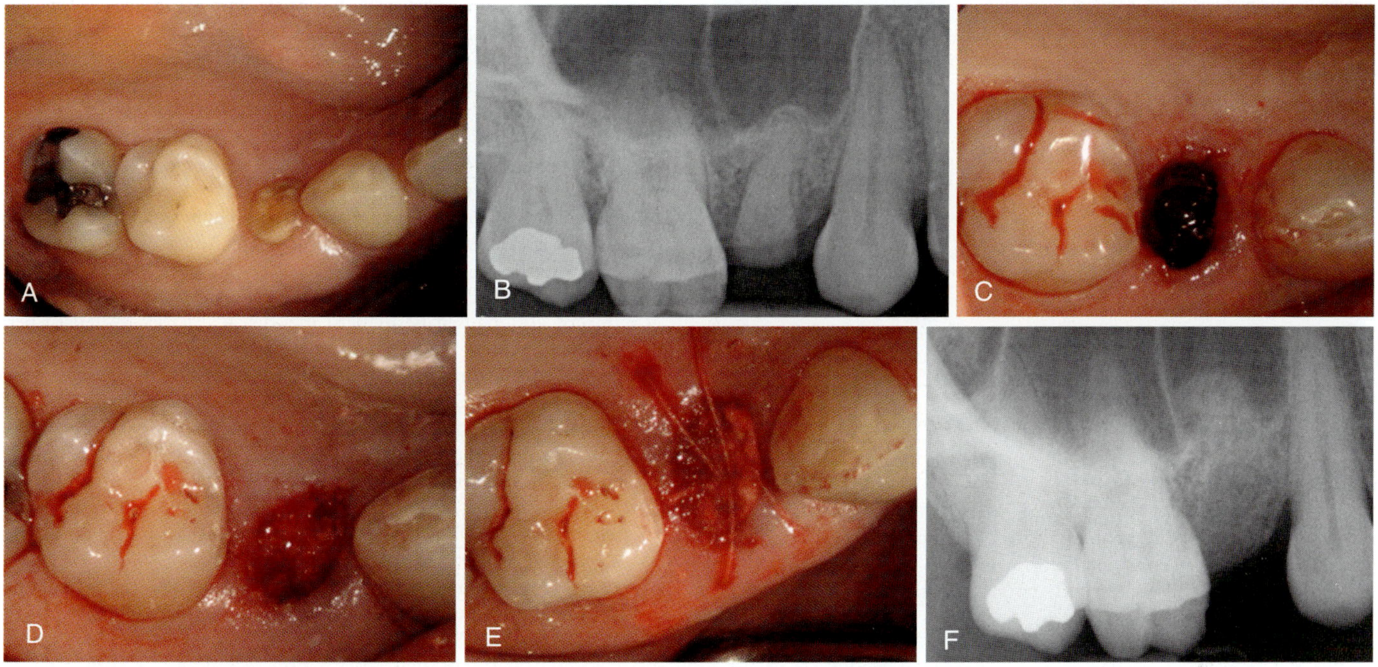

• **Fig. 21.10** **(A)** A clinical view of a second maxillary premolar with severe decay and an inadequate crown for proper restoration. **(B)** A radiograph showing absence of inadequate root and crown restoration to preserve this tooth. **(C)** A clinical picture demonstrating extraction site. **(D)** A clinical picture showing placement of graft material in the socket of extraction site. **(E)** A clinical picture showing placement of resorbable membrane and sutures over the graft material to hold it in the extraction site. **(F)** A postoperative radiograph showing completed socket preservation at the site of extraction.

F represent more challenging cases in which endodontic surgery alone may have a reduced prognosis but, with GTR and/or GBR techniques, the prognosis may be improved.

Socket Preservation

Socket preservation is the procedure used to maintain bone volume after an extraction of a tooth. Generally, bone volume will decrease as a result of resorption processes after a tooth is extracted. The socket preservation procedure is used to minimize this effect and generally involves placement of a biomaterial in the socket in order to delay the resorption process.

Indication

Indications for socket preservation include delayed placement of implants that require the need for reducing bone resorption process, as well as any patient needs that require the need for bone to be sustained. Socket preservations are typically performed with autografts, allografts, xenografts, or alloplasts.

Contraindications

Contraindication to socket preservation include acute infections/medical conditions that may affect proper healing.[37] Patient with uncontrolled diabetes, ongoing radiation therapy, and heavy smokers are also in the contraindications category as poor candidates for socket preservation because of their poor healing capability.[38] Patients with allergies to socket preservation graft material, more specifically synthetic material, are also obviously contraindicated for this procedure.

Procedure

Socket preservation first begins by extracting a tooth. Once the tooth has been extracted the chosen graft material is placed into the socket and the wound is sealed with primary closure[39] (Fig. 21.10).

Study Questions

6. What cells travel faster than other periodontal derived cells?
   a. Epithelium
   b. Connective tissue
   c. Both
7. Does a barrier prevent periodontal derived cells from apical migration?
   a. Yes
   b. No
8. What are the contraindications for GTR and GBR in endodontics?
   a. Any medical condition incompatible with the procedure
   b. Active infection at the site
   c. Poor oral hygiene
   d. All of the above
   e. None of the above
9. Which of the following are recommended in GTR and GBR in endodontics?
   a. The membrane should extend 2 to 3 mm past the margins of the bony crypt and supported with the bone graft material
   b. The membrane should be entirely covered when suturing the tissue
   c. Use a restorable membrane
   d. All of the above
10. What is the indication for socket preservation?
    a. Delayed placement of implants that require the need for reducing bone resorption process
    b. Any patient that requires the need for bone to be sustained
    c. None of the above
    d. A and B

ANSWERS

Answers Box 21

1 f. All of the above
2 d. A and B
3 d. A and B
4 d. A and B
5 d. A and B
6 a. Epithelium
7 a. Yes
8 d. All of the above
9 d. All of the above
10 d. A and B

References

1. Langer B, Stein S, Wagenberg B: An evaluation of root resections. A ten-year study, *J Periodontol* 52:719, 1981.
2. Green EN: Hemisection and root amputation, *J Am Dent Assoc* 112(4):511–518, 1986.
3. Carnevale G, Di Febo G, Tonelli MP, et al.: A retrospective analysis of the periodontal-prosthetic treatment of molars with interradicular lesions, *Int J Periodontics Restorative Dent* 11(3):189–205, 1991.
4. Basten CH, Ammons Jr WF, Persson R: Long-term evaluation of root-resected molars: a retrospective study, *Int J Periodontics Restorative Dent* 16(3):206–219, 1996.
5. Fugazzotto PA: A comparison of the success of root resected molars and molar position implants in function in a private practice: results of up to 15-plus years, *J Periodontol* 72(8):1113–1123, 2001.
6. Park SY, Shin SY, Yang SM, Kye SB: Factors influencing the outcome of root resection therapy in molars: a 10-year retrospective study, *J Periodontol* 80(1):32–40, 2009.
7. Orkin DA, Reddy J, Bradshaw D: The relationship of the position of crown margins to gingival health, *J Prosthet Dent* 57:421–424, 1987.
8. Block PL: Restorative margins and periodontal health: a new look at an old perspective, *J Prosthet Dent* 57:683–689, 1987.
9. Bader JD, Rozier RG, McFall WT, Ramsey DL: Effect of crown margins on periodontal conditions in regularly attending patients, *J Prosthet Dent* 65:75–79, 1991.
10. Gunay H, Seeger A, Tschernitchek H, Geurtsen W: Placement of the preparation line and periodontal health – a prospective 2 year clinical study, *Int J Periodontics Restorative Dent* 20:171–181, 2000.
11. Tarnow DP, Magner AW, Fletcher P: The effect of the distance from the contact point to the crest of bone on the presence or absence of the interproximal dental papilla, *J Periodontol* 63:995–996, 1992.
12. Rosenberg ES, Garber DA, Evian C: Tooth lengthening procedures, *Compend Continuing Educ Dent* 1:161–172, 1980.
13. Becker W, Ochsenbein C, Becker BE: Crown lengthening: the periodontal- restorative connection, *Compend Contin Educ Dent* 19:239–240, 242, 244–246 passim; quiz 256, 1998.
14. Moghaddam AS, Radafshar G, Taramsari M, Darabi F: Long-term survival rate of teeth receiving multidisciplinary endodontic, periodontal and prosthodontic treatments, *J Oral Rehabil* 41:236–242, 2014.
15. Pilalas I, Tsalikis L, Tatakis DN: Prerestorative crown lengthening surgery outcomes: a systematic review, *J Clin Periodontol* 43:1094–1108, 2016.
16. Heithersay GS: Combined endodontic-orthodontic treatment of transverse root fractures in the region of the alveolar crest, *Oral Surg Oral Med Oral Pathol* 36(3):404–415, 1973.
17. Simon JH: Root extrusion. Rationale and techniques, *Dent Clin North Am* 28(4):909–921, 1984.
18. Pontoriero R, Celenza Jr F, Ricci G, Carnevale G: Rapid extrusion with fiber resection: a combined orthodontic-periodontic treatment modality, *Int J Periodontics Restor Dent* 7(5):30–43, 1987.
19. Chien M, Patel R: Immediate surgical extrusion. In Schwartz R, Canakapalli V, editors: *Best practices in endodontics: a desk reference*, Chicago, 2015, Quintessence, pp 275–281.
20. American Association of Endodontists: *An annotated glossary of terms used in endodontics*, ed 8, Chicago, 2015, American Association of Endodontists.
21. Andreasen JO, Borum MK, Jacobsen HL, Andreasen FM: Replantation of 400 avulsed permanent incisors. 4. Factors related to periodontal ligament healing, *Endod Dent Traumatol* 11:76, 1995.
22. Sigurdsson A, Bourguignon C: Luxation injuries. In *A clinical guide to dental traumatology*, St. Louis, 2007, Elsevier Inc, pp 72–98.
23. Andersson L, Bodin I, Sorensen S: Progression of root resorption following replantation of human teeth after extended extraoral storage, *Endod Dent Traumatol* 5(1):38–47, 1989.
24. Torabinejad M, Dinsbach N, Turman M, White S, et al.: Survival of intentionally replanted teeth and implant-supported single crowns: a systemic review, *J Endod* 41:992–998, 2015.
25. Peer M: Intentional replantation: a "last resort" treatment or a conventional treatment procedure? Nine case reports, *Dent Traumatol* 20(1):48–55, 2004.
26. Becker BD: Intentional replantation techniques: a critical review, *J Endod* 44(1):14–21, 2018.
27. Tsukiboshi M: Autogenous tooth transplantation: a reevaluation, *Int J Periodont Restor Dent* 13:120–149, 1993.
28. Tsukiboshi M, Yamauchi N, Tsukiboshi Y. Long-term Outcomes of Autotransplantation of Teeth: A Case Series. *J Endod* 45(12S): S72–S83, 2019.
29. Rankow HJ, Krasner PR: Endodontic applications of guided tissue regeneration in endodontic surgery, *J Endod* 22(1):34–43, 1996.
30. Nalyor J, Mines P, Anderson A, Kwon D: The use of guided tissue regeneration techniques among endodontists: a web-based survey, *J Endodontics* 37(11):1495–1498, 2011.
31. Corbella S, Taschieri S, Elkabbany A, et al.: Guided tissue regeneration using a barrier membrane in endodontic surgery, *Swiss Dental Journal SSO* 126:13–25, 2016.
32. von Arx T, Cochran DL: Rationale for the application of the GTR principle using a barrier membrane in endodontic surgery: a proposal of classification and literature review, *Int J Periodont Restor Dent* 21:127–139, 2001.
33. Dietrich T, Zunker P, Dietrich D, Bernimoulin J-P: Apicomarginal defects in periradicular surgery: classification and diagnostic aspects, *Oral Surg Oral Med Oral Pathol Oral Radiol Endod* 94, 2002. 233–229.
34. Hargreaves KM, Cohen S, Berman LH: *Cohen's pathways of the pulp*, ed 10, St. Louis, 2011, Mosby Elsevier.
35. Wang HL, Al Shammari KF: Guided tissue regeneration-based root coverage utilizing collagen membranes: technique and case reports, *Quintessence Int* 33:715–721, 2002.
36. Wang HL, Carroll WJ: Guided bone regeneration using bone grafts and collagen membranes, *Quintessence Int* 32:504–515, 2001.
37. Darby I, Chen S, De Poi R: Ridge preservation: what is it and when should it be considered, *Australian Dental J* 53:11–21, 2007.
38. Serino G, Biancu S, Lezzi G, Piattelli A: Ridge preservation following tooth extraction using a polylactide and polyglycolide sponge as space filler: a clinical and histological study in humans, *Clinical Oral Implants Research* 14:651–658, 2003.
39. Irinakis T, Tabesh M: Preserving the socket dimensions with bone grafting in single sites: an esthetic surgical approach when planning delayed implant placement, *J Oral Implantol* 3:156–163, 2007.

22 Endodontic Treatment Outcomes

FRANK SETZER, SAMI CHOGLE, AND MAHMOUD TORABINEJAD

CHAPTER OUTLINE

LEARNING OBJECTIVES

After reading this chapter, the student should be able to:

1. Describe signs of successful and unsuccessful root canal treatment.
2. Describe the most common modalities used to determine success or failure.
3. State the approximate range of expected outcomes of routine, uncomplicated root canal treatment based on pretreatment conditions.
4. State predictors of success and failure.
5. Identify endodontic and nonendodontic causes of treatment failure.
6. State the outcomes of retreatment, endodontic surgery, and intentional replantation.
7. State the outcomes of fixed partial denture and single tooth implant treatments.
8. Approach treatment planning of root canal failure, recognizing the advantages and disadvantages of different treatment modalities.

Introduction

The primary goals of endodontic treatment are to provide patients with the best possible long-term outcomes regarding function, comfort, and esthetics. From a biologic perspective, this encompasses the prevention or cure of apical periodontitis. Prevention will be the focus for treating teeth presenting with pulpal inflammation, such as irreversible pulpitis. This can be achieved by maintaining aseptic conditions utilizing hygienic protocols and rubber dam isolation to prevent any oral microorganisms or bacteria present in caries from entering the root canal system during or after root canal treatment.

The objective for treating teeth with infection present within the root canal system is to significantly reduce the microbial load and to prevent recontamination.[1-3] This is achieved by a disinfecting phase, including thorough mechanical instrumentation, antimicrobial irrigation, and medication, as well as a sealing phase including root canal filling and placing permanent restoration. Complete root filling should largely eliminate the habitat for microorganisms, so that any residual microorganisms after treatment can be expected to perish as a result of the harsh environmental conditions of a well-sealed root canal root canal system, or at least rendered dormant. Finally, restorations preventing coronal leakage should disallow bacterial recontamination and achieve functional and esthetic rehabilitation.

Optimal outcomes are dependent on attaining these technical goals. However, as a result of the complexity of root canal systems,[4,5] less than perfect instrumentation, and root filling techniques, as well as the impossibility to render permanent restorations leakage free indefinitely, the guaranteed elimination of microorganisms from the root canal systems cannot be achieved under certain circumstances.

The purposes of this chapter are to (1) define success and failure, (2) describe methods used for the evaluation of endodontic outcomes, (3) provide outcome rates, including success and survival, (4) explain the signs and symptoms of negative outcomes, (5) discuss factors influencing outcomes, and (6) compare the outcomes of initial nonsurgical root canal treatment with those of nonsurgical retreatment, surgical retreatment (endodontic surgery), and alternative treatments, such as single tooth implants.

Definitions of Success and Failure

A successful outcome of root canal treatment may have a different meaning to different stakeholders involved in the treatment, including patients, dentists, and third-party payers.[6]

Patients will expect the elimination of symptoms, comfortable chewing function, satisfying esthetics, reassurance that symptoms may not recur, and that their tooth does not pose a risk of causing systemic disease. Insurance companies may judge the outcome by the access to care provided, the quality of care, cost efficiency, and the longevity of the treatment rendered.

Dentists are primarily concerned with the delivery of optimal care, predictable elimination of disease as measured clinically and radiographically, and fair compensation. In addition, they engage in aligning all stakeholders' expectations. Dentists should also reevaluate the technical quality of treatment and the long-term outcome in terms of preventing and eliminating apical periodontitis.

For endodontically treated teeth with previously vital pulps and no preexisting apical lesion, success entails that the tooth remains asymptomatic and no periapical pathosis develops after treatment. Failure will involve new symptoms and/or the appearance of a periapical lesion. For a tooth with a diagnosis of pulp necrosis, the outcome of the treatment is considered successful if the tooth remains asymptomatic and a preexisting apical periodontitis heals, respectively, no new apical lesion develops during follow-up. The presence of symptoms and/or a new or enlarging lesion is considered failure of the treatment.

Recently the American Association of Endodontists has proposed the following alternatives to the terms "success" and "failure":

- Healed—Functional, asymptomatic teeth with no or minimal radiographic periradicular pathosis.
- Nonhealed—Nonfunctional, symptomatic teeth with or without radiographic periradicular pathosis.
- Healing—Teeth with periradicular pathosis that are asymptomatic and functional, or teeth with or without radiographic periradicular pathosis that are symptomatic but for which the intended function is not altered.
- Functional—A treated tooth or root that is serving its intended purpose in the dentition.

Determination of success or failure may be difficult because of the nature and complexity of the periapical healing process itself and as a result of difficulties in observation. Many asymptomatic endodontically treated teeth demonstrate varying degrees of apical lesions radiographically. The clinician must judge whether a tooth is on a pathway to success or to failure and then decide together with the patient on a proper course of action if indicated.

When to Evaluate

Recommended follow-up periods have ranged from 6 months to 5 years.[7-12] Six months is a widely accepted and reasonable early follow-up interval for most situations. It is important to determine at what point of a healing process the outcome of treatment will be unlikely to reverse its course, and when treatment can be judged predictably as either success or failure, without a further need for follow-up.

A radiographic lesion that remains unchanged or increased in size after 1 year of follow-up is unlikely to ever resolve, and hence considered to be unsuccessful. If after 6 months a periapical lesion is still present, albeit smaller, it is likely to be in progress of healing, and further follow-up is indicated. Larger periradicular lesions will take longer to heal than smaller lesions. Unfortunately, apparent success may revert to failure later (often as a result of reinfection through coronal leakage), yet, late healing may also occur. Therefore an endodontic evaluation, including a patient history, clinical examination, and radiography of endodontically treated teeth should be part of every comprehensive patient examination.

Methods for Evaluation of Endodontic Outcomes

The evaluation process of successful endodontic therapy is complicated by the lack of direct correlation between measures of the disease process and its clinical manifestation. The clinician must therefore assimilate various metrics of information including patient history, clinical findings, and radiographic examinations to determine endodontic treatment outcomes. Evaluation of endodontic outcomes follows the same diagnostic pathway as for initial treatment (see Chapter 4). Biopsy of periradicular tissues during endodontic surgery provides a histologic diagnosis, another method for evaluation of success or failure of root canal treatment. This method is not routinely used and is an impractical approach to determine clinical outcomes of initial nonsurgical root canal treatments.

Patient History

Complaints of new, persistent, or worsening symptoms after root canal treatment has been completed may indicate failure. Persistence of signs (e.g., sinus tract opening) or symptoms long after endodontic therapy had been completed indicate primary and continuing disease. However, emergence of new signs or symptoms months or years after root canal treatment usually result from secondary posttreatment disease such as leakage secondary to absence of suitable coronal restoration. Symptoms related to discomfort or pain on chewing, aching, and so forth are generally an indication of periradicular inflammation or infection regardless of the evidence of radiographic lesion. It must be remembered that bony healing takes time and that a tooth that feels "different" on biting may be en route to healing; this should be confirmed clinically and radiographically. Pain on release may indicate a cracked tooth. A bad taste may indicate a draining abscess. Occasionally a patient reports sensitivity to cold or heat; this is most likely related to an adjacent untreated tooth but could be an indication of a missed vital canal in a treated tooth.

Clinical Examination

Presence of persistent signs or symptoms is usually an indication of disease and failure. However, absence of symptoms does not signify success. Periapical pathosis without significant symptoms is usually present in teeth before and after root canal treatment until healing has occurred.[13] There is little correlation between the presence of pathosis and corresponding symptoms; yet when adverse signs or symptoms are evident, there is a strong likelihood that a pathosis is present.[14] Persistent signs (e.g., swelling, probing defect, or sinus tract) or symptoms usually indicate failure.

Common clinical success criteria include the following[14]:

- No signs of swelling, infection, or inflammation
- Disappearance of sinus tract (separate or through periodontal ligament space)
- No soft tissue defects or pathologic probing depths

As part of the overall assessment of the tooth after endodontic therapy it is crucial to evaluate the current restoration and the periodontal attachment apparatus. A defective/missing restoration as well as active periodontal disease have been significantly associated with loss of an endodontically treated tooth.[15]

Radiographic Findings

Based on the interpretation of radiographs, the outcome of each treatment can be classified as success, failure, or questionable status. To be able to accurately compare radiographs made at different times, it is important that they are made in a reproducible fashion and with minimal distortion. The best way to ensure reproducibility is with paralleling radiographic devices. Teeth with multiple roots or canals should be examined using both straight-on- and off-angle periapical views.

Radiographic success is the absence of an apical radiolucent lesion. This means that a resorptive lesion present at the time of treatment has resolved or, if there was no lesion present at the time of initial treatment, none has developed. Thus radiographic success is evident by the elimination or lack of development of an area of rarefaction for a minimum of 1 year after treatment (Fig. 22.1).

Radiographic failure is the persistence or development of pathosis radiographically. Specifically, whether this is a radiolucent lesion that has remained the same, has enlarged, or has developed since treatment (Fig. 22.2). Nonfunctional, symptomatic teeth with or without radiographic lesions are considered failure (nonhealed).

Radiographically unknown status indicates a state of uncertainty. This classification includes teeth with pathosis that are asymptomatic and functional. The radiolucent lesion in these teeth has neither become larger nor significantly decreased in size. Teeth with radiolucencies that were treated elsewhere and for which there are no prior radiographs for comparison are often assigned to this category (Fig. 22.3).

A shortcoming of radiographic evaluation is that radiographs may not be made or interpreted in standardized ways. As early as 1966, Bender et al.[14] noted that radiographic interpretation is often subject to personal bias and that a change in angulations can often give a completely different appearance to the lesion, making it appear either smaller or larger. Also, different observers may not agree on what they see in a radiograph and the same observer may disagree with himself if asked to review the same radiograph at a different lime period.[16]

Ørstavik et al.[17] suggested the use of the periapical index (PAI) for radiographic evaluation of the outcome of root canal treatment. The PAI relies on the comparison of the radiographs with a set of five radiographic images reported by Brynolf in 1967.[18] These images represent a radiographically healthy periapex (score 1) to a large periapical lesion (score 5). Each of the preoperative and recall radiographs is assigned a score according to its resemblance to one of the five reference images. The outcome of treatment using PAI can be classified as "healing" if the lesion size is reduced, "healed" if the lesion has been eliminated, or "developing" if a

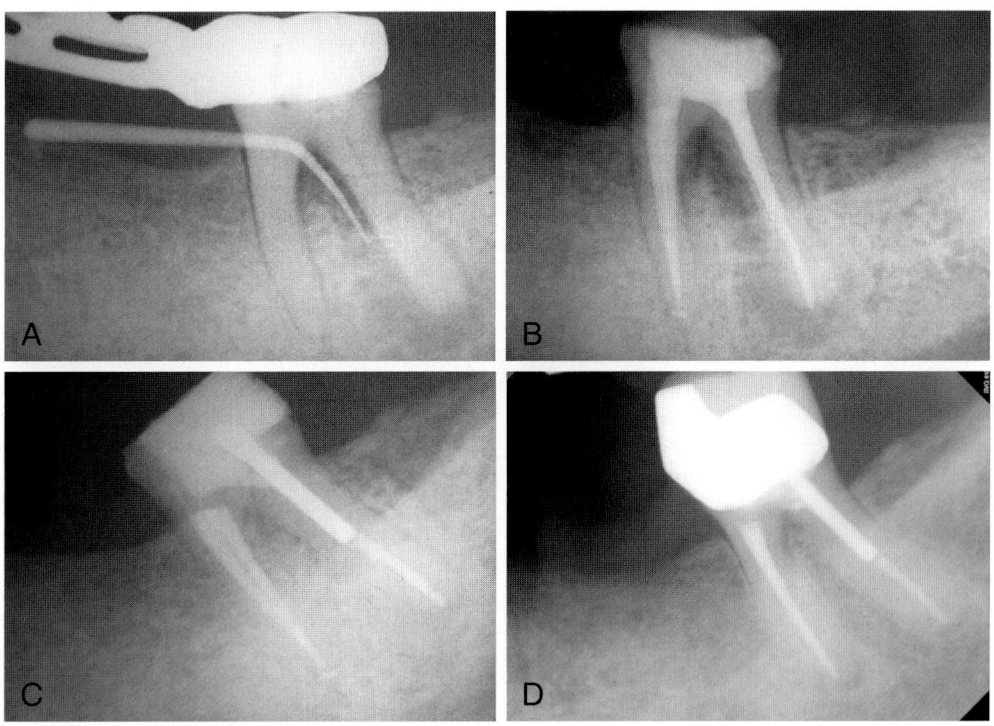

• **Fig. 22.1** Success. **(A)** The initial radiograph shows the presence of bone loss from the crest of the ridge around the apex of the distal root. A sinus tract is traced. Periodontal probing demonstrates deep pocketing. There is no response to pulpal vitality tests. **(B)** Root canal treatment completed. **(C)** A 12-year recall radiograph shows resolution of the radiolucency, build-up, and post. **(D)** A 12-year recall radiograph demonstrates healthy apical tissues. The patient wears a removable partial denture.

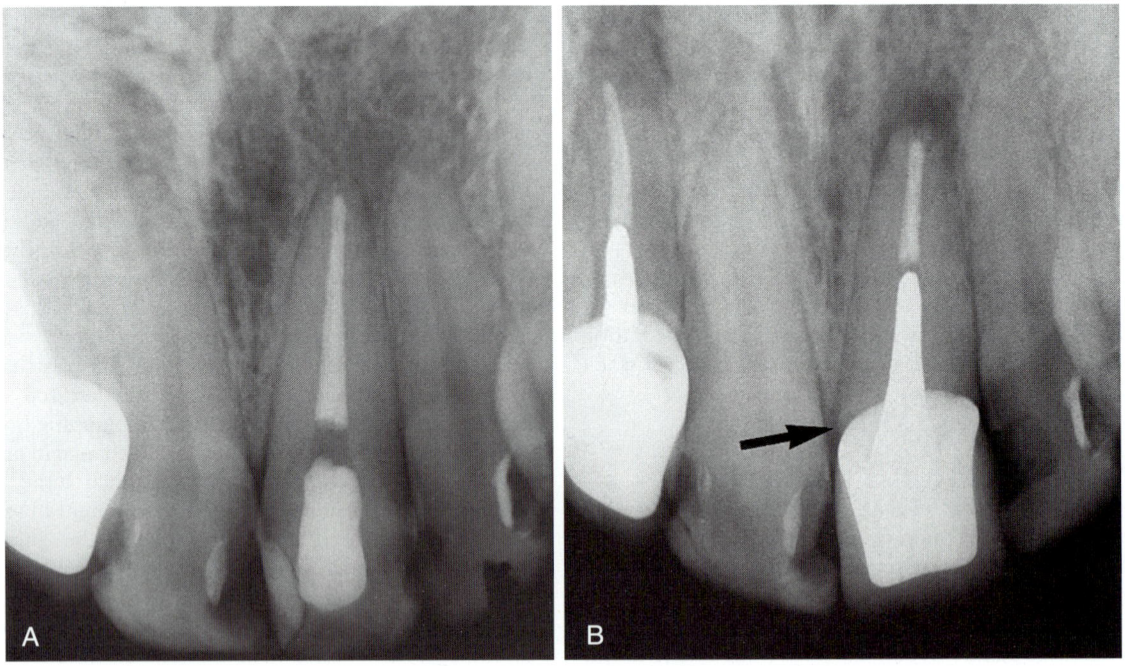

• **Fig. 22.2** Failure. **(A)** Apparently adequate root canal treatment. The tooth was restored later with a post and core and crown. **(B)** The patient reports persistent discomfort after 2 years. A periradicular radiolucency indicates failure, probably a result of coronal leakage at a defective margin *(arrow)*.

new lesion has formed. Although accurate and reproducible, complete healing using the PAI may take up to 4 or 5 years especially after endodontic surgeries evidenced by a larger number of "slow" healers compared with the "late" failures. Others have commonly used the terms healed, healing, and diseased instead of success and failure because of the potential of the latter to confuse patients.[19]

Cone beam computed tomography (CBCT) with high resolution three-dimensional (3D) imaging technique has demonstrable value in diagnosis and outcomes assessment for endodontic patients (see Chapter 3). The 3D image allows a precise evaluation without the superimposition of surrounding anatomic structures. Recent studies comparing 2D and 3D images have reported a significant increase in uncertain healing and unsatisfactory healing at the 1-year follow-up period owing to higher and more precise detection of bone lesions that may not be visible with two-dimensional radiology.[20-22] Currently, the routine use of CBCT is not recommended[23-24] owing to its higher radiation dosage. However, with constant improvements in hardware and software algorithms CBCT will increasingly become an essential diagnostic and assessment tool for the clinician. The increased sensitivity and resolution may require a reevaluation of criteria for acceptable radiographic periapical healing.

Histologic Examination

The ideal outcome through histologic assessment would necessitate reconstitution of periradicular structures and an absence of inflammation (Fig. 22.4). This is both impractical and impossible without surgery. Additionally, there is uncertainty about the degree of correlation between histologic findings and negative radiographic appearance. Two histologic investigations of teeth treated with root canals in cadavers reached very different conclusions. Brynolf[18] concluded that almost all root canal treated teeth showed some periradicular inflammation despite the appearance of successful treatment on radiographs. In contrast, Green el al.[25] observed that most root canal treated teeth with radiographically normal periapex were indeed free of inflammation histologically. Thus with current technology such as the noninvasive CBCT, the clinical and radiographic evaluation appear to be the more practical means of assessing degree of healing after endodontic treatment.

Success Rates

As is the case for other dental and medical procedures, unfortunately, not all endodontic treatments are successful. Recognition, acceptance, and management of treatments that do not resolve and heal can be difficult and often involve a complex set of factors. Historically, the popular belief has been that the success and survival rates for root canal treatment are between 80% and 95%. However, general percentages should be taken with caution, and each case should be individually assessed to determine the percentage probability of success.

Torabinejad et al.[26] performed a systematic review of the literature pertaining to success and failure of nonsurgical root canal therapy and assigned levels of evidence (LOE) to the studies. In the previous 40 years, 306 articles have been published related to the outcome of nonsurgical root canal treatment. Fifty-one studies included at least 100 teeth; meta-analysis of these studies suggested an overall radiographic success rate of 81.5% over a period of 5 years. Others who assessed the 4- to 6-year outcomes of initial endodontic treatment have reported similar overall healing rates.[27] In another systematic review, Torabinejad and colleagues[28] compared the outcomes of endodontically treated teeth with those of single implant crowns, fixed dental prostheses (FPD), and no treatment after extraction. Success data in that review consistently ranked implant therapy as superior to endodontic treatment, which in turn was ranked as superior to FPD (Table 22.1).

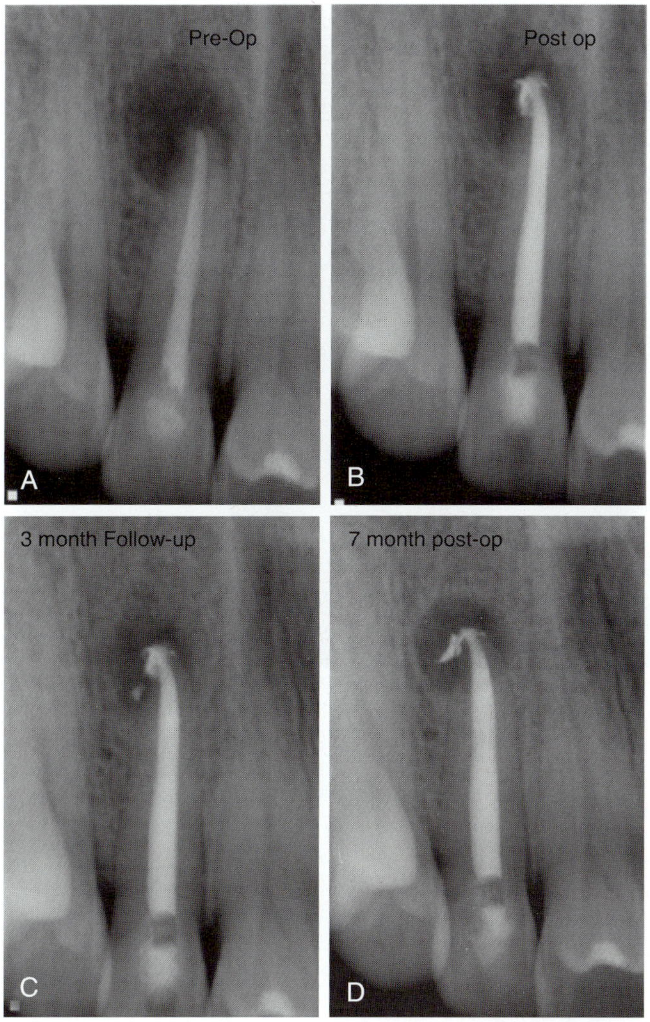

• **Fig. 22.3** Uncertainty. **(A)** Obturation demonstrating voids and coronal leakage likely all contributed to failure. The tooth is suitable for nonsurgical retreatment and a new permanent restoration. **(B)** Postoperative image after retreatment. **(C)** Three-month recall, the patient reports absence of symptoms. The radiolucent lesion is decreasing in size but has not resolved. **(D)** Seven-month recall, despite a new restoration, the lesion has remained and stays in within the same proportions.

However, very different criteria for success are used in implant dentistry, endodontics, and prosthodontics; therefore such comparisons lack validity. Comparison of survival rates is much more meaningful and were recorded at 97% in same study.[28]

Survival Rates

Long-term survival rates for endodontically treated teeth include tooth retention or survival. Introduced by Friedman and Mor[19] in 2004 the term "functional retention" is frequently used to indicate retention of the tooth in the absence of signs and symptoms regardless of a radiographic lesion. Several very large studies have all reported extremely high long-term survival rates for teeth with root canal treatment: Lazarski et al.[29] reported 94% functional survival for 44,613 cases at 3.5 years in the United States; Salehrabi and Rotstein[30] reported 97% survival for 1.1 million patients at 8 years in the United States; and Chen and colleagues[31] reported 93% survival for 1.5 million teeth at 5 years in Taiwan. Teeth with root canal treatments have remarkably high long-term survival rates.

These rates of survival of endodontically treated teeth allow a better comparison with alternative treatments such as FPD and single implant-supported restorations. The previously mentioned systematic review shows that endodontic and implant treatments resulted in superior ≥6 year survival rates compared with extraction and replacement with an FPD.[28] Torabinejad et al.[28] as well as Iqbal and Kim[32] reported similar findings when they compared the survival rates of restored endodontically treated teeth with those of implant-supported restorations. Doyle and colleagues[33] additionally reported that although similar in failure rates, the implant group showed a longer time to tooth function and a higher incidence of postoperative complications requiring intervention. Furthermore, a recent systematic review reported that implant survival rates do not exceed those of even compromised but adequately root canal treated and maintained teeth.[34] Therefore the importance to maintaining the natural dentition through evidence-based dentistry cannot be overemphasized.

Patient-Based Outcomes

In the current age of patient-centered care, patients' perspectives of their health status are gaining importance in identifying needs, treatment planning, and ultimately in evaluating outcomes from health care. Today definitions of health include psychologic measures of well-being as well.[35] Anticipation and experience of root canal associated pain are major sources of fear for patients and a very important concern of dentists. A recent systematic review found that the severity of pretreatment root canal associated pain was moderate, dropped substantially within 1 day of treatment, and continued to drop to minimal levels in 7 days.[36] Overall satisfaction ratings for root canal treatment are extremely high, generally above the 90th percentile.[37] Satisfaction is higher when endodontic treatment is provided by specialists, probably a reflection of effective communication and efficient management. Initial costs for root canal treatment and restoration are substantially lower than for replacement with an implant single crown or FDP.[28,38]

Recent studies on patient-based outcomes have focused on the Quality of Life metrics. These instruments have mostly been adapted from medicine for application to dentistry, such as the Oral Health Related Quality of Life instruments (OHQoL). Liu et al.[39] reported a longitudinal study on the OHQoL for 279 patients after endodontic treatment using the Oral Health Impact Profile (OHIP) tool of assessment, which was shown to be both sensitive and responsive to endodontic treatment and useful in understanding patients' perspectives of outcomes.

A larger study involving over 1250 patients in a practice-based research network suggests that 3 to 5 years after initial root canal therapy a small percentage (5%) of patients experience persistent pain, of which <2% are not attributable to odontogenic causes that may adversely affect their quality of life.[40] Endodontic nonsurgical retreatment has also shown to significantly improve patients' quality of life and chewing ability over time, with a success rate of 90.4% after 2 years.[41] Future studies from patients' own perspectives could expand our understanding of the prognostic factors and the consequences of root canal treatment.

Postoperative Complications

As with all dental procedures, complications may occur after root canal treatment. However, the incidence of long-term postoperative complications appears to be lower than for the alternatives, single tooth implants and fixed dental prostheses.[33,42] The 10-year

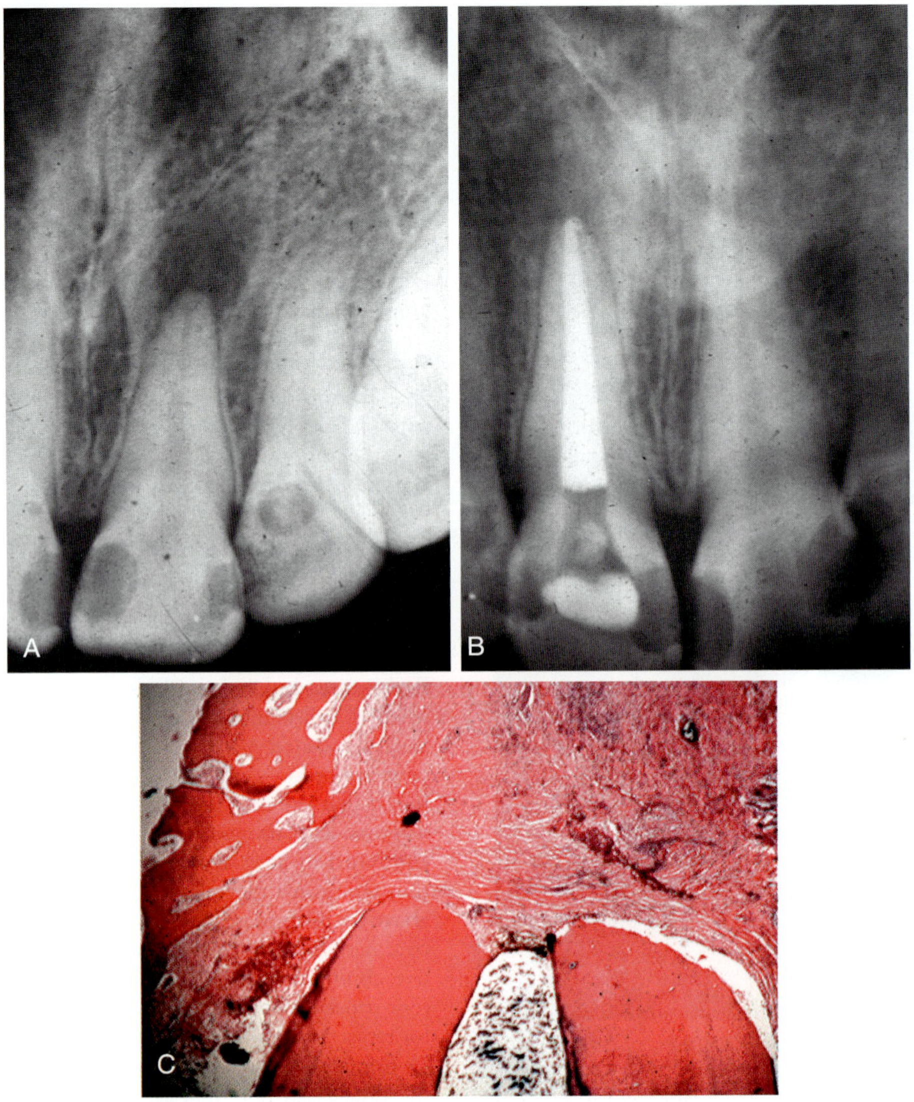

• **Fig. 22.4** **(A)** A periapical radiograph revealed an apical radiolucency on the central incisor. **(B)** A periapical film taken 6 months later shows resolution of most of the apical radiolucency. Despite radiographic change, the patient remained symptomatic, and surgery had to be performed. **(C)** Histologic examination of this tooth shows resolution of most of the inflammatory cells near the apex. (Courtesy of Dr. A. Khayat.)

complication rate for retained root canal treated teeth is approximately 4%, compared with approximately 18% for retained single tooth implant restorations.[33] Typical complications include symptoms, swelling, and the need for retreatment.[33] In endodontics, complications are recorded as failures according to the criteria described previously; in other disciplines, complications are generally not recorded as failures.

Prognostic Indicators

The classic landmark study published by Larz Strindberg in 1956 related treatment outcomes to biologic and therapeutic factors.[43] Factors now considered to be predictors of success and failure include (1) apical pathosis, (2) bacterial status of the canal, (3) extent and quality of the obturation, and (4) quality of the coronal restoration. The role of these factors should be discussed with the patient before and after treatment.

Several investigations have reported factors that result in a slightly less favorable prognosis: the presence of periradicular lesions and larger lesion size;[38,44] the presence of bacteria in the canal before obturation;[45] and obturations that are short, long, contain voids, or lack density.[46-50] Some evidence suggests that the use of a calcium hydroxide intracanal medicament may improve the prognosis.[51-53] The quality of the coronal restoration plays a key role in the outcomes of root canal treatment.[54-56]

Factors such as the tooth type, age and gender of the patient, and obturation technique have minimal if any influence on the prognosis.[51-53,57] Most medical conditions have no significant bearing on the prognosis.[58] However, patients with insulin dependent diabetes mellitus have a significantly lower healing rate after root canal therapy in teeth with apical lesions.[59] Interestingly, diabetes mellitus, hypertension, and coronary artery disease are associated with an increased risk of extraction after root canal treatment.[60] Although this finding does not indicate causality, the systemic disease burden has broad effects on the patient's welfare, morbidity, and behavior. Obviously, a patient with a complex medical history, serious illness, or disability may present a high degree of difficulty in management and demands high levels of experience and

TABLE 22.1 Percentages of Pooled and Weighted Survival and Success Rates of Dental Implants, Root Canal Treatment, and Three- or Four-Unit Bridges Over 2 to 4, 4 To 6, And 6+ Years

Procedure	Success (%)	Survival (%)
2-4 years		
Dental implant (pooled)	98 (95-99)	95 (93-97)
Dental implant (weighted)	99 (96-100)	96 (94-97)
Root canal treatment (pooled)	90 (88-92)	94
Root canal treatment (weighted)	89 (88-91)	—
Three-unit bridge (pooled)	79 (69-87)	94
Three-unit bridge (weighted)	78 (76-81)	—
4-6 years		
Dental implant (pooled)	97 (96-98)	97 (95-98)
Dental implant (weighted)	98 (97-99)	97 (95-98)
Root canal treatment (pooled)	93 (87-97)	94 (92-96)
Root canal treatment (weighted)	94 (92-96)	94 (91-96)
Three-unit bridge (pooled)	82 (71-91)	93
Three-unit bridge (weighted)	76 (74-79)	—
6+ years		
Dental implant (pooled)	95 (93-96)	97 (95-99)
Dental implant (weighted)	95 (93-97)	97 (96-98)
Root canal treatment (pooled)	84 (82-87)	92 (84-97)
Root canal treatment (weighted)	84 (81-87)	97 (97-97)
Three-unit bridge (pooled)	81 (74-86)	82
Three-unit bridge (weighted)	80 (79-82)	—

expertise. However, root canal treatment may greatly benefit some patients by preventing the need for high-risk extractions or other surgical procedures; such patients include those with bleeding disorders, those who have undergone head and neck irradiation, and those treated with high-dose bisphosphonates.

Study Questions

1. Which of the following criteria WILL NOT be considered part of a truly successful outcome at a 1-year follow-up?
   a. No clinical signs of swelling, infection, or inflammation
   b. Disappearance of a sinus tract
   c. Decrease of a radiolucency in size
   d. No soft tissue defects or pathologic probing depths
   e. No clinical symptoms experienced by the patient
2. Which of the following statements about the radiographic detection of periapical pathosis is UNTRUE?
   a. The sensitivity of detecting apical periodontitis with CBCT imaging is higher than with conventional digital radiography
   b. Any apical periodontitis in the mandible will be detectable on radiographs if it exceeds 3 mm in diameter
   c. If radiographs at follow-up are taken at a different angulation than the postoperative control, the actual healing progression may be misjudged
   d. Different observers may disagree on the interpretation of periapical radiolucencies
   e. The same observer may disagree with him/herself on the interpretation of periapical radiolucencies if viewed at different times
3. Based on systematic reviews and meta-analyses, which of the following outcome ranges does not reflect the associated procedure?
   a. Success of root canal treatment with a diagnosis of irreversible pulpitis: 90% to 100%
   b. Success of root canal treatment with a diagnosis of apical periodontitis: 75% to 85%
   c. Success of nonsurgical retreatment: 75% to 85%
   d. Success of endodontic microsurgery: 55% to 65%
   e. Survival of single-unit implants: 90% to 100%
4. Which of the following factors WOULD NOT be considered to be a predictor of success and failure for endodontic treatment?
   a. Type of root filling material
   b. Presence or absence of apical pathosis
   c. Extent and quality of the root filling
   d. Bacterial status of the root canal system
   e. Quality of the coronal restoration
5. Which of the following statements about the PAI is INCORRECT?
   a. The PAI relies on the comparison with a set of five radiographic images reported by Brynolf in 1967
   b. The outcome of treatment using PAI can be classified as "healing" if the lesion size is reduced
   c. The outcome of treatment using PAI can be classified as "healed" if the lesion has been eliminated
   d. The outcome of treatment using PAI can be classified as "developing" if a new lesion has formed
   e. The PAI grades in 4 stages from healthy periapex (score 1) to a large periapical lesion (score 4)

Causes of Nonhealed, Failed Root Canal Treatment

The outcome of endodontic therapy largely depends on the management of infection.

The presence of newly introduced, persistent, or recurrent microorganisms is the primary cause of endodontic pathology.[61] Ideally, after chemomechanical instrumentation, the root canal system should be free of microorganisms.[62]

The prevention of microbial infection of the root canal system is the primary goal for the treatment of teeth with a vital pulp status. This necessitates proper isolation, disinfection of the operative field, and aseptic root canal treatment techniques to reduce the risk of contamination and to achieve a superior prognosis. If the pulp was necrotic, or the tooth previously endodontically treated, and an apical pathology was present, the removal of microorganisms, toxins, metabolites, antigens, and byproducts is essential but may be challenging.

The location and nature of the microorganisms, the complexity of the root canal system, technical aspects of endodontic treatment, and the quality of the permanent restoration all play an important role as potential reasons for treatment failure.

Unfortunately, the complexity of the root canal system with all its ramifications may make microorganisms inaccessible to mechanical disruption or the antimicrobial effects of disinfectants, medications, and root canal filling materials.[63,64] The larger part of infected root canal systems may probably contain residual microorganisms after root canal treatment; however, the environmental conditions of a well-sealed root canal system after appropriate chemomechanical débridement are expected to eliminate them, or at the least leave them in a dormant state.

Hence, chemomechanical disinfection will primarily aim at a reduction of microbial counts by a combination of mechanical instrumentation with copious and frequent disinfecting solutions, such as sodium hypochlorite.[65] Interappointment medication with calcium hydroxide may further reduce the number of microorganisms,[66] accelerate healing, and reduce inflammation.[51,52]

Common errors leading to persistent microbial presence and ultimately failure include (1) errors in diagnosis and treatment planning; (2) lack of knowledge of pulp and/or root anatomy, resulting in missing canals or other areas of the root canal during treatment; (3) inadequate débridement and/or disinfection of the root canal system; (4) operative errors; (5) deficiencies of the root filling; (6) the absence of cuspal coverage in posterior teeth, allowing for increased fracture rates; (7) excessive removal of tooth structure, predisposing teeth to fracture; and (8) coronal leakage through inadequate temporary or permanent restorations. Understanding these preoperative, operative, and postoperative factors plays an essential role in assessing the reasons for treatment failure and the best options for its management.

Preoperative Causes

Misdiagnosis, errors in treatment planning and decision making, inadequate case selection (i.e., treatment beyond a clinician's skill levels and expertise), as well as the treatment of a tooth with a poor initial prognosis may be a reason for failure of endodontic treatment. Diagnosis should be based on all available information: the patient's medical and dental history, chief complaint, signs and symptoms, as well as a current, comprehensive endodontic evaluation, including visual inspection, percussion, palpation, probing, sensitivity tests, and radiographic evaluation (see Chapter 4). The radiographic evaluation should include periapical films from different mesiodistal angulations and may include bite wing radiographs or three-dimensional projections, such as a limited field of view CBCT (see Chapter 3). Together with the clinical examination, the radiographic evaluation may aid in identifying complexities in the root canal system, such as additional canals (Fig. 22.5) and canal anatomy, root dilacerations and curvatures, fractures (Fig. 22.6), external or internal resorption, periodontal defects, and/or the presence of periapical pathologies.

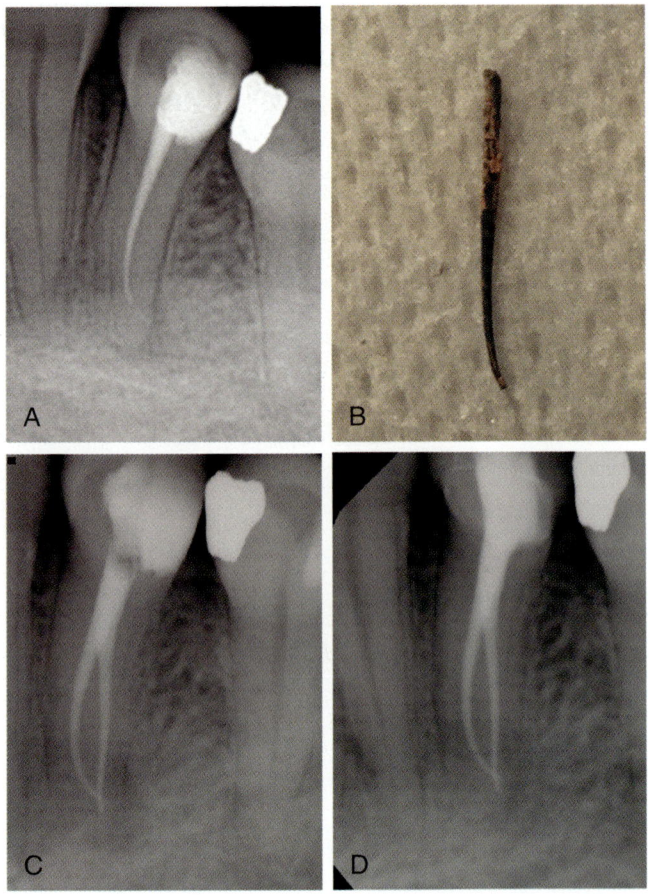

• **Fig. 22.5** **(A)** Double periodontal ligament visible mesially in the mandibular first premolar indicates the presence of a division in the canal or the root or additional canals. **(B)** Original root filling material with plastic carrier removed. **(C)** A postoperative radiograph revealed a midroot split and two canals. **(D)** Six-month recall, permanent restoration and resolution of apical periodontitis, indicative of healing.

Particular microorganisms, such as *Enterococcus faecalis*, demonstrate special survival qualities, including the ability to form biofilms.[67-69] The arrangement of bacteria in biofilms may pose significant challenges for effective elimination,[70] with an estimated 1000-fold greater resistance to antimicrobial agents than corresponding planktonic forms of bacteria.[71] Although apical periodontitis is usually in response to intraradicular infection, there are situations, such as an acute apical abscess, where microorganisms are present in the periapical tissues. In certain situations, extraradicular biofilms or cohesive bodies within the periapical lesion itself can be found, rendering these microorganisms inaccessible to intraradicular treatment strategies, with actinomyces,[72] or *Propionibacterium propionicum*[73] being common examples.

Lastly, the nature of the periapical lesion may play a role in the healing process. Most periapical pathologies are inflammatory in

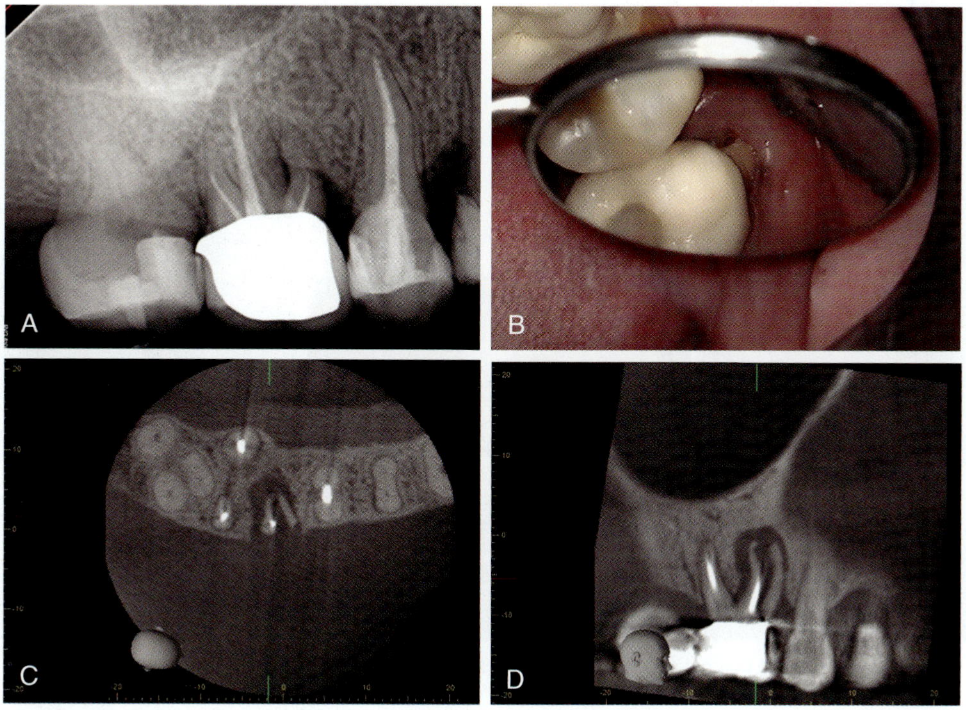

• **Fig. 22.6** Indicators of vertical root fracture. **(A)** Isolated bone loss on mesiobuccal root. **(B)** Clinical observation of fracture line. **(C)** Cone beam computed tomography (CBCT) confirmation of separated root fragments. **(D)** CBCT confirmation of J-shaped lesion. (CBCT acquisition for treatment planning of root resection; courtesy of Dr. Rami Elsabee.)

kind,[74] histologically 50% being described as granulomas, 35% as abscesses, and 15% as cysts. Of the cysts, approximately 40% were identified as pocket cysts, where the epithelial-lined cavity is connected to the root canal system through the apical foramen. These lesions are expected to heal after nonsurgical endodontic treatment.[74] However, the remaining 60% are true cysts, which are more likely to heal only after extraction or surgical endodontic treatment, as they are disconnected from the root canal system and enclosed by epithelial lining in its entirety.[74] It is currently not possible to differentiate clinically between periapical cysts and granulomas, nor between periapical pocket and true cysts. Nevertheless, larger lesions (radiographically 200 mm^2 or greater) were shown more likely to be cysts.[75,76]

Operative Causes

Many failures result from errors in operative procedure (see Chapter 18). The thorough débridement and/or disinfection of the root canal system in its entirety together with a well sealing root filling and permanent restoration are the means during endodontic treatment to prevent or eliminate apical periodontitis and to achieve success. Advancements in endodontic instruments and techniques have greatly improved the ease and completeness of chemomechanical cleaning. Rotary nickel-titanium file systems and new activation techniques for irrigation solutions have helped to clean more predictably. In comparison to stainless steel hand instrumentation rotary nickel-titanium files are more flexible and prepare root canals more centered and rounder. However, clinicians must follow proper protocols to avoid failure. A straight-line access cavity allowing for unobstructed approach to the canal orifices provides for safer canal instrumentation and reduces the risk of missing canals. If pulp horns are not removed, pulpal tissues, bacteria, debris, and filling materials may remain in the coronal pulp space and may result in persistent infection or tooth discoloration. Underextended access preparations may limit instrument maneuverability, posing a risk of insufficient cleaning and instrument fracture. However, overly large access cavities should also be avoided to reduce excessive loss of tooth structure, which may weaken the tooth, increase the risk of fracture and perforation, and complicate restoration.[77-78]

The difficulty level of the endodontic treatment may strongly affect the quality of the outcome. Significant deviations from the normal tooth or root form, extreme (>30°) or S-shaped curvatures, canal division in the middle or apical third, or very long roots (>25 mm) may increase the likelihood of perforations with subsequent leakage or mechanical irritation, and development of a lesion.[79] Although perforations have had a better prognosis since repair materials such as mineral trioxide aggregate (MTA) or bioceramics became available,[80] some may require endodontic surgery.[81] Other possible complications may be related to open apices (>1.5 mm in diameter), decreased canal visibility on radiographs, calcified canals, internal and external resorptions, as well as history of trauma.

Calcified and/or missed canals may be difficult to visualize on periapical radiographs; however, the use of CBCT imaging may allow for a clear detection. Clinically, the pulp floor should be carefully inspected after removal of decay and any existing restoration to identify missed or calcified canals.

Sjögren et al. demonstrated a 94% periapical healing rate in teeth with apical periodontitis if the root filling was extended to within 0 to 2 mm of the radiographic apex.[11] Confining endodontic procedures and materials to within the canal space facilitates repair of periradicular tissues.[46,82] However, if the apical area was underinstrumented more than 2 mm from the root-end, this outcome decreased

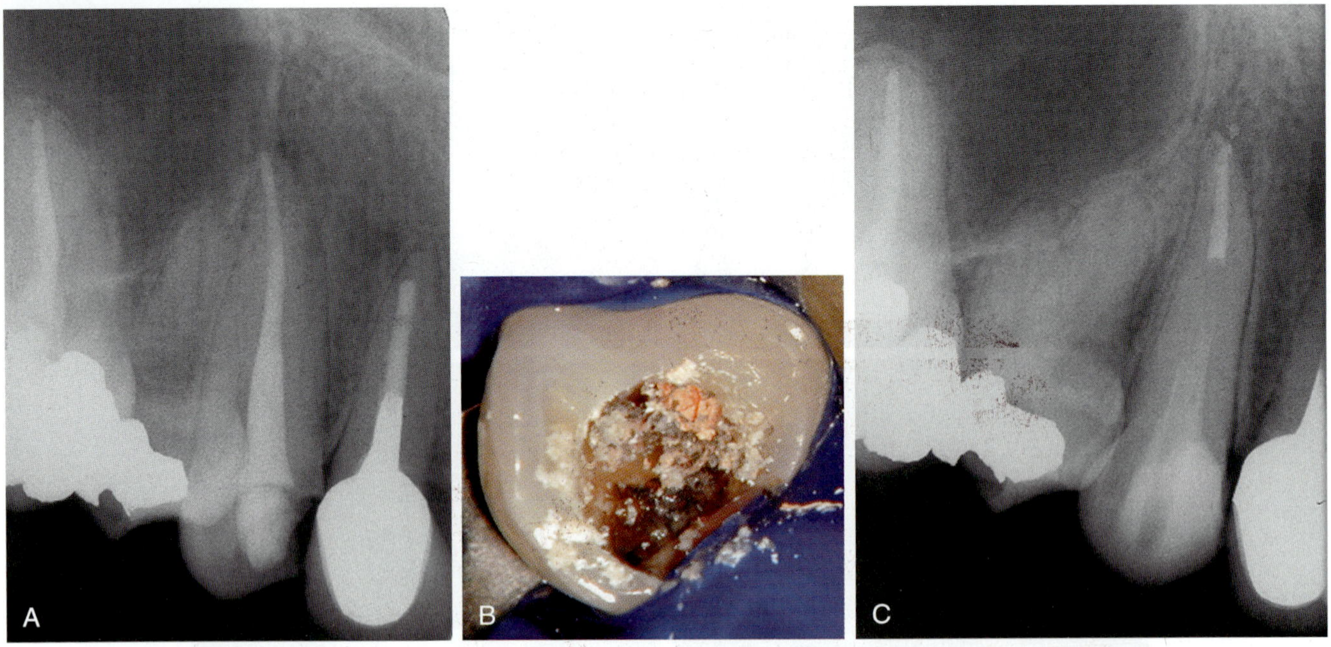

• **Fig. 22.7 (A)** Lack of coronal seal resulted in clinical symptoms and a periapical lesion in the maxillary right cuspid. **(B)** A clinical photograph shows lack of permanent restoration and coronal decay. **(C)** After retreatment of the previous root canal treatment and placement of a C-fiber post, the coronal access to the root canal treated tooth was sealed permanently. (Courtesy of Dr. D. Roland.)

to 68%.[11,50] On the other hand, overinstrumentation with overfilling of root canal filling materials may also promote foreign-body reactions,[83] periradicular hemorrhage, and induce extraradicular infection by transferring microorganisms from the canal to the periapical tissues, possibly compromising the outcome.[84]

Postoperative Causes

The restoration of the tooth after root canal treatment should be with a high-quality, durable coronal restoration that permanently protects and seals the tooth, preventing ingress and apical percolation of microorganisms and salivary contaminants (Fig. 22.7).[50-56,62-66,85-89]

Coronal leakage at any time after the completion of the root canal treatment may pose the risk of recontamination and subsequently failure of the endodontic procedure. The coronal seal must be guaranteed by a temporary restoration immediately after the completion of the root canal treatment and then for the lifetime of the tooth by a permanent restoration.

The permanent restoration may be placed immediately after the root filling is completed, or as early as possible thereafter. Rubber dam isolation in a saliva-free environment must be used whenever the actual root filling is exposed during the restoration process. Orifice sealants or barrier materials may be useful to minimize any risk of recontamination during the restoration process.[90] Any temporary restorations and cotton pellets must be completely removed before restoration.[61] Gutta-percha and sealer should be removed from the floor of the access cavity. No space should remain between the root filling and the buildup and/or restoration, as any such space provides a potential habitat for bacterial colonization and growth.

Errors throughout this restorative process may compromise success. This may include excessive dentin removal during instrumentation or for posts weakening the teeth and increasing its susceptibility to fracture (Fig. 22.8),[77] or perforations occurring during placement of the post. Full coronal coverage (i.e., with a crown or an onlay) has been shown to improve the prognosis for posterior teeth by reducing the incidence of fracture. However, for anterior teeth with enough tooth structure remaining, full coronal coverage does not increase the longevity of the tooth. On the contrary, preparing anterior endodontically treated teeth for a crown may remove too much remaining tooth structure, weaken the tooth, and result in a less favorable prognosis. Composite restorations and/or ceramic veneers are preferred for anterior teeth.

Outcomes of Treatments After Failure of Initial Nonsurgical Endodontics

For decades the primary goal of dentistry was to preserve the natural dentition, trying to save teeth with pulpal and/or periodontal diseases and, if hopeless teeth needed to be extracted, to replace them with fixed or removable prostheses. Although this may seem to lay out straight-forward decision making, treatment planning arguably has become more complex with the availability of dental implants. Both the preservation of endodontically treated teeth with appropriate permanent restoration as well as implant restorations demonstrate excellent and predictable outcomes to maintain the patient's oral health and dentition. The clear majority of teeth with endodontic treatment will heal without any further intervention. In case of failure of primary endodontic treatment, however, clinicians have the following treatment options: (1) nonsurgical retreatment, (2) surgical retreatment, (3) extraction and replacement with a single tooth implant, (4) extraction and replacement using a fixed dental prosthesis, (5) intentional replantation or autotransplantation, and (6) extraction without replacement.[91]

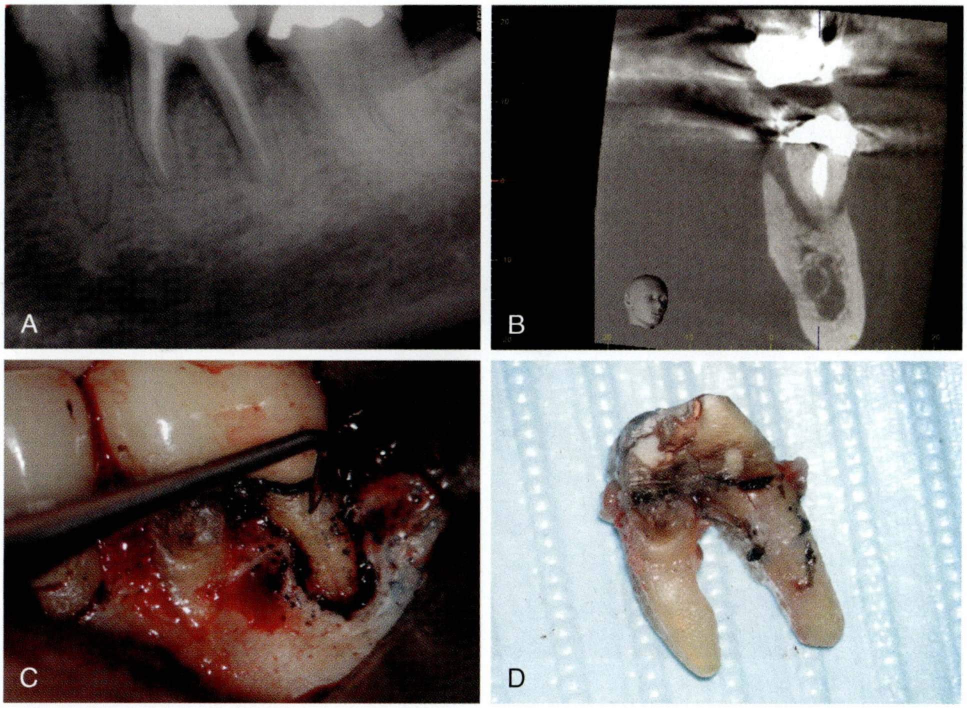

• **Fig. 22.8 (A)** Overenlargement of the coronal thirds. Bone loss in furcation and along distal root. **(B)** Cone beam computed tomography (CBCT) confirmation of extent of vertical bone loss. **(C)** Clinical confirmation after flap elevation. **(D)** Extracted tooth. (Courtesy of Dr. Rami Elsabee.)

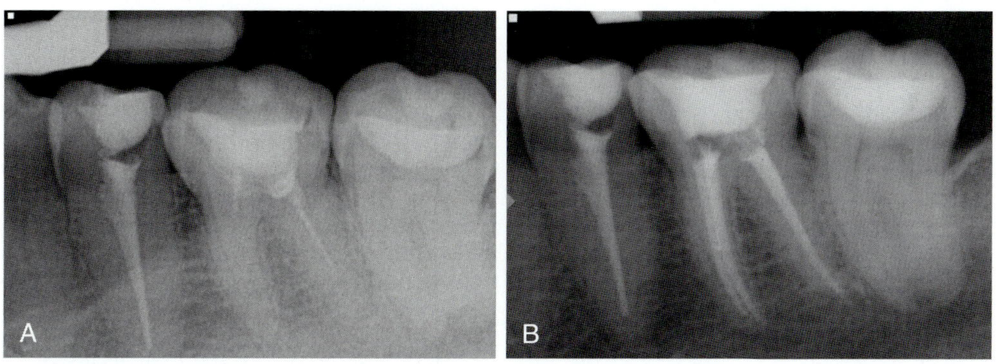

• **Fig. 22.9 (A)** A preoperative periapical radiograph shows the first mandibular molar with inadequate root canal treatment. The patient presents with clinical symptoms. **(B)** Postoperative radiograph after nonsurgical retreatment; patient is asymptomatic.

Nonsurgical Retreatment

Nonsurgical endodontic retreatment is the first treatment choice for most failed endodontic cases. The success rate of nonsurgical retreatment ranged between 40% and 100% according to a systematic review that identified 31 clinical studies since 1970 (Fig. 22.9).[92] The prospective Toronto study reported a "healed" rate of endodontic retreatment cases of 81%.[93] A systematic review and meta-analysis of nonsurgical retreatment reported an overall weighted pooled success rate of 77.2% based on data from 17 studies from 1961 to 2005.[94] In teeth with apical periodontitis the overall success was reduced to 65%, and of those with lesions larger than 5 mm in diameter to 41%.[94] However, it was mentioned that the follow-up periods for larger lesions might not have been long enough to demonstrate complete healing.[94] The technical quality of the initial endodontic treatment may negatively affect the outcome of nonsurgical retreatment if the entire root canal system is not accessible for complete reinstrumentation and disinfection during retreatment caused by obstacles left behind from the initial root canal treatment.[95] Unfortunately, to date, no higher level evidence outcome study on nonsurgical retreatment exists that included today's standard modern treatment techniques, such as nickel-titanium instrumentation, the dental operating microscope, or modern diagnostic tools such as CBCT imaging. Hence, it is unknown if there are changes in the success rates with recent endodontic technologies.

Endodontic Surgery

A systematic review of studies investigating the outcome of surgical endodontics found success rates ranging from 37% to 91%, depending on the operator and the specific techniques used for

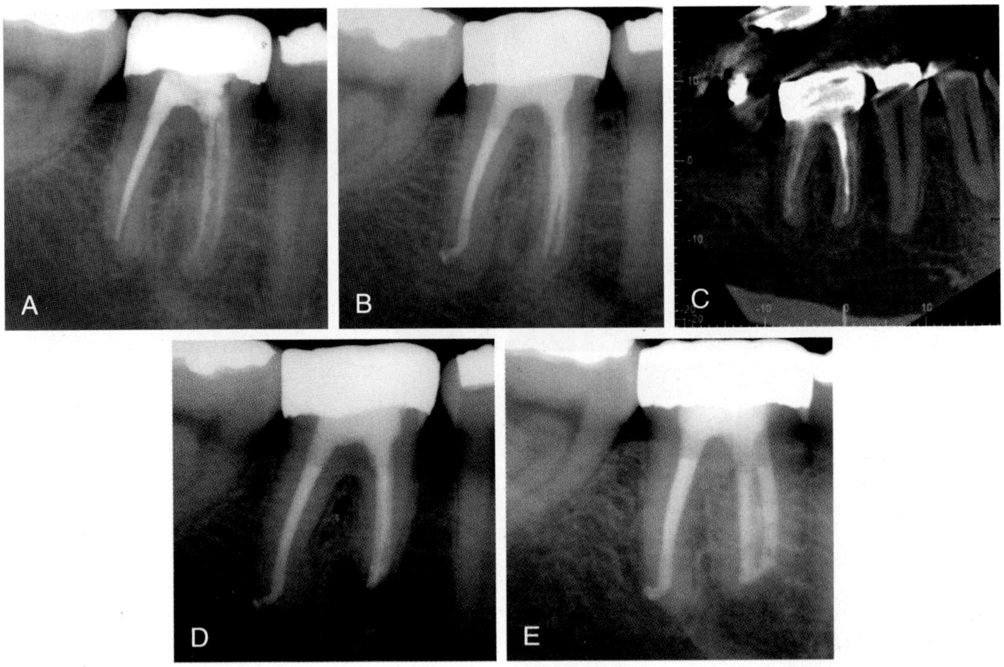

• **Fig. 22.10** **(A)** Insufficient root canal treatment of a first mandibular lower molar. **(B)** Cone beam computed tomography (CBCT) for treatment planning. **(C)** Patient remains symptomatic 3 months after nonsurgical retreatment. **(D)** Postoperative radiograph after endodontic microsurgery. **(E)** A recall radiograph 18 months later shows complete resolution of the periradicular lesion. The patient remained asymptomatic since the surgical procedure. (Courtesy of Dr. Tom Schloss.)

the surgical procedures.[96] Unfortunately, many studies reporting the success and failure of periapical surgery were identified as case series or other studies with a low level of evidence.[97] Torabinejad and colleagues performed a systematic review comparing the clinical and radiographic outcomes of nonsurgical retreatment with those of surgical retreatment.[98] The study concluded that nonsurgical retreatment provided more favorable long-term outcomes than endodontic surgery.[98]

A number of systematic reviews and meta-analyses have since then documented that the outcome of surgical retreatment very much depends on the techniques used for the procedures. Traditional, now obsolete techniques using a straight surgical handpiece, beveled root resection, and often a retrograde filling with amalgam demonstrated weighted pooled success rates of 59.0%.[99] On the other hand, the use of loupes, ultrasonic root-end preparation, and more biocompatible filling materials such as intermediate restorative material (IRM), SuperEBA, or MTA increased this outcome to 86% of periapical healing.[100] Endodontic microsurgery, which uses the same tools and techniques, but replaces loupes with a dental operating microscope capable of providing high magnification, demonstrated even higher success rates ranging from 91.4% to 94.4% for true endodontic lesions based on several meta-analyses (Fig. 22.10).[99,101-103] However, another systematic review and meta-analysis described lower outcome rates for teeth undergoing endodontic surgery compared with single unit implants.[104] Moreover, if the tooth is also periodontally compromised, surgical outcome was also reported to be significantly lower.[105]

Endodontic surgery should be reserved for teeth with failed nonsurgical retreatment, or situations where nonsurgical retreatment may be precluded for technical reasons,[98] as it appears that the success rate for a conventional retreatment is very high.[106]

Single Tooth Implant

The introduction of dental implants into modern dentistry provided great benefits for patients and allowed for functional, durable, and esthetic tooth replacement, leading to significant changes in endodontic, periodontic, and prosthodontic treatment planning and decision-making.[107] Implant-supported restorations have obviated the need for crown preparations on intact abutment teeth for fixed partial dentures (Fig. 22.11), and allowed fixed prosthodontic restorations even in the absence of suitable natural teeth as abutments.[108,109]

Comparisons between the outcome of endodontically treated teeth and dental implants are challenging as a result of the multifactorial nature of both treatment modalities, short-term versus long-term outcome, and the differences in outcome assessment. The implant field lacks a singular definition of success. Guidelines of the Academy of Osseointegration described "the desired outcome of successful implant therapy" as "not only the achievement of the therapeutic goal but the maintenance of a stable, functional and esthetically acceptable tooth replacement for the patient."[110] As a substitute of defined outcome criteria, survival of the implant unit is used frequently.[107]

Success and survival rates for single tooth implants are now generally very high. The aforementioned systematic review and meta-analysis by Iqbal and Kim included 55 studies investigating dental implants and 13 studies investigating endodontically treated teeth with various follow-up periods.[32] At the earliest point of comparison at 1 year, implant survival was higher at 97.5% compared with tooth survival of 96.9%. This trend showed reversal at long-term after 6 years when implant survival had declined to 94.2% and endodontically treated teeth were retained at 97.2%. However, over all time periods, 95.0% of implants and 94.0% of endodontically treated teeth survived.[32] Torabinejad et al. also have reported survival rate of 97% for both procedures.[28]

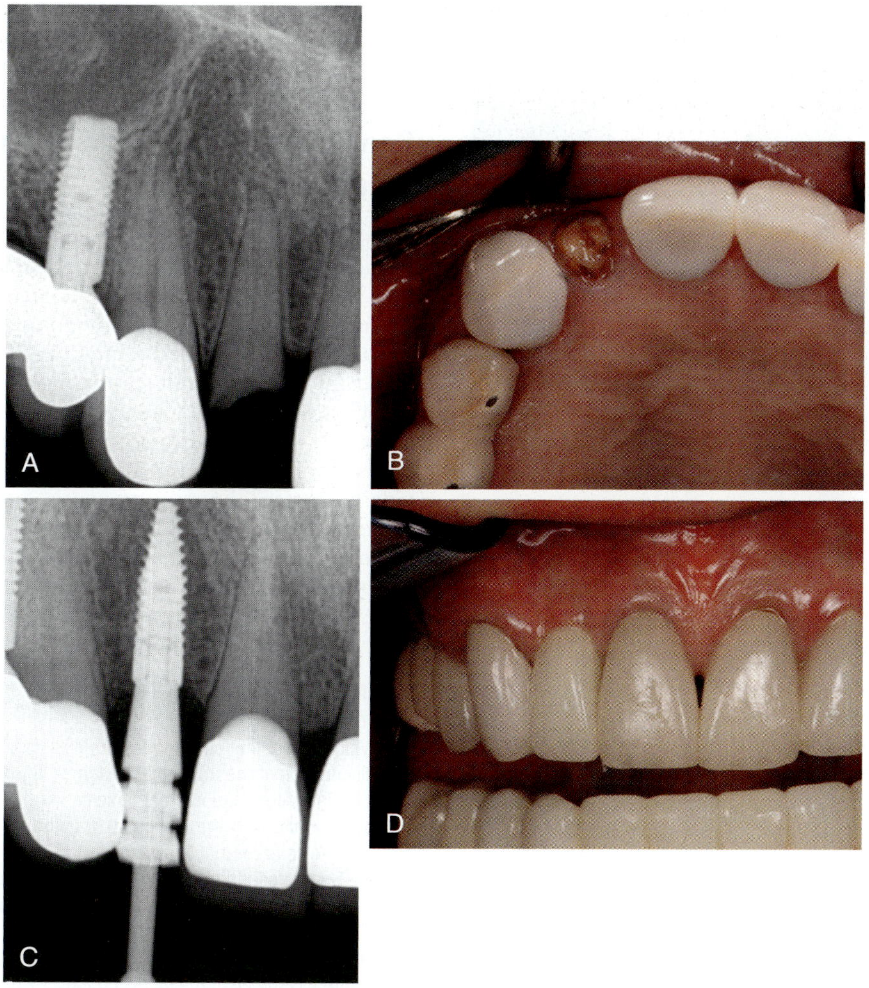

• **Fig. 22.11** **(A)** A periapical radiograph shows a maxillary right lateral incisor with extensive loss of coronal tooth structure, insufficient crown-to-root ratio, and unfavorable, tapered root form. **(B)** Corresponding clinical image demonstrates tooth structure loss at soft tissue level. The tooth was deemed nonrestorable. Note narrow space between central incisor and canine. **(C)** Radiograph showing ideal implant positioning and transfer abutment alignment. **(D)** Clinical situation at 1-year recall. (Courtesy of Dr. Santiago Jané Ceballos.)

In Doyle et al.'s study, 196 single implants were matched with 196 endodontically treated teeth, followed-up for up to 10 years, and then compared based on the outcome variables 'success', 'survival with intervention', 'survival without intervention', as well as 'failure'.[33] Results demonstrated identical failure rates at 6.1%. Tooth success was reported at 82.1%, and dental implants success at 73.5%. The rate for survival with need for intervention was higher for dental implants (17.9%) than for natural teeth (2.6%), confirming high complication rates often observed for implant restorations. Although overall degrees of satisfaction with minimal pain and discomfort have been generally observed for both procedures,[111] it is now agreed upon that restored natural teeth outlast dental implant restorations in comparable situations, Endodontic and implant success and survival rates are, however, substantially superior to those for fixed dental prostheses (Table 22.1). Vahdati et al. recently compared the survival outcome of nonsurgical root canal treatment and single-tooth implants in 170 patients who received both treatments.[112] The study confirmed Doyle and coworkers, with both treatments demonstrating a 95% survival rate with a mean 7.5-year follow-up, and a significantly higher number of adjunct and additional treatments, number of appointments, elapsed time before the final restoration, number of prescribed medications, as well as cost of treatment for single-tooth implants compared with nonsurgical root canal treatment.[112]

Both options, the preservation of a natural tooth and implant (re-)placement, should be seen as complementary and not as competing procedures.[32]

The decision to retain or to extract an individual tooth will be based on findings regarding the endodontic status, periodontal condition, remaining tooth structure, caries, root morphology, the condition of the adjacent teeth and the opposing arch, the occlusion, and esthetic parameters.[113] If in the long-term a tooth is potentially compromised in regard to prosthodontic, periodontal, or endodontic reasons, it needs to be taken into consideration that multiple risk factors may accumulate and that the risk of long-term failure may increase.[114]

Fixed Dental Prostheses

Before implant dentistry the preparation of teeth as abutments for fixed or removable partial dentures was common after the extraction of hopeless teeth. However, an increased incident rate for caries as well as pulpal and periodontal problems was

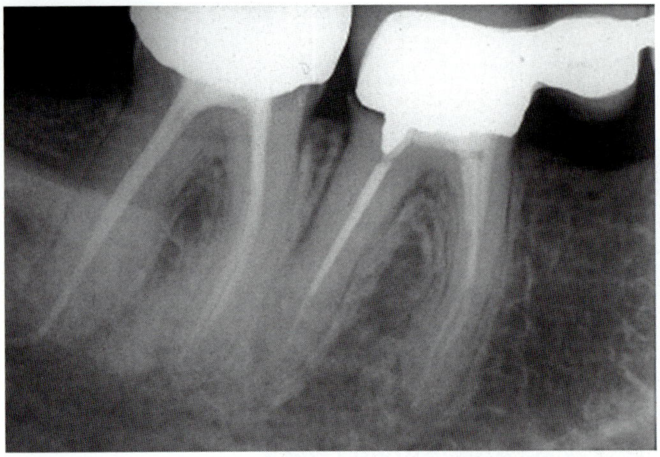

• **Fig. 22.12** Restored mandibular right molars have developed pulpal and periapical problems, in addition to caries under the margins of the crowns. Coronal leakage likely contributed to the development of the new periapical lesions.

reported, in addition to complications such as ceramic or root fractures (Fig. 22.12).[115] Success and survival rates for fixed dental prostheses have been reported as 48% to 95%. A meta-analysis of the literature demonstrated a 10-year survival of 87% and a 15-year survival rate of 69% for fixed dental prostheses.[116] Other reports also demonstrated similar results.[28,117,118] A systematic review comparing endodontically treated teeth with implant single crowns and fixed dental prostheses reported a success rate of only 82% at more than 6 years (see Table 22.1). As discussed previously, treatment planning in prosthodontics has changed significantly since the introduction of dental implants.[119] Implant-supported prostheses are now broadly preferred to tooth-supported prostheses.

Replantation and Transplantation

Replantation is the reinsertion of a tooth into its alveolus after careful, deliberate extraction of the tooth for the purpose of extraoral surgical retreatment.[120] Replantation is indicated when there is no other treatment alternative to maintain a strategic tooth, particularly in situations where the proximity of anatomic details, such as the infra-alveolar nerve or adjacent root structures prohibit direct endodontic surgery (Fig. 22.13). Replanted teeth are often successful long-term[103,121-123] but require careful case selection (see Chapter 21).

Transplantation is the transfer of a tooth from one alveolar socket to another in the same patient.[120,124,125] The clinical procedures involved include socket preparation, extraction, transplantation, and stabilization. When transplantation is appropriately indicated and performed, these teeth may have a good prognosis.[91,126-129] Ankylosis and resorption are the most common failure modes of intentionally replanted and autotransplanted teeth.

Extraction Without Replacement

Limited information is available about beneficial or harmful effects of extracting and not replacing individual teeth, including any potential psychosocial and/or economic effect. Few adverse effects were described for a shortened or even an interrupted dental arch. However, it is undebated that the loss of visible teeth without replacement has a tremendous adverse psychosocial effect.[28]

Reasons for Extraction of Endodontically Treated Teeth

Only a small proportion of endodontically treated teeth are extracted. Of these, very few are extracted for endodontic reasons.[29-31] Common reasons for extraction are decay, periodontal disease, nonrestorability, prosthodontic failure, and tooth or root fracture.[15,29-31,130] Added complexity of any additional adjunctive procedure may also result in further complications and higher associated risks, which may increase treatment costs and compromise a patient's willingness to accept endodontic treatment and tooth preservation.[131] However, after the belief that dental implants provide for better long-term prognosis compared with natural teeth has now been rejected by various comparative studies, a renewed call to revisit the long history of successful tooth maintenance for the preservation of the natural dentition has emerged.[132] After all, a missing tooth will be irreversibly gone, and extraction should be only considered after thorough deliberation.[107] Thus it is critical

Study Questions

6. Which one of the following factors WILL NOT complicate adequate disinfection of the root canal system?
   a. Virulence of the microorganisms
   b. Complexity of the root canal system
   c. Choice of rotary file system
   d. Separated instrument in the root canal system
   e. Quality of the permanent restoration all play an important role in as potential reasons for treatment failure
7. Errors that can lead to persistent microbial presence and endodontic failure include all of the following EXCEPT one. Mark this EXCEPTION.
   a. Inaccurate diagnosis
   b. Presence of tertiary dentin
   c. Missed canals
   d. Inadequate débridement and/or disinfection of the root canal system
   e. Inadequate temporary or permanent restorations
8. What is the most significant challenge posed by the presence of bacteria in a biofilm?
   a. Reduced immune response from host
   b. Increased bacterial load in apical area
   c. File separation from torsional fatigue
   d. Greater resistance to antimicrobial agents
   e. Higher potential for type I allergic reaction
9. What is the LEAST common reason for extraction of endodontically treated teeth?
   a. Inadequate endodontics
   b. Periodontal disease
   c. Prosthodontic failure
   d. Root fracture
   e. Higher success for implants compared with natural teeth
10. Vahdati et al. recently compared the survival outcome of nonsurgical root canal treatment and single-tooth implants in 170 patients who received both treatments. What was the significance noted with single-tooth implants?
   a. Higher number of adjunct and additional treatments
   b. Longer elapsed time before the final restoration
   c. Higher number of prescribed medications
   d. Higher cost of treatment
   e. All the above

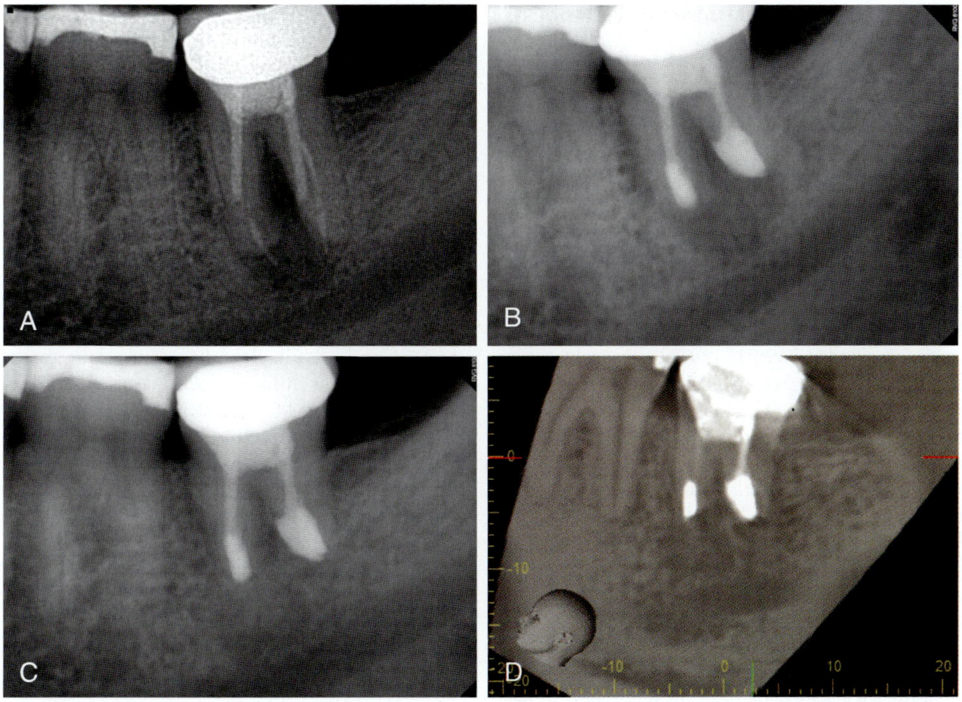

• **Fig. 22.13** **(A)** A periapical radiograph shows a mandibular second left molar with periradicular radiolucency. The previous root filling is overextended in both roots, the position of the post in the distal root and the extent of the bone loss are indicative of a post perforation. **(B)** Situation after intentional replantation using bioceramic putty as root-end filling and post perforation repair material during the extraoral procedure. **(C)** A radiograph 24 months later shows complete healing of the periradicular tissues. **(D)** Cone beam computed tomography (CBCT) confirmation of the periradicular healing.

ANSWERS

Answer Box 22

1 c. Decrease of a radiolucency in size
2 b. Any apical periodontitis in the mandible will be detectable on radiographs if it exceeds 3 mm in diameter
3 d. Success of endodontic microsurgery: 55% to 65%
4 a. Type of root filling material
5 e. The PAI grades in 4 stages from healthy periapex (score 1) to a large periapical lesion (score 4)
6 c. Choice of rotary file system
7 b. Presence of tertiary dentin
8 d. Greater resistance to antimicrobial agents
9 a. Inadequate endodontics
10 e. All the above

that the current situation as well as all potential future risk factors are being carefully considered during comprehensive patient assessment and treatment planning.[113,131,133]

References

1. Sundqvist G: *Bacteriological studies of necrotic dental pulps, odontol dissertation no 7*, Umeå, Sweden, 1976, University of Umeå.
2. Bergenholtz G: Micro-organisms from necrotic pulp of traumatized teeth, *Odontol Rev* 25:347, 1974.
3. Kantz WE, Henry CA: Isolation and classification of anaerobic bacteria from intact pulp chambers of non-vital teeth in man, *Arch Oral Biol* 19:91, 1974.
4. Hess W: The permanent dentition. I. In Hess W, Zürcher E, editors: *The anatomy of the root-canals of the teeth*, London, 1925, John Bale, Sons & Danielsson.
5. Davis SR, Brayton SM, Goldman M: The morphology of the prepared root canal: a study utilizing injectable silicone, *Oral Surg Oral Med Oral Pathol* 34:642, 1972.
6. Anderson MH: Use of evidence-based data by insurance companies, *J Evid Base Dent Pract* 4:120, 2004.
7. Reit C: Decision strategies in endodontics: on the design of a recall program, *Endod Dent Traumatol* 3:233, 1987.
8. Ørstavik D: Time-course and risk analyses of the development and healing of chronic apical periodontitis in man, *Int Endod J* 29:150, 1996.
9. Adenubi JO, Rule DC: Success rate for root fillings in young patients, *Br Dent J* 141:237, 1976.
10. Byström A, Happonen RP, Sjögren U, et al.: Healing of periapical lesions of pulpless teeth after endodontic treatment with controlled asepsis, *Endod Dent Traumatol* 3:58, 1987.
11. Sjögren U, Hägglund B, Sundqvist G, et al.: Factors affecting the long-term results of endodontic treatment, *J Endod* 16:498, 1990.
12. Molven O, Halse A: Success rates for gutta-percha and Kloroperka N-Ø root fillings made by undergraduate students: radiographic findings after 10-17 years, *Int Endod J* 21:243, 1988.
13. Lin LM, Pascon EA, Skribner J, et al.: Clinical, radiographic, and histologic study of endodontic treatment failures, *Oral Surg Oral Med Oral Pathol* 71:603, 1991.
14. Bender IB, Seltzer S, Soltanoff W: Endodontic success—a reappraisal of criteria. 1, *Oral Surg Oral Med Oral Pathol* 22:780, 1966.
15. Vire DE: Failure of endodontically treated teeth: classification and evaluation, *J Endod* 17:338, 1991.

16. Goldman M, Pearson AH, Darzenta N: Endodontic success: who's reading the radiograph? *Oral Surg Oral Med Oral Pathol* 33:432, 1972.
17. Ørstavik D, Kerekes K, Eriksen HM: The periapical index: a scoring system for radiographic assessment of apical periodontitis, *Endod Dent Traumatol* 2:20, 1986.
18. Brynolf I: A histological and roentgenological study of the periapical region of human upper incisors, *Odontol Rev* 18(Suppl II):1–33, 1967.
19. Friedman S, Mor C: The success of endodontic therapy—healing and functionality, *J Calif Dent Assoc* 32:493, 2004.
20. von Arx T, Janner SF, Hänni S, Bornstein MM: Agreement between 2D and 3D radiographic outcome assessment one year after periapical surgery, *Int Endod J* 49:915, 2016.
21. Schloss T, Sonntag D, Kohli MR, Setzer FC: A comparison of 2- and 3-dimensional healing assessment after endodontic surgery using cone-beam computed tomographic volumes or periapical radiographs, *J Endod* 43:1072, 2017.
22. Patel S, Dawood A, Mannocci F, et al.: Detection of periapical bone defects in human jaws using cone beam computed tomography and intraoral radiography, *Int Endod J* 42:507, 2009.
23. European Society of Endodontology, Patel S, Durack C, et al.: European Society of Endodontology position statement: the use of CBCT in endodontics, *Int Endod J* 47:502, 2014.
24. AAE and AAOMR Joint Position Statement: Use of cone beam computed tomography in endodontics 2015 update. Special committee to revise the joint AAE/AAOMR position statement on use of CBCT in endodontics, *Oral Surg Oral Med Oral Pathol Oral Radiol* 120:508, 2015.
25. Green TL, Walton RE, Taylor JK, et al.: Radiographic and histologic periapical findings of root canal treated teeth in cadaver, *Oral Surg Oral Med Oral Pathol Oral Radiol Endod* 83:707, 1997.
26. Torabinejad M, Kutsenko D, Machnick TK, et al.: Levels of evidence for the outcome of nonsurgical endodontic treatment, *J Endod* 31:637, 2005.
27. Friedman S, Abitbol S, Lawrence HP: Treatment outcome in endodontics: the Toronto Study—phase 1: initial treatment, *J Endod* 29:787, 2003.
28. Torabinejad M, Anderson P, Bader J, et al.: The outcomes of endodontic treatment, single implant, fixed partial denture and no tooth replacement: a systematic review, *J Prosthet Dent* 98:285, 2007.
29. Lazarski MP, Walker WATTI, Flores CM, et al.: Epidemiological evaluation of the outcomes of nonsurgical root canal treatment in a large cohort of insured dental patients, *J Endod* 27:791, 2001.
30. Salehrabi R, Rotstein I: Endodontic treatment outcomes in a large patient population in the USA: an epidemiological study, *J Endod* 30:846, 2004.
31. Chen S, Chueh L, Hsiao CK, et al: An epidemiologic study of tooth retention after nonsurgical endodontic treatment in a large population in Taiwan, *J Endod* 33:226,
32. Iqbal MK, Kim S: For teeth requiring endodontic therapy, what are the differences in the outcomes of restored endodontically treated teeth compared to implant-supported restorations? *Int J Oral Maxillofac Implants* 221(Suppl):96, 2007.
33. Doyle SL, Hodges JS, Pesun IJ, et al.: Retrospective cross sectional comparison of initial nonsurgical endodontic treatment and single-tooth implants, *J Endod* 32:822, 2006.
34. Levin L, Halperin-Sternfeld M: Tooth preservation or implant placement: a systematic review of long-term tooth and implant survival rates, *J Am Dent Assoc* 144:1119, 2013.
35. Locker D: Concepts of health, disease and quality of life. In Slade GD, editor: *Measuring oral health and quality of life*, ed 11, North Carolina, 1997, University of North Carolina Chapel Hill.
36. Pak JG, White SN: Pain prevalence and severity before, during, and after root canal treatment: a systematic review, *J Endod* 37:429, 2011.
37. Dugas NN, Lawrence HP, Teplitsky P, et al.: Quality of life and satisfaction outcomes of endodontic treatment, *J Endod* 28:819, 2002.
38. Kim SG, Solomon C: Cost-effectiveness of endodontic molar retreatment compared with fixed partial dentures and single-tooth implant alternatives, *J Endod* 37:321, 2011.
39. Liu P, McGrath C, Cheung GS: Improvement in oral health-related quality of life after endodontic treatment: a prospective longitudinal study, *J Endod* 40:805, 2014.
40. Vena DA, Collie D, Wu H, PEARL Network Group, et al.: Prevalence of persistent pain 3 to 5 years post primary root canal therapy and its impact on oral health-related quality of life: PEARL Network findings, *J Endod* 40:1917, 2014.
41. He J, White RK, White CA, et al.: Clinical and patient-centered outcomes of nonsurgical root canal retreatment in first molars using contemporary techniques, *J Endod* 43:231, 2017.
42. Goodacre CJ, Bernal G, Rungcharassaeng K, et al.: Clinical complications in fixed prosthodontics, *J Prosthet Dent* 90:31, 2003.
43. Strindberg LL: The dependence of the results of pulp therapy on certain factors, *Acta Odontol Scand* 14:175, 1956.
44. Chugal NM, Clive JM, Spangberg LS: A prognostic model for assessment of the outcome of endodontic treatment: effect of biologic and diagnostic variables, *Oral Surg Oral Med Oral Pathol Oral Radiol Endod* 91:342, 2001.
45. Sjögren U, Figdor D, Persson S, et al.: Influence of infection at the time of root filling on the outcome of endodontic treatment of teeth with apical periodontitis, *Int Endod J* 30:297, 1997.
46. Seltzer S, Bender IB, Turkenkopf S: Factors affecting successful repair after root canal therapy, *J Am Dent Assoc* 67:651, 1963.
47. Bergenholtz G, Lekholm U, Milthon R, et al.: Influence of apical overinstrumentation and overfilling on re-treated root canals, *J Endod* 5:310, 1979.
48. Ørstavik D, Hörsted-Bindslev P: A comparison of endodontic treatment results at two dental schools, *Int Endod J* 26:348, 1993.
49. De Moor RJ, Hommez GM, De Boever JG, et al.: Periapical health related to the quality of root canal treatment in a Belgian population, *Int Endod J* 33:113, 2000.
50. Chugal NM, Clive JM, Spangberg LS: Endodontic infection: some biologic and treatment factors associated with outcome, *Oral Surg Oral Med Oral Pathol Oral Radiol Endod* 96:81, 2003.
51. Katebzadeh N, Sigurdsson A, Trope M: Radiographic evaluation of periapical healing after obturation of infected root canals: an in vivo study, *Int Endod J* 33:60, 2000.
52. Katebzadeh N, Hupp J, Trope M: Histological periapical repair after obturation of infected root canals in dogs, *J Endod* 25:364, 1999.
53. Weiger R, Rosendahl R, Lost C: Influence of calcium hydroxide intracanal dressings on the prognosis of teeth with endodontically induced periapical lesions, *Int Endod J* 33:219, 2000.
54. Safavi KE, Dowden WE, Langeland K: Influence of delayed coronal permanent restoration on endodontic prognosis, *Endod Dent Traumatol* 187:1987, 1987.
55. Ray HA, Trope M: Periapical status of endodontically treated teeth in relation to the technical quality of the root filling and the coronal restoration, *Int Endod J* 28:12, 1995.
56. Chugal NM, Clive JM, Spangberg LS: Endodontic treatment outcome: effect of the permanent restoration, *Oral Surg Oral Med Oral Pathol Oral Radiol Endod* 104:576, 2007.
57. Stabholz A: Success rate in endodontics, *Alpha Omegan* 83:20, 1990.
58. Storms JL: Factors that influence the success of endodontic treatment, *J Can Dent Assoc (Tor)* 35:83, 1969.
59. Fouad AF, Burleson J: The effect of diabetes mellitus on endodontic treatment outcome: data from an electronic patient record, *J Am Dent Assoc* 134:43, 2003.
60. Wang C, Chueh L, Chen S, et al.: Impact of diabetes mellitus, hypertension, and coronary artery disease on tooth extraction after nonsurgical endodontic treatment, *J Endod* 37:1, 2011.
61. Kakehashi S, Stanley HR, Fitzgerald R: The effects of surgical exposures of dental pulps in germ free and conventional laboratory rats, *Oral Surg Oral Med Oral Pathol* 20:340, 1965.

62. Grossman LI: Endodontic failures, *Dent Clin North Am* 16:59, 1972.
63. Mandel E, Machtou P, Friedman S: Scanning electron microscope observation of canal cleanliness, *J Endod* 16:279, 1990.
64. Dalton BC, Ørstavik D, Phillips C, et al.: Bacterial reduction with nickel-titanium rotary instrumentation, *J Endod* 24:763, 1998.
65. Bystrom A, Sundqvist G: Bacteriologic evaluation of the effect of 0.5 percent sodium hypochlorite in endodontic therapy, *Oral Surg Oral Med Oral Pathol* 55:307, 1983.
66. Sjögren U, Figdor D, Spångberg L, et al.: The antimicrobial effect of calcium hydroxide as a short-term intracanal dressing, *Int Endod J* 24:119, 1991.
67. Love RM: Enterococcus faecalis – a mechanism for its role in endodontic failure, *Int Endod J* 34:399, 2001.
68. Evans M, Davies JK, Sundqvist G, Figdor D: Mechanisms involved in the resistance of *Enterococcus faecalis* to calcium hydroxide, *Int Endod J* 35:221, 2002.
69. Figdor D, Davies JK, Sundqvist G: Starvation survival, growth and recovery of *Enterococcus faecalis* in human serum, *Oral Microbiol Immunol* 18:234, 2003.
70. Svensäter G, Bergenholtz G: Biofilms in endodontic infections, *Endod Topics* 9:27, 2004.
71. Chavez de Paz LE: Redefining the persistent infection in root canals: possible role of biofilm communities, *J Endod* 33:652, 2007.
72. Schaal KP, Lee HJ: Actinomycete infections in humans - a review, *Gene* 115:201, 1992.
73. Sundqvist G, Reuterving CO: Isolation of *Actinomyces israelii* from periapical lesion, *J Endod* 6:602, 1980.
74. Ramachandran Nair PN, Pajarola G, Schroeder HE: Types and incidence of human periapical lesions obtained with extracted teeth, *Oral Surg Oral Med Oral Pathol Oral Radiol Endod* 81:93, 1996.
75. Lalonde ER: A new rationale for the management of periapical granulomas and cysts: an evaluation of histopathological and radiographic findings, *J Am Dent Assoc* 80:1056, 1970.
76. Natkin E, Oswald RJ, Carnes LI: The relationship of lesion size to diagnosis, incidence, and treatment of periapical cysts and granulomas, *Oral Surg Oral Med Oral Pathol* 57:82, 1984.
77. Trope M, Maltz DO, Tronstad L: Resistance to fracture of restored endodontically treated teeth, *Endod Dent Traumatol* 1:108, 1985.
78. Salis SG, Hood JA, Stokes AN, et al.: Patterns of indirect fracture in intact and restored human premolar teeth, *Endod Dent Traumatol* 3:10, 1987.
79. Seltzer S, Sinai I, August D: Periodontal effects of root perforations before and during endodontic procedures, *J Dent Res* 49:332, 1970.
80. Torabinejad M, Parirokh M, Dummer PMH: Mineral trioxide aggregate and other bioactive endodontic cements: an updated overview - part II: other clinical applications and complications, *Int Endod J* 51:284, 2018.
81. Hartwell GR, England MC: Healing of furcation perforations in primate teeth after repair with decalcified freeze-dried bone: a longitudinal study, *J Endod* 19:357, 1993.
82. Wu MK, Wesselink PR, Walton RE: Apical terminus location of root canal treatment procedures, *Oral Surg Oral Med Oral Pathol Oral Radiol Endod* 89:99, 2000.
83. Seltzer S, Soltanoff W, Sinai I, et al.: Biologic aspects of endodontics. Part 3. Periapical tissue reactions to root canal instrumentation, *Oral Surg Oral Med Oral Pathol* 26:534, 1968.
84. Seltzer S: *Endodontology*, ed 2, Philadelphia, 1988, Lea & Febiger.
85. Smith CS, Setchell DJ, Harty FJ: Factors influencing the success of conventional root canal therapy: a five-year retrospective study, *Int Endod J* 26:321, 1993.
86. Swanson K, Madison S: An evaluation of coronal microleakage in endodontically treated teeth. I. Time periods, *J Endod* 13:56, 1987.
87. Magura ME, Kafrawy AH, Brown Jr CE, et al.: Human saliva coronal microleakage in obturated root canals: an in vitro study, *J Endod* 17:324, 1991.
88. Khayat A, Lee SJ, Torabinejad M: Human saliva penetration of coronally unsealed obturated root canals, *J Endod* 19:458, 1993.
89. Alves J, Walton R, Drake D: Coronal leakage: endotoxin penetration from mixed bacterial communities through obturated, post-prepared root canals, *J Endod* 24:587, 1998.
90. Malik G, Bogra P, Singh S, Samra RK: Comparative evaluation of intracanal sealing ability of mineral trioxide aggregate and glass ionomer cement: an in vitro study, *J Conserv Dent* 16:540, 2013.
91. Torabinejad M, White SN: Endodontic treatment options after unsuccessful initial root canal treatment: Alternatives to single-tooth implants, *J Am Dent Assoc* 147:214–220, 2016.
92. Paik S, Sechrist C, Torabinejad M: Levels of evidence for the outcome of endodontic retreatment, *J Endod* 30:745, 2004.
93. Farzaneh M, Abitbol S, Friedman S: Treatment outcome in endodontics: the Toronto study—phases I and II: orthograde retreatment, *J Endod* 30:627, 2004.
94. Ng YL, Mann V, Gulabivala K: Outcome of secondary root canal treatment: a systematic review of the literature, *Int Endod J* 41:1026, 2008.
95. Gorni FG, Gagliani MM: The outcome of endodontic re-treatment: a 2-yr follow-up, *J Endod* 30:1, 2004.
96. Friedman S: The prognosis and expected outcome of apical surgery, *Endod Topics* 11:219, 2005.
97. Mead C, Javidan-Nejad S, Mego M, et al.: Levels of evidence for the outcome of endodontic surgery, *J Endod* 31:19, 2005.
98. Torabinejad M, Corr R, Handysides R, et al.: Outcomes of nonsurgical retreatment and endodontic surgery: a systematic review, *J Endod* 35:930, 2009.
99. Setzer FC, Shah S, Kohli M, et al.: Outcome of endodontic surgery: a meta-analysis of the literature—part 1: comparison of traditional root-end surgery and endodontic microsurgery, *J Endod* 36:1757, 2010.
100. Setzer FC, Kohli M, Shah S, et al.: Outcome of endodontic surgery: a meta-analysis of the literature - part 2: comparison of endodontic microsurgical techniques with and without the use of higher magnification, *J Endod* 38:1, 2012.
101. Tsesis I, Rosen E, Taschieri S, et al.: Outcomes of surgical endodontic treatment performed by a modern technique: an updated meta-analysis of the literature, *J Endod* 39:332, 2013.
102. Kohli MR, Berenji H, Setzer FC, et al.: Outcome of endodontic surgery: a meta-analysis of the literature-part 3: comparison of endodontic microsurgical techniques with 2 different root-end filling materials, *J Endod* 44:923, 2018.
103. Torabinejad M, Dinsbach N, Turman M, et al.: Survival of intentionally replanted teeth and implant-supported single crowns: a systemic review, *J Endod* 41:992–998, 2015.
104. Torabinejad M, Landaez M, Milan M, et al.: Tooth retention through endodontic microsurgery or tooth replacement using single implants: a systematic review of treatment outcomes, *J Endod* 41:1W10, 2015.
105. Song M, Kang M, Kang DR, et al.: Comparison of the effect of endodontic-periodontal combined lesion on the outcome of endodontic microsurgery with that of isolated endodontic lesion: survival analysis using propensity score analysis, *Clin Oral Investig* 22:1717, 2018.
106. Bergenholtz G, Lekholm U, Milthon R, et al.: Retreatment of endodontic fillings, *Scand J Dent Res* 87:217, 1979.
107. Setzer FC, Kim S: Comparison of long-term survival of implants and endodontically treated teeth, *J Dent Res* 93:19, 2014.
108. Brånemark PI, Zarb GA, Albrektsson T: *Tissue-integrated prostheses: osseointegration in clinical dentistry*, Chicago, 1985, Quintessence.
109. Schroeder A, Sutter F, Buser D, et al.: *Oral implantology*, ed 2, New York, 1996, Thieme.
110. Academy of Osseointegration: Guidelines of the Academy of Osseointegration for the provision of dental implants and associated patient care, *Int J Oral Maxillofac Implants* 25:620, 2010.
111. Torabinejad M, Salha W, Lozada J, et al.: Degree of patient pain, complications, and satisfaction after root canal treatment or a single implant: a preliminary prospective investigation, *J Endod* 40, 2014. 1940–5.
112. Vahdati SA, Torabinejad M, Handysides R, Lozada J: A retrospective comparison of outcome in patients who received both nonsurgical root canal treatment and single-tooth implants, *J Endod*, 45:99–103, 2019.

113. Su H, Liao HF, Fiorellini JP, et al.: Factors affecting treatment planning decisions for compromised anterior teeth, *Int J Periodont Restor Dent* 34:389, 2014.
114. Zitzmann NU, Krastl G, Hecker H, et al.: Strategic considerations in treatment planning: deciding when to treat, extract, or replace a questionable tooth, *J Prosthet Dent* 104:80, 2010.
115. Brägger U, Aeschlimann S, Burgin W, et al.: Biological and technical complications and failures with fixed partial dentures (FPD) on implants and teeth after four to five years of function, *Clin Oral Implants Res* 12:26, 2001.
116. Scurria MS, Bader JD, Shugars DA: Meta-analysis of fixed partial denture survival: prostheses and abutments, *J Prosthet Dent* 79:459, 1998.
117. Creugers NH, Kayser AF, van 't Hof MA: A meta-analysis of durability data on conventional fixed bridges, *Commun Dent Oral Epidemiol* 22:448, 1994.
118. Walton TR: An up to 15-year longitudinal study of 515 metal-ceramic FPDs. Part 1. Outcome, *Int J Prosthodont* 15:439, 2002.
119. Curtis DA, Lacy A, Chu R, et al.: Treatment planning in the 21st century: what's new? *J Calif Dent Assoc* 30:503, 2002.
120. American Association of Endodontists: *An annotated glossary of terms used in endodontics*, ed 8, Chicago, IL, 2015, American Association of Endodontists.
121. Kingsbury Jr BC, Wiesenbaugh Jr JM: Intentional replantation of mandibular premolars and molars, *J Am Dent Assoc* 83:1053, 1971.
122. Bender IB, Rossman LE: Intentional replantation of endodontically treated teeth, *Oral Surg Oral Med Oral Pathol* 76:623, 1993.
123. Grossman LI: Intentional replantation of teeth, *J Am Dent Assoc* 72:1111, 1966.
124. Apfel H: Autoplasty of enucleated prefunctional third molars, *J Oral Surg Anesth Hosp Dent Serv* 8:289, 1950.
125. Miller HM: Transplantation; a case report, *J Am Dent Assoc* 40:237, 1950.
126. Tsukiboshi M: Autogenous tooth transplantation: a reevaluation, *Int J Periodontics Restorative Dent* 13:120, 1993.
127. Akiyama Y, Fukuda H, Hashimoto K: A clinical and radiographic study of 25 autotransplanted third molars, *J Oral Rehabil* 25:640, 1998.
128. Andreasen JO: Third molar autotransplantation relation between successful healing and stage of root development at time of grafting. Paper presented at the annual meeting of the Scandinavian Association of Oral and Maxillofacial Surgeons, August 15-19, 1990, Nyborg, Denmark.
129. Andreasen JO, Paulsen HU, Yu Z, et al.: A long-term study of 370 autotransplanted premolars. II. Tooth survival and pulp healing subsequent to transplantation, *Eur J Orthod* 12:14, 1990.
130. Fuss Z, Lustig J, Tamse A: Prevalence of vertical root fractures in extracted endodontically treated teeth, *Int Endod J* 32:283, 1999.
131. Torabinejad M, Goodacre CJ: Endodontic or dental implant therapy: the factors affecting treatment planning, *J Am Dent Assoc* 137:973, 2006.
132. Giannobile WV, Lang NP: Are dental implants a panacea or should we better strive to save teeth? *J Dent Res* 95:5, 2016.
133. White SN, Miklus VG, Potter KS, et al.: Endodontics and implants: a catalog of therapeutic contrasts, *J Evid Based Dent Pract* 6:101, 2006.

Appendix 1

Summary Table of the Root Numbers of the Permanent Maxillary Teeth

Blaine Cleghorn, and William Christie

See Appendix 4 for a list of references.

Permanent Maxillary Teeth - Number of Roots

	NUMBER OF ROOTS						No. of Studies	References	No. of Teeth	Most Common Anomaly or Variation (Number of Case Reports in Brackets)
	Most Common	1	2	3	4	Other				
Central incisors	1 Root	100%					7	Rahimi, S et al 2009 (1), Weng, X-L et al 2009 (2), Sert, S and Bayirli, GS 2004 (3), Çaliskan, MK et al 1995 (4), Vertucci, F 1984 (5), Pineda, F and Kuttler, Y 1972 (6), Barrett, MT 1925 (7)	892	Dens evaginatus (17) 2 roots and 2 canals (14) 1 root and 2 canals (10) Fusion (9) Dens invaginatus (7)
Lateral incisors	1 Root	100%					7	Weng, X-L et al 2009 (2), Sert, S and Bayirli, GS 2004 (3), Çaliskan, MK et al 1995 (4), Vertucci, F 1984 (5), Bjorndal, AM and Skidmore, AE 1983 (8), Pineda, F and Kuttler, Y 1972 (6), Barrett MT 1925 (7)	827	Dens invaginatus (58) Palatogingival groove (20) Dens evaginatus (talon cusp) (17) 2 roots and 2 canals (10) 1 root and 2 canals (10)
Canines	1 Root	100%					7	Weng, X-L et al 2009 (2), Sert, S and Bayirli, GS 2004 (3), Çaliskan, MK et al 1995 (4), Vertucci, F 1984 (5), Bjorndal, AM and Skidmore, AE 1983 (8), Pineda, F and Kuttler, Y 1972 (6), Barrett MT 1925 (7)	842	Dens invaginatus (7) 1 root and 2 canals (2) Dens evaginatus (talon cusp) (2) 2 roots (2)

Continued

	NUMBER OF ROOTS						No. of Studies	References	No. of Teeth	Most Common Anomaly or Variation (Number of Case Reports in Brackets)
	Most Common	1	2	3	4	Other				
First pre-molar										3 roots and 3 canals (26)
Caucasian & others (excluding Asian & NA Native)*	2 Roots	37.7%	56.7%	1.9%		3.7%	17	Bürklein, S et al (2017) (9), Abella, F et al 2015 (10), Bulut, DG et al 2015 (11), Gupta, S et al (2015) (12), Dababneh, R and Rodan, R 2013 (13), Ng'ang'a, RN et al 2010 (14), Atieh, MA 2008 (15), Awawdeh, L et al 2008 (16), Chaparro, AJ et al 1999 (17), Kartal, N et al 1998 (18), Zaatar, El et al 1997 (19), Pecora, JD et al 1992 (20), Vertucci, FJ and Gegauff, A 1979 (21), Carns, EJ and Skidmore, AE 1973 (22), Green, D 1973 (23), Mueller, AH 1933 (24), Barrett MT 1925 (7)	4482	Furcation groove (palatal of B root) (3) Dens evaginatus (2)
Asian & NA Native	**1 Root**	**61.8%**	**37.6%**	**0.6%**			**5**	Tian, Y-Y et al 2012 (25), Cheng, XL and Weng, YL 2008 (26), Loh, HS et al 1998 (27), Aoki, K 1990 (28), Walker, RT 1987 (29)	4981	
All studies		50.4%	46.7%	1.2%		1.7%	22	Bürklein, S et al (2017) (9), Abella, F et al 2015 (10), Bulut, DG et al 2015 (11), Gupta, S et al (2015) (12), Dababneh, R and Rodan, R 2013 (13), Ng'ang'a, RN et al 2010 (14), Atieh, MA 2008 (15), Awawdeh, L et al 2008 (16), Chaparro, AJ et al 1999 (17), Kartal, N et al 1998 (18), Zaatar, El et al 1997 (19), Pecora, JD et al 1992 (20), Vertucci, FJ and Gegauff, A 1979 (21), Carns, EJ and Skidmore, AE 1973 (22), Green, D 1973 (23), Mueller, AH 1933 (24), Barrett MT 1925 (7), Tian, Y-Y et al 2012 (25), Cheng, XL and Weng, YL 2008 (26), Loh, HS et al 1998 (27), Aoki, K 1990 (28), Walker, RT 1987 (29)	9463	

	NUMBER OF ROOTS						No. of Studies	References	No. of Teeth	Most Common Anomaly or Variation (Number of Case Reports in Brackets)
	Most Common	1	2	3	4	Other				
Second premolar	1 Root	90.5%	8.9%	0.2%		0.4%	12	Elnour, M et al 2016 (30), Abella, F et al 2015 (10), Bulut, DG et al 2015 (11), Yang, L et al 2014 (31), Zaatar, El et al 1997 (19), Pecora, JD et al 1992 (32), Sikri, VK and Sikri, P 1991 (33), Aoki, K 1990 (28), Gorlin, RJ and Goldman, HM 1970 (34), Mueller, AH 1933 (24), Barrett MT 1925 (7)	9833	3 roots and 3 canals (16) Dens evaginatus (2)
First molar	3 Roots (MB, DB and Li)*	1.8%	2.2%	95.5%	0.2%	1.4%	20	Ghobashy, AM et al 2017 (35), Khademi, A et al 2017 (36), Martins, JN et al 2016 (37), Naseri, M et al 2016 (38), Tian, X-M et al 2016 (39), Alrahabi, M and Zafar, MS 2015 (40), Nikoloudaki GE et al 2015 (41), Singh, S and Pawar, M 2015 (42), Bhuyan, AC et al 2014 (43), Guo, J et al 2014 (44), Rouhani, A et al 2014 (45), Silva, EJ et al 2014 (46), Plotino, G et al 2013 (47), Zhang, R et al 2011 (48), Zheng, Q-H et al 2010 (49), Pattanshetti, N et al 2008 (50), Rwenyonyi, CM et al 2007 (51), al Shalabi, RM et al 2000 (52), Thomas, RP, Moule, AJ and Bryant, R 1993 (53), Gray, R 1983 (54), Barrett, MT 1925 (7)	7237	3 roots (MB, DB and Palatal) and 4-5 canals (1-2 MB, DB and 2 Palatal) (26) 3 roots (MB, DB and Palatal) and 5 canals (2MB, 2DB and Palatal) (12) Taurodontism (10) Fused roots and C-shaped canal (10) 4 roots (MB, DB and 2 Palatal) and 4 canals (MB, DB and 2 Palatal) (9)

Continued

	NUMBER OF ROOTS						No. of Studies	References	No. of Teeth	Most Common Anomaly or Variation (Number of Case Reports in Brackets)
	Most Common	1	2	3	4	Other				
Second molar	3 Roots (MB, DB and Li)	5.9%	9.1%	77.6%	0.8%		17	Ghobashy, AM et al 2017 (35), Khademi, A et al 2017 (36), Martins, JN et al 2016 (37), Tian, X-M et al 2016 (39), Nikoloudaki GE et al 2015 (41), Singh, S and Pawar, M 2015 (42), Zhang, Q et al 2014 (55), Rouhani, A et al 2014 (45), Silva, EJ et al 2014 (46), Plotino, G et al 2013 (47), Kim, Y et al 2012 (56), Zhang, R et al 2011 (48), Rwenyonyi, CM et al 2007 (51), al Shalabi, RM et al 2000 (52), Libfeld, H and Rotstein, I 1989 (57), Barrett, MT 1925 (7)	6699	4 roots (MB, DB and 2 Palatal) and 4 canals (MB, DB and 2 Palatal) (57) 3 roots and 4 canals (MB, DB and 2 Palatal canals) (7) 3 roots and 5 canals (3 MB, DB and Palatal canals) (3)
Third molar	3 Roots (MB, DB and Li)	31.2%	24.1%	42.4%	2.2%	0.1%	8	Tomaszewska, IM et al 2017 (58), Rawtiya, M et al 2016 (59), Singh, S and Pawar, M 2015 (42), Sert, S et al 2011 (60), Alavi, AM 2002 (61), Sidow, SJ et al 2000 (62), Guerisoli, DM et al 1998 (63), Barrett, MT 1925 (7)	1072	4 roots (3) C-shaped canal (1)

*NA Native = North American Native

*MB = mesiobuccal, DB = distobuccal and Li = lingual.

Appendix 2

Summary Table of the Root Canal Systems of the Permanent Maxillary Teeth

Blaine Cleghorn, and William Christie

See Appendix 4 for a list of references.

Permanent Maxillary Teeth: Number of Canals

	NUMBER OF CANALS						No. of Studies	References	No. of Teeth	Most Common Anomaly or Variation (Number of Case Reports In Brackets)
	Most Common	1	2	3	4	Other				
Central incisors *2 or more canals	1 Canal	99.1%	0.9%*				9	Da Silva, EJ et al 2016 (64), Altunsoy, M et al 2014 (65), Rahimi, S et al 2009 (1), Weng, X-L et al 2009 (2), Sert, S and Bayirli, GS 2004 (3), Çaliskan, MK et al 1995 (4), Vertucci, F 1984 (5), Pineda, F and Kuttler, Y 1972 (6), Barrett MT 1925 (7)	2635	Dens evaginatus (17) 2 roots and 2 canals (14) 1 root and 2 canals (10) Fusion (9) Dens invaginatus (7)
Lateral incisors *2 or more canals	1 Canal	96.0%	4.0%*				9	Da Silva, EJ et al 2016 (64), Altunsoy, M et al 2014 (65), Weng, X-L et al 2009 (2), Sert, S and Bayirli, GS 2004 (3), Çaliskan, MK et al 1995 (4), Vertucci, F 1984 (5), Bjorndal, AM and Skidmore, AE 1983 (8), Pineda, F and Kuttler, Y 1972 (6), Barrett MT 1925 (7)	2531	Dens invaginatus (58) Palatogingival groove (20) Dens evaginatus (talon cusp) (17) 2 roots and 2 canals (10) 1 root and 2 canalsa(10)
Canines *2 or more canals	1 Canal	95.6%	4.4%*				10	Da Silva, EJ et al 2016 (64), Altunsoy, M et al 2014 (65), Somalinga, NS et al 2014 (66), Weng, X-L et al 2009 (2), Sert, S and Bayirli, GS 2004 (3), Çaliskan, MK et al 1995 (4), Vertucci, F 1984 (5), Bjorndal, AM and Skidmore, AE 1983 (8), Pineda, F and Kuttler, Y 1972 (6), Barrett MT 1925 (7)	2815	Dens invaginatus (7) 1 root and 2 canals (2) Dens evaginatus (talon cusp) (2) 2 roots (2)
First premolar										3 roots and 3 canals (20)
Caucasian & others (excluding Asian & NA Native)*	2 Canals	11.3%	85.7%	1.7%		1.4%	20	Bürklein, S et al (2017) (9), Abella, F et al 2015 (10), Gupta, S et al (2015) (12), Ok, E et al 2014 (67), Ng'ang'a, RN et al 2010 (14), Weng, X-L et al 2009 (2), Ateih, M 2008 (15), Awawdeh, L et al 2008 (16), Sert, S and Bayirli, GS 2004 (3), Kartal, N et al 1998 (18), Zaatar, EI et al 1997 (19), Çaliskan, MK et al 1995 (4), Pecora, JD et al 1991 (20), Bellizzi, R and Hartwell, G 1985 (68), Vertucci, F and Gegauff, A 1979 (21), Carns, EJ and Skidmore, AE 1973 (22), Green, D 1973 (23), Pineda, F and Kuttler, Y 1972 (6), Mueller, AH 1933 (24), Barrett, MT 1925 (7), Hess, W 1925 (69)	6368	Furcation groove (palatal of B root) (3) Dens evaginatus (2)
Asian & NA Native	2 Canals	34.2%	63.2%	0.4%		2.4%	4	Weng, X-L et al 2009 (2), Cheng, XL and Weng, YL 2008 (26), Loh, HS et al 1998 (27), Walker, RT 1987 (204)	1574	
All studies		15.8%	81.2%	1.4%		1.6%	24	Bürklein, S et al (2017) (9), Abella, F et al 2015 (10), Gupta, S et al (2015) (12), Ok, E et al 2014 (67), Ng'ang'a, RN et al 2010 (14), Weng, X-L et al 2009 (2), Ateih, M 2008 (15), Awawdeh, L et al 2008 (16), Cheng, XL and Weng, YL 2008 (26), Sert, S and Bayirli, GS 2004 (3), Kartal, N et al 1998 (18), Loh, HS et al 1998 (27), Zaatar, EI et al 1997 (19), Çaliskan, MK et al 1995 (4), Pecora, JD et al 1991 (20), Walker, RT 1987 (29), Bellizzi, R and Hartwell, G 1985 (68), Vertucci, F and Gegauff, A 1979 (21), Carns, EJ and Skidmore, AE 1973 (22), Green, D 1973 (23), Pineda, F and Kuttler, Y 1972 (6), Mueller, AH 1933 (24), Barrett, MT 1925 (7), Hess, W 1925 (69)	7942	
Second premolar	1 or 2 Canals	47.1%	50.8%	0.8%		1.3%	19	Bürklein, S et al (2017) (9), Elnour, M et al 2016 (30), Abella, F et al 2015 (10), Ok, E et al 2014 (67), Yang, L et al 2014 (31), Jayamisha Raj, UJ and Sumitha, M 2009 (70), Weng, X-L et al 2009 (2), Sert, S and Bayirli, GS 2004 (3), Kartal, N et al 1998 (18), Zaatar, EI et al 1997 (19), Çaliskan, MK et al 1995 (4), Pecora, JD et al 1992 (32), Sikri, VK and Sikri, P 1991 (33), Bellizzi, R and Hartwell, G 1985 (68), Vertucci, F 1984 (5), Green, D 1973 (23), Pineda, F and Kuttler, Y 1972 (6), Mueller, AH 1933 (24)	5815	3 roots and 3 canals (16) Dens evaginatus (2)

First molar (three roots) *2 or more canals								3 roots (MB, DB and Palatal) and 4-5 canals (1-2 MB, DB and 2 Palatal) (26)
MB	2 Canals	40.2%	59.8%*		71	Alrahabi, M and Zafar, MS 2015 (40), Marroquin, B et al 2015 (71), Singh, S and Pawar, M 2015 (42), Bhuyan, AC et al 2014 (43), Kim, Y et al 2013 (72), Gu, Y et al 2011 (73), Peeters, HH et al 2011 (74), Somma, F et al 2009 (75), Weng, X-L et al 2009 (2), Abiodun-Solanke, IM et al 2008 (76), Alacam, T et al 2008 (77), Khraisat, A and Smadi, L 2007 (78), Rwenyonyi, CM et al 2007 (51), Eder, A et al 2006 (79), Smadi, L and Khraisat, A 2006 (80), Jung, I-Y et al 2005 (81), Scott, AE and Apicella, MJ 2004 (82), Sert, S and Bayirli, GS 2004 (3), Alavi, AM et al 2002 (61), Schwarze, T et al 2002 (83), Wasti, F et al 2001 (84), al Shalabi, RM et al 2000 (52), Weine, FS et al 1999 (85), Imura, N et al 1998 (86), Çaliskan, MK et al 1995 (4), Thomas, RP, Moule, AJ and Bryant, R 1993 (53), Pecora, JD et al 1992 (87), Kulild, JC and Peters, DD 1990 (88), Gilles, J and Reader, A 1990 (89), Vertucci, F 1984 (5), Gray, R 1983 (54), Acosta Vigouroux SA and Trugeda Bosaans, SA 1978 (90), Seidberg, BH et al 1973 (91), Pineda, F and Kuttler, Y 1972 (6), Sykaras, SN and Economou, PN 1971 (92), Weine, FS 1969 (93), Okamura, T 1927 (94), Hess, W 1925 (69), Zürcher, E 1925 (95), Moral, H 1914 (96), Ghobashy, AM et al 2017 (35), Khademi, A et al 2, MS017 (36), Betancourt, P et al 2016 (97), Coelho, MS et al 2016 (98), Naseri, M et al 2016 (38), Tian, X-M et al 2016 (39), Guo, J et al 2014 (44), Silva, EJ et al 2014 (46), Abuabara, A et al 2013 (99), Plotino, G et al 2013 (47), Reis, AG et al 2013 (100), Kim, Y et al 2012 (56), Lee, J-H et al 2011 (101), Zhang, R et al 2011 (48), Zheng, Q-H et al 2010 (49), Abiodun-Solanke, IM et al 2008 (76), Pattanshetti, N et al 2008 (50), Hartwell, G et al 2007 (102), Wolcott, J et al 2002 (103), Buhrley, LJ et al 2002 (104), Sempira, HN and Hartwell, GR 2000 (105), Stropko, JJ 1999 (106), Zaatar, El et al 1997 (19), Fogel, HM, Peikoff, MD and Christie, WH 1994 (107), Weller, RN and Hartwell, GR 1989 (108), Neaverth, EJ et al 1987 (109), Hartwell, G and Bellizzi, R 1982 (110), Pomeranz, HH and, Fishelberg, G 1974 (111), Slowey, RR 1974 (112), Nosonowitz, DM and Brenner, MR 1973 (113), Seidberg, BH et al 1973 (91)	18333	3 roots (MB, DB and Palatal) and 5 canals (2MB, 2DB and Palatal) (12) Taurodontism (10) Fused roots and C-shaped canal (10) 4 roots (MB, DB and 2 Palatal) and 4 canals (MB, DB and 2 Palatal) (9)
DB	1 Canal	98.6%	1.4%*		33	Ghobashy, AM et al 2017 (35), Naseri, M et al 2016 (38), Tian, X-M et al 2016 (39), Alrahabi, M and Zafar, MS 2015 (40), Briseno-Marroquin, B et al 2015 (71), Singh, S and Pawar, M 2015 (42), Bhuyan, AC et al 2014 (43), Guo, J et al 2014 (44), Silva, EJ et al 2014 (46), Plotino, G et al 2013 (47), Kim, Y et al 2012 (56), Zhang, R et al 2011 (48), Zheng, Q-H et al 2010 (49), Abiodun-Solanke, IM et al 2008 (76), Weng, X-L et al 2009 (2), Pattanshetti, N et al 2008 (50), Rwenyonyi, CM et al 2007 (51), Sert, S and Bayirli, GS 2004 (3), Alavi, AM et al 2002 (61), Wasti, F et al 2001 (84), al Shalabi, RM et al 2000 (52), Zaatar, El et al 1997 (19), Çaliskan, MK et al 1995 (4), Thomas, RP, Moule, AJ and Bryant, R 1993 (53), Pecora, JD et al 1992 (87), Vertucci, F 1984 (5), Gray, R 1983 (54), Hartwell, G and Bellizzi, R 1982 (110), Acosta Vigouroux SA and Trugeda Bosaans, SA 1978 (90), Pineda, F and Kuttler, Y 1972 (6), Hess, W 1925 (69), Zürcher, E 1925 (95)	8635	

Continued

Palatal	1 Canal	99.3%	0.7%*				34	Ghobashy, AM et al 2017 (35), Naseri, M et al 2016 (38), Marceliano-Alves, M et al 2016, Tian, X-M et al 2016 (39), Alrahabi, M and Zafar, MS 2015 (40), Briseno-Marroquin, B et al 2015 (71), Singh, S and Pawar, M 2015 (42), Bhuyan, AC et al 2014 (43), Guo, J et al 2014 (44), Silva, EJ et al 2014 (46), Plotino, G et al 2013 (47), Kim, Y et al 2012 (56), Zhang, R et al 2011 (48), Zheng, Q-H et al 2010 (49), Abiodun-Solanke, IM et al 2008 (76), Weng, X-L et al 2009 (2), Pattanshetti, N et al 2008 (50), Rwenyonyi, CM et al 2007 (51), Sert, S and Bayirli, GS 2004 (3), Alavi, AM et al 2002 (61), Wasti, F et al 2001 (84), al Shalabi, RM et al 2000 (52), Zaatar, El et al 1997 (19), Çaliskan, MK et al 1995 (4), Thomas, RP, Moule, AJ and Bryant, R 1993 (53), Pecora, JD et al 1992 (87), Vertucci, F 1984 (5), Gray, R 1983 (54), Hartwell, G and Bellizzi, R 1982 (110), Acosta Vigouroux SA and Trugeda Bosaans, SA 1978 (90), Pineda, F and Kuttler, Y 1972 (6), Hess, W 1925 (69), Zürcher, E 1925 (95)	8804	
Second molar (three roots) *2 or more canals										4 roots (MB, DB and 2 Palatal) and 4 canals (MB, DB and 2 Palatal) (57) 3 roots and 4 canals (MB, DB and 2 Palatal canals) (7) 3 roots and 5 canals (3 MB, DB and Palatal canals) (3)
MB	1 Canal	56.5%	43.5%*				35	Ghobashy, AM et al 2017 (35), Khademi, A et al 2017 (36), Wolf, TG et al 2017 (114), Betancourt, P et al 2016 (97), Coelho, MS et al 2016 (98), Tian, X-M et al 2016 (39), Singh, S and Pawar, M 2015 (42), Silva, EJ et al 2014 (46), Plotino, G et al 2013 (47), Reis, AG et al 2013 (100), Han, X et al 2012 (115), Kim, Y et al 2012 (56), Zhang, R et al 2011 (48), Weng, X-L et al 2009 (2), Rwenyonyi, CM et al 2007 (51), Sert, S and Bayirli, GS 2004 (3), Alavi, AM et al 2002 (61), Schwarze, T et al 2002 (83), al Shalabi, RM et al 2000 (52), Stropko, JJ 1999 (106), Imura, N et al 1998 (86), Zaatar, El et al 1997 (19), Çaliskan, MK et al 1995 (4), Eskoz, N and Weine, FS 1995 (116), Singh, C et al 1994 (117), Pecora, JD et al 1992 (87), Kulild, JC and Peters, DD 1990 (88), Gilles, J and Reader, A 1990 (89), Vertucci, F 1984 (5), Hartwell, G and Bellizzi, R 1982 (110), Pomeranz, HH and Fishelberg, G 1974 (111), Nosonowitz, DM and Brenner, MR 1973 (113), Pineda, F and Kuttler, Y 1972 (6), Hess, W 1925 (69)	8059	
DB	1 Canal	99.5%	0.5%*				21	Ghobashy, AM et al 2017 (35), Wolf, TG et al 2017 (114), Tian, X-M et al 2016 (39), Singh, S and Pawar, M 2015 (42), Silva, EJ et al 2014 (46), Plotino, G et al 2013 (47), Kim, Y et al 2012 (56), Zhang, R et al 2011 (48), Weng, X-L et al 2009 (2), Rwenyonyi, CM et al 2007 (51), Sert, S and Bayirli, GS 2004 (3), Alavi, AM et al 2002 (61), al Shalabi, RM et al 2000 (52), Zaatar, El et al 1997 (19), Çaliskan, MK et al 1995 (4), Singh, C et al 1994 (117), Pecora, JD et al 1992 (87), Vertucci, F 1984 (5), Hartwell, G and Bellizzi, R 1982 (110), Pineda, F and Kuttler, Y 1972 (6), Hess, W 1925 (69)	5053	
Palatal	1 Canal	99.8%	0.2%*				20	Ghobashy, AM et al 2017 (35), Wolf, TG et al 2017 (114), Tian, X-M et al 2016 (39), Singh, S and Pawar, M 2015 (42), Silva, EJ et al 2014 (46), Plotino, G et al 2013 (47), Kim, Y et al 2012 (56), Zhang, R et al 2011 (48), Weng, X-L et al 2009 (2), Rwenyonyi, CM et al 2007 (51), Sert, S and Bayirli, GS 2004 (3), Alavi, AM et al 2002 (61), al Shalabi, RM et al 2000 (52), Zaatar, El et al 1997 (19), Çaliskan, MK et al 1995 (4), Pecora, JD et al 1992 (87), Vertucci, F 1984 (5), Hartwell, G and Bellizzi, R 1982 (110), Pineda, F and Kuttler, Y 1972 (6), Hess, W 1925 (69)	5003	
Third molar	3 canals	9.8%	13.4%	51.5%	20.4%	2.2%	6	Rawtiya, M et al 2016 (59), Singh, S and Pawar, M 2015 (42), Weng, X-L et al 2009 (2), Alavi, AM 2002 (61), Sidow, SJ et al 2000 (62), Guerisoli, DM et al 1998 (63)	715	4 roots (3) C-shaped canal (1)

*NA Native = North American Native

Appendix 3

Summary Table of the Root Numbers of the Permanent Mandibular Teeth

Blaine Cleghorn, and William Christie

See Appendix 4 for a list of references.

Permanent Mandibular Teeth: Number of Roots

	NUMBER OF ROOTS									
	Most Common	1	2	3	4	Other	No. of Studies	References	No. of Teeth	Most Common Anomaly or Variation (Number of Case Reports In Brackets)
Central incisors	1 Root	100%					13	Verna, GR et al 2017 (118), Kamtane, S and Ghodke, M 2016 (119), Zhengyan, Y et al 2016 (120), Kayaoglu, G et al 2015 (121), Han, T et al 2014 (122), Lin, Z et al 2014 (123), Aminsobhani, M et al 2013 (124), Sert, S and Bayirli, GS 2004 (3), Çaliskan, MK et al 1995 (4), Vertucci FJ 1974 (125), Madiera MC and Hetem S 1973 (126), Pineda F and Kuttler Y 1972 (6), Barrett MT 1925 (7)	9728	Dens invaginatus (6) Dens evaginatus (talon cusp) (6) 2 canals (6)
Lateral incisors	1 Root	100%					13	Verna, GR et al 2017 (118), Kamtane, S and Ghodke, M 2016 (119), Zhengyan, Y et al 2016 (120), Kayaoglu, G et al 2015 (121), Han, T et al 2014 (122), Lin, Z et al 2014 (123), Aminsobhani, M et al 2013 (124), Sert, S and Bayirli, GS 2004 (3), Çaliskan, MK et al 1995 (4), Vertucci, FJ 1974 (125), Vertucci, FJ 1974 (125), Madiera, MC and Hetem, S 1973 (126), Pineda, F and Kuttler, Y 1972 (6), Barrett, MT 1925 (7)	9664	2 canals (5) Dens invaginatus (4)
Canines	1 Root	96.7%	3.3%				10	Soleymani, A et al 2017 (127), Shemesh, A et al 2016 (128), Zhengyan, Y et al 2016 (120), Kayaoglu, G et al 2015 (121), Han, T et al 2014 (122), Aminsobhani, M et al 2013 (124), Ouellet, R 1995 (129), Pecora, JD et al 1993 (130), Alexandersen, V 1963 (131), Barrett, MT 1925 (7)	16452	2 roots and 2 canals (8) 2 roots and 3 canals (3) 1 root and 2 canals (3)

Continued

	NUMBER OF ROOTS									
	Most Common	1	2	3	4	Other	No. of Studies	References	No. of Teeth	Most Common Anomaly or Variation (Number of Case Reports In Brackets)
First premolar	1 Root	94.3%	4.8%	0.1%	0.1%		26	Alkaabi, W et al 2017 (132), Bürklein, S et al (2017) (9), Dou, L et al 2017 (133), Abraham, SB and Gopinath, VK 2015 (134), Bulut, DG et al 2015 (11), Huang, Y-D et al 2015 (135), Kazemipoor, M et al 2015 (136), Kazemipoor, M et al 2015 (137), Kong, L-j et al 2015 (138), Llena, C et al 2014 (139), Singh, S and Pawar, M 2014 (140), Alhadainy, HA 2013 (141), Yang, H et al, 2013 (142), Yu, X et al 2012 (143), Jain, A and Bahuguna, R 2011 (144), Kheddmat, S et al 2010 (145) , Awawdeh, LA and Al-Qudah, AA 2008 (146), Rahimi, S et al 2007 (147), Iyer, VH et al 2006 (148), Sert, S and Bayirli, GS 2004 (3), Zaatar, El et al 1997 (19), Çaliskan, MK et al 1995 (4), Geider, P et al 1989 (149), Vertucci, F 1978 (150), Schulze, C 1970 (151), Barrett, MT 1925 (7)	14137	3 roots and 3 canals (5) 1 root and 2 canals (5) 1 root and 3 canals (5) Dens evaginatus (4) 2 roots and 2 canals (3) 3 canals (3) C-shaped canal (4)
Second premolar	1 Root	98.4%	1.4%	0.1%			20	Bürklein, S et al (2017) (9), Bulut, DG et al 2015 (11), Kazemipoor, M et al 2015 (136), Kazemipoor, M et al 2015 (137), lena, C et al 2014 (139), Singh, S and Pawar, M 2014 (140), Bolhari, B et al 2013 (152), Yu, X et al 2012 (143), Parekh, V et al 2011 (153), Rahimi, S et al 2009 (1), Awawdeh, LA and Al-Qudah, AA 2008 (146), Rahimi, S et al 2007 (147), Sert, S and Bayirli, GS 2004 (3), Zaatar, El et al 1997 (19), Çalişkan, MK et al 1995 (4), Geider, P et al 1989 (149), Vertucci, F 1978 (150), Zillich, R and Dowson, J 1973 (154), Visser, JB 1948 (155), Barrett, MT 1925 (7)	8002	3 canals (12) 2 roots and 2 canals (11) C-shaped canal (7) Dens evaginatus (6) 3 roots and 3 canals (6)

	NUMBER OF ROOTS									
	Most Common	1	2	3	4	Other	No. of Studies	References	No. of Teeth	Most Common Anomaly or Variation (Number of Case Reports In Brackets)
First molar										Radix entomolaris (32) 2 roots and 5 canals (3M and 2D) (20) 2 roots and 4 canals (3M and D) (10) 2 roots and 5 canals (2M and 3D) (8) 2 roots and 6 canals (3M and 3D) (7)
Caucasian & others (excluding Asian & NA Native)	2 Roots (M&D)	0.2%	96.3%	3.5%			28	Madani, ZS et al 2017 (156), Mohammadzadeh Akhlaghi, N et al 2017 (157), Celikten, B et al 2016 (158), Martins, JN et al 2016 (37), Rodrigues, CT et al 2016 (159), Peiris, R et al 2015 (160), Chourasia, HR et al 2012 (161), Colak, H et al 2012 (162), Chandra, SS et al 2011 (163), Al-Qudah, AA and Awawdeh, LA 2009 (164), Schafer, E et al 2009 (165), Pattanshetti, N et al 2008 (50), Reuben, J et al 2008 (166), Shahi, s et al 2008 (167), Ahmed, HA et al 2007 (168), Peiris, R et al 2007 (169), Al-Nazhan, S 1999 (170), Sperber, GH and Moreau, JL 1998 (171), Zaatar, El et al 1998 (172), Zaatar, El et al 1997 (19), Rocha, LF et al 1996 (173), Younes et al 1990 (174), Curzon, MEJ 1974 (175), Curzon, MEJ 1973 (176), de Souza-Freitas, JA et al 1971 (177), Skidmore, AE and Bjorndal, AM 1971 (178), Barrett, MT 1925 (7)	9639	
Asian & NA Native	2 Roots (M&D)	0.4%	77.5%	22.1%			17	Zhang, X et al 2015, Jang, J-K et al 2013 (179), Kim, S-Y et al 2013 (180), Zhang, R et al 2011 (181), Huang, CC et al 2010 (182), Wang, Y et al 2010 (183), Chen, G et al 2009 (184) Gulabivala, K et al 2002 (185), Gulabivala, K et al 2001 (186), Yew, S and Chan, K 1993 (187), Morita, M 1990 (188), Harada, Y et al 1989 (189), Onda, S et al 1989 (190), Walker, R 1988 (191), Reichart, PA and Metah, D 1981 (192), Curzon, MEJ 1974 (175), de Souza-Freitas, JA et al 1971 (177)	11632	

Continued

	NUMBER OF ROOTS									
	Most Common	1	2	3	4	Other	No. of Studies	References	No. of Teeth	Most Common Anomaly or Variation (Number of Case Reports In Brackets)
All studies	2 Roots (M&D)	0.3%	86.0%	13.7%			45	Madani, ZS et al 2017 (156), Mohammadzadeh Akhlaghi, N et al 2017 (157), Celikten, B et al 2016 (158), Martins, JN et al 2016 (37), Rodrigues, CT et al 2016 (159), Peiris, R et al 2015 (160), Chourasia, HR et al 2012 (161), Colak, H et al 2012 (162), Chandra, SS et al 2011 (163), Al-Qudah, AA and Awawdeh, LA 2009 (164), Schafer, E et al 2009 (165), Pattanshetti, N et al 2008 (50), Reuben, J et al 2008 (166), Shahi, s et al 2008 (167), Ahmed, HA et al 2007 (168), Peiris, R et al 2007 (169), Al-Nazhan, S 1999 (170), Sperber, GH and Moreau, JL 1998 (171), Zaatar, El et al 1998 (172), Zaatar, El et al 1997 (19), Rocha, LF et al 1996 (173), Younes et al 1990 (174), Curzon, MEJ 1974 (175), Curzon, MEJ 1973 (176), de Souza-Freitas, JA et al 1971 (177), Skidmore, AE and Bjorndal, AM 1971 (178), Barrett, MT 1925 (7), Zhang, X et al 2015, Jang, J-K et al 2013 (179), Kim, S-Y et al 2013 (180), Zhang, R et al 2011 (181), Huang, CC et al 2010 (182), Wang, Y et al 2010 (183), Chen, G et al 2009 (184) Gulabivala, K et al 2002 (185), Gulabivala, K et al 2001 (186), Yew, S and Chan, K 1993 (187), Morita, M 1990 (188), Harada, Y et al 1989 (189), Onda, S et al 1989 (190), Walker, R 1988 (191), Reichart, PA and Metah, D 1981 (192), Curzon, MEJ 1974 (175), de Souza-Freitas, JA et al 1971 (177)	21271	

	NUMBER OF ROOTS									
	Most Common	1	2	3	4	Other	No. of Studies	References	No. of Teeth	Most Common Anomaly or Variation (Number of Case Reports In Brackets)
Second molar	2 Roots (M&D)	23.2%	53.7%	1.8%	0.1%		27	Madani, ZS et al 2017 (156), Pawar, AM et al 2017 (193), Akhaghi, NM et al 2016 (194), Celikten, B et al 2016 (158), Kim, SY et al 2016 (195), Martins, JN et al 2016 (37), Shemesh, A et al 2015 (196), Silva, EJNL et al 2013 (197), Zare Jahromi, M et al 2013 (198), Zhang, R et al 2011 (181), Zheng, Q et al 2011 (199), Neelakantan, P et al 2010 (200), Al-Qudah, AA and Awawdeh, LA 2009 (164), Rahimi, S et al 2008 (201), Ahmed, HA et al 2007 (168), Peiris, R et al 2007 (169), Cheung, LHM et al 2006 (202), Gulabivala, K et al 2002 (185), Gulabivala, K et al 2001 (186), Zaatar, El et al 1997 (19), Rocha, LF da Costa et al 1996 (173), Manning, SA 1990a (203), Onda, S et al 1989 (190), Walker, RT 1988 (204), Weine, FS et al 1988 (205), Kotoku, K 1985 (206), Barrett, MT 1925 (7)	13932	C-shaped canal (19) Taurodontism (18) Fusion with a paramolar (7) 3 roots (MB, MLi, and D) and 3 canals (6) 1 root and 1 canal (6)
Third molar	2 Roots (M&D)	42.8%	53.3%	3.7%	0.1%	0%	10	Somasundaram, P et al 2017 (207), Park, J-B et al 2013 (208), Kuzekanani, M et al 2012 (209), Sert, S et al 2011 (60), Gulabivala, K et al 2002 (185), Gulabivala, K et al 2001 (186), Sidow, SJ et al 2000 (62), Guerisoli, DM et al 1998 (63), Ogiwara, I et al 1981 (210), Barrett, MT 1925 (7)	14001	Highly variable; variation is the norm

Appendix 4

Summary Table of the Root Canal Systems of the Permanent Mandibular Teeth

Blaine Cleghorn, and William Christie

Permanent Mandibular Teeth: Number of Canals

	NUMBER OF CANALS						No. of Studies	References	No. of Teeth	Most Common Anomaly or Variation (Number of Case Reports In Brackets)
	Most Common	1	2	3	4	Other				
Central incisors	1 Canal	84.3%	15.6%			0.1%	23	Verna, GR et al 2017 (118), Da Silva, EJ et al 2016 (64), Zhengyan, Y et al 2016 (120), Kayaoglu, G et al 2015 (121), Altunsoy, M et al 2014 (65), Han, T et al 2014 (122), Lin, Z et al 2014 (123), Liu, J et al 2014 (211), Aminsobhani, M et al 2013 (124), Sert, S and Bayirli, GS 2004 (3), Gomes, BP et al 1996 (212), Çaliskan, MK et al 1995 (4), Karagöz-Kücükay, I 1994 (213), Walker RT 1988 (214), Kaffee I et al 1985 (215), Bellizzi R and Hartwell G 1983 (216), Warren, EM and Laws, AJ 1981 (217), Miyoshi S et al 1977 (218), Vertucci FJ 1974 (125), Madiera MC and Hetem S 1973 (126), Pineda F and Kuttler Y 1972 (6), Laws AJ 1971 (219), Barrett MT 1925 (7)	14045	Dens invaginatus (6) Dens evaginatus (talon cusp) (6) 2 canals (6)
Lateral incisors	1 Canal	79.1%	20.8%			0.1%	23	Verna, GR et al 2017 (118), Da Silva, EJ et al 2016 (64), Zhengyan, Y et al 2016 (120), Kayaoglu, G et al 2015 (121), Altunsoy, M et al 2014 (65), Han, T et al 2014 (122), Lin, Z et al 2014 (123), Liu, J et al 2014 (211), Aminsobhani, M et al 2013 (124), Sert, S and Bayirli, GS 2004 (3), Gomes, BP et al 1996 (212), Çaliskan, MK et al 1995 (4), Walker, RT 1988 (214), Karagöz-Kücükay, I 1994 (213), Kaffe, I et al 1985 (215), Warren, EM and Laws, AJ 1981 (217), Bellizzi, R and Hartwell, G 1983 (216), Miyoshi, S et al 1977 (218), Vertucci, FJ 1974 (125), Madiera, MC and Hetem, S 1973 (126), Pineda, F and Kuttler, Y 1972 (6), Laws, AJ 1971 (219), Barrett, MT 1925 (7)	13748	2 canals (5) Dens invaginatus (4)

	NUMBER OF CANALS						No. of Studies	References	No. of Teeth	Most Common Anomaly or Variation (Number of Case Reports In Brackets)
	Most Common	1	2	3	4	Other				
Canines * 2 or more canals	1 Canal	91.2%	8.8%*				20	Soleymani, A et al 2017 (127), Da Silva, EJ et al 2016 (64), Shemesh, A et al 2016 (128), Zhengyan, Y et al 2016 (120), Kayaoglu, G et al 2015 (121), Altunsoy, M et al 2014 (65), Han, T et al 2014 (122), Somalinga, NS et al 2014 (66), Aminsobhani, M et al 2013 (124), Vaziri, P et al 2008 (220), Sert, S and Bayirli, GS 2004 (3), Caliskan, MK et al 1995 (4), Pecora, JD et al 1993 (130), Kaffee I et al 1985 (215), Vertucci, F 1984 (5), Bellizzi, R and Hartwell, G 1983 (216), Miyoshi, S et al 1977 (218), Green, D 1973 (23), Pineda, F and Kuttler, Y 1972 (6), Barrett, MT 1925 (7)	14377	2 roots and 2 canals (8) 2 roots and 3 canals (3) 1 root and 2 canals (3)
First premolar * 2 or more canals	1 Canal	72.2%	28.9%*				40	Alkaabi, W et al 2017 (132), Bürklein, S et al (2017) (9), Dou, L et al 2017 (133), Zhang, D et al 2017 (221), Abraham, SB and Gopinath, VK 2015 (134), Chen, J et al 2015 (222), Huang, Y-D et al 2015 (135), Kazemipoor, M et al 2015 (136), Kazemipoor, M et al 2015 (137), Llena, C et al 2014 (139), Ok, E et al 2014 (67), Shetty, A et al 2014 (223), Singh, S and Pawar, M 2014 (140), Alhadainy, HA 2013 (141), Liu, N et al 2013 (224), Yang, H et al, 2013 (142), Baroudi, K et al 2012 (225), Yu, X et al 2012 (143), Jain, A and, Bahuguna, R 2011 (144), Parekh, V et al 2011 (153), Rahimi, S et al 2007 (147), Kheddmat, S et al 2010 (145) , Velmurugan, N and Sandhya, R 2009 (226), Awawdeh, LA and Al-Qudah, AA 2008 (146), Lu, T-Y et al 2006 (227), Sert, S and Bayirli, GS 2004 (3), Yoshioka, T et al 2004 (228), Zaatar, EI et al 1997 (19), Çaliskan, MK et al 1995 (4), Sabala, CL et al 1994 (229), Baisden, MK et al 1992 (230), Geider, P et al 1989 (149), Walker, RT 1988 (231), Miyoshi, S et al 1977 (218), Vertucci, F 1978 (150), Green, D 1973 (23), Zillich, R and Dowson, J 1973 (154), Pineda, F and Kuttler, Y 1972 (6), Mueller, AH 1933 (24), Barrett, MT 1925 (7)	13086	3 roots and 3 canals (5) 1 root and 2 canals (5) 1 root and 3 canals (5) Dens evaginatus (4) 2 roots and 2 canals (3) 3 canals (3) C-shaped canal (4)

Continued

	NUMBER OF CANALS						No. of Studies	References	No. of Teeth	Most Common Anomaly or Variation (Number of Case Reports In Brackets)
	Most Common	1	2	3	4	Other				
Second premolar * 2 or more canals	1 Canal	84.2%	15.8%*				25	Bürklein, S et al (2017) (9), Kazemipoor, M et al 2015 (136), Kazemipoor, M et al 2015 (137), Llena, C et al 2014 (139), Shetty, A et al 2014 (223), Singh, S and Pawar, M 2014 (140), Ok, E et al 2014 (67), Bolhari, B et al 2013 (152), Baroudi, K et al 2012 (225), Yu, X et al 2012 (143), Parekh, V et al 2011 (153), Rahimi, S et al 2009 (1), Awawdeh, LA and Al-Qudah, AA 2008 (146), Rahimi, S et al 2007 (147), Hasheminia, M and Hashemi, A 2005 (232), Sert, S and Bayirli, GS 2004 (3), Zaatar, El et al 1997 (19), Çalişkan, MK et al 1995 (4), Geider, P et al 1989 (149), Miyoshi, S et al 1977 (218), Vertucci, F 1978 (150), Green, D 1973 (23), Zillich, R and Dowson, J 1973 (154), Pineda, F and Kuttler, Y 1972 (6), Barrett, MT 1925 (7)	8733	3 canals (12) 2 roots and 2 canals (11) C-shaped canal (7) Dens evaginatus (6) 3 roots and 3 canals (6)
First molar (Two Roots) * 2 or more canals										Radix entomolaris (32) 2 roots and 5 canals (3M and 2D) (20) 2 roots and 4 canals (3M and D) (10) 2 roots and 5 canals (2M and 3D) (8) 2 roots and 6 canals (3M and 3D) (7)
Mesial	2 Canals	3.1%	95.7%	1.1%		0.2%	23	Mohammadzadeh Akhlaghi, N et al 2017 (157)Ja, ng, J-K et al 2013 (179), Kim, S-Y et al 2013 (180), Wang, Y et al 2010 (183), Al-Qudah, AA and Awawdeh, LA 2009 (164), Reuben, J et al 2008 (166), Jung, I-Y et al 2005 (81), Sert, S and Bayirli, GS 2004 (3), Gulabivala, K et al 2002 (185), Gulabivala, K et al 2001 (186), Wasti, F et al 2001 (84), Al-Nazhan, S 1999 (170), Zaatar, El et al 1998 (172), Zaatar, El et al 1997 (19), Rocha, LF et al 1996 (173), Çaliskan, MK et al 1995 (4), Yew, S and Chan, K 1993 (187), Goel, NK et al 1990 (233), Fabra-Campos, H 1985 (234), Vertucci, F 1984 (5), Hartwell, G and Bellizzi, R 1982 (110), Pineda, F and Kuttler, Y 1972 (6), Skidmore, AE and Bjorndal, AM 1971 (178)	6428	

	NUMBER OF CANALS						No. of Studies	References	No. of Teeth	Most Common Anomaly or Variation (Number of Case Reports In Brackets)
	Most Common	1	2	3	4	Other				
Distal	1 Canal	68.7%	31.3%*				24	Mohammadzadeh Akhlaghi, N et al 2017 (157), Wang, Y et al 2010 (183), Filpo-Perez, C et al 2015 in press (235), Jang, J-K et al 2013 (179), Kim, S-Y et al 2013 (180), Al-Qudah, AA and Awawdeh, LA 2009 (164), Pattanshetti, N et al 2008 (50), Reuben, J et al 2008 (166), Sert, S and Bayirli, GS 2004 (3), Gulabivala, K et al 2002 (185), Gulabivala, K et al 2001 (186), Wasti, F et al 2001 (84), Al-Nazhan, S 1999 (170), Zaatar, EI et al 1998 (172), Zaatar, EI et al 1997 (19), Rocha, LF et al 1996 (173), Çaliskan, MK et al 1995 (4), Yew, S and Chan, K 1993 (187), Goel, NK et al 1990 (233), Fabra-Campos, H 1985 (234), Vertucci, F 1984 (5), Hartwell, G and Bellizzi, R 1982 (110), Pineda, F and Kuttler, Y 1972 (6), Skidmore, AE and Bjorndal, AM 1971 (178)	6569	
First molar (Three Roots) * 2 or more canals										
Mesial	2 Canals	2.8%	97.2%*				8	Mohammadzadeh Akhlaghi, N et al 2017 (157), Rodrigues, CT et al 2016 (159), Kim, S-Y et al 2013 (180), Wang, Y et al 2010 (183), Al-Qudah, AA and Awawdeh, LA 2009 (164), Gulabivala, K et al 2002 (185), Gulabivala, K et al 2001 (186), Yew, S and Chan, K 1993 (187)	928	
Distobuccal	1 Canal	98.3%	1.7%*				8	Mohammadzadeh Akhlaghi, N et al 2017 (157), Rodrigues, CT et al 2016 (159), Kim, S-Y et al 2013 (180), Wang, Y et al 2010 (183), Al-Qudah, AA and Awawdeh, LA 2009 (164), Gulabivala, K et al 2002 (185), Gulabivala, K et al 2001 (186), Yew, S and Chan, K 1993 (187)	928	
Distolingual	1 Canal	100%					9	Mohammadzadeh Akhlaghi, N et al 2017 (157), Rodrigues, CT et al 2016 (159), Kim, S-Y et al 2013 (180), Chourasia, HR et al 2012 (161), Wang, Y et al 2010 (183), Al-Qudah, AA and Awawdeh, LA 2009 (164), Gulabivala, K et al 2002 (185), Gulabivala, K et al 2001 (186), Yew, S and Chan, K 1993 (187)	936	
Second molar (two roots) * 2 or more canals										C-shaped canal (19) Taurodontism (18) Fusion with a paramolar (7) 3 roots (MB, MLi, and D) and 3 canals (6) 1 root and 1 canal (6)

Continued

	NUMBER OF CANALS						No. of Studies	References	No. of Teeth	Most Common Anomaly or Variation (Number of Case Reports In Brackets)
	Most Common	1	2	3	4	Other				
Mesial	2 Canals	16.5%	84.0%*				14	Akhaghi, NM et al 2016 (194), Kim, SY et al 2016 (195), Silva, EJNL et al 2013 (197), Neelakantan, P et al 2010 (200), Al-Qudah, AA and Awawdeh, LA 2009 (164), Sert, S and Bayirli, GS 2004 (3), Gulabivala, K et al 2002 (185), Gulabivala, K et al 2001 (186), Zaatar, El et al 1997 (19), Rocha, LF da Costa et al 1996 (173), Çaliskan, MK et al 1995 (4), Weine, FS et al 1988 (236), Vertucci, F 1984 (5), Hartwell, G and Bellizzi, R 1982 (110)	3293	
Distal	1 Canal	88.2%	11.8%				14	Akhaghi, NM et al 2016 (194), Kim, SY et al 2016 (195), Silva, EJNL et al 2013 (197), Neelakantan, P et al 2010 (200), Al-Qudah, AA and Awawdeh, LA 2009 (164), Sert, S and Bayirli, GS 2004 (3), Gulabivala, K et al 2002 (185), Gulabivala, K et al 2001 (186), Zaatar, El et al 1997 (19), Rocha, LF et al 1996 (173), Çaliskan, MK et al 1995 (4), Weine, FS et al 1988 (205), Vertucci, F 1984 (5), Hartwell, G and Bellizzi, R 1982 (110)	3293	
Third molar	2-3 Canals	6.9%	32.9%	51.0%	9.3%	2.2%	3	Somasundaram, P et al 2017 (207), Sidow, SJ et al 2000 (62), Guerisoli, DM et al 1998 (63)	420	Highly variable; variation is the norm

References

1. Rahimi S, Shahi S, Yavari HR, et al.: A stereomicroscopy study of root apices of human maxillary central incisors and mandibular second premolars in an Iranian population, *J Oral Sci* 51(3):411–415, 2009.
2. Weng XL, Yu SB, Zhao SL, et al.: Root canal morphology of permanent maxillary teeth in the Han nationality in Chinese Guanzhong area: a new modified root canal staining technique, *J Endod* 35(5):651–656, 2009.
3. Sert S, Bayirli GS: Evaluation of the root canal configurations of the mandibular and maxillary permanent teeth by gender in the Turkish population, *J Endod* 30(6):391–398, 2004.
4. Çalişkan M, Pehlivan Y, Sepetçioğlu F, et al.: Root canal morphology of human permanent teeth in a Turkish population, *J Endod* 21(4):200–204, 1995.
5. Vertucci FJ: Root canal anatomy of the human permanent teeth, *Oral Surg Oral Med Oral Pathol* 58(5):589–599, 1984.
6. Pineda F, Kuttler Y: Mesiodistal and buccolingual roentgenographic investigation of 7,275 root canals, *Oral Surg Oral Med Oral Pathol* 33(1):101–110, 1972.
7. Barrett M: The internal anatomy of the teeth with special reference to the pulp and its branches, *Dent Cosmos* 67:581–592, 1925.
8. Bjørndal AM, Skidmore AE: *Anatomy and morphology of permanent teeth*, Iowa City, 1983, University of Iowa College of Dentistry.
9. Burklein S, Heck R, Schafer E: Evaluation of the root canal anatomy of maxillary and mandibular premolars in a selected german population using cone-beam computed tomographic data, *J Endod* 43(9):1448–1452, 2017.
10. Abella F, Teixido LM, Patel S, et al.: Cone-beam computed tomography analysis of the root canal morphology of maxillary first and second premolars in a spanish population, *J Endod* 41(8):1241–1247, 2015.
11. Bulut DG, Kose E, Ozcan G, et al.: Evaluation of root morphology and root canal configuration of premolars in the Turkish individuals using cone beam computed tomography, *Eur J Dent* 9(4):551–557, 2015.
12. Gupta S, Sinha DJ, Gowhar O, et al.: Root and canal morphology of maxillary first premolar teeth in north Indian population using clearing technique: an in vitro study, *J Conserv Dent* 18(3):232–236, 2015.
13. Dababneh R, Rodan R: Anatomical landmarks of maxillary bifurcated first premolars and their influence on periodontal diagnosis and treatment, *J Int Acad Periodontol* 15(1):8–15, 2013.
14. Ng'ang'a RN, Masiga MA, Maina SW: Internal root morphology of the maxillary first premolars in Kenyans of African descent, *East Afr Med J* 87(1):20–24, 2010.
15. Atieh MA: Root and canal morphology of maxillary first premolars in a Saudi population, *J Contemp Dent Pract* 9(1):46–53, 2008.
16. Awawdeh L, Abdullah H, Al-Qudah A: Root form and canal morphology of Jordanian maxillary first premolars, *J Endod* 34(8):956–961, 2008.

17. Chaparro AJ, Segura JJ, Guerrero E, et al.: Number of roots and canals in maxillary first premolars: study of an Andalusian population, *Endod Dent Traumatol* 15(2):65–67, 1999.
18. Kartal N, Ozcelik B, Cimilli H: Root canal morphology of maxillary premolars, *J Endod* 24(6):417–419, 1998.
19. Zaatar EI, al-Kandari AM, Alhomaidah S, al-Yasin IM: Frequency of endodontic treatment in Kuwait: radiographic evaluation of 846 endodontically treated teeth, *J Endod* 23(7):453–456, 1997.
20. Pecora J, Saquy P, Sousa Neto M, Woelfel J: Root form and canal anatomy of maxillary first premolars, *Braz Dent J* 2:87–94, 1991.
21. Vertucci FJ, Gegauff A: Root canal morphology of the maxillary first premolar, *J Am Dent Assoc* 99(2):194–198, 1979.
22. Carns EJ, Skidmore AE: Configurations and deviations of root canals of maxillary first premolars, *Oral Surg Oral Med Oral Pathol* 36(6):880–886, 1973.
23. Green D: Double canals in single roots, *Oral Surg Oral Med Oral Pathol* 35(5):689–696, 1973.
24. Mueller A: Anatomy of the root canals of the incisors, cuspids and bicuspids of the permanent teeth, *J Am Dent Assoc* 20:1361–1386, 1933.
25. Tian YY, Guo B, Zhang R, et al.: Root and canal morphology of maxillary first premolars in a Chinese subpopulation evaluated using cone-beam computed tomography, *Int Endod J* 45(11):996–1003, 2012.
26. Cheng XL, Weng YL: Observation of the roots and root canals of 442 maxillary first premolars, *Shanghai Kou Qiang Yi Xue* 17(5):525–528, 2008.
27. Loh HS: Root morphology of the maxillary first premolar in Singaporeans, *Aust Dent J* 43(6):399–402, 1998.
28. Aoki K: Morphological studies on the roots of maxillary premolars in Japanese, *Shikwa Gakuho* 90(2):181–199, 1990.
29. Walker RT: Root form and canal anatomy of maxillary first premolars in a southern Chinese population, *Endod Dent Traumatol* 3(3):130–134, 1987.
30. Elnour M, Khabeer A, AlShwaimi E: Evaluation of root canal morphology of maxillary second premolars in a Saudi Arabian subpopulation: an in vitro microcomputed tomography study, *Saudi Dent J* 28(4):162–168, 2016.
31. Velmurugan N, Parameswaran A, Kandaswamy D, et al.: Maxillary second premolar with three roots and three separate root canals—case reports, *Aust Endod J* 31(2):73–75, 2005.
32. Pecora J, Sousa Neto M, Saquy P, Woelfel J: In vitro study of root canal anatomy of maxillary second premolars, *Braz Dent J* 3(2):81–85, 1992.
33. Sikri VK, Sikri P: Maxillary second premolar: configuration and deviations of root canals, *J Indian Dent Assoc* 62(3):46–49, 1991.
34. Gorlin R, Goldman H: *Thoma's oral pathology*, ed 6, St. Louis, 1970, CV Mosby.
35. Ghobashy AM, Nagy MM, Bayoumi AA: Evaluation of root and canal morphology of maxillary permanent molars in an Egyptian population by cone-beam computed tomography, *J Endod* 43(7):1089–1092, 2017.
36. Khademi A, Zamani Naser A, Bahreinian Z, et al.: Root morphology and canal configuration of first and second maxillary molars in a selected Iranian population: a cone-beam computed tomography evaluation, *Iran Endod J* 12(3):288–292, 2017.
37. Martins JN, Mata A, Marques D, Carames J: Prevalence of root fusions and main root canal merging in human upper and lower molars: a cone-beam computed tomography in vivo study, *J Endod* 42(6):900–908, 2016.
38. Naseri M, Safi Y, Akbarzadeh Baghban A, et al.: Survey of anatomy and root canal morphology of maxillary first molars regarding age and gender in an iranian population using cone-beam computed tomography, *Iran Endod J* 11(4):298–303, 2016.
39. Tian XM, Yang XW, Qian L, et al.: Analysis of the root and canal morphologies in maxillary first and second molars in a chinese population using cone-beam computed tomography, *J Endod*, 2016.
40. Alrahabi M, Sohail Zafar M: Evaluation of root canal morphology of maxillary molars using cone beam computed tomography, *Pak J Med Sci* 31(2):426–430, 2015.
41. Nikoloudaki GE, Kontogiannis TG, Kerezoudis NP: Evaluation of the root and canal morphology of maxillary permanent molars and the incidence of the second mesiobuccal root canal in greek population using cone-beam computed tomography, *Open Dent J* 9:267–272, 2015.
42. Singh S, Pawar M: Root canal morphology of South Asian Indian maxillary molar teeth, *Eur J Dent* 9(1):133–144, 2015.
43. Bhuyan AC, Kataki R, Phyllei P, Gill GS: Root canal configuration of permanent maxillary first molar in Khasi population of Meghalaya: an in vitro study, *J Conserv Dent* 17(4):359–363, 2014.
44. Guo J, Vahidnia A, Sedghizadeh P, Enciso R: Evaluation of root and canal morphology of maxillary permanent first molars in a North American population by cone-beam computed tomography, *J Endod* 40(5):635–639, 2014.
45. Rouhani A, Bagherpour A, Akbari M, et al.: Cone-beam computed tomography evaluation of maxillary first and second molars in Iranian population: a morphological study, *Iran Endod J* 9(3):190–194, 2014.
46. Silva EJ, Nejaim Y, Silva AI, et al.: Evaluation of root canal configuration of maxillary molars in a Brazilian population using cone-beam computed tomographic imaging: an in vivo study, *J Endod* 40(2):173–176, 2014.
47. Plotino G, Tocci L, Grande NM, et al.: Symmetry of root and root canal morphology of maxillary and mandibular molars in a white population: a cone-beam computed tomography study in vivo, *J Endod* 39(12):1545–1548, 2013.
48. Zhang R, Yang H, Yu X, et al.: Use of CBCT to identify the morphology of maxillary permanent molar teeth in a Chinese subpopulation, *Int Endod J* 44(2):162–169, 2011.
49. Zheng QH, Wang Y, Zhou XD, et al.: A cone-beam computed tomography study of maxillary first permanent molar root and canal morphology in a Chinese population, *J Endod* 36(9):1480–1484, 2010.
50. Pattanshetti N, Gaidhane M, Al Kandari AM: Root and canal morphology of the mesiobuccal and distal roots of permanent first molars in a Kuwait population-a clinical study, *Int Endod J* 41(9):755–762, 2008.
51. Rwenyonyi CM, Kutesa AM, Muwazi LM, Buwembo W: Root and canal morphology of maxillary first and second permanent molar teeth in a Ugandan population, *Int Endod J* 40(9):679–683, 2007.
52. al Shalabi RM, Omer OE, Glennon J, et al.: Root canal anatomy of maxillary first and second permanent molars, *Int Endod J* 33(5):405–414, 2000.
53. Thomas RP, Moule AJ, Bryant R: Root canal morphology of maxillary permanent first molar teeth at various ages, *Int Endod J* 26(5):257–267, 1993.
54. Gray R: The maxillary first molar. In Bjørndal AM, Skidmore AE, editors: *Anatomy and morphology of permanent teeth*, Iowa City, 1983, University of Iowa College of Dentistry.
55. Zhang Q, Chen H, Fan B, et al.: Root and root canal morphology in maxillary second molar with fused root from a native Chinese population, *J Endod* 40(6):871–875, 2014.
56. Kim Y, Lee SJ, Woo J: Morphology of maxillary first and second molars analyzed by cone-beam computed tomography in a Korean population: variations in the number of roots and canals and the incidence of fusion, *J Endod* 38(8):1063–1068, 2012.
57. Libfeld H, Rotstein I: Incidence of four-rooted maxillary second molars: literature review and radiographic survey of 1,200 teeth, *J Endod* 15(3):129–131, 1989.
58. Tomaszewska IM, Leszczynski B, Wrobel A, et al.: A micro-computed tomographic (micro-CT) analysis of the root canal morphology of maxillary third molar teeth, *Ann Anat*, 2017.
59. Rawtiya M, Somasundaram P, Wadhwani S, et al.: Retrospective study of root canal configurations of maxillary third molars in Central India population using cone beam computed tomography Part-I, *Eur J Dent* 10(1):97–102, 2016.

60. Sert S, Sahinkesen G, Topcu FT, et al.: Root canal configurations of third molar teeth. A comparison with first and second molars in the Turkish population, *Aust Endod J* 37(3):109–117, 2011.
61. Alavi AM, Opasanon A, Ng YL, Gulabivala K: Root and canal morphology of Thai maxillary molars, *Int Endod J* 35(5):478–485, 2002.
62. Sidow SJ, West LA, Liewehr FR, Loushine RJ: Root canal morphology of human maxillary and mandibular third molarsm, *J Endod* 26(11):675–678, 2000.
63. Guerisoli DM, de Souza RA, de Sousa Neto MD, et al.: External and internal anatomy of third molars, *Braz Dent J* 9(2):91–94, 1998.
64. da Silva EJ, de Castro RW, Nejaim Y, et al.: Evaluation of root canal configuration of maxillary and mandibular anterior teeth using cone beam computed tomography: an in-vivo study, *Quintessence Int* 47(1):19–24, 2016.
65. Altunsoy M, Ok E, Nur BG, et al.: A cone-beam computed tomography study of the root canal morphology of anterior teeth in a Turkish population, *Eur J Dent* 8(3):302–306, 2014.
66. Somalinga Amardeep N, Raghu S, Natanasabapathy V: Root canal morphology of permanent maxillary and mandibular canines in Indian population using cone beam computed tomography, *Anat Res Int*1–7, 2014.
67. Ok E, Altunsoy M, Nur BG, et al.: A cone-beam computed tomography study of root canal morphology of maxillary and mandibular premolars in a Turkish population, *Acta Odontol Scand*1–6, 2014.
68. Bellizzi R, Hartwell G: Radiographic evaluation of root canal anatomy of in vivo endodontically treated maxillary premolars, *J Endod* 11(1):37–39, 1985.
69. Hess W: *The anatomy of the root-canals of the teeth of the permanent dentition, part 1*, New York, 1925, William Wood and Co.
70. Jayasimha Raj U, Mylswamy S: Root canal morphology of maxillary second premolars in an Indian population, *J Conserv Dent* 13(3):148–151, 2010.
71. Briseno-Marroquin B, Paque F, Maier K, et al.: Root canal morphology and configuration of 179 maxillary first molars by means of micro-computed tomography: an ex vivo study, *J Endod* 41(12):2008–2013, 2015.
72. Kim Y, Chang SW, Lee JK, et al.: A micro-computed tomography study of canal configuration of multiple-canalled mesiobuccal root of maxillary first molar, *Clin Oral Investig* 17(6):1541–1546, 2013.
73. Gu Y, Lee JK, Spangberg LS, et al.: Minimum-intensity projection for in-depth morphology study of mesiobuccal root, *Oral Surg Oral Med Oral Pathol Oral Radiol Endod* 112(5):671–677, 2011.
74. Peeters HH, Suardita K, Setijanto D: Prevalence of a second canal in the mesiobuccal root of permanent maxillary first molars from an Indonesian population, *J Oral Sci* 53(4):489–494, 2011.
75. Somma F, Leoni D, Plotino G, et al.: Root canal morphology of the mesiobuccal root of maxillary first molars: a micro-computed tomographic analysis, *Int Endod J* 42(2):165–174, 2009.
76. Abiodun-Solanke IM, Dosumu OO, Shaba PO, Ajayi DM: Prevalence of additional canals in maxillary first molars in a Nigerian population, *J Contemp Dent Pract* 9(7):81–88, 2008.
77. Alacam T, Tinaz AC, Genc O, Kayaoglu G: Second mesiobuccal canal detection in maxillary first molars using microscopy and ultrasonics, *Aust Endod J* 34(3):106–109, 2008.
78. Khraisat A, Smadi L: Canal configuration in the mesio-buccal root of maxillary first molar teeth of a Jordanian population, *Aust Endod J* 33(1):13–17, 2007.
79. Eder A, Kantor M, Nell A, et al.: Root canal system in the mesiobuccal root of the maxillary first molar: an in vitro comparison study of computed tomography and histologym, *Dentomaxillofac Radiol* 35(3):175–177, 2006.
80. Smadi L, Khraisat A: Root canal morphology of the mesiobuccal root in maxillary first molars of a Jordanian population, *Gen Dent* 54(6):413–416, 2006.
81. Jung IY, Seo MA, Fouad AF, et al.: Apical anatomy in mesial and mesiobuccal roots of permanent first molars, *J Endod* 31(5):364–368, 2005.
82. Scott Jr AE, Apicella MJ: Canal configuration in the mesiobuccal root of the maxillary first molar: a descriptive study, *Gen Dent* 52(1):34–36, 2004.
83. Schwarze T, Baethge C, Stecher T, Geurtsen W: Identification of second canals in the mesiobuccal root of maxillary first and second molars using magnifying loupes or an operating microscope, *Aust Endod J* 28(2):57–60, 2002.
84. Wasti F, Shearer AC, Wilson NH: Root canal systems of the mandibular and maxillary first permanent molar teeth of south Asian Pakistanis, *Int Endod J* 34(4):263–266, 2001.
85. Weine FS, Hayami S, Hata G, Toda T: Canal configuration of the mesiobuccal root of the maxillary first molar of a Japanese subpopulation, *Int Endod J* 32(2):79–87, 1999.
86. Imura N, Hata GI, Toda T, et al.: Two canals in mesiobuccal roots of maxillary molars, *Int Endod J* 31(6):410–414, 1998.
87. Pecora JD, Woelfel JB, Sousa Neto MD, Issa EP: Morphologic study of the maxillary molars. Part II: Internal anatomy, *Braz Dent J* 3(1):53–57, 1992.
88. Kulild JC, Peters DD: Incidence and configuration of canal systems in the mesiobuccal root of maxillary first and second molars, *J Endod* 16(7):311–317, 1990.
89. Gilles J, Reader A: An SEM investigation of the mesiolingual canal in human maxillary first and second molars, *Oral Surg Oral Med Oral Pathol* 70(5):638–643, 1990.
90. Acosta Vigouroux SA, Trugeda Bosaans SA: Anatomy of the pulp chamber floor of the permanent maxillary first molar, *J Endod* 4(7):214–219, 1978.
91. Seidberg BH, Altman M, Guttuso J, Suson M: Frequency of two mesiobuccal root canals in maxillary permanent first molars, *J Am Dent Assoc* 87(4):852–856, 1973.
92. Sykaras S, Economou P: Root canal morphology of the mesiobuccal root of the maxillary first molar, *Oral Res Abstr*2025, 1971.
93. Weine FS, Healey HJ, Gerstein H, Evanson L: Canal configuration in the mesiobuccal root of the maxillary first molar and its endodontic significance, *Oral Surg Oral Med Oral Pathol* 28(3):419–425, 1969.
94. Okamura T: Anatomy of the root canals, *J Am Dent Assoc* 14:632–636, 1927.
95. Zürcher E: *The anatomy of the root-canals of the teeth of the deciduous dentition and of the first permanent molars, part 2*, New York, 1925, William Wood and Co.
96. Moral H: *Ueber Pulpaausgüsse*, Deutsche Monatsschrift für Zahnheilkunde, 1914.
97. Betancourt P, Navarro P, Munoz G, Fuentes R: Prevalence and location of the secondary mesiobuccal canal in 1,100 maxillary molars using cone beam computed tomography, *BMC Med Imaging* 16(1):66, 2016.
98. Coelho MS, Parker JM, Tawil PZ: Second mesiobuccal canal treatment in a predoctoral dental clinic: a retrospective clinical study, *J Dent Educ* 80(6):726–730, 2016.
99. Abuabara A, Baratto-Filho F, Aguiar Anele J, et al.: Efficacy of clinical and radiological methods to identify second mesiobuccal canals in maxillary first molars, *Acta Odontol Scand* 71(1):205–209, 2013.
100. Reis AG, Grazziotin-Soares R, Barletta FB, et al.: Second canal in mesiobuccal root of maxillary molars is correlated with root third and patient age: a cone-beam computed tomographic study, *J Endod* 39(5):588–592, 2013.
101. Lee JH, Kim KD, Lee JK, et al.: Mesiobuccal root canal anatomy of Korean maxillary first and second molars by cone-beam computed tomography, *Oral Surg Oral Med Oral Pathol Oral Radiol Endod* 111(6):785–791, 2011.
102. Hartwell G, Appelstein CM, Lyons WW, Guzek ME: The incidence of four canals in maxillary first molars: a clinical determination, *J Am Dent Assoc* 138(10):1344–1346, 2007.
103. Wolcott J, Ishley D, Kennedy W, et al.: Clinical investigation of second mesiobuccal canals in endodontically treated and retreated maxillary molars, *J Endod* 28(6):477–479, 2002.

104. Buhrley LJ, Barrows MJ, BeGole EA, Wenckus CS: Effect of magnification on locating the MB2 canal in maxillary molars, *J Endod* 28(4):324–327, 2002.
105. Sempira HN, Hartwell GR: Frequency of second mesiobuccal canals in maxillary molars as determined by use of an operating microscope: a clinical study, *J Endod* 26(11):673–674, 2000.
106. Stropko JJ: Canal morphology of maxillary molars: clinical observations of canal configurations, *J Endod* 25(6):446–450, 1999.
107. Fogel HM, Peikoff MD, Christie WH: Canal configuration in the mesiobuccal root of the maxillary first molar: a clinical study, *J Endod* 20(3):135–137, 1994.
108. Weller RN, Hartwell GR: The impact of improved access and searching techniques on detection of the mesiolingual canal in maxillary molars, *J Endod* 15(2):82–83, 1989.
109. Neaverth EJ, Kotler LM, Kaltenbach RF: Clinical investigation (in vivo) of endodontically treated maxillary first molars, *J Endod* 13(10):506–512, 1987.
110. Hartwell G, Bellizzi R: Clinical investigation of in vivo endodontically treated mandibular and maxillary molars, *J Endod* 8(12):555–557, 1982.
111. Pomeranz HH, Fishelberg G: The secondary mesiobuccal canal of maxillary molars, *J Am Dent Assoc* 88(1):119–124, 1974.
112. Slowey RR: Radiographic aids in the detection of extra root canals, *Oral Surg Oral Med Oral Pathol* 37(5):762–772, 1974.
113. Nosonowitz DM, Brenner MR: The major canals of the mesiobuccal root of the maxillary 1st and 2nd molars, *N Y J Dent* 43(1):12–15, 1973.
114. Wolf TG, Paque F, Woop AC, et al.: Root canal morphology and configuration of 123 maxillary second molars by means of micro-CT, *Int J Oral Sci* 9(1):33–37, 2017.
115. Han X, Yang H, Li G, et al.: A study of the distobuccal root canal orifice of the maxillary second molars in Chinese individuals evaluated by cone-beam computed tomography, *J Appl Oral Sci Revista FOB* 20(5):563–567, 2012.
116. Eskoz N, Weine FS: Canal configuration of the mesiobuccal root of the maxillary second molar, *J Endod* 21(1):38–42, 1995.
117. Singh C, Sikri VK, Arora R: Study of root canals and their configuration in maxillary second permanent molar, *Indian J Dent Res* 5(1):3–8, 1994.
118. Verma GR, Bhadage C, Bhoosreddy AR, et al.: Cone beam computed tomography study of root canal morphology of permanent mandibular incisors in indian subpopulation, *Pol J Radiol* 82:371–375, 2017.
119. Kamtane S, Ghodke M: Morphology of mandibular incisors: a study on CBCT, *Pol J Radiol* 81:15–16, 2016.
120. Zhengyan Y, Keke L, Fei W, et al.: Cone-beam computed tomography study of the root and canal morphology of mandibular permanent anterior teeth in a Chongqing population, *Ther Clin Risk Manag* 12:19–25, 2016.
121. Kayaoglu G, Peker I, Gumusok M, et al.: Root and canal symmetry in the mandibular anterior teeth of patients attending a dental clinic: CBCT study, *Braz Oral Res* 29, 2015.
122. Han T, Ma Y, Yang L, et al.: A study of the root canal morphology of mandibular anterior teeth using cone-beam computed tomography in a Chinese subpopulation, *J Endod* 40(9):1309–1314, 2014.
123. Lin Z, Hu Q, Wang T, et al.: Use of CBCT to investigate the root canal morphology of mandibular incisors, *Surg Radiol Anat*, 2014.
124. Aminsobhani M, Sadegh M, Meraji N, et al.: Evaluation of the root and canal morphology of mandibular permanent anterior teeth in an Iranian population by cone-beam computed tomography, *J Dent (Tehran)* 10(4):358–366, 2013.
125. Vertucci FJ: Root canal anatomy of the mandibular anterior teeth, *J Am Dent Assoc* 89(2):369–371, 1974.
126. Madeira MC, Hetem S: Incidence of bifurcations in mandibular incisors, *Oral Surg Oral Med Oral Pathol* 36(4):589–591, 1973.
127. Soleymani A, Namaryan N, Moudi E, Gholinia A: Root canal morphology of mandibular canine in an iranian population: a CBCT assessment, *Iran Endod J* 12(1):78–82, 2017.
128. Shemesh A, Levin A, Katzenell V, et al.: Root anatomy and root canal morphology of mandibular canines in Israeli population, *Refuat Hapeh Vehashinayim (1993)* 33(1):19–23, 2016. 60.
129. Ouellet R: Mandibular permanent cuspids with two roots, *J Can Dent Assoc* 61(2):159–161, 1995.
130. Pecora JD, Sousa Neto MD, Saquy PC: Internal anatomy, direction and number of roots and size of human mandibular canines, *Braz Dent J* 4(1):53–57, 1993.
131. Alexandersen V: Double-rooted human lower canine teeth. In Brothwell D, editor: *Dental anthropology*, Oxford, 1963, Pergamon Press, pp 235–244.
132. Alkaabi W, AlShwaimi E, Farooq I, et al.: A micro-computed tomography study of the root canal morphology of mandibular first premolars in an Emirati population, *Med Princ Pract* 26(2):118–124, 2017.
133. Dou L, Li D, Xu T, et al.: Root anatomy and canal morphology of mandibular first premolars in a Chinese population, *Sci Rep* 7(1):750, 2017.
134. Abraham SB, Gopinath VK: Root canal anatomy of mandibular first premolars in an Emirati subpopulation: A laboratory study, *Eur J Dent* 9(4):476–482, 2015.
135. Huang YD, Wu J, Sheu RJ, et al.: Evaluation of the root and root canal systems of mandibular first premolars in northern Taiwanese patients using cone-beam computed tomography, *J Formos Med Assoc* 114(11):1129–1134, 2015.
136. Kazemipoor M, Poorkheradmand M, Rezaeian M, Safi Y: Evaluation by CBCT of root and canal morphology in mandibular premolars in an Iranian population, *Chin J Dent Res* 18(3):191–196, 2015.
137. Kazemipoor M, Hajighasemi A, Hakimian R: Gender difference and root canal morphology in mandibular premolars: a cone-beam computed tomography study in an Iranian population, *Contemp Clin Dent* 6(3):401–404, 2015.
138. Kong LJ, Wan K, Liu DG: Double roots of mandibular premolar in full-mouth periapical films, *Chin Med Sci J* 30(3):174–178, 2015.
139. Llena C, Fernandez J, Ortolani PS, Forner L: Cone-beam computed tomography analysis of root and canal morphology of mandibular premolars in a Spanish population, *Imaging Sci Dent* 44(3):221–227, 2014.
140. Singh S, Pawar M: Root canal morphology of South Asian Indian mandibular premolar teeth, *J Endod* 40(9):1338–1341, 2014.
141. Alhadainy HA: Canal configuration of mandibular first premolars in an Egyptian population, *J Adv Res* 4(2):123–128, 2013.
142. Yang H, Tian C, Li G, et al.: A cone-beam computed tomography study of the root canal morphology of mandibular first premolars and the location of root canal orifices and apical foramina in a Chinese subpopulation, *J Endod* 39(4):435–438, 2013.
143. Yu X, Guo B, Li KZ, et al.: Cone-beam computed tomography study of root and canal morphology of mandibular premolars in a western Chinese population, *BMC Med Imaging* 12:18, 2012.
144. Jain A, Bahuguna R: Root canal morphology of mandibular first premolar in a Gujarati population - an in vitro study, *Dent Res J (Isfahan)* 8(3):118–122, 2011.
145. Khedmat S, Assadian H, Saravani AA: Root canal morphology of the mandibular first premolars in an Iranian population using cross-sections and radiography, *J Endod* 36(2):214–217, 2010.
146. Awawdeh LA, Al-Qudah AA: Root form and canal morphology of mandibular premolars in a Jordanian population, *Int Endod J* 41(3):240–248, 2008.
147. Rahimi S, Shahi S, Yavari HR, et al.: Root canal configuration of mandibular first and second premolars in an Iranian population, *J Dent Res Dent Clin Dent Prospects* 1(2):59–64, 2007.
148. Iyer VH, Indira R, Ramachandran S, Srinivasan MR: Anatomical variations of mandibular premolars in Chennai population, *Indian J Dent Res* 17(1):7–10, 2006.
149. Geider P, Perrin C, Fontaine M: Endodontic anatomy of lower premolars- apropos of 669 cases, *J Odontol Conserv*(10)11–15, 1989.
150. Vertucci FJ: Root canal morphology of mandibular premolars, *J Am Dent Assoc* 97(1):47–50, 1978.

151. Schulze C: Developmental abnormalities of teeth and jaws. In Gorlin R, Goldman H, editors: *Thoma's oral pathology*, ed 6, St. Louis, 1970, CV Mosby Co, pp 106–107.
152. Bolhari B, Assadian H, Fattah T: Evaluation of the root canal morphology of mandibular second premolars in an Iranian population, *J Dent (Tehran)* 10(6):516–521, 2013.
153. Parekh V, Shah N, Joshi H: Root canal morphology and variations of mandibular premolars by clearing technique: an in vitro study, *J Contemp Dent Pract* 12(4):318–321, 2011.
154. Zillich R, Dowson J: Root canal morphology of mandibular first and second premolars, *Oral Surg Oral Med Oral Pathol* 36(5):738–744, 1973.
155. Visser J: *Beitrag zur Kenntnis der menschlichen zahnwurzelformen, medical dissertation*, Universität Zürich, 1948.
156. Madani ZS, Mehraban N, Moudi E, Bijani A: Root and canal morphology of mandibular molars in a selected Iranian population using cone-beam computed tomography, *Iran Endod J* 12(2):143–148, 2017.
157. Mohammadzadeh Akhlaghi N, Khalilak Z, Vatanpour M, et al.: Root canal anatomy and morphology of mandibular first molars in a selected Iranian population: an in vitro study, *Iran Endod J* 12(1):87–91, 2017.
158. Celikten B, Tufenkci P, Aksoy U, et al.: Cone beam CT evaluation of mandibular molar root canal morphology in a Turkish Cypriot population, *Clin Oral Investig* 20(8):2221–2226, 2016.
159. Rodrigues CT, Oliveira-Santos C, Bernardineli N, et al.: Prevalence and morphometric analysis of three-rooted mandibular first molars in a Brazilian subpopulation, *J Appl Oral Sci revista FOB* 24(5):535–542, 2016.
160. Peiris R, Malwatte U, Abayakoon J, Wettasinghe A: Variations in the root form and root canal morphology of permanent mandibular first molars in a Sri Lankan population, *Anat Res Int* 2015:803671, 2015.
161. Chourasia HR, Meshram GK, Warhadpande M, Dakshindas D: Root canal morphology of mandibular first permanent molars in an Indian population, *Int J Dent* 1–6, 2012.
162. Colak H, Ozcan E, Hamidi MM: Prevalence of three-rooted mandibular permanent first molars among the Turkish population, *Nigerian J Clin Pract* 15(3):306–310, 2012.
163. Chandra SS, Chandra S, Shankar P, Indira R: Prevalence of radix entomolaris in mandibular permanent first molars: a study in a South Indian population, *Oral Surg Oral Med Oral Pathol Oral Radiol Endod* 112(3):e77–82, 2011.
164. Al-Qudah AA, Awawdeh LA: Root and canal morphology of mandibular first and second molar teeth in a Jordanian population, *Int Endod J* 42(9):775–784, 2009.
165. Schafer E, Breuer D, Janzen S: The prevalence of three-rooted mandibular permanent first molars in a German population, *J Endod* 35(2):202–205, 2009.
166. Reuben J, Velmurugan N, Kandaswamy D: The evaluation of root canal morphology of the mandibular first molar in an Indian population using spiral computed tomography scan: an in vitro study, *J Endod* 34(2):212–215, 2008.
167. Shahi S, Yavari HR, Rahimi S, Torkamani R: Root canal morphology of human mandibular first permanent molars in an Iranian population, *J Dent Res Dent Clin Dent Prospects* 2(1):20–23, 2008.
168. Ahmed HA, Abu-bakr NH, Yahia NA, Ibrahim YE: Root and canal morphology of permanent mandibular molars in a Sudanese population, *Int Endod J* 40(10):766–771, 2007.
169. Peiris R, Takahashi M, Sasaki K, Kanazawa E: Root and canal morphology of permanent mandibular molars in a Sri Lankan population, *Odontology / the Society of the Nippon Dental University* 95(1):16–23, 2007.
170. Nazhan S: Incidence of four canals in root-canal-treated mandibular first molars in a Saudi Arabian sub-population, *Int Endod J* 32(1):49–52, 1999.
171. Sperber GH, Moreau JL: Study of the number of roots and canals in Senegalese first permanent mandibular molars, *Int Endod J* 31(2):117–122, 1998.
172. Zaatar EI, al Anizi SA, al Duwairi Y: A study of the dental pulp cavity of mandibular first permanent molars in the Kuwaiti population, *J Endod* 24(2):125–127, 1998.
173. Rocha LF, Sousa Neto MD, Fidel SR, et al.: External and internal anatomy of mandibular molars, *Braz Dent J* 7(1):33–40, 1996.
174. Younes SA, al-Shammery AR, el-Angbawi MF: Three-rooted permanent mandibular first molars of Asian and black groups in the Middle East, *Oral Surg Oral Med Oral Pathol* 69(1):102–105, 1990.
175. Curzon ME: Miscegenation and the prevalence of three-rooted mandibular first molars in the Baffin Eskimo, *Community Dent Oral Epidemiol* 2(3):130–131, 1974.
176. Curzon ME: Three-rooted mandibular permanent molars in English Caucasians, *J Dent Res* 52(1):181, 1973.
177. de Souza-Freitas JA, Lopes ES, Casati-Alvares L: Anatomic variations of lower first permanent molar roots in two ethnic groups, *Oral Surg Oral Med Oral Pathol* 31(2):274–278, 1971.
178. Skidmore AE, Bjørndal AM: Root canal morphology of the human mandibular first molar, *Oral Surg Oral Med Oral Pathol* 32(5):778–784, 1971.
179. Jang JK, Peters OA, Lee W, et al.: Incidence of three roots and/or four root canals in the permanent mandibular first molars in a Korean sub-population, *Clin Oral Investig* 17(1):105–111, 2013.
180. Kim SY, Kim BS, Woo J, Kim Y: Morphology of mandibular first molars analyzed by cone-beam computed tomography in a Korean population: variations in the number of roots and canals, *J Endod* 39(12):1516–1521, 2013.
181. Zhang R, Wang H, Tian YY, et al.: Use of cone-beam computed tomography to evaluate root and canal morphology of mandibular molars in Chinese individuals, *Int Endod J* 44(11):990–999, 2011.
182. Huang CC, Chang YC, Chuang MC, et al.: Evaluation of root and canal systems of mandibular first molars in Taiwanese individuals using cone-beam computed tomography, *J Formos Med Assoc* 109(4):303–308, 2010.
183. Wang Y, Zheng QH, Zhou XD, et al.: Evaluation of the root and canal morphology of mandibular first permanent molars in a western Chinese population by cone-beam computed tomography, *J Endod* 36(11):1786–1789, 2010.
184. Chen G, Yao H, Tong C: Investigation of the root canal configuration of mandibular first molars in a Taiwan Chinese population, *Int Endod J* 42(11):1044–1049, 2009.
185. Gulabivala K, Opasanon A, Ng YL, Alavi A: Root and canal morphology of Thai mandibular molars, *Int Endod J* 35(1):56–62, 2002.
186. Gulabivala K, Aung TH, Alavi A, Ng YL: Root and canal morphology of Burmese mandibular molars, *Int Endod J* 34(5):359–370, 2001.
187. Yew SC, Chan K: A retrospective study of endodontically treated mandibular first molars in a Chinese population, *J Endod* 19(9):471–473, 1993.
188. Morita M: Morphological studies on the roots of lower first molars in Japanese, *Shikwa Gakuho* 90(6):837–854, 1990.
189. Harada Y, Tomino S, Ogawa K, et al.: Frequency of three-rooted mandibular first molars. Survey by x-ray photographs, *Shika Kiso Igakkai Zasshi* 31(1):13–18, 1989.
190. Onda S, Minemura R, Masaki T, Funatsu S: Shape and number of the roots of the permanent molar teeth, *Bull Tokyo Dent Coll* 30(4):221–231, 1989.
191. Walker RT: Root form and canal anatomy of mandibular first molars in a southern Chinese population, *Endod Dent Traumatol* 4(1):19–22, 1988.
192. Reichart PA, Metah D: Three-rooted permanent mandibular first molars in the Thai, *Community Dent Oral Epidemiol* 9(4):191–192, 1981.
193. Pawar AM, Pawar M, Kfir A, et al.: Root canal morphology and variations in mandibular second molar teeth of an Indian population: an in vivo cone-beam computed tomography analysis, *Clin Oral Investig*, 2017.

194. Akhlaghi NM, Abbas FM, Mohammadi M, et al.: Radicular anatomy of permanent mandibular second molars in an Iranian population: a preliminary study, *Dent Res J (Isfahan)* 13(4):362–366, 2016.
195. Kim SY, Kim BS, Kim Y: Mandibular second molar root canal morphology and variants in a Korean subpopulation, *Int Endod J* 49(2):136–144, 2016.
196. Shemesh A, Levin A, Katzenell V, et al.: Prevalence of 3- and 4-rooted first and second mandibular molars in the Israeli population, *J Endod* 41(3):338–342, 2015.
197. Silva EJ, Nejaim Y, Silva AV, et al.: Evaluation of root canal configuration of mandibular molars in a Brazilian population by using cone-beam computed tomography: an in vivo study, *J Endod* 39(7):849–852, 2013.
198. Zare Jahromi M, Jafari Golestan F, Mashhadi Esmaeil M, et al.: Root and canal morphology of mandibular second molar in an Iranian population by clearing method, *J Dent (Shiraz)* 14(2):78–81, 2013.
199. Zheng Q, Zhang L, Zhou X, et al.: C-shaped root canal system in mandibular second molars in a Chinese population evaluated by cone-beam computed tomography, *Int Endod J* 44(9):857–862, 2011.
200. Neelakantan P, Subbarao C, Subbarao CV, Ravindranath M: Root and canal morphology of mandibular second molars in an Indian population, *J Endod* 36(8):1319–1322, 2010.
201. Rahimi S, Shahi S, Lotfi M, et al.: Root canal configuration and the prevalence of C-shaped canals in mandibular second molars in an Iranian population, *J Oral Sci* 50(1):9–13, 2008.
202. Cheung LH, Low D, Cheung GSP: Root morphology—a study of the mandibular second molar of ethnic Chinese, *Ann R Australas Coll Dent Surg* 18:47–50, 2006.
203. Manning SA: Root canal anatomy of mandibular second molars. Part I, *Int Endod J* 23(1):34–39, 1990.
204. Walker RT: Root form and canal anatomy of mandibular second molars in a southern Chinese population, *J Endod* 14(7):325–329, 1988.
205. Weine FS, Pasiewicz RA, Rice RT: Canal configuration of the mandibular second molar using a clinically oriented in vitro method, *J Endod* 14(5):207–213, 1988.
206. Kotoku K: Morphological studies on the roots of Japanese mandibular second molars, *Shikwa Gakuho* 85(1):43–64, 1985.
207. Somasundaram P, Rawtiya M, Wadhwani S, et al.: Retrospective study of root canal configurations of mandibular third molars using CBCT- Part-II, *J Clin Diagn Res* 11(6):ZC55–ZC59, 2017.
208. Park JB, Kim N, Park S, Ko Y: Evaluation of number of roots and root anatomy of permanent mandibular third molars in a Korean population, using cone-beam computed tomography, *Eur J Dent* 7(3):296–301, 2013.
209. Kuzekanani M, Haghani J, Nosrati H: Root and canal morphology of mandibular third molars in an Iranian population, *J Dent Res Dent Clin Dent Prospects* 6(3):85–88, 2012.
210. Ogiwara I, Adachi M, Morita T: Morphological characteristics of Japanese mandibular third molars- roots number and accessory root (author's transl), *Shikwa Gakuho* 81(5):889–898, .
211. Liu J, Luo J, Dou L, Yang D: CBCT study of root and canal morphology of permanent mandibular incisors in a Chinese population, *Acta Odontol Scand* 72(1):26–30, 2014.
212. Gomes BP, Rodrigues HH, Tancredo N: The use of a modelling technique to investigate the root canal morphology of mandibular incisors, *Int Endod J* 29(1):29–36, 1996.
213. Karagoz-Kucukay I: Root canal ramifications in mandibular incisors and efficacy of low-temperature injection thermoplasticized gutta-percha filling, *J Endod* 20(5):236–240, 1994.
214. Walker RT: The root canal anatomy of mandibular incisors in a southern Chinese population, *Int Endod J* 21(3):218–223, 1988.
215. Kaffe I, Kaufman A, Littner MM, Lazarson A: Radiographic study of the root canal system of mandibular anterior teeth, *Int Endod J* 18(4):253–259, 1985.
216. Bellizzi R, Hartwell G: Clinical investigation of in vivo endodontically treated mandibular anterior teeth, *J Endod* 9(6):246–248, 1983.
217. Warren EM, Laws AJ: The relationship between crown size and the incidence of bifid root canals in mandibular incisor teeth, *Oral Surg Oral Med Oral Pathol* 52(4):425–429, 1981.
218. Miyoshi S, Fujiwara J, Tsuji YT, Yamamoto K: Bifurcated root canals and crown diameter, *J Dent Res* 56(11):1425, 1977.
219. Laws AJ: Prevalence of canal irregularities in mandibular incisors: a radiographic study, *N Z Dent J* 67(309):181–186, 1971.
220. Vaziri FB, Kasraee S, Abdolsamadi HR, et al.: Root canal configuration of one-rooted mandibular canine in an Iranian population: an in vitro study, *J Dent Res Dent Clin Dent Prospects* 2(1):28–32, 2008.
221. Zhang D, Chen J, Lan G, et al.: The root canal morphology in mandibular first premolars: a comparative evaluation of cone-beam computed tomography and micro-computed tomography, *Clin Oral Investig* 21(4):1007–1012, 2017.
222. Chen J, Li X, Su Y, et al.: A micro-computed tomography study of the relationship between radicular grooves and root canal morphology in mandibular first premolars, *Clin Oral Investig* 19(2):329–334, 2015.
223. Shetty A, Hegde MN, Tahiliani D, et al.: A three-dimensional study of variations in root canal morphology using cone-beam computed tomography of mandibular premolars in a South Indian population, *J Clin Diagn Res* 8(8):ZC22–24, 2014.
224. Liu N, Li X, Liu N, et al.: A micro-computed tomography study of the root canal morphology of the mandibular first premolar in a population from southwestern China, *Clin Oral Investig* 17(3):999–1007, 2013.
225. Baroudi K, Kazkaz M, Sakka S, Tarakji B: Morphology of root canals in lower human premolars, *Niger Med J* 53(4):206–209, 2012.
226. Velmurugan N, Sandhya R: Root canal morphology of mandibular first premolars in an Indian population: a laboratory study, *Int Endod J* 42(1):54–58, 2009.
227. Lu TY, Yang SF, Pai SF: Complicated root canal morphology of mandibular first premolar in a Chinese population using the cross section method, *J Endod* 32(10):932–936, 2006.
228. Yoshioka T, Villegas JC, Kobayashi C, Suda H: Radiographic evaluation of root canal multiplicity in mandibular first premolars, *J Endod* 30(2):73–74, 2004.
229. Sabala CL, Benenati FW, Neas BR: Bilateral root or root canal aberrations in a dental school patient population, *J Endod* 20(1):38–42, 1994.
230. Baisden MK, Kulild JC, Weller RN: Root canal configuration of the mandibular first premolar, *J Endod* 18(10):505–508, 1992.
231. Walker RT: Root canal anatomy of mandibular first premolars in a southern Chinese population, *Endod Dent Traumatol* 4(5):226–228, 1988.
232. Hasheminia M, Hashemi A: Frequency of canal configuration in maxillary first premolars and mandibular second premolars, *J Isfahan Dent School* 1(3&4):59–64, 2005.
233. Goel NK, Gill KS, Taneja JR: Study of root canals configuration in mandibular first permanent molar, *J Indian Soc Pedod Prev Dent* 8(1):12–14, 1991.
234. Fabra-Campos H: Unusual root anatomy of mandibular first molars, *J Endod* 11(12):568–572, 1985.
235. Filpo-Perez C, Bramante CM, Villas-Boras MH, et al.: Micro-computed tomographic analysis of the root canal morphology of the distal root of mandibular first molar, *J Endod* 41(2):231–236, 2015.
236. Weine FS: The C-shaped mandibular second molar: incidence and other considerations. Members of the Arizona Endodontic Association, *J Endod* 24(5):372–375, 1998.

Index

Note: Page numbers followed by "f" indicate figures "t" indicate tables, and "b" indicate boxes.

D

N

O